Textbook of Genitourinary Surgery

Textbook of Genitourinary Surgery

VOLUME 1

EDITED BY

H.N.Whitfield MA, MB, MChir, FRCS, FEBU
Institute of Urology and Nephrology,
48 Riding House Street, London W1P 7PN

W.F.Hendry MD, ChM, FRCS
St Bartholomew's Hospital, London EC1A.
Also at 149 Harley Street, London W1N 2DE

R.S.Kirby MA, MD, FRCS
St George's Hospital, London SW17 0QT.
Also at 149 Harley Street, London W1N 2DE

J.W.Duckett MD
Formerly Professor of Urology and Director of Pediatric Urology,
Children's Hospital of Philadelphia, Philadelphia, PA 19104, USA

Foreword by John Blandy

Second Edition

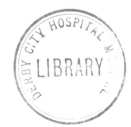

**Blackwell
Science**

© 1998 by
Blackwell Science Ltd
Editorial Offices:
Osney Mead, Oxford OX2 0EL
25 John Street, London WC1N 2BL
23 Ainslie Place, Edinburgh EH3 6AJ
350 Main Street, Malden
  MA 02148 5018, USA
54 University Street, Carlton
  Victoria 3053, Australia

Other Editorial Offices:
Blackwell Wissenschafts-Verlag GmbH
Kurfürstendamm 57
10707 Berlin, Germany

Blackwell Science KK
MG Kodenmacho Building
7–10 Kodenmacho Nihombashi
Chuo-ku, Tokyo 104, Japan

First published 1985
  (by Churchill Livingstone)
Second edition 1998

Set by Setrite Typesetters, Hong Kong
Printed and bound in Italy
by Vincenzo Bono srl, Turin

The Blackwell Science logo is a
trade mark of Blackwell Science Ltd,
registered at the United Kingdom
Trade Marks Registry

A catalogue record for this title
is available from the British Library

ISBN 0-632-03774-1

Library of Congress
Cataloging-in-publication Data

Textbook of genitourinary surgery/
  edited by Hugh Whitfield—[et al.]
  —2nd ed.
      p.   cm.
  Includes bibliographical references
  and index.
  ISBN 0-632-03774-1
  1. Genitourinary organs—Surgery.
  I. Whitfield, Hugh N.
  [DNLM: 1 Urogenital System—surgery.
  2. Urogenital Diseases—surgery.
  WJ 168 T355 1997]
RD571.T49   1997
617.4′6—dc20
DNLM/DLC
for Library of Congress   96-27776
                                      CIP

The right of the Author to be identified as
the Author of this Work has been asserted
in accordance with the Copyright, Designs
and Patents Act 1988.

DISTRIBUTORS

Marston Book Services Ltd
PO Box 269
Abingdon, Oxon OX14 4YN
(Orders: Tel: 01235 465500
        Fax: 01235 465555)

USA
Blackwell Science, Inc.
Commerce Place
350 Main Street
Malden, MA 02148 5018
(Orders: Tel: 800 759 6102
                781 388 8250
        Fax: 781 388 8255)

Canada
Login Brothers Book Company
324 Saulteaux Cresent
Winnipeg, Manitoba R3J 3T2
(Orders: Tel: 204 224-4068)

Australia
Blackwell Science Pty Ltd
54 University Street
Carlton, Victoria 3053
(Orders: Tel: 3 9347 0300
        Fax: 3 9347 5001)

For further information on
Blackwell Science, visit our website:
www.blackwell-science.com

Contents

Section 9: Neoplastic Diseases

Section 9a: Epidemiology and Pathology

Section 9b: Renal Cell Carcinoma

Section 9c: Urothelial Tumours

Section 9d: Carcinoma of the Prostate

Section 9e: Genital Tumours

Section 10: Endocrine Disorders

Section 11: Andrology

Section 11a: Impotence

List of Contributors

G.M. Aber *Green Leaves, Seabridge Lane, Newcastle, Staffs ST5 3LS*

P. Abrams *Consultant Urological Surgeon, Department of Urology, Southmead Hospital, Bristol BS10 5NB*

R. Ackermann *Professor and Chairman, Department of Urology, Heinrich-Heine-University, Moorenstr 5, 40225, Düsseldorf, Germany*

R. Ahlawat *Associate Professor, Department of Urology and Rental Transplantation, Sanjay Gandhi Post Graduate Institute of Medical Science, Lucknow 226014, India*

P. Alken *Professor and Chairman, Department of Urology, Mannheim Hospital, University of Heidelberg, Theodor-Kutzer-Ufer 1-3, 68135 Mannheim, Germany*

J.T. Andersen *Consultant Urologist, Department of Urology, Frederiksberg Hospital, University of Copenhagen, DK-2000 Frederiksberg, Denmark*

J. Anderson *Senior Lecturer/Honorary Consultant Genitourinary Physician, St Bartholomew's Hospital, West Smithfield, London EC1A 7BE*

F. Aragona *Professor of Urology, Department of Urology, University of Padova, Istituto di Urologia, Monoblocco Ospedaliero, Via Giustiniani 2, 35128 Padova, Italy*

Y. Aso *President and Professor Emeritus, Fujieda Mun. General Hospital, 4-1-11 Surugadai, Fujieda-shi, Shizuoka 426, Japan*

S.A. Awad *Department of Urology, Dalhousie University, Room 5014 Centennial Building, Victoria General Hospital, 1278 Tower Road, Halifax, Nova Scotia, Canada B3H 27Y9*

J. Spencer Barthold *Associate Professor of Urology, Children's Hospital of Michigan, 3901 Beaubien Blvd, Detroit, MI 48201, USA*

L. Beeley *3 Newland Road, Droitwich, Worcestershire WR9 7AF*

R.D. Bellah *Chief, Ultrasound Division, Department of Radiology, The Children's Hospital of Philadelphia, 34th Street and Civic Center Boulevard, Philadelphia, PA 19104, USA*

M. Bhandari *Professor and Director of Urology and Renal Transplant, Sanjay Gandhi Post Graduate Institute of Medical Sciences, Lucknow 226014, India*

Sir N. Blacklock *42 Western Way, Alverstoke, Gosport, Hants PO12 2NQ*

L. Boccon-Gibod *Chirurgien des Hôpitaux, Chef de Service Clinique Urologieque de l'Hôpital Bichat, 46 rue Henri Huchard, 75788 Paris, France*

C. Boshoff *Lecturer in Medical Oncology, School of Medicine and Dentistry, The Royal London Hospital, London E1 1BB*

W.G. Bowsher *Consultant Urological Surgeon, Royal Gwent Hospital, Cardiff Road, Newport, Gwent NP9 2UB*

P. Boyle *Division of Epidemiology and Biostatistics, European Institute of Oncology, Via Ripamonti 332/10, 20141 Milan, Italy*

A.F. Brading *University Lecturer in Pharmacology, Department of Pharmacology, Mansfield Road, Oxford OX1 3QT*

J.D. Briggs *Consultant Physician, The Renal Unit, Western Infirmary, Dumbarton Road, Glasgow, G11 6NT*

K.E. Britton *Professor of Nuclear Medicine, St Bartholomew's Hospital, West Smithfield, London EC1A 7BE*

E. Broseta *Consultant Urological Surgeon, Department of Urology, Hospital Universitari La Fe, Avenida de Campanar 21, 46009 Valencia, Spain*

C.C. Carson *Department of Urology, UNC School of Medicine, 427 Burnett Womack Building, Chapel Hill, NC 27599/7235, USA*

P.C. Cartwright *Associate Professor of Surgery, Primary Children's Medical Center, University of Utah, 100 No Medical Drive, Suite 2200, Salt Lake City, UT 84113, USA*

W.R. Cattell *99 Harley Street, London W1N 1DF*

D.M. Chaput de Saintonge *Clinical Skills Centre, The Robin Brook Centre, St Bartholomew's Hospital, West Smithfield, London EC1A 7BE*

T.J. Christmas *Consultant Urological Surgeon, Department of Urology, Charing Cross Hospital, Fulham Palace Road, London W6 8RF*

David W. Cohen *Former Fellow in Urologic Oncology, Memorial Sloan-Kettering Cancer Center, Middletown Urologic Associates, 25 Myrtle Avenue, Middletown, New York 10940, USA*

F.H. Comhaire *Professor of Endocrinology, Department of Endocrinology, State University of Gent, De Pintelaan 185, B9000 Gent, Belgium*

C.E. Constantinou *Associate Professor, Stanford University Medical School, Stanford CA 94305, USA*

C.L. Coogan *Rush Presbyterian St Luke's Medical Center, Department of Urology, 1653 West Congress Parkway, Chicago, IL 60612-3833, USA*

J.A. Cook *Consultant in Clinical Genetics, Centre for Human Genetics, Sheffield Children's Hospital, Sheffield S20 2TH*

A.G.A. Cowie *Consultant Urologist, Eastbourne District General Hospital, King's Drive, Eastbourne, East Sussex BN21 2UD*

M. Dawahra *Service d'Urologie et Chirurgie de la Transplantation Hôpital Édouard Herriot, Place d'Arsonval 69437 Lyon, Cedex 03, France*

C. Dawson *Consultant Urologist, Edith Cavell Hospital, Bretton Gate, Peterborough PE3 9GZ*

E. DeAntoni *University of Colorado Health Sciences Center, Campus Box C319, 4200 East Ninth Avenue, Denver, CO 80262, USA*

D.P. Dearnaley *Senior Lecturer and Consultant, Institute of Cancer Research and Royal Marden NHS Trust, Downs Road, Sutton, Surrey*

W. De Sy *Professor Urology, Department of Urology, University Hospital, De Pintelaan, 185, B-9000 Gent, Belgium*

C.J. Devine *Eastern Virginia Medical School, Norfolk General Hospital, 600 Gresham Drive, Norfolk, VA 23507, USA*

M.D. Dinneen *Consultant Urological Surgeon, Chelsea and Westminster Hospital, 369 Fulham Road, London SW10 9NH*

J.S. Dixon *Department of Anatomy, The Chinese University of Hong Kong, Shatin New Territories, Hong Kong*

J.C. Djurhuus *Institute of Experimental Clinical Research, University of Åarhus, Skejoy Sygehus, DK-8200 Åarhus N, Denmark*

K. Dowell *Park Hospital, Sherwood Lodge Drive, Arnold, Nottingham NG5 8RX*

J-M. Dubernard *Service d'Urologie et Chirurgie de Transplantation, Hôpital Édouard Herriot, Place d'Arsonval, 69437 Lyon, Cedex 03, France*

J.W. Duckett *Formerly Professor of Urology and Director of Pediatric Urology, Children's Hospital of Philadelphia, Philadelphia PA 19104, USA*

I. Eardley *Leeds General Infirmary, Great George Street, Leeds LS1 3EX*

J.L. Edens *Federal Department of Justice, Federal Prison Camp, Seymour Johnson Airforce Base, Caller Box 8004, Building 3681, Goldsboro, NC 27533-8004, USA*

F. Eisenberger *Katharinenhospital, Kriegsbergstr. 60, D 70174 Stuttgart, Germany*

S.J. Eykyn *Consultant Clinical Microbiologist, Department of Microbiology, St Thomas' Hospital, Lambeth Palace Road, London SE1 7EH*

W.R. Fair *Chief Urology Service, Department of Surgery, Cornell University Medical College, Memorial Sloan-Kettering Cancer Centre, 1275 York Avenue, Rm C1061, NY 10021, USA*

G.A. Farrow *Suite 14-214 Eaton Wing, Toronto General Hospital, 200 Elizabeth Street, Toronto, Ontario M5G 2C4, Canada*

D. Felsen *Associate Research Professor of Pharmacology (Urology) Department of Urology, The New York Hospital Cornell Medical Centre, 1300 York Avenue, New York NY 10021, USA*

S. Fishel *Park Hospital, Sherwood Lodge Drive, Arnold, Nottingham NG5 8RX*

C. Fisher *Consultant and Head of Histopathology, Royal Marsden NHS Trust, Fulham Road, London SW3 6JJ*

C.J. Fowler *Consultant in Uroneurology, The National Hospital for Neurology and Neurosurgery, Queen Square, London WC1N 3BG*

J.D. Frank *Consultant Paediatric Urologist, Bristol Royal Hospital for Sick Children, St Michael's Hill, Bristol BS2 8BJ*

J.B. Gajewski *Associate Professor, Department of Urology, Dalhousie University, Room 5014, Centennial Building, Victoria General Hospital, 1278 Tower Road, Halifax, Nova Scotia, Canada B3H 2Y9*

M.A. Ghoneim *Professor of Urology, Director, Urology and Nephrology Centre, Mansoura, Egypt*

K.M. Gil *Department of Psychology, University of North Carolina, Caller Box 3270, David Hall, Chapel Hill, NC 27599-3270, USA*

D.A. Goldfarb *Department of Urology, Cleveland Clinic Foundation, 9500 Euclid Avenue, Cleveland, OH 44195, USA*

J.A. Gosling *Chairman, Department of Anatomy, The Chinese University of Hong Kong, Shatin New Territories, Hong Kong*

S. Green *Park Hospital, Sherwood Lodge Drive, Arnold, Nottingham NG5 8RX*

G.E. Griffin *Professor of Infectious Diseases and Medicine, St George's Hospital Medical School, Blackshaw Road, Tooting, London SW17 0QT*

F.A. Gulmi *Clinical Assistant Professor of Urology, State University of New York, Health Sciences Center of Brooklyn, Attending Urologist, Brookdale University Hospital and Medical Center, Brooklyn, New York 11212, USA*

T. Hald *Department of Urology, Herlev Hospital, 2730 Herlev, Denmark*

T.B. Hargreave *University Department of Surgery/Urology, Western General Hospital, Crewe Road, Edinburgh EH4 2XU*

J.V. Harney *Consultant Urologist, Manchester Royal Infirmary, Oxford Road, Manchester MI3 5WL*

W.F. Hendry *Genitourinary Surgeon, St Bartholomew's and The Royal Marsden Hospitals, London. Also at 149 Harley Street, London W1N 2DE*

P.M. Higgins *Windrush House, Aldsworth, Cheltenham, Gloucester GL54 3QY*

J. Hofbauer *Department of Urology, University of Vienna, Wahringer Gürtel 18-20, A-1090 Vienna, Austria*

S.A.V. Holmes *Consultant Urologist, St Mary's Hospital, Milton Road, Portsmouth PO3 6AD*

A. Horwich *Director of Clinical Research and Development, The Royal Marsden NHS Trust, Downs Road, Sutton, Surrey SM2 5PT*

J.E. Husband *Department of Diagnostic Radiology, The Royal Marsden NHS Trust, Downs Road, Sutton, Surrey SM2 5PT*

J.F. Jiménez-Cruz *Head of Department of Urology, Hospital Universitari La Fe, Avenida de Campanar 21, 46009 Valencia, Spain*

U. Jonas *Klinik fur Urologie, Medizinische Hochschule Hannover, Hannover 61 D-30623, Germany*

G.H. Jordan *Eastern Virginia Medical School, Norfolk General Hospital, 600 Gresham Drive, Norfolk, VA 23507, USA*

K.T. Kadesky *8210 Walnut Hill Lane, Suite 208, Dallas, TX 75231, USA*

B.S. Kaplan *Director of Nephrology, Professor of Pediatrics, Division of Nephrology, Room 3380-Wood Building, Children's Hospital of philadelphia, 34th Street and Civic Center Blvd, Philadelphia PA 19104, USA*

P. Kaplan *Senior Paediatrician, Division of Clinical Metabolism, The Children's Hospital of Philadelphia, 34th Street and Civic Center Blvd, Philadelphia PA 19104, USA*

M.A. Keating *8 Orlando, Florida 32806, USA*

P. Kincaid-Smith *Director of Nephrology, Epworth Hospital, Erin Street, Richmond, Victoria 3121, Australia*

L.R. King *Department of Surgery, Division of Urology, 2211 Lomas Blvd. NE, Albuquerque, New Mexico 87131-5341, USA*

R.S. Kirby *Consultant Urologist to St George's Hospital, London. Also at 149 Harley Street, London W1N 2DE*

N.W. Kour *10/107 Kour Surgery Mount Elizabeth Medical Centre, 3 Mount Elizabeth Road, Singapore 228510*

S.A. Kramer *Head, Section of Pediatric Urology Mayo Clinic and Mayo Foundation, 200 1st Street, Rochester, MN 55905, USA*

M.R. Laftavi *Service d'Urologie et Chirurgie de Transplantation, Hôpital Édouard Herriot, Place d'Arsonval, 69437 Lyon, Cedex 03, France*

H.P. Lambert *Emeritus Professor of Microbial Diseases, St George's Hospital Medical School, London SW17 0RE*

N. Lameire *Professor of Medicine, Renal Division, Department of Internal Medicine, University Hospital, De Pintelaan 185, B-9000 Gent, Belgium*

S-S. Lee *Tri-Service General Hospital, Department of Urology, Department of Surgery, Section 3, Tin-Chow Road, Taipei, Taiwan, Republic of China*

L.A. Levine *Director of Reconstructive Urology, Rush Presbyterian St Luke's Medical Center, Department of Urology, 1653 West Congress Parkway, Chicago, Ill 60612-3833, USA*

D.A. Levison *Professor of Pathology, Department of Pathology, Ninewells Hospital and Medical School, University of Dundee, Dundee DD1 9SY*

J.A. Libertino *Chairman, Institute of Urology, Lahey Hitchcock Medical Center, Burlington, MA 01805, USA*

T.F. Lue *Department of Urology UCSF, Box 0738, San Francisco, CA 94143-0738, USA*

J. Lunec *Senior Lecturer and Assistant Director, Cancer Research Unit, Medical School, University of Newcastle upon Tyne, Newcastle upon Tyne DD1 9SY*

D.F. Lynch Jr *Professor of Urology, Eastern Virginia School of Medicine, Sentara Cancer Institute, River Pavilion 203, 600 Gresham Drive, Norfolk, VA 23507, USA*

P. Maisonneuve *Division of Epidemiology and Biostatistics, European Institute of Oncology, Via Ripamonti 332/10, 20141 Milan, Italy*

A. Mansoor *2386 NW Marshall Street, Portland, OR 97210, USA*

M. Marberger *Professor and Chairman, Department of Urology, Kilink fur Urologie der Universität Wien, Allgemeines Krankenhaus, Währinger, Eürtel 15-20, Germany*

S. Marina *Instituto de Reproducción CEFER (Centro Medico Teknon), c/Marquesa de Vilallonga 12, 08017 Barcelona, Spain*

V.R. Marshall *Department of Surgery, Flinders Medical Centre, Bedford Park, South Australia 5042, Australia*

X. Martin *Service d'Urologie et Chirurgie de la Transplantation Hôpital Édouard Herriot, Place d'Arsonval, 69437 Lyon Cedex 03, France*

R. Maskell *Woodcroft House, Chalton, Horndean, Waterlooville, Hants PO8 0BD*

J.W. McAninch *University of California, San Francisco General Hospital, Room 3a 18, San Francisco, CA 94110, USA*

K.A. McCammon *Eastern Virginia Medical School, Norfolk General Hospital, 600 Gresham Drive, Norfolk, VA 23507, USA*

D.R. McMahon *Pediatric Urology, Children's Hospital, Medical Center, Akron, OH 44302, USA*

J.K. Mellon *Senior Lecturer in Urology, University of Newcastle upon Tyne, Newcastle upon Tyne NE2 4HH*

A. Morales *Professor of Urology and Oncology, Queen's University, Kingston, Ontario, Canada K7L 2V7*

D. Mortimer *Scientific Director, Sydney IVF, 4 O'Connell Street, Sydney, NSW 2000, Australia*

J.L. Mostwin *Associate Professor of Urology, Marburg 401C, The Johns Hopkins Medical Institutions, 600 N Wolfe Street, Baltimore, MD 21287-2411, USA*

P.D.E. Mouriquand *Honorary Senior Lecturer, Institute of Child Health, Consultant in Paediatric Urology, Great Ormond Street Hospital for Children NHS Trust, London WC1N 3JH*

A.R. Mundy *Institute of Urology and Nephrology, 48 Riding House Street, London W1P 7PN*

P. Napalkov *Division of Epidemiology and Biostatistics, European Institute of Oncology, Via Ripamonti 332/10, 20141 Milan, Italy*

S.A.A. Naqvi *Professor Of Urology, Sindh Institute of Urology and Transplantation (SIUT), Dow Medical College and Civil Hospital, Karachi-74200, Pakistan*

P.A. Nash *10 Anglo Road, Greenwich, NSW 2065, Australia*

J.H. Naudé *Department of Urology, Groote Schuur Hospital, Observatory 7925, Cape Town, South Africa*

D.E. Neal *Professor of Surgery, The Medical School, University of Newcastle, Newcastle upon Tyne NE2 4HH*

J.G. Noble *Department of Urology, Radcliffe Oxford Hospitals, Oxford OX2 6HE*

A.C. Novick *Chairman, Department of Urology, The Cleveland Clinic Foundation, 9500 Euclid Avenue, Cleveland OH 44106, USA*

R.T.D. Oliver *Sir Maxwell Joseph Professor in Medical Oncology, The Royal London Hospital School of Medicine and Dentistry, Whitechapel, London E1 1BB*

P.H. O'Reilly *Consultant Urological Surgeon, Department of Urology, Stepping Hill Hospital, Stockport SK2 7JE*

G. Passerini Glazel *Professor of Urology, Department of Urology, University of Padova, Istituto di Urologia, Monoblocco Ospedaliero, Via Giustiniani 2, 35128 Padova, Italy*

C. Pavone *Institute of Urology, University of Palermo Polyclinic Hospital, Via del Vespro 129, 90127 Palermo, Italy*

M. Pavone-Macaluso *Institute of Urology, University of Palermo Polyclinic Hospital, Via del Vespro 129, 90127, Palermo, Italy*

L.M. Pérez *Division of Urologic Surgery, University of Alabama at Birmingham, The Children's Hospital, 1600 Seventh Avenue South, Birmingham, AL 35233, USA*

K. Persson *Department of Clinical Pharmacology, Lund University Hospital, S-221 85 Lund, Sweden*

P.C. Peters *Department of Urology, University of Texas, Southwestern Medical Center, 5323 Harry Hines Boulevard, Dallas, Texas 75235, USA*

J.P. Pryor *Institute of Urology, Lisler Hospital, Chelsea Bridge Road, London SW1W 8RM*

R. Ravi *Department of Urology, Ground Floor, KGV Building, St Bartholomew's Hospital, West Smithfield, London EC1A 7BE*

S. Raz *924 Westwood Boulevard, Suite 520, Los Angeles, CA 90024-2910, USA*

J.F. Redman *Professor and Chairman, Department of Urology, University of Avkansas College of Medicine, Little Rock, AR 72205, USA*

J.M. Reynard *Senior Registrar, Department of Urology, Royal London Hospital, London E1 1BB*

R.H. Reznek *Professor of Diagnostic Imaging, Academic Department of Radiology, St Bartholomew's Hospital, West Smithfield, London EC1A 7ED*

J.P. Richie *Harvard Medical School, Brigham and Women's Hospital, 45 Francis Street, ASB II-3, Boston MA 02115, USA*

D. Rickards *Department of Radiology, University College London Hospitals, London W1N 8AA*

A.M.K. Rickwood *Consultant Urological Surgeon, Alder Hey Children's Hospital, Eaton Road, Liverpool L12 2AP*

S.A.H. Rizvi *Sindh Institute of Urology and Transplantation Dow (SIUT) Medical College and Civil Hospital, Karachi-74200, Pakistan*

J.H. Ross *Department of Urology, Cleveland Clinic Foundation, 9500 Euclid Ave, Cleveland, OH 44195, USA*

G. Rümenapf *Mineral Metabolism and Endocrine Research Laboratory, University Hospital, D-91023 Erlangen, Germany*

P.F. Schellhammer *Professor and Chairman, Department of Urology, Eastern Virginia School of Medicine, Sentara Cancer Institute, River Pavilion 203, 600 Gresham Drive, Norfolk VA 23507, USA*

S.M. Schlossberg *Eastern Virginia Medical School, Norfolk General Hospital, 600 Gresham Drive, Norfolk, VA 23507, USA*

A.S. Schmidt *Raueneggstr. 4, 88121 Ravensburg, Germany*

A.S. Schmiedl *Mineral Metabolism and Endocrine Research Laboratory, University Hospital, D-91023 Erlangen, Germany*

B.J. Schmitz-Dräger *Professor of Urology, Heinrich-Heine-University Moorenstr 5, 40225 Dusseldorf, Germany*

S.L. Schulman *Assistant Professor of Pediatrics, Children's Hospital of Philadelphia, 34th Street and Civic Center Blvd, Philadelphia, PA 19104, USA*

P.O. Schwille *Professor of Experimental Surgery and Urology, Mineral Metabolism and Endocrine Research Laboratory, University Hospital, D-91023 Erlangen, Germany*

V. Serretta *Division of Urology, Civic Hospital, USL 6, 90127 Palermo, Italy*

R.P. Sessions *427 Burnett Womack Building, University of North Carolina, Chapel Hill, NC 27599-7235, USA*

B.P. Setchell *Department of Animal Science, University of Adelaide (Waite Campus), Glen Osmond, 5064 Adelaide, Australia*

P.J.R. Shah *Senior Lecturer and Honorary Consultant Urologist, Institute of Urology and Nephrology, University College London Medical School, 48 Riding House Street, London W1P 7PN*

L.M.D. Shortliffe *Stanford University, Medical Center, Department of Urology, Stanford, CA 94305-5118, USA*

A. Simpson *Department of Microbiology, St Bartholomew's Hospital Medical College, West Smithfield, London EC1A 7BE*

M. Smans *International Agency for Research on Cancer, 150 Cours Albert Thomas, F-69372 Lyons Cedex 08, France*

B.W. Snow *Professor of Surgery, University of Utah Primary Children's Medical Center, 100 No Medical Drive, Suite 2200, Salt Lake City, Ut 84113, USA*

H.McC. Snyder *Division of Urology, 34th Street and Civic Center Boulevard, Children's Hospital, Philadelphia, PA 19104, USA*

M.J. Speakman *Department of Urology, Musgrove Park Hospital, Taunton TA1 5DA*

O. Sperling *Professor of Chemical Pathology and Director of Clinical Biochemistry, Beilinson Campus, Rabin Medical Center, Petah-Tikva 49100, Israel*

W.D. Steers *Associate Professor of Urology, University of Virginia, Health Sciences Center, Box 422, Charlottesville, VA 22908, USA*

C.G. Stief *Department of Urology, Medizinische Hochschule Hannover, D-30623, Hannover, Germany*

S. Tabaqchali *Professor of Medical Microbiology, St Bartholomew's Medical College, West Smithfield, London EC1A 7BE*

A. Tajima *Department of Urology, Faculty of Medicine, University of Tokyo, 7-3-1 Hongo, Bunkyo-Ku, Tokyo 113, Japan*

R.N. Thin *Consultant Physician, Department of Genitourinary Medicine, St Thomas' Hospital, Lambeth Palace Road, London SE1 7EH*

D.F.M. Thomas *Department of Paediatric Surgery, Clinical Sciences Building, St James's University Hospital Trust, Leeds LS9 7TF*

S. Thornton *Park Hospital, Sherwood Lodge Drive, Arnold, Nottingham NG5 8RX*

P.A. Trott *Consultant Pathologist, Department of Histology/Cytology, Royal Marsden Hospital, Fulham Road, London SW3 6JJ*

W.H. Turner *Department of Urology, Princess Royal Hospital, The Saltshouse Road, Hull HU8 9HE*

R.G. Uzzo *Department of Urology, The New York Hospital, Cornell University Medical Center, 525 East 68th Street, NY 10021, USA*

J.D. van Gool *Paediatric Nephrologist, Paediatric Renal Centre, University Children's Hospital, PO Box 18009, 3501 CA Utrecht, The Netherlands*

E.D. Vaughan Jr *Urologist-in-Chief, Department of Urology, The New York Hospital, Cornell University Medical Center, 525 East 68th Street, New York 10021, USA*

D.G. Vidt *Senior Physician, Department of Nephrology and Hypertension, The Cleveland Clinic Foundation, 9500 Euclid Avenue, Cleveland, OH 44195-5242, USA*

G.R. Wahle *Department of Urology, Indiana University Medical Center, University Hospital 1725, 550 North University Boulevard, Indianapolis, IN 46202-5250, USA*

D.M.A. Wallace *Consultant Urologist, Queen Elizabeth Hospital, Edgbaston, Birmingham B15 2TH*

S. Walter *Professor of Urology, Department of Urology, Odense University Hospital, DK-5000 Odense, Denmark*

H. Watanabe *Professor and Chairman, Department of Urology, Kyoto Prefectural University of Medicine, Kawaramachi-Hirokoji, Kyoto 602, Japan*

S.W. Waxman *West Kansas Urology Associates 2501 E, 13th Street Hayes Kansas 67601 USA*

Judith A.W. Webb *Consultant Radiologist, St Bartholomew's Hospital, West Smithfield, London EC1A 7BE*

G.D. Webster *Professor of Urology, Duke University Medical Center, Box 3146, Durham, NC 27710, USA*

R.H. Whitaker *21 High Street, Great Shelford, Cambridge CB2 5EH*

H.N. Whitfield *Institute of Urology and Nephrology, 48 Riding House Street, London W1P 7PN*

D.J. Wilkinson *Consultant Anaesthetist, Department of Anaesthesia, St Bartholomew's Hospital, West Smithfield London EC1A 7BE*

G. Williams *Department of Urology, Hammersmith Hospital, Du Cane Road, London W12 0HS*

E-M. Wong *Senior Registrar, Department of Anaesthesia, St Bartholomew's Hospital, West Smithfield, London EC1A 7BE*

M. Yajima *Department of Urology, St Marianna University, School of Medicine, 2-16-1 Sugao, Miyamae-Ku, Kawasaki 213, Japan*

J.M. Zelin *Consultant Genitourinary Physician, Department of Genitourinary Medicine, St Bartholomew's Hospital, West Smithfield, London EC1A 7BE*

E.J. Zingg *Department of Urology, University of Bern, Inselspital, CH 3010 Bern, Switzerland*

Foreword

This is a truly comprehensive textbook of urology. Each authority has been selected regardless of national boundaries and they reflect the practice and the opinions of many different schools of urology, not merely of one country or even one continent. The result is an international view of urology which will be as useful to the resident who has just started specialist surgical training as to his or her chief with many years of experience, whether they work in Manchester or Moshi.

In no other surgical specialty have advances been so rapid or have touched on so many basic principles. Every month brings something new to understand which, for the experienced urologist often requires a refresher course in basic science, or even an introduction to a branch of science that did not exist 30 years ago. For the newcomer to urology this book fills in the background to the principles of anatomy, physiology, physics and pharmacology which are specific to our specialty.

To handle such a diverse and precious cargo must have called for immense skill and effort, and Hugh Whitfield, Bill Hendry, Roger Kirby and the late John Duckett are to be congratulated on bringing their argosy safely into harbour. They have been well served by their crew. The publishers here set a new standard for textbook publication which will be difficult to emulate. David Gardner, the artist, has broken the long tradition of surgical illustration which felt obliged to depict each bolt on every polished retractor with laborious realism. What the surgeon needs is a map, not a photograph and these images set a new standard of accuracy and clarity; they explain, amplify and decorate the text and make this book truly a delight to open. When Vesalius persuaded Titian to illustrate his masterpiece he was breaking new ground. Whitfield *et al.* and Gardner have achieved no less.

JOHN BLANDY
London 1998

Preface to the Second Edition

The last edition of the *Textbook of Genitourinary Surgery* was published in 1985. Since then there have been enormous changes in urological practice and in the ways in which medical education is delivered. The advent of the CD-Rom and the internet have persuaded some people to question the role of a traditional textbook. However, the new technology has brought with it some disadvantages. Information overload has made it harder to discriminate between proven facts and untested speculations. There is therefore an even more pivotal role for a textbook in which the basics of our specialty are expounded by authors who have established international reputations. We are indebted to all our friends and colleagues who have devoted their time, energy and expertise to contribute to this textbook.

There are many people who have helped us to produce this book. We all have hard-working and patient secretaries.

To them we owe a great debt of gratitude. Our long-suffering and supportive wives and families have shown tolerance and forbearance when our work on the book has intruded on them. Our publishers have given us great support, in particular Rebecca Huxley and Jan East, who, between them, have drawn together all the strands of production.

A very special tribute must go to John Duckett. The sadness that we all felt at his untimely death in February 1997 comes back to us as we see the project for which he had worked so hard come to fruition. He was a giant of a man and the paediatric section of this book was his inspiration; he chose the authors and had reviewed the first proofs. We dedicate this textbook to his memory and trust that he would feel that it is a worthy tribute.

H.N.W., W.F.H., R.S.K..
London 1998

Preface to the First Edition

With the enormous changes in urological practice that have occurred in recent years, we felt that this new *Textbook of Genitourinary Surgery* required an entirely fresh approach. The conventional division of urology on an organ-by-organ basis suffers from the drawback that the effect of disease of one organ on the function of the genitourinary tract as a whole is not emphasized, and it is for this reason that we have designed this new book on a pathological rather than an anatomical basis. We believe that this approach is more relevant to urological practice since it reflects the way in which patient management is orientated.

We are fortunate to have persuaded so many eminent contributors to write on topics on which they have very special expertise. We have aimed to combine a broad background knowledge with clear indications of the preferred lines of management. Inevitably in a book of this size, some areas of overlap exist, and where two authors have expressed differing opinions we believe that readers can either decide for themselves where the truth lies, or appreciate that there remain areas in genitourinary surgery where there is room for more than one view.

During the preparation of this book we have relied heavily on the forbearance of our wives and families. The book was conceived and largely developed during evening meetings at Ristorante Campana, Marylebone High Street, where inspiration from the kitchen sustained us. We have also enjoyed much help, advice and cooperation from our publishers. Finally we are deeply indebted to our hardworking secretaries, Mrs Philippa Stanger and Mrs Sally Lisanti.

H.N.W., W.F.H.
London, 1985

Section 1
Investigations

1 Principles of Urological Investigations

H.N. Whitfield and R.S. Kirby

Introduction

Urology encompasses the investigation and management of a range of diseases that affect the upper and lower urinary tracts as well as those that involve the male genital system. This *Textbook of Genitourinary Surgery* reviews the latest developments in this specialty and the present chapter reviews the principles underlying the investigations that urologists order on a day-to-day basis.

Good urological practice depends on the availability of high quality diagnostic facilities. Giant strides have been made over the last two decades. Just as in treatment, where the emphasis in all surgical disciplines has been to reduce morbidity by developing minimally invasive techniques, so the same philosophy drives the search for new methods of diagnosis. Many of the investigations which were routinely carried out such as intravenous urography and arteriography have now been replaced in many situations. Intravenous urography is no longer considered the method of choice for the investigation of patients with lower urinary tract symptoms. Arteriography is rarely used now for the diagnosis of renal carcinoma and Doppler studies have largely replaced angiography in the identification of renal artery stenosis. The onus upon the urologist now is to keep abreast of all diagnostic advances and to choose for the individual patient the investigation(s) which will provide an accurate, safe and economic diagnostic pathway. The scientific assessment of any new technique is as important in diagnosis as in therapy.

The demarcation that used to exist between investigations to define anatomy and those to identify function has become blurred. Image processing and computer-aided diagnosis have opened up new opportunities for converting images to provide functional information.

Image acquisition, storage and transmission

It is outside the scope of a urological textbook to cover the details of the technological innovations which can be employed in diagnostic imaging. Digital imaging in radiology was first introduced in nuclear medicine. It is now possible to represent digitally images from ultrasound and conventional X-rays; computed tomography (CT) and magnetic resonance imaging (MRI) have always required digital imaging. In effect, all images are viewed in analog form, and it is in the storage that images are divided up into pixels as a sequence of binary digits or bits. Picture archiving and communication symptoms (PACS) enable digital images to be handled electronically. An integral part of data storage is archiving, and although the volume of data is staggering, storage systems with gigabyte (10^9 bytes) and terabyte (10^{12} bytes) capacities have been developed. The reporting of images can also benefit from new technology. The use of such techniques can be extended into teaching and distance teleradiology. The interested reader is referred to a recent overview 'Imaging and information management: computer systems for a changing healthcare environment' [1].

Ultrasound

Ultrasound technology has revolutionized much of urological imaging and has the added advantage of being relatively economic. The debate continues, however, about who can most appropriately perform such investigations. No single solution is right for every situation; residual urine volume estimation, for example, can be assessed easily and accurately after only minimal training; the definition of renal pathology often requires the experience of a highly trained radiologist. Transrectal ultrasound (TRUS) of the prostate is performed by urologists in some countries, by radiologists in others and by either in yet others; because digital rectal examination (DRE) is an essential adjunctive procedure, urologists may be better able to exploit the full potential of this investigation.

The addition of Doppler, colour Doppler and power Doppler to standard ultrasound has raised the level of sophistication to the point at which anatomy and function can both be assessed. Even those parts of the genitourinary tract which are accessible for clinical examination can often be more accurately investigated by ultrasound, (e.g. the prostate and testes), even to the extent that new pathological processes are being identified. The use of contrast agents in colour Doppler sonography of mass lesions of the genitourinary tract may herald a further significant step forward in diagnostic ultrasound [2].

Diagnosis of upper urinary tract obstruction

It has been suggested that it is possible to distinguish between an obstructive and a non-obstructive hydonephrosis using diuresis duplex Doppler sonography. In a recent publication Mallek et al. reported a prospective study in 26 patients (48 kidneys) with suspected chronic upper urinary tract obstruction [3]. All patients underwent both diuretic renography and duplex Doppler sonography before and after the administration of frusemide. They calculated resistive indices before and after the administration of frusemide and concluded that diuresis duplex Doppler sonography was a useful discriminator, particularly in kidneys in which diuretic renography failed to define whether or not obstruction was present. However, other studies have emphasized that in the diagnosis of acute upper urinary tract obstruction duplex Doppler sonography is an insensitive tool compared to standard intravenous urography [4,5].

Diagnosis of renal artery stenosis

Although Doppler ultrasound has been advocated as an accurate method of evaluating renal artery stenosis this technique has not yet found an established place as the investigation of choice [6]. The method is still observer dependent and although agreement in the interpretation of wave form morphology was found by Kliewer et al. they concluded that the analysis of Doppler wave form morphology could not be used to predict the presence or severity of renal artery stenosis [7].

Other renal pathologies

Doppler sonography has been used as a diagnostic tool for predicting chronic rejection in renal transplant patients. However, Deane found that the diagnostic use of changes to intrarenal flow velocities in chronic rejection was limited [8]. Colour flow Doppler sonography for evaluating urinary stone fragmentation during extracorporeal shockwave lithotripsy was investigated by Hobarth et al. [9]; they suggested that the number of shock waves could be reduced by 20% compared with a control group. The intraoperative use of colour Doppler has also been recommended both at open operation in patients undergoing conservative renal surgery for patients with renal tumours and in laparoscopic nephrolithotomy [10]. Further developments in Doppler ultrasound are eagerly awaited.

Lower urinary tract

The measurement of residual urine volume by ultrasound is now standard practice in all urological departments. Transrectal ultrasonography has also become established as an accurate, economical and readily available method of investigating prostatic diseases. The quality of prostate imaging has progressively improved with the advent of higher frequency probes combined with grey scale imaging. The zonal anatomy that was first proposed by McNeal can be clearly demonstrated and the ability to take biopsies from predetermined sites whether they be hypoechoic, isoechoic or hyperechoic is equally important. Prostate volume can be measured, but there are very significant potential inaccuracies [11]. Colour Doppler has added little or nothing to the accuracy of the investigation but may be valuable for the diagnosis of inflammatory conditions such as prostatitis. Computer-assisted diagnosis has also been investigated and the suggestion has been made that carcinoma of the prostate is more accurately diagnosed in this way [12].

The use of echo-contrast agents has been investigated by Watanabe et al. [2]. Such materials contain microbubbles and although at an early stage of development, the evidence so far suggests that there could be a significant enhancement of colour Doppler signals which will improve the accuracy of imaging in the urinary tract.

Computed tompography

Computed tomography has an established place in urological investigation in both the upper and lower urinary tract. A major technical advance has been the development of spiral CT which enables three-dimensional imaging to be performed. This can be particularly useful in deciding whether a renal tumour is suitable for conservative parenchyma-saving surgery. The relationship of the tumour to the collecting system and the arteriovenous anatomy can be demonstrated [13] (Figs 1.1 and 1.2).

Local staging of bladder and particularly prostatic tumours is less easy. CT and MRI scanning unfortunately lack the necessary resolution to identify the micrometastases that are frequently present [14]. Currently the most accurate staging modality in terms of predicting treatment responses is histological examination of transurethral biopsies in the case of bladder tumours and transrectal biopsies for prostate cancer. Much work is currently devoted to the identification of molecular prognostic indicators which will provide an indication of future likely biological behaviour of a given tumour.

Although CT scans can show thickening of the bladder wall it is not possible to differentiate between T1, T2 and T3a tumours with any degree of reliability. Even when the tumour spreads outside the bladder to an adjacent organ,

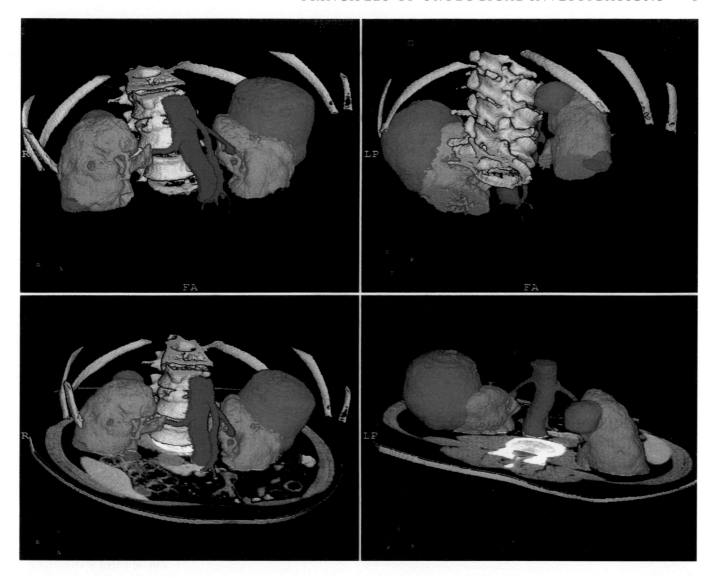

Fig.1.1 Three-dimensional reconstruction of bilateral renal tumours. (Courtesy of Mr M. Singh and Dr I. Mootosamy.)

invasion cannot be identified reliably. Even the absence of a fat plain between the bladder and an adjacent organ is not necessarily evidence of invasion [15]. Many factors influence the accuracy of CT. The equipment itself, the use of intravenous contrast medium, the body habitus of the patient, previous radiotherapy and the experience of the radiologist all contribute to a variability in the accuracy of staging.

Magnetic resonance imaging

It was hoped that the added sophistication of MRI would overcome some of the drawbacks of CT. Images can be obtained in multiple plains and new techniques are being developed using intravenous contrast medium, fat/water suppression techniques, different strength magnets and dedicated coils [16].

In the upper urinary tract MRI has been used to investigate parenchymal renal disease, cysts, angiomyolipomas and renal tumours [17–21].

Screening investigations

When ordering investigations in a particular patient, a number of general considerations need to be taken into account. In the case of a screening test, such as, for example, prostate-specific antigen (PSA), the accuracy with which the test is able to correctly identify affected individuals is known as the sensitivity, while the ability of the test to accurately exclude unaffected individuals is described as the specificity. In general, enhancement of the former results in impairment of the latter, and vice versa. As a result the selection of a cut-off point, (4 ng/ml in the

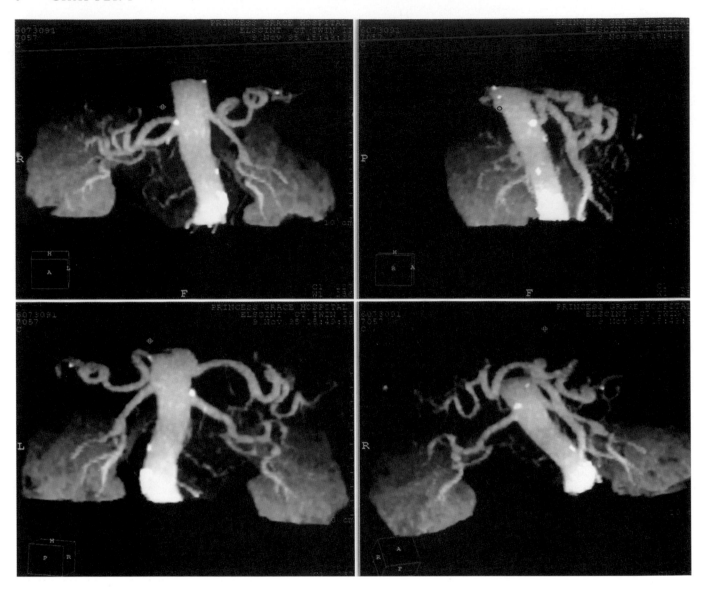

Fig.1.2 Three-dimensional reconstruction of arterial supply to bilateral renal tumours in the same patient as Fig.1.1. (Courtesy of Mr M. Singh and Dr I. Mootosamy.)

case of PSA) reflects a compromise between the twin paradigms of 100% sensitivity and 100% specificity. The overall performance of a test can be best expressed as a receiver operating curve in which sensitivity is plotted against specificity. The nearer the curve is to the top of the right-hand corner of such a plot the closer that test is to perfection.

In addition, other related factors need to be taken into account: those patients who test positive but do not have the disease (false positives) and those who test negative but in fact suffer from the disorder (false negatives) pose a particular problem for the clinician. In this respect the reproducibility (i.e. test/retest reliability) of the particular investigation may be relevant. For example, measurements of post-void residual urine are so lacking in reproducibility that the information gained from a single evaluation is of limited clinical value.

Diagnostic pathways

Disorders of the lower urinary tract constitute by far the most prevalent causes of urological symptoms in men beyond middle age. Around 43% of men over 65 suffer symptoms of bladder outflow obstruction and about half of these (i.e. one man in four) have consequent impairment of their quality of life. The predominant cause of lower urinary tract symptoms is benign prostatic hyperplasia (BPH) which is present in histological form in 70% of 70-year-old men. As this is seldom a cause of mortality, but so often a cause of morbidity, symptom assessment together with quality of life evaluation have become pre-eminent in treatment decisions in this disease area.

Symptoms associated with bladder outflow obstruction caused by BPH include frequency, nocturia, urgency and less commonly urge incontinence (so-called irritative symptoms). In addition patients often complain of hesitancy, poor flow and a sensation of incomplete bladder emptying (obstructive symptoms). Of these, the last two correlated most strongly with the eventual need for operative invervention in the Baltimore longitudinal study of ageing [22]. Madsen [23]

and Iversen and Boyarsky and colleagues [24] were the first to attempt to quantitate BPH-associated symptoms, but their scoring symptoms were never validated. The American Urological Association (AUA) subsequently conceived a score that was validated and included a global question that assessed the degree of 'bother' that resulted from the symptoms [25]. This scoring system has subsequently been endorsed by the International Consensus Committee on BPH and has been termed the International Prostate Symptom Score (IPPS) (Fig. 1.3, see also Chapter 36, p. 511)).

International Prostate Symptom Score (I-PPS)

Patient Name: Date:	Not at all	Less than 1 time in 5	Less than half the time	About half the time	More than half the time	Almost always	Your score
1 Incomplete emptying Over the past month, how often have you had a sensation of not emptying your bladder completely after you finish urinating?	0	1	2	3	4	5	
2 Frequency Over the past month, how often have you had to urinate again less than two hours after you finished urinating?	0	1	2	3	4	5	
3 Intermittency Over the past month, how often have you found you stopped and started again several times when you urinated?	0	1	2	3	4	5	
4 Urgency Over the past month, how often have you found it difficult to postpone urination?	0	1	2	3	4	5	
5 Weak stream Over the past month, how often have you had a weak urinary stream?	0	1	2	3	4	5	
6 Straining Over the past month, how often have you had to push or strain to begin urination?	0	1	2	3	4	5	

	None	1 time	2 times	3 times	4 times	5 times or more	
7 Nocturia Over the past month, how many times did you most typically get up to urinate from the time you went to bed at night until the time you got up in the morning	0	1	2	3	4	5	
Total I-PSS Score							

Quality of life due to urinary symptoms	Delighted	Pleased	Mostly satisfied	Mixed-about equally satisfied and dissatisfied	Mostly dissatisfied	Unhappy	Terrible
If you were to spend the rest of your life with your urinary condition just the way it is now, how would you feel about that?	0	1	2	3	4	5	6

The International Prostate Symptom Score (I-PSS) is based on the answers to seven questions concerning urinary symptoms. Each question is assigned points from 0 to 5 indicating increasing severity of the particular symptom. the total score can therefore range from o to 35 (asymptomatic to very symptomatic).

Although there are presently no standard recommendations into grading patients with mild, moderate or severe symptoms, patients can be tentatively classified as follows: 0–7 = **mildly symptomatic**; 8–19 = **moderately symptomatic**; 20–35 = **severely symptomatic**.

The International Consensus Committrr (ICC) recommends the use of only a single question to assess a patient's quality of life. The answers to this question range from 'delighted' to 'terrible' or 0 to 6. Although this single question may or may not capture the global impact of BPH symptoms on quality of life, it may serve as a valuable starting point for a doctor - patient conversation.

Fig.1.3 The International Prostate Symptom Score.

Currently most clinicians utilize either the AUA symptom score or IPSS in men presenting with BPH and take the value into account before making treatment decisions. In these circumstances there are, however, two other important considerations: first the need to exclude carcinoma of the prostate and secondly the confirmation of the presence of obstruction and the estimation of its severity.

The exclusion of prostate cancer

The glycoprotein PSA is exclusively produced by the epithelial cells of the prostate. Its function is that of a protease to liquify semen after ejaculation. In health only a small proportion (around one-thousandth) of secreted PSA is absorbed in the circulation. Of the fraction that is absorbed a fraction remains unbound as 'free' PSA, while the remainder is bound either to antichymotrypsin or to α-macroglobulin. The resultant total measurable PSA is generally less than 4.0 ng/ml, but values above this cut-off point are frequently encountered, not only in prostate cancer but also in BPH, and to a lesser extent in prostatitis. Recently it has been discovered that the amount of 'free' PSA is diminished in patients with prostate cancer compared with those with normal or benign conditions [26]. A free:total ratio of < 0.15 may therefore indicate the likely presence of prostate cancer and can be considered, like a total PSA value of > 4.0 ng/ml, as an indication for a TRUS-guided biopsy of the prostate.

The reproducibility of multiple PSA determinations in the same individual depends upon the assay employed; there is a variation of up to 25%. Levels can be altered by prostatic perturbations, especially biopsy, and to a minor extent by sexual activity; DRE, however, does not significantly affect serum PSA values. In a given individual whenever possible the same PSA assay should be employed to reduce the variability and to obtain a clearer picture of the so-called 'PSA velocity' — that is the change in PSA over time [27].

The diagnosis of bladder outflow obstruction

Although bladder outflow obstruction is by far the commonest cause of lower urinary tract symptoms in the male, before any invasive therapy is contemplated the presence of obstruction should be verified and the severity assessed. Although the intravenous urogram has been used historically in this context, its role has now largely been usurped by the combined use of transabdominal ultrasound and uroflowmetry. The combination of a significantly reduced flow rate and the presence of a post-voiding residue carries a high probability of the presence of obstruction. Although values of the latter parameter are very variable [28], uroflow values do have reasonably good test/retest reliability [29]. It should be remembered, however, that bladder contractility is an essential component of voiding. Conditions such as diabetes, which are associated with damage to the parasympathetic innervation of the detrusor, may result in a reduced uroflow and impaired bladder emptying without obstruction being present. In these circumstances pressure–flow urodynamics are required to confirm the presence of low-pressure/low-flow voiding.

Location of the precise level of the lower urinary tract obstruction may also be important. Although in practice the prostate is most often implicated, urethral strictures (membranous, bulbar or anterior) and bladder neck dyssynergia all need to be considered as differential diagnoses and require very different treatment. In the case of a suspected urethral stricture, retrograde urethrography (Fig. 1.4) is required to demonstrate the site of narrowing. Although some still advocate urethroscopy as a diagnostic (and simultaneously therapeutic) manoeuvre, occasionally a stricture can be convoluted and difficult to instrument without the prior knowledge of the particular anatomy that a preoperative urethrogram affords.

Diagnostic cystoscopy, while an essential component of a work-up for haematuria (macroscopic or microscopic), is not regularly required for the investigation of a patient with lower urinary tract symptoms. In patients with atypical symptoms, however, especially associated with sterile pyuria, a cystoscopy and bladder biopsy may provide crucial confirmatory evidence of serious conditions such as transitional cell carcinoma *in situ* or tuberculosis.

Neurophysiological investigations

Although many neurological conditions can masquerade as bladder outflow obstruction as a result of BPH, most are associated with other neurological signs and symptoms that provide a clue to the diagnosis. Occult neuropathic lesions of the bladder are in fact rather unusual. Those that do occur are usually lower motor neurone lesions of the cauda equina or pelvic plexus, caused, for example, by a prolapsed intervertebral disc or a previous abdomino-perineal resection of the rectum. In either circumstance urethral sphincter electromyography will usually reveal prolonged and polyphasic motor units characteristic of reinnervation. Other, more complex neurophysiological tests such as sacral reflex latencies and cortical-evoked responses, although technically feasible, are of less practical diagnostic value.

Confirming the diagnosis of lower urinary tract malignancy

The two dominant malignancies of the lower urinary tract are transitional cell carcinoma (TCC) and adenocarcinoma

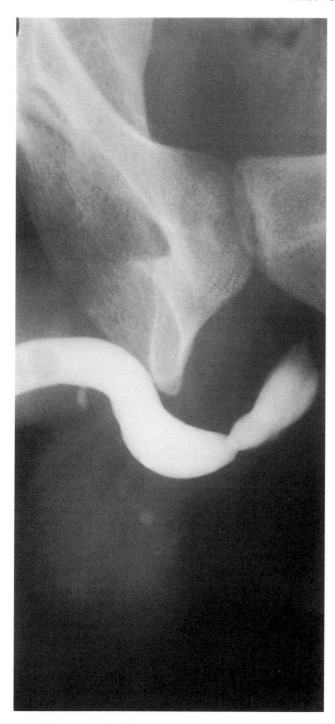

Fig.1.4 A retrograde urethrogram demonstrating a tight stricture of the bulbar urethra.

of the prostate. The former is generally suspected on the basis of a history of haematuria, the latter by the finding of a suspicious DRE or a raised PSA. In either circumstance the diagnosis of cancer should be confirmed histologically before treatment is initiated. In the case of prostate cancer this is achieved by systematic ultrasound-guided biopsy with targeted sampling of any hypoechoic areas; in TCC transurethral resection of the tumour and sampling of the underlying muscle to assess invasion is required. Histopathological examination of sampled tissue provides vital information concerning tumour grade which is essential not only for treatment decisions but also carries prognostic significance. It should be appreciated, however, that pathological grading of needle biopsy specimens, especially in prostate cancer, not infrequently underestimates the final grading value in the subsequent surgical specimen.

Staging of bladder tumours and prostate cancer

Treatment decisions in both bladder and prostate cancer depend not only on tumour grade but also critically on tumour stage. To this end imaging investigations are ordered with two aims: first to exclude distant metastases, secondly to assess the local tumour stage. Distant metastases may be detected by chest X-rays and CT as well as with bone scanning. Recently the prospect of molecular staging using polymerase chain reaction technology to detect cells in the bone marrow or circulation capable of producing mRNA encoding PSA has arisen [30]. At the time of writing, however, this is still investigational but could well prove an invaluable staging tool.

Conclusion

The role of a urologist, just as of any clinician, is to be the coordinator of the management strategy for any individual patient. The urologist must be the person to decide the most appropriate investigations, the sequence of those investigations and the treatment to be pursued on the basis of the results. Although a truism it is worth repeating the much quoted but often neglected principle that an investigation is only worth while if management decisions will be influenced by the outcome.

The urologist must also on occasions act as the gatekeeper, and resist change for the sake of change and avoid oversophistication of simple issues. Acute renal colic, a common urological emergency, can best be investigated by emergency intravenous urography; pressures either to 'simplify' by using a plain abdominal X-ray and ultrasound or to 'sophisticate' by using reformatted non-contrast helical CT, must be resisted [31].

The accuracy of diagnostic techniques available to the urologist makes the investigation of urological pathology in patients of all ages a safe and accurate science rather than simply a clinical estimate.

References

1 Greenes RA, Bauman RA, eds. *Imaging and Information*

Management: Computer Systems for a Changing Healthcare Environment. Radiol Clin Noth Am 1996;**34**:3.

2 Watanabe H, Saitoh M, Orikasa S *et al.* Efficacy of an echo contrast agent, SH/TA-508, in color Doppler sonography of mass lesions. *Urol Oncol* 1995;**1**:215–22.

3 Mallek R, Bankier AA, Etele-Hainz A, Kletter K, Mostbeck GH. Distinction between obstructive and non-obstructive hydronephrosis: value of diuresis duplex Doppler sonography. *Am J Roentgenol* 1996; **166**(1):113–17.

4 Deyoe LA, Cronan JJ, Breslaw BH, Ridlen MS. New techniques of ultrasound and color Doppler in the prospective evaluation of acute renal obstruction. Do they replace the intravenous urogram? *Abdominal Imaging* 1995;**20**(1):58–63.

5 Tublin ME, Dodd GD III, Verdile VP. Acute renal colic: diagnosis with duplex Doppler ultrasound. *Radiology* 1994; **193**(3):697–701.

6 Miralles M, Cairols M, Cotillas J, Gimenez A, Santiso A. Value of Doppler parameters in the diagnosis of renal artery stenosis. *J Vasc Surg* 1996;**23**(3):428–35.

7 Kliewer MA, Tupler RH, Hertzberg BS *et al.* Doppler evaluation of renal artery stenosis: intraobserver agreement in the interpretation of waveform morphology. *Am J Roentgenol* 1994;**162**(6):1371–6.

8 Deane C. Doppler and color Doppler ultrasonography in renal transplants: chronic rejection. *J Clin Ultrasound* 1992;**28**(8): 539–44.

9 Hobarth K, Maier A, Hofbauer J, Marberger M. Color flow Doppler sonography for extracorporeal shockwave lithotripsy. *J Urol* 1993;**150**(6):1768–70.

10 Van Cangh PJ, Abi Aad AS, Lorge F *et al.* Laparoscopic nephrolithotomy: the value of intracorporeal sonography and color Doppler. *Urology* 1995;**45**(3):516–19.

11 Nathan MS, Seenivasagam K, Mei Q *et al.* Transrectal ultrasonography: why are estimates of prostate volume and dimension so inaccurate? *Br J Urol* 1996;**77**:401–7.

12 De le Rosette JJMCH, Giesen RJB, Huynen RG *et al.* Computerized analysis of transrectal ultrasonography images in the dectection of prostate carcinoma. *Br J Urol* 1995;**75**:485–91.

13 Chernoff DM, Silverman SG, Kikinis R *et al.* Three-dimensional imaging and display of renal tumours using spiral CT: a potential aid to partial nephrectomy. *Urology* 1994;**43**(1):125–9.

14 Rifkin MD, Zerhouni EA, Gatsonis CA *et al.* Comparison of magnetic resonance imaging and ultrasonography in staging early prostate cancer. *N Engl J Med* 1990;**323**(10):621–6.

15 Husband JE. Review: staging bladder cancer. *Clin Radiol* 1992;**46**:153–9.

16 Persad T, Kabala J, Gillatt D *et al.* Magnetic resonance imaging in the staging of bladder cancer. *Br J Urol* 1993;**71**:566–73.

17 Harmon WJ, King BF, Lieber MM. Renal oncocytoma: magnetic resonance imaging characteristics. *J Urol* 1996;**155**(3):863–7.

18 Nishi T. Magnetic resonance imaging of autosomal recessive polycystic kidney disease *in uretero. J Obstet Gynaecol* 1995;**21**(5):471–4.

19 Hauser M, Krestin GP, Hagspiel KD. Bilateral solid multifocal intra-renal and peri-renal lesions: differentiation with ultrasonography, computed tomography and magnetic resonance imaging. *Clin Radiol* 1995;**50**(5):288–94.

20 Parks CM, Kellett MJ. Staging renal cell carcinoma. *Clin Radiol* 1994;**49**(4):223–30.

21 Silverman JM, Friedman ML, Van Allan RJ. Detection of main renal artery stenosis using phase-contrast cine MR angiography. *Am J Roentgenol* 1996;**166**(5):1131–7.

22 Arrighi H, Guess H, Metter E, Fozard J. Symptoms and signs of prostatism as risk factors for prostatectomy. *Prostate* 1990;**16**:253–61.

23 Madsen P, Iversen P. A point scoring system for selecting operative candidates. In: Hinman FJ, ed. *Benign Prostatic Hypertrophy.* New York: Springer Verlag, 1983:763–5.

24 Boyarsky S, Jones G, Paulson DF, Front CR. A new look at bladder neck obstruction by the Food and Drug Administration regulators. Guidelines for investigation of benign prostatic hypertrophy. *Trans Am Assoc Genito-Urin Surg* 1977;**68**: 29–32.

25 Barry M, Fowler F, O'Leary M *et al.* Correlation of the American Urological Association Symptom index with self-administered versions of the Madsen–Iversen, Boyarsky and Maine medical assessment with program symptom indexes. *J Urol* 1992;**148**:1558–63.

26 Christensson A, Bjork T, Nilsson O *et al.* Serum prostate specific antigen complexed to alpha-1-antichymotrypsin as an indicator of prostate cancer. *J Urol* 1993;**150**:100–5.

27 Carter B, Pearson K, Metter J *et al.* Longitudinal evaluation of prostate specific antigen levels in men with and without prostate cancer. *J Am Med Assoc* 1993;**267**:2215–20.

28 Dunsmir W, Feneley M, Corry D, Bryan J, Kirby RS. The day-to-day variation (test–retest reliability) of residual urine measurement. *Br J Urol* 1996;**77**:192–3.

29 Feneley M, Dunsmir W, Pearce J, Kirby RS. Reproducibility of uroflow measurement: experience during a double-blind, placebo-controlled study of doxazosin in benign prostatic hyperplasia. *Urology* 1996;**47**:658–63.

30 Katz AE, Olsson MD, Raffo AJE. Molecular staging of prostate cancer with the use of an enhanced reverse transcriptase-PCR assay. *Urology* 1994;**43**:765–75.

31 Sommer FG, Jeffrey RB, Rubin GD *et al.* Detection of ureteral calculi in patients with suspected renal colic: value of reformatted noncontrast helical CT. *Am J Roentgenol* 1995;**165**:509–13.

2 Basic Uroradiological Investigations
Judith A.W.Webb

Radio-opaque contrast media

Radio-opaque contrast media may be given either intra-vascularly—for intravenous urography (IVU), computed tomography (CT) or angiography—or may be introduced directly into the urinary tract through a needle or catheter—for urethrography, micturating cystography or antegrade and retrograde pyelography. The currently used contrast agents (Table 2.1) all depend for their radio-opacity on a tri-iodinated benzene ring. The ionic monomers in use since the 1950s are sodium or meglumine salts which ionize to give high osmolality solutions. At the commonly used concentrations of 300 mg I/ml these agents have an osmolality approximately five times that of plasma. Recently, lower osmolality agents have been developed. The most commonly used are monomers which do not ionize in solution (non-ionic monomers) and others are dimers, both ionic and non-ionic. The osmolality of the

Table 2.1 Radio-opaque contrast media.

	Non-proprietary name	Proprietary name
High osmolality		
Ionic monomers	Iothalamate	Conray
(ratio 1.5 media)	Diatrizoate	Hypaque, Urografin, Angiografin,Renografin
	Metrizoate	Triosil, Isopaque
Iodamide	Uromiro	
	Ioxithalamate	Telebrix, Vasobrix
	Ioglicate	Rayvist
Low osmolality		
Non-ionic	Iopamidol	Niopam, Isovue
monomers	Iohexol	Omnipaque
(ratio 3.0 media)	Iopromide	Ultravist
	Ioversol	Optiray
Ionic dimers	Ioxaglate	Hexabrix
(ratio 3.0 media)		
Non-ionic dimers	Iotrolan	Isovist
(ratio 6.0 media)	Iodixanol	Visipaque

non-ionic monomers at a concentration of 300 mg I/ml is approximately twice that of plasma. The low osmolality ionic monomers are considerably more expensive than the higher osmolality agents, by a factor of four to five times in Europe and approximately 10 times in the USA.

Excretion

Contrast media given intravascularly are rapidly distributed throughout the extracellular fluid [1–3]. Over 90% is then excreted through the kidneys in the first 24 h [1]. At the doses used in diagnostic radiology, excretion is by glomerular filtration [1,2,4,5].

Radiographs or CT scans obtained immediately after intravascular contrast medium is given show opacification of the renal parenchyma, the nephrogram. When contrast medium is given intra-arterially or early images are obtained at CT, opacification of the renal cortex is seen to precede opacification of the remaining renal parenchyma. The so-called cortical or angiographic nephrogram is largely produced by contrast medium in the vascular tree. The homogeneous nephrogram seen on later angiographic and CT images and at urography is produced largely by filtered contrast medium in the lumen of the proximal convoluted tubules [6]. Nephrogram density depends on glomerular filtration rate and plasma contrast concentration and is at its peak immediately after contrast medium injection. Larger doses of contrast medium produce nephrograms of increased density [7]. Since the nephrogram is a proximal rather than a distal tubular phenomenon, it is not affected by dehydration [8].

As contrast medium passes along the renal tubules, it is concentrated so that contrast medium density in the pelvicalyceal system, the pyelogram, is considerably greater than nephrogram density. Pyelogram density depends on the concentration of contrast medium in the urine and on the degree of distension of the pelvicalyceal system [9]. It can be increased by increasing the contrast medium dose, within certain limits, or by dehydration [4,9,10]. The lower osmolality agents produce less osmotic diuresis and are associated with increased contrast medium concentrations in the urine, but the detectable effect on pyelogram density is minimal [11,12].

Adverse effects

General effects

Intravascular contrast medium often produces a sensation of warmth or flushing, mild nausea or a metallic taste in the mouth. These minor effects may be considered to be normal and are all commoner with the higher osmolality agents. About 5% of patients given ionic agents and 1% given non-ionic agents experience significant side effects [13–15]. Most reactions are of moderate severity and involve bronchospasm, vomiting, urticaria, angioneurotic oedema and hypotension. More serious side effects, including cardiac arrhythmias, cardiac arrest, convulsions and loss of consciousness, occur in 0.01% of individuals receiving ionic agents and approximately 5–10 times less in individuals receiving non-ionic agents [15–17]. Death occurs in between one in 40 000 and one in 75 000 receiving an ionic agent [13,18] and with non-ionic agents appears to be four to five times less common [17]. The cause of contrast medium reactions is incompletely understood. Activation of the complement system and release of histamine and vasoactive agents are considered to be important [19].

The risk of a contrast medium reaction is increased if there is a history of previous reaction to contrast medium, asthma, significant allergy or heart disease [17,20]. In such at-risk subjects a non-ionic agent should always be used. Where there is a history of contrast medium reaction, asthma or significant allergy, steroid premedication should be given before intravascular contrast medium. To be effective it must be given at least 12 h (preferably 24 h) before contrast medium. A typical regimen would be prednisolone 20 mg three times daily for 2 days, starting 24 h before the planned contrast medium injection.

Contrast medium injections should be given in a setting where full resuscitation facilities are available. Most contrast medium reactions occur in the first 10–15 min after contrast medium injection and the patient should be monitored during this period. Management of reactions is symptomatic. In addition, in all severe reactions, intravenous hydro-cortisone should be given [21].

Renal effects

If renal function is normal, intravascular contrast media produce no adverse effects on renal function. When renal function is impaired, there is an approximately 10% risk of causing a rise in serum creatinine which is usually reversible [22]. The risk of producing a deterioration in renal function is increased by the use of large contrast medium doses, by dehydration and by diabetes mellitus [23].

Plain films and plain renal tomography

Plain films are used to detect urinary tract calcifications and may also show the renal outlines. A full-length film of the abdomen taken on inspiration and a coned view of the renal area taken on expiration are a good combination. A calcification overlying the kidney is intrarenal if it maintains its relationship to the renal poles on these films. It may also be necessary to obtain an oblique film of the kidney or plain renal tomography to confirm that a calcification is intrarenal.

Plain films also show calcifications along the line of the ureters, which usually cross the lumbar transverse processes before curving into the pelvis. However, plain films have only a sensitivity of 50–77% for the detection of ureteric calculi [24–26]. Problems arise with small low-density or lucent calculi and where calculi overlie bone (Fig. 2.1a) or are hidden by overlying bowel. The specificity of plain films alone is also poor, particularly in the pelvis, where phleboliths and arterial calcifications may mimic ureteric stones. Phleboliths usually lie below the line of the ischial spines and are rounded with a lucent centre. However, to make a confident diagnosis of a ureteric calculus a contrast medium examination, usually IVU, is almost always necessary (Fig. 2.1b).

The kidneys and psoas muscles are usually seen outlined by lucent retroperitoneal fat on plain films. However, the renal outline is usually not seen with sufficient certainty for accurate renal measurement; this should be obtained either by ultrasonography (US) or IVU.

Plain renal tomography is a very important additional method of detecting renal calculi, especially in the common situation where there is overlying bowel or where the calculi are of low density. Plain tomography often shows calculi unsuspected on plain films, for example Schwartz *et al.* [27] detected unsuspected calculi in nearly 40% of patients being investigated for haematuria or suspected renal colic. Plain tomography is also helpful in showing that calcifications overlying the kidney are intrarenal, where plain films alone are equivocal. The combination of plain films and plain renal tomography is more sensitive than renal US in the detection of opaque renal calculi [28].

Intravenous urography

Technique

Although dehydration is no longer considered necessary, some fluid restriction before urography, for example to not

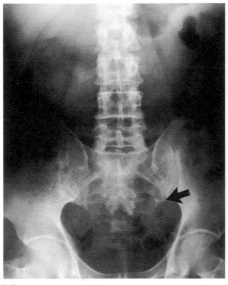
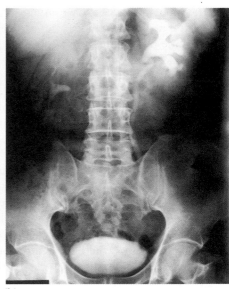

Fig. 2.1 (a) A 7 mm calcification overlying the lower left sacrum (arrowed), shown at urography (b) to lie in the ureter and to be causing hold up.

(a)

(b)

more than 500 ml in the preceding 4 h, is usually recommended. When renal function is impaired the patient must be well hydrated to minimize the potential for contrast medium nephrotoxicity.

After preliminary plain films, the intravenous contrast medium is given. A dose of 300 mg I/kg is used if renal function is normal and is given as a bolus injection over about 1 min. With impaired renal function a high-dose technique (600 mg I/kg) is used. Cost considerations have slowed the introduction of the low osmolality non-ionic contrast media for urography [29]. They are more comfortable for the patient, have less risk of side effects and it is to be hoped that eventually they will entirely replace higher osmolality agents for IVU. Low osmolality agents

should always be used in patients at risk of contrast medium reaction or nephrotoxicity (see p. 12).

A coned film of the renal area immediately after the contrast medium is given shows the nephrogram best. A coned film of the renal area 5 min after contrast medium should show filling of the pelvicalyceal systems. In adults, provided there is no evidence of obstruction or any other contraindication (e.g. aortic aneurysm, recent surgery), ureteric compression is applied at pelvic brim level. This distends the pelvicalyceal systems so that their detailed anatomy can be assessed on a film obtained when ureteric compression has been in place for 5 min (Fig. 2.2). Ureteric compression is not used in children. Following the release of ureteric compression, a full-length film will show the

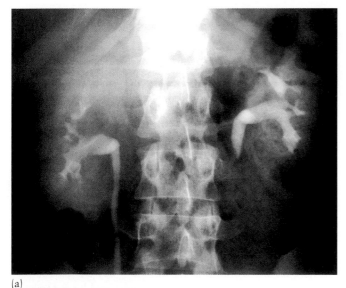
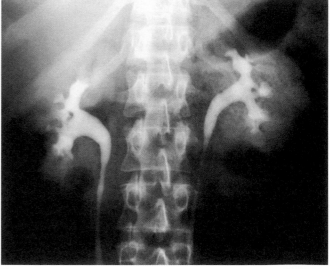

(a)

(b)

Fig. 2.2 (a) A poorly distended pelvicalyceal system before compression is applied. (b) Detailed normal pelvicalyceal anatomy can be well seen when ureteric compression is applied.

ureters and bladder (Fig. 2.3). A further full-length film taken after voiding allows the assessment of upper tract drainage and bladder emptying.

Additional films may be helpful in particular circumstances. Tomography of the nephrogram phase is helpful to search for masses not altering the renal contour (e.g. in patients with haematuria) (Fig. 2.4). Tomography is also useful when the kidneys are obscured by overlying bowel or are only faintly opacified when renal function is impaired. Oblique views of the kidneys with ureteric compression applied are helpful when pelvicalyceal anatomy is unclear or when abnormalities are suspected (e.g. papillary necrosis, medullary sponge kidney, tuberculosis). A prone film may help to show the mid and lower ureter, and oblique films or fluoroscopy of the ureters may be necessary to show whether calcifications overlying them are intraureteric. Oblique views of the bladder are helpful when it is unclear whether lucency overlying the bladder represents an intraluminal mass or gas in overlying bowel. Delayed films are often necessary if there is obstruction, but should not be obtained too frequently. The 'rule of eight' is a useful guide—thus if there is no pelvicalyceal

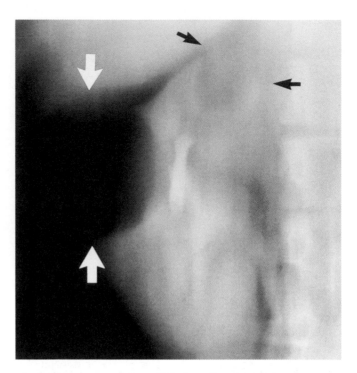

Fig. 2.4 Tomogram of the right kidney showing a 2.5 cm upper pole mass not deforming the renal contour (black arrows) as well as a lateral 6.5 cm mass (white arrows) causing a defect in the renal outline.

filling with contrast medium by 15 min, the next film need not be taken until 2 h [30].

Special techniques

Emergency urography

When ureteric colic or acute pelviureteric junction (PUJ) obstruction is suspected, limited emergency urography should be done at the time when the patient has pain. After preliminary plain films, contrast medium is injected and a full-length film is obtained 15 min later. If there is hold up at vesicoureteric junction level, a full-length post-micturition film should also be obtained (Fig. 2.5). If there is obstruction, delayed films should be obtained to define the site of the hold up.

Frusemide urography

This is useful in the diagnosis of PUJ obstruction [31]. If PUJ obstruction is suspected before the urogram, a high-dose technique is used (600 mg I/kg). After the full-length film, 40 mg frusemide is given intravenously and a further full-length film is obtained 15 min later. In PUJ obstruction the affected system increases in size appreciably and fails to drain (Fig. 2.6), while normal systems have washed out by the post-frusemide film. The method is also a useful

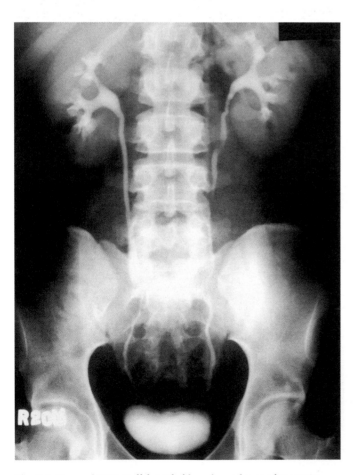

Fig. 2.3 Normal IVU. Full-length film after release of ureteric compression showing anatomy of the pelvicalyceal systems, ureters and bladder.

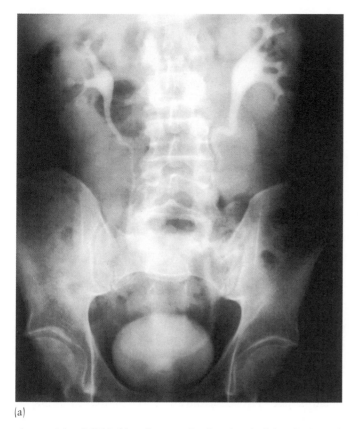

(a)

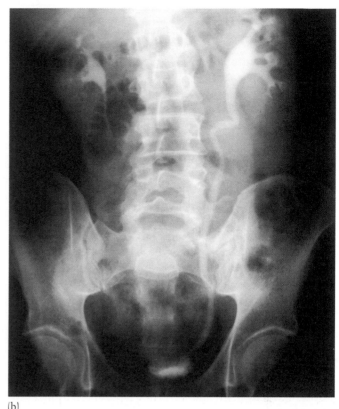

(b)

Fig. 2.5 (a) A full bladder obscures the distal end of the obstructed left ureter. Hold up at the left vesicoureteric junction, caused by a small opaque stone, can be well seen after voiding (b).

Fig. 2.6 Left pelviureteric junction obstruction. (a) A slightly full, left pelvicalyceal system in a patient with left loin pain. (b) After frusemide the left pelvicalyceal system dilates and the right system washes out.

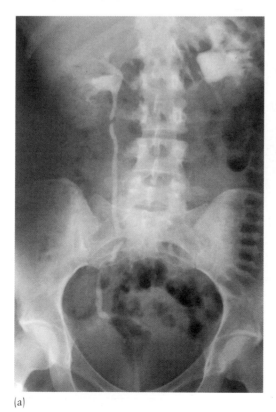

(a)

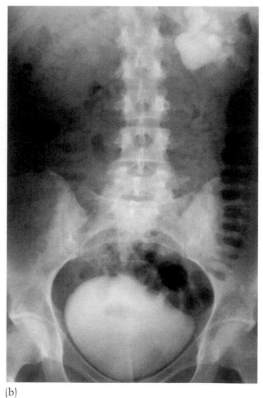

(b)

adjunct during urography. If there is a large renal pelvis and it is unclear whether it is obstructed, 40 mg frusemide should be given intravenously and a full-length film obtained 15 min later to assess drainage.

Assessment

The urogram films should be studied systematically.
1 The *plain films* should be checked for calcifications.
2 The *nephrogram film* should be used to assess renal position, measure the kidneys, check the renal outline and detect masses and scars. The kidneys usually lie with the upper pole medial to the lower poles. Renal length measurement at urography is an overestimate (usually by about 20–25%) because of radiographic magnification [32]. In adults, normal kidney length approximates to the first 3.5 lumbar vertebrae and their intervening disc spaces [33]. A kidney measuring less than 11 cm is considered to be small. Parenchymal thickness should be assessed by measuring the distance between a line joining the tips of the papillae and the renal outline (Fig. 2.7), which should be uniform. This is the best method to detect scars.
3 The *pelvicalyceal system* should be assessed with and without compression. It is important to check that the calyces have all filled and that they have sharp fornices on the films without ureteric compression. Filling defects in the pelvicalyceal system and abnormal contrast medium collections in the papillae should be sought.
4 The *ureters* should be assessed for position, filling

defects, strictures and calculi. Drainage of the pelvicalyceal systems and ureters should be assessed on the post-micturition films.
5 The *bladder* should be assessed for size, position, wall thickness, filling defects and emptying.

Indications

IVU was formerly the usual first renal imaging method but this role has been challenged by US and to a lesser extent by nuclear medicine and CT. None the less, IVU retains its pre-eminent position in a variety of settings [34] because of its ability to:
1 provide a rapid overview of urinary tract anatomy (see Fig. 2.3);
2 detect and localize calcifications in the urinary tract (see Fig. 2.1);
3 show the detailed anatomy of the pelvicalyceal system and ureter, as well as demonstrating the renal parenchyma and bladder.

A variety of renal diagnoses can only be made by assessing the calyces and the overlying parenchyma together (Table 2.2 and Fig. 2.8). Thus blunted calyces are associated with focal parenchymal thinning in focal reflux nephropathy (Fig. 2.9), diffuse parenchymal thinning if there is ureteric obstruction, and no overlying parenchymal loss in papillary necrosis.

The major indications for IVU in urological practice are in patients with haematuria, stone disease or suspected obstruction.

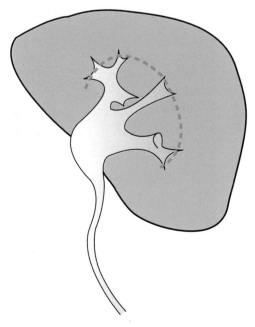

Fig. 2.7 Assessment of renal parenchymal thickness on the urogram. (Redrawn with permission from Cattell WR, Webb JAW, Hilson AJW. *Clinical Renal Imaging* (1989) John Wiley & Sons, Ltd.)

Table 2.2 Differential diagnosis of renal disease.

1 Calyceal/papillary abnormality without parenchymal loss:
    papillary necrosis
    medullary sponge kidney
    tuberculosis
    megacalyces
    calyceal cyst

2 Calyceal/papillary abnormality with associated focal parenchymal scarring:
    focal reflux nephropathy (chronic atrophic pyelonephritis)
    stone disease with previous infundibular obstruction

3 Focal parenchymal scarring without calyceal/papillary abnormality:
    infarct
    post-trauma

4 Calyceal/papillary abnormality with diffuse parenchymal thinning:
    obstructive or post-obstructive atrophy
    diffuse high-pressure reflux nephropathy

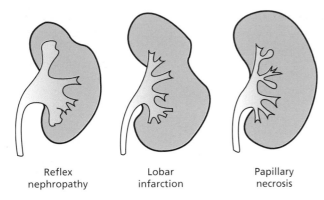

| Reflex nephropathy | Lobar infarction | Papillary necrosis |

Fig. 2.8 Diagram illustrating the differentiation of focal reflux nephropathy (blunted calyces, overlying scars), infarction (normal calyx, overlying scar) and papillary necrosis (blunted calyces, contrast tracks and pools in the papillae, normal overlying parenchyma).

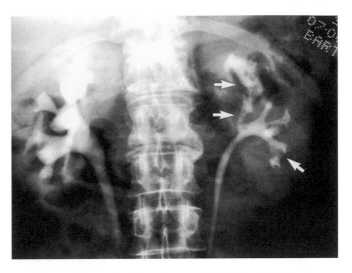

Fig. 2.10 Transitional cell carcinoma of the left pelvicalyceal system with multiple small lucent filling defects in the upper and lower calyces (arrowed).

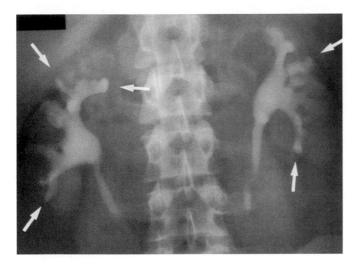

Fig 2.9 Focal reflux nephropathy showing multiple blunted calyces with overlying parenchymal thinning.

Haematuria

It has been suggested that US should replace IVU as the first imaging method in haematuria [35,36]. Although US is a more sensitive detector of renal masses than is IVU with tomography [37], other major concerns in patients with haematuria are calculus disease and transitional cell carcinoma of the upper tract (Fig. 2.10). Other causes of haematuria which may also be identified by renal imaging are papillary necrosis (Fig. 2.11), tuberculosis and renal infarcts. Only urography can define upper tract anatomy sufficiently well to show the subtle abnormalities in transitional cell carcinoma and to detect and localize urinary tract calculi. Urography remains the method of choice to detect upper tract causes of haematuria, combined with cystoscopy for bladder assessment. If both IVU and cystoscopy are negative, a cross-sectional imaging

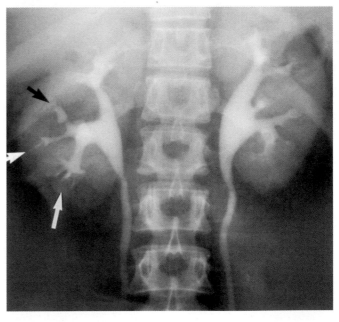

Fig. 2.11 Papillary necrosis in sickle cell trait. Note the blunted calyx (black arrow), the contrast medium pool in the calyx (short white arrow) and the contrast medium tracks arising from the calyces (long white arrow).

method (US or CT) should be used to check for small renal masses not detected by IVU.

Stone disease

Urography is the best method of detecting opaque urinary tract calculi, measuring them accurately and localizing them to the calyces, pelvis, ureter or bladder. IVU allows

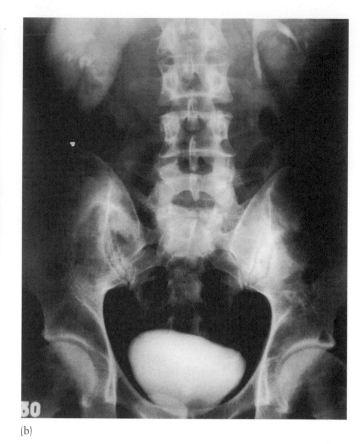

(a)

(b)

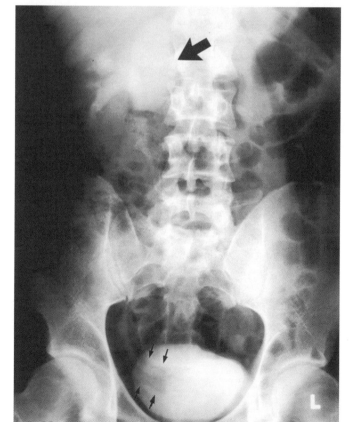

(c)

Fig. 2.12 Calculus at the right vesicoureteric junction causing acute obstruction. (a) Calculus (arrowed). (b) Dense right nephrogram and delayed right pelvicalyceal filling. (c) Filling of a mildly dilated pelvicalyceal system and ureter to the level of the calculus. There is oedema around the vesicoureteric junction (small black arrows) and contrast medium in the gallbladder (large black arrow). (Reprinted by permission of Cattell WR, Webb JAW, Hilson AJW. *Clinical Renal Imaging* (1989) John Wiley & Sons, Ltd.)

some assessment of the degree of obstruction, either in acute obstruction by the typical increasingly dense nephrogram, or in chronic obstruction from the degree of secondary dilatation and hold up. Urography also shows urinary tract anatomy in sufficient detail to allow treatment decisions to be made; such as whether drainage after extracorporeal shockwave lithotripsy (ESWL) will be adequate, or whether percutaneous nephrolithotomy can be performed and, if so, by what route [38,39].

Obstruction

In suspected ureteric colic, urography remains the method of choice in most centres. It is both sensitive and specific (87% and 100% in Svedstrom's series [24]) and widely available. US and plain films in the hydrated subject may have a high sensitivity (95% [26]) but have a much lower specificity (67%) in the diagnosis of calculous obstruction of the ureter. In Dalla Palma's series [26], 40% of patients would have required IVU as well as the initial US and plain film. The typical urographic appearance in ureteric colic is of delayed pelvicalyceal filling with contrast medium with an increasingly dense nephrogram. Delayed films typically show mild dilatation of the ureter to the level of hold up at the calculus (Fig. 2.12).

In many situations where chronic renal obstruction is suspected or must be excluded (e.g. renal failure, prostatism, pelvic tumour), US is now the method of choice to check for pelvicalyceal dilatation [40]. Urography still has a role in diagnosing the cause of obstruction in some patients and in detecting some of the US false positives, caused, for example, by vesicoureteric reflux, distensible systems or congenital variants. Frusemide urography (see p. 12) is helpful if pelviureteric junction obstruction is suspected.

Other indications

1 *Urinary tract infection* (UTI): urography has also been challenged by US in the investigation of adults with UTI [41]. US is a good method for checking for evidence of complicating obstruction in patients with UTI which is not responding normally to antibiotics. In patients with proven recurrent UTI, after the acute episode it is important to check for conditions which may predispose to renal damage or relapsing infection — for example calculi, papillary necrosis, medullary sponge kidney (Fig. 2.13), scars or calyceal cysts. Urography, not US, should be used in this setting.

2 *Local loin trauma*: to check for function on the affected side, and anatomy and function on the uninjured side, as well as showing the effects of the injury.

3 *Unexplained pyuria and persistent unexplained proteinuria* (not caused by nephritis or the nephrotic syndrome): to check for reflux nephropathy, papillary necrosis or tuberculosis.

4 *Renal impairment* (with serum creatinine 300 μmol or less and no evidence of obstruction on US): to detect reflux nephropathy, papillary necrosis, infarcts.

5 *Congenital urinary tract anomalies*: the ureteric anatomy in duplex kidney and complex fusion and rotation anomalies can be rapidly elucidated (Fig. 2.14).

6 *Prospective renal transplant donors*: to check for normal renal anatomy.

7 Postoperative follow-up after ureteric surgery.

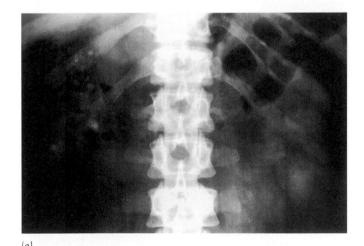

(a)

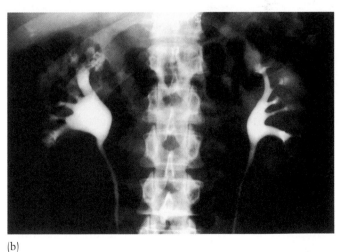

(b)

Fig. 2.13 Medullary sponge kidney. (a) Plain film showing papillary nephrocalcinosis. (b) Multiple contrast medium pools and streaks in the affected papillae. (Reproduced with permission from Webb J. Imaging Urinary Tract Infection. In: Cattell WR, ed. *Urinary Tract Infection*. Oxford University Press, Oxford, 1996.

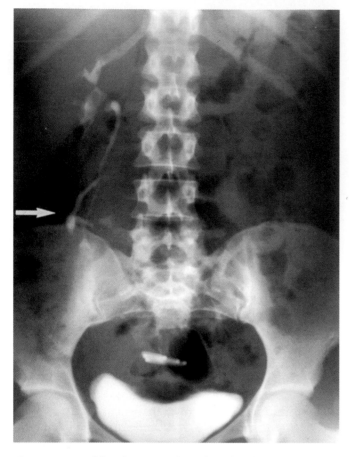

Fig. 2.14 Crossed fused ectopia where the pelvicalyceal system of the ectopic kidney can be well seen (arrowed).

Micturating cystourethrography and cystography

Indications

In children, micturating cystourethrography (MCU) remains an important part of the evaluation of UTI. It is the method of choice to detect vesicoureteric reflux and to assess its degree [42]. This diagnosis is particularly important in children under the age of 5 years who are at the greatest risk of developing scars. MCU is also used to check urethral anatomy, particularly in males with UTI, in whom it is important to detect posterior urethral valves.

In adults the use of MCU alone has declined and MCU is no longer indicated in the routine evaluation of adult UTI. MCU or cystography are indicated:
1 if vesicoureteric reflux is suspected or if there is loin pain during voiding or unexplained ureteric dilatation, especially of the lower ureters, at IVU;
2 in the assessment of bladder outflow obstruction not considered due to prostatic hypertrophy in males, combined with ascending urethrography (see below);

3 if bladder fistula (e.g. vesicocolic, vesicovaginal) is suspected;
4 if tumour in a bladder diverticulum is suspected; US shows bladder diverticula but cystography is a more sensitive method of detecting tumours or filling defects within them;
5 if urethral diverticulum is suspected in a female.

When bladder function is abnormal, it is usually more helpful to perform pressure–flow videocystography, in which bladder pressure and urine flow rate are recorded at the same time as images of the bladder and urethra are obtained.

Technique

The bladder is emptied and contrast medium at a strength of approximately 150 mg I/ml (e.g. Urografin 150, Hypaque 25) is infused into the bladder. Intermittent fluoroscopy is used during bladder filling to check for vesicoureteric reflux or bladder leaks. Images of the full bladder are obtained, with lateral and oblique views when a fistula is suspected. Following the removal of the catheter, adults void in the erect oblique position and small children in the supine oblique position. Further images of the bladder and urethra are obtained during voiding (Fig. 2.15). To reduce radiation exposure it is preferable to use video or 100 mm film to record the images. Adults should also be assessed for their

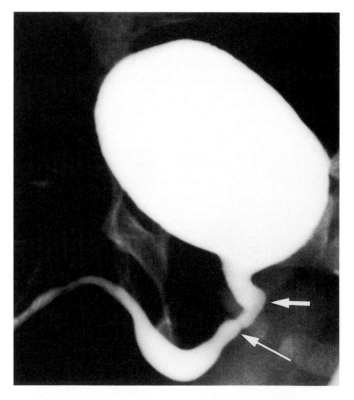

Fig. 2.15 Normal micturating cystogram in a male child. Note the verumontanum (short arrow) and level of the external sphincter (long arrow).

ability to stop voiding and of the male posterior urethra or the female urethra to then empty ('milk back').

In patients not taking antibiotics, antibiotic prophylaxis is prescribed following MCU to prevent UTI (e.g. in adults, nitrofurantoin 100 mg immediately and then 50 mg tds for 2 days). Contrast medium allergy is not usually a problem with MCU because contrast medium entering the bloodstream is only a very remote possibility. However, if there has been a serious previous contrast medium reaction, steroid prophylaxis and a non-ionic contrast medium are appropriate.

Urethrography

Male

In the adult male, urethrography is indicated when urethral stricture is suspected or in suspected urethral trauma. Less commonly it may be used to evaluate a patient with a penile mass or fistula.

Technique

Urethrography should not be performed if there is urethral infection or if there has been urethral instrumentation within the preceding week [43]. The bladder is emptied and contrast medium at a strength of approximately 150 mg I/ml (e.g. Urografin 150 or Hypaque 25) is used. The external meatus is occluded with either a Knutssons'

clamp, with the tapered tip firmly introduced into the external meatus, or a Foley catheter with the balloon inflated in the fossa navicularis. The patient lies obliquely with the lower leg flexed at the hip and knee and the penis is gently stretched over the flexed thigh. Contrast medium is injected and films are obtained when the anterior urethra is distended. Because the injection is against the external sphincter, distension of the posterior urethra is poor. To examine the posterior urethra, contrast medium injection is continued to fill the bladder and, after removal of the filling catheter or clamp, the patient voids in the erect oblique position. Further films of the anterior and posterior urethra are obtained. The descending study demonstrates the functional significance of any strictures (Fig. 2.16).

Following the procedure haematuria is not unusual. Contrast medium intravasation into the veins can occur during the procedure and intermittent fluoroscopy is important so that contrast medium injection can be stopped if this occurs. Contrast medium intravasation and haematuria after urethrography are both more common in patients with urethral strictures [44].

Female

Urethrography is technically more difficult in the female than the male because of the difficulties in occluding the external meatus. It is indicated if a urethral diverticulum is suspected but cannot be detected at MCU or on the post-

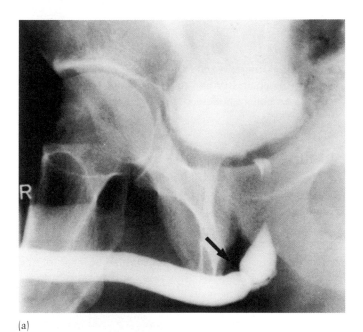

(a)

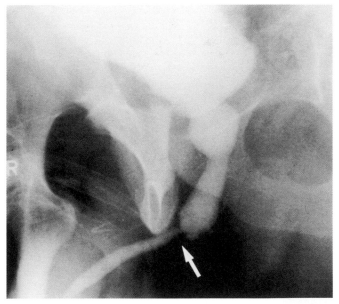

(b)

Fig. 2.16 Bulbar urethral stricture. (a) An ascending study shows a tight stricture in the bulbar urethra (arrowed); the posterior urethra is poorly seen. (b) A descending study shows marked dilatation of the urethra to the level of the stricture (arrowed).

void IVU film. The technique uses a modified Foley catheter with the balloon at the bladder neck. A second balloon is passed over the catheter to sit against the external meatus. The catheter tip is occluded and there are side holes between the two balloons. Contrast medium passes through these to distend the urethra [45].

Ileal loopography

Indications

Ileal loopography is undertaken:
1 to demonstrate loop anatomy and function;
2 to check for free reflux into the upper tracts (especially if an obstruction is suspected) (Fig. 2.17);
3 to outline upper tract anatomy, particularly in patients who have had a cystectomy for bladder cancer and are at risk of developing upper tract transitional cell carcinoma (Fig. 2.18).

Technique

The loop is catheterized with a Foley catheter and the balloon is inflated just deep enough to the abdominal wall to occlude the stoma. Contrast medium, at a concentration of

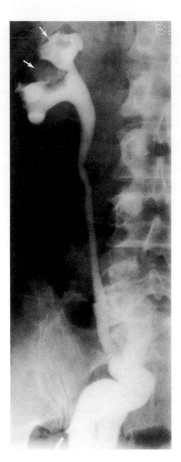

Fig. 2.18 Right pelvicalyceal transitional cell tumour (arrowed) shown at ileal loopography in a patient who had had a cystectomy for bladder carcinoma.

150 mg I/ml (Urografin 150 or Hypaque 25) is injected. Loop anatomy, distensibility and peristalsis and reflux into the upper tracts can be assessed and films obtained to show these.

Antegrade pyelography

Antegrade pyelography involves introducing a needle into the pelvicalyceal system and injecting contrast medium to outline the pelvicalyceal system and ureter. It is usually used when the collecting system is dilated to define the site and cause of obstruction. It is now generally preferred to retrograde ureterography in this situation because of the lower risk of introducing infection, and because it is a preliminary to placing a drainage catheter percutaneously into the obstructed system (percutaneous nephrostomy). Once a drainage catheter has been placed, this maybe used to introduce contrast medium for antegrade studies. Antegrade pyelography is also used when performing antegrade pressure-perfusion studies (Whitaker test, see Chapter 8).

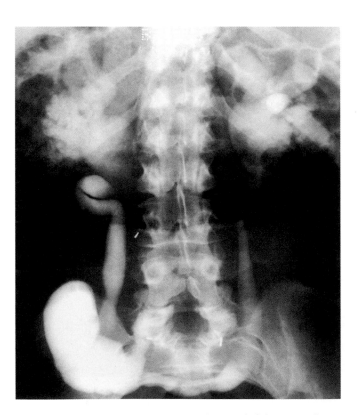

Fig. 2.17 Ileal loopogram in patient with spina bifida. Free reflux into the dilated upper tracts indicates there is no obstruction at the ureteric insertions into the loop.

Technique

The platelet count and clotting screen should be checked before the procedure, which is performed under local anaesthesia, is started. Imaging guidance may be either by ultrasound or by fluoroscopy following renal opacification by intravenous contrast medium. This should be given an appropriate time before the procedure if the system is obstructed. With the patient in the prone oblique position, a fine needle (20 or 22 gauge) is passed through the renal parenchyma to enter a calyx using a subcostal approach. The patient holds his or her breath for each needle pass. When the needle enters the collecting system, contrast medium in a concentration of 150 mg I/ml (e.g. Urografin 150) can be injected to outline pelvicalyceal and ureteric anatomy (Fig. 2.19).

Haematuria is common following antegrade pyelography but is usually transient. If an infected system is punctured, bacteraemia or septicaemia may occur. Under these circumstances antibiotics should be given, a drainage

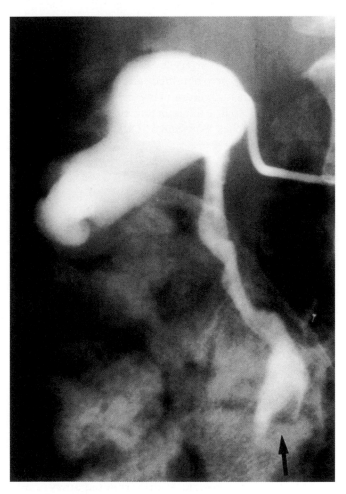

Fig. 2.19 Antegrade pyelogram performed through a nephrostomy catheter outlines an obstructed right ureter to the level of a lucent filling defect (arrowed) caused by a uric acid stone.

catheter should be placed and the diagnostic antegrade study should be deferred until the infection has settled.

Retrograde ureterography

Retrograde ureterography is now used relatively infrequently. The antegrade route is generally preferred for delineating the cause of a ureteric obstruction because of the reduced incidence of infection.

Indications

1 To demonstrate ureteric or pelvicalyceal anatomy when this has been incompletely shown at IVU, particularly in patients with haematuria and when IVU suggests a possible filling defect.
2 In suspected obstruction if the pelvicalyceal systems are slightly distended only or are not dilated.
3 To show the lower extent of a ureteric obstruction when the upper end has been shown by antegrade pyelography.
4 To demonstrate a ureteral fistula.
5 As a preliminary to puncture of a non-dilated pelvicalyceal system or to ureteric stent placement.

Technique

A bulb-tip catheter is placed in the distal ureter and contrast medium is injected. Fluoroscopic control should be used and overdistension of the pelvicalyceal system, which can lead to rupture, should be avoided. Films of the pelvicalyceal system and ureter in more than one projection should be obtained (Fig. 2.20).

Vascular studies and interventional angiographic procedures

Renal angiography and digital subtraction angiography

Principles

In conventional renal angiography, contrast medium is injected directly into the aorta or renal arteries and high-resolution images are recorded on X-ray film. In digital subtraction angiography (DSA), images are recorded using an image intensifier [46]. A preliminary image (mask) is obtained and is subtracted from the image obtained after contrast medium. In this way the unwanted structures (bone, bowel, etc.) are removed from the contrast image. Patient movement degrades the image. The technique requires a cooperative patient who can hold his or her breath. Smooth muscle relaxants are used to stop bowel movement and abdominal compression is also helpful. The image of the arterial tree so obtained is enhanced

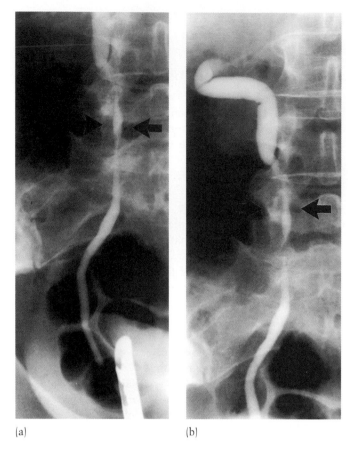

(a)   (b)

Fig. 2.20 Right retrograde pyelogram showing extrinsic stricturing of the right ureter (arrowed) by retroperitoneal fibrosis.

electronically to produce the diagnostic image. Initially DSA techniques were used after intravenous contrast medium injection Even with bolus injection into the superior vena cava or right atrium the results were often unsatisfactory with only the major renal vessels being adequately visualized, and problems arising from the overlapping of multiple vessels. More recently the DSA technique has been used with intra-arterial contrast medium injections. The resultant images have excellent contrast resolution but less good spatial resolution so that small intrarenal vessels are less well shown than with conventional film methods. The technique has the advantages that:

1 contrast medium doses are approximately 25-50% of those used with conventional angiography which reduces the potential for contrast nephrotoxicity (see p. 10);

2 smaller catheters can be used with lower complication rates and some procedures can therefore be performed on outpatients;

3 images are viewed rapidly during the procedure, which is helpful during interventional procedures such as angioplasty, embolization, etc.

For many indications the DSA method of image recording has replaced conventional film techniques; the latter may still be required when detailed examination of the small intrarenal vessels is necessary.

Technique

Before angiography the patient fasts for 4 h and takes no fluid for 2 h. A preliminary clotting screen is only performed if the patient is on anticoagulants or if a clotting abnormality is suspected. The technique is performed under local anaesthesia but preliminary sedation (e.g. diazepam 10 mg orally) may be helpful if the patient is anxious.

The retrograde femoral route is usual. The Seldinger technique is used with direct puncture of the artery, passage of a guidewire through the needle, and subsequent introduction of the arterial catheter over the guidewire after the needle has been removed.

An aortogram should always be performed first because there are multiple renal arteries in 20–30% of individuals [47] (Fig. 2.21). Selective injection into one of several arteries supplying the kidney may give the false impression of pathology in the part of the kidney supplied by the other artery or arteries. The aortogram is usually performed through a pigtail catheter with multiple side holes positioned at the renal artery level. Rapid sequence images (e.g. 2 images/s) are obtained after injection of low osmolality contrast medium. The early films are best for examining the renal arteries before they are obscured by other aortic branches. Subsequently there is a nephrogram

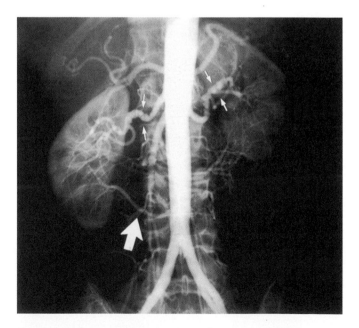

Fig. 2.21 Midstream aortogram. Note the accessory artery supplying the right lower pole (large arrow) and beaded appearance, typical of fibromuscular hyperplasia, affecting both renal arteries (short arrows). (Courtesy of Dr J.E. Dacie.)

phase when renal parenchymal opacification is maximal and a venous phase which is maximal 5–10 s after contrast injection. Views in oblique projections are often helpful so that the renal artery, which runs posteriorly from the aorta in a plane oblique to the horizontal, can be examined parallel to the film.

To perform a selective study of the renal arteries, the pigtail catheter is removed over the guidewire and a selective renal catheter is introduced. Selective renal catheters have a hooked shape so that they can be introduced into the renal artery orifice for direct injection of small amounts of non-ionic contrast medium.

Renal transplant angiography is usually performed with a catheter placed in the appropriate common iliac artery following puncture of the contralateral femoral artery. Oblique, and sometimes lateral, projections are necessary and DSA is favoured. Selective catheterization of the transplant artery may sometimes be used.

Bruising and haematoma formation are common after angiography but, with experienced radiologists, serious complications are rare. Local complications include arterial dissection and thrombosis, pseudoaneurysm or arterio-venous fistula formation, damage to adjacent structures, particularly nerves, and distal embolism from a thrombus formed on the catheter, or from atheroma dislodged by the catheter. The systemic and renal complications of contrast medium are discussed on page 12.

Renal venography

The diagnoses of renal thrombosis and of tumour extension into the renal veins and inferior vena cava can now almost always be made by an appropriate combination of ultrasound with Doppler, CT and, if available, magnetic resonance imaging (MRI). Renal venography is therefore now used infrequently. The technique involves retrograde catheterization of the vena cava from the femoral vein. Contrast medium can be injected into the vena cava to obtain a cavogram, and selective renal vein catheterization and contrast medium injection can also be performed.

Interventional angiographic procedures

Interventional angiographic procedures are usually performed under local anaesthesia using DSA. Angioplasty [48] is used to dilate renal artery stenoses (Fig. 2.22). The method involves introducing a catheter incorporating a balloon across the stenotic arterial segment and inflating the balloon. This is believed to produce dilatation by rupturing the intima and stretching the media and adventitia. The associated risk of arterial and renal damage is considerably higher than that for arteriography alone and it is essential that a surgeon is available to deal with possible complications. A recent development is the use of intra-arterial stents to improve the results of angioplasty; this technique is currently being assessed [49,50].

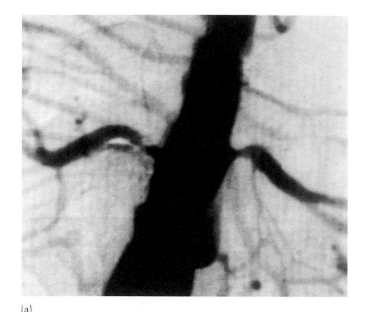

(a)

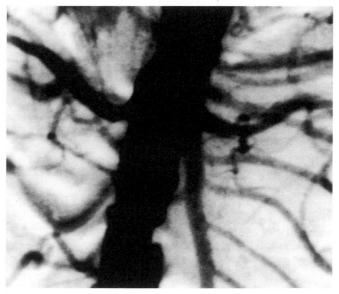

(b)

Fig. 2.22 DSA aortograms. (a) Bilateral proximal renal artery stenoses typical of atheroma. (b) Appearances following bilateral angioplasty. (Reproduced with permission from Raine AEG, Ledingham JGG. Renal and Renovascular Hypertension. Weatherall *et al.* (eds.) *Oxford Textbook of Medicine.* 3e Oxford University Press, 1996, Chap. 15.28 and Dr J.E. Dacie.)

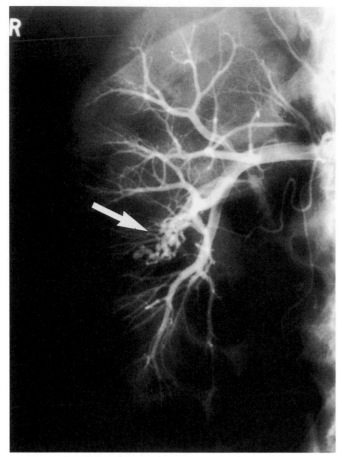

(a)

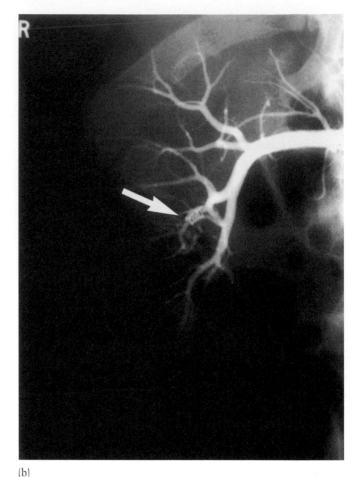

(b)

Fig. 2.23 Right pelvicalyceal haemangioma which caused haematuria in a 31-year-old male. (a) A selective right renal arteriogram showing a leash of abnormal arteries (arrowed). (b) After embolization the steel coil is seen (arrowed) with no filling of the abnormal arteries. (Courtesy of Abercrombie JF, Holmes SAV, Ball AJ. Diagnosis and Management of Renal Angioma. *Journal of the Royal Society of Medicine* (1992) **95**, 625–627 and Dr JE Dacie.)

Embolization is used to control renal bleeding in a variety of situations.
1 Spontaneous, from congenital arteriovenous malformations (Fig. 2.23).
2 Post-traumatic, often iatrogenic, for example following biopsy and percutaneous interventional procedures.
3 Advanced renal neoplasm for symptomatic relief.

The renal artery is selectively catheterized and the branch supplying the bleeding lesion is also catheterized — this may necessitate coaxial catheters. A variety of embolic materials may be injected, for example steel coils, polyvinyl alcohol foam particles or haemostatic gelatin sponge. When large renal segments or the whole kidney is embolized the patient may develop loin pain and fever. Antibiotics are recommended after infarction of large renal tumours because of the risk of secondary infection.

Indications for renal angiography

Renal angiography is now almost exclusively used for vascular diagnosis and intervention. Its former role in the diagnosis and assessment of renal cysts and masses has been replaced by the combination of ultrasound and CT. Indications for its use are listed here.
1 *Diagnosis and treatment of renal artery stenosis* (RAS). Renal angiography is principally used to detect RAS in hypertensive patients in whom it is suspected clinically. Atheromatous RAS usually affects the proximal one-third of the renal artery and is eccentric (see Fig. 2.22). It may affect the renal ostium. Fibromuscular dysplasia affects the distal two-thirds of the renal artery and may affect the segmental branches. In the commonest form of fibromuscular dysplasia, medial fibroplasia, there is a 'string of beads' appearance caused by alternating stenotic and aneurysmal areas of vessel (see Fig. 2.21). The best results with angioplasty are obtained in fibromuscular dysplasia with 90% immediate technical success and cure in 40–60% [51,52]. With atheroma, initial technical success is approximately 75% provided the stenosis is non-ostial, but only 20% with ostial stenosis [51]. Long-term cure is usually in the range 20–30% [51,53,54]. Angioplasty may

also be used to preserve renal function in patients with renal failure and RAS; success is achieved in approximately 50% [55,56].

2 *Diagnosis and treatment of renal haemorrhage.* Angiography is indicated to detect a bleeding source in patients with unexplained haematuria who have normal imaging (IVU plus ultrasound or CT) and cystoscopy. Suitable lesions such as arteriovenous malformations may be embolized (see Fig. 2.23). It is also indicated to localize and treat bleeding following trauma or bleeding from inoperable renal tumours.

3 *Renal transplants: preoperative and postoperative assessment.* Angiography is a part of the preoperative assessment of renal donors. Aortography with supine oblique projections usually provides adequate assessment of the renal arteries. Hypertension or impaired renal function after transplantation may be caused by RAS and angiography, preferably using the DSA technique, is indicated.

4 *Other indications.* These include:

(a) providing a preoperative 'road map' when conservative renal surgery is planned for a renal tumour (e.g. in a single kidney) or when tumour surgery is likely to be complicated by a congenital anomaly (e.g. horseshoe kidney);

(b) detection of an abnormality in the small intrarenal vessels (e.g. aneurysms in suspected polyarteritis nodosa).

References

1 Denneberg T. Clinical studies on kidney function with radioactive sodium diatrizoate. *Acta Med Scand Suppl* 1965;**442**:1.

2 Bonati F, Felder E, Tirone P. Iopamidol: new preclinical and clinical data. *Invest Radiol* 1980;**15**:S310–16.

3 Mutzel W, Speck U. Pharmacokinetics and biotransformation of iohexol in the rat and the dog. *Acta Radiol Suppl* 1980;**362**:111–15.

4 Cattell WR, Fry IK, Spencer AG, Purkiss P. Excretion urography. I. Factors determining the excretion of Hypaque. *Br J Radiol* 1967;**40**:561–71.

5 Wolf KJ, Steidle B, Skutta T, Mutzel W. Iopromide—clinical experience with a new non-ionic contrast medium. *Acta Radiol Diagnos* 1983;**24**:55–62.

6. Sherwood T. The physiology of intravenous urography. In: *Scientific Basis of Medicine Annual Reviews*. London: Athlone Press, 1971:336–48.

7 Doyle FH, Sherwood T, Steiner RE, Breckenridge A, Dollery CT. Large dose urography. Is there an optimum dose? *Lancet* 1967;**2**:964–6.

8 Saxton HM. Review article. Urography. *Br J Radiol* 1969;**42**: 321–46.

9 Fry IK, Cattell WR, Spencer AG, Purkiss P. Excretion urography. II. The relation between Hypaque excretion and the intravenous urogram. *Br J Radiol* 1967;**40**:572–80.

10 Sherwood T, Doyle FH, Breckenridge A, Dollery CT, Steiner RE. Value of fluid deprivation in large dose urography. *Lancet* 1968;**2**:754–5.

11 Dalla Palma L, Rossi M, Stacul F, Agostini R. Iopamidol in urography. *Urol Radiol* 1982;**4**:1–3.

12 Lalli AF, Williams B, Maynard E. Iohexol in urography. *Urol Radiol* 1983;**5**:95–7.

13 Shehadi WH. Adverse reactions to intravascularly administered contrast media. *Am J Roentgenol* 1975;**124**:145–52.

14 Schrott KM, Behrends B, Clauss W, Kaufmann J, Lehnert J. Iohexol in excretory urography. *Fortschr Med* 1986;**104**: 153–6.

15 Palmer FJ. The RACR survey of intravenous contrast medium reactions. Final report. *Australas Radiol* 1988;**32**:426–8.

16 Ansell G. Adverse reactions to contrast agents. *Invest Radiol* 1970;**5**:374–84.

17 Katayama H, Yamaguchi K, Kozuka T *et al.* Adverse reactions to ionic and non-ionic contrast media. *Radiology* 1990; **175**:621–8.

18 Hartman GW, Hattery RR, Witten DM, Williamson B. Mortality during excretory urography: Mayo Clinic experience. *Am J Roentgenol* 1982; **139**:919–22.

19 Lasser EC. Contrast media for urography. In: Pollack HM, ed. *Clinical Urography*. Philadelphia: WB Saunders, 1990:23–36.

20 Ansell G, Tweedie MCK, West CR, Price Evans DL, Couch L. The current status of reactions to intravenous contrast media. *Invest Radiol* 1980;**15**:S32.

21 Ansell G. Adverse reactions profile: 8. Intravascular iodinated radiocontrast media. *Prescribers J* 1993;**33**:82–8.

22 Berns AS. Nephrotoxicity of contrast media. *Kidney Int* 1989;**36**:730–40.

23 Byrd L, Sherman RL. Radiocontrast-induced acute renal failure. *Medicine* 1979;**58**:270–9.

24 Svedstrom E, Alanen A, Nurmi M. Radiologic diagnosis of renal colic: the role of plain films, excretory urography and sonography. *Eur J Radiol* 1990;**11**:180–3.

25 Mutgi A, Williams JW, Nettleman M. Renal colic: utility of the plain abdominal roentgenogram. *Ann Int Med* 1991;**151**: 1589–92.

26 Dalla Palma L, Stacul F, Bazzochi M *et al.* Ultrasonography and plain film versus intravenous urography in ureteric colic. *Clin Radiol* 1993;**47**:333–6.

27 Schwartz G, Lipschitz S, Becker JA. Detection of renal calculi: the value of tomography. *Am J Roentgenol* 1984;**143**:143–5.

28 Middleton WD, Dodds WJ, Lawson TL, Foley WD. Renal calculi: sensitivity for detection with US. *Radiology* 1988;**167**: 239–44.

29 Grainger RG. Annotation: radiological contrast media. *Clin Radiol* 1987;**38**:3–5.

30 Talner LB. Urinary obstruction. In: Grainger RG, Allison DJ, eds. *Diagnostic Radiology*, 2nd edn. Edinburgh: Churchill Livingstone, 1992:1269–88.

31 Whitfield HN, Britton KE, Hendry WF, Wickham JEA. Frusemide intravenous urography in the diagnosis of pelviureteric junction obstruction. *Br J Urol* 1979;**51**:445–8.

32 Lewis E, Ritchie WGM. A simple ultrasonic method for assessing renal size. *J Clin Ultrasound* 1980;**8**:417–20.

33 Batson RG, Keats TE. The roentgenographic determination of normal adult kidney size as related to vertebral height. *Am J Roentgenol* 1972;**116**:737–9.

34 Pollack HM, Banner MP. Current status of excretory urography. *Urol Clin North Am* 1985;**12**:585–601.

35 Spencer J, Lindsell D, Mastorakou I. Ultrasonography compared

with intravenous urography in the investigation of adults with haematuria. *Br Med J* 1990; **301**:1074–6.

36 Aslaksen A, Gadeholt G, Gothlin JH. Ultrasonography versus intravenous urography in the evaluation of patients with microscopic haematuria. *Br J Urol* 1990;**55**:144–7.

37 Warshauer DM, McCarthy SM, Street L *et al.* Detection of renal masses: sensitivities and specificities of excretory urography/linear tomography, US and CT. *Radiology* 1988;**169**:363–5.

38 Van Arsdalen KN, Banner MP, Pollack HM. Radiographic imaging and urologic decision-making in the management of renal and ureteric calculi. *Urol Clin North Am* 1990;**17**:171–90.

39 Choyke PL. The urogram: are rumours of its death premature? *Radiology* 1992;**184**:33–6.

40 Webb JAW. Ultrasonography in the diagnosis of renal obstruction. *Br Med J* 1990;**301**:944–6.

41 Spencer J, Lindsell D, Mastorakou I. Ultrasonography compared with intravenous urography in the investigation of urinary tract infection in adults. *Br Med J* 1990;**301**:221–3.

42 Blickman JG, Taylor GA, Lebowitz RL. Voiding cysto-urethrography: the initial radiologic study in children with urinary tract infection. *Radiology* 1985;**156**:659–62.

43 McCallum RW. The adult male urethra. Normal anatomy, pathology and method of urethrography. *Radiol Clin North Am* 1979;**17**:227–44.

44 McLennan BL, Becker JA, Robinson T. Venous extravasation at retrograde urethrography: precautions. *J Urol* 1971;**106**: 412–3.

45 Greenberg M, Stone D, Cochran ST *et al.* Female urethral diverticula: double-balloon catheter study. *Am J Roentgenol* 1981;**136**:259–64.

46 Hillman BJ. Digital radiology. *Radiol Clin North Am* 1985;**23**: 211–26.

47 Boijsen E. Angiographic studies of the anatomy of single and multiple renal arteries. *Acta Radiol Suppl* 1959;**183**:1.

48 Gruntzig A, Kuhlmann U, Vetter W *et al.* Treatment of renovascular hypertension with percutaneous transluminal dilatation of a renal artery stenosis. *Lancet* 1978;**1**:801–2.

49 Rees CR, Palmaz JC, Becker GJ *et al.* Palmaz stent in atherosclerotic stenoses involving the ostia of the renal arteries: preliminary report of a multicenter study. *Radiology* 1991;**181**:507–14.

50 Wilms GE, Peene PT, Baert AL *et al.* Renal artery stent placement with use of the Wallstent endoprosthesis. *Radiology* 1991;**179**:457–62.

51 Sos TA, Pickering TG, Sniderman K *et al.* Percutaneous transluminal angioplasty in renovascular hypertension due to atheroma or fibromuscular dysplasia. *N Engl J Med* 1983;**309**:274–9.

52 Geyskes GG. Treatment of renovascular hypertension with percutaneous transluminal angioplasty—in depth review. *Am J Kid Dis* 1988;**12**:253–65.

53 Colapinto RF, Stronell RD, Harries Jones EP *et al.* Percutaneous transluminal dilatation of the renal artery: follow-up studies on renovascular hypertension. *Am J Roentgenol* 1982;**139**: 727–32.

54 Geyskes GG, Puylaert GBAJ, Oei HY, Dorhout Mees EJ. Followup study of 70 patients with renal artery stenosis treated by percutaneous transluminal dilatation. *Br Med J* 1983;**287**: 333–6.

55 Bell GM, Reid J, Buist TAS. Percutaneous transluminal angioplasty improves blood pressure and renal function in renovascular hypertension. *Q J Med* 1987;**241**:393–403.

56 Martin LG, Casarella WJ, Gaylord GM. Azotaemia caused by renal artery stenosis: treatment by percutaneous angioplasty. *Am J Roentgenol* 1988;**150**:839–44.

3   Transrectal Ultrasound of the Prostate

H. Watanabe

Introduction

The idea of transrectal ultrasonography (TRUS) was proposed by Wild and Reid [1] in the very early stage of the development of medical ultrasound, even before the appearance of contact compound scanning. Only the contour of the rectal wall could, however, be visualized by the primitive machine at that time.

The first clinically useful sonograms of the prostate were obtained by an original transrectal scanner 10 years afterwards by Watanabe et al. [2]. They designed special equipment for transrectal scanning with the subject in the sitting position [3,4], determined various applications and established the method as a new systematic diagnostic procedure.

In the 1980s, TRUS spread rapidly in the USA and European countries as the best imaging modality for the prostate. Lee [5] was a leader of this new tide with his term 'hypoechoic lesion', as he called it. The names of Resnick [6], Pontes [7], Scardino [8], Peeling [9] and Cooner [10] can also be mentioned as early contributors to the development of this procedure.

Interventional techniques [11,12] and colour Doppler sonography [13] were also introduced in the 1980s. Currently, TRUS is employed commonly throughout the world in daily clinics as an indispensable routine step for prostatic diagnosis.

Method

Transrectal probes can be divided into two categories according to their mechanism: (i) mechanical; or (ii) electronic. The mechanical scanner has a single round oscillating disc, which is rotated mechanically by a motor, while the electronic scanner consists of multiple (usually 64–128) small rectangular discs set in parallel, which are driven electronically one by one at very high speed. Colour Doppler sonography is feasible only with electronic scanners. Usually, mechanical scanners are suitable for radial scanning, which provides horizontal sections of the prostate, whereas electronic scanners are preferable for linear scanning to obtain sagittal sections.

Recently, however, to meet the demand for simultaneous visualization of both sections, several kinds of biplane transrectal probes have become commercially available. Some of these probes contain two sets of electronic transducers, for linear and convex types, respectively, whereas others employ a mechanical system switching between horizontal and vertical directions of a single transducer moving pendulously.

In general, these scanners are set inside a tube-shaped probe for insertion into the rectum. The tip of the probe is wrapped with a rubber balloon (condom) and contact with the rectal wall is maintained by inflation of the balloon with water. The probe is held either in the hand or by a tripod and is introduced with the patient in the lithotomy position or recumbent. However, chair-type equipment with the subject in a sitting position [3] is more efficient and allows higher standards of reproducibility. This equipment consists of a chair, in the seat of which a hole has been made to allow the passage of a special intra-corporeal probe, which is set up beneath it. The tip of the probe is wrapped in a disposable rubber balloon combined with a mat on the seat. The examinee is requested to sit on the chair and the anus is positioned above the top of the probe. The probe is inserted into the rectum smoothly by rotating a handle attached to the chair. This method is useful for daily routine work, especially for prostatic screening by ultrasound [14,15].

Size measurement of the prostate can be achieved accurately by TRUS [16]. To determine prostatic volume, two kinds of estimation are employed.

1 *Planimetry*. This is the standard estimation method. Each of the horizontal sections taken at certain distances (usually 5 mm apart) of insertion of the probe are measured by a roller planimeter or a computer. The estimated volume can be determined by the sum of the areas multiplied by the distance of insertion. This method is much more precise than ellipsoid volumetry but has a tendency to produce slightly low estimates (Salami effect) [17].

2 *Ellipsoid volumetry.* This is another, but less accurate, method of estimating prostatic volume. The depth, length and height of the prostate are measured independently by TRUS. The volume is then calculated by the formula used to calculate the volume of ellipsoids.

Normal prostate

The prostate is visualized anterior to the rectum where the transducer is located. Strong linear echo patterns from the pubic bone in front of the prostate and from the ischial bones on both sides are visible. The linear continuous echo patterns caused by the prostatic capsule are called capsular echoes and the homogeneously distributed echo patterns caused by the prostatic tissue are known as internal echoes.

In a tomogram of a normal adult, the prostate has a slender triangular or semilunar pattern, with the antero-posterior (AP) diameter far shorter than the transverse diameter. The shape of the prostate is symmetrical. The capsular echoes are smooth, continuous and thin, while the internal echoes are fine and regular. Of these characteristics, the slender, symmetrical and homogeneous findings are extremely important (Fig. 3.1).

In horizontal sections of the normal prostate, the peripheral zone [18] occupies the major area. The transition zone [18] is delineated only in sections from the upper part.

The prostatic volume of normal subjects increases rapidly from the age of 10 to 20 years and then decreases after the age of 20 [19] (Fig. 3.2).

Benign prostatic hypertrophy

The most important contribution of TRUS must be the

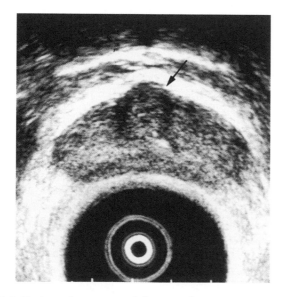

Fig. 3.1 Horizontal sonogram of the normal prostate. Arrow, urethra and surrounding muscle.

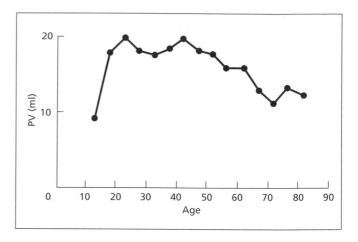

Fig. 3.2 Mean prostatic volume in 5 year steps by age ($n = 346$).

diagnosis of benign prostatic hypertrophy (BPH). In this disease, neither the size of the prostate nor the histological findings will indicate directly the degree of obstruction [20]. No examination except TRUS can tell at a glance how large the adenoma has become and how intense the obstruction from it is.

In patients with BPH, a section of the prostate is enlarged symmetrically, most noticeably along the AP diameter. The shape of the prostate is semilunar in the early stages and is nearly round or oval in the advanced stages (Fig. 3.3). The capsular echoes are even, continuous and thick; there are increased internal echoes, giving the impression of a compact substance. However enlarged the prostate may be, the symmetry and evenness of the capsular echoes are always maintained (Table 3.1). Hypertrophied adenoma inside the prostate can be delineated if it has developed sufficiently.

The horizontal section of the prostate should be round when BPH is present: the rounder the section, the more advanced the BPH. This evidence was quantified by the theory of the presumed circle area ratio (PCAR) [20], which indicates how the prostate evolves towards a circular shape in BPH.

The PCAR is the ratio of the area of the maximum horizontal section of the prostate to the area of a presumed circle, the circumference of which equals the circumference of the maximum horizontal section. Figure 3.4a shows the maximum horizontal section of the prostate obtained by ultrasound examination. The circumference is defined as L and the area as S. Figure 3.4b shows the presumed circle having the same circumference, L. Its area can be defined as S', and can be determined by the following formula:

$$S' = \pi \left(\frac{L}{2\pi} \right)^2.$$

The PCAR is represented as S/S'. A PCAR of 1.0 means

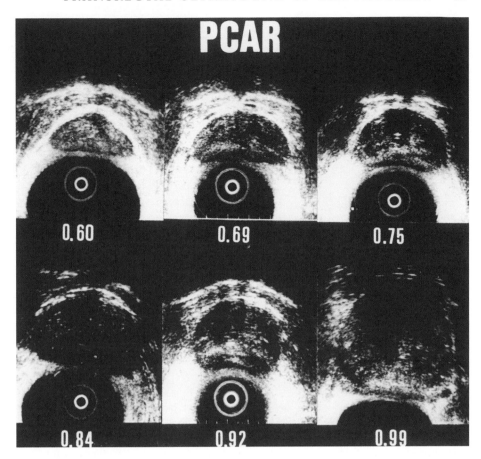

Fig. 3.3 Presumed circle area ratio (PCAR) in the various prostates. The diagnosis of BPH should be made only in cases having a PCAR of more than 0.75.

Table 3.1 Diagnostic criteria in transrectal sonography for the prostate.

Findings	Diseases			
	Normal	Hypertrophy	Cancer	Prostatitis
Shape of section	Triangular or semilunar	Enlarged Nearly round	Irregular Deformed	Enlarged in acute cases, deformed in chronic cases
Anteroposterior diameter	Short	Elongated	Elongate but with some exceptions	Usually short
Superoinferior diameter	Short	Elongated, associated with anteroposterior diameter	Occasionally elongated and unbalanced	Usually short
Symmetry	Present	Present	Absent	Absent
Change of shape on each level	Little	Little	Marked	Little
Capsular echoes				
Thickness	Thin	Thick	Irregular if invaded	Irregular
Continuity	Present	Present	Absent	Usually present
Unevenness	Absent	Absent	Present	Present
Internal echoes				
Density	(+)	(++)	(+)	(++) in chronic cases
Quality	Orderly	Orderly	Disorderly but occasionally disappear (hypoechoic lesion)	Disorderly

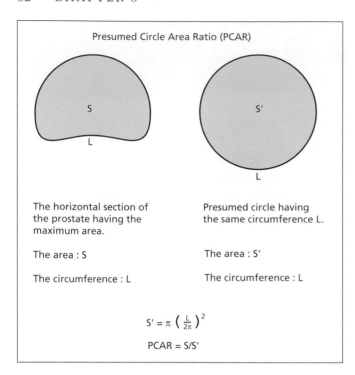

Presumed Circle Area Ratio (PCAR)

The horizontal section of the prostate having the maximum area.

The area : S

The circumference : L

Presumed circle having the same circumference L.

The area : S'

The circumference : L

$$S' = \pi \left(\frac{L}{2\pi} \right)^2$$

$$PCAR = S/S'$$

Fig. 3.4 Calculation of PCAR.

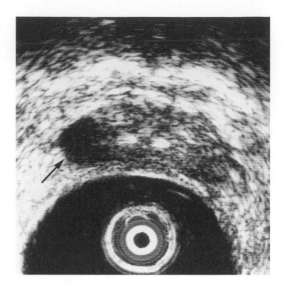

Fig. 3.5 Horizontal sonogram of the prostate with early prostatic cancer. Arrow, hypoechoic lesion (1.2 cm in diameter).

that the section is a circle. The PCARs of various prostates are shown in Fig. 3.3.

Pathological residual urine is only caused by BPH when the PCAR is more than 0.75. If the PCAR is below 0.75, the cause of the urinary disturbance should not be sought in the prostate. TRUS enhances this capacity of exclusion, whether the cause of the urinary disturbance is from the prostate or not.

In our clinic, indication for surgery in BPH patients is reserved strictly for cases having a PCAR of more than 0.80 and a residual urine volume of more than 30 ml. The outcome from surgery in cases selected in this way was evaluated by the American Urological Association (AUA) score system. Symptoms improved in 97% of cases after surgery [21].

TRUS only indicates the possibility of malignancy in prostatic cancer, but makes the final diagnosis in BPH.

Prostatic cancer

When interpreting sonograms attention should primarily be directed towards changes in prostatic shape. It is a recent trend that attention is only paid to the internal echoes in order to detect small foci of cancer. However, deformity of the prostate frequently appears even in cases of very early cancer [4].

Changes in internal echoes in cases of prostatic cancer (PC) are mainly present as hypoechoic lesions (Fig. 3.5). In some cases of PC, however, the internal echoes occasion-

ally disappear (see Table 3.1). Some advanced large cancer foci appear as hyperechoic areas, although every small cancer focus without exception shows hypoechoic signs.

It is also undoubtedly a mistake to think that any 'black' part in the prostate means malignancy. In ultrasonography, a 'black' region only means that there is no difference in acoustic impedence in that region, whether the tissue is hard or soft.

Our results of a study of the accuracy of ultrasound for detecting PC showed a sensitivity of 97.1% in 102 outpatients. The sensitivity and specificity in 3479 cases in our mass-screening programme were 86.3 and 91.4%, respectively, and those in an official blind test supported by the Ministry of Health and Welfare in Japan, performed by 21 urologists, were 64.2 and 76.2%, respectively. In this official test, particularly, the discrepancy in efficacy among physicians having different experience in reading scans was prominent. There was a sensitivity of 80.0% and a specificity of 78.3% by five physicians who had read more than 3000 scans, and a sensitivity of 59.5% and a specificity of 76.3% by 16 physicians who had read less than that number.

An irregularity or discontinuity of the capsular echoes suggests malignant invasion in cases of PC. However, the irregularity of the capsular echoes is occasionally caused by artefacts. Prostatic calculi generate acoustic shadows, which cause discontinuities in the capsular echoes. In addition, at the posterolateral corner of the prostate, the resolution of TRUS becomes worse, because the ultrasonic beam is projected in a direction parallel to the capsule. These drawbacks can be compensated for by skill in reading the scans, making sure that attention is paid to the overall section of the prostate.

The sensitivity of TRUS on extracapsular invasion confirmed by pathology was 89% in our blind test in 31 cases. The rate of coincidence of staging between ultrasound and pathology was 65.2% by nine senior readers in the official blind test supported by the Ministry of Health and Welfare in Japan.

The monitoring of the effect of treatment or drug administration is easily performed by periodic measurements of prostatic volume by TRUS [22]. A striking result was obtained from monitoring prostatic volume after castration in cases of PC. This kinetic study showed that prostatic volume reduced exponentially after castration according to a formula and that the prognosis of individual patients could be predicted accurately, by calculating a factor in the formula [23].

The value of screening for PC has not yet been confirmed. However, in our long-term prostatic mass-screening project in progress since 1975 [14], using a special mobile unit with TRUS equipment [15], the detection rate of PC in the apparently normal Japanese male population over the age of 55 years was 0.6%. One must keep in mind that the prevalence of PC in Japan is only 20% of that in western countries. The establishment of a practical screening system using a combination of TRUS and prostate-specific antigen (PSA) assay is expected to be more sensitive than TRUS alone.

Prostatitis

The ultrasonic findings of acute prostatitis are characteristic: an expanded round shape of the prostate on the horizontal section, with reduced internal echoes, suggesting oedema.

In contrast, findings in chronic prostatitis are varied and irregular, resulting in difficulty of diagnosis. It is evident from our investigations, however, that the clinical situation of chronic prostatitis is not the same throughout its course. Intermittently, once every few months to a few years, there are acute episodes in the chronic process. Ultrasonic findings in these acute stages are similar to those in acute prostatitis and the same treatment as for acute prostatitis is, in fact, also very effective at this stage. When the acute stage regresses, ultrasonic findings also return to the former state. For this reason, TRUS is thought to be a suitable means for monitoring the clinical course of chronic prostatitis, and timely intervention in the acute stage may be feasible by examinations at regular intervals.

A sonolucent zone [24], which is a sign that the prostatic capsule resembles a 'double' shape (Fig. 3.6), has been said to be a characteristic finding of chronic prostatitis. Recently developed transrectal colour Doppler sonography [13] has proved that the sign is caused by the dilated vein plexus around the prostate.

In 1993, magnetic resonance angiography was developed,

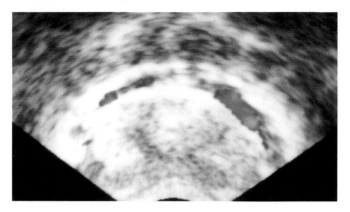

Fig. 3.6 Colour Doppler sonogram of the prostate with chronic prostatitis. A sonolucent zone is obvious along the anterior margin of the prostate, showing bloodflow inside it by Doppler signals.

a new system visualizing slow bloodflow by the maximum intensity projection method in magnetic resonance imaging (MRI). Employing this system, a remarkable pathological dilatation of veins inside the whole small pelvis, including the prostatic and perivesical plexus, was detected in many cases of so-called prostatism. We proposed that this type of disease was caused primarily by such venous congestion inside the pelvis, and could be called intrapelvic venous congestion syndrome (IVCS) [25]. There is a possibility that the large majority of cases diagnosed as prostatitis to date might belong to this new syndrome. A sonolucent zone on TRUS may be one of the features of this phenomenon of venous congestion. Further studies on the pathogenesis of the syndrome are expected.

Interventional ultrasound

Interventional ultrasound is a technique of puncture guided by ultrasound. Interventional ultrasound for the prostate was turned into practical use in the 1980s [25,26]. Ultrasound-guided selective biopsy is now thought to be the only way to confirm a small cancer nodule, which was displayed as a hypoechoic lesion on TRUS [27]. For that reason, TRUS and interventional ultrasound by TRUS are accepted widely as associated techniques.

Electronic linear probes have usually been employed for needle guidance [25], but recently developed 'biplane' probes are recommended (Fig. 3.7).

Interventional ultrasound is also employed during some treatment. During the procedure for cryoprostatectomy, the ice-ball formation is clearly represented by TRUS [28]. In the same manner, monitoring of transurethral resection of the prostate (TURP) is easily possible. Transperineal radioactive seed implantation for prostatic cancer [29] is performed under direct monitoring by TRUS alone.

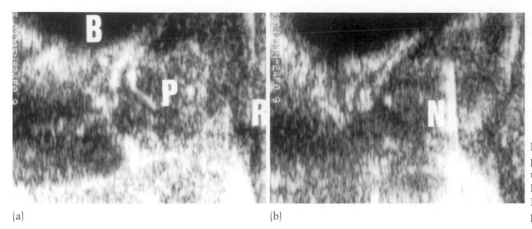

(a)   (b)

Fig. 3.7 Puncture of the prostate with interventional ultrasound. (a) Before puncture: B: urinary bladder; P: prostate; R: rectum. (b) During needle puncture: N: needle.

Seminal vesicles

TRUS was the first modality to show the total shape of the human seminal vesicles in vivo [30]. The seminal vesicles appear on the horizontal tomogram as two symmetrical spindle shapes behind the bladder. Cancer invasion into the seminal vesicles can be detected [31] (Fig. 3.8).

The size of the seminal vesicles changes remarkably before and after ejaculation [32]. A shrinkage of the organ was observed after hormone treatment for prostatic cancer [33].

Seminal vesicle puncture as an application of interventional ultrasound is a very informative means of diagnosis. Needle biopsy may prove cancer invasion from the prostate [34]. In almost all cases of haematospermia examined, some bleeding, either fresh or stale, was observed on seminal vesicle puncture [34]. It is therefore thought that bleeding in this disease may not be from the prostate as formerly stated, but from the seminal vesicles.

References

1 Wild JJ, Reid JM. Progress in techniques of soft tissue examination by 15MC pulsed ultrasound. In: Kelly E, ed. *Ultrasound in Biology and Medicine.* Washington DC: American Institute of Biological Sciences, 1957:30–48.
2 Watanabe H, Kato H, Kato T *et al.* Diagnostic application of ultrasonotomography for the prostate. Jpn J Urol 1968;**59**: 273–9.
3 Watanabe H, Igari D, Tanahashi Y, Harada K, Saitoh M. Development and application of new equipment for transrectal ultrasonography. *J Clin Ultrasound* 1974;**2**:91–8.
4 Watanabe H, Igari D, Tanahashi Y, Harada K, Saitoh M. Transrectal ultrasonotomography of the prostate. *J Urol* 1975; **114**:734–9.
5 Lee F, Gray JM, McLeary RD et al. Transrectal ultrasound in the diagnosis of prostate cancer: location, echogenicity, histopathology, and staging. *Prostate* 1985;**7**:117–29.
6 Resnick MI, Willard JW, Boyce WH. Recent progress in ultrasonography of the bladder and prostate. J Urol 1977; **117**:444–6.
7 Pontes JE, Ohe H, Watanabe H, Murphy GP. Transrectal ultrasonography of the prostate. *Cancer* 1984;**53**:1369–72.
8 Carter SStC, Scardino PT, Shinohara K, eds. Advances in urologic ultrasound. *Urol Clin North Am* 1989;**16**(4).
9 Peeling WB, Griffiths GJ, Evans KT, Roberts EE. Diagnosis and staging of prostatic cancer by transrectal ultrasonography. A preliminary study. *Br J Urol* 1979;**51**:565–9.
10 Cooner WH, Mosley BR, Rutherford CL Jr *et al.* Clinical application of transrectal ultrasonography and prostate specific antigen in the search for prostate cancer. *J Urol* 1988; **139**:758–61.
11 Watanabe H, Makuuchi M, eds. *Interventional Real-Time Ultrasound.* Tokyo: Igaku-shoin, 1985.
12 Holm HH, Kristensen JK, eds. *Interventional Ultrasound.* Copenhagen: Munksgaard, 1985.
13 Miyashita H, Watanabe H, Inaba T *et al.* Application of 2D

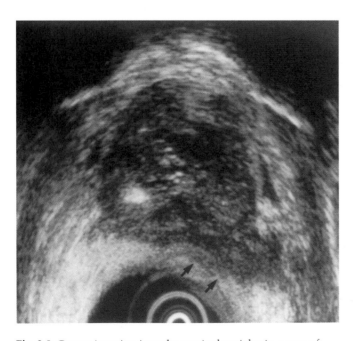

Fig. 3.8 Cancer invasion into the seminal vesicles in a case of advanced prostatic cancer (arrow).

Doppler color flow mapping to the prostate. *Jpn J Med Ultrason* 1987;**14**(Suppl. 1):1013–14.

14 Watanabe H, Saitoh M, Mishina T *et al.* Mass screening program for prostatic diseases with transrectal ultrasono-tomography. *J Urol* 1977;**117**:746–8.

15 Watanabe H, Ohe H, Inaba T *et al.* A mobile mass screening unit for prostatic disease. *Prostate* 1984;**5**:559–65.

16 Watanabe H, Igari D, Tanahashi Y, Harada K, Saitoh M. Measurements of size and weight of prostate by means of transrectal ultrasonotomography. *Tohoku J Exp Med* 1974; **114**:277–85.

17 Dähnert WF. Determination of prostate volume with transrectal US for cancer screening. *Radiology* 1992;**183**:625–7.

18 Stamey TA, ed. *Monogr Urol* 1988;**9**(3).

19 Mori Y. Measurement of the normal prostate size by means of transrectal ultrasonotomography. *Jpn J Urol* 1982;**73**: 767–81.

20 Watanabe H. Natural history of benign prostatic hypertrophy. *Ultrasound Med Biol* 1986;**127**:567–71.

21 Watanabe H. Diagnosis of benign prostatic hypertrophy by ultrasound and outcome from surgery. *Akt Urol* 1993;**24**(Suppl. 1):127–30.

22 Kojima M, Watanabe H, Ohe H, Miyashita H, Inaba T. Kinetic evaluation of the effect of LHRH analog on prostatic cancer using transrectal ultrasonotomography. *Prostate* 1987;**10**: 11–17.

23 Ohe H, Watanabe H. Kinetic analysis of prostatic volume in treating prostatic cancer and its predictability for prognosis. *Cancer* 1988;**62**:2325–9.

24 Peeling WB, Griffiths GJ. Imaging of the prostate by ultrasound. *J Urol* 1984;**132**:217–24.

25 Saitoh M, Watanabe H, Ohe H. Ultrasonically guided punc-ture for the prostate and seminal vesicles with transrectal

real-time linear scanner. *J Kyoto Pref Univ Med* 1981;**90**: 47–53.

26 Holm HH, Gammelgaard J. Ultrasonically guided precise needle placement in the prostate and the seminal vesicles. *J Urol* 1981;**125**:385–7.

27 Abe M, Hashimoto T, Matsuda T, Saitoh M, Watanabe H. Prostatic biopsy guided by transrectal ultrasonography using real-time linear scanner. *Urology* 1987;**29**:567–9.

28 Tanahashi Y, Igari D, Harada K. Cryoprostatectomy under ultrasonic control. In: White D, Brown RE, eds. *Ultrasound in Medicine*, Vol. 3A. New York: Plenum Publishing, 1977: 413–17.

29 Holm HH, Juul N, Pedersen JF, Hansen H, Stroyer I. Transperineal ^{125}iodine seed implantation in prostatic cancer guided by transrectal ultrasonography. *J Urol* 1983;**130**: 283–6.

30 Tanahashi Y, Watanabe H, Igari D, Harada K, Saitoh M. Volume estimation of the seminal vesicles by means of transrectal ultrasonotomography: a preliminary report. *Br J Urol* 1975; **47**:695–702.

31 Pontes JE, Eisenkraft S, Watanabe H *et al.* Preoperative evaluation of localized prostatic carcinoma by transrectal ultrasonography. *J Urol* 1985;**134**:289–91.

32 Tanahashi Y. Seminal vesicles. In: Watanabe H, Holmes JH, Holm HH, Goldberg BB, eds. *Diagnostic Ultrasound in Urology and Nephrology*. Tokyo: Igaku-shoin, 1981: 141–17.

33 Terasaki T, Kojima M, Kamoi K *et al.* Effect of LHRH analog on the seminal vesicles evaluated by transrectal sonography. *Prostate* 1993;**23**:115–21.

34 Abe M, Watanabe H, Kojima M, Saitoh M, Ohe H. Puncture of the seminal vesicles guided by a transrectal real-time linear scanner. *J Clin Ultrasound* 1989;**17**:173–8.

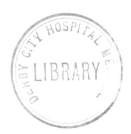

4   Renal, Bladder and Genital Ultrasound
D.Rickards

Ultrasound technique

Ultrasound is non-invasive and provides excellent anatomical and functional information of renal, vesical, testicular and penile anatomy. The blind spot of the urinary tract to ultrasound is the mid-ureter which is difficult to see because of overlying gas-filled bowel. Little functional information is gained and the detail of the pelvicalyceal system afforded by excretory urography (EU) is not matched by ultrasound. As a screening modality, ultrasound has replaced EU and competes as a diagnostic modality. It is the guidance method of choice for biopsy of renal or retroperitoneal lesions.

Kidneys

The liver and spleen provide acoustic windows and are used as references for echogenicity. The kidneys are scanned in all planes with 3.5 to 5 MHz probes. A Doppler scan identifies abnormal bloodflow and is of particular use in the transplant kidney. Indications for US in the kidneys are:
1 to differentiate solid from cystic masses;
2 to identify dilatation of the collecting system;
3 to monitor renal size and parenchymal changes in transplant kidneys;
4 to guide biopsy and interventional techniques;
5 to measure intrarenal bloodflow.

The echogenicity of the renal cortex is slightly less than that of the spleen or liver. It is interrupted by the renal pyramids, which appear as a series of conical structures with their base oriented towards the surface of the kidney. The renal sinus is highly reflective due to renal sinus fat, and in normally hydrated patients no separation of the collecting system can be defined (Fig. 4.1). Colour Doppler allows imaging of the renal vasculature (Fig. 4.2) and normal indices derived from the spectral waveform are shown in Table 4.1. Power Doppler is more sensitive than colour Doppler in defining flow, but does not colour encode the direction of flow (Fig. 4.3).

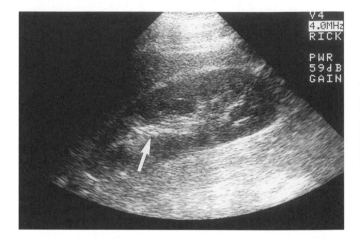

Fig. 4.1 Normal longitudinal scan of the right kidney. The renal outline is clearly defined and there is no separation seen in the echogenic renal sinus (arrow).

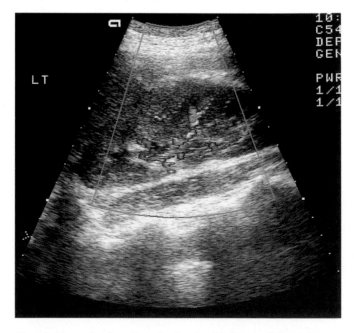

Fig. 4.2 Normal colour Doppler longitudinal scan of the right kidney.

Table 4.1 Normal colour Doppler indices of the renal vessels.

Indices	Range
Peak systolic velocity	60–140 cm/s
Pulsatility index	0.7–1.4
Resistance index	0.56–0.7

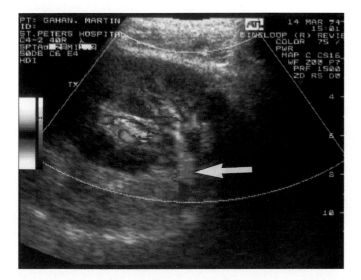

Fig. 4.3 Normal power Doppler scan of the right kidney. The renal artery (arrow) is clearly seen.

Bladder

The bladder should be comfortably distended. The bladder is a transonic structure and the lateral and posterior bladder walls are well seen. The anterior bladder wall is less well seen (Fig. 4.4). Transabdominal scanning can be used to calculate bladder volume using planimetric methods. Bladder ultrasound done before and after micturition and combined with uroflowmetry is called an ultrasound cystodynamogram (USCD). Post-micturition residuals can be measured and this test provides basic urodynamic information. Bladder filling can be expedited with intravenous frusemide. Endoscopic vesical ultrasound is invasive and is combined with cystoscopy. Excellent definition of the bladder wall provides accurate local staging of urothelial malignancy.

Testicles

Contact scanning with 7.5-10 MHz probes is preferable to probes requiring some form of acoustic stand-off to image the near field. The normal testicle is a homogeneous olive-shaped structure and flow in the capsular vessels and within the testicle can be seen on colour Doppler (Fig. 4.5). The rete testes is usually not obvious, but can be prominent and mimic disease (Fig. 4.6). Varicoceles are more pronounced with the patient standing. Warm contact jelly is essential to avoid provoking the cremasteric reflex which causes the testicles to migrate cranially making the examination more difficult.

Penis

Contact scanning using 7.5 or 10 MHz linear array probes is ideal. The corpora are paired structures of homogeneous reflectivity in which the cavernosal arteries can be seen. The corpus spongiosum has a similar echogenicity to the corpora. The urethra can be scanned whilst saline is instilled into it. Ultrasound is sensitive in depicting anterior urethral pathology. Vascular assessment of the cavernosal arteries and dorsal artery is performed after the intracorporeal administration of a vasodilator, either prostaglandin E_1 or papaverine (Fig. 4.7).

Kidneys

Congenital anomalies

Ultrasound is useful in establishing the diagnosis of congenital renal disease. Unilateral renal agenesis leads to compensatory hypertrophy of the contralateral kidney which may not be normal, with malrotation and ectopia being common. Anomalies of the genital tract (e.g. bicornuate uterus and the VATER association) should be positively sought and excluded. Malposition of the splenic flexure of the colon in left renal agenesis due to absence of the phrenicocolic ligament is a diagnostic pointer in unrecognized cases. In renal hypoplasia there is a quantitative decrease in the amount of renal tissue, with otherwise normal features. The contralateral kidney shows

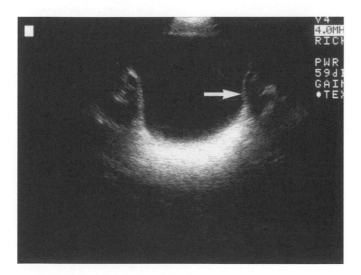

Fig. 4.4 Transverse scan of the normal bladder. The iliopsoas muscles are seen laterally (arrow).

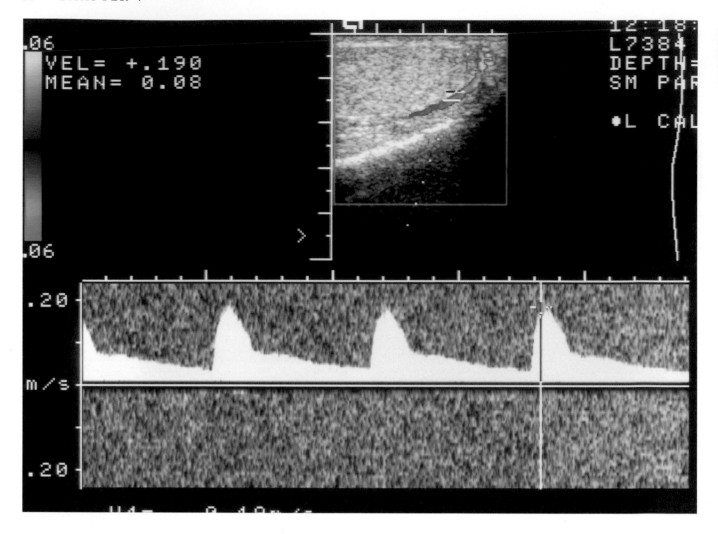

Fig. 4.5 Colour Doppler scan of a normal testicle with normal capsular flow.

compensatory hypertrophy. The hypoplastic kidney is smooth in outline, has a small renal artery and a normal ureter. Ectopic kidneys may be difficult to define with ultrasound as bowel gas frequently obscures the view.

Renal duplication (Fig. 4.8) associated with duplex ureters is of clinical importance because of ectopic ureterovesical junctions and the attendant complications. Obstruction to an upper moeity is manifest on ultrasound by dilatation of its calyces. In a horseshoe kidney, ultrasound will determine whether functioning renal tissue or fibrous tissue crosses anteriorly over the midline (Fig. 4.9). The ureters pass anteriorly over the lower poles sometimes precipitating hydronephrosis. Ectopic kidneys that cross the midline commonly fuse with the inferior aspect of the orthotopic kidney. The ureters insert normally.

Normal variants

The normal renal outline can be interrupted to resemble a renal tumour. Ultrasound will differentiate between a tumour and the following.
1 Dromedary hump. This occurs on the lateral aspect of the left kidney and is due to the proximity of the spleen (Fig. 4.10).
2 Fetal lobulation. This may persist into adult life and needs to be differentiated from pyelonephritic scarring which always occurs opposite a calyx.
3 Hypertrophy of a column of Bertin. This is due to excess invagination of the normal cortical parenchyma, which may displace calyces simulating a mass lesion.

Benign lesions

Cystic disease

The classification of cystic disease is well known. In adult polycystic disease, ultrasound is sensitive at detecting small cysts in the early stages of the disease and will also

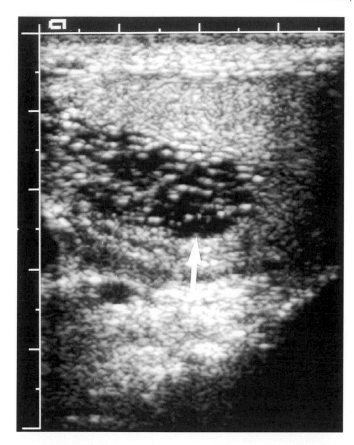

Fig. 4.6 Longitudinal scan of a normal testicle with a prominent rete testis (arrow).

detect associated cysts in the liver, spleen, pancreas and ovaries (Fig. 4.11). Pelvicalyceal obstruction, coexistent malignancy and infection are very difficult to diagnose.

Computed tomography (CT) rarely contributes further to the ultrasound appearances. Differentiation from the tuberous sclerosis complex can be difficult.

Simple renal cysts are usually cortical in position and an incidental finding unless they cause pain or reach sufficient size to present as a flank mass. They can rupture and be complicated by haemorrhage or infection. Ultrasound is the simplest method of confirming the diagnosis (Fig. 4.12), often as a sequel to an abnormality noted on EU. Essential US criteria are:

1 a smooth and sharply marginated wall;
2 an anechoic lesion;
3 posterior echo enhancement.

If these criteria are fulfilled then no further investigation is required. On the other hand a solid component, multiple septae, irregularity of the wall (Fig. 4.13) or calcification necessitate further evaluation and CT is the usual next step. The only exception is thin septae within the cyst or minimal calcification confined to the wall of the cyst and not associated with any other abnormality, in which case a benign aetiology can be assumed.

Multilocular renal cysts are rare. They consist of well-defined masses containing multiple non-communicating fluid-filled locules. Their importance is that they must be distinguished from several different conditions including benign cystic nephroma, cystic hamartoma, cystic Wilm's tumour and renal cell carcinoma. Cysts associated with medullary sponge kidney are medullary in position and are small, although multiple cortical cysts have been described. Ultrasound clearly defines them.

Complex cysts are those that do not fit all the criteria for simple cysts and because of the threat of malignancy, further investigation is essential. Ultrasound-guided aspir-

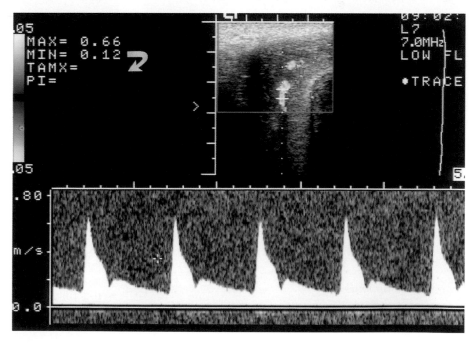

Fig. 4.7 Colour Doppler scan of the base of the penis. The cavernosal artery lies between the Doppler gate. There is a maximum flow of 0.66 m/s (arrow) in systole with a flow in diastole of 0.12 m/s.

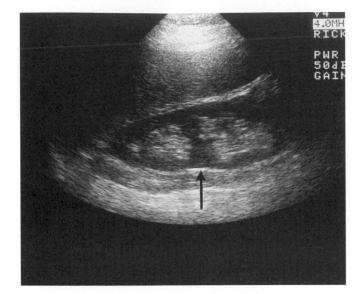

Fig. 4.8 Longitudinal scan of the right kidney. The echogenic renal sinus is divided into two (arrow) and the patient has a duplex collecting system.

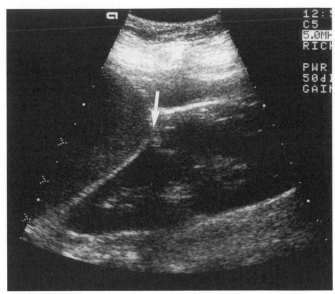

Fig. 4.10 Dromedary hump. The spleen (arrow) is indenting the posterolateral aspect of the left kidney which can give the appearance of a tumour on EU.

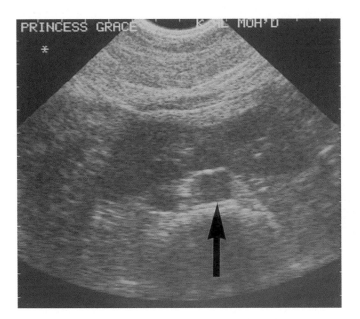

Fig. 4.9 Transverse scan of the upper abdomen. Lying in front of the aorta (arrow) is a soft tissue mass which represents normal renal tissue crossing the midline in a patient with a horseshoe kidney.

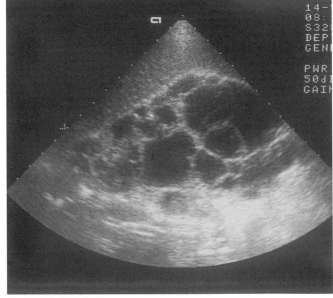

Fig. 4.11 Adult polycystic disease. In this right kidney there are numerous cysts of different sizes, characteristic of polycystic disease.

ation is valuable, though surgical exploration is the only definitive diagnostic procedure.

Benign renal tumours

Renal adenomas are invariably asymptomatic cortical lesions which can be multiple and are increasingly diagnosed incidentally with ultrasound as homogeneous mass lesions. No increased flow is seen with colour Doppler. Oncocytomas are not diagnostic on ultrasound. Angiomyolipomas are characteristic. A focal lesion with well-defined borders and markedly increased echogenicity is typical (Fig. 4.14). This is because of the large number of fat–muscle interfaces that are highly reflective.

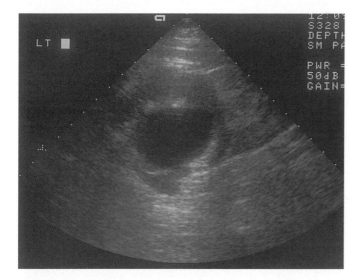

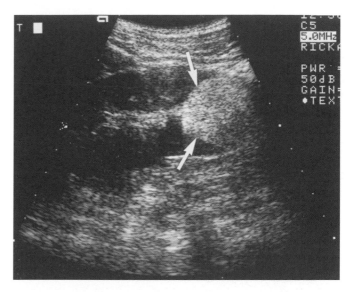

Fig. 4.12 Longitudinal scan of the right kidney. There is a well-defined cystic lesion in the upper pole that has all the characteristic of a benign renal cyst.

Fig. 4.14 Longitudinal scan of the left kidney. There is a well-defined echogenic mass lesion in the lower pole (arrows), which is characteristic of an angiomyolipoma.

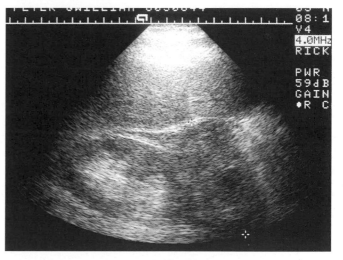

Fig. 4.13 Complex cysts of the right kidney. The cyst has an irregular and thickened wall. Although there are no internal echoes, needle aspiration of this lesion proved that it was an abscess.

Fig. 4.15 Longitudinal scan of the right kidney. There is an echogenic mass lesion in the lower pole (between calipers); this is an adenocarcinoma.

Malignant renal tumours

Renal adenocarcinomas are echogenic in 75% of cases. Necrosis within a tumour or cystic hypernephromas (3% of cases) will demonstrate echo-poor areas. There is no correlation between echogenicity and vascularity. Tumour masses may displace the collecting system and obliterate the renal sinus and perinephric fat planes (Fig. 4.15). The tumour is staged by looking for an extension of the tumour thrombus into the renal vein and inferior vena cava (Fig. 4.16), retroperitoneal lymph node status and the presence of hepatic metastases. The contralateral kidney must be assessed. Duplex Doppler aids the diagnosis of vascular involvement.

Transitional cell tumours are often very small, multiple and lie within the normally echogenic renal sinus, therefore ultrasound has a limited role. Larger lesions can be seen and are predominately echogenic. Necrosis or haemorrhage within transitional cell tumours is uncommon. Where ultrasound and CT is of value is in differ-

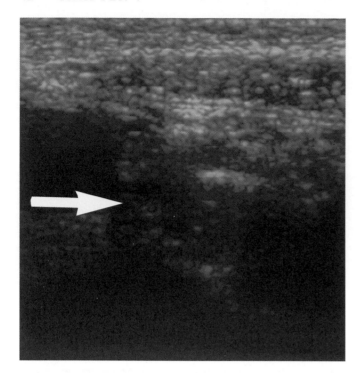

Fig. 4.16 Longitudinal scan showing an endovenous extension of tumour within the inferior vena cava (arrow) in a patient with a renal adenocarcinoma.

entiating a tumour from non-opaque calculi or blood clot. CT can stage a tumour more effectively.

Renal lymphoma can cause generalized renal enlargement, multiple focal masses (45%), a solitary mass (15%) or diffuse infiltration (10%). The echo pattern is usually hypoechoic in relation to normal renal parenchyma. The renal sinus is often largely obliterated with consequent loss of its echogenicity. In addition, there may be perirenal infiltration with nodular or conglomerate masses.

Renal calculi and obstruction

Irrespective of the chemical composition, stones appear echogenic and cast an acoustic shadow (Fig. 4.17). Small stones (less than 5 mm) may not be visualized and can be lost within the normally echogenic renal sinus. Medially situated stones within the renal pelvis may be obscured by the transverse process of the adjoining vertebral body. In patients presenting with acute renal colic, a plain film of the abdomen combined with ultrasound will define the degree of pelvicalyceal dilatation and the position of the obstructing calculus in up to 80% of patients, potentially replacing the EU. The attendant lack of ionizing radiation is important, especially in those patients who are recurrent stone formers. Identical ultrasound appearances for calculi are to be expected from cysts containing milk of calcium and sloughed papillae in papillary necrosis.

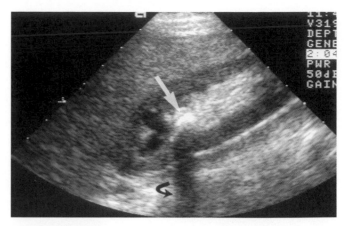

Fig. 4.17 Longitudinal scan of the right kidney. There is an echogenic focus within the collecting system (arrow) associated with acoustic shadowing (white curved arrow); this is due to a renal stone.

Obstruction to the upper urinary tract can be unilateral, bilateral, acute or chronic and ultrasound has an important role in defining the situation. Pelvicalyceal dilatation is the cardinal ultrasound feature of obstruction which can be graded from 0 to 4, where grade 0 is normal, grade 1 is minimal dilatation of the calyces and renal pelvis (Fig. 4.18) and grade 4 is gross dilatation (Fig. 4.19). In acute obstruction, the resistive index (RI) is raised to more than 0.7 and this finding has a specificity of 88% in differentiating the presence or absence of obstruction

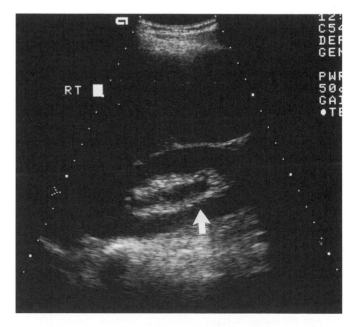

Fig. 4.18 Longitudinal scan of the right kidney. There is a slight separation of the renal sinus (arrow) indicating early hydronephrosis.

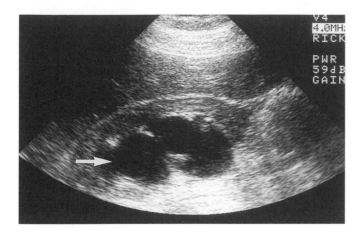

Fig. 4.19 Gross hydronephrosis of the right kidney (arrow). There is some thinning of the renal cortex.

(Fig. 4.20). The cause of obstruction must also be looked for. Retroperitoneal lesions causing obstruction will only be seen if large, but distal ureteric lesions are well seen through the full bladder (Fig. 4.21).

Renal parenchymal disease

In acute pyelonephritis, an increase in renal size, often with a generalized decrease in echogenicity, is typical. Acute lobar nephronia produces a focal mass with a decrease in cortical echogenicity and can mimic an abscess or tumour. Predisposing factors such as calculi and obstruction should be excluded.

A renal abscess appears as a complex, predominately solid and hypoechoic mass that frequently contains a necrotic element. The abscess wall is typically irregular and there may be involvement of the perinephric tissues. Gas may be present within the lesion. Needle aspiration under ultrasound control is diagnostic. Percutaneous drainage may be necessary.

In acute tubular necrosis, ultrasound is commonly performed to exclude obstruction. The kidneys are either normal or slightly large with increased cortical echogenicity and accentuated corticomedullary differentiation. Resistance indices on colour Doppler are often high. Acute cortical necrosis results in the renal cortex becoming initially hypoechoic, then hyperechoic as calcification develops.

Chronic pyelonephritis causes localized cortical loss with disruption of the normal corticomedullary junction in the early stages, usually in the upper pole, due to reflux nephropathy. Global cortical loss and small kidneys is the end stage. Ultrasound appearances in acute glomerulonephritis are non-specific. An abnormally reflective renal cortex implies active interstitial disease. Xanthogranulomatous pyelonephritis is the result of chronic renal infection where the renal parenchyma is partially (focal or tumefactive xanthogranulomatous pyelonephritis) or completely replaced by lipid-laden foam cells. It is frequently associated with obstruction and chronic urinary tract infections with *Proteus mirabilis*. Nephrolithiasis is seen in 75% of cases. Nephrolithiasis and a decrease in parenchymal echogenicity are usual. There may be evidence of longstanding obstruction. The focal form is difficult to distinguish from a neoplasm.

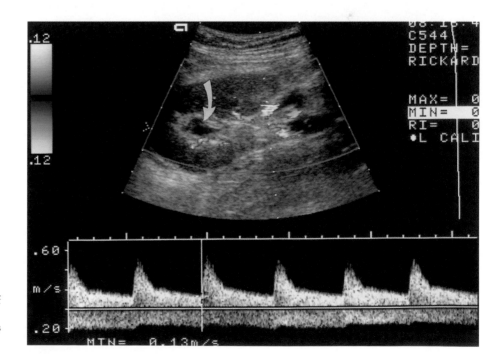

Fig. 4.20 Colour Doppler scan of the right kidney in a patient with acute obstruction. There is slight dilatation of the collecting system (arrow). The RI is 0.75. This suggests that the dilatation is due to obstruction.

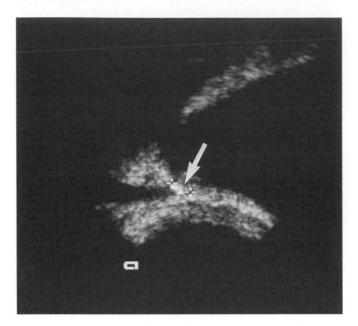

Fig. 4.21 Transverse scan of the bladder demonstrating a small obstructing calculus at the vesicoureteric junction (arrow).

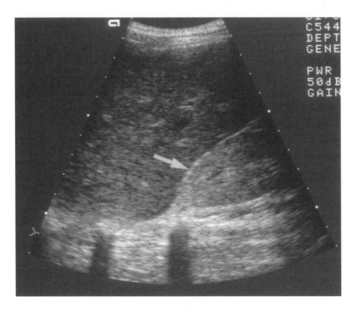

Fig. 4.22 Longitudinal scan of the upper pole of the right kidney. There is generalized increased echogenicity when compared to the liver and loss of the normal corticomedullary differentiation (arrow).

Renal vascular disease

Renal artery thrombosis presents with acute loin pain and haematuria. Echogenic material is visible within the renal arterial lumen on ultrasound and Doppler flow is absent. Wedge-shaped infarcts within the renal parenchyma are commonplace. The diagnosis of renal artery stenosis before irreversible changes occur depends on colour Doppler spectral analysis. Sampling of the main renal artery is performed and an increase in systolic velocity to greater than 1.5 m/s, spectral broadening and an increase in maximum diastolic flow are indicative of renal artery stenosis. Ratios of greater than 3.5 between peak systolic flows in the adjacent aorta to the renal artery are also sensitive in the diagnosis. Aortic aneurysms commonly originate below the level of the renal arteries, but when they involve the renal arteries, intrarenal flow can be compromised. Findings similar to renal artery stenosis can be expected.

In renal vein thrombosis, the kidney is hypoechoic in the acute stages becoming echogenic at about 10 days. There is often loss of corticomedullary differentiation with disorganization of the intrarenal architecture and poor visualization of the medullary pyramids. A patchy echogenic pattern eventually ensues. A reflective mass within the lumen of the expanded vein is typical. Absence of the normal venous Doppler signal is further evidence.

Renal trauma

The role of imaging is dependent on whether the patient is haemodynamically stable or unstable at presentation. Unstable patients with penetrating injuries often require urgent surgical management and radiological evaluation is therefore limited but may still have a role. The presence or absence of haematuria is of limited use as severe renal trauma can result in complete disruption of the vascular pedicle leading to non-function of the kidney. Ultrasound is valuable in detecting associated injuries, e.g. splenic trauma and perinephric abnormalities.

Renal failure

Two specific questions need answering in the initial assessment in a patient presenting with renal failure.
1 Is it acute or chronic?
2 Is there evidence of obstruction?
US usually provides the answer to both. Renal size and parenchymal echogenicity distinguishes acute from chronic failure and pelvicalyceal dilatation assesses obstruction. This has replaced high-dose EU.

There are potential pitfalls. Accurate measurement of renal size can be difficult in the obese. The end-stage kidney may not be seen. Pelvicalyceal dilatation is not synonymous with obstruction. Dilatation can occur in other conditions, e.g. reflux nephropathy. Conversely, a normal pelvicalyceal system does not always exclude either acute or chronic obstruction. For instance, acute calculus obstruction may not show dilatation in the early stages, and in retroperitoneal fibrosis there may never be dilatation.

Renal transplant

A postoperative baseline ultrasound is done to compare with subsequent images. Minimal dilatation of the pelvicalyceal system and a slight increase in renal size are normal findings. The pyramids appear more prominent due to the superficial location of the transplant. A small perinephric collection of fluid is not uncommon in the immediate postoperative period.

Acute rejection is characterized by:

1 a decrease in corticomedullary differentiation;
2 an increase in renal size and change in shape from elliptical to spherical;
3 decreased echogenicity of the renal sinus;
4 enlargement of the renal pyramids.

These findings distinguish acute rejection from acute tubular necrosis and cyclosporin toxicity where the ultrasound is normal.

The accuracy of ultrasound in this context varies between 52 and 85%. Duplex Doppler demonstrates an increase in vascular resistance and consequently a decrease or even reversal of end diastolic flow in acute rejection. It is also of value in screening for renal artery stenosis.

Ureteric obstruction can be caused by a blood clot, calculus, fungus ball or stricture of extrinsic compression by a pelvic mass (e.g. haematoma). Ureteric dilatation can occur in acute rejection as well as in obstruction or reflux. Postoperative fluid collections (e.g. urinoma, lymphocele, haematoma) are identified and drained under ultrasound control.

Ureter and upper urinary tract obstruction

The majority of the ureter is not easily visualized with ultrasound. Through a full bladder, the distal ureter is easily seen and the proximal 3 cm can reliably be imaged.

Ureteric tumours appear as filling defects within expanded ureters. Endoluminal high-frequency probes are now available that will accurately define the nature of these lesions and stage them. This necessitates retrograde or antegrade ureteric catheterization. Ureteric tuberculosis causing strictures and schistosomiasis causing dilatation and calcification can be imaged, but is not specific. Retroperitoneal fibrosis appears as an echogenic mass encasing the aorta and inferior vena cava and differs from lymphadenopathy which is echo-poor.

The dilatation of the pelvicalyceal systems and ureters during pregnancy is usually bilateral, but asymmetrical and more pronounced on the right. Ultrasound cannot differentiate between obstructed and unobstructed dilated ureters. Resistive indexes from colour Doppler-derived spectral waveforms may help, but clinical symptoms and marked differences in the degree of dilatation between both sides is helpful. Ultrasound is used to guide any drainage procedure to obviate the risk of radiation to the developing fetus. Pelviureteric junction obstruction on ultrasound shows a grossly dilated pelvicalyceal system with no ureteric filling. Lasix-induced diuresis invokes further dilatation and sometimes flank pain.

Bladder

A USCD is the initial investigation of choice in any patient with symptoms of a voiding disorder. Bladder volumes are measured before and after micturition using the standard technique described by Poston [1], i.e. the bladder volume in millilitres is 0.7 HDW (where D is the depth in the sagittal plane; H is the maximum diameter in the sagittal plane; and W is the maximum transverse diameter in the transverse plane; all measurements are in centimetres). Voided volumes of less than 200 ml are of little clinical relevance, so it is important to establish by ultrasound that the bladder is sufficiently full. Overfull bladders are to be avoided as such a state will inhibit micturition. Once the full bladder has been scanned and its volume measured, the patient voids into a standard flow rate machine having been asked to void as normally as possible and not to try and impress with superimposed abdominal straining. Immediately after voiding, the bladder is rescanned and any residual urine measured. If there is a large residue (100 ml or more), the bladder should be rescanned after a second void and that residual assessed. Uroflowmetry provides:

1 maximum flow rate;
2 average flow rate;
3 voided volume;
4 time to peak flow;
5 voiding time.

A bell-shaped curve is seen in normal uroflowmetry with a maximum flow rate of 30–50 ml/s. Prostate dimensions can be measured on suprapubic scanning. The following patterns may be seen.

1 *Normal flow rate—complete bladder emptying.* A normal USCD does not exclude abnormalities of bladder function. Early prostate outflow obstruction is compensated for by the bladder generating higher voiding pressures to establish complete bladder emptying at normal flow rates. It will be in the later stages of bladder decompensation that flow rates will deteriorate and residual urine volumes will be seen. Instability (involuntary bladder contraction) will not be excluded. Bladder wall hypertrophy, if present, should suggest outflow obstruction even if the rest of the USCD is normal.

2 *Low flow rate—complete bladder emptying.* This combination will be commonly seen in the following conditions.

   (a) Outflow obstruction (see Chapter 7). The bladder wall may be thickened and the elevation of the bladder base may be due to prostatomegaly (Fig. 4.23). Acquired diverticula are further evidence of high-pressure voiding. When these findings are seen in association with large residuals and dilated upper tracts (Fig. 4.24), high-

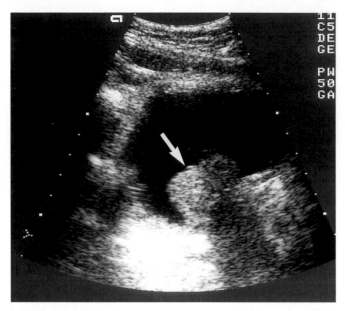

Fig. 4.23 Sagittal scan of the bladder. There is irregular elevation of the bladder base due to an enlarged prostate (arrow); there is also hypertrophy of the bladder wall.

pressure chronic retention is likely, an important diagnosis because of renal impairment. Other causes of outflow obstruction (e.g. urethral stricture, bladder neck dyssynergia) cannot be excluded.

(b) Poorly functioning bladder without outflow obstruction. This is seen in women who are infrequent voiders (so-called cameloid bladders). The bladder becomes chronically overdistended and the bladder muscle (detrusor) is subsequently damaged.

3 *High flow rate—complete bladder emptying.* This can be seen in normal patients who augment micturition with abdominal straining. It is also seen in detrusor instability without obstruction; such patients void with high pressures.

4 *Low flow rate—incomplete emptying.* This is characteristic of decompensated outflow obstruction. The detrusor can only manage to generate sufficient pressures to overcome the outflow resistance for so long, it decompensates and a residual is left. These patients characteristically feel the need to void a few minutes after the initial void as the detrusor recovers. This pattern is also seen in patients with poor detrusors and no outflow obstruction.

5 *Intermittent flow rate—variable emptying.* Such flow patterns are characteristic of patients in whom voiding is predominately by abdominal pressure, the detrusor having all but failed. The effectiveness of the abdominal straining will determine how much of a residual is left.

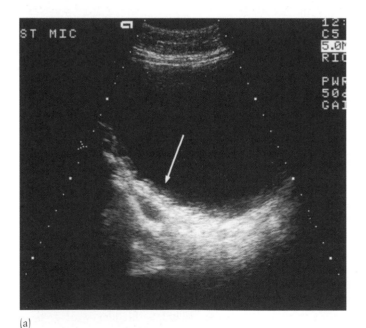

(a)

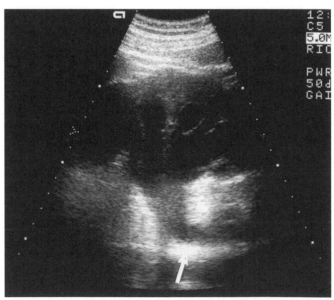

(b)

Fig. 4.24 (a) Transverse scan of the full bladder. There is hypertrophy of the bladder wall and numerous small diverticula (arrow). (b) Longitudinal scan of the left kidney in the same patient. There is dilatation of the collecting system and ureter (arrow). The combination of bladder wall hypertrophy, symmetrical upper tract dilatation and incomplete emptying is characteristic of high-pressure chronic retention of urine.

The USCD is most useful in the follow-up of patients who have undergone transurethral resection of the prostate (TURP) for outflow obstruction or urethral repositioning procedures in the treatment of stress incontinence. As a diagnostic test it is limited, being unable to differentiate between an overactive detrusor in the presence of obstruction and a normal patient, etc. More invasive but definitive urodynamic studies have to be performed. In our unit, USCD is used as an initial test of lower tract function in all symptomatic patients. This gives some idea as to which patients need to go on to formal urodynamic studies. It is extensively used to monitor the effect of treatment of any kind of lower tract obstruction, whether it be prostate mediated or due to urethral stricture. USCD also affords the advantage of defining other pelvic pathology which may be significant in determining the cause of lower tract function and pelvic pain.

Bladder calculi are usually the result of outflow obstruction. Stones that pass into the bladder from the upper urinary tract should easily be passed urethrally unless there is associated outflow obstruction. Stones appear as discrete echogenic masses associated with posterior acoustic shadowing and are mobile (Fig. 4.25). Underlying prostatic outflow obstruction should be sought by performing a USCD. A blood clot may be mobile or adherent to the bladder wall (Fig. 4.26); they appear as echogenic intravesical masses, often with a discrete urine–blood clot fluid level.

The bladder is the most common site of urothelial malignancy. Vesical ultrasound can be performed endoscopically at the time of cystoscopy or suprapubically.

Endoscopic ultrasound can define all tumours except carcinoma *in situ*. T1 tumours are echo-poor masses that cause no interruption of the underlying bladder wall. T2 lesions infiltrate the echo-dense bladder wall and T3a tumours involve the entire thickness of the bladder wall (Fig. 4.27). The differential diagnoses are:

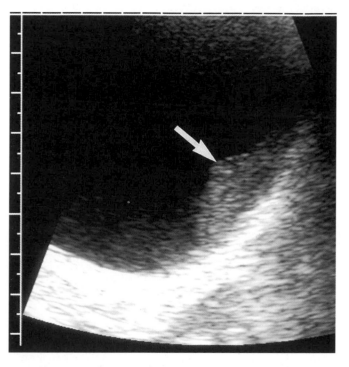

Fig. 4.26 Transverse scan of the bladder. There is a mass adjacent to the bladder wall, but the bladder wall is intact. This is adherent blood clot (arrow).

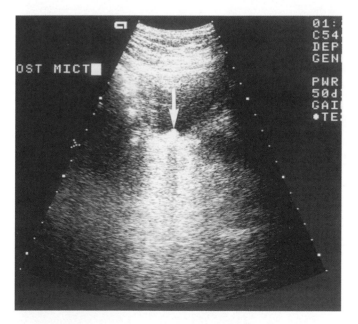

Fig. 4.25 Transverse scan of the bladder post-micturition. There is an echogenic focus seen posteriorly (arrow) associated with acoustic shadowing due to a bladder stone.

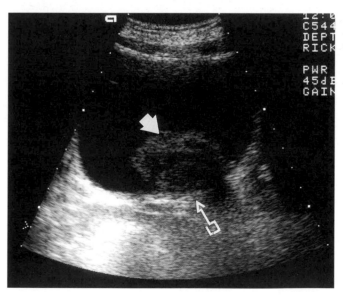

Fig. 4.27 Transverse scan of the bladder. There is a mass lesion infiltrating the bladder (arrow) and involving the bladder wall (open arrow). This is due to an infiltrating bladder carcinoma, a T3a tumour.

1 bladder wall trabeculation;

2 oedema;

3 focal chronic cystitis.

As a staging modality, ultrasound is invasive and of limited usefulness.

Bladder diverticula are congenital or acquired. Acquired diverticula are more common in males, are usually paraureteric and associated with vesicoureteric reflux. They can be associated with renal dysplasia and megaureter. They are thin-walled, containing very little muscle. Acquired diverticula are virtually always associated with outflow tract obstruction and 85% arise just lateral and superior to the ureteric orifice. Very little muscle is present in their walls and they can achieve enormous sizes. Calculi commonly form in them because of stasis and there is a 5% association between diverticula and transitional cell tumour.

Ultrasound can rapidly confirm the presence of a diverticulum and to what extent it empties following micturition. In some patients the diverticulum might transiently increase in size as a functioning detrusor voids into it rather than through an obstructed lower tract. The position and size of the orifice can help preoperative planning. The most important use of ultrasound is to detect complications, i.e. a stone or tumour. It is not always possible to endoscopically assess a diverticulum.

Simple ureteroceles arise at the normal ureteric orifice, whilst ectopic ureteroceles can arise anywhere in the lower urogenital tract. They are often associated with upper tract dilatation, but not always. They are easily seen on both suprapubic and transrectal ultrasonography (TRUS) and appear as a 'cyst within a cyst'.

There are numerous reports of foreign objects, ranging from light bulbs to £50 notes, that have been inserted urethrally into the bladder. Ultrasound can detect the presence of these objects, often found incidentally in the assessment of patients with haematuria or urinary tract infections. Surgeons are also prone to leaving things in bladders, for example bits of retrograde catheters, etc. In obese patients or those with peritonism in whom palpation of the abdomen is not possible, ultrasound is very useful in determining whether the bladder is full enough to allow safe suprapubic catheterization. Blind catheterization in such cases can be complicated by bowel damage.

Scrotum and testicles

The testicle is a superficial structure and is easily palpated, and much scrotal pathology is clinically obvious. The role of imaging is to confirm clinical suspicions and evaluate equivocal findings.

Indications for scrotal ultrasound

Investigation of a scrotal swelling

Ultrasound is the method of choice to demonstrate testicular tumours. On ultrasound, seminomas are usually uniformly echo-poor (Fig. 4.28), sometimes containing areas of necrosis (Fig. 4.29). Teratoma occurs in a slightly younger age group and in contrast tend to have a mixed or often bizarre echo pattern, often with cystic changes together with echogenic areas. Calcification is a feature. Both tumour types are commonly associated with a hydrocele. Embryonal cell and choriocarcinoma are the other two types of germ cell tumour and tend to be highly aggressive malignancies. Occasionally, these tumours may undergo spontaneous regression, resulting in a fibrous scar. It is not possible on ultrasound alone to distinguish confidently between tumour types or to be definitive about the diagnosis of malignancy. Benign disease, for example haematocele and chronic granulomatous orchitis, simulate a tumour.

Secondary deposits in the testes are more common in older age groups. The kidney and prostate are common primary sites. Leukaemia and lymphoma may also involve the testis and usually appear diffusely echo-poor.

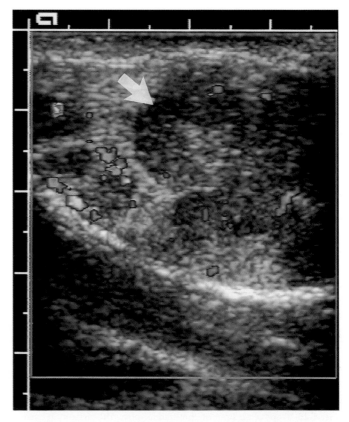

Fig. 4.28 Testicular scan. The testicle is heterogeneous with numerous echo-poor lesions (arrow) due to a seminoma.

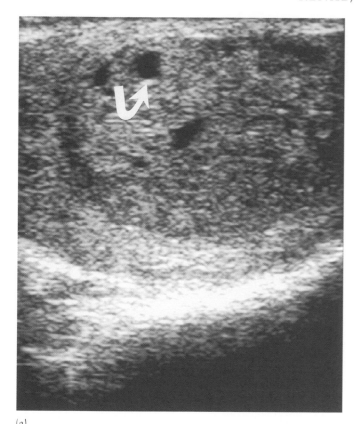

(a)

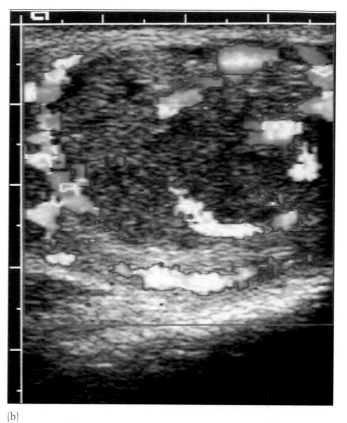

(b)

Fig. 4.29 (a) Testicular scan. There is disruption of the normal echo pattern of the testicle with cystic areas within it (arrow) due to a teratoma. (b) A colour Doppler scan of the same patient showing considerable increased bloodflow within the lesion characteristic of primary testicular malignancy.

Extratesticular scrotal tumours that involve the epididymis are rare. The majority are adenomatoid tumours which are usually well defined and have an echo pattern similar or greater than the testis.

Hydroceles are either congenital or acquired. The former usually resolve spontaneously. The latter may result from trauma, although an underlying neoplasm must always be excluded. On ultrasound, hydroceles are transonic and surround the testicle (Fig. 4.30). Internal echoes will be seen in haematoceles and pyoceles. Epididymal cysts and spermatoceles are well defined, transonic and occasionally multiple (Fig. 4.31). Ultrasound confirms their location, assesses their size and can be used to monitor their progress.

Investigation of scrotal pain

In epididymo-orchitis, the epididymis is enlarged and echo-poor and 20% of patients will have associated changes in the testis. There may be an associated hydrocele. In chronic epididymitis, the epididymis appears echogenic and the

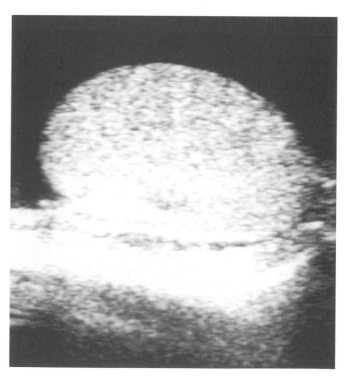

Fig. 4.30 Scrotal scan showing a normal testicle surrounded by fluid due to a hydrocele.

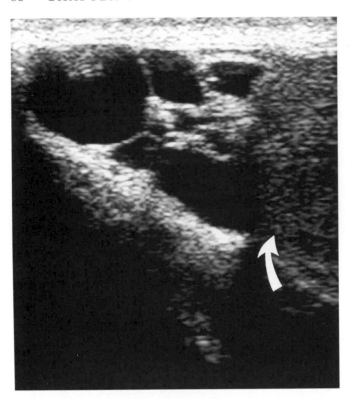

Fig. 4.31 Scrotal scan showing multiple cystic lesions in the head of the epididymis. The upper pole of the testicle is seen (arrow).

tunica albuginea is thickened. Inflammatory disease can be complicated by abscess formation in either the testis or epididymis.

Varicoceles appear as serpiginous echo-poor structures surrounding the testicle and are more than 2 mm in diameter. On colour Doppler and with the patient performing valsalva, flow within the varicocele will be seen (Fig. 4.32). Testicular torsion causes ultrasound abnormalities within 1 h of onset. The testicle is uniformly enlarged and echo-poor. The epididymis may be enlarged and a hydrocele is often associated. The appearances are very similar to acute epididymo-orchitis, but can be differentiated from it with Doppler studies of the testicular vessels. In suspected torsion, radioisotopes show a photon-deficient area surrounded by activity, a classic appearance. Ultrasound needs to be performed within the first hour if the testis is to be salvaged.

Investigation of scrotal trauma

Scrotal trauma may cause the following problems.
1 Testicular rupture. There is disruption of the normal testicular outline and echo pattern. Actual fracture lines within the testicle are rarely identified.
2 Scrotal haematoma. Blood within the scrotal soft tissues causes thickening of the scrotal wall. With resolution and liquefaction of the haematoma, echo-poor areas are seen.

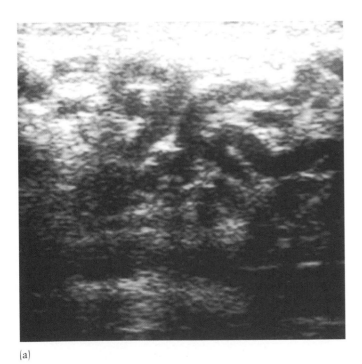

(a)

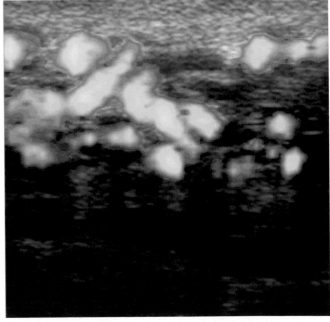

(b)

Fig. 4.32 (a) Scrotal scan showing multiple serpiginous structures due to a varicocele. (b) Power Doppler scan during valsalva showing considerable bloodflow within the veins.

3 Acute haematoceles are due to haemorrhage within the tunica vaginalis, forming a relatively echo-poor collection separate from the testis.

Investigation of subfertility

Subfertility and, in the extreme form, infertility, is associated with:
1 varicoceles, see p. 50;
2 testicular atrophy. The testicles are small, relatively echo-poor and can be slightly irregular in outline (Fig. 4.33). It is difficult to recognize small tumours in atrophic testicles.

Investigation of an ectopic testicle

Undescended testes can be unilateral or bilateral. The normal descent of the testes from the abdomen to the scrotum is interrupted and is commonly sited in the inguinal canal (70%). In the remainder, it is found high in the scrotum, the abdomen or lower pelvis. If it cannot be palpated, both ultrasound and CT may locate it. If these fail, testicular venography or angiography are performed, but there are technical problems. Even in expert hands, there is a 20% failure rate of left testicular vein

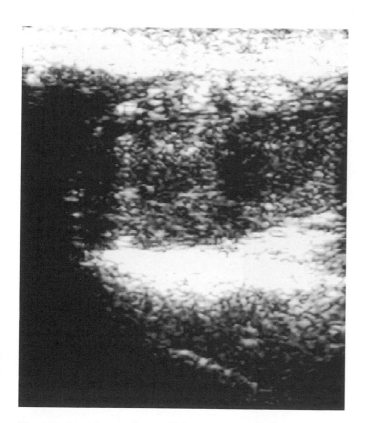

Fig. 4.33 Scrotal scan of a small, heterogeneous testicle which was avascular on colour Doppler. This is testicular atrophy due to mumps.

catheterization and 50% on the right. Unilateral or bilateral anorchia must also be considered in the differential diagnosis of an empty scrotum.

Penis

Indications for penile imaging

Penile trauma

Penile rupture is uncommon and only 200 cases have been reported. It only occurs in the erect penis as a result of direct blunt trauma that abnormally bends the penis, usually during coitus. Plain films may show dystrophic calcification within the corpora. Cavernosonography, ultrasound and magnetic resonance imaging (MRI) are indicated if rupture is not clinically obvious. At cavernosonography, extravasation of contrast associated with a defect in the corpora are seen. Recognition of the precise site of injury helps plan surgery. Cavernosonography can be complicated by increased fibrosis from extravasated contrast. Ultrasound is difficult because clot fills the rupture and small tears may be missed. On T_1-weighted MRI, vascular sinusoids are readily distinguished from the avascular tear.

Investigation of impotence

General

Careful history taking should identify the majority of patients with non-organic impotence. Details should be taken of past medical events or traumatic episodes. Medication and cigarette habits should be altered as appropriate. Physical examination will identify patients with gross anatomical, hormonal, vascular or neurogenic problems and blood testing should be done to check blood sugar, testosterone levels, prolactin levels and thyroid function. Clinical evaluation is important; patients with a psychogenic history should have counselling and those who are not prepared to undergo surgery should not have contrast studies. Further investigation should obtain objective evaluation of the penile vasculature and classify the aetiology of the impotence into one of four clinically useful groups.
1 Arterial disease.
2 Venous leakage.
3 A combination of 1 and 2.
4 Normal penile vasculature.
    Colour Doppler ultrasound and cavernosometry are the most widely used investigations. Doppler ultrasound will diagnose whether there is sufficient inflow of arterial blood in response to vasoactive agents for erection, whether there is a leak in the veins or whether there is a possible

combination of both arteriogenic and venogenic causes of impotence; it should be the first line of investigation. Cavernosometry will document the degree of venous leakage and the anatomy of the draining veins, but is only performed once it is known that there is no arterial insufficiency.

Vasoactive agents

All tests of erectile function are performed before and after the injection of vasoactive (smooth muscle relaxant) agents into the corpora. The most commonly used agent is papaverine hydrochloride which can be used in combination with phentolamine. Prostaglandin E_1 may be effective when other agents fail and is now the agent of choice because it is less painful to inject and associated with less complications, especially priapism. All vasoactive agents carry the risk of priapism and the dose administered to an individual patient should take account of the clinical picture. If papaverine is used, an initial dose of 30 mg can be supplemented by another dose of 30 mg should there be no response to the initial dose. Prostaglandin E_1 comes in ready-made doses of 20 µg.

Vasoactive agents are injected directly into the corpora through a 25 gauge needle. If performing colour Doppler ultrasound, the needle is placed in the base of one corpus cavernosum as it is held by the thumb and index finger of the hand. Tourniquets are not used, but dispersion of the vasoactive agent is improved if the base of the penis is massaged.

Erectile grade

Although there will be subjective variability, the quality of the erection obtained after injection of the vasoactive agent should be graded:

Grade 0: no response;
Grade 1: tumescence but no deviation from the vertical;
Grade 2: tumescence but less than 90° deviation;
Grade 3: normal response, suitable for penetration.

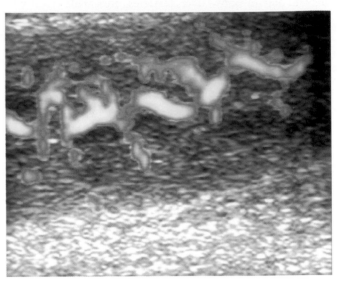

Fig. 4.34 Power Doppler scan of the penis showing a cavernosal artery and its branches. The cavernosal artery is tortuous due to arteriosclerosis.

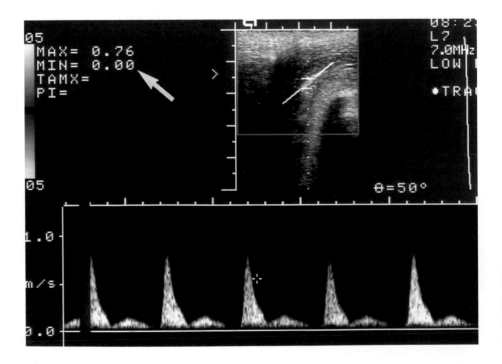

Fig. 4.35 Colour Doppler ultrasound of the proximal cavernosal artery following the injection of prostaglandin E_1. Flow within the vessel is 0.76 m/s in systole with no flow in diastole (arrow).

Colour Doppler imaging

Colour Doppler imaging is capable of visualizing bloodflow over the entire field of the ultrasound image and encoding the bloodflow velocity according to a colour scale. It can document the number of cavernosal arteries, their tortuosity (Fig. 4.34) and the presence of abnormal collateral vessels. Colour Doppler imaging assists the identification of the origin of the cavernosal arteries and allows for an accurate angle correction from the colour Doppler signal yielding a true velocity value on duplex imaging. Because the vessels can be more readily imaged, more data can be obtained and changes in arterial waveform easily monitored as the erection develops.

The technique involves three basic steps.
1 Scan the flaccid penis; attempts should be made to pick up the cavernosal arteries and identify any areas of fibrosis or Peyronie's disease.
2 Inject the papaverine.
3 Scan the cavernosal arteries at the base of the penis bilaterally every 4 min for 16 min.

The following measurements should be documented.
1 Maximal inflow velocity (m/s).
2 Lowest end diastolic velocity.
3 Erectile grade.
4 Diameter of the cavernosal artery.

Immediately following the injection there is a reduction in resistance leading to an increased velocity of flow in both systole and diastole, seen on analysis of the spectral waveform. As intracorporeal pressure rises, the flow in diastole decreases and is usually retrograde at full erection in the normal subject. A 75% increase in the diameter of the caversonal arteries demonstrates good vessel compliance. Normal indices are:

1 maximum inflow velocity greater than 0.35 m/s (Fig. 4.35);
2 lowest end diastolic velocity less than 0.05 m/s;
3 grade 3 erection.

Criteria for the diagnosis of arterial disease where there is failure to achieve a grade 3 erectile response are any of the following.
1 Maximum inflow velocity less than 0.35 m/s at the origin of the cavernosal artery (Fig. 4.36).
2 A difference between the left and right cavernosal arteries of >0.12 m/s.
3 An absent or nearly absent cavernosal artery on colour Doppler imaging.
4 A local stenosis demonstrated on colour Doppler imaging and confirmed by a sharp velocity gradient on duplex imaging.

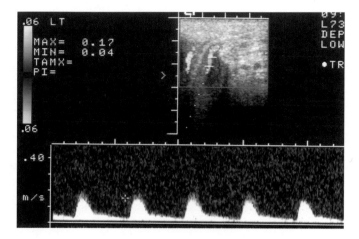

Fig. 4.36 Colour Doppler scan following the injection of prostaglandin E_1. Maximum flow achieved in systole was 0.17 m/s; this indicates arterial insufficiency causing impotence.

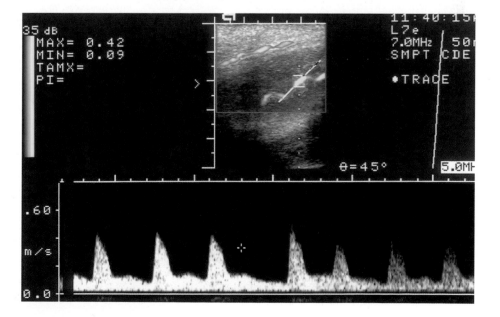

Fig. 4.37 Power Doppler scan of the cavernosal artery following the injection of prostaglandin E_1. Flow in systole is normal at 0.42 m/s, but flow in diastole is elevated at 0.09 m/s, this indicates a venous leak causing impotence.

5 An abnormal collateral flow.

Venous leakage should not be assessed by colour Doppler imaging if the arterial inflow is inadequate.

Criteria for the diagnosis of venous leakage are as follow.
1 A sustained end diastolic velocity of greater than 0.05 m/s for at least 5 min of the study (Fig. 4.37).
2 A failure to achieve a grade 3 erection.
3 Normal arterial inflow.

Reference

1 Poston GL, Joseph AEA, Riddle PR. The accuracy of ultrasound in the measurement of bladder volumes. *Br J Urol* 1983; **55**: 361–3.

Further reading

Bookstein J. Cavernosal venoocclusive insufficiency in male impotence: valuation of degree and location. *Radiology* 1987; **164**:175–8.

Bosniak MA. The current radiological approach to renal cysts. *Radiology* 1986;**158**:1–10.

Bosniak MA, Megibow AJ, Mitnick JS, Lefleur RS, Gordon R. CT of ureteral obstruction. *Am J Roentgenol* 1982;**138**:1107–13.

Carris CK, Schmidt JD. Emphysematous pyelonephritis. *J Urology* 1977; **118**:457.

Chisholm GD. Obstructive uropathy. In: O'Rielly PH, ed. *Postgraduate Surgery Lectures*, Vol. 2. London: Butterworths, 1974:51–66.

Davidson AJ. *Renal Parenchymal Disease*. Philadelphia: WB Saunders, 1982.

Eardley I, Vale J, Holmes S, Patel A, Kirby RS. Pharmacocavernometry in the assessment of erectile impotence. *J R Soc Med* 1990;**83**:22–4.

Frick MP, Feinberg SB, Sibley RK, Idstrom ME. Ultrasound in acute transplant rejection. *Radiology* 1981;**138**:657–60.

Fry IK, Cattell WR. Radiological investigation of renal disease. In: Black DAK, Jones NF, eds. *Renal Disease*. Oxford: Blackwell Scientific Publications, 1979:257–66.

Grainger RG, Longstaff AJ, Parsons MA. Xanthogranulomatous pyelonephritis: a reappraisal; 80 personal cases. *Lancet* 1982;**I**:1398–401.

Hodson CJ. The radiological contribution toward the diagnosis of chronic pyelonephritis. *Radiology* 1967;**88**:857–71.

Jackman RJ, Stevens GM. Benign haemorrhagic renal cyst. *Radiology* 1974;**110**:7–13.

Krane RJ, Goldstein I, de Tejada IS. Medical progress, impotence. *N Engl J Med* 1989; **321**:1648–59.

Krysewicz S, Mellinger BC. The role of imaging in the diagnostic evaluation of impotence. *Am J Radiol* 1989;**153**:1133–9.

Laing PC, Jeffrey RB, Wing VW. Ultrasound versus excretory urography in evaluating acute flank pain. *Radiology* 1985; **154**:613–16.

Lalli AF. Retroperitoneal fibrosis and inapparent obstructive uropathy. *Radiology* 1977;**122**:339–42.

Leopold GR, Woo VL, Scheilble FW, Nachtsheim D, Gosnick BB. High resolution ultrasonography of scrotal pathology. *Radiology* 1979;**131**:719–22.

Lue TF, Tanagho EA. Physiology of erection and pharmacological management of impotence. *J Urol* 1987;**137**:829–36.

Minford JE, Davies P. The urographic appearances in acute and chronic retroperitoneal fibrosis. *Clin Radiol* 1984;**35**: 51–6.

Mueller SC, Wallenberg-Pachaly H, Voges GE, Schild HH. Comparison of selective internal iliac pharmacoangiography, penile brachial index and duplex sonography with pulsed Doppler analysis for the evaluation of vasculogenic (arteriogenic) impotence. *J Urol* 1990;**143**:928–32.

Pollack HM, Wein AJ. Imaging of renal trauma. *Radiology* 1989;**172**:297–308.

Quam JP, King BF, James EM *et al.* Duplex and color Doppler sonographic evaluation of vasculogenic impotence. *Am J Radiol* 1989;**153**:1141–7.

Rose JG, Gillenwater JY. Pathophysiology of ureteral obstruction. *Am J Physiol* 1972;**225**:830–7.

Rosen MP, Greenfield AJ, Walker TG *et al.* Arteriogenic impotence: findings in 195 impotent men examined with selective internal pudendal angiography. *Radiology* 1990;**174**: 1043–8.

Rosenfield AT, Siegelk NJ. Renal parenchymal disease: histopathologic–sonographic correlation. *Am J Roentgenol* 1981;**137**:793–8.

Sherwood T. The dilated upper urinary tract. *Radiol Clin North Am* 1979;7:333–40.

Waltzer WC. The urinary tract in pregnancy. *J Urol* 1981;**125**: 271–6.

Wespes E, Declour C, Struyven J *et al.* Pharmaco-cavernometry-cavernography in the diagnosis of impotence. *Br J Urol* 1986;**58**:429–33.

Whitaker RH. Methods of assessing obstruction in dilated ureters. *Br J Urol* 1973;**45**:15–22.

5 Computed Tomography and Magnetic Resonance Imaging in Urology

R.H.Reznek and J.E.Husband

Introduction

Over the past decade, both computed tomography (CT) and magnetic resonance imaging (MRI) have undergone great technological developments enabling far more rapid imaging and substantially improving the quality of the images. CT has become a vital component of urological diagnosis, particularly in evaluation of the kidney and ureters, and remains unsurpassed in evaluating lesions containing fat and calcium. In a relatively short time, MRI has proved to be unequivocally superior to CT in investigating pelvic pathology, particularly for staging neoplasms of the bladder and prostate. As always, factors such as cost, availability and the likely impact on the management of the patient must be considered in combination with the accuracy of each technique in deciding on the appropriate role of CT and MRI in the investigation of patients with urological disease.

Technical principles

Computed tomography

CT and conventional radiography generate X-rays in much the same way. CT differs in that it uses a more sensitive X-ray detection system than photographic film, either gas or crystal detectors, and then uses a computer to manipulate the data obtained from the detectors. The outstanding advantage of CT is that it can detect very small differences in X-ray absorption values so that whereas the range of densities recorded on standard film is approximately 20, that on CT is about 2000. Although other planes are sometimes practicable, horizontal (axial) sections are by far the most commonly used. The section level and thickness to be imaged are selected before scanning and is usually between 1.0 and 10 mm. The data computer then calculates the attenuation (absorption) value of each pixel and the data from each set of exposures are reconstructed into an image. The attenuation values are expressed on an arbitrary scale (Hounsfield units) with water density being 0, air density being –1000 and bone density being +1000 units. The range and level of densities to be displayed can be selected by computer controls. The range of densities visualized on a particular image is known as the 'window width' and the mean level as the 'window level' or 'window centre'.

Detection and evaluation of renal pathology almost always requires intravenous injection of iodinated contrast medium. However, scans without contrast medium are also performed to detect calcification or calculi and to evaluate the nature of cystic lesions. Scans performed only after the intravenous administration of contrast medium may mask these abnormalities.

Recently, 'spiral' or 'helical' CT has been developed whereby the patient is scanned continuously while the table is moving. This allows a large volume of the body to be scanned while the breath is held, eliminating motion artefact and breathing misregistration. This new development is likely to provide many advantages in evaluation of the kidney, including the evaluation and characterization of small renal masses, and in patients with suspected renal trauma.

Magnetic resonance imaging

MRI depends on the phenomenon that protons of certain elements behave like small spinning bar magnets and when placed in a strong magnetic field will align themselves with the magnetic force. Hydrogen nuclei (protons) in water molecules and lipids are responsible for producing images at the field strengths used in medical imaging. When a radiofrequency (RF) pulse is applied at an appropriate (resonant) frequency, some protons alter alignment, flipping through a preset angle and rotate in phase with each other. When the RF pulse is removed, the protons realign (or relax) to their original position and in so doing induce a very weak radio signal, which can be detected by coils placed around the patient. An image representing the distribution of the hydrogen protons can be built up. The signal strength depends on the density of the protons and two relaxation times, T_1 and T_2. T_1 depends on the time the spinning protons take to return to the axis of the magnetic field following removal of the RF pulse; T_2 depends on the time the protons take to dephase. The T_1 and T_2 weighting of an image can be selected by altering the timing and sequences of the RF pulses.

Until quite recently, MRI has been a relatively slow process requiring long scan times, when compared to CT, and unavoidable biological movement has degraded the image quality. However, techniques for limiting the effect of such motion (e.g. shorter scan times, electronic gating devices) have been developed and are likely to prove extremely useful, particularly for scanning the abdomen.

Contrast agents depend on magnetic and paramagnetic properties to produce contrast. The most widely used is gadolinium diethylenetriamine penta-acetic acid (DTPA) which dramatically decreases the T_1 relaxation time.

Kidneys

CT, with its superb contrast sensitivity, allowing distinction between tissues of only minor differences in density, and its cross-sectional display, has made a substantial impact on diagnostic renal imaging. Nevertheless, intravenous urography (IVU) and ultrasound remain the first imaging investigations of choice in the evaluation of most renal problems with specific indications for CT that have evolved over recent years. The direct multiplanar imaging capability of MRI, together with its superior contrast resolution, have made it an extremely useful method too for evaluation of the kidney. Until very recently, MRI was limited by slow image-acquisition times and respiration-related artefacts, but the use of new breath-hold techniques is likely to increase the application of MRI in the evaluation of renal abnormalities [1]. The inability to demonstrate calcification reliably with MRI remains problematic. Thus, as with CT, the next few years will see the gradual evolution of indications for MRI in the evaluation of patients with renal pathology.

Cystic disease

Simple cysts

A renal space-occupying lesion must meet the following criteria on CT to be termed a simple cyst:
1 its contents have an attenuation value close to that of water;
2 the density of the contents is homogeneous;
3 its wall is almost indiscernible;
4 it is sharply demarcated from the surrounding renal parenchyma;
5 the contents do not increase in attenuation value after intravenous injection of contrast medium.

All renal space-occupying lesions detected on urography are further evaluated with ultrasonography (US). When all the US criteria for a benign renal cyst are rigorously applied, it is generally accepted that the accuracy for the well-performed ultrasound examination for diagnosing benign cysts is close to 100% [2]. A space-occupying lesion is considered indeterminate when it fails to meet all the criteria of a simple cyst or those of a solid mass. About 20% of all cystic lesions evaluated on ultrasound are interpreted as lacking one or more of the criteria for a benign renal cyst and thus become indeterminate [3]. CT is then indicated to determine whether the space-occupying lesion does represent a simple benign cyst or whether further investigation is required.

Common causes of such indeterminate cystic lesions on ultrasound include calcification, septation and multiple or clustered renal cysts.

Calcification. Although calcification is most often associated with benign simple cysts, the risk of malignancy of a calcified lesion approaches 20% [4,5]. As calcium reflects sound, precluding a complete US examination, all calcified cystic lesions must be evaluated by CT [2,6]. There have been several attempts to distinguish between benign and malignant patterns of calcification. A calcified mass is considered benign on CT if:
1 there is only a small amount of calcification in the wall;
2 there is no associated soft tissue mass;
3 the centre is entirely of water density;
4 no portion of the mass enhances after intravenous injection of contrast medium [5,7].

If the calcification is thick or irregular, or if the centre of the space-occupying lesion is not the density of water, or any portion of the mass enhances after intravenous contrast medium injection, then further evaluation such as cyst puncture is indicated [5–9].

Septation. One or more septations within a cystic mass are commonly detected on ultrasound and may be a manifestation of healing or organization of haemorrhage within a cyst. If the septa are thin (1 mm or less), smooth and attached to the walls without associated thickened elements, they are of no clinical consequence [7,10]. As it is often difficult to identify the margins of the cyst adequately at the site of attachment, further evaluation with CT of septate cysts detected on ultrasound is usually indicated.

About 5–8% of simple cysts may appear indeterminate on CT [6,8] as they do not fulfil all the necessary criteria. Such lesions require further investigation, usually image-guided percutaneous aspiration or biopsy.

Multiple cysts. Multiple or simple cysts clustered in one portion of the kidney have been termed localized renal cystic disease and they can be extremely difficult to distinguish from a multiloculated renal cell carcinoma or multilocular cystic nephroma either on ultrasound or CT [7,11,12]. In this latter condition, there is replacement of a portion of one kidney by multiple cysts scattered diffusely through the parenchyma without a distinct encapsulated renal mass. If the CT criteria for a benign cyst are carefully applied (to distinguish it from a multiloculated cystic renal neoplasm) then renal biopsy or surgery can be avoided [2]. However, follow-up CT scans should be obtained before final diagnosis of localized renal cystic disease [12].

Acquired cystic disease of dialysis

This develops in up to 90% of patients undergoing haemodialysis or peritoneal dialysis for more than 3 years [13,14]. About 16% of these patients will develop renal tumours [13] and about 7% of patients will develop renal adenocarcinomas [14–17].

Ultrasound studies are often difficult to perform and interpret as the kidneys are often small, distorted and surrounded by echogenic fat. In addition, calcification frequently occurs either in the cyst wall or in the interstitium [18]. There is thus general agreement that CT is the method of choice for examining the native kidneys as it has a higher sensitivity than ultrasound for detecting small solid lesions [13–18].

Adult polycystic disease

CT is occasionally indicated in patients with known adult polycystic disease because there is a clinical suspicion that the cysts have become infected or haemorrhagic. The detection of these complications relies on demonstrating that a cyst (or cysts) has an increased density. However, as the attenuation values of these cysts vary with the presence of proteinaceous mucoid material, these complications may be extremely difficult to detect. However, CT does provide an indication of the most appropriate cysts to aspirate percutaneously.

Von Hippel–Lindau disease

Renal cysts and neoplasms (carcinomas and adenomas) are frequently seen in patients with von Hippel–Lindau disease [19,20]. Screening for the development of renal neoplasms is best performed with CT [19,20] as the renal carcinomas may be small, less than 2 cm in size, and can even occur within the cysts [19,20].

On MRI, simple cyst fluid has a long T_1 and T_2 relaxation time (Fig. 5.1). They are thus seen as localized and clearly delineated, rounded structures of low signal intensity on T_1-weighted and high signal intensity on T_2-weighted images. Cysts do not enhance after administration of gadolinium DTPA. Cysts complicated by haemorrhage or infection will have a variable appearance depending on the precise nature of their contents.

Renal neoplasms

Staging renal cell carcinomas

On CT, a renal cell carcinoma is seen as a mass of density similar to that of the surrounding renal parenchyma on unenhanced scans. Injection of intravenous contrast medium leads to inhomogeneous enhancement of these tumours, which usually remain of lower attenuation than the surrounding cortex (Figs 5.2 and 5.3). The interface between the tumour and normal renal tissue is typically indistinct. Evaluation of the patency of the renal veins and inferior vena cava requires intravenous administration of contrast medium (see Figs 5.2 and 5.3). On MRI, a renal carcinoma is typically inhomogeneous in signal intensity (see Fig. 5.3). MRI offers particular advantages in the evaluation of renal venous and inferior vena caval patency for which intravenous contrast medium is not required.

Over the past decade, CT has become the most widely used imaging technique for staging renal cell carcinomas. Incremental dynamic or spiral scans after intravenous injection of a bolus of contrast medium are required. Ultrasound is also used to stage the renal carcinoma and has some advantages over CT in staging, such as the detection of tumour extension into the suprahepatic inferior cava and right atrium, and the demonstration of the relationship of tumour in the right upper pole of the kidney to the liver. However, in a high proportion of cases overlying bowel gas precludes adequate US visualization of the renal vessels, the infrahepatic inferior cava and the retroperitoneum [21,22]. Ultrasound is also inferior to CT for detecting muscle invasion [23]. Increasingly, MRI is proving to be a valuable method for staging renal carcinomas and seems to be at least as accurate as CT for staging [24,25].

Two systems for clinical staging of renal carcinomas are in use, the Robson and TNM classification of the International Union Against Cancer (UICC). The Robson classification is widely used in the UK and is referred to in this text.

The overall accuracy rate for CT in staging renal cell carcinomas varies between 72 and 91% [26,27]. Recent reports record an overall accuracy for MRI of between 80 and 96% [24,25].

Both CT and MRI can distinguish between the normal perirenal fascia and fat. Nevertheless, early perinephric extension of tumour remains extremely difficult to detect and although both CT and MRI are superior to ultrasound, failure to distinguish between stage I and II accounts for more than 50% of staging errors [27,28] and neither

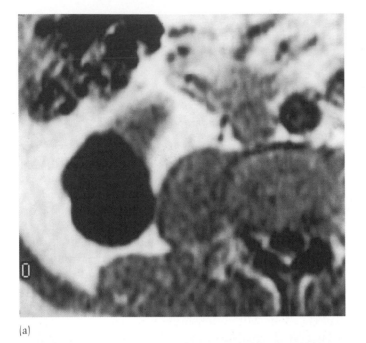

(a)

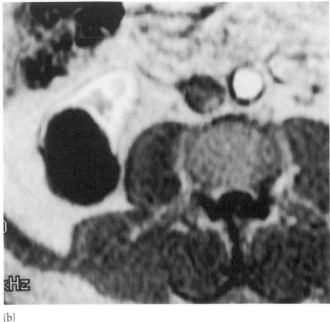

(b)

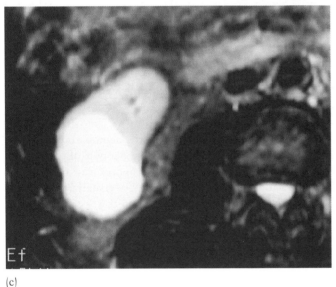

(c)

Fig. 5.1 MRI of a benign renal cyst. (a) Spin-echo T_1-weighted sequence showing typical well-defined, uniform low signal intensity of benign cyst. (b) T_1-weighted image after injection of gadolinium DTPA at the same level as (a), showing enhancement of the renal parenchyma but not of the renal cyst. (c) T_2-weighted sequence of the same cyst showing the typical appearance of its very high signal intensity contents.

technique is able to detect microinvasion through the renal capsule [25,27,28].

The accuracy of both CT and MRI for distinguishing between stage I and III is, however, extremely high. The sensitivity of CT in detecting invasion of the renal vein is about 80% and invasion of the inferior vena cava about 90% [26,27]. MRI has certain advantages over CT: (i) intravenous contrast medium is not required; (ii) the technique is not affected by respiration in assessing the veins; and (iii) the multiplanar imaging capability makes it superior to CT for imaging the full extent of thrombus in the inferior vena cava (see Fig. 5.3). Fewer false-positive results are recorded with MRI [25]. Close to 100% accuracy

has been reported for the detection of inferior vena cava thrombus [25] and 80% accuracy for detection of right atrial thrombus [29].

The recent development of spiral (helical) CT may greatly improve the accuracy of CT in staging renal cell carcinomas as all the data can be acquired on a single breath-hold and 3D reconstruction of the volume scanned is possible. However, the accuracy of this technique in detecting venous invasion is unlikely to exceed that of MRI.

Both CT and MRI rely on showing an increase in nodal size for the detection of lymph node infiltration, and neither can distinguish between enlarged hyperplastic

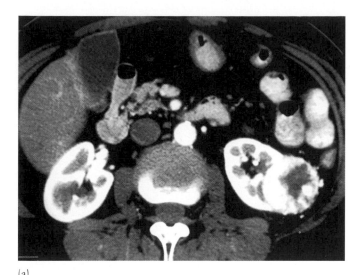

(a)

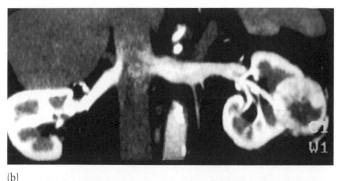

(b)

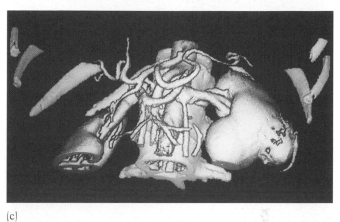

(c)

Fig. 5.2 Spiral (helical) CT of renal cell cancer. (a) Axial spiral CT scan following intravenous injection of contrast medium showing typical inhomogeneous enhancement of a large left renal cell carcinoma. (b) Coronal reconstruction showing the patency of the renal veins bilaterally. The contrast medium has not yet opacified the inferior vena cava. (c) 3D reconstruction in an oblique plane showing the left renal mass and the venous structures.

nodes and adenopathy [25,27]. Conversely, neither method detects normal-sized nodes infiltrated with neoplastic tissue. The sensitivity of CT in lymph node staging has been shown to be between 82 and 89% [26,27] and the results of MRI are similar [25,28].

Stage IV tumours are accurately diagnosed by both CT and MRI. Using strict criteria, direct invasion of adjacent organs is diagnosed with similar specificity and accuracy with both techniques [25,27,28], although 97–100% accuracy for visceral invasion using MRI has recently been reported [30], which is higher than has been achieved by CT. Disseminated haematogenous spread to the adrenal glands, bone and intrathoracic lymph nodes is well depicted by both CT and MRI [31], but spread to the lungs is more appropriately detected on CT.

CT has also proved useful for the detection of recurrent renal cell carcinomas [31] as the renal bed is extremely well demonstrated. Postoperative fibrosis seldom causes confusion on images obtained on modern scanners, and loops of bowel which fall into the renal fossa are opacified with contrast medium and easily distinguished from recurrent disease. The frequency of follow-up examinations will depend on the approach of the clinician, the stage of the initial lesion and on the likelihood of recurrence based on the completeness of resection.

Benign renal neoplasms

Angiomyolipoma (AML)

CT or MRI diagnosis of AML is dependent on the detection of fat within the tumour (Fig. 5.4). Most AMLs contain areas of fat detectable on CT or MRI, but rarely an AML contains no macroscopic areas of fat and is indistinguishable from a renal cell carcinoma [32]. Vascular and smooth muscle components of the tumour have the same density as soft tissue and haemorrhage may also be detected in tumours that have bled. Massive haemorrhage from an AML may obscure the presence of fatty elements and prevent an accurate CT or MRI diagnosis. Although MRI may also detect fat within an AML and so provide a definitive diagnosis [33,34], it has not been shown to have a better accuracy when compared with CT [32].

Oncocytoma

This is an extremely rare benign neoplasm. CT and MRI may suggest the possibility of an oncocytoma, but a definitive diagnosis requires surgery [31,35]. On CT, an oncocytoma often appears as a well-defined homogeneous solid mass, occasionally containing calcification [36]. Almost one-third of cases will exhibit a central scar, generally with a stellate configuration. Except for the scar,

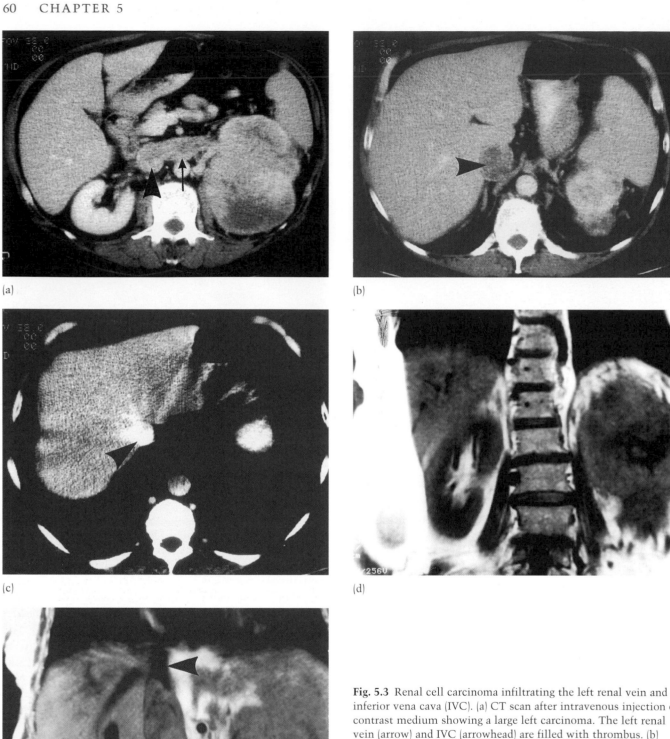

(a)

(b)

(c)

(d)

(e)

Fig. 5.3 Renal cell carcinoma infiltrating the left renal vein and inferior vena cava (IVC). (a) CT scan after intravenous injection of contrast medium showing a large left carcinoma. The left renal vein (arrow) and IVC (arrowhead) are filled with thrombus. (b) Axial scan taken slightly above (a) showing the IVC filled with thrombus (arrowhead). (c) Scan through the liver on the same patient showing the contrast-filled IVC (arrowhead) at the level of the middle hepatic vein. (d) T_1-weighted coronal MRI scan in the same patient showing the large left renal tumour. (e) T_1-weighted coronal MRI scan in a plane anterior to (d) showing the normal signal void in the patient's IVC (arrowheads). The low signal intensity of the thrombus can be seen to fill the left renal vein and the IVC to a level below the entrance of the hepatic vein into the IVC.

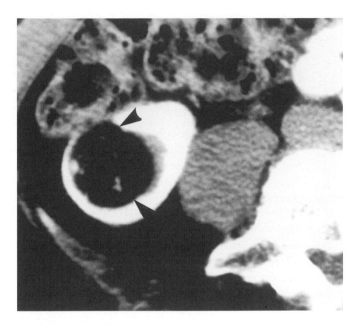

Fig. 5.4 A CT scan following intravenous injection of contrast medium, showing a large space-occupying lesion of very low density (arrowheads) equal to that of the surrounding perirenal fat. The appearance is characteristic of a benign AML.

the tumour often enhances uniformly after injection of intravenous contrast medium [37]. On MRI a homogeneous mass is seen [36] with the central scar appearing as an area of high intensity on T_2-weighted images and low signal intensity on T_1-weighted images [38]. Although, as in CT,

the scar is suggestive, it is not pathognomonic of an oncocytoma and a similar appearance can be seen in a MRI of a renal cell carcinoma [39].

Detection of small renal space-occupying lesions

The widespread use of CT and ultrasound has greatly increased the early detection and diagnosis of small renal tumours [40–43]. Both these imaging methods detect lesions that may not be shown by urography [42] and their high sensitivity results in the increased detection of benign lesions, particularly renal cysts, complicated or uncomplicated, and AMLs.

If a small renal mass is suspected, the CT scan has to be performed with great care, using thin sections (5 mm or thinner at 5 mm intervals) to characterize the lesion optimally. Size alone cannot be used as a reliable determinant of the nature of a renal tumour (Fig. 5.5). The traditional view that a renal tumour less than 3 cm in diameter is benign has not been supported by numerous reports of small renal neoplasms metastasizing and causing death, even though it has been well established that the number of metastasizing tumours increases with the size of the primary lesion [43,44]. If the attenuation values are less than 20–25 Hounsfield units and the mass is round, smooth and homogeneous, and does not enhance after injection of contrast medium, then it is considered a cyst [35]. If the lesion is shown to enhance after injection of contrast medium, a diagnosis of a solid tumour is established

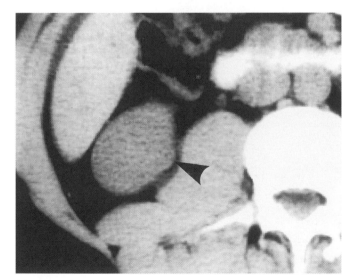

(a)

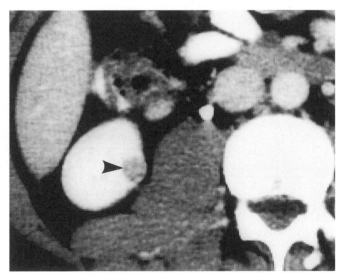

(b)

Fig. 5.5 A very small renal cell carcinoma. (a) CT scan without contrast medium showing a slight irregularity on the medial surface of the left kidney (arrowhead). (b) CT scan at the same level as (a) showing some enhancement of a small solid lesion after intravenous injection of contrast medium (arrowhead). This proved to be an 8 mm renal cell carcinoma.

[45,46]. In about 90% of cases such a solid tumour will be malignant [35]. However, specific efforts should always be made on CT to demonstrate small amounts of fat within the lesion as radiologically detectable fat is highly suggestive of an AML [47]. Exceptions have been documented including Wilms' tumour [48], teratoma and, exceptionally rarely, a renal adenocarcinoma [49]. Thus the probability that a renal mass with radiologically detectable fat represents anything other than an AML remains exceedingly low [50].

Needle aspiration or biopsy has a very limited role in the evaluation of these small lesions [35,51] as equivocal or even normal results are of no real value, especially as they can be difficult to target and thus there is a higher possibility of sampling error. In general, needle aspiration or biopsy has not proved to be very helpful [43,46]. Nevertheless, biopsy could be tried to help establish a diagnosis in a lesion that is highly suspicious for neoplasm, in order to justify surgery in poor surgical-risk patients [35].

Until recently, limitations to MRI have been considered to hamper its ability to detect and characterize small renal masses. However, recently developed approaches to MRI imaging (breath-hold imaging and fat suppression) appear to dramatically enhance the ability of MRI to depict renal mass lesions [52]. In the study reported by Semelka *et al.* [52] MRI and CT were shown to be comparable in the detection and characterization of small cysts and small renal tumours (<2 cm). Despite these encouraging results, further larger studies are necessary before MRI can be considered as reliable as CT in the detection and evaluation of small renal masses [1].

Evaluating the lucent pelvic filling defect

Calculi

CT plays a major part in the differential diagnosis of non-opaque pelvicalyceal filling defects. CT has the advantage of far greater contrast resolution or density discrimination than plain radiography and can distinguish calculi from other non-opaque filling defects in almost every instance [53,54]. Tumours of all types will have soft tissue attenuation values (30–50 Hounsfield units) and although blood clots may have a higher density than unopacified urine or renal parenchyma their density does not approach that of urinary tract calculi [54–56] (Fig. 5.6). All reported non-opaque urinary calculi examined by CT have been of high density [54–56]. The increased attenuation of non-opaque calculi is directly related to the increased density of the calculus [57] and does not indicate calcium content [56]. Differentiation among calculi of various compositions has been attempted by CT but has not proved reliable because the CT densities of different calculi overlap [56,58,59].

Transitional cell tumours

Most commonly, tumours appear as sessile intraluminal

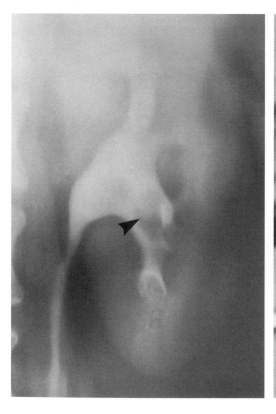
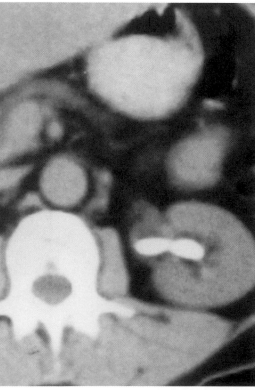

Fig. 5.6 Lucent calculus. (a) IVU showing a filling defect in the left renal pelvis (arrowhead). The plain film showed no evidence of a radio-opaque calculus. (b) Axial non-contrast CT scan through the level of the left renal pelvis showing a dense calculus.

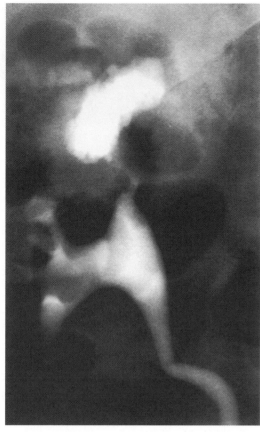

(a)

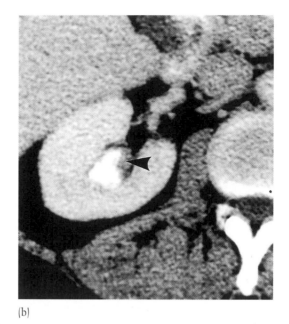

(b)

Fig. 5.7 Transitional cell tumour. (a) IVU showing narrowing of the right upper pole infundibulum and dilatation of the upper pole calyx. The margins of the calyx are irregular. (b) Post-contrast CT scan through the level of the dilated calyx showing a small sessile tumour with irregular margins (arrowhead).

masses [60] (Fig. 5.7). Other patterns include concentric or eccentric ureteral (or pelvic) wall thickening and least commonly a large infiltrating renal mass.

When presenting as a sessile filling defect, the tumour is usually sufficiently different from other causes of pelvicalyceal filling defects to allow diagnosis [61]. The frequent local effects of the urothelial tumour are easily recognized on CT, such as infundibular stenosis resulting in calyceal dilatation, and focal or diffuse non-filling of the pelvicalyceal system [62]. The more invasive pattern of transitional cell carcinomas may mimic a renal cell carcinoma but a renal cell carcinoma is usually hypervascular, whereas a transitional cell carcinoma is hypovascular and shows less enhancement after intravenous injection of contrast medium. Also, transitional cell carcinomas are typically centrally located, expand centrifugally and invade the renal parenchyma preserving the renal contour, whereas renal cell carcinomas tend to be eccentric and distort the renal outline [63].

CT can help to stage the transitional cell carcinoma [64], particularly in the advanced stages of the disease, but cannot differentiate between tumours limited to the urothelial mucosa and invasion of the muscle wall [20].

To date MRI has not been used frequently in the diagnosis and management of transitional cell tumours as the detection of tumour is far better accomplished with other techniques. On T_1-weighted images, the tumour has similar or slightly lower signal intensity than normal renal parenchyma. T_2-weighted images show a slight increase in signal intensity [65]. As in renal cell carcinomas, MRI is useful for detecting vascular invasion [66].

Inflammatory disease of the kidney

Uncomplicated acute pyelonephritis in the adult generally does not require any imaging. CT may, however, be required in patients who fail to respond to antibiotics, or when surgical or percutaneous intervention is being considered to drain a superimposed abscess and ultrasound has failed to yield sufficient information [67]. Ultrasound has been shown to be less sensitive than CT in the demonstration of renal and perirenal inflammatory pathology [68–71].

Acute pyelonephritis

With severe infection there may be generalized or focal swelling of the kidneys. On the precontrast scan, there may be, in a small percentage of patients, areas of increased parenchymal density. On the post-contrast scans one or more well-defined wedge-shaped or streaky areas of low density, are seen within the renal parenchyma [67,69,72]. These hypodense zones are thought to be due to a combination of focal ischaemia, obstructed tubules and interstitial inflammation [72].

Intrarenal and perirenal abscess

CT is accurate in the detection, localization and delineation of the extent of intrarenal abscesses and also in the demonstration of perinephric and paranephric extension [67,69]. Typically, an abscess on CT will be seen as an area of low attenuation that does not meet the criteria for a simple cyst and the centre of which does not enhance after intravenous injection of contrast medium. Most commonly, in over 85% of cases, there is abnormal enhancement of the surrounding inflamed parenchyma and inflammatory changes in the perirenal fat [69,73]. The wall will usually be thickened and irregular. Rarely, an abscess will resemble a simple cyst but with the fluid content having a CT number higher than that of water. Thickening of Gerota's and/or the lateroconal fascia, and extension of the inflammation into one of the pararenal spaces [67,69], is frequently seen (Fig. 5.8). A renal abscess may rupture into the perirenal and pararenal spaces and will occasionally extend through the transversalis fascia into the flank (Fig. 5.9).

MRI has been used infrequently to demonstrate renal abscesses and shows a hypointense inhomogeneous pattern on T_1-weighted images with a similarly inhomogeneous but increased intensity pattern on T_2-weighted images [74,75].

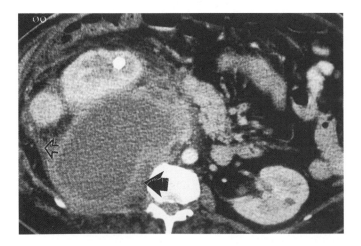

Fig. 5.8 Perirenal abscess. A CT scan showing a large fluid-filled, thick-walled perirenal abscess infiltrating the right psoas muscle (arrow). A calculus can be seen within the collecting system causing collecting system dilatation and there is thickening of Gerota's fascia (open arrow).

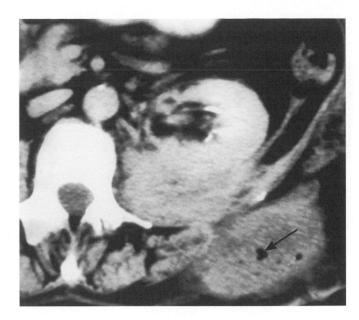

Fig. 5.9 A CT scan showing the extension of a left perirenal abscess through the posterior abdominal wall into the subcutaneous fat. Pockets of air are seen within the subcutaneous component of the abscess (arrow).

Pyonephrosis and xanthogranulomatous pyelonephritis

Both CT and US are accurate methods for demonstrating pyonephrosis [76–78]. The findings on non-contrast-enhanced CT include a dilated collecting system filling with fluid (usually with Hounsfield units slightly above water), debris and sometimes a fluid–debris level [67,78]. MRI will also show low signal intensity dilated calyces on T_1-weighted images and a corresponding high signal intensity on T_2-weighted images [67]. Unfortunately, on both CT and MRI, the appearances may be indistinguishable from other causes of collecting system dilatation.

CT is recommended in cases of xanthogranulomatous pyelonephritis suspected on IVU or ultrasound because of its ability to demonstrate perinephric and paranephric extension accurately [79,80]. The usual CT appearances of diffuse xanthogranulomatous pyelonephritis include: (i) a large central calculus occupying most of the renal pelvis; (ii) poor excretion of contrast medium; (iii) multiple, non-enhancing rounded areas within the renal contours with attenuation values slightly lower than that of urine, corresponding to dilated calyces; and (iv) frequent perinephric involvement [79–81] (Fig. 5.10). Focal involvement (tumefactive xanthogranulomatous pyelonephritis) may also occur.

MRI of xanthogranulomatous pyelonephritis will also show the dilated calyces, abscesses and perinephric involvement [74,82] but has the disadvantage of not showing the obstructing calculus or the parenchymal calcification [67].

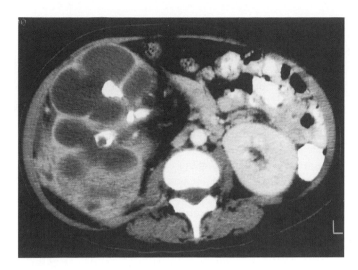

Fig. 5.10 Xanthogranulomatous pyelonephritis. A post-contrast CT scan showing a large central calculus occupying a contracted right renal pelvis, multiple non-enhancing low-density rounded areas corresponding to dilated calyces, marked parenchymal thinning and extension of the perinephric space posteriorly. This appearance is characteristic of xanthogranulomatous pyelonephritis.

Renal trauma

There are several advantages to the use of CT for evaluating renal trauma: (i) it is more sensitive, specific and accurate than urography or angiography in defining the extent of renal injuries [83,84]; (ii) associated abdominal injuries, particularly hepatic, splenic and retroperitoneal are optimally displayed; and (iii) any underlying renal abnormality can be shown. CT is frequently employed as the initial diagnostic study, especially in large trauma centres, where multiple-system injuries are common [85]. In patients with suspected isolated renal trauma, who are clinically stable, an IVU may be all that is required for management.

CT can demonstrate a wide spectrum of renal damage from minor injuries through to the effects of severe renal trauma. The recent introduction of spiral (helical) CT has several advantages. It allows substantially shorter scanning times (on occasions requiring only 30 s), better demonstration of the renal vessels, and will allow the use of smaller amounts of intravenous contrast medium.

CT is very helpful in the detection of pre-existing congenital or acquired renal abnormalities which predispose to renal injury even when the trauma is relatively mild.

The restrictive environment of most MRI units precludes a significant role in the seriously injured patient.

CT appearances

Renal contusion, haemorrhage and infarction. Renal contusion causes delayed excretion of contrast medium. This is thought to be due to a delayed tubular transit secondary to oedema and may be segmental or global. A haematoma appears on CT as a focal area of high density relative to the renal parenchyma which does not enhance after intravenous administration of contrast medium and is poorly marginated. Infarction due to occlusion of intrarenal vessels produces a sharply marginated, wedge-shaped area of non-enhancement of the renal parenchyma after intravenous contrast medium injection.

Subcapsular haematoma. Haemorrhage confined by the renal capsule often has a lenticular shape on CT, results in flattening of the kidney and separation from Gerota's fascia by fat. When acute, a haematoma is of high density and subsequently the density decreases with time.

Laceration and fractures. Corticomedullary lacerations with or without communication with the collecting system are readily shown on CT. CT is extremely sensitive in detecting urine extravasation. A fracture is seen as transection of the kidney with urine extravasation and haemorrhage.

Renal artery occlusion and avulsion. Renal artery occlusion resulting from acceleration and deceleration injuries leading to subintimal dissection and thrombosis causes an absent nephrogram on contrast-enhanced CT. Collateral circulation contributes to a 'cortical rim' of enhancing parenchyma (Fig. 5.11). Avulsion of the renal

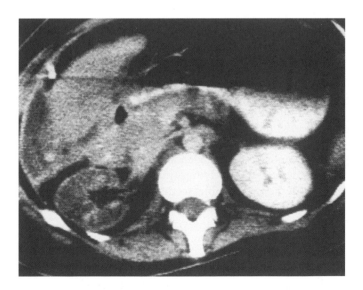

Fig. 5.11 Post-traumatic renal artery occlusion. A post-contrast CT scan showing a normal nephrogram of the left kidney. The right kidney shows a typical 'rim nephrogram' due to renal artery occlusion in which a collateral circulation contributes to a rim of enhancing parenchyma while much of the parenchyma remains unenhanced.

artery shows a similar rim nephrogram and a large, dense perirenal haematoma.

Renal failure, obstruction and the retroperitoneum

Ultrasound is highly sensitive in detecting collecting system dilatation and for identifying obstruction as a cause of renal failure. It is now extremely unusual for ultrasound to fail to demonstrate the kidneys adequately for technical reasons such as obesity. However, in those rare instances in which ultrasound, for technical reasons fails to exclude collecting system dilatation, CT has a part to play. Non-enhanced CT scans show the dilated collecting system and ureters as low-density structures with attenuation values approximating that of water. After intravenous injection of, the dilated collecting system opacifies. Potential pitfalls in the ultrasound diagnosis of hydronephrosis, such as the presence of parapelvic cysts or large calculi, are readily identified on CT. CT will detect pelvicalyceal dilatation with a reported accuracy close to 100% [53].

Ultrasound is often not effective in identifying the cause of ureteric obstruction as the retroperitoneum is obscured by bowel gas, and CT or MRI are then indicated to demonstrate the site and aetiology of ureteric obstruction [1]. Contrast-enhanced CT should be avoided when a ureteric calculus is suspected as it may otherwise be obscured. However, contrast enhancement is useful for the detection of tumours because the normal ureteral wall is often be more readily visualized. Delayed scans (30–60 min or more after injection) to allow filling of the obstructed ureter often allows a clearer definition of the site of obstruction.

As in the renal pelvis, CT is extremely valuable in demonstrating 'lucent' calculi in the ureter and distinguishing them from ureteric urothelial tumours as a cause of obstruction. CT is useful for staging ureteric tumours as it can distinguish localized from advanced disease with more than 95% accuracy [86].

Both MRI and CT are well suited to the demonstration of retroperitoneal causes of extrinsic ureteric obstruction, most commonly lymphadenopathy. As both techniques rely on demonstrating lymph node enlargement to detect pathology, neither is able to distinguish between benign and malignant disease, and their accuracies are comparable [87–90]. The main advantages of MRI are its ability to display vascular anatomy without the need for intravenous contrast medium and its superior soft tissue contrast resolution. However, MRI also has several significant limitations when compared with CT, the most important being the current absence of an optimal MRI oral contrast medium so that differentiating lymph nodes from bowel loops may be difficult. In general, too, MRI at present is still more expensive and less readily available than CT. CT has the important advantage of allowing image-guided percutaneous biopsy. Thus contrast-enhanced CT remains the procedure of choice for the initial evaluation of the retroperitoneum [20,53].

Both CT and MRI have been shown to be extremely accurate in demonstrating idiopathic retroperitoneal fibrosis [91,92]. The CT findings are non-specific but are often suggestive of the diagnosis. A fibrous sheet or a bulky mass envelopes the aorta, the inferior vena cava, the iliac vessels and the ureter, without significant displacement of these structures. The process rarely extends cephalad to the renal vessels and may be localized to the pelvis. The size of the mass may depend on the stage of the disease and CT has been shown to be an effective method of monitoring the evolution of the disease with or without steroid treatment [93]. The periaortic mass is also readily identified on MRI and the ability to demonstrate patent vascular structures without administration of contrast medium facilitates the identification of even quite small masses, often difficult to identify on CT (Fig. 5.12). It has been proposed that MRI may be of value in distinguishing between malignancy and retroperitoneal fibrosis by identifying areas of proton-deficient fibrosis [91,94]. However, this has not been substantiated in a sufficiently large series and all patients with periaortic masses require biopsy.

CT remains the imaging method of choice for the demonstration of other retroperitoneal causes of extrinsic ureteric obstruction, whether inflammatory such as Crohn's disease or a psoas abscess or primary neoplastic causes such as liposarcoma or leiomyosarcoma, as experience with MRI in these conditions is still limited [20,53].

Staging bladder cancer

Several factors which influence the prognosis of patients with bladder cancer may be assessed by imaging techniques. These include tumour size, growth pattern, depth of bladder wall infiltration and the presence of metastases in lymph nodes and distant blood-borne sites. Today the imaging methods most frequently employed to stage the primary tumour are CT and MRI.

Primary tumour staging

Cystoscopic evaluation, which forms the basis of clinical staging, is highly accurate in the assessment of superficial non-invasive lesions because the tumour can be completely resected and the depth of penetration of the bladder wall examined pathologically. However, in patients with more advanced disease, clinical staging is subject to error and inaccuracies may be as high as 50% [95,96]. Understaging is more common than overstaging and in one series 40% of patients were understaged whereas overstaging only accounted for 20% of errors [97]. Such errors in estimating

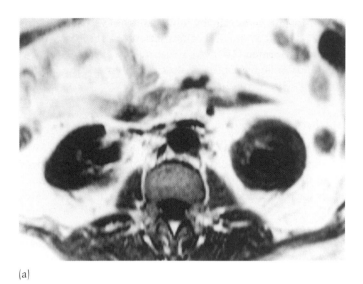

(a)

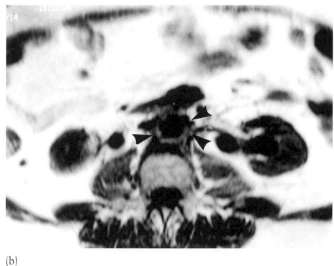

(b)

(c)

Fig. 5.12 MRI of retroperitoneal fibrosis. (a) T_1-weighted MRI showing bilateral fluid of low signal within the dilated collecting system. The normal signal void is seen in the aorta. (b) T_1-weighted scan in the same patient at a level below (a) showing a rim of soft tissue of low signal intensity surrounding the aorta (arrowheads). (c) T_2-weighted scan at the same level as (a) showing a high signal intensity of fluid in the dilated collecting system. The periaortic fibrosis is also of low signal intensity (arrowheads).

the extent of invasive disease make decisions on management difficult, and for this reason imaging has assumed a key role in staging the primary tumour.

Computed tomography

CT is widely used for staging primary bladder tumours and for evaluating retroperitoneal and pelvic lymph nodes. During the 1980s several studies were undertaken comparing CT staging with pathological staging and with reported accuracies for CT ranging from 64 to 92% [98,99]. It was generally recognized that the major advantage of CT was the ability to distinguish tumours confined to the bladder wall (stage T3a or less) from those extending into the perivesical fat (T3b) and that the accuracy of CT increases with advancing disease. Although CT can demonstrate thickening of the bladder wall, the technique cannot distinguish the stage of superficial tumours and is,

therefore, an unreliable method for assessing T1, T2 and T3a lesions.

Advances in CT over recent years have included improvements in image quality and the development of fast scanning techniques. Together with the routine use of intravenous contrast medium these advances have rendered CT a highly accurate method of delineating invasive tumours (Fig. 5.13). However, even using current CT technology, there are significant drawbacks to the technique, mainly due to lack of tissue characterization and to the limitations of spatial resolution. For example, several studies have included patients who have been previously treated with radiotherapy in whom fibrosis of the bladder wall is indistinguishable from the tumour [98,100]. This leads to errors of overstaging. Understaging usually results from the inability to detect microscopic or minimal perivesical tumour extension and from the inability to diagnose early organ invasion. These limitations

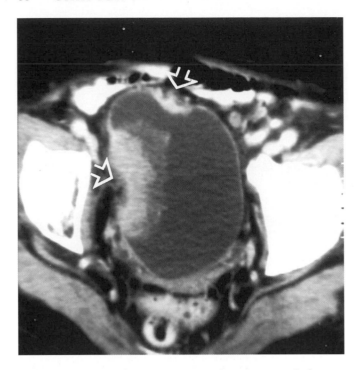

Fig. 5.13 A CT scan showing extravesical tumour spread of bladder cancer (arrow). The tumour shows marked enhancement following the injection of intravenous contrast medium.

may in part be overcome by new scanning systems utilizing spiral technology since reconstruction of data in any plane can be performed [101]. At present, however, insufficient information is available to allow comment on the clinical value of such technological advances.

Magnetic resonance imaging

MRI is well suited to the evaluation of pelvic cancer. Most of the information on staging bladder cancer has been obtained using the body coil but recent developments such as dedicated surface coils are currently being evaluated [102]. Endorectal coils may also have a place in staging tumours at the bladder base but are unlikely to be of value in patients with advanced disease due to the limited field of view.

Bladder tumours are low signal lesions on T_1-weighted images and relatively high signal lesions on T_2-weighted images (Fig. 5.14). Both T_1- and T_2-weighted sequences are required for evaluating bladder cancer [103,104]. T_1-weighted images are needed for assessing perivesical tumour spread and T_2-weighted images are valuable for assessing the depth of penetration of the bladder wall [104]. Although new sequences are continually being introduced, the major goal of these developments is to reduce scanning

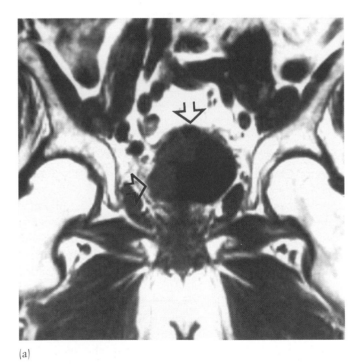

(a)

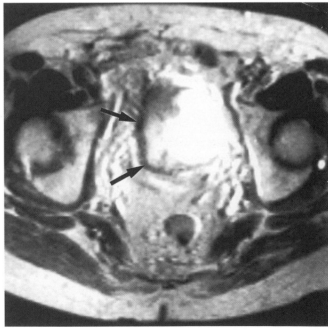

(b)

Fig. 5.14 MRI scan of bladder cancer. (a) T_1-weighted image in the coronal plane showing a right-sided bladder tumour as a relatively low signal intensity (SI) (arrow) mass. Note the extravesical spread on the right. (b) T_2-weighted image in the same patient showing the tumour as a mass of intermediate SI. The bladder wall has a low SI (arrow) and the urine has a high SI.

times and the basic concept of providing images with T_1 and T_2 information remains unchanged. Other sequences such as fat/water-suppression techniques may prove useful for evaluating tumours in certain situations and the use of intravenous contrast medium is also being investigated. Two recent studies suggest that contrast enhancement of bladder tumours may be particularly helpful for staging early lesions [105,106]. This is because the tumour enhances to a greater degree than muscle. This permits the detection of muscular invasion because the low signal wall is interrupted by enhancing tumour. Contrast enhancement may also be helpful for detecting early organ invasion, but at present there is insufficient information to confirm this observation.

Comparison of MRI and CT

Comparison of MRI with CT shows that MRI has several major advantages over CT. T_2-weighted sequences and contrast-enhanced T_1-weighted sequences are superior to CT for staging early lesions confined to the bladder. MRI has a staging accuracy of 69–89% (mean 85%) which is significantly better than CT [107].

Images in the sagittal and coronal plane may demonstrate tumour spread beyond the bladder which cannot be readily appreciated in the transaxial plane on CT. This will probably be best demonstrated in patients with lesions at the bladder base or dome when partial volume averaging on CT may make interpretation difficult. The inherent superior contrast resolution of MRI may also facilitate the diagnosis of adjacent organ invasion.

Over recent years major studies have been reported comparing the accuracy of MRI with CT in the same patients. The overall accuracy of MRI ranges from 72 to 96% which is a similar range to that reported for CT [103–105]. However, in several studies in which both CT and MRI have been carried out on the same patients, the advantages of MRI can be readily appreciated. Furthermore, in the early studies few patients with superficial lesions were included which tended to mask the advantages of MRI.

Despite the superior contrast resolution of MRI compared with CT and its multiplanar capability, MRI has important limitations in the assessment of bladder cancer. As with CT, a major constraint relates to tissue characterization. Thus, at present, it seems unlikely that oedema and fibrosis can be reliably distinguished from tumour within the bladder wall and errors of overstaging are therefore likely to remain [108]. Understaging of microscopic disease also persists due to the constraints of spatial resolution inherent in all imaging systems.

As MRI and CT continue to develop during the 1990s both techniques are likely to be used effectively for evaluation of patients with bladder cancer and the technique of choice will depend upon local preferences and the availability of scanner time.

Staging prostate cancer

Although diagnostic imaging has a part to play in the diagnosis of prostate cancer, its most important application is for staging proven disease. Abdominal and transrectal ultrasound (TRUS), CT and MRI have all been vigorously studied during recent years and it is now clear that MRI and TRUS are superior to CT.

The normal prostate is elegantly demonstrated with MRI (Fig. 5.15). The inner prostate, which is a combination of the smooth muscle of the internal sphincter, periurethral glandular tissue, verumontanum and the transitional zone is seen on MRI as a central portion of relatively low signal on T_2-weighted images. The outer zone of the prostate is composed entirely of glandular tissue and comprises the central and peripheral zones. On T_2 weighting the peripheral zone has a high signal whereas the central zone and inner prostate have a lower signal intensity. The fibromuscular stroma anteriorly has a uniformly low signal. On T_1 weighting, the zonal anatomy of the prostate cannot be appreciated and the whole gland returns a homogeneous low signal. Zonal anatomy with imaging correlates well with the site of origin of benign and malignant disease. Benign prostatic hypertrophy, which exclusively develops from the transition zone, is well demonstrated on MRI and the characteristic appearance with whirls and nodules in the central gland is readily appreciated [109] (Fig. 5.16).

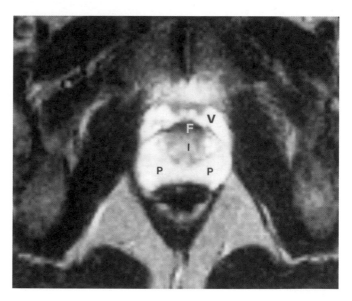

Fig. 5.15 MRI scan showing a normal prostate on a T_2-weighted image. F, anterior fibromuscular band; I, inner prostate; P, peripheral zone; V, periprostatic venous plexus.

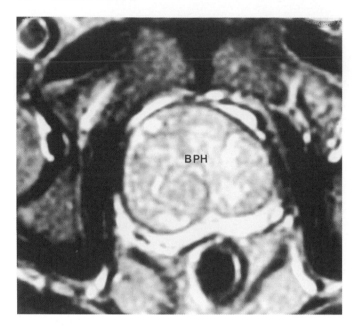

Fig. 5.16 MRI scan showing benign prostatic hypertrophy (BPH) on a T_2-weighted image. The enlarged inner prostate shows the characteristic features of benign prostatic hypertrophy.

Since the majority of carcinomas arise in the peripheral zone, these may also be well shown on MRI as low signal lesions which contrast to the high signal of the normal peripheral gland on T_2 weighting [110] (Fig. 5.17). However, not all low signal lesions within the peripheral zone are tumours and tumours may also develop within the central

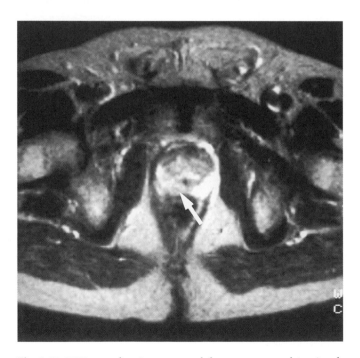

Fig. 5.17 MRI scan showing cancer of the prostate as a low signal intensity lesion in the peripheral zone on a T_2-weighted image (arrow).

zone, which are difficult to identify due to the low signal of this portion of the prostate.

Both T_1- and T_2-weighted images should be obtained for staging prostatic cancer. As in bladder cancer, the T_1-weighted images are most useful for demonstrating spread beyond the prostatic capsule into the periprostatic fat or adjacent structures because tumour has a low signal compared to the high signal of periprostatic fat. T_2-weighted images are valuable for determining the extent of the tumour within the gland as well as assessing the integrity of the venous plexus surrounding the prostate. Intravenous contrast medium (gadolinium DTPA) has not been widely used yet in the investigation of prostatic cancer, but a recent study demonstrated that contrast enhancement using a dynamic scanning technique improves the definition of the extent of disease compared with conventional images in 50% of cases [111] (Fig. 5.18). Contrast enhancement may also be valuable for assessing adjacent organ invasion such as involvement of the seminal vesicles.

Although axial scans are usually obtained initially, sagittal scans may be helpful for diagnosing bladder or rectal invasion and may also be helpful for confirming seminal vesicle involvement. Coronal scans are seldom useful unless volume measurements of the gland are required.

In the early days of clinical MRI excellent results for staging prostatic cancer were reported with accuracy rates between 80 and 90% [110,112,113]. However, as more experience was gained and larger numbers of patients studied, the results of MRI were less impressive. The largest series to date is a multicentre study of 230 patients in whom both MRI and TRUS were compared [113]. MRI examinations were carried out using a body coil, but even so the results of this study demonstrated that MRI was superior to TRUS in the evaluation of both localized and advanced disease, with an overall accuracy for MRI of 69% compared with 59% for TRUS. MRI was, not surprisingly, more accurate in patients with advanced disease with an accuracy of 77% compared with an accuracy of 57% in patients with localized tumours. Although the results of this study are disappointing when compared with earlier results, the patients entered into the study were all considered to have early surgically resectable disease, thus tending to bias the results towards a reduction in accuracy compared with earlier studies in which patients with gross disease were included. It should also be borne in mind that both MRI and TRUS are considerably more accurate than clinical examination alone and both techniques are therefore a useful adjunct to tumour staging.

The introduction of endorectal surface coils are likely to have a major role in tumour staging of prostatic cancer. The main advantage of the endorectal coil is an improvement in the signal 1:1 noise ratio and improved spatial resolution.

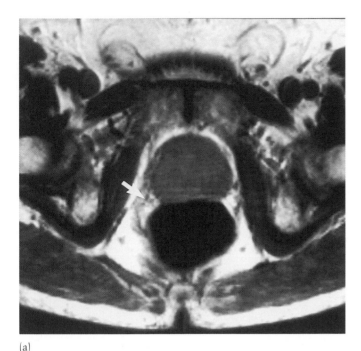

(a)

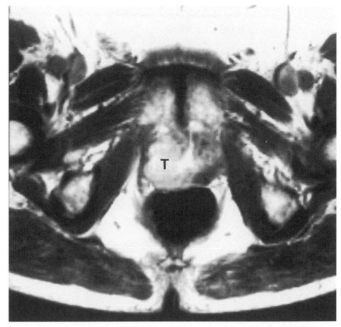

(b)

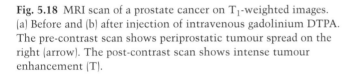

Fig. 5.18 MRI scan of a prostate cancer on T_1-weighted images. (a) Before and (b) after injection of intravenous gadolinium DTPA. The pre-contrast scan shows periprostatic tumour spread on the right (arrow). The post-contrast scan shows intense tumour enhancement (T).

However, the field of view is limited and although good views of the prostate gland and seminal vesicles are obtained, lymph nodes of the pelvis cannot be assessed. The improved demonstration of prostatic cancer and an increased accuracy of tumour staging of 16% was demonstrated by Schnall *et al.* in a recent study [114] in which the results of staging using an endorectal coil were compared with the use of a body coil.

CT scanning has little to offer in imaging primary prostate tumours because the internal anatomy of the gland cannot be appreciated and the fat plane around the prostate is difficult to delineate. At present, MRI and TRUS are the techniques of choice. To date, MRI appears to be superior to TRUS in staging and as MRI technology advances further it is likely to have an increasingly prominent role in the evaluation of these patients. A further advantage of MRI compared with TRUS is the ability to assess lymph node status at the same examination.

Other aspects of bladder and prostate cancer

Lymph node evaluation

Over the last decade lymphography has been superseded by CT and MRI for staging pelvic lymph node metastases.

However, these techniques can only demonstrate a metastasis if the lymph node is enlarged and benign causes of enlargement cannot be distinguished from tumours. Despite such limitations, CT and MRI have been shown to be as effective as lymphography in the demonstration of metastatic disease in patients with prostate and bladder cancer with accuracy rates ranging from 70 to 90% [103,115–117]. Although guidelines for the upper limit of normal and pelvic lymph nodes have been suggested, these have been arbitrary and have varied from 1 to 1.5 cm in the short axis diameter. Recently, we have drawn up new guidelines for the measurement of normal nodes within the pelvis (external iliac: 9 mm; obturator: 8 mm; internal iliac: 7 mm). These measurements are considerably less than criteria commonly adopted and the use of these new guidelines may help to reduce the high false-negative rates for staging lymph node disease [118].

On CT, enlarged lymph nodes appear as soft tissue structures which may show enhancement with intravenous contrast medium. On MRI, enlarged lymph nodes have similar signal characteristics to the primary tumour. Thus, on T_1 weighting, enlarged lymph nodes appear as low signal masses, whereas on T_2 weighting they appear as relatively high signal masses. The size criteria used to assess pelvic lymph nodes on CT should also be used for MRI and in most patients an enlarged lymph node can be demonstrated equally well by both techniques. However, on some occasions an enlarged lymph node may be better appreciated by MRI than CT due to the differences in signal characteristics between vessels and the tumour, and due to the ability to demonstrate enlarged nodes in the coronal plane as well as the axial plane.

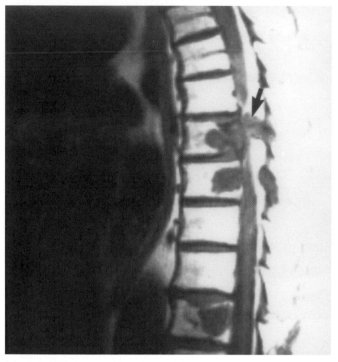

(a)

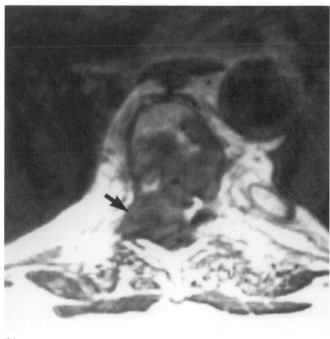

(b)

Fig. 5.19 (a) MRI scan in the sagittal plane of the lower thoracic and upper lumbar spine showing low signal intensity bone marrow metastases at the levels of T8, T9 and T12. The normal marrow has a high signal due to fat. (b) The deposit in T8 (arrow) has produced expansion of the vertebral body causing spinal cord compression.

Distant metastases

In general, CT and MRI are only used to detect distant metastases in patients with clinical features suggestive of tumour spread. It is beyond the scope of this text to review all the sites of distant metastases, but special reference is made to the demonstration of spinal metastatic disease in prostate cancer. Because of the propensity of prostate carcinoma to expand bone, spinal cord compression is common. This is elegantly demonstrated on MRI and the technique has important advantages over conventional myelography, which include the ability to demonstrate the extent of disease as well as the presence of multiple sites of compression [119] (Fig. 5.19).

Follow-up studies

Imaging continues to have a role in the assessment of bladder and prostate cancer following radical treatment, whether this is by surgery, radiotherapy, hormone therapy or chemotherapy. Such images are often difficult to interpret due to the effect of the treatment, such as radiotherapy on normal and abnormal tissue, and the presence of scar tissue following surgery. The most

pertinent clinical question posed is whether the technique can distinguish recurrent tumours from fibrosis induced by treatment. Such a distinction cannot be made reliably with CT on the basis of X-ray attenuation as both the tumour and fibrosis have similar values.

In the early days of MRI it was hoped that tumours could be reliably distinguished from fibrosis because fibrosis returns a low signal intensity on T_2-weighted images compared with a tumour which returns a relatively high signal. A gross tumour may be recognized but identification of small areas of recurrent disease within an area of fibrosis is impossible.

Localization of undescended testis

Several small series have suggested that both CT and MRI are sensitive techniques for the preoperative localization of low undescended testis [120,121]. Studies in the use of CT have shown close to 100% accuracy in the localization of impalpable testes, and similar levels of accuracy with MRI using standard spin-echo sequences have been achieved [120,121]. The multiplanar imaging capability and improved contrast resolution of MRI may, however, provide distinct advantages over CT. Neither technique has proved reliable in the identification of high or intra-abdominal testes.

References

1 Dunnick NR. Renal lesions. Great strides in imaging. *Radiology* 1992;**182**:305–6.

2 Hartman DS, Aronson S, Frazer H. Current status of imaging indeterminate renal masses. *Radiol Clin North Am* 1991;**23**:475–96.

3 Pollack HM, Banner MP, Arger PH *et al.* The accuracy of gray-scale renal ultrasonography in differentiating cystic neoplasms from benign cysts. *Radiology* 1982;**143**:741–5.

4 Amis ES, Cronan JJ, Yoder IC *et al.* Renal cysts: curios and caveats. *Urol Radiol* 1982;**4**:199–209.

5 Patterson J, Lohr D, Briscoe P *et al.* Calcified renal masses. *Urology* 1987;**39**:353–6.

6 Balfe DM, McClennan BL, Stanley RJ *et al.* Evaluation of renal masses considered indeterminate on computed tomography. *Radiology* 1982;**142**:421–8.

7 Bosniak MA. The current radiological approach to renal cysts. *Radiology* 1986;**158**:1–10.

8 Curry NS, Reinig J, Schabel SI *et al.* An evaluation of the effectiveness of CT vs other imaging modalities in the diagnosis of atypical renal masses. *Invest Radiol* 1984;**19**: 447–52.

9 Love L, Yedlicka J. Computed tomography of internally calcified renal cysts. *Am J Roentgenol* 1985;**145**:1225–7.

10 Rosenberg ER, Korobkin M, Foster W *et al.* The significance of septations in a renal cyst. *Am J Roentgenol* 1985;**144**:593–5.

11 Hartman DS, Davis CJ, Sanders RC *et al.* The multiloculated renal mass: considerations and differential features. *Radiographics* 1987;**7**:29–52.

12 Levine E, Huntrakoon M. Unilateral renal cystic disease: CT findings. *J Comput Assist Tomogr* 1989;**13**:273–6.

13 Grantham JS, Levine E. Acquired cystic disease: replacing one kidney disease with another. *Kidney Int* 1985;**28**:99–105.

14 Jabour BA, Ralls PW, Tang WW *et al.* Acquired cystic disease of the kidneys; computed tomography and ultrasonography in appraisal in patients on peritoneal and haemodialysis. *Invest Radiol* 1987;**22**:728–32.

15 Ishikawa I, Saito Y, Shikura N *et al.* Ten year prospective study on the development of renal cell carcinoma in dialysis patients. *Am J Kidney Dis* 1990;**16**:452–8.

16 Matson MA, Cohen EP. Acquired cystic disease: occurrence, prevalence and renal cancers. *Medicine* 1990;**611**:217–26.

17 Levine E, Shisher SL, Grantham JJ, Wetzel LH. Natural history of acquired renal cystic disease in dialysis patients: a prospective longitudinal CT study. *Am J Roentgenol* 1991;**156**:501-6.

18 Dunnick NR. Renal cystic disease. In: Husband JES, ed. *CT Review*. Edinburgh: Churchill Livingstone, 1989;123–35.

19 Levine E, Colins DL, Horton WA, Schmenke RN. CT screening of the abdomen in von Hippel–Lindau disease. *Am J Roentgenol* 1982;**139**:505–10.

20 McClennan BL, Rabin DN. Kidney. In: Lee JKT, Sagel SS, Stanley RJ, eds. *Computed Body Tomography with MRI Correlation*, 2nd edn. New York: Raven Press, 1989: 755–849.

21 Webb JAW, Murray A, Bary PR, Hendry WF. The accuracy and limitation of ultrasound in the assessment of venous extension in renal carcinoma. *Br J Urol* 1987;**60**:14–17.

22 Levine E, Maklad NF, Rosenthal SJ, Lee KR, Weigel J. Comparison of computed tomography and ultrasound in abdominal staging of renal cancer. *Urology* 1980;**16**:317–22.

23 Cronan JJ, Zeman RK, Rosenfeld AT. Comparison of computerized tomography, ultrasound and angiography in staging renal cell carcinoma. *J Urol* 1982;**127**:712–14.

24 Kabala JE, Penry B, Chadwick D. Magnetic resonance imaging of renal masses. *Br J Radiol* 1990;**63**:15.

25 Hricak H, Thoeni RF, Carroll PR *et al.* Detection and staging of renal neoplasm. A measurement of MR imaging. *Radiology* 1988;**166**:643–9.

26 London NM, Messios N, Kinder RB *et al.* A prospective study of the value of conventional CT, dynamic CT, ultrasonography and arteriography for staging renal cell carcinoma. *Br J Urol* 1989;**64**:209–17.

27 Johnson CD, Dunnick NR, Cohan RC, Illescas FF. Renal adenocarcinoma: CT staging of 100 tumors. *Am J Roentgenol* 1987;**148**:59–63.

28 Fein AB, Lee JKT, Balfe DM *et al.* Diagnosis and staging of renal cell carcinoma: a comparison of MR imaging and CT. *Am J Roentgenol* 1987;**148**:749.

29 Roubidoux MA, Dunnick NR, Sostman HD, Leder RA. Renal carcinoma. Detection of venous extension with gradient-echo MR imaging. *Radiology* 1992;**182**:269–72.

30 Kabala JE. Magnetic resonance imaging of renal cell carcinoma. *Clin MRI* 1992;**2**:9–11.

31 Birnbaum BA, Bosniak MA. CT and MRI of renal cell carcinoma. In: Goldman SM, Gatewood OMB, eds. *CT and MRI of the Genitourinary Tract in Contemporary Issues in Computed Tomography*. New York: Churchill Livingstone, 1990:25–42.

32 Williamson B. CT and MRI of benign renal neoplasms. In: Goldman SM, Gatewood OMB, eds. *CT and MRI of the Genitourinary Tract in Contemporary Issues in Computed Tomography*. New York: Churchill Livingstone, 1990:43–58.

33 Choyke PL, Kressel HY, Pollack HM *et al.* Focal renal masses: magnetic resonance imaging. *Radiology* 1984;**152**:471.

34 Newhouse JH, Markisz JA, Kazam E. Magnetic resonance of the kidneys. *Cardiovasc Intervent Radiol* 1989;**8**:351.

35 Bosniak MA. The small (≤3.0 cm) renal parenchymal tumor: detection, diagnosis and controversies. *Radiology* 1991;**179**: 307–17.

36 Sohn HK, Kim SY, Seo HS. MR imaging of a renal oncocytoma. *J Comput Assist Tomogr* 1987;**11**:6.

37 Quinn MJ, Hartman DS, Friedman AL. Renal oncocytoma: new observations. *Radiology* 1984;**153**:49.

38 Ronsinger MB, Kenney PJ, Morgan DE, Bernreuter WK, Litinsky JJ. Gadolinium-enhanced MR imaging of renal masses. *Radiographics* 1992;**12**:1097–16.

39 Ball DS, Friedman AC, Hartman DS *et al.* Scar sign of renal oncocytoma: magnetic resonance imaging appearance and lack of specificity. *Urol Radiol* 1986;**8**:46.

40 Smith SJ, Bosniak MA, Megibow AJ *et al.* Renal cell carcinoma: earlier discovery and increased detection. *Radiology* 1989;**170**:699–703.

41 Amendola MA, Bree BL, Pollack HM. Small renal cell carcinoma: resolving a diagnostic dilemma. *Radiology* 1988;**166**:637–41.

42 Warshauer DM, McCarthy SM, Street L *et al.* Detection of renal masses: sensitivities and specificities of excretory urography/linear tomography and CT. *Radiology* 1988;**169**: 363–5.

43 Curry NS, Schabel SI, Betswill WC Jr. Small renal neoplasms: diagnostic imaging, pathologic features and clinical course. *Radiology* 1986;**158**:113–17.

44 Medeiros LJ, Gelb AB, Weiss CM. Low grade renal cell carcinoma: a clinicopathologic study of 53 cases. *Am J Surg Pathol* 1987;**11**:633–42.

45 Bosniak MA. The current radiologic approach to renal cysts. *Radiology* 1986;**158**:1–10.

46 Levine E, Huntrakoon M, Wetzel LH. Small renal neoplasms:

clinical pathological and imaging features. *Am J Roentgenol* 1989;**153**:69–73.

47 Bosniak MA, Megibow AJ, Hulnick DA, Horii S, Raghavendra BN. CT diagnosis of renal angiomyolipoma: the importance of detecting small amounts of fat. *Am J Roentgenol* 1988;**151**:497–501.

48 Parvey LS, Warner RM, Callihan TR, Magill HL. CT demonstration of fat tissue in malignant renal neoplasms: atypical Wilms' tumors. *J Comput Assist Tomogr* 1981;**5**:851–4.

49 Strotzer M, Lehrer KB, Becker K. Detection of fat in a renal cell carcinoma mimicking angiomyolipoma. *Radiology* 1993;**188**:427–8.

50 Davidson AJ, Davis CJ. Fat in renal adenocarcinoma. Never say never. *Radiology* 1993;**188**:316.

51 Amiss ES, Cronan JJ, Pfister RC. Needle puncture of cystic renal masses: a survey of the Society of Uroradiology. *Am J Roentgenol* 1987;**148**:297–9.

52 Semelka RC, Shoenut JP, Kroeker MA, McMahon RG, Greenberg HM. Renal lesions: controlled comparison between CT and 1.5 MR imaging with nonenhanced and gadolinium enhanced fat-suppressed spin-echo and breath-hold flash techniques. *Radiology* 1992;**182**:425–30.

53 Moss AA, Bush WH. The kidneys. In: Moss AA, ed. *Computed Tomography of the Body with Magnetic Resonance Imaging*, Vol. 3. Philadelphia: WB Saunders, 1992:933–1020.

54 Pollack HM, Arger PH, Banner MP, Mulhern CB, Coleman BG. Computed tomography of renal pelvic filling defects. *Radiology* 1981;**138**:645–51.

55 Segal AJ, Spataro RR, Linke CA, Frank IN, Rabinowitz R. Diagnosis of non-opaque calculi by computed tomography. *Radiology* 1978;**129**:447.

56 Federle MP, McAninch JW, Kaizer JA *et al*. Computed tomography of urinary calculi. *Am J Roentgenol* 1981;**136**:255.

57 Brown RC, Leoning SA, Ehrhardt JC, Hawtrey CE. Cystine calculi are radio-opaque. *Am J Roentgenol* 1980;**135**:565.

58 Newhouse JH, Prieu EL, Amiss ES Jr, Dretter SP, Pfister RC. Computed tomography analysis of urinary calculi. *Am J Roentgenol* 1984;**142**:545–8.

59 Hillman BJ, Drach SW, Tracey P, Gaines JA. Computed tomographic analysis of renal calculi. *Am J Roentgenol* 1984;**142**:549–52.

60 Baron RL, McLennan BL, Lee JKT, Lawson TL. Computed tomography of transitional cell carcinoma of the renal pelvis and ureter. *Radiology* 1982;**144**:125–30.

61 Parienty RA, Ducellier R, Pradel J *et al*. Diagnostic value of CT numbers in pelvicalyceal filling defects. *Radiology* 1982;**145**:743–7.

62 Gatewood OMB, Goldman SM, Marshall FF, Siegelman SS. Computed tomography of transitional carcinoma of the kidney. In: Siegelman SS, Gatewood OMB, Goldman SM, eds. *Computed Tomography of the Kidneys and Adrenals*, Vol. 3. New York: Churchill Livingstone, 1984:81–111.

63 Leder RA, Dunnick NR. Transitional cell carcinoma of the pelvicalices and ureter. *Am J Roentgenol* 1990;**155**:713–22.

64 Cholankeril JV, Freundlich R, Ketyer S, Spirito AL, Napolitano J. Computed tomography in urothelial tumors of renal pelvis and related filling defects. *Comput Tomogr* 1986;**10**:263–72.

65 Jaffe J, Friedman AC, Seidmon EJ *et al*. Diagnosis of ureteral stump transitional cell carcinoma by CT and MR imaging. *Am J Roentgenol* 1987;**149**:741–2.

66 Hricak H, Theoni RF, Carroll PF *et al*. Detection and staging of renal neoplasms and reassessment of MR imaging. *Radiology* 1988;**166**:643–9.

67 Goldman SM, Fishman EK, Soulen MC. CT and MRI of inflammatory disease of the kidney. In: Goldman SM, Gatewood OMB, eds. *CT and MRI of the Genitourinary Tract in Contemporary Issues in Computed Tomography*. New York: Churchill Livingstone, 1990:59–95.

68 Oyen R, Baert AL, Marchal G. CT and US in acute inflammatory kidney disease. In: *Proceedings of 17th International Congress of Radiology*, Paris, 1989.

69 Soulen MC, Fishman EK, Goldman SM, Gatewood OMB. Bacterial renal infection: role of CT. *Radiology* 1989;**171**:703–7.

70 Moreham HT, Weiner SN, Hoffman-Tretin JC. Inflammatory disease of the kidney. *Semin Ultrasound CT and MR* 1986;**7**:246–60.

71 Jeffrey RB. Bacterial renal infection: role of CT [Letter]. *Radiology* 1989;**173**:574.

72 Gold RP, McClennan BL, Rottenberg RR. CT appearance of acute inflammatory disease of the renal interstitium. *Am J Roentgenol* 1983;**141**:343–9.

73 Soulen MC, Fishman EK, Goldman SM. Bacterial renal infection: role of CT [Letter]. *Radiology* 1989;**173**:575.

74 Lipuma JP. Magnetic resonance of the kidney. *Radiol Clin North Am* 1984;**22**:925–64.

75 Hamlin DJ, Ackerman N, Kaude JV *et al*. Magnetic resonance imaging of renal abscess in an experimental animal model. *Acta Radiol Diagnost* 1985;**26**:315.

76 Piccirillo M, Rigsby CM, Rosenfeld AT. Sonography of renal inflammatory disease. *Urol Radiol* 1987;**9**:66.

77 Yocker IC, Lindfors KK, Pfister RC. Diagnosis and treatment of pyonephrosis. *Radiol Clin North Am* 1984;**22**:407.

78 Soulen ML, Fishman, EK, Goldman SM. Sequelae of acute renal infections: CT evaluation. *Radiology* 1989;**173**:423–6.

79 Goldman SM, Hartman DS, Fishman EK *et al*. CT of xanthogranulomatous pyelonephritis. Radiologic–pathologic correlation. *Am J Roentgenol* 1984;**142**:963–9.

80 Subramanyam BR, Megibow AJ, Raghavendra BN, Bosniak MA. Diffuse xanthogranulomatous pyelonephritis: analysis of computed tomography and sonography. *Urol Radiol* 1982;**4**:5.

81 Varma DG, Rojo JR, Thomas R, Walker PD. Computed tomography of xanthogranulomatous pyelonephritis. *J Comput Assist Tomogr* 1985;**9**:241–7.

82 Mulopulos GP, Patel SK, Pessis D. MR imaging of xanthogranulomatous pyelonephritis. *J Comput Assist Tomogr* 1986;**10**:154.

83 Nicolaisen GS, McAninch JW, Marshall GA, Bluth RF, Carroll PR. Renal trauma: evaluation of the indications for radiographic assessment. *J Urol* 1985;**133**:183–7.

84 Steinberg DL, Jeffrey RB, Federle MP, McAninch JW. The computerized tomography appearances of renal pedicle injury. *J Urol* 1984;**132**:1163–4.

85 Fanney DR, Casillas J, Murphy BJ. CT in the diagnosis of renal trauma. *Radiographics* 1990;**10**:29–46.

86 Baron RL, McClennan BL, Lee JKT, Lanson TL. Computed tomography of transitional cell carcinoma of the renal pelvis and ureter. *Radiology* 1982;**144**:125.

87 Dooms GL, Hricak H, Crooks LE, Higgins CB. Magnetic resonance imaging of the lymph nodes: comparison with CT. *Radiology* 1984;**153**:179.

88 Ellis JH, Bies JR, Kopecky KK *et al*. Comparison of NMR and

CT imaging in the evaluation of metastatic retroperitoneal lymphadenopathy from testicular carcinoma. *J Comput Assist Tomogr* 1984;**8**:709.

89 Lee JKT, Heiken GP, Ling D, Glazer HS, Balfe DM. Magnetic resonance imaging of abdominal and pelvic lymphadenopathy. *Radiology* 1984;**153**:181.

90 Dooms GC, Hricak H, Mosely ME *et al.* Characterization of lymphadenopathy by magnetic resonance relaxation times: preliminary results. *Radiology* 1985;**155**:691.

91 Brooks AP, Reznek RH, Webb JAW. Magnetic resonance imaging in idiopathic retroperitoneal fibrosis: measurement of T_1 relaxation time. *Br J Radiol* 1990;**63**:842–4.

92 Dalla Palma L, Rocca Rossetti S, Pozzi-Mucelli RS, Rizzatto S. Computed tomography in the diagnosis of retroperitoneal fibrosis. *Urol Radiol* 1981;**3**:77–83.

93 Brooks AP, Reznek RH, Webb JAW, Baker LRI. Computed tomography in the follow-up of retroperitoneal fibrosis. *Clin Radiol* 1987;**38**:597–601.

94 Yancey JM, Kaude JV. Diagnosis of perirenal fibrosis by MR imaging. *J Comput Assist Tomogr* 1988;**12**:335.

95 Whitmore WF, Batata MA, Ghoneim MA, Grabstald H, Unal A. Radical cystectomy with or without prior irradiation in the treatment of bladder cancer. *J Urol* 1977;**118**:184–7.

96 Jager N, Radeke HW, Adolphs HD *et al.* Value of intravesical sonography in tumour classification of bladder carcinoma. *Eur Urol* 1986;**12**:76–84.

97 Skinner DG, Tift JP, Kaufman JJ. High dose short course preoperative radiation therapy and immediate single stage radical cystectomy with pelvic node dissection in the management of bladder cancer. *J Urol* 1982;**127**:671.

98 Neuerburg JM, Bohndorf K, Sohn M *et al.* Urinary bladder neoplasms: evaluation with contrast-enhanced MR imaging. *Radiology* 1989;**172**:739.

99 Morgan CL, Calkins RF, Cavalcanti EJ. Computed tomography in the evaluation, staging and therapy of carcinoma of the bladder and prostate. *Radiology* 1981;**140**:751–61.

100 Vock P, Haertel M, Fuchs WA *et al.* Computed tomography in staging of carcinoma of the urinary bladder. *Br J Urol* 1982;**54**:158–63.

101 Ney DR, Fishman EK, Kawashima A, Robertson DD Jr, Scott WW. Comparison of helical and serial CT with regard to three-dimensional imaging of musculoskeletal anatomy. *Radiology* 1992;**185**:865.

102 Barentsz JO, Lemmens JAM, Ruijs SHJ *et al.* Carcinoma of the urinary bladder: MR imaging with a double surface coil. *Am J Roentgenol* 1988;**151**:107–12.

103 Husband JES, Olliff JFC, Williams MP, Heron CW, Cherryman GR. Bladder cancer: staging with CT and MR imaging. *Radiology* 1989;**173**:435–40.

104 Rholl KS, Lee JKT, Heiken J, Ling D, Glaser HS. Primary bladder carcinoma: evaluation with MR imaging. *Radiology* 1987;**163**:117–21.

105 Tachibana M, Baba S, Deguchi N *et al.* Efficacy of gadolinium-diethylenetriaminepentaacetic acid enhanced magnetic resonance imaging for differentiation between superficial and muscle-invasive tumour of the bladder: a comparative study with computed tomography and transurethral ultrasonography. *Radiology* 1991;**181**:910.

106 Tanimoto A, Yuasa Y, Imai Y *et al.* Bladder tumor staging: comparison of conventional and gadolinium-enhanced dynamic MR imaging and CT. *Radiology* 1992;**185**:741–7.

107 Barentsz J, Ruijs SHJ, Strijk SP. The role of MR imaging in carcinoma of the bladder. *Am J Roentgenol* 1993;**160**: 937–47.

108 Husband JE. Staging bladder cancer. *Clinical Radiology* 1992;**46**:153–9.

109 Schiebler ML, Tomaszewski JE, Bezzi M *et al.* Prostatic carcinoma and benign prostatic hyperplasia: correlation of high-resolution MR and histopathologic finding. *Radiology* 1989;**172**:131–7.

110 Bezzie M, Kressel HY, Allen KS *et al.* Prostatic carcinoma: staging with MR imaging at 1.5T. *Radiology* 1988;**169**:339–46.

111 Brown G, Husband JE, MacVicar D. Dynamic contrast enhancement in MR imaging of prostatic carcinoma [Abstract]. In: *79th Scientific Assembly and Annual Meeting of the Radiological Society of North America*, 1993:843.

112 Biondetti PR, Lee J, Ling D *et al.* Clinical stage B prostate carcinoma: staging with MR imaging. *Radiology* 1987;**162**: 325–9.

113 Rifkin MD, Zerhouni EA, Gatsonis CA *et al.* Comparison of magnetic resonance imaging and ultrasonography in staging early prostate cancer: results of a multi-institutional co-operative trial. *N Engl J Med* 1990;**323**:621–6.

114 Schnall MD, Imai Y, Tomaszewski J *et al.* Prostate cancer: local staging with endorectal surface coil MR imaging. *Radiology* 1990;**178**:777–80.

115 Beyer HK, Funk PLJ, Brackins-Romero J, Uhlenbrock D. Wertigkeit der Kernspintomographie bei dere Diagnostik und Stadienbestimmung von Harnblasenneoplasmen. *Digitale Bilddiagn* 1985;**5**:167–72.

116 Bryan PJ, Butler HE, LiPuma JP *et al.* CT and MR imaging in staging bladder neoplasms. *J Comput Assist Tomogr* 1987;**11**:96–101.

117 Amendola MA, Glaser GM, Grossman HB *et al.* Staging of bladder carcinoma: MRI–CT–surgical correlation. *Am J Roentgenol* 1986;**146**:1179–83.

118 Vinnecombe SJ, Husband JE, Nicolson V, Norman A. CT evaluation of normal pelvic lymph nodes [Abstract]. In: *79th Scientific Assembly and Annual Meeting of the Radiology Society of North America*, 1993:1102.

119 Williams MP, Cherryman GR, Husband JE. Magnetic resonance imaging in suspected metastatic spinal cord compression. *Clinical Radiology* 1989;**40**:286–90.

120 Wolverson MK, Houttuin E, Heiberg E, Sundaram M, Shields JB. Comparison of computed tomography with high resolution real-time ultrasound in the localization of impalpable undescended testis. *Radiology* 1983;**146**:133.

121 Fritzsche PJ, Hricak H, Kogan BA, Winkler ML, Tanagho EA. Undescended testis: value of MR imaging. *Radiology* 1987; **164**:169.

6 Renal Radionuclide Studies

K.E.Britton

Introduction

The preservation and improvement of renal function is one of the fundamental purposes of genitourinary surgery.

Radionuclide images are to function as X-ray films are to structure. Both pictures are obtained using ionizing radiation. This radiation is called X-rays when it originates from the orbiting electron shells of certain atoms, and γ-rays when it comes from the nucleus of certain atoms, hence the term 'nuclear medicine'. The atoms which emit γ-rays are part of a class of atoms called radionuclides. When such radionuclides are administered and taken up by organs in the body, the γ-rays penetrate the body wall and are detectable externally by a gamma camera, hence the term 'radionuclide imaging'.

A gamma camera is usually made up of a single large crystal with many detectors behind it. They feed a display system where the position from which the γ-ray pulse came is recorded as well as the number of pulses. The more pulses, the brighter the image. Thus, for example, a radioactive tracer taken up by bone will be displayed as an image of the lumbar spine simply by sitting the patient with his or her back to the camera. The advantage of this for the patient is evident. The resulting picture is a 2D representation of the distribution of a particular function of an organ or system which takes up the radioactive tracer, and is called a scan or 'static' image — in this case a 'bone scan' of the skeletal system.

The gamma camera also allows serial images to be taken so that the manner in which the distribution of activity changes with time may be displayed — a 'dynamic' study. The data are at the same time collected, stored and analysed using an on-line computer to give measurements of the quantities of activity at different sites and the tracer passage times, 'transit times', through selected regions of interest. Before the advent of the gamma camera, dynamic studies were recorded using scintillation detector probes placed over the body, and graphs of activity against time were obtained without images, e.g. renography. Samples may also have been taken from the patient at a series of times after injection of a radioactive tracer and the activities measured *in vitro* in a sample counter, as in a 'clearance' study.

Radionuclide studies of the kidney and renal outflow tract enable various functions to be measured objectively. Thus they enhance intuitive, subjective or visual assessments and help to demonstrate where such assessments are misleading. Serial measurements may be made to detect any change in function during the observation of patients in whom surgery is not yet thought to be indicated. The presence or absence of significant obstruction of outflow may be determined. The amount of function that will be lost through partial or total nephrectomy may be estimated before operation and this knowledge should help in deciding between a restorative and an ablative operation. The documentation of improvement in renal function gives a reliable indicator of the success of surgery. The techniques of radionuclide investigation generally involve no more than an intravenous injection for the patient and the absorbed radiation dose is typically much less than that given during X-ray studies of the kidney.

Measurement of total renal function

The kidney has many functions particularly designed to conserve and maintain the internal environment through salt and water balance, acid and osmolar control, and the production of and response to various hormones. However, the overall renal function that dominates the clinical assessment of how the kidneys are working is the kidneys' ability to remove substances from the blood. This may be termed the *uptake* function of the kidney. As the anatomical site of uptake is different for different compounds, Smith [1] categorized the various functions of the kidney thus: (i) effective renal plasma flow (ERPF); (ii) glomerular filtration (GFR); and (iii) tubular function. This separation led to the incorrect view that each of these functions was in some way discrete and independent of the others whereas, in reality, the kidney has a hierarchy of interacting control systems which interrelate renal plasma flow (RPF), glomerular filtration and tubular function through autoregulation, tubuloglomerular balance and the juxtaglomerular apparatus. Thus these functions occurring at anatomically separate sites are, in physiological terms, interdependent.

A number of assumptions are made and have to be adhered to when renal function is measured using radionuclides. There should be steady-state conditions. Anxiety and unexpected noise or pain cause fluctuations in renal bloodflow. Severe fluid depletion or overhydration, changes of posture and alterations in concentrations of drugs affecting renal function should be avoided during the test. Unsteady-state conditions may be obtained shortly after surgery, anaesthesia, renal biopsy or X-ray contrast studies. For the radionuclide measurement of overall renal function, it is assumed that the kidneys are the only exit from the body for the radiopharmaceutical and that the compound used does not undergo metabolism.

Measurement of GFR

Physiological basis

The properties of an ideal agent with which to measure GFR include the absence of binding to plasma constituents, the absence of reabsorption or secretion by renal tubules, and ease of technique and assay. [51Cr] ethylenediamine tetra-acetic acid (EDTA) (51Cr: gamma energy 0.32 MeV, half-life 27.8 days) and [99mTc] diethylenetriamine penta-acetic acid (DTPA) (99mTc: gamma energy 0.14 MeV, half-life 6 h) are preferred. Neither of these compounds shows significant plasma protein binding in humans and, provided the best preparations of [99mTc] DTPA are used [2], neither shows tubular uptake.

Whichever radiopharmaceutical compound is used, the measurement of overall renal function depends on the following relationship:

Rate of uptake of tracer by the kidneys
= Rate of loss of tracer from the blood.

The rate of loss of a compound from the blood is called its clearance, and the rate of uptake by the kidneys is determined by measuring the amount that appears in the urine collected over a time period, given by $(U \times V)/t$, that is urinary concentration times urine volume passed per unit time. The imagined volume of blood cleared totally of the compound per unit time, C, times the plasma concentration, P, of the compound is the rate of loss of the compound from the blood. When these are equated [3]:

$$C \times P = (U \times V)/t$$

thus

$$C = (U \times V)/(P \times t).$$

The classic technique of constant infusion and urine collection may be used with a radiopharmaceutical instead of inulin, but an alternative approach which avoids urine collection is now favoured. In this circumstance, clearance is redefined as the amount lost per unit time to the kidneys, not to urine.

The rate of uptake of a radiopharmaceutical by the kidneys per unit time, $Q(t)$, is equal to the rate of supply of the radiopharmaceutical in plasma from the blood flowing to the kidneys. This is given by the product of RPF and its plasma concentration $P(t)$ at the time of measurement. The fraction that is taken up by the kidneys depends on their efficiency, E, in extracting the radiopharmaceutical from the plasma. Thus the rate of uptake of a compound by the kidney equals $(RPF \times P(t) \times E)$. Therefore:

$$Q(t) = RPF \times P(t) \times E.$$

The product of rate of loss of radiopharmaceutical from the plasma, λ, and the dose of radiopharmaceutical administered, D, gives the amount of tracer lost from the plasma per unit time. Thus:

$$D \times \lambda = Q(t) = RPF \times P(t) \times E.$$

For a purely filtered agent, the extraction efficiency, E, is the fraction of bloodflow that is filtered, and this is the filtration fraction given by (GFR/RPF). Thus, for a purely filtered agent:

$$D \times \lambda = Q(t) = RPF \times P(t) \times (GFR/RPF),$$

therefore:

$$D \times \lambda = Q(t) = GFR \times P(t)$$

and

$$GFR = D \times \lambda /P(t).$$

Thus in order to measure the GFR it is necessary to know the dose of [51Cr] EDTA or [99mTc] DTPA that is administered, its rate of loss or 'washout' from the blood and the change of plasma activity of the tracer with time.

Single shot technique

About 4 MBq (100 μCi) of [51Cr] EDTA or 80 MBq (2 mCi) of [99mTc] DTPA may be used for the measurement of GFR.

The patient is prepared for intravenous injection and care is taken *not* to displace air from the syringe and needle before injection. All the activity, which has been measured accurately, must be injected intravenously and blood drawn back and reinjected to wash out the syringe. Extravasation of activity invalidates the test. After injection the needle and syringe are saved so that the exact activity injected may be measured by the difference. The residual contents of the syringe and needle are washed and rewashed into a 100 ml volumetric flask. This is made up to the meniscus with water and shaken. An accurately measured sample is taken.

In order to prepare the standard, an aliquot, approximately 0.5 ml, is taken using a sterile needle and syringe, previously weighed empty, from the stock solution from which the injection was prepared. After reweighing, the difference gives the weight of the standard, S.

The aliquot is flushed into a 1000 ml volumetric flask. The syringe is washed and rewashed into the flask with water and the volume made up to the meniscus with water. Alternatively the standard may be prepared and transferred to the volumetric flask using an accurate automatic 1 ml pipette but this would break the sterility of the stock solution. The volumetric flask is stoppered well and mixed by shaking.

Samples are taken from the patient typically at 2, 3, 4 and 5 h, and at 24 h if there is oedema or renal failure, into heparin tubes which are inverted several times and labelled with the patient's name and time since injection or time of sampling.

Measurement is made of a weighed standard representing the activity injected, tubes representing background activity and the plasma samples.

The values for GFR together with an error estimate are printed out both uncorrected and corrected for body surface area. The mathematical approach used in the computer programme may be single or double exponential analysis [4–6] performed conventionally or using the technique of Nimmon et al. [7]:

$$GFR = (D \times 0.693)/(P_0 \times T_{1/2})$$

where D is the activity injected, P_0 is the plasma sample activity extrapolated back to time zero and $T_{1/2}$ is the half-life of clearance.

Compartmental models carry with them a number of important assumptions which must be fully recognized. The compartment must be fully mixed at the time that the exchange process is considered, and this requires that the rate of mixing of a tracer in a compartment must be very rapid as compared with the rate of exchange between compartments. These assumptions are evidently not quite true and are not at all well held when there is oedema or when renal function is poor. They impose a limitation on the accuracy of the technique. Nevertheless, the results are acceptable given normal biological variation and the lack of any precise definition of particular thresholds of renal function on which particular clinical decisions are based.

Single sample approach

A number of alternative approaches have been developed in attempts to simplify the technique of measurement of GFR even further. These simplifications are particularly appropriate when GFR is to be monitored serially over a period of time in one patient. Perhaps the best approach is to undertake a full measurement of GFR in the most accurate way possible first, collecting data for the simpler approach at the same time and then using the simpler approach for repeat studies. The serum creatinine should be measured on the first occasion as, given a constant muscle bulk and catabolic state, a doubling of serum creatinine is associated with a halving of GFR. However, such conditions may not apply and there is a moderate error on the chemical determination of creatinine. Estimation of radioactivity in vitro is about 100 times more sensitive than chemical estimation.

The basis of the single plasma sample approach depends on the fact that the volume of distribution of the tracer in the steady state, V, is given by the dilution of the activity of the administered dose, D (administered volume × activity) in the plasma at the time of sampling, $P(t)$. Thus:

$$V = D/P(t).$$

There is a moment of equilibrium when the rate of movement of tracer from the plasma to the extracellular fluid is just balanced by the rate of return of tracer from the extracellular fluid. At this time, the rate of loss of tracer from the kidney will be proportional to its volume of distribution, V (GFR $\propto V$).

In adults the moment of equilibrium is about 3 h for [^{51}Cr] EDTA [8,9]. A standard graph is constructed using the values of GFR and V at 3 h obtained during studies on a series of patients using the full single shot technique. In this way, knowing the activity of a single plasma sample taken at 3 h and the dose administered (determined as described in the section on technique), V is given and the GFR is read off directly from the graph. One formula for the relationship is given by Constable et al. [9]:

$$GFR = 24.5 \ (V - 6.2)^{1/2} - 67 \ ml/min \ (SD \pm 4)$$

where V is the distribution of [^{51}Cr] EDTA in litres. The errors are greater than for the single shot method but it appears satisfactory for repeated studies in patients whose GFR is over 30 ml/min.

Effective renal plasma flow

The same basic techniques apply to the measurement of ERPF using ^{125}I or ^{131}I orthoiodohippurate (^{125}I-OIH or ^{131}I-OIH) as to the measurement of GFR. Because of the more rapid excretion of ^{131}I-OIH, sampling times are earlier than for GFR, typically at 7, 17, 30, 44, 60 and 120 min.

$$ERPF = (D \times 0.693)/(P_0 \times T_{1/2})$$

where D and P_0 apply to ^{131}I-OIH and are determined in the manner indicated for GFR. However, because of the shorter clearance period for ^{131}I-OIH, the use of external monitoring is much more feasible. The rate of clearance (washout rate) may be monitored externally with a detector placed over the chest, head or shoulder and this continuous record may be calibrated by taking one or two blood plasma samples at time intervals which must be measured and indicated accurately on the chart record. The simplest index of all is to plot the slope of the 7 and 17 min samples or points on the externally recorded graph on semi-logarithmic paper and measure this estimate of the rate of clearance. This may be followed daily as an index of renal function, for example in the early days after renal transplantation. It is unaffected by the presence or otherwise of oliguria.

The moment of equilibrium for the single plasma sample method for ^{131}I-OIH is 44 min [10–12]. One formula is:

$$ERPF = 120\ (V + 56)^{1/2} - 936\ ml/min\ (SD \pm 46)$$

where V represents the volume distribution of ^{131}I-OIH at 44 min. A more complex, but more accurate, formula with V in litres is:

$$ERPF = 1126\ (1 - e^{-0.008(V - 7.8)})\ ml/min.$$

The preparation of ^{131}I-OIH should be such that the free iodine content should be less than 1% and the content of iodobenzoic acid contaminant less than 0.2%, both of these being excreted much more slowly than ^{131}I-OIH. The solution of ^{131}I-OIH should be kept in a dark glass bottle and stored at 4°C.

The documentation of the state of overall renal function is a necessary part of any evaluation of a patient before and after surgery and the serial assessment of overall renal function is required during long-term follow-up.

Renal imaging

The gamma camera computer system

The technical problem consists essentially of determining the quantity and distribution of radioactivity in an organ under study at a particular time and in measuring how this changes with time. ^{99m}Tc is a radionuclide with a half-life of 6 h which gives off γ-rays of 0.14 MeV energy as it disintegrates. When combined in a radiopharmaceutical such as [^{99m}Tc] mercapto acetyl triglycine (MAG$_3$) and injected, these γ-rays penetrate the body. Some γ-rays interact with the tissue and are scattered, travelling with a lower energy at different angles (Compton scattering). These are rejected by the electronic settings of the gamma camera. Others pass directly through the body. In front of the face of the camera is fixed a lead sheet (collimator) — 4 cm thick — in which many thousands of parallel holes reduce the entrance of γ-rays other than those travelling normal (directly at right angles) to the face of the camera. These are detected by their interaction with the crystal behind the collimator.

Technique and interpretation

The patient requires hydration with about 200 ml fluid at least 30 min before the test so that the urine flow during the test is 1–4 ml/min. The patient should receive a reassuring explanation of the test before entering the renography room. The patient should be studied reclining, for example, in a modified dental chair. The supine position may be preferred since the kidneys are less likely to descend, but positioning of the camera is difficult. The sitting position, particularly sitting forward, and the standing position allow the kidneys to drop and move anteriorly, making positioning and quantitation less reliable. The reclining position is a suitable compromise. The gamma camera is positioned so that its face is set back about 20° off the vertical plane. The patient sits on a comfortable backless chair with side arms and reclines back against the camera face. With the arm abducted, the injection of the chosen radiopharmaceutical is given in less than 1 ml, rapidly into a deep antecubital vein. Alternatively, a 'butterfly' needle with a sterile extension tube and three-way tap may be used. The injectate is introduced into the extension tube and flushed in using 10–20 ml saline. This system also allows access for a subsequent injection of 40 mg frusemide for the diuresis technique. Data are collected for 20 min or longer if the pelvis is not visualized and for at least 10 min after an injection of frusemide if that technique is used. Frusemide (40 mg) should not be injected before 18 min have elapsed in the adult, but it may be necessary to wait for 30 min in a child (0.5 mg/kg body weight administered).

Images on transparent film (analogue images) are usually collected at 30 s intervals for the first 180 s, and then at 5 min intervals for the remainder of the study. The following features should be noted.

1 The length of time the activity in the left ventricular cavity is visible — prolonged with renal impairment.
2 The patency and tortuosity of the aorta and possible aneurysm.
3 Whether the times of arrival and tracer distribution are equal in the two kidneys; prolongation on one side may occur with an inflow disorder.
4 The site and position of the kidneys relative to the liver and spleen, and any possible space-occupying lesion between.
5 Whether the cortical outline of each kidney is complete; is there a possible scar due to infection, infarction or tumour?
6 Whether there are any defects in the parenchyme, and any possible tumour, cyst or parenchymal infection or scar.

A dilated calyx should fill at the pelvic retention stage but not if it contains a stone. A cyst in the parenchyme will not show any tracer uptake, whereas a vascular tumour may show initial tracer activity which may persist for longer than that in adjacent normal tissue and be followed by a focal defect in the distribution of activity due to the absence of normal nephrons.

Corticopelvic transfer will normally be seen to occur as the tracer moves from parenchyme to pelvis as the lateral edge of the kidney, noted on the 1–2 min frames, appears to move medially as the test progresses. Pelvic, calyceal and/or ureteric retention of tracer occurs when the capacity of these structures has increased through dilatation but cannot be used to distinguish whether obstruction is or is not present. The ureter should not be considered to have retained tracer unless its whole length or that down to a block can be seen to persist over several images. Blobs of activity in the ureter are of no clinical significance. The bladder is usually visualized at the end of the test. A ureterocele or a diverticulum of the bladder may be observed.

Consider the events following a rapid intravenous injection of a small volume of [^{99m}Tc] MAG$_3$ and its effect on a gamma camera placed externally over the region of each kidney and over the chest. Within 15 s, 10% of the injected dose arrives at each kidney as a bolus, as each receives about 10% of the cardiac output. Since the mean renal artery to renal vein passage time is about 8 s and since about 65% of MAG$_3$ is taken up with each passage of blood, the quantity in the kidney rises rapidly and then more slowly as recirculated MAG$_3$ in lower concentrations enters. Meanwhile, the bolus that arrived with the first circulation, having been taken up by the proximal tubules of the cortical and juxtamedullary nephrons and secreted within a few seconds, progresses in quanta along the lumens of the million nephrons of each kidney. The quanta of the bolus move along collecting ducts to enter the pelvis, pass through in 20 s and move down the ureter. A sharp fall in activity is thus recorded and a peak is formed in the activity–time curve recorded over the kidney region. This activity–time curve is called a renogram.

It is easy to confirm that the first arrival of activity in the bladder coincides approximately with the peak of the normal renogram. The fact that the renogram has a sharp peak implies that the quanta of the bolus pass through the majority of nephrons in approximately the same time. This in turn implies some form of local nephron control. The bladder appearance time of about 3 min for injected MAG$_3$ is true not only for the bolus arriving with the first circulation, but also for each subsequent package of recirculated MAG$_3$ taken up by the kidney. Thus, after the peak, the activity in the kidney declines progressively more slowly, because progressively smaller packages are entering 3 min previously from the blood. The third phase that follows the peak is thus not an excretory phase, but a record of the quantity of MAG$_3$ remaining in the kidney, reflecting falling input and continuing transit of activity as well as its loss.

The renogram is a crude representation of the kidney curve, which is the ideal activity–time curve that would be obtained just from the kidney. The renogram may thus be considered to be a composite curve: one component of this is the kidney curve and the other component is the variation of activity with time of non-kidney tissue and blood in the renal region of interest. The activity–time curve of this latter component has, after about 90 s of tracer mixing following intravenous injection, the same shape as a record of the change of tracer activity with time obtained with a detector over the left ventricle. This non-kidney curve is called the blood clearance curve, somewhat inaccurately as it differs slightly from the activity–time curve obtained from a series of blood samples. Nevertheless, it is the representation of non-kidney activity with which each renogram may be compared. If the renogram differs from the blood clearance curve, the difference represents some function in the kidney from which the renogram was obtained. It is clear that the kidney curve is the recording of physiological and clinical interest. As the renograms more or less conceal the kidney curves depending on the level of renal function, so their understanding and interpretation is more difficult.

It may not be appreciated that the terms 'vascular spike', 'secretory' phase and 'excretory' phase introduced by Winter [13] have no relation to the bloodflow to the kidney, its secretory ability, nor its urinary output of tracer and so these terms misled many workers. In particular, absence of the so-called excretory phase does *not* mean obstruction to outflow.

It was thought that measurements made from the renogram indicated measurements of renal function, when in fact they were merely descriptive of the renogram curve itself. Thus measurement of, for example, the height of an inflection point, the peak and the time taken for the curve to fall to half peak height, enabled one to reconstruct the curve crudely but there should have been no expectation that these values would have physiological significance. It is necessary to seek out and derive from the renogram those features which represent clinically relevant functions of the kidney, i.e. the *uptake function* and the *transit function*.

On visual inspection a normal pair of renograms are characterized by their symmetry. A normal renogram curve has a steeply rising part usually lasting 20–30 s and ending with an apparent discontinuity of the slope. This is called the first phase and is absent in the renogram when it is corrected for tissue and blood background. The renogram then rises over the next few minutes towards peak and this is called the second phase. If there is no peak to the renogram, as is the case in certain diseases, it can be said that the second phase continues to rise. After the second phase is the peak, which should be sharp. The record descends after the peak in a normal renogram and this is called the third phase. If there is no peak (as in disease) then there is no third phase (Fig. 6.1).

An abnormal renogram is characterized by loss of the sharpness of the peak and alteration of either the second or third phase, or both of these. Absence of the second phase does not necessarily mean absence of renal function; absence of the third phase certainly does not necessarily mean obstruction to outflow. Differences in peak time between two renograms of over 1 min are of clinical significance only if either the second or third phase of the renogram with the delayed peak are impaired.

Small rapid fluctuations seen in the second or third phases are statistical in nature. When there are fluctuations in renal bloodflow, for example due to anxiety, sudden noise or discomfort, an unsteady state occurs and larger irregularities occur. These last over 2 min and return to the line of the third phase. Since ureteric peristalsis is about two to four contractions per minute and as an increase in resistance to flow in the ureter leads to a rise in distending pressure and reduced force but increased frequency of peristalsis, these irregularities are *not* due to ureteric 'spasm'. Hydronephrosis or reflux of urine may also be associated with large alterations, rising above and descending below the line, of the third phase.

The report of an abnormal renogram should be in two parts, the description and the interpretation in the individual clinical context. In describing the abnormal renogram, the first phase should be ignored. The second phase may be called 'absent', 'impaired', 'normal' and/or 'continuing to rise' when no peak occurs. The third phase may be called 'absent', 'impaired' or 'normal'. The time to peak varies non-linearly with the state of hydration and urine flow. It is indirectly related to the rate of salt and water reabsorption by the nephrons and to the state of the pelvis. It is a crude index of the tracer transit through the parenchyme and pelvis. Normal peak times vary from 2.0 to 4.5 min with a mean of 3.7 min at a urine flow of 1 ml/min.

If renograms without third phases are symmetrically abnormal, prerenal or renal parenchymal disorder is the most likely explanation. If renograms without third phases are asymmetrical, then bilateral outflow disorder is more likely. In the context of bilateral outflow obstruction, the kidney that should be operated upon first to relieve the outflow obstruction is that with the better uptake function [14]. A successful operation is followed by an improvement in the rate of rise of the second phase; however, the third phase may remain absent for weeks or even months after a successful operation. If the renogram curve continues to rise and renal function is moderate or good, then an injection of 40 mg frusemide intravenously at about 18 min after the start will cause the curve to fall rapidly if the resistance to outflow is trivial [15]. This apparent holdup may also be overcome by standing the patient up and then repositioning, but the frusemide injection is more reliable in the reclining patient (see p. 89).

Renal function in a patient with hydronephrosis cannot be judged by the cortical thickness seen on intravenous urography (IVU), because the cortical thickness is not uniform. A grossly inaccurate underassessment of function may be made from IVU if the central cortical thinning is taken as representative, because normal nephrons are often present in the poles. Anatomical information is gained from the IVU through black and white contrast, whereas renography gives a grey scale related to renal function which is summarized graphically.

Computer analysis

Renal input

The activity–time curve representing the input of activity to the kidney may be obtained from a region of interest (ROI) set over the left ventricle. Due to the interference of the vertebral column, using an ROI over the aorta gives a rather poor input curve when viewed from the back.

Renal background

Controversy has ranged over the most appropriate way to

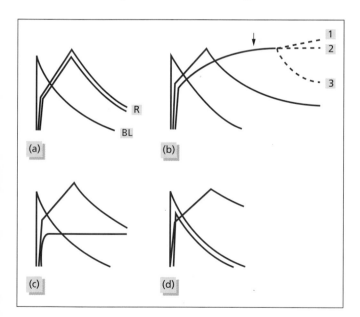

Fig. 6.1 Renography: vertical axis, activity; horizontal axis, time. (a) Normal pair of renograms, R, and blood clearance Bl. (b) One renogram has an impaired second phase that continues to rise, and no third phase, compatible with inflow or outflow disease. ↓ injection of frusemide, 1 outflow obstruction, 2 equivocal result, 3 normal response. (c) One renogram runs horizontally indicating renal function is present since it differs from the blood clearance curve. (d) One renogram from a nephrectomy site is the same shape as the blood clearance curve.

make a correction for activity in non-renal tissue anterior and posterior to the kidney, when an ROI is drawn around each kidney. No method is perfect but familiarity with any chosen method and its sources of error is more important than following the latest fashion. A number of points can be made. Using [^{99m}Tc] MAG$_3$, background correction is probably not needed until the activity in one or both kidneys is less than 20% of normal. As the environment of one kidney is different from another (liver on the right, stomach and spleen on the left), a single ROI to represent the background is insufficient and two regions should be used. An ROI is drawn from just superior to each kidney to close to the midline, avoiding the aorta, or in a C shape around the lateral circumference of each kidney, avoiding potentially unrepresentative areas such as the central aorta, renal pelvis and ureters. An alternative technique is to use the blood background activity determined by deconvolution analysis to make the correction.

Separation of parenchyme from pelvis

In order to measure the parenchymal transit time, which is important in the assessment of obstructive nephropathy, it is necessary to separate all elements of the pelvicalyceal system from the parenchyme. The conventional count distribution image does not easily enable such separation, particularly when there is cortical scarring or thinning and/or calyceal clubbing. This separation may be achieved by creating a 'mean time' image. Each pixel of the matrix containing the kidney may be analysed serially so that the activity–time curve of just that pixel (a 'minirenogram') may be obtained. The mean time of that activity–time curve may be obtained by the transformation:

$$t = (\sum_i t_i N_i)/(\sum_i N_i)$$

where N_i is the number of counts between the time t_i and t_{i+1}.

Longer mean times may be shown as higher intensities. As no activity reaches the calyces and pelvis until 2.5 min or more, the pelvis and calyces are easily identified as high intensities and a generous ROI can be drawn around them to exclude them. This ROI is then superimposed on an ROI drawn around the kidney taken 1.5–2 min before any activity has left the kidney. The difference gives a pure parenchymal area. An activity–time curve is then generated from this parenchymal area (and from the whole kidney for comparison) for subsequent deconvolution analysis.

Deconvolution analysis and the impulse retention function

This technique is a mathematical way of saying that if one considers a system as a black box and if one knows what goes into and comes out of a system then one can determine what has happened in the system. This approach is usually applied to time relationships. An analogy may be made with fluid flowing in a stream to which an injection of dye is made upstream. If the flow in the stream is smooth, the spread of dye as monitored downstream would be relatively small compared with that in a stream which is turbulent where the dye would be well mixed up, and thus spread out. There is clearly a relationship between the degree of spread of dye noted at the monitor site and the characteristics of flow in the stream. Each particle of a dye could be considered to have taken its own path length or path time to reach the monitor site; path lengths and path times depend on the flow characteristics. Thus a range, frequency/distribution or spectrum of transit times relates the shape of the dye distribution at the output to the characteristics of the flow in the tube.

This example can be generalized to state that if the shape of the activity–time or concentration–time curve representing the 'system content' and the input or the output curve of the system is known, then, by deconvolution analysis, the spectrum of transit times through the system can be obtained. This spectrum is the frequency with which numbers of molecules of the test substance take a particular distribution of time paths through the system. Thus, deconvolution analysis applied to the kidney input and the kidney parenchyme or whole kidney activity–time curves will give the mean and distribution of parenchymal or whole kidney tracer transit times.

Another way of looking at this spectrum of transit times is that it is the result that would have been obtained if a spike injection of the tracer had been given directly into the renal artery. The response of the kidney to this single input is called the impulse retention function. Thus deconvolution analysis, in effect, allows one to obtain results of an intra-arterial spike injection into the organ of interest from an ordinary non-spike injection given non-invasively into a vein, and the impulse retention function is the 'renogram' consequent upon a spike injection into the renal artery.

The impulse retention function is shown in Fig. 6.2. The spike input calculated by deconvolution analysis is shown on the left, the height of the vertical axis represents activity and the horizontal axis, time. In a kidney made up of a million nephrons, the spike of activity is split into a million quanta, each taking approximately 180 s to pass through the lumens of the nephrons and 20 s to pass through the pelvis, giving a whole kidney mean transit time of 200 s. During this time the total activity in the kidney remains constant, as shown idealized in Fig. 6.2a. The time of 180 s represents the tracer's mean transit time. In fact the renal blood pool means that there is vascular transit of some activity giving an early spike to the impulse retention function labelled v, for vascular activity. This may be excluded by computer analysis by extrapolating

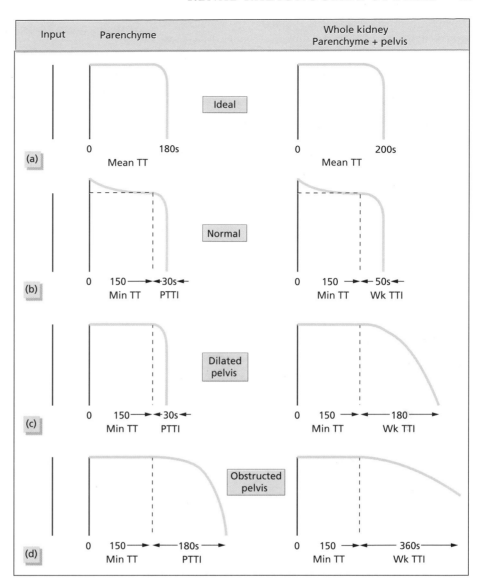

Fig. 6.2 The impulse retention function (see text). (a) Normal parenchyma and whole kidney impulse retention function representing the mean transit time, TT. (b) Division of mean transit time into minimum transit time and the parenchymal transit time index (PTTI) for the parenchyma, and the whole kidney transit time index (WkTTI) for the whole kidney. (c) Results in the dilated unobstructed pelvis. (d) Results in the dilated obstructed pelvis.

back from the plateau part of the impulse retention function. The minimal transit time, 150 s, is the shortest transit time and is given by the point of downward sloping of the impulse retention function indicated at the vertical dotted line. Transit times longer than minimal are shown as lasting 30 s in the parenchyma, and this part of the impulse retention function gives the parenchymal transit time index (PTTI). Transit times longer than minimal are shown as lasting 50 s in the parenchyma plus pelvis, and this part of the impulse retention function gives the whole kidney transit time index (WkTTI). Thus the mean transit time equals the minimum transit time plus the PTTI. When the pelvis is dilated but not obstructed the PTTI is unchanged, whereas the pelvic transit time is prolonged causing an increased WkTTI (Fig. 6.2c). Only when there is significant outflow resistance causing obstructive nephropathy is the PTTI increased as shown in Fig. 6.2d.

The reason for separating the mean transit time into the minimum transit time and the PTTI is that the subtracting of the minimum transit time increases the sensitivity of the test for obstructive nephropathy, partly because it reduces the effect of differing urine flow rates between different patients. There is a hyperbolic relationship between urine flow rate and minimum transit time, with a roughly inverse linear relationship at urine flow rates of 1–3 ml/min; the slower the urine flow, the longer the minimum transit time.

Renal output efficiency

The principal advantage for using a diuretic is that the number of equivocal cases, especially those with non-obstructed dilated collecting systems associated with indeterminate flow curves, are substantially reduced [15].

However, uncertainty still persists in kidneys with intermediate responses in diuresis renograms. This is normally encountered in patients with severely impaired renal function in whom the third phase of the renogram curve does not accurately reflect radiopharmaceutical excretion from the kidneys. This is because the shape of the third phase in a renogram curve depends on the uptake, parenchymal transit and removal rate of the radio-pharmaceutical by the kidneys, which vary with time in a way that ultimately depends on plasma concentration variations.

Britton and Brown [16] described a measurement of renal output efficiency (ROE) (the isotope removal factor) using data from OIH probe renography which related OIH output to renal function levels. This approach was adapted by Nimmon et al. [17,18] to obtain ROE in gamma camera studies using ^{99m}Tc-labelled DTPA and MAG$_3$.

The main purpose of the ROE is to provide a quantitative assessment of frusemide diuretic response independent of renal function in the management of urinary obstruction.

The ROE was determined as follows. Blood background subtraction was performed on each whole kidney activity–time curve obtained from an ROI around the kidney outline on the 90–120 s image. By using an iterative least squares technique, the integral of the blood clearance curve $P(t)$ (obtained from an ROI over the left ventricle), was fitted to a part of the rising second phase of the background-corrected kidney curve, $R(t)$, in accordance with the linear expression:

$$Y(t) = A + B \cdot \int P(t)\, dt$$

where $Y(t) = R(t)$ for $t_1 \leq t \leq t_2$; A is the intercept and B is the slope of the fitted curve.

The range of data included in the fit was determined using statistical chi-squared (χ^2) and Fisher's (F) ratio parameters. Initially, data from t_1 equal to 60 s up to the peak time t_2, or up to 6 min in the absence of a clearly defined peak, were used and the value of χ^2 was calculated. Points were then sequentially deleted starting at the highest data point until no significant change in χ^2 was detected as judged by the F ratio [17]. The resultant fitted curve $Y(t)$ corresponds to the integrated input to the kidney as a function of time. By subtraction of the background-corrected kidney curve $R(t)$ from the integrated input $Y(t)$, the curve $O(t)$ — representing the integrated output from the kidney — was obtained. ROE is the integrated output as a percentage of the integrated input and is defined by the following equation:

$$ROE\% = [O(t)/Y(t)] \times 100\ (\%).$$

In this way the response to frusemide is corrected for the level of renal function. It has been validated in clinical use [18].

Radiopharmaceuticals

A radiopharmaceutical is any compound containing radioactivity that is in a form suitable for administration to humans. Thus, for intravenous use, it must be sterile, pyrogen- and particle-free. Since the rapid decay of the radionuclide prevents prior preparation and storage of many radiopharmaceuticals and since the products are usually used within 4 h, a suitable environment and adequate quality control for preparation are essential. To this end, pharmaceutical and radiation protection skills need to be combined. The physical, staffing and legal requirements for the production of radiopharmaceuticals are one of the limitations to the general application of nuclear medicine to the speciality of genitourinary surgery. Nevertheless, the distribution of suitable radiopharmaceuticals from a central laboratory is becoming more widespread.

Radioiodinated Hippuran

Hippuran is the commercial name for ^{131}I-radioiodinated orthoiodohippurate (^{131}I-OIH) used for probe renography for many years. ^{131}I-OIH should no longer be used with the gamma camera since the administered dose needs to be 11 MBq (300 µCi) or more and this gives, by nuclear medicine standards, a high radiation dose to the bladder and kidneys, particularly when there is an outflow disorder [19]. This is due to the β-rays of ^{131}I. The γ-ray energy of ^{131}I (0.364 MeV) is also too high for the usual gamma camera collimator system described above, so resolution of detail is poor. ^{131}I-OIH may also be used to measure ERPF. ^{123}I radioiodine is the radionuclide of choice for labelling OIH. It has no β-rays, a γ-ray of 0.159 MeV energy and a half-life of 13 h. Thus it is very suitable for the gamma camera. It is expensive and its availability is limited.

[^{99m}Tc] DTPA

This compound is the previous standard radiopharmaceutical for renal work and is glomerular filtered. [^{99m}Tc] pertechnetate is eluted from the ^{99}Mo generator with saline each morning and its activity measured using an ionization chamber. DTPA is supplied in a kit form. The expiry date should be checked. [^{99m}Tc] DTPA is prepared using an aseptic technique in a laminar flow cabinet. The vial is swabbed using alcohol and 2–10 ml sodium pertechnetate containing up to 1 GBq (300 mCi) ^{99m}Tc is added and agitated gently until dissolved. The preparation is allowed to stand for 15 min and stored at 4°C until use, within 8 h. The adult dose is 400 MBq (10 mCi) and the paediatric dose is 5 MBq (150 µCi)/kg body weight. Preparations of [^{99m}Tc] DTPA vary in their suitability for use in determining GFR [2]. An example in hydronephrosis is shown in Fig. 6.3.

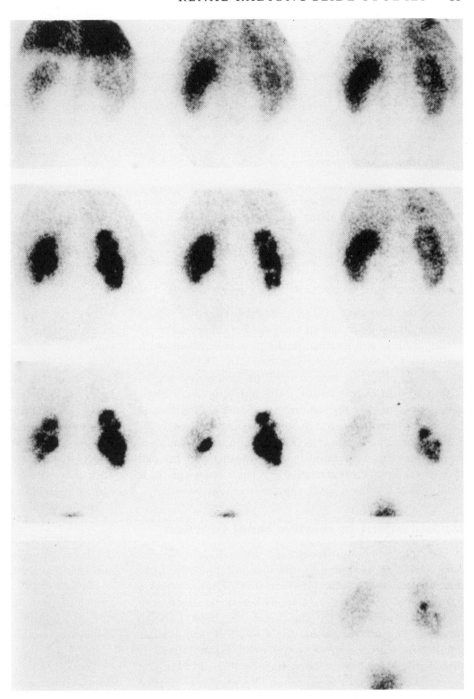

Fig. 6.3 Bilateral hydronephrosis [^{99m}Tc] DTPA study. Images: top line, 30 s, 60 s, 90 s; next line, 10 min, 5 min, 120 s; next line, 15 min, 20 min, frusemide injection, 25 min; bottom line, 35 min, 30 min. No obstructive nephropathy or obstructing uropathy. Parenchymal transit times were normal.

[^{99m}Tc] MAG$_3$

MAG$_3$ has become the standard agent for urological studies [20–23]. It is over 90% weakly protein bound in plasma so it is hardly filtered at all and is tubularly secreted, but not as avidly as ^{131}I-OIH. Its rate of clearance is similar to ^{131}I-OIH but its volume of distribution is much smaller so its clearance is less. It is related to ^{131}I-OIH as follows: ^{131}I-OIH clearance = MAG$_3$ clearance $\times$ 1.5 + 40 ml/min (SEM 8%).

Note that if the volume of distribution is not measured,

as in the Gates' method [24], MAG$_3$ clearance is very similar to ^{131}I-OIH clearance. [^{99m}Tc] MAG$_3$ clearance is about twice that of [^{99m}Tc] DTPA clearance.

[^{99m}Tc] MAG$_3$ is prepared by adding [^{99m}Tc] pertechnetate generator elute to the MAG$_3$ kit, followed by boiling the vial for 10 min in a water bath. After cooling, the contents of the vial can be taken up into four or five separate syringes. These are sealed with blind hubs and put in the freezer compartment (0–4°C) of the radiopharmacy refrigerator. In this state, the rate of production of a lipophyllic impurity which goes to the liver is reduced over a 100-fold [25]. The MAG₃ can thus be used over 8 h and not within 30 min as advised by the manufacturer. When the patient arrives, the MAG₃ syringe can be thawed under a table lamp and be ready to use by the time the patient is ready. If the preparation is poor, liver uptake will be seen. If renal function is poor, stomach activity may be seen.

[⁹⁹ᵐTc] ethylene dicysteine

This new compound has less protein-binding ability than [⁹⁹ᵐTc] MAG₃ and a higher extraction efficiency—about 71% as compared with about 66% for MAG₃ [26,27]. It does not require a boiling step. It is not yet available commercially.

[⁹⁹ᵐTc] dimercapto succinate acid

Dimercapto succinate acid (DMSA) labelled with ⁹⁹ᵐTc is a representative of a class of compounds that are taken up by the kidneys and retained in the proximal tubules with less than 5% being excreted in the urine if the correct preparation procedure is used and if the compound is used within 20 min of preparation. Without using an air bleed needle, 1–6 ml [⁹⁹ᵐTc] sodium pertechnetate solution is introduced into the kit and the vial is shaken vigorously for 8 min. It may be stored at 4°C but should be used as soon as possible. The compound binds to plasma proteins and then is taken up by filtration and tubular reabsorption. If renal function is poor, uptake by the liver may be seen.

Measurement of relative renal function

In the 'intact nephron hypothesis', Bricker [28] proposed that 'surviving nephrons of the diseased kidney largely retain their essential functional integrity'. Thus, whether a tubule is damaged or a glomerulus is damaged, the hypothesis implies that the whole nephron fails to function. For this to be so, the GFR, RPF and tubular uptake and secretion must be indissolubly interrelated. If this is true, then the filtration fraction (GFR/RPF) of one kidney is equal to that of the other. This may be confirmed experimentally [29]. Thus if one sets out the problem 'what is the GFR of the left kidney?' (Table 6.1), then the answer 20 ml/min is self-evident.

This result in turn implies that the percentage contribution of one kidney to total function is the same whether a

Table 6.1 Intact nephron hypothesis.

	Left kidney	Right kidney	Left % total
GFR (ml/min)	?	80	?
ERPF (ml/min)	100	400	20%
Filtration fraction	?	0.2	

glomerularly filtered agent or a tubularly fixed agent is used. That this is generally true has been confirmed many times using pairs of the following: ¹³¹I-OIH, [⁹⁹ᵐTc] DTPA and [⁹⁹ᵐTc] DMSA.

Finally, the hypothesis implies that functioning nephrons are working in a similar way whichever kidney they are in. This may be demonstrated by:
1 the fact that the peaks of a pair of normal renograms occur at the same time;
2 the fact that a kidney with half the normal number of nephrons (e.g. due to pyelonephritis) has a peak to its kidney curve at the same time as that of the contralateral normal kidney (in the absence of a renovascular disorder), although, of course, the amplitude of the kidney curve is less;
3 the similarity of the total and intrarenal flow distribution in the left and right kidney in essential hypertension [30].

It may be noted that situations where the intact nephron hypothesis does not hold may be created in order to investigate the control mechanism, as shown by unsteady-state conditions and by experimental alterations of the intrarenal flow distribution of one kidney only. The mechanism on which the intact nephron hypothesis is based includes tubuloglomerular balance and autoregulation. The importance of the intact nephron hypothesis is that it does not matter whether [⁹⁹ᵐTc] DTPA, [⁹⁹ᵐTc] MAG₃ or [⁹⁹ᵐTc] DMSA is used to measure relative renal function; under steady-state conditions and within experi-mental error they will give the same measurement of percentage contribution of one kidney to total renal function.

The most important measurement made using radionuclides is that of the contribution of each kidney to total renal function. This is obtained by determining the relative uptake of tracer by each kidney, which, depending on the radiopharmaceutical used, gives a direct measure of the fraction of ERPF or GFR of each kidney. The uptake by a kidney per unit time, $Q(t)$, is given by the product of the RPF, the plasma concentration of tracer $P(t)$ and the kidney's extraction efficiency E. Thus:

$$Q(t) = RPF \times P(t) \times E.$$

Considering separately the left (L) and right (R) kidneys:

$$Q(t)_L = RPF_L \times P(t) \times E_L,$$

$$Q(t)_R = RPF_R \times P(t) \times E_R$$

and dividing:

$$Q(t)_L / Q(t)_R = (RPF_L \times E_L)/(RPF_R \times E_R).$$

For I-OIH, $(RPF \times E)$ is known as the ERPF; and for DTPA, the extraction by the kidney is given by the fraction of RPF that is filtered: GFR/RPF. Thus, rearranging:

$$Q(t)_L/\text{total } Q(t) = ERPF_L/\text{total ERPF}$$
$$\text{or } GFR_L/\text{total GFR}.$$

From the intact nephron hypothesis, in steady conditions, the fraction $Q(t)_L$/total $Q(t)$ is the same whether a filtered agent such as [^{99m}Tc] DTPA or a secreted agent such as ^{131}I-OIH is used. It gives the fraction that one kidney contributes to total renal function. This fraction is more conveniently expressed as a percentage of the total.

The amount of radioactivity in the kidney, $Q(t)$, must be determined after adequate mixing in the circulation, usually after about 1.5 min, and before any has been lost through the kidney, usually about 2.5 min. Therefore the measurement of the value of $Q(t)$ is taken from each of the activity–time curves obtained for ROIs set up around each kidney, for example at 2 min. If renal function is poor or there is inflow or outflow obstruction, the timing of $Q(t)$ should be delayed until the ratio $Q(t)_L$/total $Q(t)$ becomes approximately constant, which may be as long as 6 min. Thus the percentage contribution of each kidney to total renal function is obtained. The normal variation is 42.5–57.5% of total function in each kidney and the error on the measurement is of the order of 7%, partly due to variation between the depths of each kidney. This assessment of relative renal function can be applied to any measure of overall renal function such as the single shot ERPF or GFR.

Relative renal function: usage in urology

The contribution of one kidney to total function cannot be estimated from X-ray contrast images [31,32] because their high black and white contrast is the antithesis of a grey scale. The thinness or thickness of the cortex of a kidney is so variable along its length that it is a very poor guide to function. Typically, a thin mid-section of the kidney in hydronephrosis is associated with normal-functioning nephrons at one or both poles. Thus the use of radionuclides is essential before surgery to the kidney. A restorative operation is usually indicated in adults if more than 20% of total renal function is present in a kidney with hydronephrosis, stone or renovascular disorder, whereas a nephrectomy is usually performed if less than 8% of total function remains in such a kidney, as it is unlikely for such a kidney to recover function. The percentage uptake should rise gradually after successful treatment to one kidney, assuming unchanging function in the other. The rate of improvement will depend on many factors, such as the age of the patient and the length of time that an obstruction has been present before its successful relief.

It should be noted that the uptake function is made up of two components: (i) an irreversible component which depends on the number of nephrons present and which can only change for the worse when there is destruction of nephrons, for example by infection or tumour; and (ii) a reversible component in which nephron function, such as ERPF and GFR, falls as a physiological response to some pathological process causing inflow or outflow disorder, to rise again when such a process is corrected.

To take an example, a stone obstructing the renal outflow tract will lead to a reduction in GFR through its normal physiological response to a rise in tubular and pelvic pressure; but when the stone is removed, this pressure falls and the GFR returns towards normal and may even overshoot, leading to a postoperative diuresis. However, if the obstructing stone is associated with infection in the kidney, that infection may cause nephron damage and thus loss of functioning nephrons. Such a loss of nephrons will not be made up when the infection is treated by removal of the stone and antibiotic administration, so that component of uptake function will not improve. Measurement of relative renal function cannot distinguish between these two states, but generally, the poorer the uptake, the less likely is its reversibility.

Obstructive nephropathy and uropathy

Obstructive nephropathy is the effect on renal function of an obstructing process involving the outflow tract. Assessment of its presence or absence is crucial in evaluating the need for, and timing of, surgery. An apparently obstructing process which is not affecting renal function may be reasonably watched until such time as it has resolved or until such time as evidence of the initiation of impairment of renal function is obtained. This in turn requires that a sensitive index of renal function is available for monitoring progress. Whereas previously the relative uptake function of a kidney was used as this guide, it is not sensitive enough since, for example, a kidney that is evidently completely obstructed may have normal uptake function initially. The PTTI, which is based firmly on the pathophysiology of renal outflow obstruction, is a more sensitive index of obstructive nephropathy than the uptake function and is now used in this context.

Obstructive uropathy is the effect of an obstructing process on the outflow tract. Typically, dilatation of the outflow tract proximally and the nature of the obstructing process are visualized using IVU or ultrasound. Nevertheless, these features of obstructive uropathy are static in time. When a dynamic test of the continuing presence or otherwise of the obstructing process is undertaken, for example, by antegrade perfusion pressure measurement or frusemide IVU and active obstruction to outflow is confirmed, then the term 'obstructing' uropathy is preferred by some to 'obstructive' uropathy. An obstructing process that causes a resistance to outflow sufficient to cause a rise in pressure in order to maintain urine flow is an obstructing uropathy and needs correction. If resistance to outflow is insufficient to cause a pressure rise then there is no obstructing process. In this way the meaningless phrase 'partial obstruction' is obviated.

Thus there are two fundamental processes in outflow obstruction, the resistance to outflow and the rise in pressure. The degree of resistance to outflow may be tested objectively either by the antegrade perfusion pressure method or by frusemide diuresis, whether combined with urography or with radionuclide studies. The rise in pressure may be very small but it is not 'back pressure', for pressure is equal in all directions. It arises because continuing cardiac output and glomerular filtration provide a force against which significant resistance to outflow causes a pressure rise, the consequence of which is that the pressure gradient from glomerulus to the site of resistance falls less steeply than in the absence of such a resistance to outflow. The physiological consequences of this alteration in the pressure gradient enable the presence of an obstruction to be assessed using the PTTI.

Physiological basis

Tubuloglomerular balance is the term used to describe the interrelationship between tubular reabsorption and glomerular filtration. The more salt that is filtered, the more salt is reabsorbed in proportion. The proximal tubular reabsorption of salt and water occurs in two main ways: (i) by active transport through the cell, under the control of natriuretic hormones; and (ii) by passive movement through the 'tight' junctions and along the intercellular spaces.

Fromter et al. [33] demonstrated in the rat kidney that up to 60% of filtered salt and water could be reabsorbed passively. In the human, a smaller percentage of the filtered salt and water reabsorbed by the tubule depends on passive forces. Earley and Friedler [34] demonstrated the importance of peritubular capillary pressure in the control of salt and water reabsorption. The many studies in this field [35] demonstrate that a fall in peritubular capillary pressure relative to intratubular pressure enhances salt and water reabsorption (as occurs in renovascular disorder) and that a rise in intratubular pressure relative to peritubular capillary pressure similarly enhances salt and water reabsorption (as occurs with resistance to outflow).

One consequence of both situations is that the rate of tubular movement of a non-reabsorbable solute is slower than before, and thus the renal parenchymal transit time of such a solute is prolonged. Therefore, prolongation of the parenchymal transit times of the radioactively labelled non-reabsorbable tracers [99mTc] MAG$_3$ and [99mTc] DTPA is a clear indication of a raised intrarenal and pelvic pressure consequent on the presence of significant outflow obstruction. Such prolongation of nephron transit time in the presence of outflow obstruction is well established in stop–flow studies in animals where lissamine green was used as the non-reabsorbable solute [36].

In this way the problem of the diagnosis of outflow obstruction is transduced into that of measuring parenchymal transit time [37,38] and the PTTI. A normal PTTI excludes obstructive nephropathy. A prolonged PTTI may be due to either renal ischaemia or to obstructive nephropathy. In the former, the pelvic transit time is normal as there is no outflow disorder whereas, in the latter, the pelvic transit time and thence the whole kidney transit time is prolonged due to any outflow disorder (see Fig. 6.2). When both the PTTI and the pelvic transit time are more prolonged than normal there is obstructive nephropathy.

The kidney contains two populations of nephrons. The cortical nephrons mainly conserve salt and have the property of autoregulation, that is the ability to maintain a constant renal bloodflow and GFR in the face of physiological changes in blood pressure [39]. Cortical nephron autoregulation depends on the renin-containing juxtaglomerular apparatus. The juxtamedullary nephrons mainly conserve water and their bloodflow is directly related to the prevailing perfusion pressure. Loss of the non-autoregulating juxtamedullary nephrons, 'obstructive atrophy', is a typical consequence of a persistent pressure rise due to a prolonged increase of outflow resistance, and causes a loss of urinary concentrating ability.

Parenchymal transit time index

The technical, physiological and analytical basis for obtaining the PTTI has been described above and in Fig. 6.2. The normal range is from 40 to 140 s and a normal kidney has a PTTI of about 70 s. There is a borderline range from 140 to 156 s and PTTI is abnormal if it is over 156 s. These ranges apply to an obstructing process sited at the pelvis and proximal ureter. If the obstructing process is thought to be in the distal ureter or ureterovesical junction, then, empirically, the normal range has been found to be 0–125 s and an abnormal PTTI is over 130 s [38,40,41]. This may be due to the effect of the extra capacity and compliance of the obstructed ureter reducing the pressure gradient slightly as compared with an obstructing process at the pelviureteric junction.

In the presence of a suspected obstruction, the PTTI is much more sensitive than the uptake function and becomes abnormally prolonged even when the uptake function is still in the normal range. This is partly because the PTTI is more directly dependent on the physiological consequence of obstruction than the uptake function, and partly because the uptake function has some error in its measurement due mainly to biological variation and to differences in renal depths in any individual. As PTTI is only time dependent, its measurement is much less influenced by structural and geometrical problems. In particular the part of a kidney overlapped by a dilated pelvis can be ignored since (in the absence of obstruction of a single dilated calyx) the parenchyme of any part of a kidney is representative of the whole, following the intact nephron hypothesis.

In the presence of outflow obstruction when both the PTTI is abnormally prolonged and the uptake function is reduced, then the PTTI becomes normal before an improvement is seen in uptake function. The adaptation to the slight reduction in pressure following relief of obstruction appears to be quicker than the 'autoregulatory' adaptation of the cortical nephrons. However, one proviso is that if the kidney has been rendered ischaemic by renal artery clamping during surgery for a difficult stone, then reduction of the PTTI to normality may take months instead of the usual few days to 3 weeks after surgery. The use of these two measurements is summarized in Table 6.2.

The pelvic transit time is normally of the order of 20–50 s [42]. Any cause of dilatation of the renal pelvis or ureter, whether due to previous obstruction to outflow now relieved, disease or previous surgery or due to present obstructing uropathy, will cause a prolongation of pelvic transit time due to the effects of turbulence of urine flow, mixing and eddying in these circumstances. Thus prolongation of the pelvic transit time does not help in the diagnosis of whether obstruction to outflow is or is not present. The WkTTI is given by the sum of the PTTI and the pelvic transit time (see Fig. 6.2). Prolongation of the WkTTI in the presence of a normal PTTI is of no clinical significance.

Use of diuretics

One way to test the degree of resistance due to a renal outflow disorder is by the induction of a diuresis. A trivial outflow resistance would be overcome by a diuresis and thus would be classified as non-obstructing (Fig. 6.3); whereas a diuresis would be ineffective if there were a significant resistance to outflow, and the outflow resistance would be classified as obstructing [15,43]. Unfortunately, three factors mitigate against the precision of this classification.
1 The degree of diuresis depends on the number of

nephrons, the state of the circulation and their response to the diuretic.
2 The effect of the diuresis depends on the capacity and compliance of the pelvis.
3 The resistance to outflow is a graded phenomenon ranging from the trivial to the severe with no definite cut-off point between.

Frusemide is the favoured diuretic since its dose–diuretic response curve does not level off in normally perfused kidneys. The higher the dose administered, the greater the response. A typical adult dose is 0.5 mg/kg body weight or 40 mg given intravenously, or 1 mg/kg body weight, up to 20 mg, for children. It is normally given at 18 min or more after the injection of a tracer; however, it is given at 30 min if there is gross ureteric dilatation. Its site of action on the nephron is the thick ascending limb (THAL) of the loop of Henle. The THAL has a unique property in the nephron in that it is the only site where the absorption of salt occurs without water, for the THAL is impermeable to water. Salt transport is active and depends directly on an active non-adenosine triphosphatase (ATPase) dependent chloride pump. The increased concentration of salt in the interstitium, which exerts an osmotic pressure, is the basic force on which the medullary concentration gradient and the conservation of water depend. Frusemide specifically inhibits this active salt transport making it a potent diuretic [44].

The diuresis induced simulates the situation seen with the antegrade perfusion pressure test [45]. The rise in pressure may be manifest as a radiologically demonstrable dilatation of the pelvis [46], as a failure to wash radioactive tracer out of the pelvis, or as a failure to cause a fall in the renal activity–time curve determined from ROIs over the kidney in the gamma camera-linked computer display [47,48] (Fig. 6.4).

There have been several attempts to quantitate the change in the radionuclide activity–time curve in response to frusemide. These include measuring the time for the activity to fall by various percentages and replotting the half-life of the falling curve on semilogarithmic paper. Kidneys with upper urinary tract dilatation have a half-life of under 10 min if not obstructed and over 20 min if obstructed, with an equivocal range in between [49]. In children, in particular with dilated ureters, an ROI should be set over the lower ureter as well as over the kidney so that a frusemide response is seen both in the ureter and the kidney. This enables the effect of reflux to be detected, or alternatively the response to voiding may be assessed. The main source of error is due to poor renal function when an insufficient diuresis may be obtained [50]. The level of renal function at which an unreliable response occurs varies, but if the kidney with the dilated outflow tract contributes less than 15% to total renal function, then a poor activity — time curve response to frusemide may not

Table 6.2 Relative uptake function and parenchymal transit time index (PTTI) in patients with renal outflow disorders.

Uptake	PTTI	Interpretation
Normal	Normal	No obstructive nephropathy
Reduced	Normal	Previous loss of nephrons No present obstructive nephropathy
Normal	Prolonged	Obstructive nephropathy present No reduction in nephron population
Reduced	Prolonged	Obstructive nephropathy present Reduced nephron function Reduced nephron population

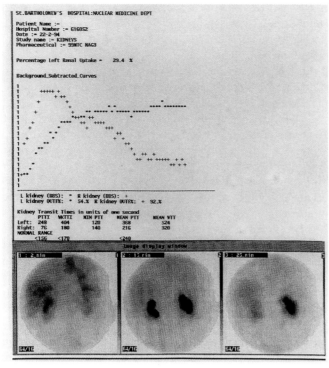

(a)

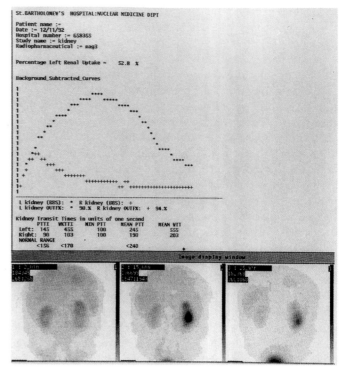

(b)

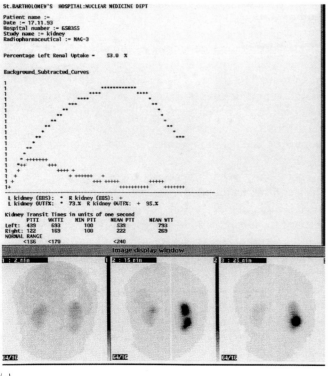

(c)

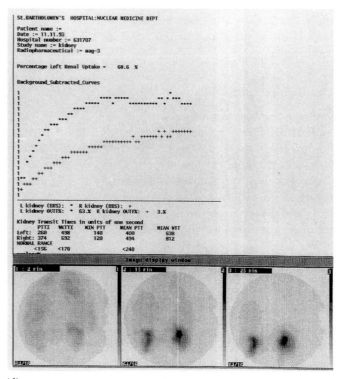

(d)

be due to an obstructing uropathy. The use of the ROE, described above, is designed to overcome this problem by relating the response to frusemide to the level of renal function [18].

A comparison of frusemide diuresis and PTTI has been performed in the same patients. All patients had a dilated outflow tract with uncertainty as to whether outflow obstruction was present [38]. For the final outcome, antegrade perfusion pressure measurement and/or frusemide urography were used to determine the presence of outflow obstruction (Table 6.3).

The study showed that the frusemide diuresis test was simpler to perform and was very satisfactory when a clear answer was obtained. The PTTI was more sensitive to the presence of an outflow obstruction than frusemide diuresis and was able to be used at lower levels of renal function. As the PTTI may be determined in the first 20 min of the renal radionuclide study and the response to frusemide over the next 10 min, a combination of the two techniques during one test, together with the ROE, is now routine and has reduced the number of equivocal results.

Table 6.3 Comparison of the parenchymal transit time index (PTTI) with frusemide diuresis in outflow disorders.

	Outflow obstruction		
	Present	Absent	Uncertain
PTTI*			
Prolonged	35	1	2
Normal	1	24	
Frusemide†			
Positive	30	0	
Negative	6	25	2

*PTTI correct in 59 of 61 cases.
†Frusemide correct in 55 of 61 cases.

Static studies

The anatomy and pathology of the kidney is best demonstrated by structural techniques of IVU, X-ray computed tomography (CT), ultrasound and nuclear magnetic resonance imaging (MRI). It is not very often necessary to obtain static images of the kidneys with radionuclides. However, it is an effective way of demonstrating whether a suspected renal lesion contains normally functioning nephrons or not, particularly within the renal parenchyma which is not well visualized with IVU. The radiopharmaceutical of choice is [99mTc] DMSA. 100 MBq (2–3 mCi) are given intravenously and imaging is performed typically 3 h later. If renal function is good, the imaging may be made earlier, and conversely imaging is delayed if renal function is poor. It is essential to take lateral and oblique views as well as posterior views to demonstrate defects in the renal parenchyma. Image enhancement may be obtained after recording the data in the computer.

Scars in the kidney appear as defects in the cortical outline on the image and these may be seen in chronic pyelonephritis even in the absence of defects in the cortical outline or calyceal clubbing on IVU [51]. Interstitial nephritis may also show defects. Small, often segmental defects are seen in patchy renal ischaemia in children with hypertension and may be taken as evidence of a renovascular disorder [52]. Renal infarcts in adults also cause segmental defects and these will be evident before indentation of the cortical outline is seen on IVU.

Masses in the kidney due to tumours, cysts, abscesses or fat cannot be identified in pathological terms, only as a defect in the [99mTc] DMSA distribution [53]. However, defects due to quite small tumours may be demonstrated by computer analysis. Conversely, a renal pseudotumour will have a normal uptake of DMSA at this site, thereby excluding a pathological tumour [54].

Fig. 6.4 (*see left-hand page*) (a) [99mTc] MAG$_3$ study in a patient with left hydronephrosis. The left kidney contributes 29% of total function, has a rising activity–time curve, an outflow efficiency of 54% (normal = >78%) and a PTTI of 248 s (normal = <156 s) and a pelvic transit time of 156 s (WkTTI–PTTI = 404–248 s). This is a typical pattern of left obstructive nephropathy. The right kidney is almost normal but with a slightly irregular third phase, a dilated pelvis (pelvic transit time = 104 s); it has a PTTI of 76 s and an outflow efficiency of 92%, which are normal. (b) [99mTc] MAG$_3$ study in a patient with left hydronephosis. The left kidney appears enlarged and contributes 53% of total function, has a delayed peak to its activity–time curve, an outflow efficiency of 90% after frusemide injection with some retention of activity, a PTTI of 145 s (just below normal) and a pelvic transit time of 310 s. This is a non-obstructive dilated pelvis. The right kidney is normal. As the PTTI was close to the upper limit of normal, the patient was followed-up. (c) [99mTc] MAG$_3$ study in the same patient as (b), 1 year later. The left kidney appears enlarged and contributes 53% of total function, has a delayed rounded peak, an outflow efficiency of 73% after frusemide injection with some retention of activity, a PTTI of 439 s and a pelvic transit time of 254 s. The right kidney remains normal. The left kidney now clearly has an obstructive nephropathy and it was operated upon. The changes due to the obstructive nephropathy are not evident just from observation of the curves and images, but the changes in the indices are diagnostic. (d) [99mTc] MAG$_3$ study in a patient with bilateral stone disease. Both curves rise, the left curve to a plateau and the right curve continuously. The right curve has an outflow efficiency of only 37%, the left one of 63% (normal = >78%), and both PTTIs are prolonged—the right PTTI is 374 s, and the left one 260 s. The right kidney contributed 31% and the left one 69% of total function. There is bilateral obstructive nephropathy, which is more severe on the right side.

[99mTc] DMSA is also used to demonstrate whether there is any residual functioning renal tissue when a kidney cannot be visualized radiologically, and in identifying the position of an ectopic kidney. The relative function of the two kidneys, or, for example, the parts of a duplex or horseshoe kidney, may be obtained by quantitating the counts in the appropriate anterior and posterior ROIs, using the geometric means and making a correction for background activity [55]. This measure of the relative functional masses of the two kidneys correlates with their relative uptake as measured by [99mTc] DTPA or radioiodinated 123I-OIH as predicted by the intact nephron hypothesis.

As [99mTc] DMSA is not, or should not be, evident in urine at 3 h, defects in the parenchyma due to dilated calyces cannot be easily distinguished from defects in the kidneys due to other causes. This is sometimes put forward as a reason for using radiopharmaceuticals such as [99mTc] gluconate or glucoheptonate which are partly bound to renal tissue and partly excreted. However, this mixture of handling responses by the kidneys makes general interpretation of the data obtained from these techniques more difficult and they give a less adequate definition of the renal parenchyme than [99mTc] DMSA. Usually an ultrasound study should precede a DMSA study. The use of [99mTc] DMSA in acute pyelonephritis and in renal transplants is given below.

An alternative approach to taking multiple views of the [99mTc] DMSA scan is through the use of single photon emission computed tomography (SPECT). This instrument, typically a computer-linked gamma camera which rotates totally around the patient, collects data which may be reconstructed to give images of slices of the distribution of radioactivity in the patient. Thus, slices of the kidney in the transverse, coronal and sagittal planes may be imaged free of the background activity of over- and underlying renal tissue [56]. This technique may enhance the demonstration of renal infarcts, scars and space-occupying lesions.

Renal parenchymal disorders

Hypertension

In essential hypertension, the ERPF is reduced equally to each kidney and the cortical nephron flow is reduced, whereas the juxtamedullary nephron flow is maintained. Renal disease that causes hypertension is called a renovascular disorder. Renovascular hypertension may be defined as being present in those patients in whom an occlusive lesion or lesions of the *large* or *small* renal arteries or arterioles are associated with a particular pattern of renal function and in whom angioplasty, surgical repair or bypass of the lesion or nephrectomy relieves the

hypertension. If no surgery is undertaken the diagnosis must remain in doubt, although the functional pattern may be typical. The crux of the matter is whether successful surgery to one or both kidneys will cause relief of hypertension.

The physiological consequence of a reduction in perfusion pressure associated with a narrowing of a renal artery or arteriole is increased salt and water reabsorption in the proximal tubules due to the reduction in peritubular capillary pressure relative to the intratubular luminal pressure. Thus [99mTc] DTPA and [99mTc] MAG₃ as non-reabsorbable solutes take longer to traverse the length of the nephrons. The consequence of this is a delay in the peak of the renogram of the kidney with a renovascular disorder relative to that of the other kidney, and a prolongation of the mean transit time of the renal parenchyma. The normal mean transit time is under 240 s. Values over 240 s, together with a normal pelvic transit time, under conditions of normal hydration, are suggestive of a renovascular disorder [57]. A relative prolongation of the mean transit time of one kidney of over 60 s compared with the other kidney is also likely in a unilateral renovascular disorder. An established renovascular disorder is associated with a reduction of uptake function below 42% of the total.

When considering whether a small kidney should be removed because it is thought to be causing hypertension, it is recognized that nephrectomy results in control of hypertension in about 25% of cases. Which 25% is now determinable by demonstrating the prolonged mean transit time or delayed peak of renovascular disorder. Nephrectomy of small kidneys without renovascular disorder will not relieve hypertension. Another requirement is that the other kidney is normal, which requires that it has an ERPF of over 300 ml/min, in order to demonstrate that it has not itself developed a renovascular disorder as a consequence of the hypertension.

Angiotensin II is an important intrarenal regulatory agent that affects autoregulation, reabsorption of salt and the tone of the efferent arterioles of the juxtamedullary nephrons. The oral administration of captopril (25 mg), therefore, is being used as a stress test to expose renovascular disorders. The patient should be off oral diuretics for 3 days as salt depletion predisposes to a hypotensive response to captopril. It is not the induction of hypotension that is the captopril stress but the inhibition of intrarenal and circulating angiotensin-converting enzyme (ACE). Blood pressure is monitored before the administration of captopril and then at 5 min intervals. If the blood pressure falls by 10 mmHg diastolic then the renal radionuclide study is commenced, otherwise it is started an hour after the administration.

If a functionally significant renovascular disorder is present, a number of changes occur. First, the shape of the activity–time curve has a far more impaired second phase, a further delayed peak and maybe no third phase at all. Second, the relatively function tends to fall on the side of the affected kidney. Third, the mean parenchymal transit time increases by more than 10%. If renovascular disorder is not present, then there is no change in the activity–time curve or relative function and the mean parenchymal transit time either remains unchanged or falls slightly [58,59]. A positive captopril study predicts a good response to angioplasty or surgical intervention provided that the other kidney has a normal plasma flow and function. The captopril test can also be used to follow-up patients after intervention to show that there is no evidence of restenosis or to demonstrate restenosis if it occurs.

With the increasing use of captopril and related ACE inhibitors in the management of patients with hypertension, heart failure and/or renal impairment, the captopril test is also being applied to such patients to see if there is a beneficial or adverse effect on renal function. The captopril renogram is compared with the previous baseline and if there is evidence of deterioration in the activity–time curve, function or transit time then it is likely that captopril or other ACE inhibitors will not have a beneficial effect. If, however, there is an improvement as compared with baseline then ACE inhibitors are considered to be of benefit. This is particularly so in diabetic nephropathy [59].

Acute pyelonephritis and other inflammatory disorders

Acute pyelonephritis, particularly in children and young adults, typically causes a star-shaped defect in the renal parenchyma imaged with [99mTc] DMSA. This is due to the microabscesses, but this defect is not seen in every case [60]. The distribution of transit times through the kidney is also disturbed so that the peak of the renogram appears flattened. Both these features recover on resolution of the acute infection and the absence of residual scarring may be confirmed with subsequent [99mTc] DMSA imaging.

The current practice for the demonstration of acute infection by imaging is to use [99mTc] hexamethyl propylene amine oxine (HMPAO)-radiolabelled white cells. The white cells are harvested in 20–30 ml of blood according to the method of Solanki et al. [61] and are labelled with [99mTc] HMPAO. The cells are reinjected and images are taken at 1 h, 3 h and, if necessary, the next morning, including the site of suspected infection and the whole of the abdomen and thorax. Increasing uptake with time at the site of the abnormality is consistent with acute inflammation. It is not specific for infection. [99mTc] HMPAO white cells are normally secreted into the small intestine and caecum, and so images showing bowel activity taken after 4 h are not abnormal. Inflammatory bowel disease will show up on the 1 h images, as will most acute infections. Some chronic bone infections may not be demonstrated and patients who have had long-term antibiotics may have lost the leucotaxins from the site of their infection and therefore no longer attract white cells. Alternative non-specific agents such as [111]In- and 99mTc-radiolabelled human immunoglobulin G (HIG) have been used [62] as well as 99mTc-labelled monoclonal antibodies against granulocytes [62].

Very recently, a 99mTc-radiolabelled derivative of the antibiotic ciprofloxacin, known as Infecton, has been used to image infection since this antibiotic binds to living bacteria [63]. It is potentially a more specific approach to imaging infection than the use of white cells or HIG since these latter are deposited at any site of active inflammation.

Acute renal failure

Radionuclides have a limited but important role in the management of acute renal failure. The clinical diagnosis, the importance of the nephrogram on IVU and the demonstration of pelvic dilatation by ultrasound in this context are familiar ground. One use of renography is to help distinguish a prerenal from a renal problem. This it cannot do by itself, but if the uptake of tracer by the two kidneys is disproportionately better than one would expect from observations of the concurrent blood urea and serum creatinine, then a prerenal element is very likely. Whether there is a prerenal element or not, good renal uptake shows that potentially recoverable renal function is present, even though oliguria may be profound or persistent.

A second use is to distinguish a prerenal or renal problem from a postrenal one. This depends on the clinical principle that in acute renal failure, a prerenal cause (shock, blood or fluid depletion, septicaemia, etc.) would involve each kidney to the same extent so that the activity–time curves recorded during renography would rise symmetrically. In acute renal failure due to acute glomerulonephritis, the same principle would hold. Only if the acute renal failure was superimposed on pre-existing asymmetrical renal disease would this simple clinical approach break down. Postrenal outflow obstruction due to cancer of the cervix, bladder, prostate, etc., or stones, usually affects one kidney more severely than the other and so the activity–time curves rise asymmetrically. The kidney that was obstructed for longer has the more slowly rising curve due to its poorer uptake function. The distinction between prerenal, renal and postrenal causes of acute renal failure is thus made because activity–time curves rise symmetrically in the former two conditions and asymmetrically in the latter.

It cannot be overemphasized that a continuously rising activity–time curve from a kidney does not of itself mean outflow obstruction as, as described above, it may be due to a prolonged parenchymal transit time of tracer due to ischaemia. When renal function is poor, the use of frusemide to distinguish a renal from postrenal cause is unreliable. ROE helps here. Parenchymal and pelvic transit time studies may be useful down to a GFR of about 8 ml/min.

When bilateral outflow obstruction is diagnosed as the cause of an apparently acute or chronic renal failure, Sreenevasan's dictum applies. From his personal series of over 1000 cases of renal stone disease he demonstrated that one should normally relieve the obstruction of the better functioning kidney first, that is the kidney with the better uptake function as demonstrated by renography [14]. This is primarily because the kidney with the better uptake function recovers more quickly after relief of outflow obstruction than the poorer functioning kidney, so that the clinical situation stabilizes sooner. Which kidney is better functioning is not reliably determined by IVU or ultrasound, as the black and white contrast of IVU does not allow function determination, and cortical thickness is an unreliable guide.

In both prerenal and postrenal causes of acute renal failure, the improvement in function of each kidney may be followed serially. The test is undertaken between dialyses and, being an 'instant' assessment of relative renal function, it is unaffected by recent dialysis.

Renal transplantation

There are many ways of assessing the progress of renal transplants. If radionuclide techniques are to be used, they must be undertaken seriously and frequently with baseline studies after surgery rather than as a last refuge investigation when things go wrong.

The viability of the transplant immediately after surgery is most simply tested by giving an intravenous bolus of 375 MBq (10 mCi) [99mTc] pertechnetate. The blush of activity in the transplant confirms the integrity of the vascular anastomoses. The suitable positioning of a mirror will allow the patient to see for the first time that there is a successfully functioning kidney, with psychotherapeutic benefit. A 'black hole' where the transplant should be indicates a failure of the anastomosis or, less often, a poorly viable kidney with a poor chance of recovery. If some recovery occurs, the final GFR is unlikely to be better than 25 ml/min [64].

The strategy for studying the renal transplant depends on asking two questions: 'Is the transplant's function improving each day?' Failure to continue to improve means that a complication is supervening. This leads to asking, 'Why is the transplant failing to improve?' The first question is usually answered using biochemical tests such as serum and urinary creatinine and sodium tests, although the equilibrium time in the body and the delay in the return of biochemical results may mean that the findings represent those of the previous day. The alternative is to use a simple estimate of ERPF such as the 7–17 min 131I-OIH clearance. An injection of 131I-OIH is given intravenously. The injection site and a corresponding contra-lateral site are monitored to check that the injection is, in fact, intravenous, since many transplant patients have poor veins. Either by taking blood samples at 7 and 17 min or by a continuous recording using a probe over the chest, the results are plotted on semilogarithmic paper and the half-life of the clearance obtained. A reduction in $T_{1/2}$ each day indicates that the transplant is improving, a failure to improve indicating the onset of a problem but not the nature of the problem. Serial monitoring of the perfusion index (PI, see below) is an alternative.

To determine the cause of the failure of a transplant to improve, a study is usually undertaken using [99mTc] MAG$_3$. The computer-linked gamma camera with a medium resolution, low-energy collimator is placed anteriorly over the transplant. A bolus injection of up to 150 MBq (4 mCi) [99mTc] MAG$_3$ is given intravenously. Images are recorded continuously for the first 30 s and then at 2, 5, 10, 15, 20 and 10 min and also from the bladder and catheter bag. In the computer, using a 64 × 64 matrix, data are recorded at one frame per second for 30 s and then at one frame per minute.

Observation of the images enables certain deductions to be made. A normally functioning cadaver transplant will show an early vascular blush with an even distribution of activity, followed by the appearance of activity in the pelvis at about 5 min, and then activity in the bladder and/or catheter bag. In acute tubular necrosis, the vascular blush is maintained but the transit time of the activity through the parenchyma is grossly prolonged so that activity may not be seen in the pelvis or bladder before the end of the study. Acute rejection is demonstrated by a reduction or loss of the early vascular blush, the parenchymal transit time is prolonged but pelvis and bladder activity are evident before the end of the test. The problem is that there is considerable overlap and gradation between these states. To help to distinguish between them, quantitation of the activity–time curves of a vascular site and the transplant are undertaken. An ROI is set over the transplant, over the iliac artery distal to the anastomosis, and over a background region lateral to the kidney. The activity–time curves are superimposed (Fig. 6.5) and the PI [65] is given by the integrated iliac counts per cell to peak × 100, divided by the integrated renal counts per cell to the same peak time. The normal range for the PI is less than 150 but it is not the absolute value but how the value changes with serial studies that is important. The PI falls with an improving situation; it stops falling or rises with complications. An alternative approach is to measure the half-life of the renal activity–time curve after the peak (Fig. 6.5). Lengthening of the half-life indicates deterioration. It must be emphasized

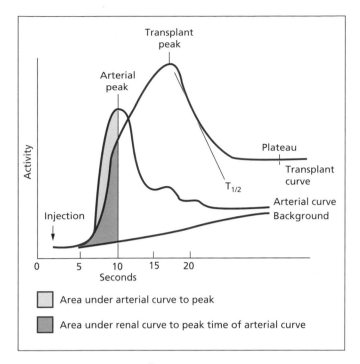

Fig. 6.5 Renal transplant [^{99m}Tc] DTPA activity–time curves.

that the trend of the values is more important than the absolute values. Renal radionuclide studies are more sensitive than Doppler studies for the diagnosis of rejection [66].

Another approach to the diagnosis of rejection has been made with several other radiopharmaceuticals related to the cellular infiltration that accompanies rejection [67]. [^{99m}Tc] colloid is taken up by the phagocytic cells and is normally used to image the liver and spleen. It is taken up by kidneys with established rejection. [^{67}Ga] citrate is carried into the rejecting kidney with white cells but its uptake is not specific. [^{111}In] platelets have been shown to be taken up during acute rejection. Unfortunately, all these tests become positive when rejection is advanced.

Partial infarction due to thrombosis of a branch of a secondary renal artery may be demonstrated as a wedge-shaped defect in a [^{99m}Tc] DMSA renal image. A defect will be seen with an abscess and this may be demonstrated by the uptake of [^{67}Ga] citrate or radiolabelled white cells.

The diagnosis of functionally significant renal artery stenosis as a cause of hypertension in renal transplantation used to be difficult using radionuclides as the previous acute tubular necrosis and rejection episodes directly affect small vessel function. Dubrovsky *et al.* [68] have demonstrated that the effect of RPF measured on and off captopril will distinguish between hypertension due to the native kidneys and that due to the transplant. If the hypertension is due to the transplant, ERPF will fall on captopril administration whereas, if it is due to the native kidneys, it will increase on captopril.

Cyclosporin toxicity cannot be distinguished from rejection as both affect the small vessels in a functionally similar way. However, given the present good donor to recipient transplant matching, a picture of 'rejection' seen in the first few days after transplantation is likely to be due to cyclosporin toxicity. A new agent, [^{99m}Tc] diamino-cyclohexane (DACH), which is cationically transported [69], as is cyclosporin, is starting to be evaluated in this context.

Urinary leakage is usually evident as extravasation of activity outside the normal confines of the renal outflow tract. Lymphoceles may be evident as a defect in activity but are better demonstrated by ultrasound. Urinary obstruction is difficult to determine as some pelvic retention of tracer is normal after ureteric anastomosis. The demonstration of a response of the [^{99m}Tc] MAG$_3$ renal images or activity–time curve to frusemide may be used to exclude significant obstruction, but absence of a response cannot be relied upon. Due to oliguria outflow resistance may be increased without pelvic dilatation and ultrasound may be misleading in this case.

Ureter imaging

The frequency of normal ureteric peristalsis is about 2–4/min. This can be determined by renal radionuclide studies with [^{99m}Tc] MAG$_3$ and the use of a space–time matrix. Up to 10 ROIs are set along the ureters and activity in each region is recorded against time during the study [70–72]. As a bolus of activity passes, so the activity in successive regions increases. This is displayed as a space–time matrix. Normal antegrade flow is shown as a series of downward sloping lines (spindle slopes), and retrograde flow as upward sloping lines. The conclusions from such studies are that ureteric peristalsis is very variable in the normal and abnormal ureter. Spindle frequency is not proportional to urine flow but spindle slope is proportional to bolus speed. Bolus size increases with urine flow rate. Episodes of 'hesitancy' or 'closure' may occur with cessation of peristalsis. Retrograde con-duction is often seen after ureteric surgery. Ureteric func-tion is particularly disordered with urinary infection but the disordered peristalsis is not different from what may occur in normal people and is not specific for infection.

The pain of ureteric colic is not due to hypercontraction of ureteric muscle against a stone. The consequences of increasing resistance to flow are an increasing frequency of ureteric peristalsis with a *decreasing* amplitude until peristalsis stops. At the same time there is an increase in the basal pressure with distension of the ureter. This distension is interpreted by the brain as colic fluctuating over several minutes, because of accommodation by the brain to the contrast stimulus as described by Sherrington in 1902 [29].

Bladder imaging

Vesicoureteric reflux

The advantages of radionuclide assessment of vesico-ureteric reflux are: (i) the low radiation dose, of the order of 10–100 times less than that from X-ray micturating cystography in children, so that serial studies may reasonably be performed; and (ii) that, using the indirect technique, catheterization of the bladder may be avoided, particularly in children in whom it may be physically and psychologically traumatic. Its main disadvantage is lack of structural detail. Thus it is proposed that, when micturating cystography is indicated, one X-ray catheter technique is used for anatomical and pathological assessment and a radionuclide study is performed at the same time. Further studies after therapy or surgery may then be undertaken using the indirect catheter-free technique.

In the direct technique, 40 MBq (1 mCi) [^{99m}Tc] colloid in a saline infusion is instilled into the bladder via a catheter. By means of a gamma camera under the supine patient, continuous recording over the kidney, ureter and bladder is made both during infusion of the activity and during subsequent micturition, increasing the chance of eliciting reflux. A good correlation with the findings of X-ray micturition cystography was found [73,74] and, in some cases, renal reflux was detected only by the radionuclide technique and vice versa.

The indirect technique is performed following the normal performance of a [^{99m}Tc] MAG$_3$ dynamic study. The patient is seated on a commode during the study and when the bladder is full of activity, he or she is encouraged to micturate. Renal reflux is detected by the sudden increase in renal activity. The technique is unsuccessful in the presence of renal impairment.

Both techniques are unreliable in detecting minor ureteric reflux but satisfactory in demonstrating renal reflux, which is thought to be more important in the aetiology of renal scarring during growth. Ureteroureteric reflux in a duplex system may also be assessed using appropriate ROIs [75].

Genital imaging

Scrotal imaging

The purpose of scrotal imaging is to avoid operation when it is unnecessary. Imaging of the scrotum is undertaken using a bolus of [^{99m}Tc] pertechnetate which arrives by the vascular system and then diffuses into extracellular fluid. The technique is not as simple as it sounds and attention to detail is required if interpretation of the results is to be reliable.

A sling is taped to each thigh to elevate the scrotum and during static imaging a thin lead shield under the scrotum helps to remove some thigh background activity in the prepubertal boy. In the adult, only abduction of the thighs is required. The penis should be taped back against the abdomen. In boys, a pinhole collimator is attached to the camera to magnify the image. In adults, a parallel hole collimator is satisfactory. In neonates, the technique is unreliable although torsion is the commonest cause of a hard scrotal swelling in this group. In order to separate the images of the two testicles, particularly if there is unilateral swelling, a thin lead strip is placed on the scrotal raphe. A 30 s dynamic study using 375 MBq (10 mCi) [^{99m}Tc] pertechnetate is followed by serial static images over the next 5 min. The indications for imaging are limited to the problem of acute pain or swelling in one half of the scrotum. It is more reliable in excluding acute torsion of the testicle than in confirming it. Clinically evident acute testicular torsion requires immediate surgery without delay for a scan.

In acute testicular torsion, the scrotal image shows a focal defect in the scrotum on the side of the torsion, surrounded by increased peripheral activity in the early stages. In epididymitis, the scrotal contents show increased activity in and around the testis, which has uptake equal to the contralateral testis. Alternative infrequent causes of a reduced uptake in the region of the testis are those of abscess and trauma where the history is different. The findings are summarized in Table 6.4 [76]. The assessment

Table 6.4 Scrotal imaging.

Condition	Dynamic study	Static images
Normal	Normal	Normal uptake equal in each testis
Complete torsion	Decreased flow relative to iliac artery	No uptake in testis
Partial torsion	Decreased flow	Increased uptake in affected testis
Trauma	Normal flow	Focal area of reduced or increased activity
Acute epididymitis	Increased flow	Increased uptake by affected testis
Chronic epididymitis	Normal flow	Reduced uptake focally
Neoplasm	Increased flow	Large testis with variable uptake
Hydrocele	Normal flow	Testis shows normal uptake with an environment of reduced uptake

of epididymal outflow obstruction is not possible with currently available radiopharmaceuticals.

Penile bloodflow

Phallography has been shown to be an effective way of distinguishing psychological impotence from vascular impotence. Vasogenic impotence can also be divided into

that due to inadequate arterial supply and that due to venous leakage (Fig. 6.6) using the radionuclide technique [77,78].

Prostate imaging

The key requirement in prostate cancer assessment is the demonstration of whether nodes are involved local to the

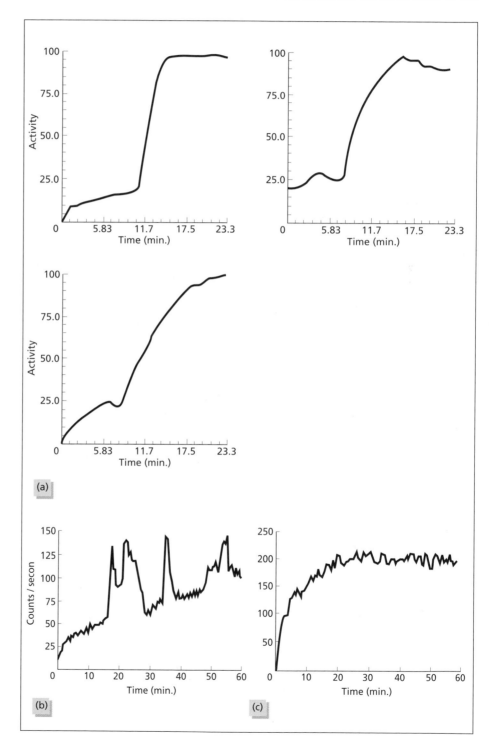

Fig. 6.6 (a) Stimulated radionuclide phallograms. Top left: normal response to intracavernous prostaglandin E with a rapid rise to a plateau. Centre left: impaired response typical of arterial vascular insufficiency with a slow rising curve. Top right: impaired response typical of arterial and venous insufficiency with a slow rising curve that starts to fall due to venous leakage. (Courtesy of *Nuclear Medicine Communications* and Dr Q.H. Siraj.) (b) Unstimulated radionuclide phallograms. There is a characteristic saw tooth pattern from the flaccid penis indicating normality. (c) Unstimulated radionuclide phallogram. There is no saw tooth pattern. The curve rises slowly and starts to fall indicating both arterial and venous vascular insufficiency. (Courtesy of *Nuclear Medicine Communications* and Dr Q.H. Siraj.)

prostate cancer. If even one node is involved the 5-year survival falls from about 85% to under 40%. X-ray, CT and MRI, which distinguish involvement in relation to size, have been shown to be relatively inaccurate as many nodes smaller than 1 cm diameter may be involved. Recently, monoclonal antibodies reacting with a prostate-membrane antigen have been labelled with [111]In [79,80] and [99m]Tc [81] to image primary prostate cancer and its related nodes using SPECT. Some success in this approach in detecting involved nodes has been obtained. Recurrent prostate cancer may also be demonstrated.

Bone imaging

Imaging the skeletal system with radionuclides has become a routine technique. In genitourinary surgery, bone imaging may provide answers to a number of questions. Is the skeleton free of metastases from genitourinary carcinoma or is there good evidence of skeletal metastases? If the latter, how are these responding to chemotherapy? Is there evidence of renal azotaemic osteodystrophy?

Physiological basis

The advantage of radionuclide imaging of bone over X-ray techniques is that it depends on the normality or otherwise of bone metabolism and this is more sensitive to bone disorders. In lumbar vertebrae, a 30% or more change in bone density has to occur due to disease before radiological change is evident on conventional views. Thus bone imaging is more sensitive but it is much less specific than radiology as many different causes of bone pathology will give the appearances of the same disorder of bone function.

The current radiopharmaceutical for bone imaging is ^{99m}Tc] methylene disphosphonate (MDP). The uptake of ^{99m}Tc] MDP depends on three factors: (i) the blood supply; (ii) the amount of extracellular fluid (ECF); and (iii) the osteoblastic activity.

$$\text{Blood supply} \rightleftharpoons \text{ECF} \rightarrow \text{Osteoid undergoing mineralization.}$$

In metastases due to carcinoma and sarcoma there is a combination of increased blood supply, local oedema and increased osteoclastic activity which is compensated for by increased osteoblastic activity leading to a focal area of increased uptake at the site of the disease. In patients with malignant disease of tissues normally present in the bone marrow, such as lymphoma or myeloma, the local inflammatory response is much less and, for example, in the pure lytic lesions of myeloma there may be no osteoblastic response and no visualization of abnormality on the bone scan. The uptake of the bone-imaging agent is critically dependent on the level of overall renal function, since over 50% of the agent is excreted in the urine. With renal impairment, both the non-bone tissue background and the uptake by bone will increase. The newer bone-imaging agents have been chosen because their more rapid renal clearance reduces this tissue background, thereby enhancing the normal signal:noise, bone:non-bone ratios. The kidneys are normally visualized on a bone scan and some major renal problems may be identified: the relative sizes and positions of the kidney, a focal defect due to a large space-occupying lesion including a calculus, loss of a part of the kidney due to an infarct or scarring, and pelvic and/or ureteric retention of tracer indicating the need for ultrasound. Minor calyceal retention of activity is commonly seen and appears to be of no significance. Bladder diverticula, extrinsic pressure on the bladder (e.g. from the uterus or prostate) and even space-occupying lesions may be demonstrable. In addition, activity is seen in ileal loops after ureteric diversion, in catheters and in collecting bags.

In severe renal disease, metastatic calcification may also be demonstrated. Two forms of renal osteodystrophy may be distinguished by bone imaging, although both may coexist and be related to the duration of dialysis. In both the 24 h uptake of ^{99m}Tc] MDP is increased above normal [82]. In the hyperparathyroid form with fibrous osteitis, increased uptake is seen mainly in the long bones whereas, in renal osteomalacia, increased uptake is mainly noted in the region of the joints, particularly of the fingers and in the costochondral junctions. In both conditions the renal images may be poorly seen due to the competition from the increased bony uptake. Avascular necrosis of the femoral head may be visualized on a three-phase bone scan.

Techniques and interpretation

[99m]Tc] MDP is prepared in the nuclear medicine department. No preparation is required for the patient and the injection of about 555 MBq (15 mCi) is given intravenously. The patient is then encouraged to drink fluids and is called back about 3 h after injection. Before imaging, the patient must empty his or her bladder. The patient lies supine on a couch. A composite series of static images are collected anteriorly and posteriorly using the gamma camera. Lateral and oblique views may also be helpful. For hip and limb disorders, a three-phase study is made. Serial images of the region of concern are taken immediately after injection followed by a blood pool image at 10 min and then the images taken at 3 h.

The report of the bone scan includes hard copies of the images and a description of the appearance of the kidneys and of focal and/or general areas of abnormally increased or decreased bone uptake. An interpretation of these findings in the clinical context is then given.

The list of bone diseases that give a focal increase in uptake is long and includes benign bone disease such as local osteoma, sites of fracture (pathological, traumatic, osteoporotic and due to stress), osteomyelitis and granulomatous diseases affecting bone such as tuberculosis, sarcoid and eosinophilic granuloma, and in association with joint disorders. The features of metastases from genitourinary cancer are their multiplicity and their predilection for the spine. A single focal area of increased uptake cannot be taken to represent a metastasis in this context, although that diagnosis is not excluded. In view of the frequency with which genitourinary carcinomas metastasize to the bone, it is cost effective to undertake bone imaging as a routine part of the general investigation of a patient before definitive surgery for cancer is undertaken. This is essential if the prostate-specific antigen is elevated.

Some metastases, particularly those in renal carcinomas, may give a focal defect in bone uptake when bone destruction overwhelms bone repair, surrounded by a ring of high uptake. Such features may also be seen with aseptic or avascular necrosis, with radiotherapy, bone

sequestration in osteomyelitis, and chronic infection (e.g. due to tuberculosis), as well as causes of osteolysis without reaction such as myeloma.

The 'superscan' is a name given to a situation where there is a very high skeletal uptake of [^{99m}Tc] MDP [83]. The vertebral body:soft tissue uptake ratio, normally about 5:1 may be about 15:1 or more. The superscan is typical of widespread metastases in prostatic carcinoma, and although asymmetry in uptake may be seen, this is not always the case. The increased uptake may be partly related to the increased phosphatase activity of the prostatic malignancy. A superscan may also be seen in acute renal failure and in renal osteodystrophy.

Serial studies (Fig. 6.7) well demonstrate the progression of disease or its response to chemotherapy or radiotherapy [84]. It should be noted that with successful therapy the bone scan tends to improve whereas the bone X-ray, often having been previously normal, becomes more abnormal due to recalcification of the destroyed tumour site.

In conclusion, bone scanning is much more sensitive

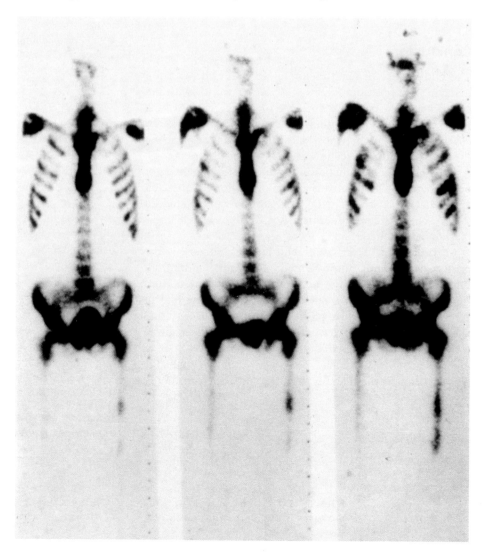

Fig. 6.7 Prostatic carcinoma progression. Bone scans at 6-weekly intervals. Anterior bone scans.

than bone X-rays to the presence of metastases from adenocarcinomas, but less specific as to the particular nature of the pathology. Bone scanning should be a routine part of the staging of genitourinary cancer, and single or equivocal areas should be accompanied by high definition X-rays. The combination of a focal area of increased activity and a normal X-ray is very suspicious of malignancy. When both are positive the X-ray findings should help to distinguish between a degenerative, infective, benign or malignant cause of the abnormality on bone scanning.

^{89}Sr is a therapeutic β-emitting radionuclide which is avidly taken up by bone at sites of high metabolic activity, such as is induced by bone metastases of prostate cancer. It may be given intravenously for therapy of intractable bone pain which is not palliatable by opiates or radiotherapy, and is available commercially as Metastron. Relief of pain occurs in up to 75% of patients and there is some anecdotal evidence of a reduction in recurrence rate in bone [85–87]. ^{153}Sm- and ^{186}Re-labelled bone-seeking agents are also being evaluated.

Conclusion

The clinical use of renal radionuclide studies depends on marrying the concept of 'How well does it work?' with the traditional view of 'What does it look like?'. Thus, asking whether there is a tumour in the right kidney is an anatomical and pathological question best answered using the high-resolution techniques of diagnostic radiology. Asking how much functioning kidney will remain after nephrectomy is performed is a pathophysiological question appropriately answered using the gamma camera. Indeed it may be considered unethical not to obtain such information before operation.

An important objective of genitourinary surgery is the preservation and improvement of renal function. Radionuclides enable the accurate measurement of that function and provide a reliable non-invasive method of assessing the significance of the renal outflow disorder and answer the question as to whether surgical relief is required to preserve renal function. The techniques of nuclear medicine are easy for the patient to undergo and give objective answers to many of the questions commonly presenting to the urologist.

References

1 Smith HW. *The Kidney: Structure and Function in Health and Disease*. Oxford: Oxford University Press, 1951.
2 Carlsen JG, Moller ML, Lund JO, Trap Jensen J. Comparison of four commercial ^{99m}Tc Sn, DTPA preparations for the measurement of glomerular filtration rate. *J Nucl Med* 1980;**21**:126–9.
3 Van Slyke DD, Rhoades CP, Hiller A, Alving AS. Relationship between urea excretion, renal blood flow, renal oxygen consumption and diuresis: the mechanism of urea excretion. *Am J Physiol* 1934;**109**:336–74.
4 Chantler C, Garnett ES, Parson V, Veall N. GFR measurement in man by single injection using ^{51}Cr EDTA. *Clin Sci* 1969;**37**:169–80.
5 Brochner-Mortensen J, Rodbro P. Selection of a routine method for determination of glomerular filtration rate in adult patients. *Scand J Clin Lab Invest* 1976;**36**:35–43.
6 Brochner-Mortensen J. Routine methods and their reliability for assessment of GFR in adults. *Dan Med Bull* 1978; **25**:181–202.
7 Nimmon CC, McAlister JM, Hickson B, Cattell WR. Study of post equilibrium slope approximation in the calculation of GFR using ^{51}Cr EDTA single injection technique. In: *Dynamic Studies with Radioisotopes in Medicine*. Vienna: International Atomic Energy Agency, 1974:249–56.
8 Fisher M, Veall N. Glomerular filtration rate estimation based on a single blood sample. *Br Med J* 1975;**2**:542.
9 Constable AR, Hussein MM, Albrecht MP, Joekes AM. Renal clearance determined from single plasma samples. In: Hollenberg NK, Lange S, eds. *Radionuclides in Nephrology*. Stuttgart: Georg Thieme, 1980:61–6.
10 Tauxe WN, Maher FT, Taylor WF. ERPF estimation from theoretical volumes of distribution of intravenously injected ^{131}I-orthoiodohippurate. *Mayo Clin Proc* 1971;**46**:524–31.
11 Tauxe WN, Dubovsky EV, Kidd T. New formulae for the calculation of effective renal plasma flow by the single plasma sample method. In: Joekes AM, Constable AR, Brown NJG, Tauxe WN, eds. *Radionuclides in Nephrology*. London: Academic Press, 1982:119–24.
12 Constable AR, Hussein MM, Albrecht F *et al*. Single sample estimates of renal clearance. *Br J Urol* 1979;**51**:84–7.
13 Winter CC. *Radioisotope Renography*. Baltimore: Williams & Wilkins, 1963.
14 Sreenevasan G. Bilateral renal calculi. *Ann R Coll Surg Engl* 1974;**55**:3–12.
15 O'Reilly PH, Testa HJ, Lawson RS, Farrar DJ, Edwards EC. Diuresis renography in equivocal urinary tract obstruction. *Br J Urol* 1978;**50**:76–80.
16 Britton KE, Brown NJG. The value of obstructive nephropathy of the hippuran output curve derived by computer analysis of the renogram. In: *The Proceedings of the International Symposium on Dynamic Renal Studies with Radioisotopes in Medicine*. Vienna: International Atomic Energy Agency, 1971:263–75.
17 Nimmon CC, Britton KE, Al-Nahhas A *et al*. Tc-99m MAG$_3$ (mercapto acetyl triglycine), a renal pharmaceutical for routine use. In: *The Proceedings of Dynamic Functional Studies in Nuclear Medicine in Developing Countries*. Vienna: International Atomic Energy Agency, 1989:163-75.
18 Chaiwatatanarat T, Padhy AK, Bomanji J *et al*. Validation of renal output efficiency as an objective quantitative parameter in the evaluation of upper urinary tract obstruction. *J Nucl Med* 1993;**34**:845–8.
19 Elliott AT, Britton KE. A review of the physiological parameters in the dosimetry of ^{123}I and ^{131}I-labelled Hippuran. *Int J Appl Radiat Isot* 1978;**29**:571–3.
20 Taylor A, Eshima D, Fritzberg AR *et al*. Comparison of iodine-131 and technetium 99m MAG3 renal imaging in volunteers. *J Nucl Med* 1986;**27**:795–803.
21 Jafri RA, Britton KE, Nimmon CC *et al*. Tc-99m MAG3:

comparison with I-123 and I-131 orthoiodohippurate in patients with renal disorder. *J Nucl Med* 1988;**29**:147–58.

22 Al Nahhas AA, Jafri RA, Britton KE *et al*. Clinical experience with Tc-99m MAG3, mercaptoacetyltriglycine, and a comparison with Tc-99m DTPA. *Eur J Nucl Med* 1988;**14**:453–62.

23 Pickworth FE, Vivian GC, Franklin K, Brown EF. ^{99m}Tc mercapto acetyl triglycine in paediatric renal tract disease. *Br J Radiol* 1992;**65**:21–9.

24 Gates GF. Glomerular filtration rate, estimation from fractional renal accummulation of Tc-99m DTPA (stannous). *Am J Radiol* 1982;**138**:565–70.

25 Solanki K, Al Nahhas A, Britton KE. Cold Tc-99m MAG3. In: Schmidt HAE, Buraggi GL, eds. *Trends and Possibilities in Nuclear Medicine*. Stuttgart: Schattauer Verlag, 1989:443–6.

26 Jamar F, Stoffel M, Van Nerom C *et al*. Clinical evaluation of kit labelled Tc-99m L,L-ethylene dicysteine in renal transplant patients. *Eur J Nucl Med* 1993;**20**:831 (Abs).

27 Kabasakal T, Turoglu T, Onsel C *et al*. Comparative continuous infusion renal clearance of Tc-99m EC, Tc-99m MAG3 and I-131 OIH. *Eur J Nucl Med* 1993;**20**:831 (Abs).

28 Bricker NS, Morrin PAF, Kime SW. The pathological physiology of chronic Bright's disease. An exposition of the intact nephron hypothesis. *Am J Med* 1960;**28**:77–98.

29 Britton KE, Brown NJG. *Clinical Renography*. London: Lloyd Luke, 1971:60–86, 172–82.

30 Gruenewald SM, Nimmon CC, Nawaz MK, Britton KE. A non-invasive gamma camera technique for the measurement of intrarenal flow distribution in man. *Clin Sci* 1981;**61**:385–9.

31 Saxton MM, Urography. *Br J Radiol* 1969;**42**:321–46.

32 Banner MP, Pollack HM. Evaluation of renal function by excretory urography. *J Urol* 1979;**124**:437–43.

33 Fromter G, Rumrich G, Ullrich KJ. Phenomenologic description of Na^+, Cl^- and HCO_3^- absorption from proximal tubules of the rat kidney. *Pflugers Arch* 1973;**343**:189–220.

34 Earley LE, Friedler RM. Effects of combined renal vasodilation and pressor agents on renal haemodynamics and tubular reabsorption of sodium. *J Clin Invest* 1966;**43**:542–60.

35 De Wardener HE. Control of sodium reabsorption. *Am J Physiol* 1978;**235**:163–73.

36 Rector FC, Brunner FP, Seldin DW. Mechanism of glomerular balance. *J Clin Invest* 1966;**45**:590–602.

37 Britton KE, Nimmon CC, Whitfield HN, Hendry WF, Wickham JEA. Obstructive nephropathy: successful evaluation with radionuclides. *Lancet* 1981;**2**:900–2.

38 Britton KE, Nawaz MK, Whitfield HN *et al*. Obstructive nephropathy: comparison between parenchymal transit time index and frusemide diuresis. *Br J Urol* 1987;**59**:127–32.

39 Britton KE. Renin and renal autoregulation. *Lancet* 1968;**2**:329–33.

40 Whitfield HN, Britton KE, Nimmon CC, Hendry WF. Renal transit time measurements in the diagnosis of ureteric obstruction. *Br J Urol* 1981;**53**:445–8.

41 Britton KE, Nimmon CC, Whitfield HN. The assessment of obstructive nephropathy by parenchymal transit time analysis in patients with a dilated ureter. In: Joekes AM, Constable AR, Brown NJG, Tauxe WN eds. *Radionuclides in Nephrology*. London: Academic Press, 1982:151–4.

42 Britton KE, Nimmon CC, Whitfield HN *et al*. The evaluation of obstructive nephropathy by means of parenchymal retention functions. In: Hollenberg NK, Lange S, eds. *Radionuclides in Nephrology*. Stuttgart: Georg Thieme, 1980:164–72.

43 O'Reilly PH, Lupton EW, Testa HJ *et al*. The dilated non obstructed renal pelvis. *Br J Urol* 1981;**53**:205–9.

44 Burg MB, Green N. Function of the thick ascending limb of Henle's loop. *Am J Physiol* 1973;**224**:659–68.

45 Whitaker RM. An evaluation of 170 diagnostic pressure flow studies of the upper urinary tract. *J Urol* 1979;**121**:602–4.

46 Whitfield HN, Britton KE, Hendry WF, Wickham JEA. Frusemide intravenous urography in the diagnosis of pelvi ureteric junction obstruction. *Br J Urol* 1979;**51**:445–8.

47 Koff SA, Thrall JH, Keyes JWJR. Diuretic radionuclide urography. *J Urol* 1979;**122**:451–4.

48 Stage KH, Lewis S. Use of the radionuclide washout test in evaluation of suspected upper urinary tract obstruction. *J Urol* 1981;**125**:379–82.

49 Ash JM, Kass EM, Gilday DL. Diuretic renal scans in paediatric hydronephrosis. *J Nucl Med* 1979;**20**:623–7.

50 Kletter K, Nürnberger N. Diagnostic potential of diuresis renography limitations by the severity of hydronephrosis and by impairment of renal function. *Nucl Med Commun* 1989;**10**:51–61.

51 Davies ER, Roberts JBM, Meney NM, Seadden G. Renal scintigraphy in pyelonephritis. *Proc R Soc Med* 1971;**64**:63–4.

52 Gordon I, Stringer DA, de Bruyn R *et al*. Technetium 99m DMSA scan—a sensitive index of renal perfusion in hypertension. In: Joekes AM, Constable AR, Brown NJG, Tauxe WN, eds. *Radionuclides in Nephrology*. London: Academic Press, 1982:205–10.

53 Bingham JB, Maisey MN. An evaluation of the use of ^{99m}Tc dimercapto succinate (DMSA) as a static imaging agent. *Br J Radiol* 1978;**51**:599–607.

54 Carty AT, Short MD, O'Connell MA. The diagnosis of renal pseudotumours. *Br J Urol* 1975;**47**:495–8.

55 Taylor A. Quantitation of renal function with static imaging agents. *Semin Nucl Med* 1982;**12**:330–44.

56 Buscombe JR, Hilson AJW, Hall ML *et al*. Looking for renal scans with Tc-99m DMSA SPECT: is it worth it? *J Nucl Med* 1993;**34**:138P.

57 Al Nahhas A, Marcus AJ, Bomanji J *et al*. Validity of the mean parenchymal transit time as a screening test for the detection of functional renal artery stenosis in hypertensive patients. *Nucl Med Commun* 1989;**10**:807–15.

58 Fommei E, Ghione S, Hilson AJW *et al*. Captopril radionuclide test in renovascular hypertension: a European multicentre study. *Eur J Nucl Med* 1993;**20**:617–24.

59 Datseris IE, Bomanji JB, Brown EA *et al*. Captopril renal scintigraphy in patients with hypertension and chronic renal failure. *J Nucl Med* 1994;**35**:251–4.

60 Handmaker H. Nuclear renal imaging in acute pyelonephritis. *Semin Nucl Med* 1982;**12**:246–53.

61 Solanki KK, Mather SJ, Janabi M Al, Britton KE. A rapid method for the preparation of Tc-99m hexametazine labelled leucocytes. *Nucl Med Commun* 1988;**9**:753–61.

62 Pons F, Moya F, Herranz R *et al*. Detection and quantitative analysis of joint activity inflammation with ^{99m}Tc-polyclonal human immunoglobulin G. *Nucl Med Commun* 1993;**14**:225–31.

63 Solanki KK, Bomanji J, Siraj Q *et al*. Tc-99m 'Infecton'—a new class of radiopharmaceutical for imaging infection. *J Nucl Med* 1993;**34**:119P.

64 Sherman RA, Byun KJ. Nuclear medicine in acute and chronic renal failure. *Semin Nucl Med* 1982;**12**:265–79.

65 Hilson AJW, Maisey MN, Brown CB, Ogg CS, Berwick MS.

Dynamic renal transplant imaging with Tc-99m DTPA (Sn) supplemented by a transplant perfusion index in the management of renal transplants. *J Nucl Med* 1978;**19**: 994–1000.

66 Al-Nahhas AA, Kedar R, Morgan SH *et al.* Cellular versus vascular rejection in transplant kidneys, correlation of radionuclide and Doppler studies with histology. *Nucl Med Commun* 1993;**14**:761–5.

67 George EA. Radionuclide diagnosis of allograft rejection. *Semin Nucl Med* 1982;**12**:379–86.

68 Dubrovsky EV, Curtis JJ, Luke RG *et al.* Captopril as a predictor of curable hypertension in renal transplant recipients. In: Bischof-Delaloye A, Blaufox MD, eds. *Radionuclides in Nephrology*. Basel: Karger, 1986:117–23.

69 Padhy AK, Solanki KK, Bomanji J *et al.* Clinical evaluation of Tc-99m diaminocyclohexane, a renal tubular agent with cationic transport: results in healthy human volunteers. *Nephron* 1993;**65**:294–8.

70 Muller-Schauenberg W. The nuclear medicine space–time matrix approach to ureteral motility. In: Lutzeyer W, Hannappel J, eds. *Urodynamics: Upper and Lower Urinary Tract*, Vol. II. Berlin: Springer Verlag 1985:154–67.

71 Lewis CA, Coptcoat MJ, Carter SSC *et al.* Radionuclide imaging of ureteric peristalsis. *Br J Urol* 1989;**63**:144–8.

72 Lepej J, Kliment J, Horak V *et al.* A new approach in radionuclide imaging to ureteric peristalsis using ^{99m}Tc MAG$_3$ and condensed images. *Nucl Med Commun* 1991;**12**:397–417.

73 Maizels M, Weiss S, Conway JJ, Firlit CF. Urological neurology and urodynamics. The cystometric nuclear cystogram. *J Urol* 1979;**121**:203–5.

74 Conway JJ, Kruglik GC. Effectiveness of direct and indirect radionuclide cystography in detecting vesico ureteric reflux. *J Nucl Med* 1976;**17**:81–7.

75 O'Reilly PH, Lawson RS, Shields RA *et al.* A radioisotope method of assessing uretero-ureteric reflux. *Br J Urol* 1978;**50**:164–8.

76 Lopez-Majano V, Salvatore M. Testicular imaging. *Nucl Med Commun* 1981;**2**:221–5.

77 Siraj QH, Bomanji J, Akhtar MA *et al.* Quantitation of pharmacologically-induced penile erections: the value of radionuclide phallography in the objective evaluation of erectile haemodynamics. *Nucl Med Commun* 1990;**14**:445–58.

78 Siraj QH, Hilson AJW, Bomanji J, Ahmed H. A pilot study of flaccid penile blood flow patterns in normal subjects and patients with erectile dysfunction. *Nucl Med Commun* 1993;**14**:976–82.

79 Abdel-Nabi N, Wright GL, Gulfo JV *et al.* Monoclonal antibodies and radioimmunoconjugates in the diagnosis and treatment of prostate cancer. *Semin Urol* 1992;**10**:45–54.

80 Texter JH, Neal CE. Current applications of immunoscintigraphy in prostate cancer. *J Nucl Med* 1993;**34**(Suppl.): 549–53.

81 Feneley MR, Chengazi VU, Kirby RS, Granowska M, Britton KE. Clinical Evaluation of Radioimmunoscintigraphy for Imaging Prostate Malignancy. *Br J Urol* 1996;**77**:373–381.

82 Fogelman I, Bessent RG, Turner JG *et al.* The use of whole body retention of Tc-99m diphosphonate in the diagnosis of metabolic bone disease. *J Nucl Med* 1978;**19**:270–5.

83 Constable AR, Cranage RW. Recognition of the superscan in prostatic bone scintigraphy. *Br J Radiol* 1981;**54**:122–5.

84 Fitzpatrick JM, Constable AR, Sherwood T *et al.* Serial bone scanning: the assessment of treatment in carcinoma of the prostate. *Br J Urol* 1978;**50**:555–61.

85 Lewington VJ, McEwan AJ, Ackery DM *et al.* A prospective randomised double blind crossover study to examine the efficacy of strontium-89 in pain palliation in patients with advanced prostate cancer metastatic to the bone. *Eur J Cancer* 1991;**27**:954–8.

86 Laing AH, Ackery DM, Bayly RJ *et al.* Strontium-89 chloride for pain palliation in prostatic skeletal malignancy. *Br J Radiol* 1991;**64**:816–22.

87 Breen SL, Powe JE, Porter AT. Dose estimation in strontium-89 radiotherapy of metastatic prostatic carcinoma. *J Nucl Med* 1992;**33**:1316–23.

7 Urodynamic Studies of the Lower Tract
J.T.Andersen and S.Walter

Introduction

The general purpose of urodynamic studies is to provide objective and accurate information on the pathophysiology of the lower urinary tract in patients with symptoms suggesting dysfunction of the bladder and/or urethra. Studies of bladder behaviour in the filling phase (cystometry) were reported in the last decades of the nineteenth century. Measurement of pressure and flow was introduced by von Garrelts in 1957 [1], and the last four decades have brought sophisticated electronic computerized equipment for neurophysiological studies of the lower urinary tract.

The widespread interest in the treatment of incontinence and other lower urinary tract disorders led to the formation of the International Continence Society (ICS) in 1971. The society is multidisciplinary, including urologists, gynaecologists, nurses, engineers, geriatricians, physiotherapists, neurologists, neurosurgeons, health economists and any other disciplines with an interest in lower urinary tract dysfunction. The membership of the society now exceeds 1300 people from 38 countries. In 1973 the society realized the global need for uniform standards and terms in order to help clinical investigators compare their results with those from other centres. The ICS has published a series of recommendations which should be used in dealing with lower urinary tract function. The methods, definitions and units in this chapter conform to the standards proposed by the ICS [2].

Terminology

The bladder and urethra may behave differently during the storage and micturition phases. Lower urinary tract dysfunction may be caused by:
1 disturbances of the pertinent nervous or psychological control system;
2 disorders of muscle function;
3 structural abnormalities.

In order to be clinically useful, urodynamic diagnoses should correlate with the patients' symptoms and signs.

Bladder function during storage of urine

This may be described according to: (i) detrusor activity; (ii) bladder sensation; (iii) bladder capacity; and (iv) bladder compliance.

Detrusor activity

Detrusor activity is interpreted from the measurement of detrusor pressure. Detrusor activity may be normal or overactive.
1 *Normal detrusor function.* This is characterized by an increase in bladder volume during the filling phase without a significant rise in pressure (accommodation). No involuntary contractions occur despite provocation.
2 *Overactive detrusor function.* This is characterized by involuntary detrusor contractions during the filling phase, which may be spontaneous or provoked and which the patient cannot completely suppress. Involuntary detrusor contractions may be provoked by rapid filling, alterations of posture, coughing, walking, jumping and other triggering procedures. The term 'unstable detrusor' is used for overactive detrusor function, whether symptomatic or asymptomatic. The presence of uninhibited detrusor contractions does not necessarily imply a neurological disorder. Detrusor hyperreflexia is defined as overactivity due to disturbance of the nervous control mechanisms, i.e. evidence of a relevant neurological disorder.

Bladder sensation

Bladder sensation can be classified broadly as follows.
1 Normal.
2 Increased (hypersensitive).
3 Reduced (hyposensitive).
4 Absent.

Bladder capacity

The term capacity must be qualified. Maximum cystometric capacity is the volume registered during cystometry at which the patient feels he or she can no longer delay micturition in the presence of bladder sensation. The functional bladder capacity (voided volume) is the largest volume assessed from a frequency–volume chart (urinary diary).

Compliance

Compliance indicates the change in volume for a change in pressure ($\Delta V/\Delta p$). At the present time there are insufficient data to define normal, high and low compliance.

Urethral function during storage of urine

The urethral closure mechanism during storage may be normal or incompetent.
1 The normal urethral closure mechanism maintains a positive urethral closure pressure during filling, even in the presence of increased abdominal pressure.
2 The incompetent urethral closure mechanism is defined as one which allows leakage of urine in the absence of a detrusor contraction. Leakage may occur whenever intravesical pressure exceeds intraurethral pressure (genuine stress incontinence) or when there is an involuntary fall in urethral pressure.

The voiding phase

During voiding, the detrusor may be in one of three states.
1 *Acontractile.* The acontractile detrusor cannot be demonstrated to contract during urodynamic studies. Detrusor areflexia is defined as acontractility due to an abnormality of the nervous control.
2 *Underactive.* Detrusor underactivity is defined as a detrusor contraction of inadequate magnitude and/or duration to effect bladder emptying within a normal time span.
3 *Normal.* Normal detrusor contractility effects complete bladder emptying in the absence of obstruction.

Urethral function during micturition may be normal or obstructive, either due to overactivity or mechanical obstruction. The most commonly encountered form of overactive urethral function during micturition is detrusor–external sphincter dyssynergia or detrusor–sphincter dyssynergia describing a detrusor contraction concurrent with involuntary contraction of the urethral and/or periurethral striated muscle.

Urinary incontinence

Urinary incontinence is an involuntary loss of urine which is objectively demonstrable and a social or hygienic problem. The loss of urine through channels other than the urethra is called extraurethral incontinence. Urinary incontinence involves the presence of a symptom, a sign and a condition. The symptom indicates the patient's statement of involuntary urine loss; the sign is the objective demonstration of urine loss; and the condition is the urodynamic demonstration of urine loss.

Urge incontinence

Urge incontinence is the involuntary loss of urine associated with a strong desire to void. It may be subdivided into motor urge incontinence, which is associated with an overactive detrusor function, and sensory urgency, which is not due to inhibited detrusor contractions but reflects bladder hypersensitivity.

Stress incontinence

Stress incontinence is indicated by a patient's statement of involuntary loss of urine during physical exertion. The sign of stress incontinence involves the observation of loss of urine from the urethra with physical exertion (e.g. coughing). The condition of genuine stress incontinence is involuntary loss of urine when the intravesical pressure exceeds the maximum urethral pressure but in the absence of detrusor activity.

Other types of incontinence

Reflex incontinence. This is the loss of urine due to detrusor hyperreflexia and/or involuntary urethral relaxation in the absence of sensation, usually associated with the desire to micturate. This condition is only seen in patients with neuropathic bladder/urethral disorders.

Overflow incontinence. This is the involuntary loss of urine associated with overdistension of the bladder.

Enuresis. This means any involuntary loss of urine. If it is used to denote incontinence during sleep, it should always be qualified with the adjective nocturnal.

Post-micturition dribble and continuous leakage. These are other symptomatic forms of incontinence.

Investigations

History taking

Lower urinary tract symptoms can be based on a variety of functional and structural abnormalities. It is important to assess the symptoms in detail in order to reach a final diagnosis. In general, lower urinary tract symptoms are overlapping and non-specific. Patients with infection can have frequency of urination, as can patients with overactive detrusor function. Conversely, patients with infection and patients with overactive bladder function may be without these symptoms. Normal micturition depends on a normally functioning nervous system and an intact lower urinary tract. Symptoms can be assessed by asking the patient, or perhaps better by having the patient fill in a questionnaire. The questionnaire can review previous urological diseases, a family history of urological disorders, previous surgery, medical diseases, neurological history and current medication. The doctor can then review the positive responses. Nevertheless, a questionnaire will not give the entire history, but it will help highlight and focus on the patient's problems.

After history taking the patient is instructed to fill in a voiding chart at home comprising a diary of micturition and incontinence episodes over 3–7 days.

Voiding charts

Before any invasive diagnostic procedures are undertaken, it is mandatory to get an impression of the patient's fluid intake and voiding habits. This information is easily obtained from the frequency/volume chart. The following variables are registered: the single micturition volume, the average micturition volume, the number of voidings during 24 h and the distribution of the voidings during the day and night. The 24 h diuresis is also registered.

It is very important that the patient is carefully instructed in measuring the fluid intake and the voided volumes. Abnormal voiding patterns may be: small single volumes during the day and night, normal voiding volumes and variable small volumes during the daytime, as well as normal single volumes and increased 24 h volumes. The voiding diary can monitor the effect of medication on renal function and urine production. If the patient also fills in incontinence episodes, one has nearly obtained a full urodynamic examination in a non-invasive way. The voiding chart can also be used for control of treatment and as a part of treatment, for example when using biofeedback or behavioural therapy.

The pad test

Pad testing is a simple objective non-invasive procedure for detecting and quantifying urinary leakage, especially stress urinary incontinence [3]. Several test procedures have been described. The ICS recommended a standardized 1 h pad-weighing test [2] for scientific purposes. It is performed according to Fig. 7.1. The increase in the weight of the pad is a measure of the urine loss. An increase in the weight of the pad of less than 1 g is not considered a sign of incontinence.

The pad-weighing test is useful in screening for urinary

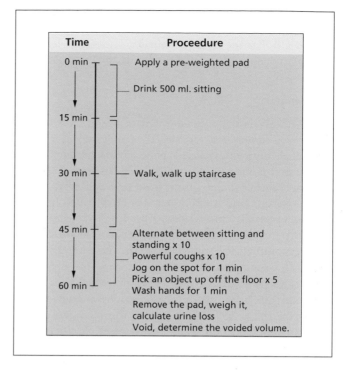

Fig. 7.1 Test schedule for the 1 h pad-weighing test (reproduced from [4] with permission).

incontinence and/or quantifying urine leakage [5]. It helps in the choice of therapy or in assessing treatment outcome. The reliability of the different tests is good. Tests done over longer periods, e.g. 24 hours, are superior to the shorter ones in screening.

Pitfalls are vaginal discharge, voluntary voiding in the pad and excessive perspiration. The pad test should not be performed during a menstrual period.

Other tests

A number of pad-weighing tests have been described with varying duration, fluid load and provocative manoeuvres. A very useful one is performed with a standardized volume of 50 or 75% of the maximum cystometric bladder capacity [6]. Cystometry is first performed, and after the patient has voided the instilled volume the bladder is refilled to 50 or 75% of the capacity and the patient is asked to do the provocative manoeuvres. Some clinics use a longer test of 12, 24 or 48 h. During the examination the patient is asked to change the pad every hour and to do the weighing herself or himself.

Normal values

In continent women, the 1 h pad-weighing test may show a weight gain from 1 to 2 g due to perspiration or fluor vaginalis. In mild urinary incontinence the urine loss is

2–10 g/h; moderate urinary incontinence is a urine loss of 10–50 g/h; and severe urinary incontinence is a loss of more than 50 g/h. For the 24 h home pad test, leakage less than 8 g is not considered to reflect incontinence.

Uroflowmetry

Uroflowmetry is the measurement of the urinary flow by means of a flowmeter. Urinary flow may be described in terms of the flow rate defined as the voided volume per unit of time and is measured in millilitres per second. Besides absolute values for maximum flow rate and average flow rate, important information can also be obtained from the flow curve pattern and whether the flow is continuous or intermittent. The urine flow represents the net outcome of bladder contractility, opening of the bladder neck and urethral conductivity. Several types of electronic flowmeters are available. The two most widely used types are based on either the deceleration of a rotating disk caused by the urine stream where the electrical energy necessary to maintain a constant speed of rotation is proportional to the flow rate, or a gravitational principle using continuous measurement of the weight or volume of the voided urine. Although the sensitivity varies from one flowmeter to another, both types are sufficiently accurate for clinical purposes.

Uroflowmetry must allow measurement of the patient's voiding in privacy, and as artefacts due to inhibition or anxiety during the first measurement are frequently encountered, the performance of multiple flow rates is recommended [7]. Electronic flowmeters for multiple flow measurements in the patient's home are now available.

A diagram of a continuous flow with the recommended ICS nomenclature is shown in Fig. 7.2. Normally, the urine flow rate rises rapidly to a plateau of the maximum flow rate followed by a gradual decline in the flow rate until the bladder is empty. The maximum flow rate (Q_{max}) is the parameter which best differentiates normal people from those with voiding disorders. In men under the age of 40 years, the normal maximum flow rate is greater than 15 ml/s with a continuous reduction in maximum flow rate in the range of 2 ml/s per 10 years of age after the age of 50. In normal females the maximum flow rate is greater than 20 ml/s.

The maximum flow rate is dependent on the voided volume. Q_{max} increases with increasing voided volume up to 150–200 ml, and the reproducibility of Q_{max} is best in the range of voided volumes between 200 and 400 ml. In order to overcome the volume dependency of the registered maximum flow rate, nomograms have been constructed for both men and women [8,9].

Alternatively, a flow clinic can be set up for the registration of multiple voidings in order to circumvent the unreliability of a single flow rate measurement [7]. The residual urine volume is conveniently obtained after uroflowmetry using ultrasound scanning.

Important information can also be obtained from the configuration of the flow curve (Fig. 7.3). A plateau-like (box-shaped) flow curve suggests a rigid urethral obstruction (e.g. urethral stricture). Conversely, a long flow curve with reduced Q_{max} and terminal dribbling is characteristic of an elastic obstruction as seen in benign prostatic obstruction. Intermittent flow curves may suggest either voiding by abdominal straining, poor detrusor contractility or overactive urethral function, such as detrusor–sphincter dyssynergia. However, it must be emphasized that clinical diagnosis cannot be based on flow curves alone. A normal flow curve can never rule out significant dysfunction of the lower urinary tract. Nevertheless, uroflowmetry is an extremely useful non-invasive investigation both for patient screening and follow-up.

Residual urine

The residual urine is the amount of urine left in the bladder after incomplete voiding. The amount of residual urine may vary from a few millilitres to several litres, and in a single person the residual urine volume may vary considerably between voidings. Residual urine is only of clinical significance if it causes symptoms or deterioration of bladder or renal function.

Residual urine is caused by underactive detrusor function either due to poor detrusor contractility as seen in myogenic decompensation or, more often, in conditions with a poorly sustained detrusor contraction, which is most frequently secondary to infravesical obstruction. Other causes of poor detrusor contractility are infrequent voiding or neurogenic bladder dysfunction.

Residual urine volume should routinely be registered

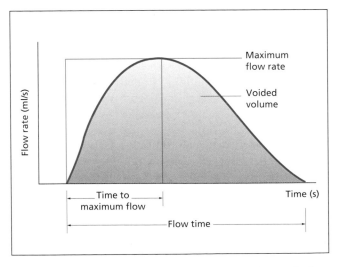

Fig. 7.2 Diagram of a continuous urine flow recording with the ICS recommended nomenclature.

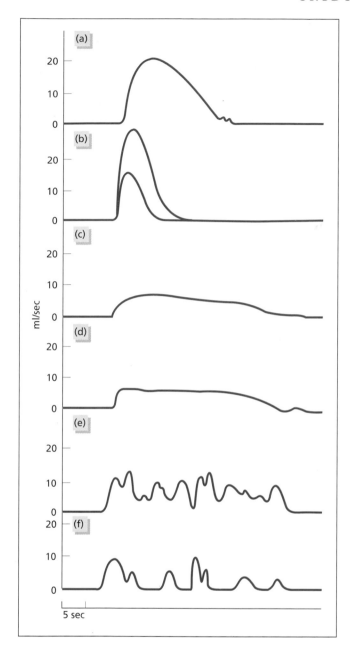

Fig. 7.3 Different configurations of flow curves. (a) Normal male. (b) Normal female (small/larger volume). (c) Prolonged flow curve with reduced maximum flow rate as seen in obstructive benign prostatic hypertrophy. (d) Box-shaped flow curve with reduced maximum flow rate as seen in urethral stricture. (e) Fluctuating flow curve as seen with abdominal straining. (f) Intermittent flow curve as seen in detrusor–sphincter dyssynergia or an underactive detrusor with abdominal straining.

non-invasively by transabdominal ultrasound scanning of the bladder region after voiding. A clinically useful formula for the estimation of residual urine by ultrasound is: height × breadth × depth × 0.7. When more invasive procedures such as cystometry or pressure–flow studies are indicated, the residual urine volume can be obtained by

catheterization. In patients with benign prostatic obstruction, a large day-to-day variation in residual urine volume has been demonstrated [10]. For daily clinical practice, very exact determination of the residual volume is not necessary. Vesicoureteric reflux and larger bladder diverticula may also lead to significant volumes of residual urine.

Cystometry

Cystometry is the method by which the pressure/volume relationship of the bladder is measured during bladder filling. Cystometry is used to assess detrusor activity, bladder sensation, bladder capacity and bladder compliance. The following pressure parameters are recorded during cystometry:

1 P_{ves}: intravesical pressure, that is the pressure within the bladder;

2 P_{abd}: abdominal pressure, that is the pressure surrounding the bladder. The abdominal pressure is usually estimated from rectal or, less commonly, extraperitoneal pressure recorded from the prevesical space;

3 P_{det}: detrusor pressure, that is the component of intravesical pressure which is created by forces in the bladder wall (passive and active);

4 P_{det}: $P_{ves} - P_{abd}$.

Bladder sensation is usually assessed during cystometry by questioning the patient in relation to the fullness of the bladder during cystometry. Commonly used descriptive terms are: volume at first sensation, volume at which urgency occurs and the volume at which the patient feels he or she can no longer delay micturition (maximum cystometric capacity).

Bladder and rectal pressures can be measured either by using fluid-filled lines connected to pressure transducers or by using catheter-tip transducers. For bladder filling, isotonic saline at room temperature or 37°C is most frequently used. The ICS recommends the following terms [2] to be used for the ranges of filling rate.

1 Slow-fill cystometry — up to 10 ml/min.

2 Medium-fill cystometry — 10–100 ml/min.

3 Rapid-fill cystometry — over 100 ml/min.

Medium-fill cystometry is most frequently used, although the filling rate of the bladder is far above physiological filling rates.

The outcome of the cystometric investigation is dependent on several variables such as bladder filling rate, temperature of the filling medium and the position of the patient (supine/sitting/standing). These details should be reported along with the result of the cystometric investigation and taken into consideration in the interpretation of the cystometric findings.

The normal cystometrogram is characterized by the accommodation of the bladder to increasing filling volumes without any significant rise in detrusor pressure. First sensation of fullness usually occurs at 150–200 ml filling volume, urgency at 300–400 ml and maximum cystometry capacity at 350–500 ml. At maximum cystometric capacity, the healthy person is able voluntarily to elicit a detrusor contraction and subsequently to suppress the contraction. Provocative manoeuvres such as coughing or change of posture do not elicit uninhibited detrusor contractions.

In the investigation of patients with neurological disorders, the filling cystometrogram has been referred to as the 'reflex hammer of the urologist'.

The presence of uninhibited detrusor contractions during bladder filling is abnormal (Fig. 7.4). When there is no evidence of neurological disease the term detrusor instability (unstable bladder) is used. Detrusor instability is frequently encountered in prostatic infravesical obstruction and female urge incontinence, and the instability is probably responsible for the associated symptoms of urinary frequency, nocturia, urgency and urge incontinence. With evidence of neurological disease, the term detrusor hyperreflexia is used. It is important to stress that if a diagnosis is to be made, the result of a cystometrogram must be taken in conjunction with the clinical findings and other investigations. The maximum cystometric bladder

capacity is usually reduced with the presence of overactive detrusor function. It should be emphasized that bladder behaviour during filling cystometry may be quite different from bladder behaviour during voiding, and no conclusions about possible disorders of the voiding phase can be drawn from a filling cystometry.

Hypersensitive bladders (e.g. cystitis, interstitial cystitis, radiation cystitis) are characterized by the occurrence of first sensation at a low filling volume, and a gradual rise in bladder pressure during filling without phasic contractions (reduced bladder compliance). In autonomic neuropathy (e.g. diabetic cystopathy) bladder sensation is either severely impaired or absent. Bladder sensation is also absent in patients with damage to the peripheral innervation of the bladder (infrasacral bladder paresis).

Bladder compliance (Δ volume/Δ pressure) is an expression for the stiffness of the bladder wall. Low compliance (stiff bladder wall) is frequently found after long-lasting chronic cystitis, tuberculous cystitis and radiation cystitis. Abnormally high bladder compliance (flaccid bladder) is frequently found in myogenic decompensated bladder dysfunction (chronic overdistension, infrequent voider), in diabetic autonomic cystopathy and in infrasacral bladder paresis.

Cystometry may be performed as a solitary procedure or in conjunction with other procedures, most frequently electromyography (EMG) of the striated urethral or anal sphincter. Filling cystometry may also be combined with registration of urethral pressure (urethrocystometry) and pharmacological testing, either by the administration of parasympathomimetics (bethanechol or urocholine) or parasympatholytics (anticholinergics).

Ambulatory monitoring of intravesical pressure has gained increasing popularity in recent years. The use of microtip transducers and tape recorders for continuous monitoring permits assessment of bladder behaviour during daily physical activities. This method has given extra information on the presence of overactive detrusor function especially in female patients with urge incontinence or mixed incontinence.

Pitfalls in the interpretation of cystometric investigations are numerous. The most important are pressure artefacts due to coughing, movement of the patient, speech or poor patient cooperation during the cystometric investigation. The distinction between phasic pressure rises (detrusor overactivity) and gradual pressure rises (reduced bladder compliance) may be difficult. Again, the clinical impression and the outcome of other diagnostic modalities may then be taken into consideration before making a final diagnosis.

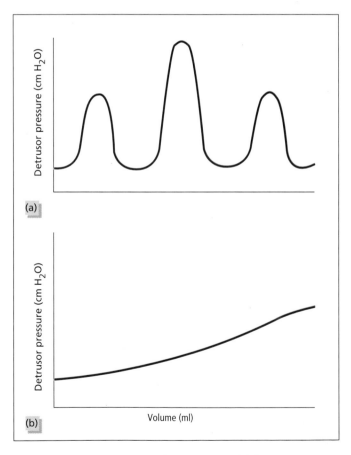

Fig. 7.4 Cystometric tracings demonstrating: (a) detrusor instability with typical phasic detrusor contraction; (b) reduced bladder compliance with a gradual increase in detrusor pressure.

Urethral closure pressure profile

The urethral closure pressure profile (UCPP) is a measurement designed to give information about the urethral length and to supply a graphic recording of the pressure within the urethra and along its length. Many factors may influence the urethral pressure profile: (i) the smooth and striated muscle activity; (ii) the fibroelastic tension of the urethral wall; (iii) the cavernous tissue; and (iv) the bloodflow through the vessels in the urethral mucosa. The UCCP represents a sum of all these factors at the time the investigation is performed.

Technique

Brown and Wickham [11] were the first to describe the technique of perfusion urethral pressure profilometry. They used a saline-perfused catheter with side holes. The perfusion rate should be over 1 ml/min and this serves to keep the catheter eyes unplugged by the urethral mucosa (Fig. 7.5).

The patient is told about the procedure and the examination is performed with the patient resting in the supine, sitting or standing position. The pressure-measuring catheter is placed in the bladder under sterile conditions. If the bladder is not empty, the bladder is drained through the catheter. The bladder is filled to a fixed volume. The catheter is then withdrawn at a constant speed. When the side holes appear at the bladder neck the urethral closure pressure measurement starts, and when the side holes appear at the external urethral meatus the profile measurement is completed. The perfusion rate is normally between 2 and 10 ml/min, usually 5 ml/min, and the catheter retraction rate is 1 cm/min.

Microcatheters with tip transducers allow the recording of very rapid intraurethral pressure changes, and if the

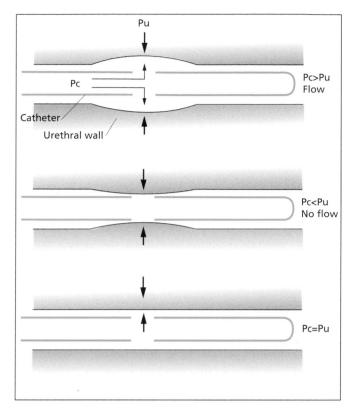

Fig. 7.5 The method of measuring the urethral closure pressure profile (UCPP) (reproduced from [11] with permission). Pu, urethral pressure. Pc, pressure in catheter lumen.

microtip catheter has several pressure transducers, pressure changes at different points in the bladder and urethra can be measured. With simultaneous measurement of the intraurethral pressure (P_{ura}) and the intravesical pressure

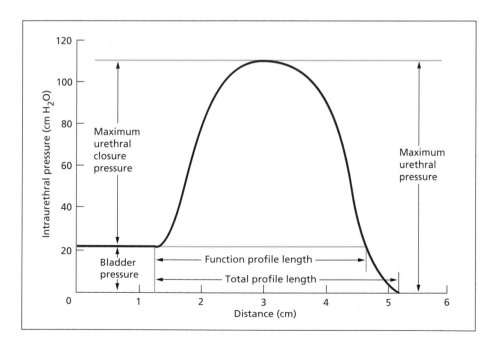

Fig. 7.6 Parameters and terms in the UCPP according to the ICS [2].

(P_{ves}) it is possible to determine the urethral pressure difference — the urethral closure pressure.

P_{ura} difference = P_{ura} − P_{ves}.

The zero reference point for the pressures is the upper level of the symphysis pubis, and the bladder pressure should be measured at the same time as the UCPP. Various parameters of the UCPP have been defined by the ICS (Fig. 7.6). The maximal urethral pressure is the maximal pressure of the measured profile. The maximal urethral closure pressure is the difference between the maximal urethral pressure and the bladder pressure at the same time. The functional profile length is the length of the urethra along which the urethral pressure exceeds the bladder pressure. The total profile length is the length of the urethra from the bladder neck to the external urethral meatus [12,13].

Stress urethral closure pressure profile

This test is performed with two pressure transducers. The proximal one measures the bladder pressure while the distal one measures the urethral pressure. When the catheter is withdrawn from the urethra the patient is asked to cough several times at fixed intervals. In a normal patient without incontinence the increased intravesical pressure exceeds the urethral pressure (Fig. 7.7).

In a patient with genuine stress urinary incontinence a failure of pressure transmission is often seen. The pressure transmission rate is bladder pressure/urethral pressure. Measurement of the urethral pressure profile can be criticized. The urethral outflow resistance is measured in a static position and not during the dynamic phase of micturition, which is far more important.

It is very difficult to exclude artefacts from detrusor contraction even if the intravesical pressure is measured simultaneously. The patient's cooperation is important when performing resting urethral profilometry and artefacts can be due to pelvic muscle contractions.

The range of normal values (Table 7.1) is dependent on the technique used, the size and type of catheter, the rate of perfusion and retraction, the position of the patient and the bladder, pelvic floor muscle activity and the patient's age [14]. There is a great inter- and intra-individual variation of the measured values. The catheter should be about 4–8 Ch.

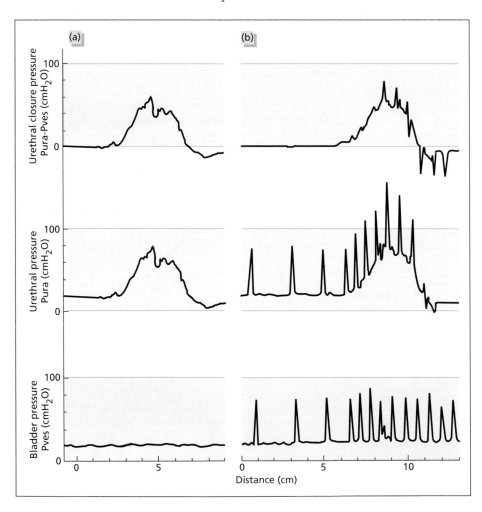

Fig. 7.7 Urethral pressure profiles (a) at rest and (b) during coughs in a continent woman (reproduced from [4] with permission).

Table 7.1 The reference values of the closure pressure profile.

Women (premenopausal)		Men	
Maximal urethral pressure	50–80 cmH$_2$O	Maximal urethral pressure	70–90 cmH$_2$O
Maximum closure pressure	40–70 cmH$_2$O	Maximum closure pressure	50–70 cmH$_2$O
Functional length	3 cm	Length of bladder neck to maximum	< 4 cm
Pressure transmission rate	>100 %	pressure (presphincteric length)	

The fluid bridge test

The fluid bridge test was described by Brown and Sutherst [15,16] in order to diagnose stress urinary incontinence with a very simple apparatus. First the UCPP is performed. When the exact urethral length and the position of the bladder neck are known, a double lumen catheter is placed just below the bladder neck. The catheter has an end hole and side holes. The end hole is in the bladder and the side holes are in the bladder neck position. The patient is asked to cough and if the bladder neck becomes incompetent, the fluid bridge is established between the bladder and the test point and the pressure in the bladder and the urethral pressure will momentarily become equal. The test is designed to demonstrate stress urinary incontinence (Figs 7.8 and 7.9).

Pressure–flow studies

The most important urodynamic examination of the voiding phase is the pressure–flow study with simultaneous measurement of intravesical pressure and urinary flow rate. These parameters are usually supplemented with recordings of the intra-abdominal pressure and the detrusor pressure (intravesical pressure – intra-abdominal pressure). The study can be combined with EMG recording from the pelvic floor. In some instances the study is performed during fluoroscopy or combined with video cystourethrography.

The purpose of the pressure–flow study is to obtain an impression of the vesical and urethral changes during micturition. Information is obtained on the influence of detrusor contractility on the voiding, abdominal pressure contribution and the relation between bladder pressure,

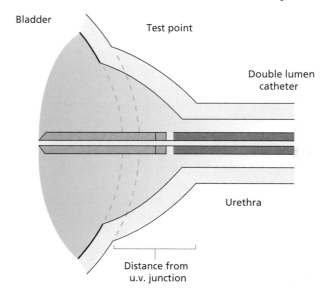

Fig. 7.8 The principle of the fluid bridge test (reproduced from [16] with permission).

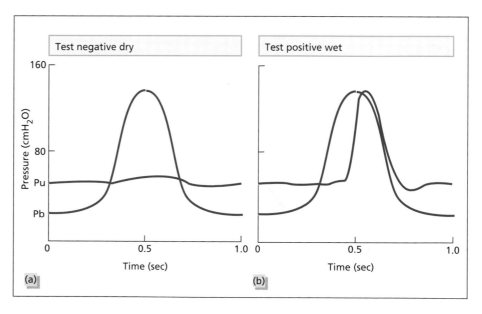

Fig. 7.9 (a) Negative and (b) positive results of the fluid bridge test. Pb, bladder pressure; Pu, urethral pressure (reproduced from [16] with permission).

flow rate and opening of the bladder neck and relaxation of the pelvic floor. The pressure–flow study provides diagnostic information on outflow resistance and/or dysfunction of the detrusor and sphincter as well as in some cases on urinary incontinence.

Technique

The intravesical pressure can be measured by a thin (3.5 F) suprapubic catheter or a transurethral catheter. The transurethral catheter is preferred in most cases because of its easy insertion, but the suprapubic route gives a better measurement of urethral function during voiding (Fig. 7.10).

Intra-abdominal pressure can be measured either using a nasogastric tube, or from within the prevesical space (space of Retzius) or in the rectum. The intrarectal catheter is most commonly used. The catheter can be perfused, or a balloon catheter or a microtip transducer catheter can be used. In most cases an open-end perfused catheter is used. The pressures in urodynamic examinations are given in centimetres of water (cmH2O).

When using perfused catheters, all manometer lines and pressure transducers should be filled with physiological saline free of air bubbles. The external pressure transducers should be at the level of the bladder, i.e. the upper edge of the symphysis pubis. The examination can be performed in the lying, sitting or the standing position.

The ICS nomenclature of parameters during pressure–flow studies is shown in Fig. 7.11. In many cases a nomogram [17] of the relation between detrusor pressure and flow can give additional information, whether obstruction is present or not (Abrams–Griffiths nomogram) (Fig. 7.12).

Normal values in the pressure–flow examination are dependent on the population studied and the technique used [18–20]. Pitfalls in the pressure–flow study are the lack of privacy during voiding, measuring with catheters and in some cases obstruction of the catheter, especially the rectal catheter which easily blocks with faeces.

Denervation–supersensitivity testing

Peripheral denervation leads to supersensitivity of the end organ to its specific neurotransmitter according to the law of Cannon [21]. This is also the case for the detrusor muscle, which becomes supersensitive to cholinergic stimulation after peripheral, parasympathetic denervation. Denervation testing is based on measuring the intravesical pressure response to a subcutaneous injection of carbachol or bethanechol in a standardized set-up. The test was first described by Lapides et al. [22] who used repetitive filling cystometries to a volume of 100 ml at 10, 20 and 30 min after subcutaneous injection of bethanechol. The test was modified by Glahn [23] who monitored the bladder pressure at a filling volume of 100 ml over 30 min after subcutaneous injection of 0.25 mg carbacholine. In Glahn's modification, a pressure rise above 20 cmH2O after 30 min indicated a positive test result, indicating supersensitivity secondary to peripheral parasympathetic denervation of the detrusor muscle. The denervation test will usually first be positive 1–2 weeks after bladder denervation, but in some patients the maximum response cannot be demonstrated until several months after the denervation.

False-negative test results may be seen in premature testing, myogenic detrusor underactivity, during concurrent anticholinergic medication and in patients with strictly unilateral denervation.

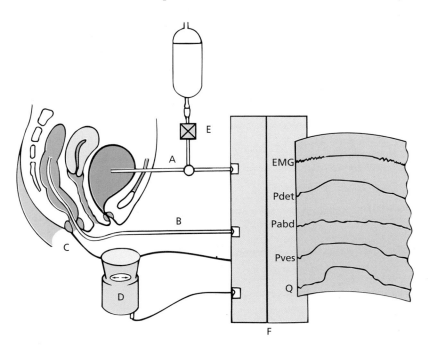

Fig. 7.10 Schematic instrumental set-up for pressure–flow studies. A=intravesical pressure recording; B=abdominal pressure recording; C=electromyography (EMG) from the anal sphincter muscle; D=flowmeter; E=infusion pump; F=tranducers, amplifiers, electronic subtraction device; Pves=total intravesical pressure; Pabd=abdominal pressure; Pdet=detrusor pressure=intravesical pressure − abdominal pressure; Q=flow rate. Reproduced with permission from *Scand J Urol Nephrol*.

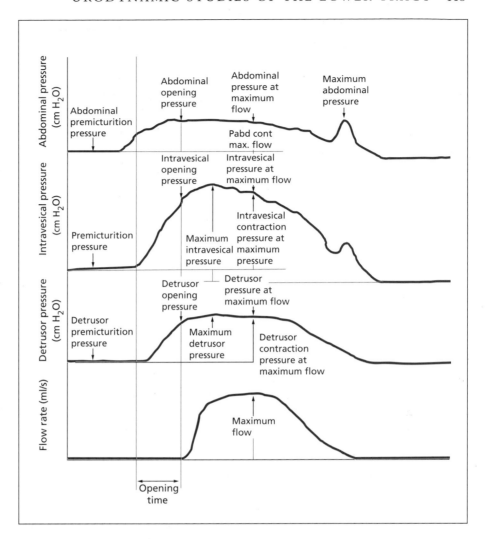

Fig. 7.11 A pressure–flow examination with nomenclature according to the ICS [2].

False-positive tests may be due to concurrent cholinergic medication, impaired renal function or reduced bladder compliance. Denervation testing only supplies indirect evidence of detrusor denervation. Neurophysiological testing, using evoked responses or sacral reflex latency measurements, provides more specific information on lesions or impairment of the peripheral innervation of the bladder.

Neurophysiological investigations

Electromyography

Electromyography (EMG) is the study of electrical potentials generated by the depolarization of muscle. EMG of the striated urethral and anal sphincters and of the pelvic floor musculature is used clinically to diagnose lesions of the innervation of the pertinent muscles (denervation) and disturbances of the coordination between detrusor activity and sphincter activity in both the storage and the voiding phases. Previously, EMG activity in the striated external anal sphincter muscles was regarded as being representative of the activity in the urethral sphincter, as both sphincters are innervated by the pudendal nerve. However, the sphincters may contract independently both in healthy people and in patients [24]. Therefore, it is essential to record EMG activity directly from the periurethral striated musculature in the study of neurogenic disorders of the lower urinary tract.

Muscle action potentials may be detected either by needle electrodes or by surface electrodes. Needle electrodes permit recording of individual motor unit action potentials, whereas surface electrodes detect the action potentials from groups of adjacent motor units underlying the recording surface. In the female, the needle is inserted 1 cm lateral to the external urinary meatus into the urethral sphincter. In the male, the needle is inserted via the perineum towards the bulbocavernosus muscle. Correct placement of the needles is checked by monitoring the EMG signal during voluntary contraction of the pelvic floor.

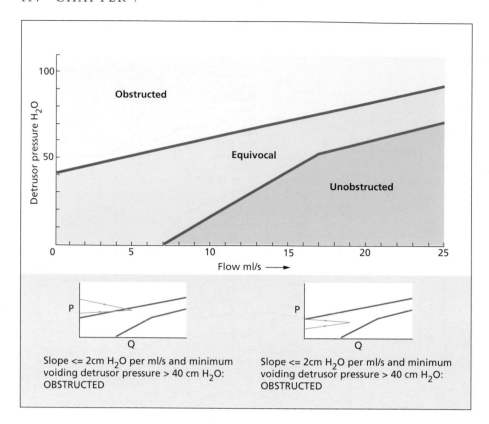

Slope <= 2cm H$_2$O per ml/s and minimum voiding detrusor pressure > 40 cm H$_2$O: OBSTRUCTED

Slope <= 2cm H$_2$O per ml/s and minimum voiding detrusor pressure > 40 cm H$_2$O: OBSTRUCTED

Fig. 7.12 The pressure–flow nomogram [17].

Surface EMG can be obtained either via a ring electrode mounted on a urethral catheter or, in the female, via vaginal surface electrodes mounted on a sponge, picking up the EMG signal from the anterior vaginal wall adjacent to the urethral striated sphincter. Surface EMG from the pelvic floor musculature can be obtained via disposable surface ECG electrodes mounted on both sides of the anus. This technique is especially useful in children in the diagnosis of pelvic floor spasticity and also during biofeedback treatment for this condition. EMG from the anal sphincters can be obtained via surface electrodes mounted on a sponge which is placed in the anal canal.

In daily urological clinical practice sphincter EMG is rarely performed as a solitary procedure, but more often in conjunction with filling cystometry or pressure–flow studies. The urethral ring electrode can only be used for filling studies.

In the neurologically intact person the resting EMG activity is very low when the bladder is empty, but during filling there is a gradual increase in sphincter EMG activity (the holding pattern). Immediately prior to voiding the urethral striated sphincter is relaxed, as can be seen by a rapid disappearance of sphincter EMG activity. Any sphincter EMG activity during voiding is abnormal unless the patient is attempting to inhibit micturition. The finding of increased sphincter EMG activity during voiding accompanied by characteristic simultaneous detrusor pressure and flow changes is referred to as detrusor–sphincter dyssynergia.

Recording of sphincter EMG activity is important in the diagnosis of neurogenic bladder dysfunctions, where involvement of the sphincter musculature is suspected. EMG recording is also important for the diagnosis of psychogenic retention of urine and in bladder-emptying disturbances in children, especially the so-called spastic sphincter syndrome (Hinman–Allen syndrome).

In cases of non-neurogenic, functional overactivity of the external sphincter musculature, EMG can also be used therapeutically during biofeedback. Here, the EMG signal is demonstrated to the patient either visually on an oscilloscope or audibly via a loudspeaker. Excellent results have been reported using this technique for functional overactivity of the external striated sphincter with associated bladder-emptying problems.

Nerve conduction studies, reflex latency measurements and evoked responses

These are highly specialized neurophysiological tests which can be used for the detection of autonomic neuropathy with slowing of nerve conduction and an increase of reflex latencies. These studies are time consuming and very few centres employ them routinely.

Sensory testing

Sensory testing is most frequently performed during cystometry by recording the patient's subjective registration of first sensation of fullness or urgency. However, sensation in the bladder and urethra can be assessed semi-objectively by the measurement of urethral and/or vesical sensory thresholds to a standard applied stimulus such as a known electrical current. The registration of electrical sensory thresholds is, however, still regarded as a research investigation.

Conclusion

The urodynamic investigation outlined in this chapter have been widely practised for many years and should now be regarded as routine urological functional investigations. Our knowledge of the physiology and pathophysiology of voiding disorders has increased significantly by the widespread use of urodynamic studies and now forms a rational basis for patient care in the majority of dysfunctions of the lower urinary tract. The choice of investigation will depend on the nature of the clinical problem. Clinical decision-making, however, should not only be based on the outcome of urodynamic studies but also on clinical findings and other investigations.

References

1 Von Garrelts B. Intravesical pressure and urinary flow during micturition in normal subjects. *Acta Chir Scand* 1957;**114**: 49–66.

2 Abrams P, Blaivas JG, Stanton SL, Andersen JT. The standardisation of terminology of lower urinary tract function. *Scand J Urol Nephrol* 1988 *Suppl;***114**:5–19.

3 Sutherst J, Brown M, Shawer M. Assessing the severity of urinary incontinence in women by weighing perineal pads. *Lancet* 1981;**1**:1128–30.

4 Andersen JT, Djurhuus JC, Nordling J, Walter S, Mortensen SO, eds. *Methods in Clinical Urodynamics. Urinary Incontinence in Women*. Copenhagen: Dantec, 1991.

5 Lose G, Versi E. Pad-weighing tests in the diagnosis and quantification of urinary incontinence. *Int Urogyn J* 1992; **3**:324–8.

6 Lose G, Rosenkilde P, Gammelgaard, J, Schroeder T. Pad-weighing test performed with standardized bladder volumen. *Urology* 1988;**32**:78–80.

7 Abrams P. The urine flow clinic. In: Fitzpatrick JM, ed. *Non-Surgical Treatment of BPH*. London: Churchill Livingstone,. 1992:33–43.

8 Siroky MB, Olsson CA, Krane RJ. The flow rate nomogram: 2. Clinical correlation. *J Urol* 1980;**123**:208–10.

9 Haylen BT, Parys BT, Anyaegbunan WI, Ashby D, West CR. Urine flow rates in male and female urodynamic patients compared with the Liverpool nomograms. *Br J Urol* 1990;**65**: 483–7.

10 Bruskewitz RC, Iversen P, Madsen PO. The value of postvoid residual urine determination in evaluation of prostatism. *Urology* 1982;**20**:602–4.

11 Brown M, Wickham JEA. The urethral pressure profile. *Br J Urol* 1969;**41**:211–17.

12 Abrams PH, Martin S, Griffiths DJ. The measurement and interpretation of urethral pressures obtained by the method of Brown and Wickham. *Br J Urol* 1978;**50**:33–8.

13 Harrison NW, Constable AR. Urethral pressure measurement; a modified technique. *Br J Urol* 1970;**42**:229–33.

14 Sørensen S. Urethral pressure variations in healthy and incontinent women. *Neurourol Urodyn* 1992;**11**:549–91.

15 Brown M, Sutherst JR. A test for bladder neck competence: the fluid-bridge test. *Urol Int* 1979;**34**:403–9.

16 Sutherst JR, Brown M. Detection of urethral incompetence: erect studies using the fluid-bridge test. *Br J Urol* 1981;**53**: 360–3.

17 Abrams PH, Griffiths DJ. The assessment of prostatic obstruction from urodynamic measurements and residual urine. *Br J Urol* 1979;**51**:129–34.

18 Frimodt-Møller C, Hald T. Clinical urodynamics. Methods and results. *Scand J Urol Nephrol* 1973 *Suppl;***15**:143–55.

19 Andersen JT, Jacobsen O, Worm-Petersen J, Hald T. Bladder function in healthy elderly males. *Scand U Urol Nephrol* 1978;**12**:123–7.

20 Walter S, Olesen KP, Nordling J, Hald T. Bladder function in urologically normal middle aged females. *Scand J Urol Nephrol* 1979;**13**:249–58.

21 Cannon WB. A law of denervation. *Am J Med Sci* 1939;**198**: 737–9.

22 Lapides J, Friend CR, Ajemian EP, Reus WF. A new test for neurogenic bladder. *J Urol* 1962;**88**:245–7.

23 Glahn BE. Neurogenic bladder diagnosed pharmacologically on the basis of denervation supersensitivity. *Scand J Urol Nephrol* 1970;**4**:13–24.

24 Nordling J, Meyhoff HH. Dissociation of urethral and anal sphincter activity in neurogenic bladder dysfunction. *J Urol* 1979;**122**:352–6.

8   Urodynamic Studies of the Upper Tract

R.H.Whitaker

Introduction

There are three broad categories of equivocal obstruction. First, the initial impression on an intravenous urogram (IVU) or renogram may suggest that the system is obstructed but it is subsequently shown that it is not obstructed. Second, is the opposite to this when obstruction is not suspected, despite the dilatation, but is later proved to be present. The third category is when all studies show that there is a degree of obstruction which is not severe but the clinical significance of it is uncertain. Over the last 20 years upper urinary tract dynamic studies have proved to be of enormous value to the author and others [1–8] in distinguishing between these three categories.

In most patients in whom dilatation of the upper urinary tract is discovered, there is no problem in arriving at the correct diagnosis and deciding upon the appropriate management. However, in a few patients, studies such as IVU, micturating cystourethrography (MCU) or even retrograde ureteropyelography are not able to determine whether or not there is a clinically significant degree of obstruction (Figs 8.1 and 8.2). Such patients with equivocal obstruction were often inadequately investigated until the advent of renography and upper tract perfusion studies and, in many, an operation was performed for symptoms and signs rather than in the certain knowledge that obstruction was present. It is probable that many inappropriate operations were undertaken before these tests were available and, no doubt, in a few, the original condition was inadvertently worsened. Witnessing the occasional failed pyeloplasty is sufficiently salutary evidence that there is no place for an inappropriate or unnecessary operation. There is an obligation to ensure that obstruction is truly present before undertaking an operation to relieve it.

In the early days of upper urinary tract dynamic studies there was great reluctance to puncture the pelvicalyceal system for diagnostic purposes, but such techniques are now regarded as minimally invasive and present no great technical challenge to the modern radiologist and urologist.

It is of historical interest that accurate dynamic studies of the upper urinary tract predate by many years the modern investigations that are performed on the lower urinary tract. Kiil [9] provided invaluable information concerning normal and abnormal urine transport in the renal pelvis in the 1950s, long before routine lower tract urodynamic assessment was popular. Clinical applications of Kiil's early work were introduced by Backlund and Reuterskiold [10] and Johnston [11] and then, in the early 1970s, a simple clinical test was established [1].

For a while such urodynamic assessment promised to be the main, if not the only, means of assessing equivocal obstruction, but renography was becoming more sophisticated and was offering an alternate, and often complementary, way of assessing the problem [12]. Perhaps the most important achievement of all these newer studies was to introduce for the first time the idea that not all dilated systems are obstructed. Shopfner [13] had already stated this but his wisdom and foresight had largely been ignored. The findings of patients with conditions that fit within the spectrum of dysplastic and post-obstructive diseases are now well recognized, largely as a result of their documentation by dynamic studies.

Principles of dynamic assessment

Essentially, a urodynamic assessment measures the pressure and flow and uses the relationship of these two parameters to calculate the resistance of the system. Thus, obstruction, in the form of a raised resistance, is present when the pressure proximal to the site of suspected obstruction is raised or the flow through it is lowered. The more usual situation is a combination of raised pressure and lowered flow.

What remains in doubt to this day is the clinical significance of a relatively small rise in resistance. Thus, the renogram and pressure study can tell us that there is a degree of obstruction but they give no absolute indication as to whether an operation is essential. It seems clear enough that it is the abnormally high pressure that causes

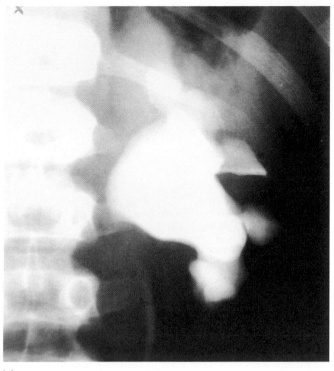

(a)

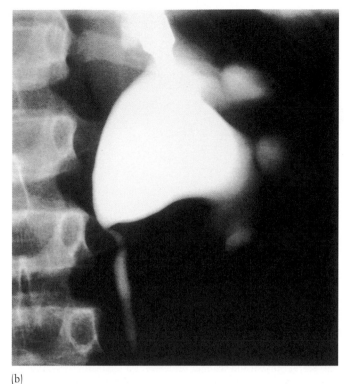

(b)

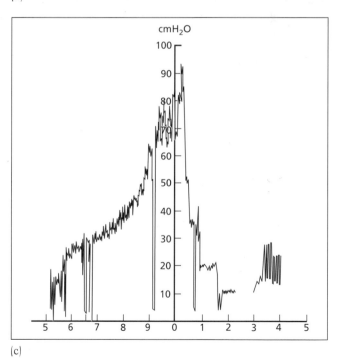

(c)

Fig. 8.1 An 8-year-old boy had his left kidney explored for suspected pelviureteric obstruction. It was deemed normal at the time and no pyeloplasty was performed. He presented later with further symptoms of pain and was studied with (a) an IVU and (b) a pressure–flow study, which showed (c) a renal pelvic pressure of over 65 cmH_2O at 10 ml/min. A pyeloplasty was then performed successfully.

the renal damage in obstruction but what remains debatable is whether a relentless small rise in pressure is more or less damaging than short periods of more obvious higher pressure. Furthermore, compliance of the upper tract must also be considered. It takes longer to raise the pressure in a compliant system than it does in a non-compliant system when they are both obstructed to the same extent. In this situation the length of duration of the diuresis must be taken into account. In addition, the efficacy of peristalsis must be assessed. Kiil [9] showed that the pressure in the normal renal pelvis is kept low by the removal of boluses from the pelvis by coaptive peristalsis. In a dilated system this is no longer true and a rise in pressure from early obstruction can be more harmful to a

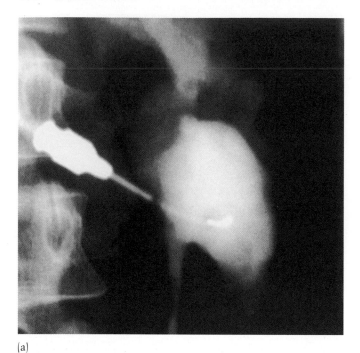

(a)

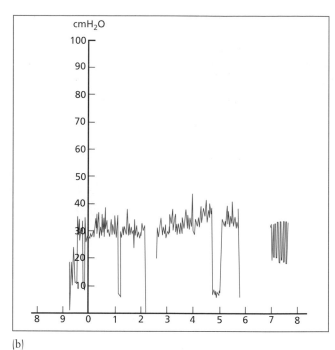

(b)

Fig. 8.2 A 30-year-old woman underwent a left Anderson–Hynes pyeloplasty 7 years previously. Her symptoms were temporarily relieved but then returned and were not helped by two balloon dilatations of the pelviureteric junction. We were asked to study the patient. A pressure–flow study (a) showed a perfectly adequate pelviureteric junction and the renal pressure (b) was only 9 cmH$_2$O at 10 ml/min. It was then clear that no further pyeloplasty would help her.

dilated system than it would be in a system with effective peristalsis.

Patient assessment

Once the presence of dilatation has been established, nowadays usually by an ultrasound examination, it is then necessary to decide whether an obstruction is present and, if so, to determine its site — usually the pelviureteric or ureterovesical junction. An IVU continues to be an exceedingly useful study and answers most of the questions. However, if any doubt remains then renography and a pressure–flow study are strongly recommended (see Figs 8.1 and 8.2). These together will assess the renal function and drainage and quantify the degree of obstruction.

Having established that obstruction is present other factors must then be taken into account before deciding that an operation is necessary. A small degree of obstruction in an elderly patient, for instance, may lead to such a slow deterioration in renal function that the risks of the operation may outweigh the benefit. The same degree of obstruction in a child would probably be a perfectly good justification for an operation. Compliance in a dilated system may be so good that, despite a degree of obstruction, only a very prolonged diuresis would lead to the development of deleterious renal pelvic pressures. On

occasion there is no obvious operation to relieve the obstruction or the patient may have had so many previous operations that a further surgical attack may be unwise. As with any study the results of renography and pressure–flow studies must be interpreted in the light of signs, symptoms and all the other tests that have been performed.

Practical aspects of pressure–flow studies

Although undoubtedly invasive, the principle of this type of study is simple [14]. A cannula, mounted on a needle, is introduced percutaneously into the renal pelvis, proximal to the site of suspected obstruction, and the pressure is measured whilst the system is perfused at a fixed flow rate (see Figs 8.1b and 8.2a). Several methods for introducing the flow and measuring the pressure have been described but the author has always measured the pressure as a *back pressure* via the same needle through which the flow is administered. Others workers have preferred two needles — one for flow and the other for pressure measurement.

It is essential that the bladder pressure is measured simultaneously as the slightest abnormality of bladder function can have a marked effect on the ability of the ureter to empty into the bladder [15]. An analysis of the pressures at a known flow rate, usually 10 ml/min, allows the degree of obstruction to be assessed accurately. General anaesthesia may be needed in young children; in virtually all other patients local anaesthesia is perfectly adequate. Fluoroscopy is essential if maximal information is to be gained and ultrasound can be useful for guiding the needle into the upper tract.

Equipment

A constant infusion pump provides the flow of saline or contrast medium into the renal pelvis and the pressure is measured and recorded by means of a pressure transducer and chart recorder. Details of the equipment that the author has used for many years have been described elsewhere [14].

Procedure

The only preliminary investigation is urinary culture to ensure that the urine is sterile for at least a week beforehand. Antibiotic cover is not routinely used. The procedure is explained to the patient as cooperation is essential in terms of lying still and holding the breath as requested. A urethral catheter is introduced. The patient lies horizontal on the X-ray table, at first supine whilst the intravenous contrast medium is given to show up the kidney for puncture and a sedative such as diazepam is administered. A plain X-ray is taken, then the patient is turned prone for the puncture.

The renal and bladder pressure lines are connected to the measuring apparatus and a baseline is established level with the kidney outside the body. All further pressures are in reference to this level. The initial normal resting pressure in the empty bladder is approximately 5–8 cmH$_2$O. The cannula is secured and 30% Urografin is perfused at 10 ml/min. The tip of the cannula is easily adjusted so that it lies unobstructed within the renal pelvis. Extravasation, though rare, is easily detected by fluoroscopy. Passage of the contrast medium is followed by intermittent fluoroscopy and compared with the pressure changes.

The end point of the study is achieved when there is a steady pressure and the system is judged as full by fluoroscopy (see Figs 8.1b and 8.2a). In the presence of severe obstruction the pressure may continue to rise. At equilibrium the contrast medium is entering the bladder at the same rate as it is being perfused. A falsely low pressure may be obtained if the procedure is abandoned before equilibrium is reached. Overfilling of the bladder should be avoided as it may lead to an excessive rise in pressure in the kidney. If this occurs the bladder is simply drained via the catheter and the pressures re-recorded. Rising pressures in the kidney, even with a less than full bladder, can indicate abnormal bladder activity. Pressures should then be measured with the bladder draining freely to analyse this more carefully. If high pressures are seen with a flow of 10 ml/min it is worth observing the pressures at a lower flow such as 5 ml/min.

At the end of the procedure the fluid is aspirated from the kidney and the cannula removed. The cannula is then perfused away from the patient to estimate its resistance because the pressure that it generates by itself at the flow rate that was used must be subtracted when the final result is calculated. The patient is kept quiet for 12 h before discharge from hospital. Haematuria is monitored during this time and is rarely more than minor. A little soreness is usual but infection after the procedure is most uncommon.

Calculation and interpretation of the result

To calculate the pressure drop across the site of suspected obstruction it is necessary to subtract both the resistance of the cannula and the bladder pressure from the renal pelvic pressure. Intra-abdominal pressure can be discounted as it is equally applied to the kidney and the bladder. A high pressure drop, in excess of 20 cmH$_2$O, indicates an obstructed system (see Fig. 8.1c); the higher the pressure above this level, the greater the degree of severity of obstruction. Patients with such pressures are considered for operation. Between 12 and 20 cmH$_2$O the resistance is somewhat greater that normal, but within this range it is debatable whether operative intervention is needed. This is the third category of equivocal obstruction as described in the introduction of this chapter. Below 12 cmH$_2$O there is no obstruction (see Fig. 8.2b).

A high renal pressure with a low differential between the bladder and kidney indicates abnormal bladder function for which appropriate action should be taken. A final combination may be a high renal pelvic pressure, a high bladder pressure and a high differential pressure between the two. This suggests a true obstruction between the kidney and bladder but in association with abnormal bladder behaviour. This may be seen after an unsatisfactory reimplant of a ureter in a boy whose urethral valve has been destroyed or in a patient with a neuropathic bladder. It is in situations such as these that the pressure study provides invaluable information that would be difficult to obtain by other means.

These discriminating levels have been decided upon after several hundred studies in both patients and animal models. Clearly, intermittent obstruction will be missed if the obstruction is not present at the time of the study. Such patients are best diagnosed by an IVU during an attack of pain.

In general there is an inclination to operate on children earlier rather than later in the assumption that they have more to lose in terms of renal function over the years. Whereas an elderly patient with an equivocal pressure and a compliant system could probably be left alone with little deterioration in function.

Accuracy of obstruction assessment

Several hundred pressure studies over a period of 20 years in patients and various animal and inanimate models have convinced the author that these studies provide an accurate assessment of obstruction and that they are of prognostic value provided that conditions are stable. Because there is no other quantitative study with which to compare them there must remain a little doubt as to whether they can be regarded as the gold standard against which all other studies should be judged.

An assessment of their long-term value has been published [16,17]. A follow-up for 5–10 years of 63 patients showed that no patient with a low pressure treated conservatively showed deterioration in renal function, whilst all but one patient with high pressure showed deteriorating function. Others have endorsed the efficacy of the studies [5–8,18].

These studies are criticised as being invasive, which is a fair comment, but the author contends that a short test that is both safe and accurate is better than an inappropriate operation with the risks of worsening the problem. No patient investigated by us has had a complication following the study that has led to the need for intervention. Workers have reported false-negative or false-positive results suggesting that the pressures are not to be believed. If the study is performed correctly with care to avoid underfilling, excessive extravasation or cannula blockage it is difficult to explain an inaccurate result. It is, of course, easily understandable that the clinical picture can change and thus a single pressure study may not reflect what will happen at a later date in this situation.

A further criticism is that the initial flow of 10 ml/min is unphysiological. This, however, is not the case. Even in small children we have found that unobstructed systems can tolerate this flow with ease. Furthermore, in extremes of diuresis individual normal kidneys can reach this level of flow. It is sometimes said that pressure levels of between 12 and 22 cmH$_2$O are frequently found and, because these levels are indeterminate, the test has failed. This is certainly not true as such levels indicate early, but not necessarily clinically significant, obstruction. Although such borderline pressures would be expected to occur often in a group of patients with difficult diagnostic problems, in fact there were very few patients with these levels out of the whole of the author's group.

Diuretic renography

For many years there has been a search for alternative techniques to replace these invasive pressure–flow studies and much investigation has taken place into the benefits of diuresis renography. There are those who believe that renography can give an accurate assessment of obstruction [19–21] and others who still hold that the quantitative assessment that is provided by a pressure study is essential in the really difficult diagnostic problem [4,6,8]. The author believes that the two studies are complementary, in that they each look at different aspects of obstruction. As renography does not directly measure pressure and flow it is clear that it can never quantitatively assess the degree of obstruction, but it is more than capable of detecting defects in the normal transit of flow through the system and excellent at measuring the degree of deterioration in renal function that has been caused by an obstruction. Thus by performing both studies in the difficult situation, the maximal information is obtained and a logical approach can be taken to the problem.

When the ability of renography to detect accurately the presence or absence of obstruction was reviewed in a series of difficult diagnostic problems, it was found that the renogram failed to give a satisfactory answer in a quarter of patients, assuming that the pressure–flow study had given an accurate assessment [22]. Others have also found a lack of correlation between the tests due to a lack of standardization of renography technique [23]. It was clear that poorly functioning kidneys or even kidneys with an early limited ability to respond to a diuresis could easily give a false-positive answer when asked to diagnose obstruction. Other, ill-understood factors may also be involved. Alternatively, systems that are grossly dilated may allow such poor mixing of the isotope that an impression of obstruction is given when none is present. The author believes, controversially, that false-negative scans can occasionally be seen in early obstruction in a solitary kidney or where there is equal obstruction in both kidneys.

The search for more sophistication in renography continues [19–21]; in the meantime most clinicians will perform combined studies, including renography and urography, in the majority of patients and keep the pressure–flow study for the fewer really difficult diagnostic problems.

References

1 Whitaker RH. Methods of assessing obstruction in dilated ureters. *Br J Urol* 1973;**45**:5–22.
2 Whitaker RH. Investigating wide ureters with ureteral pressure flow studies. *J Urol* 1976;**116**:81–2.
3 Whitaker RH. An evaluation of 170 diagnostic pressure flow studies of the upper urinary tract. *J Urol* 1979;**121**:602–4.
4 Whitaker RH. The diagnosis of upper urinary tract obstruction. *Postgrad Med J* 1990;**66**(Suppl. 1):25–30.
5 Bouchot O, Le Normand L, Couteau E, Buzelin JM. The Whitaker test. Its reliability and place in the study of congenital malformative uropathies. *Ann Urol Paris* 1989; **23**: 58–64.
6 Clayman RV, Basler JW, Kavoussi L, Picus DD. Ureteronephroscopic endopyelotomy. *J Urol* 1990;**144**:246–51.
7 Gotoh M, Yoshikawa Y, Nagai T *et al.* Urodynamic evaluation

of results of endopyelotomy for ureteropelvic junction obstruction. *J Urol* 1993;**150**:1444–7.

8 Kashi SH, Irving HC, Sadek SA. Does the Whitaker test add to antegrade pyelography in the investigation of collecting system dilatation in renal allografts? *Br J Radiol* 1993;**66**:877-81.

9 Kiil F. *The Function of the Ureter and Renal Pelvis*. Oslo: Oslo University Press, 1957.

10 Backlund L, Reuterskiold AG. The abnormal ureter in children. I. Perfusion studies on the wide nonrefluxing ureter. *Scand J Urol Nephrol* 1969;**3**:219–28.

11 Johnston JH. The pathogenesis of hydronephrosis in children. *Br J Urol* 1969;**41**:724–34.

12 Koff SA, Whitaker RH. Recent advances in the diagnosis of upper urinary tract obstruction. In: Whitaker RH, Woodard JR, eds. *Pediatric Urology*. London: Butterworths, 1985:154–66.

13 Shopfner CE. Ureteropelvic junction obstruction. *Am J Roent Rad Ther* 1966;**98**:148–59.

14 Whitaker RH. The Whitaker test. Symposium on advances in laboratory and intraoperative diagnostic techniques. *Urol Clin North Am* 1979;**6**:529–39.

15 Whitaker RH. The ureter in posterior urethral valves. *Br J Urol* 1973;**45**:395–403.

16 Witherow RO'N, Whitaker RH. The predictive accuracy of antegrade pressure flow studies in equivocal upper tract obstruction. *Br J Urol* 1981;**53**:496–9.

17 Wolk FN, Whitaker RH. Late follow-up of dynamic evaluation of upper urinary tract obstruction. *J Urol* 1982;**128**:346–7.

18 Ryan PC, Maher K, Hurley GD, Fitzpatrick JM. The Whitaker test: experimental analysis in a canine model of partial ureteric obstruction. *J Urol* 1989;**141**:387–90.

19 English PJ, Testa HJ, Lawson RS, Carroll RNP, Edwards EC. Modified method of diuresis renography for the assessment of equivocal pelviureteric junction obstruction. *Br J Urol* 1987;**59**:10–14.

20 Reiners C, Kropfl D, Rubben H. Diagnosis of urine transport disorders. Diuresis renography. *Urologe A* 1993;**32**:133–40.

21 Bahar RH, Elgazzar AH, Abu Zidan FM *et al*. The predictive value of Tc-99m DTPA renography in obstructive uropathy using animal model. *Am J Physiol Imaging* 1990;**5**:107–11.

22 Whitaker RH, Buxton-Thomas M. A comparison of pressure flow studies and renography in equivocal upper urinary tract obstruction. *J Urol* 1984;**131**:446–9.

23 Conway JJ. 'Well-tempered' diuresis renography: its historical development, physiological and technical pitfalls, and standardization technique protocol. *Semin Nucl Med* 1992;**22**:74–84.

Section 2
Paediatric Disorders

9 Embryology of the Urinary Tract
J.A.Gosling and J.S.Dixon

Development of the kidney and ureter

The permanent kidney and ureter are derived from two distinct embryological components, namely, the metanephrogenic blastema (cap) and the ureteric bud. The latter develops from the mesonephric duct and its growth induces the formation of the metanephrogenic blastema in the caudal extremity of the nephrogenic cord.

About 28 days (4–5 mm crown–rump length, CRL) after fertilization, cells in the dorsomedial wall of the mesonephric duct begin to proliferate and give rise to a diverticulum, the ureteric bud (Fig. 9.1). The portion of the mesonephric duct which lies between the ureteric bud and the cloaca is renamed the common excretory duct. The free end of the ureteric bud grows first in a dorsal direction and then, at about 30 days (6 mm CRL), it turns cranially and comes into apposition with the caudal end of the nephrogenic cord (Fig. 9.2).

Meanwhile, the attachment of the ureteric outgrowth to the mesonephric duct also migrates, first dorsally and then dorsolaterally. As a consequence, the lengthening ureteric bud, which initially lies dorsomedial to the mesonephric duct, is now situated on the lateral aspect of the duct (Fig. 9.3).

The closed end of the ureteric bud, as it invades the nephrogenic cord, induces condensation of the adjacent mesoderm to form the metanephrogenic blastema around the ureteric bud (Fig. 9.4). The presence of the ureteric bud is essential for this differentiation and absence of the outgrowth is invariably associated with renal agenesis. Once formed, the metanephrogenic blastema in its turn induces changes in the ureteric bud, causing it to expand and subdivide at its cranial end (Figs 9.5 and 9.6). During

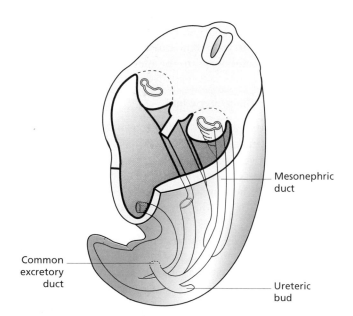

Fig. 9.1 Ureteric bud (5.5 mm CRL embryo). This diverticulum makes its appearance as an outgrowth from the cells in the genu of the mesonephric duct.

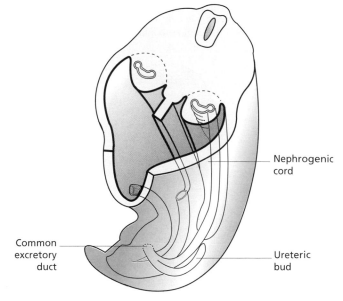

Fig. 9.2 Growth of the ureteric bud (6.0 mm CRL embryo). The ureteric bud grows rapidly in a dorsal direction towards the caudal end of the nephrogenic cord.

125

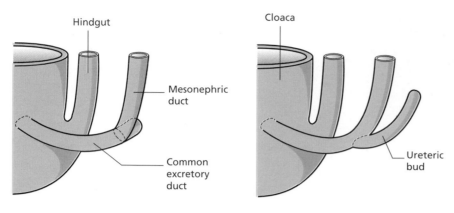

Fig. 9.3 Mesonephric duct and ureter. The ureteric bud arises as an outgrowth of cells on the dorsomedial aspect of the mesonephric duct (left); continued growth carries the ureter into a dorsal position (right).

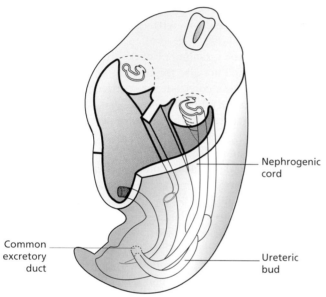

Fig. 9.4 Metanephrogenic blastema (6.5 mm CRL embryo). The cranial end of the ureteric bud contacts the nephrogenic cord and induces the formation of the metanephrogenic blastema.

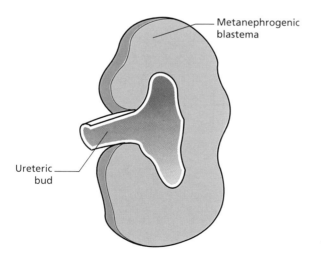

Fig. 9.5 The developing kidney induces the ureteric bud to undergo subdivision, the first of which gives rise to two approximately equal branches.

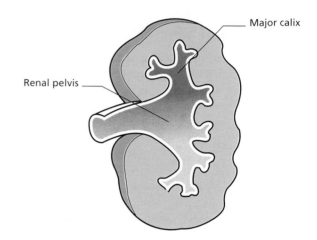

Fig. 9.6 The ureter continues to subdivide from these two branches, the branching taking place more rapidly at the poles than in the interpolar region. This results in the development of the characteristic shape of the kidney.

the period from 32 to 37 days (7–11 mm CRL), continued growth of the ureteric bud causes the metanephrogenic blastema to ascend dorsal to the mesonephros.

Subdivision of the ureteric bud

The first partial division of the expanded cranial end of each ureteric bud occurs at 33–35 days (9 mm CRL) and gives rise to two approximately equal branches (Fig. 9.5). These branches undergo further subdivision (Fig. 9.6), a process which continues until the time of birth and ultimately results in the formation of the renal pelvis, major and minor calyces and collecting ducts of approximately one million nephrons per kidney. The remaining parts of each nephron are derived from the mesoderm of the metanephrogenic blastema.

Positional changes of the upper urinary tract

Originally, the metanephros lies at the level of the upper sacral segments and receives its arterial supply from branches of the lateral sacral arteries. As the nephric elements ascend, the ventral surfaces rotate medially through approximately 90° carrying the upper ureters to the medial aspects of the kidneys (Fig. 9.7). Each kidney receives segmental vessels during its ascent, the definitive artery being established at about the eighth week (25 mm CRL). This developmental pattern explains the blood supply of the adult ureter which receives its vessels from several different segmental vessels.

At birth, the lower poles of the kidneys lie at the level of the iliac crest. During subsequent skeletal growth, the lumbosacral angle increases as the lumbar curve of the vertebral column becomes pronounced. These changes, associated with an increase in bulk of the psoas major muscle, produce the prominent paravertebral gutter evident in the adult. As a consequence, the orientation of the kidney changes so that its ventral surface now faces anterolaterally and its lower pole lies lateral to the upper pole. During the development of the upper urinary tract, important changes occur at the vesical end of the ureter.

Development of the bladder, ureters and urethra

Cloacal membrane and cloaca

Approximately 15 days after fertilization, cells differentiate from the primitive streak and migrate between the ectoderm and endoderm. This intermediate layer forms the intra-embryonic or secondary mesoderm and, in most regions, converts the bilaminar embryonic plate into a trilaminar structure. However, in the caudal part of the embryo adjacent to the attachment of the connecting stalk, mesoderm fails to excavate between the ectoderm and endoderm. The persistence of this bilaminar region results in the formation of the cloacal membrane (Fig. 9.8).

The increase in thickness of the embryonic plate which accompanies the development of the intra-embryonic mesoderm causes the dorsal surface of the embryo to bulge in to the amniotic cavity. The cranial and caudal extremities of the embryo bend ventrally to form the head and tail folds and during these changes, part of the endoderm lining of the yolk sac is carried into these cranial and caudal folds to form the foregut and the hindgut, respectively (Fig. 9.9). As the tail fold continues to enlarge, the connecting stalk and contained allantois are displaced on to the ventral aspect of the embryo. Similar positional changes affect the cloacal membrane which moves from its original position to a ventral location at the base of the tail fold and connecting stalk (Fig. 9.10). The hindgut undergoes slight dilatation and receives the termination of the allantois. At this stage of development, the cloaca can be defined as that part of the hindgut which lies caudal to the attachment of the allantois. Mesoderm adjacent to the cloacal membrane produces bilateral elevations, the urethral folds. These folds border a midline surface depression, the external cloaca or proctodaeum, which is floored in by the cloacal membrane (Fig. 9.11). The cloacal membrane retreats caudally because of subsequent growth

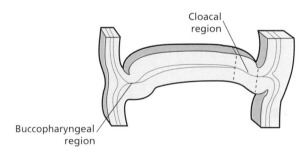

Fig. 9.8 Trilaminar embryonic plate. An intermediate layer of secondary mesoderm separates the endoderm and ectoderm except in the buccopharyngeal and cloacal regions.

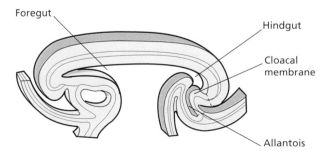

Fig. 9.9 Folding of the embryo. Continued growth and ventral flexion of the embryo results in marked positional changes.

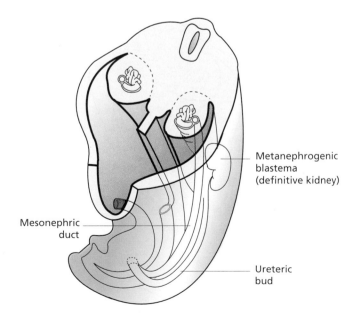

Fig. 9.7 Definitive kidney (10 mm CRL embryo). The ureter has induced the formation of the definitive kidney which lies dorsal to the mesonephric duct.

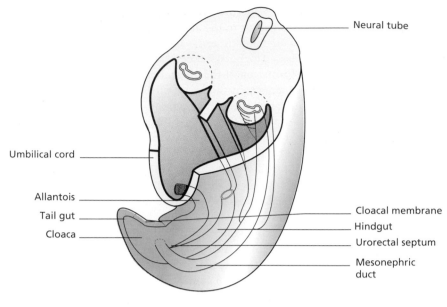

Fig. 9.10 The cloaca (4.5 mm CRL embryo). The cloacal membrane is located at the base of the connecting stalk. The mesonephric duct opens into the cloaca ventral to the urorectal septum.

This mesoderm extends in the curvature of the embryo towards the cloacal membrane and forms the urorectal septum of the hindgut. This septum grows caudally into the lumen of the cloaca parallel to its dorsal wall (Fig. 9.12). As the urorectal septum extends towards the cloacal membrane, the growth of the lateral attachments of the septum to the side walls of the cloaca outstrip its central part. Thus, the caudal part of the septum forms a free margin, the concave edge of which is directed towards the cloacal membrane. The lateral sides of the urorectal septum reach the cloacal membrane by the 10 mm CRL stage and the complete partitioning of the cloaca into the

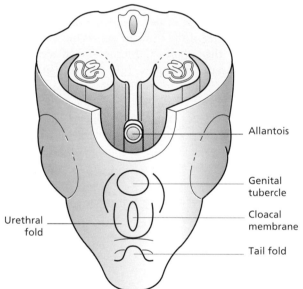

Fig. 9.11 Urethral folds (5.5 mm CRL embryo). The relationship between the genital tubercle, the urethral folds and the cloacal membrane is illustrated.

of both the cranial (strictly ventral) end of the urethral folds (the genital tubercle) and of the anterior abdominal wall. This process is also enhanced by regression of the tail fold. Consequently, the cloacal membrane, stopping short of its original dorsal position, comes to face caudally.

Division of the cloaca

The cloaca begins to be partitioned into smaller dorsal and larger ventral compartments about 28 days (4–5 mm CRL) after fertilization. This process of division is produced by growth of mesoderm from the rostral limit of the allantois.

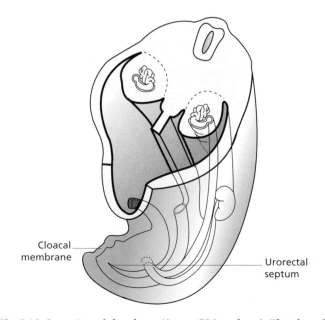

Fig. 9.12 Septation of the cloaca (9 mm CRL embryo). The cloacal membrane faces caudally and is approached by the urorectal septum.

primitive urogenital sinus ventrally and the rectum dorsally is usually established at 12 mm CRL (Fig. 9.13). Immediately prior to complete septation, a channel connecting the rectum and primitive urogenital sinus is situated on the cranial aspect of the cloacal membrane. Persistence of this interconnection (the cloacal duct) occurs due to failure of further growth by the urorectal septum and results in a fistula between the definitive rectum and urethra. On reaching the cloacal membrane, the urorectal septum divides it into a ventral urogenital membrane and dorsal anal membrane. The anal and urogenital openings are formed by the independent involution of these membranes, a process which is usually complete as early as the 18 mm CRL stage. As indicated previously, the mesonephric duct opens into the ventral part of the lateral cloacal wall. The line of growth of the urorectal septum lies dorsal to these openings so that by the 8 mm CRL stage, the ducts already terminate into the urogenital sinus portion of the partially divided cloaca (see Fig. 9.10).

Formation of the bladder and urethra

As the urorectal septum grows towards the cloacal membrane, the partially formed primitive urogenital sinus begins to undergo changes which lead to the formation of the bladder and the primitive urethra. The primitive urogenital sinus receives the allantois and the common excretory ducts and is limited caudally by the urogenital part of the cloacal membrane (see Fig. 9.13). These attachments, in effect, anchor the primitive urogenital

sinus so that, as the position of each structure changes with respect to the other, the sinus is caused to undergo corresponding changes in size and shape. Initially, the cloacal membrane lies at the root of the connecting stalk, subsequent growth causing these two structures to separate as the anterior abdominal wall develops.

Since the primitive urogenital sinus is fixed to the connecting stalk by the allantois, the ventral wall of the urogenital sinus must increase in order to accommodate these positional changes. Failure of this process will give rise, after breakdown of the urogenital membrane, to the condition known as ectopia vesicae. Thus, at this stage of development, the sinus is attached to the umbilicus by the allantois. As the posterior abdominal wall elongates, the associated common excretory duct and attached ureter draw the adjacent part of the primitive urogenital sinus in a dorsal direction. That portion lying between the terminations of the common excretory ducts and the allantois undergoes dilatation and forms the vesicourethral canal (see Fig. 9.13). It is from this structure that the urinary bladder develops. At this stage, the urogenital sinus is defined as the part of the primitive sinus which lies caudal to the attachments of the common excretory ducts. This sinus is subdivided into the narrow pelvic and dilated phallic parts (Fig. 9.14), and the subsequent fate of the latter is intimately related to the development of the external genitalia.

To summarize, in the female, the vesicourethral canal gives rise to the bladder and urethra, the contribution of the definitive urogenital sinus being confined to the formation

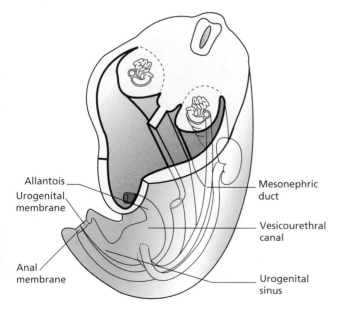

Fig. 9.13 Formation of bladder. The vesicourethral canal becomes dilated to form the bladder. In the female it also gives rise to the whole urethra but in the male it forms only the proximal prostatic urethra.

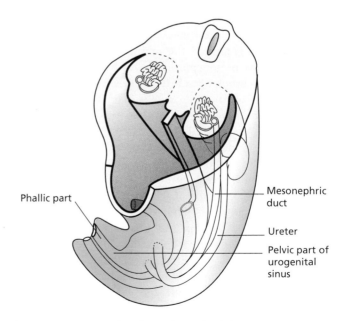

Fig. 9.14 Formation of male urethra. The definitive urogenital sinus dilates in its phallic portion giving rise to the spongy urethra.

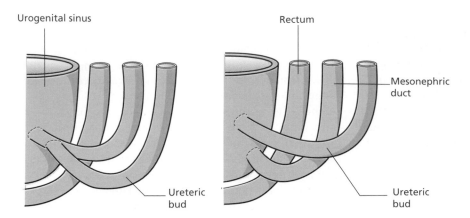

Urogenital sinus
Rectum
Mesonephric duct
Ureteric bud
Ureteric bud

Fig. 9.15 The fate of the common excretory duct. Differential growth results in the incorporation of the common excretory duct into the urogenital sinus. Thus the ureter gains a separate opening into the sinus, cranial and lateral to that of the mesonephric duct.

of the vestibule. In the male, the vesicourethral canal forms the bladder and proximal urethra as far as the terminations of the ejaculatory ducts, the definitive urogenital sinus forming the remainder of the urethra.

Contribution of the common excretory ducts and terminal ureters

As development proceeds, the attachment of the ureteric bud migrates first dorsally and then dorsolaterally relative to the mesonephric duct.

Concomitant with these positional changes, the common excretary duct shortens due to the absorption of its distal extremity into the wall of the vesicourethral canal. The latter process continues with the result that the ureter opens separately into the vesicourethral canal through an orifice placed lateral to that of the mesonephric duct (Fig. 9.15). Continued growth results in further separation of the ureters and mesonephric ducts and by 17 mm CRL, a well-defined trigone can be distinguished (Fig. 9.16). The ureters open into the bladder at the craniolateral angles of the trigone while the mesonephric ducts, which remain closely apposed to each other, open into the definitive urethra. The terminal parts of the mesonephric ducts open on the surface at a midline elevation, the müllerian tubercle, situated on the dorsal wall of the urethra.

In that the common excretory ducts and terminal ureters contribute to the wall of the definitive bladder and urethra, the endoderm of the vesicourethral canal is supplemented by a mesodermal component which forms the trigone and posterior urethral wall. This mesodermal contribution extends distally as far as the mesonephric ducts. The embryological origin of the epithelium of the trigone has not, however, been established with certainty. Some authorities suggest that the mesodermal components of this part of the bladder wall give rise to the epithelial lining. Others consider that the epithelium of the vesicourethral canal (of endodermal origin) migrates to cover those regions derived from the absorption of the common excretory ducts and ureters. Separation of the

ureters from the mesonephric ducts is accompanied by marked changes in the shape of the vesicourethral canal. That portion destined to become the bladder undergoes a marked dilatation and projects from the anterior abdominal wall into the peritoneal cavity.

The distal portion remains narrow and represents the segment of the vesicourethral canal which will develop into the urethra.

Development of the ovary and female genital tract

During the fifth week genital ridges make their appearance as thickenings of coelomic epithelium on the medial side of each mesonephros. These thickenings, together with the mesonephros, constitute the urogenital ridge (see Fig. 9.10). In developing from the undifferentiated gonad, the

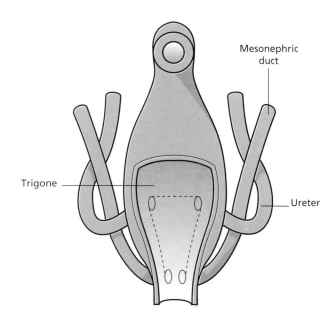

Mesonephric duct
Trigone
Ureter

Fig. 9.16 Trigone (17 mm CRL embryo). The separation of the mesonephric ducts and ureters produces the trigone, which forms an integral part of the urogenital sinus.

primordial germ cells of the ovary remain in a cortical position close to the epithelium covering the genital ridge. The primitive sex cords and the mesonephric tubules usually regress leaving remnants, the epo-ophoron and paro-ophoron. During weeks 8–20 the primordial germ cells undergo repeated divisions to provide the adult complement of oogonia. During this differentiation and growth the ovary gradually projects further into the coelomic cavity and displaces the regressing mesonephros in a dorsolateral direction (see Fig. 9.13). The original attachment of the ovary to the mesonephros becomes reduced to a mesentery, the mesovarium. The displaced mesonephros consists of a dorsolateral portion with regressing tubules and a ventrolateral tubal part containing the mesonephric and paramesonephric (müllerian) ducts.

From the caudal end of the ovary, a band of mesoderm extends across the abdominal wall into the inguinal region. This continues into the labia majora through the future inguinal canal and forms the gubernaculum. As the uterus develops, the gubernaculum becomes attached to the junction between the body of the uterus and uterine tube. The cranial portion of the gubernaculum forms the ovarian ligament; the caudal part becomes the round ligament of the uterus.

Uterine tubes, uterus and vagina

During the sixth week, the paramesonephric ducts develop as groove-like invaginations of the coelomic epithelium. Each invagination extends caudally as a solid rod growing parallel to the mesonephric duct. The rod of epithelial cells acquires a lumen from the cranial end; the opening into the coelomic cavity persists as the ostium of the uterine tube.

Each paramesonephric duct extends towards the midline and continues growing in a caudomedial direction to fuse with its contralateral counterpart. The caudal end of the fused ducts contacts the dorsal wall of the urogenital sinus to form an elevation, the müllerian tubercle. The fused paramesonephric ducts form the uterovaginal canal. Initially a septum divides the cavity and this normally disappears during the 12th week. The cranial part of the uterovaginal canal forms the uterus—the unfused portions of the paramesonephric ducts forming the uterine tubes (Fig. 9.17). Many uterine abnormalities can be explained in terms of incomplete fusion of the paired paramesonephric ducts. The uterovaginal canal contacts the dorsal wall of the urogenital sinus at the müllerian tubercle and induces the formation of the distal portion of the vagina. Hence, the proximal three-quarters of the vaginal epithelium is derived from the mesoderm of the uterovaginal canal and the remainder from the endoderm of the urogenital sinus.

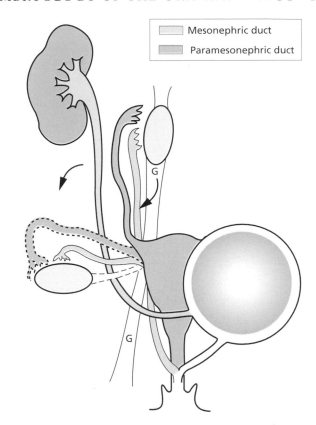

▢	Mesonephric duct
▬	Paramesonephric duct

Fig. 9.17 Schematic diagram showing the descent of the ovary and associated paramesonephric duct which forms the uterine tube. The gubernaculum (G) is also indicated.

Development of the testis and male genital tract

In developing from the undifferentiated gonad, the male gonadal blastema makes its appearance during the sixth week (15 mm CRL) of intrauterine life. Fibrous tissue subdivides the blastema into a series of sex cords and these are subsequently separated from the germinal epithelium by a dense layer of fibrous tissue, the tunica albuginea. Primordial germ cells are included in the sex cords and the latter form a network extending into the mesorchium (analogous to the mesovarium) as the rete testis. The sex cords later become canalized to form the seminiferous tubules; those of the rete testis joining with some of the mesonephric tubules (efferent ductules) to bring the rete into communication with the mesonephric duct.

As in the female, the caudal end of the gonad is attached to a prominent band of connective tissue, the gubernaculum (Fig. 9.18). The gubernaculum extends downwards, running across the abdominal wall to terminate in the genital swelling. During growth of the pelvis and trunk the gubernaculum undergoes little change in length and, as a consequence, the testis appears to descend relative to the

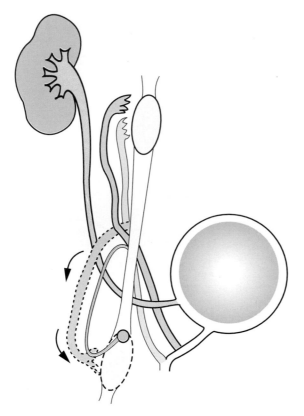

Fig. 9.18 Schematic diagram showing the descent of the testis and mesonephric duct.

body wall. By the third month, the testis lies on the posterior aspect of the anterior abdominal wall in the region of the inguinal canal. A pouch of peritoneum, the processus vaginalis, follows the gubernaculum through the inguinal canal into the scrotum during the sixth month of intrauterine life. During the seventh month the testis traverses the inguinal canal. It lies behind, but projects into, the processus vaginalis and reaches the scrotal sac by the end of the eighth month. The lower part of the processus persists as the tunica vaginalis while the upper part is obliterated, usually at the time of birth.

Epididymis and ductus deferens

As previously noted, the cranial part of the mesonephric duct is connected to the seminiferous tubules of the testis by some of the mesonephric tubules forming the efferent ductules. That part of the mesonephric duct which receives the efferent ductules becomes elongated and convoluted to form the epididymis.

The closed cranial portion of the mesonephric duct persists as the appendix of the epididymis. The remainder of the mesonephric duct increases in thickness and gives rise to the ductus deferens. Close to its termination the ductus becomes dilated and forms the ampulla. From this region a diverticulum appears which subsequently develops into the seminal vesicle. The terminal part of the mesonephric duct which connects the seminal vesicle and ductus to the prostatic urethra becomes the ejaculatory duct.

In the male the paramesonephric ducts undergo degenerative changes. However, the cranial end persists to form the appendix of the testis; the caudal end is thought to give rise to the prostatic utricle.

10 Perinatal Urology
D.F.M. Thomas and J.A. Cook

Introduction

Malformations of the urogenital tract are common, accounting for an estimated one-third of all congenital anomalies. Whilst malformations such as bladder exstrophy and prune belly syndrome are immediately evident in the neonatal period, most non-lethal uropathies are undetectable at birth and previously came to light only when patients presented with symptoms or complications in later childhood or adult life. Other anomalies, such as unilateral renal agenesis, were often destined to remain undetected throughout the individual's lifetime unless they were discovered as incidental findings during autopsy or during the investigation of unrelated conditions. During the last decade, however, this pattern of presentation has been transformed by the introduction into routine obstetric practice of high-resolution ultrasound imaging of the fetus. Paediatric urologists face the task of trying to establish how best to apply the information derived from prenatal ultrasound to the benefit of the affected infant. The guiding aims of postnatal urological management can be summarized as:

1 preservation of renal function;
2 prevention of morbidity, particularly urinary infection.
To these can be added a third,
3 minimizing invasive intervention in healthy infants.

Normal development of the fetal urinary tract

The kidney has its origins in the metanephrosis, the most caudal of the three blocks of intermediate mesoderm. The pronephros, a rudimentary non-functional kidney, undergoes complete regression in humans. The mesonephros is destined to give rise to the epididymis and ejaculatory ducts in the male, but undergoes regression in the female. Development of the primitive fetal kidneys is stimulated by the penetration of the metanephros by the ureteric bud, an outgrowth of the mesonephric duct, during the fifth week of gestation. Within the metanephros, branching of

the ureteric bud results in the formation of the intrarenal collecting tubules, the calyces and the renal pelvis. Branching of the intrarenal component of the ureteric bud is virtually complete by the 15th week of gestation and thus precedes the most active period of nephrogenesis which occurs between 20 and 36 weeks. Eight to 12 generations of nephrons are represented in the normal fetal kidney but the creation of new nephrons ceases after around 36 weeks and their number thereafter (approximately one million in a normal kidney) remains fixed for life.

Fetal urine is produced from around the eighth week of gestation onwards and at this early stage the fetal kidney's major role appears to be in contributing urine to the amniotic fluid. In fetal life the principal excretory and homeostatic functions of the kidney are undertaken by the placenta and even the fetus with bilateral renal agenesis, which is in effect dialysed by the placenta, can survive normally to term. At birth the concentrations of creatinine, urea and electrolytes in the fetal blood mirror those in the maternal circulation. In the absence or virtual absence of fetal urine, however, the ensuing oligohydramnios is associated with pulmonary hypoplasia and compression deformities which occur because the developing fetus has been deprived of the physical support of amniotic liquor. Although severe oligohydramnios and the underlying renal parenchymal damage do not threaten survival *in utero*, severe oligohydramnios is a sensitive predictor of early postnatal demise — either from pulmonary hypoplasia or renal failure [1]. Intermediate degrees of oligohydramnios, however, correlate less closely with fetal outcome [2].

In the early stages of gestation fetal urine consists essentially of a sodium-rich plasma filtrate. Throughout fetal life renal bloodflow as a percentage of cardiac output is much lower than in postnatal life, whilst conversely renal vascular resistance is much higher. Amniotic fluid reaches its maximum volume of around 1000 ml at 38 weeks' gestation and at this stage fetal urine contributes about 90% of the amniotic fluid volume [3]. Ultrasound measurements of fetal bladder volume and frequency of bladder emptying indicate that in the third trimester the rate of urine production is much higher than in early postnatal life. This high urine flow rate through the upper tracts during the later stages of pregnancy may constitute a form of diuretic stress, which might account for some examples of the relatively common ultrasound appearance of mild upper tract dilatation which reverts to normality in infancy and early childhood.

Abnormal development of the fetal urinary tract

Geneticists define a 'sequence' as a pattern of abnormalities which derive from a single initial abnormality. In the urinary tract, examples include the Potter sequence due to the mechanical moulding effect of prolonged oligohydramnios. Features include a characteristic facies consisting of a flattened nose, recessed chin, a prominent fold running downwards and outward from the inner canthus and folded flattened ears which are often low set. Pulmonary hypoplasia and limb defects such as talipes equinovarus also form part of this sequence. In a survey of 80 cases [4] of the Potter sequence, 21% were attributed to bilateral renal agenesis, 48% to cystic dysplasia, 25% to obstructive uropathy and a small percentage to other causes. Prune belly syndrome (dilated urinary tract, deficient abdominal wall musculature, bilateral cryptorchidism) is another example of a sequence believed to have its origins in a single abnormality, i.e. urethral obstruction.

Regardless of whether or not they are subsequently associated with a 'sequence', most initial abnormalities can be attributed to one of four pathological mechanisms.

1 *Intrinsic abnormalities of the metanephros.* Absence of the metanephric mesoderm or catastrophic faults in its early development probably account for some cases of renal agenesis.

2 *Ureteric bud anomalies.* The crucial role of the ureteric bud in inducing orderly differentiation of the metanephric blastema has been highlighted by the embryological studies of Douglas Stephens. According to Stephens [5], a ureteric bud arising from an abnormal or ectopic site on the mesonephric duct is more likely to penetrate the peripheral zone of the metanephros, giving rise to dysplasia. In contrast, a normally sited ureteric bud fuses with the healthy central zone to stimulate the normal process of differentiation. The ureteric bud hypothesis fits neatly with clinical observations in duplex systems in which the parenchyma of the upper pole, drained by an ectopic ureter, is usually dysplastic. Studying 51 duplex kidneys, Mackie and Stephens [6] found a close correlation between the extent of renal dysplasia and the degree of ureteral ectopia. Citing a further study contrasting the pattern of renal damage seen in obstructive uropathy with the characteristics of hypoplasia and dysplasia associated with

vesicoureteric reflux, Sommer and Stephens [7] highlighted the importance of the interaction between the ureteric bud and the metanephric mesenchyme.

3 *Fetal obstructive uropathy.* Obstruction is a potent insult to the normal development of the fetal urinary tract. As early as 1971, Beck [8] demonstrated that complete ligation of the proximal ureter in the fetal lamb in the first half of gestation resulted in the characteristic features of renal dysplasia. In contrast, experimentally induced obstruction in the second half of gestation resulted in hydronephrosis and cortical thinning in an otherwise recognizable kidney. The pathophysiology of fetal obstructive uropathy has been studied in depth by Harrison and colleagues in San Francisco [9,10]. Having developed a model of experimental infravesical obstruction associated with pulmonary hypoplasia and renal dysplasia, Harrison demonstrated the ability of intrauterine decompression to reverse some of these pathological processes. Unfortunately the findings of animal studies cannot be directly translated to the clinical setting. Experimentally induced obstruction is acute in onset, severe in nature and introduced at a relatively late stage in gestation into a urinary tract which has previously developed normally. In contrast, human fetal uropathies are generally the outcome of a more gradual obstructive process which frequently dates from an early stage in gestation.

4 *Vesicoureteric reflux* (VUR). The relationship between fetal VUR and renal dysplasia has not been investigated experimentally in a fetal model. As a result of the experimental work of Hodson *et al.* [11] and Ransley *et al.* [12], in conjunction with clinical studies, it is now widely believed that at normal voiding pressures sterile reflux does not give rise to renal scarring. But whilst the 'water hammer' effect of sterile VUR does not appear to be important in postnatal life the impact of sterile urine on the fetal kidney and its involvement in the aetiology of congenital reflux-related dysplasia cannot be discounted.

At a more fundamental level, congenital abnormalities of the urogenital tract can occur as sporadic defects of embryogenesis, as genetically determined anomalies confined to the urinary tract or as part of a syndrome or a complex of multiple anomalies. For this reason whenever a urinary tract abnormality is detected prenatally, a detailed anomaly scan is required to look for possible congenital abnormalities in other systems. In addition, consideration must be given to the possible need for an invasive procedure to karyotype the fetus. In part this decision is guided by the probability of finding a chromosomal disorder.

Ferguson-Smith and Yates [13], studying the karyotypes of 682 fetuses with renal abnormalities, noted that the overall risk of a chromosomal abnormality with an isolated renal defect was three times the maternal age-related risk. If additional malformations were present this risk rose dramatically to 30 times the age-related risk. In their study, the likelihood of a chromosomal abnormality did not correlate with the severity of the renal pathology nor was it influenced by whether the pathology was unilateral or bilateral in distribution. Twelve per cent of all urological abnormalities, including renal agenesis, hydronephrosis and multicystic kidney, were associated with an underlying chromosomal abnormality. Isolated abnormalities of the urinary tract, however, carried a low (3%) risk of chromosomal abnormalities whereas the incidence of chromosomal abnormalities rose to 34% if there were coexistent abnormalities in other systems. In a study undertaken in our centre [14], renal anomalies were associated with serious coexistent disease in 14 (26%) out of 54 fetuses with bilateral uropathy compared with only two (3%) of 72 cases of unilateral uropathy.

From our experience the discovery of an isolated unilateral lesion generally carries a good prognosis and karyotyping would normally be reserved for cases in which there is severe bilateral uropathy or evidence of coexistent anomalies in other systems. Rapid fetal karyotyping can be performed by chorionic villus sampling or by amniocentesis. Some of the more common chromosomal abnor-

malities associated with renal defects are listed in Table 10.1.

Prenatal detection

Sensitivity

Modern high-resolution ultrasound imaging in experienced hands can yield a wealth of detailed information on the fetus. In most centres it is now possible to identify virtually 100% of normal fetal kidneys at 17–19 weeks, the current timing of routine fetal anomaly scans in the UK. Severely dilated systems can often be identified as early as 12–14 weeks. It is becoming increasingly clear, however, that although ultrasound at 17–19 weeks is a sensitive tool for the detection of the majority of lethal congenital anomalies of the urinary tract, many cases of fetal uropathy associated with anomalies at the non-lethal end of the spectrum are not picked up because they have not given rise to detectable dilatation in the second trimester. In routine clinical practice prenatal ultrasound imaging is best regarded as a screening tool that serves two important purposes.

Table 10.1 Chromosomal anomalies associated with renal abnormalities.

Chromosomal anomaly renal findings	Frequency of	Renal findings
Turner syndrome, 45X	60–80%	Horseshoe kidney, double renal pelvis
Trisomy 18 (Edwards syndrome)	70%	Horseshoe kidney, ectopic kidney, double ureter, polycystic kidney, hydronephrosis
Trisomy 13 (Patau syndrome)	60–80%	Polycystic kidney, hydronephrosis, horseshoe kidney, duplicated ureters
18q-	40%	Horseshoe kidney
4p- (Wolf–Hirschorn syndrome)	33%	Hypospadias, polycystic kidneys, hydronephrosis, agenesis
Cat eye syndrome (extra marker chromosome from 22)	Common	Renal agenesis
Trisomy 9 mosaic	Common	Polycystic kidneys, posterior urethral valves
Trisomy 21 (Down syndrome)	3–7%	Renal agenesis, horseshoe kidney
Triploidy	Uncertain	Cystic dysplasia, hydronephrosis
Trisomy 9p		Hydronephrosis, horseshoe kidney, hypospadias
Trisomy 20p		Hypospadias, renal malformations
5p- (cri-du-chat syndrome)		Hypospadias, renal agenesis
9p-		Hydronephrosis
13q-		Hypospadias, renal hypoplasia
XXXXX		Renal dysplasia

1 Detecting lethal fetal uropathy at a stage in gestation when termination of pregnancy is a feasible and legal option (the possible role of fetal intervention in such cases is considered below).

2 Identifying significant forms of non-lethal uropathy which merit investigation in early postnatal life.

Incidence of prenatally detected uropathy

The frequency with which congenital abnormalities of the urinary tract are identified on prenatal ultrasound is governed by two factors.

1 The gestational age at which obstetric ultrasound is routinely performed. For example in the prospective study reported by Helin and Persson [15] in which 11 986 pregnancies were scanned at 17 and 33 weeks, a total of 33 urinary tract anomalies were identified. Of these, however, only three (9%) were evident on the 17-week scan. In the remaining 30 cases dilatation was not apparent until the second scan at 33 weeks. Studying the functional outcome in 35 cases of prenatally detected pelviureteric junction (PUJ) obstruction in infants scanned in the second trimester [16], we noted that in 11 cases (31%) the fetal kidneys had appeared normal on ultrasound during the second trimester and it was only in later pregnancy that dilatation became apparent. Even in posterior urethral valves, potentially the most severe form of obstructive uropathy consistent with survival, second trimester ultrasound appearances may be entirely normal. Dineen et al. [17], reviewing 19 cases of prenatally detected posterior urethral valves at the Hospital for Sick Children, Great Ormond Street, London, noted that second trimester ultrasound had failed to detect 16 (84%) of the cases. In our experience [18] the detection rate was higher, but nevertheless 14 (45%) of 31 prenatally detected cases of posterior urethral valves managed in our centre had non-dilated urinary tracts in the second trimester.

2 The definition of 'abnormality', i.e. the degree of dilatation regarded as signifying genuine pathology.

Although some anomalies (e.g. multicystic dysplastic kidney, severe hydronephrosis, etc.) are immediately evident on ultrasound, in many instances the reported 'abnormality' consists of mild or moderate dilatation confined to the renal pelvis or pelvis and calyces. In an ongoing study intended to establish the incidence, natural history and clinical significance of mild dilatation, Chitty et al. [19] reported an incidence of 0.62% (a total of 84 in 13 500 deliveries). Rosendahl [20] found a renal pelvis with an anteroposterior diameter of greater than 1 cm in 0.48% of fetuses. In Leeds, a combination of routine second trimester ultrasound combined with later ultrasound for selective obstetric indications, identified significant urinary tract anomalies in 78 out of 46 775 fetuses, i.e. an incidence of 1:600 [14].

In summary, current data suggest that the overall incidence of detectable dilatation is of the order of 1:100 fetuses, whilst the incidence of significant uropathies for which postnatal intervention or termination of pregnancy might be indicated is of the order of 1:500.

Fetal surgery

The scientific rationale for intrauterine drainage procedures derives largely from the detailed experimental work of Harrison [9,10] and his colleagues in San Francisco in the early 1980s. 1982 saw the first reported case of fetal surgery in humans [21]. A fetus with posterior urethral valves was delivered via hysterotomy and underwent bilateral cutaneous ureterostomies at 21 weeks' gestation. The pregnancy then continued until 35 weeks when the infant was delivered, but died from pulmonary hypoplasia within the first few hours of life despite adequate decompression of the upper tracts. Undeterred, obstetricians across the world then began to embark on fetal intervention on a largely uncontrolled and unreported basis. Where results have been reported, they have been uniformly disappointing. For example, the Fetal Surgery Registry [22] reported an overall mortality rate of 59% in 73 cases. Enthusiasm for the technique is waning. Mandell et al. [23] identified 24 publications on fetal intervention in the literature between 1982 and 1985, but only seven between 1985 and 1989, two of which had a cautionary message and two consisted of single case reports. With the aim of improving selection criteria, the San Francisco group and others have explored the possible use of fetal urinary biochemical markers as a guide to the severity of renal functional damage. Data derived from 40 fetuses [24] indicated that a fetal urinary sodium level of < 100 mmol/l, chloride < 90 mmol/l and osmolality > 210 mosml/l were sensitive predictors of survival. More recently, Mandelbrot et al. [2] have identified fetal urinary β_2-microglobulin as another useful marker of postnatal renal function.

Techniques employed to drain the fetal urinary tract have included the following.

1 Vesicoamniotic shunting, i.e. ultrasound-guided percutaneous placement of a pigtail stent into the fetal bladder.

2 Hysterotomy and open surgery. Of eight cases treated by the San Francisco group [3] in this fashion, two were stillborn and two died of pulmonary hypoplasia despite fetal surgery. One of the four survivors was in chronic renal failure at the time of reporting, but three infants treated in utero were alive and well; i.e. an overall success rate of 38%.

3 Fetoscopy and placement under vision of a purpose-designed expandable wire mesh suprapubic stent. This technique is currently being evaluated in primates [25] prior to possible use in humans.

Coplen et al. [26] have reported the outcome of

attempted shunting procedures in eight fetuses of whom four were liveborn after successful drainage *in utero*. Of these four infants, three had evidence of diminished renal function and were predicted to require renal transplantation during childhood whilst the fourth had evidence of salt-losing nephropathy. In Leeds [18] we have treated three liveborn infants with documented posterior urethral valves who have undergone vesicoamniotic shunting. Of these one died of severe renal insufficiency in the neonatal period, one has undergone renal transplantation at 3 years of age and the third is predicted to require renal transplantation.

The published results coupled with anecdotal evidence from a number of centres indicate that whilst fetal surgery may be capable of preventing some neonatal deaths from pulmonary hypoplasia, the severe degree of associated renal dysplasia is usually irreversible by the time of treatment in the late second trimester (Fig. 10.1).

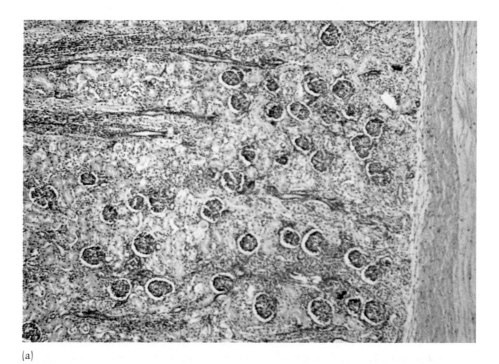

(a)

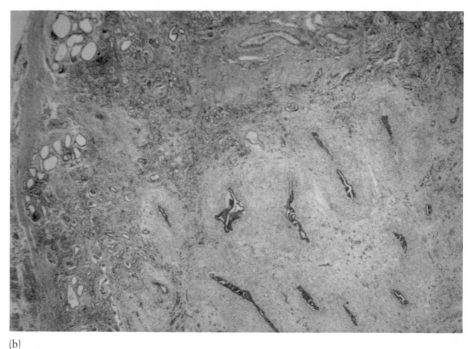

(b)

Fig. 10.1 (a) Normal histological appearances of the renal cortex in a fullterm newborn infant. (b) Nephron-depleted, dysplastic renal cortex in a fullterm newborn infant with lethal pulmonary hypoplasia associated with severe urethral obstruction.

Specific genetic considerations

Renal agenesis

The birth incidence of bilateral renal agenesis is of the order 15:100 000. The true underlying incidence of renal agenesis is more difficult to gauge because the anomaly frequently remains undetected. One estimate, however, puts the incidence of unilateral renal agenesis at 3:1000 [27]. Bilateral renal agenesis is a lethal condition and a reliable prenatal diagnosis is therefore important. Characteristic ultrasound findings include profound oligohydramnios, failure to visualize the kidneys and absence of urine in the fetal bladder. In experienced hands the diagnosis can be made with a high degree of accuracy and Romero et al. [28] , for example, reported a positive diagnosis in 100% of cases by 24 weeks' gestation.

Renal agenesis probably represents a heterogeneous group of disorders and autosomal recessive, autosomal dominant, X-linked recessive and multifactorial patterns of inheritance have all been postulated. Some of the genetic syndromes most commonly associated with renal agenesis and dysgenesis are listed in Table 10.2. A male:female ratio of 1.67:1 has been reported for unilateral agenesis and 3.37:1 for bilateral agenesis. The empirical recurrence risk in siblings is 3.5%. When the index case is female this figure rises to 6.98% [29] in siblings. Renal agenesis occurring in conjunction with other abnormalities, increases the risk in siblings to 12.5%. The recurrence risk of isolated renal agenesis is such that prenatal screening should be offered in future pregnancies. Roodhoft et al. [27] found asymptomatic malformations in 7.4% of parents of children with bilateral renal agenesis or dysgenesis and on

this basis recommended that in addition to siblings, parents should be screened with ultrasound.

Infantile polycystic kidney disease (Potter type I disease)

This autosomal recessive condition has a quoted incidence [30] of approximately 2:100 000 and a recurrence risk of 25%. Perinatal, neonatal, infantile and juvenile types have been described [31] and the spectrum of clinical manifestation ranges from massive renal enlargement in the fetus to a predominantly hepatic presentation in older children. The severe early onset form is associated with characteristic prenatal ultrasound findings (Fig. 10.2) but the less severe forms cannot yet be diagnosed prenatally.

Adult polycystic kidney disease (Potter type III disease)

This autosomal dominant condition has an incidence of 1:1000 and a 50% recurrence risk [32]. Typically, the condition remains asymptomatic until the fourth or fifth decades. But in one study of children with polycystic kidneys presenting in the first year of life, 12.5% [33] were found to have a variant of adult polycystic kidney disease. Prenatal ultrasound findings of the adult form of polycystic kidney disease have been described [34] but it is not clear whether children in whom cysts are detected in utero have a worse prognosis. The genetic basis of polycystic disease is being intensively studied and in children with cysts detected in utero, a defect at chromosome 16p13.3. (polycystic kidney disease type 1) has been identified [35]. A second locus has been localized to chromosome 4

Table 10.2 Genetic conditions associated with renal agenesis/dysgenesis.

Condition	Inheritance	Other findings
Fraser syndrome	AR	Cryptophthalmos, syndactyly, genital malformations
Fanconi syndrome	AR	Pancytopenia, skeletal malformations
Klippel–Feil sequence	Sporadic	Fusion of cervical vertebrae
Branchio-oto-renal syndrome	AD	Ear pits, deafness, branchial cysts or fistulas
MURCS association	Sporadic	Vertebral/rib malformations, uterovaginal anomalies
Rokitansky sequence	Sporadic	Absence of uterus
Sirenomelia sequence	Sporadic	Fusion of the lower extremities
VATER association	Sporadic	Vertebral anomalies, anal atresia, tracheo-oesophageal fistulas, radial limb anomalies

AD, autosomal dominant; AR, autosomal recessive.

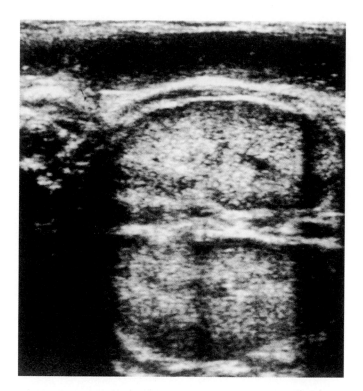

Fig. 10.2 Ultrasound appearances of massive diffuse bilateral enlargement of the fetal kidneys in infantile polycystic disease, which is autosomal recessive.

(polycystic kidney disease type 2). Over 70 different genetic syndromes have been reported in association with polycystic kidney disease and these are summarized in Table 10.3.

Multicystic dysplastic kidney

It is important to distinguish this anomaly from other forms of renal cystic disease. Multicystic dysplastic kidneys are characterized by a collection of tense non-communicating cysts with an absence of functioning renal parenchyma (Fig. 10.3). Most commonly, the lesion is associated with ureteric atresia at the level of the PUJ. Although bilateral multicystic dysplasia is invariably lethal, unilateral multicystic dysplastic kidneys are frequently asymptomatic and it is only following the advent of routine prenatal ultrasound that the relative frequency of this anomaly has been recognized. The genetic basis of multicystic dysplasia has not been adequately researched but is generally believed to represent a sporadic defect of embryogenesis rather than a genetically determined abnormality.

Ureteric duplication

This can be complete or incomplete. Estimates suggest that 5% of the general population have a variant (usually asymptomatic) of upper tract duplication. The evidence of two studies [36,37] indicates that duplication is inherited as an autosomal dominant with variable penetrance.

Pelviureteric junction obstruction

This is the single urological anomaly detected with most frequency by prenatal ultrasound (Table 10.4 and Fig. 10.4). Although PUJ obstruction is occasionally associated with specific genetic syndromes (e.g. Schinzel Giedion and Johanson Blizzard syndrome) it is generally regarded as an

Table 10.3 Genetic conditions associated with polycystic kidneys.

Condition	Inheritance	Other findings
Tuberous sclerosis	AD	Cardiac rhabdomyomas, fits, skin hamartoma, renal hamartoma
Nail–patella syndrome	AD	Dysplastic nails, hypoplastic patellae, skeletal malformations
Meckel–Gruber syndrome	AR	Encephalocele, polydactyly, genital abnormalities
Zellweger (cerebro-hepato-renal) syndrome	AR	Intrauterine growth retardation, hypotonia, high forehead, congenital heart disease, hepatomegaly
Asphyxiating thoracic dystrophy (Jeune syndrome)	AR	Skeletal dysplasia
Roberts syndrome	AR	Intrauterine growth retardation, microcephaly, cleft lip and palate, limb reduction
Oro-facial-digital syndrome type 1	X-linked dominant	Oral clefts, digital asymmetry

AD, autosomal dominant; AR, autosomal recessive.

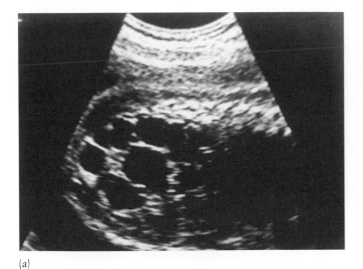

(a)

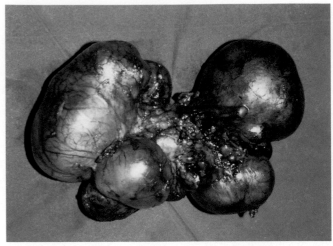

(b)

Fig. 10.3 (a) Characteristic prenatal ultrasound appearances of multicystic dysplastic kidney, i.e. multiple non-communicating cysts with an absence of recognizable cortex. (b) A nephrectomy specimen of a multicystic dysplastic kidney.

Table 10.4 Analysis of final urological diagnoses in 426 liveborn infants with significant* prenatally detected uropathy.

Diagnosis	Number	Per cent
Pelviureteric junction obstruction	150	35
Vesicoureteric reflux	83	20
Multicystic kidney	64	15
Vesicoureteric junction obstruction	42	10
Posterior urethral valves	37	9
Duplex systems	36	8
Renal agenesis	14	3
Total	426	100

*Excluding mild pelvicalyceal dilatation, crossed renal ectopia, etc.

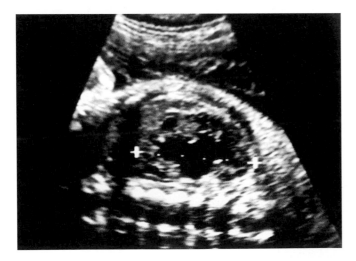

Fig. 10.4 Isolated fetal hydronephrosis. Ultrasound appearances indicate PUJ obstruction but the definitive diagnosis of obstruction requires further diagnostic imaging in postnatal life.

anomaly of sporadic occurrence. In a few families, however, the condition has been reported as behaving as an autosomal dominant [38]. The conservative management of an increasing proportion of asymptomatic prenatally detected PUJ obstructions has revealed the potential for spontaneous resolution—possibly in up to 50% of instances. Studies of asymptomatic siblings and family members may shed further light on the true recurrence risk of PUJ obstruction.

Posterior urethral valves (Fig. 10.5)

Although most cases are regarded as sporadic in aetiology,

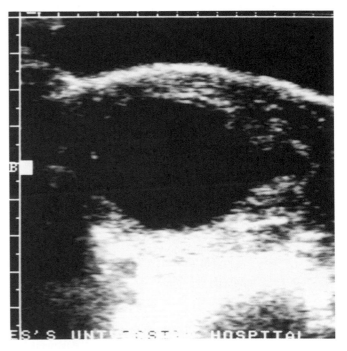

Fig. 10.5 Ultrasound appearances of dilatation of the fetal bladder and posterior urethra (posterior urethral valves).

there are rare reports of familial cases indicating a possible genetic predisposition. The literature includes cases of both twin [39] and non-twin [40] affected siblings, suggesting a polygenetic mode of inheritance. However, discordance in monozygotic twins has also been reported [41], suggesting that a random mutation may also be implicated in some cases. Although the genetic risk is low, male siblings should be screened with ultrasound postnatally.

Vesicoureteric reflux

This is a common condition with an incidence in the general population estimated at between 1 and 2% [42,43]. The familial nature of this condition is now well established and in a 10-year prospective study, Noe [44] identified VUR in 119 (34%) of 354 siblings of clinically presenting index patients. Segregation analysis suggests that VUR is the result of a single dominant gene whose effects are modified by random environmental effects.

Screening the asymptomatic siblings of affected children for possible VUR is an attractive concept, but unfortunately there are problems in selecting the ideal screening test. Ultrasound, whilst simple and non-invasive, is an unreliable modality for the detection of VUR with an unacceptably high rate of false-negative and occasional false-positive findings. The most reliable test, i.e. conventional contrast and voiding cystography, is a time consuming and invasive procedure with a significant radiation dosage — particularly to the ovaries. Studies to validate the benefits of invasive screening in asymptomatic siblings would be required before it could be advocated on a routine basis. As a practical compromise it seems reasonable to screen siblings with ultrasound in the first instance and to reserve voiding cystography for those in whom ultrasound reveals evidence of dilatation.

Bladder exstrophy

Bladder exstrophy has a low recurrence risk and an empirical risk factor of 1% is quoted in counselling.

Hypospadias

A number of studies place the incidence of isolated hypospadias at around 4:1000 live births [45,46]. There is an increased incidence amongst first-degree relatives of index cases and in one study it was found that 14% [47] of male siblings were also affected. The mechanism of inheritance is thought to be polygenic. Some of the genetic syndromes classically associated with hypospadias are listed in Table 10.5.

Postnatal diagnosis and management of fetal uropathy

A detailed account of the diagnosis and management of individual prenatally detected uropathies is beyond the scope of this chapter. Broadly speaking, however, the investigative protocol stems from a postnatal ultrasound scan performed at around 24–48 h of age when a representative fluid intake and urine output have been established. The findings of this initial scan then guide the pattern of further investigation. Anomalies such as multicystic dysplastic kidney or severe hydronephrosis, which are associated with distinctive ultrasound appearances, are then studied by a standardized sequence of diagnostic imaging. When postnatal ultrasound reveals only mild or moderate dilatation of the pelvis alone or of the pelvis and/or calyces, however, it is doubtful whether invasive investigations such as micturating cystography and isotope renography are justified. In a study [48] representing 122 child years of follow-up, we documented a low risk of urological morbidity associated with mild pelvicalyceal dilatation (pyelocalyectesis). At a mean of 4.2 years follow-up, ultrasound re-evaluation of 39 mildly dilated kidneys revealed that the appearances had reverted to normal in 69%, whilst in the remaining 31% of kidneys the dilatation was unchanged or improving.

Maizels et al. [49] have suggested that calyceal dilatation may be a more consistent marker of underlying pathology and have devised a scoring system to grade prenatally detected hydronephrosis. Opinion differs, but we believe that a non-interventionist approach to the investigation of mild pyelocalyectesis, whilst missing occasional cases of VUR, is of overall benefit by minimizing the burden of unnecessary invasive investigations in healthy infants.

Voiding cystography is undoubtedly justified, however, when the initial postnatal ultrasound demonstrates

Table 10.5 Genetic syndromes associated with hypospadias.

Condition	Inheritance	Other findings
Fraser syndrome	AR	Cryptophthalmus, renal agenesis, syndactyly
Smith–Lemli–Opitz syndrome	AR	Congenital heart disease, cleft palate, syndactyly, polydactyly
Opitz–G syndrome	AD	Characteristic face, dysphagia, hoarse voice

AD, autosomal dominant; AR, autosomal recessive.

ureteral dilatation, a thick-walled or a poorly emptying bladder. When posterior urethral valves are demonstrated, definitive treatment is usually undertaken in the neonatal period. Primary VUR detected prenatally is predominantly a feature of males (male:female ratio 5:1) [50] and is managed conservatively in the first instance.

The investigation of presumed PUJ or vesicoureteric junction obstruction is best deferred until functional imaging with isotopes can be performed more reliably at around 4–6 weeks of age. Even in the presence of high-grade obstruction, the information derived from isotope imaging rarely influences management in the first few weeks of life. Recent years have seen most centres switching from routine early pyeloplasty to a more conservative approach, reserving early pyeloplasty for the minority of cases in which there is gross hydronephrosis or isotopic evidence of significant impairment of renal function. Despite renographic evidence of obstruction, normal levels of differential renal function are retained in approximately two-thirds of cases [51,52].

Conclusion

Although the assumed benefits of routine obstetric ultrasound have been challenged, it is unlikely that obstetricians (or pregnant women) will wish to see a reversion to the pre-ultrasound era. The theoretical promise of fetal surgery has not been fulfilled and it is unlikely to have an enduring role in the management of urinary tract anomalies in the fetus. Termination of pregnancy, on the other hand, can be expected to exert a continuing impact on paediatric urological practice with the result that fewer infants at the severe end of the spectrum will find their way to paediatric urologists in postnatal life. Mild to moderate forms of fetal uropathy, which are often undetectable in the second trimester, will be identified with increasing frequency as third trimester scans become incorporated into routine obstetric practice. Despite the diminishing role of early postnatal surgical intervention, paediatric urologists will continue to have a key role in the decision-making process and the follow-up of affected infants will contribute to a growing workload in the specialty. Conversely, the involvement of adult urologists in the management of urological disease in childhood is likely to diminish.

References

1 Hobbins JC, Romero R, Grannum P et al. Antenatal diagnosis of renal anomalies with ultrasound. I. Obstructive uropathy. Am J Obstet Gynecol 1984;148:868–7.

2 Mandelbrot L, Dumez Y, Muller F et al. Prenatal prediction of renal function in fetal obstructive uropathy. J Perinat Med 1991;19 (Suppl. 1):283–7.

3 Estes JM, Harrison R. Fetal obstructive uropathy. Semin Ped Surg 1993;2(2):129.

4 Curry CJR, Jenson K, Holland J, Miller L, Hall BD. The Potter sequence: a clinical analysis of 80 cases. Am J Med Genet 1984;19:679–702.

5 Stephens FD. The pathogenesis of renal dysplasia. In: Stephens FD, ed. Congenital Malformations of the Urinary Tract. New York: Praeger, 1983; 441–62.

6 Mackie GG, Stephens FD. Duplex kidneys: a correlation of renal dysplasia with position of the ureteral orifice. J Urol 1975;114:274–80.

7 Sommer JT, Stephens FD. Morphogenesis of nephropathy with partial ureteral obstruction and vesicoureteral reflux. J Urol 1981;125:67–72.

8 Beck AD. The effect of intrauterine urinary obstruction upon the development of the fetal urinary tract. J Urol 1971;105: 784–9.

9 Harrison MR, Nakayama DR, de Lorimer AA. Correction of congenital hydronephrosis in utero II. Decompression reverses the effects of obstruction on the fetal lung and urinary tract. J Pediatr Surg 1982;17:965–74.

10 Harrison MR, Ross N, Noall R et al. Correction of congenital hydronephrosis in utero I. The model: fetal urethral obstruction produces hydronephrosis and pulmonary hypoplasia in fetal lambs. J Pediatr Surg 1983;18:247–56.

11 Hodson CJ, Maling TMJ, McManamon PJ. Reflux nephropathy. Kidney Int 1975;8:50–8.

12 Ransley PG, Risdon RA, Goldy ML. High pressure sterile vesicoureteral reflux and renal scarring: an experimental study in the pig and minipig. Contrib Nephrol 1984;39:320–43.

13 Ferguson-Smith M, Yates J. Maternal age specific rates for chromosome aberration and factors influencing them: report of a collaborative European study on 52,965 amniocenteses. Prenat Diagn 1984;4 (Special Issue):5.

14 Arthur RJ, Irving HC, Thomas DFM et al. Bilateral fetal uropathy: what is the outlook? Br Med J 1989;298:1419–20.

15 Helin I, Persson P. Prenatal diagnosis of urinary tract abnormalities by ultrasound. J Pediatr 1986;78:879–83.

16 Barker AP, Cave MM, Thomas DFM et al. Fetal PUJ obstruction: predictors of outcome. Br J Urol 1995;76: 649–52.

17 Dineen MD, Dhillon HK, Ward HC et al. Antenatal diagnosis of posterior urethral valves. Br J Urol 1993;72:365.

18 Hutton KAR, Thomas DFM. Prenatally detected posterior urethral valves: is gestational age at detection a predictor of outcome? J Urol 1994;152:698–701.

19 Chitty LS, Pembrey ME, Chudleigh PM, Campbell S. Multicentre study of antenatally calyceal dilatation detected by ultrasound. Lancet 1990;336:875.

20 Rosendahl H. Ultrasound screening for fetal urinary tract malformations: a prospective study in general population. Eur J Obstet Gynecol Reprod Biol 1990;36:27–33.

21 Harrison MR, Golbus MS, Filly RA et al. Fetal surgery for congenital hydronephrosis. N Engl J Med 1982;306:591–3.

22 Manning FA, Harrison MR, Rodeck C et al. Catheter shunts for fetal hydronephrosis and hydrocephalus. N Engl J Med 1986;315:336–40.

23 Mandell J, Peters CA, Retik AB. Current concepts in the perinatal diagnosis and management of hydronephrosis. Urol Clin North Am 1990;17:247–62.

24 Crombleholme TM, Harrison MR, Golbus MS et al. Fetal

intervention in obstructive uropathy: prognostic indicators and efficacy of intervention. *Am J Obstet Gynecol* 1990;**162**: 1239–44.

25 Estes JM, MacGillivray TE, Hedrick MH *et al*. Fetoscopic surgery for the treatment of congenital anomalies. *J Pediatr Surg* 1992;**27**:950–4.

26 Coplen DE, Hare JY, Zderic S *et al*. 10 year experience with antenatal *in utero* intervention. Abstract 5. Presented to the Section of Urology, American Academy of Pediatrics, Annual Meeting, Dallas, 1994.

27 Roodhoft AM, Birnholz J, Holmes L. Familial nature of congenital absence and severe dysgenesis of both kidneys *N Engl J Med* 1984;**310**:1341–5.

28 Romero R, Cullen M, Grannum P *et al*. Antenatal diagnosis of renal anomalies with ultrasound III. Bilateral renal agenesis. *Am J Obstet Gynecol*, 1985;**151**:38–43.

29 Carter C, Evans K, Pescia G. A family study of renal agenesis. *J Med Genet* 1979;**16**:176–88.

30 Zerres K, Hansmann R, Mallmann R, Gembruck U. Autosomal recessive polycystic kidney disease: problems of prenatal diagnosis. *Prenat Diagn* 1988;**8**:215–29.

31 Blyth H, Ockenden B. Polycystic disease of kidneys and liver presenting in childhood. *J Med Genet* 1971;**8**:257–84.

32 Dalgaard OZ. Bilateral polycystic disease of the kidneys: a follow-up of two hundred and eighty-four patients and their families. *Acta Med Scand Suppl* 1957;**328**:1–255.

33 Cole B, Conley S, Stapleton F. Polycystic kidney disease in the first year of life. *J Pediatr* 1987;**111**:693–9.

34 McHugo J, Shafi M, Rowlands D, Weaver H. Prenatal diagnosis of adult polycystic kidney disease. *Br J Radiol* 1988;**61**:1072.

35 Michaud J, Russo P, Grignon A *et al*. Expression of autosomal dominant polycystic kidney disease (ADPKD) during fetal life. *Am J Hum Genet* 1993;**53**(3):1439.

36 Whitaker J, Porteous M, Paramo P *et al*. A study of the inheritance of duplication of the kidneys and ureters. *J Urol* 1966;**95**:176–8.

37 Atwell J, Cook P, Howell C *et al*. Familial incidence of bifid and double ureters. *Arch Dis Child* 1974;**49**:390–3.

38 Atwell JD. Familial pelviureteric junction hydronephrosis and its association with a duplex pelvicaliceal system and vesicoureteric reflux. A family study. *Br J Urol* 1985;**57**:365–9.

39 Livne PM, Delaune J, Gonzales EJ. Genetic etiology of posterior urethral valves. *J Urol* 1983;**130**(4):781–4.

40 Borzi PA, Beasley SW, Fowler R. Posterior urethral valves in non-twin siblings. *Br J Urol* 1992;**70**(2):201.

41 Thomalla JV, Mitchell ME, Garett RA. Posterior urethral valves in siblings. *Urology* 1989;**33**(4):291–4.

42 Iannaccone G, Panzironi PE. Ureteral reflux in normal infants. *Acta Radiol* 1955;**44**:451–6.

43 McGovern JH, Marshall VF, Paquin A Jr. Vesicoureteral regurgitation in children. *J Urol* 1960;**83**:122–49.

44 Noe HN. The long term results of prospective sibling reflux screening. *J Urol* 1993;**148**(5):1739–42.

45 Sweet RA, Schrott HG, Kurland R *et al*. Study of the incidence of hypospadias in Rochester, Minnesota 1940–1970 and a case control comparison of possible etiologic factors. *Mayo Clin Proc* 1974;**49**:52–9.

46 Chung CS, Myrianthopoulos NC. Racial and prenatal factors in major congenital malformations. *Am J Hum Genet* 1968;**20**: 44–60.

47 Bauer SB, Retik AB, Colodny AH. Genetic aspects of hypospadias. *Urol Clinic North Am* 1981;**8**:559–64.

48 Thomas DFM, Madden NP, Irving HC *et al*. Mild dilatation of the fetal kidney: a follow-up study. *Br J Urol* 1994;**74**: 236–9.

49 Maizels M, Reisman ME, Flom LS *et al*. Grading nephroureteral dilatation detected in the first year of life: correlation with obstruction. *J Urol* 1992;**148**:609–14.

50 Elder JS. Commentary: importance of antenatal diagnosis of vesicoureteral reflux. *J Urol* 1992;**148**:(5):1750–4.

51 Ransley PG, Dhillon HK, Gordon I *et al*. The postnatal management of hydronephrosis diagnosed by prenatal ultrasound. *J Urol* 1990;**144**:584–7.

52 Madden NP, Thomas DFM, Gordon AC *et al*. Antenatally detected pelviureteric junction obstruction. Is non-operation safe? *Br J Urol* 1991;**68**:305–10.

11 Cystic and Dysplastic Kidneys

B.S.Kaplan, P.Kaplan and R.D.Bellah

Introduction

The classification of cystic and dysplastic kidney diseases has been confusing. The different terms and classifications that have been used do not always take into account associated abnormalities and variable expression. A precise diagnosis requires careful integration of many sources of information: prenatal history and fetal ultrasonography (US), family history, clinical examination, imaging studies of proband and parents, interpretation of laboratory studies (including DNA tests if available) and pathology. A precise diagnosis is required for prognosis, treatment and genetic counselling. The efforts of a multispecialty team [1] are needed for the diagnosis and management of a patient with cystic or dysplastic kidneys and abnormal urinary tract.

Prenatal diagnosis of renal abnormalities has altered the knowledge of the natural progression and treatment of some disorders. Prenatal history should include details of maternal illness, medical and recreational drug use, and exposure to environmental teratogens. Family history must include all illnesses, handicaps, deaths, miscarriages, stillbirths, parental ages, consanguinity, ethnic origins and occupations. Few genetic renal disorders are confined to the kidneys and, conversely, many syndromes have renal involvement. Therefore, it is advisable to use US to examine the kidneys and urinary tract in newborns with multiple defects.

The importance of understanding the concepts of variable expression and incomplete penetrance cannot be overemphasized. An example of variable expression is shown in Table 11.1. It is also important to draw attention to the occurrence of more than one kind of renal cystic and/or dysplastic disorder which can occur within a well-defined syndrome. In tuberosclerosis, for example, pleomorphic renal abnormalities include simple cysts, polycystic kidneys, angiomyolipomas and renal carcinomas. Single case reports of 'new' or unique family syndromes are not reviewed in this chapter.

Table 11.1 Variable expression in a kindred with branchio-oto-renal syndrome. Modified from [2] and personal observations.

	Renal/urological anomalies	Extrarenal anomalies
Father	Nil	Nil
Mother	Nil, normal urogram	Lop ears Left pre-auricular fistula Bilateral cervical fistulas Facial asymmetry
Male child	Right renal agenesis Interstitial nephritis Chronic renal failure	Bilateral pre-auricular pits Cervical fistulas Conductive hearing loss Lachrymal aplasia
Female child	Left renal agenesis Left ureteral agenesis Right renal hypoplasia Two calyces on right	Oligohydramnios Bilateral pre-auricular pits No cervical fistulas Normal ovaries and uterus Died at birth
Female child	Left renal agenesis Right renal hypoplasia Chronic renal failure	Bilateral pre-auricular pits Cervical fistulas Hearing loss Abnormal vagina Died at age 6 years

Terminology

The definitions used in this chapter are summarized in Table 11.2. A renal cyst [4,5] is an enclosed sac or nephron segment of more than 200 μm, lined by epithelium. It usually contains fluid with the chemical composition of plasma ultrafiltrate. Renal cysts may be solitary, multiple or innumerable; cortical or medullary; familial or sporadic; and may sometimes be associated with extrarenal abnormalities. A cystic kidney contains three or more cysts. Cystic kidney disease is the illness caused by a cystic kidney [5].

Polycystic kidney disease (PKD) must not be confused with multicystic kidney disease. 'Infantile' and 'adult' are not useful adjectives for polycystic kidneys because the presentation occurs also at other ages. It is more accurate to

Table 11.2 Definitions of cystic and dysplastic kidneys. Modified from [3].

Term	Definition
Simple cyst	Benign, fluid-filled cavity
Multicystic kidney	No continuity between glomeruli and calyces Kidney does not function Contralateral kidney may be normal, absent, hydronephrotic, ectopic or dysplastic Bilateral multicystic kidneys cause severe oligohydramnios
Adysplasia	Includes renal agenesis, hypoplasia and/or dysplasia
Dysplastic kidneys	Unilateral or bilateral Usually cystic, disorganized architecture Ectopic tissues (cartilage, muscle) often present May function
Renal agenesis	Unilateral or bilateral absence of kidney May be isolated or occur with multiple abnormalities
Hypoplastic kidneys	Small, have fewer calyces, may be dysplastic Include simple hypoplasia, oligomeganephronia and renal dysplasia
Simple hypoplasia	Normal renal architecture but fewer reniculi Reduced number and size of nephrons
Oligomeganephronia	Small kidneys Large glomeruli but decreased numbers
Dysgenetic kidneys	Do not develop normally Are not dysplastic, cystic or obstructed Do not contain ectopic tissue Absent proximal tubules
Dysmorphic kidneys	Abnormal shape or echo texture on imaging studies May be dysplastic
Polycystic kidneys	Many cysts in both kidneys No renal dysplasia Continuity of the lumen of the nephron from the uriniferous space to the urinary bladder
Glomerulocystic kidneys	Dilated Bowman spaces Few or no tubular cysts
Medullary sponge kidney	Dilated collecting tubules in pyramids
Medullary cystic kidneys	Progressive renal tubular atrophy Dilated tubules Interstitial and periglomerular fibrosis

use the designations of autosomal recessive and autosomal dominant polycystic kidneys. The term PKD is usually restricted to autosomal dominant PKD and autosomal recessive PKD [6]. It is clear, however, that the dominant polycystic kidney phenotype can occur in other inherited conditions (Table 11.3). The classifications of Osathanondh and Potter [21] and Blyth and Ockenden [22] are obsolete. A practical classification of renal cystic and dysplastic conditions is shown in Table 11.4.

Multicystic renal dysplasia is often used synonymously with multicystic kidney. However, cysts are not present in all dysplastic kidneys, and dysplastic elements cannot be demonstrated in all multicystic kidneys. Dysplastic kidneys may be hypoplastic (small) but not all hypoplastic kidneys are dysplastic.

Associated abnormalities

Low-set ears, pre-auricular pits, two-vessel umbilical cord and hypospadias are not sensitive pointers to a renal anomaly. However, there are anomalies that often occur in association with renal cystic or dysplastic diseases.

The oligohydramnios sequence (Potter syndrome) can be the consequence of inadequate amounts of urine due to obstructive uropathy, renal agenesis and renal cystic or dysplastic diseases. Compression of the fetus by the uterus produces the flattened Potter facies, limb deformations, a narrow, small chest and pulmonary hypoplasia. In prune belly syndrome, urethral obstruction results in the sequence of dilated bladder, absent or deficient anterior abdominal muscles, wrinkled abdomen, undescended testes and renal cystic dysplasia.

Congenital hepatic fibrosis occurs in association with recessive PKD and in other hereditary renal diseases [23,24] (Table 11.5). Evaluation of the liver by US and confirmation by biopsy may be indicated in these conditions. Genital abnormalities and unilateral or bilateral renal agenesis occur in the Mayer–Rokitansky syndrome [26,27]. In patients with associated vaginal and/or rectal atresia, the kidneys may be dysplastic, or if one kidney is affected the contralateral kidney may be absent. Genital abnormalities occur in the Townes–Brock radial–ear–anal–renal (REAR) syndrome, Fraser cryptophthalmos syndrome, ectodermal dysplasia–ectrodactyly–cleft lip/palate (EEC) syndrome, Meckel syndrome and glutaric aciduria type II. Skeletal dysplasias are often associated with a wide spectrum of renal abnormalities. Pyloric stenosis occurs in autosomal dominant PKD, autosomal recessive PKD, autosomal dominant glomerulocystic kidneys, and congenital nephrotic syndrome. There are several acrorenal syndromes with renal abnormalities and radial ray defects. The Dandy–Walker malformation or cyst is reported in the Fitch–Fryns, Ivemark, Goldston and Meckel syndromes.

Table 11.3 Conditions associated with the dominant PKD phenotype (renal clinical and imaging features).

	Chromosome locus/Inheritance		Extrarenal manifestations	References
PKD1	16p13.3	AD	Hepatic cysts, pancreatic cysts, colonic diverticula, mitral valve prolapse, berry aneurysm, inguinal hernia	Reeders *et al.* [7,8]*
PKD2	4q13-q23	AD	As PKD1	Kimberling *et al.* [9] Peters *et al.* [10]
PKD3	?	AD	As PKD1	Daoust *et al.* [11]
PKD1 and overlap connective tissue disorder	16p	Cosegregation AD	Aortic root dilatation, aortic and vertebral artery disorder aneurysms with dissection, aortic valve incompetence, pectus, pes planus, joint laxity, arachnodactyly, dolichostenomelia, high arched palate	Somlo *et al.* [12]
Tuberosclerosis complex (TSC2)	16p	AD (1 : 10 000 to 1 : 50 000)	Infantile spasms, ash-leaf macules, facial angiofibromas, shagreen patch, periungual fibromas, cortical tubers, subependymal or cortical calcifications, retinal hamartomas Renal imaging features and gross appearance resemble PKD but histopathologic features differ from PKD Renal carcinomas, angiomyolipomas	Bernstein [13] ECTSC [14] Kandt *et al.* [15]
von Hippel–Lindau syndrome	3p25-26	AD (1 : 50 000 to 1 : 60 000)	CNS and retinal hemangioblastomas, pancreatic, hepatic, epididymal cysts, pheochromocytomas, onset fourth decade, angiomas, renal carcinomas	Lamiell *et al.* [16] Latif *et al.* [17]
Oro–facial–digital type 1 syndrome		XD (rare)	Mental retardation, CNS and facial anomalies, pseudocleft upper lip, polysyndactyly Usually lethal in males	Salinas *et al.* [18]
Hajdu–Cheney syndrome		AD (rare)	Short stature, abnormal skull, distinctive facies, hoarse voice, progressive skeletal dysplasia, acro-osteolysis of terminal phalanges, loss of teeth	Kaplan *et al.* [19]* Rosenmann *et al.* [20]

AD, autosomal dominant; XD, X-linked dominant.

Simple cysts

Simple cysts are uncommon in childhood. They may be single or multiple, may occur in the cortex or the medulla, and are rarely symptomatic [28]. At sonography, a simple cyst can mimic a calyceal diverticulum or a cystic upper pole of a duplication anomaly. Simple cysts are important in the differential diagnosis of autosomal dominant PKD.

Multicystic kidney

Multicystic kidney is a congenital anomaly that results from abnormal metanephric differentiation [29]. Ureteropelvic dysplasia or atresia is usually present, the kidney is enlarged and the cysts vary in size. The pelvis and calyces cannot be demonstrated (Fig. 11.1). Microscopic examination usually shows rudimentary lobes with corticomedullary differentiation [29].

Multicystic kidney must be differentiated from obstructive cystic renal dysplasia associated with hydronephrosis and lower ureteral atresia or other forms of obstructive uropathy. Obstructive cystic renal dysplasia is seen mainly in patients with posterior urethral valves and in prune belly syndrome [29]. The pathogenesis of multicystic kidney and renal dysplasia may be similar: the term dysplasia/adysplasia recognizes the fact that combinations of multicystic kidney, renal dysplasia and renal agenesis can occur in the same patient or in any of its various forms in several different members of a kindred [30]. When one kidney is multicystic, the other may be normal, absent, hydronephrotic or ectopic, and occasionally multicystic and dysplastic [31,32]. It has been suggested that there may be a spectrum of obstructive renal dysplastic disease [33] that includes calyceal diverticulum, pyelogenous cyst, pelviureteric junction stenosis, multi-infundibular stenosis, pelvic stenosis and multicystic kidneys [34] (see Fig. 11.1).

The prevalence of multicystic kidney in live newborns is 1:4300 [35]. Neonates with bilateral multicystic kidneys die soon after birth from pulmonary hypoplasia and renal failure. Multicystic kidney can be detected by US *in utero*, by palpation or during evaluation of a urinary tract

Table 11.4 Cystic and dysplastic kidneys in neonates and children. Modified from [1].

SIMPLE RENAL CYST*	POLYCYSTIC KIDNEYS
CALYCEAL ABNORMALITIES*	Autosomal recessive
Diverticula	Autosomal recessive polycystic kidney disease (PKD)
Calyectasis	Meckel syndrome
Hydrocalycosis	Jeune syndrome
Infundibulopelvic stenosis	Renal–hepatic–pancreatic dysplasia
	Glutaric aciduria type II
MULTICYSTIC KIDNEY*	Zellweger syndrome
	Carbohydrate-deficient glycoprotein syndrome
RENAL ADYSPLASIA/DYSPLASIA	Autosomal dominant
Isolated adysplasia/dysplasia†	Autosomal dominant PKD
Sporadic	PKD1
Autosomal recessive	PKD2
Autosomal dominant	PKD3 (see ref [11])
Multifactorial inheritance	Tuberosclerosis
Adysplasia in regional defects	von Hippel–Lindau syndrome
Usually sporadic	Oro–facial–digital syndrome type I
Prune belly syndrome	Hajdu–Cheney syndrome
Posterior urethral valves (PUV)‡	?Ehlers–Danlos syndrome
Genital anomalies and renal adysplasia/dysplasia	
Adysplasia in multiple congenital abnormalities syndromes	MEDULLARY SPONGE KIDNEYS
Autosomal dominant	
Branchio-oto-renal (BOR) syndrome	MEDULLARY CYSTIC KIDNEYS
Ectodermal dysplasia, ectrodactyly, cleft lip/palate syndrome	Autosomal recessive medullary cystic kidney disease
Radial ray aplasia and renal anomalies (RRARA)§	Familial juvenile nephronophthisis
Autosomal recessive	Senior–Lorkin syndrome
Chondrodysplasias	Boichis syndrome or variant
Fanconi pancytopenia syndrome	Biedl–Bardet syndrome
Thrombocytopenia absent radius syndrome	Autosomal dominant medullary cystic disease
Radial ray aplasia and renal anomalies (RRARA)§	
Fraser syndrome	GLOMERULOCYSTIC KIDNEYS
Fryns syndrome	Isolated glomerulocystic kidneys
Usually sporadic	Associated with other kidney diseases
VACTERL ‖ (VATER)	Autosomal dominant
Adysplasia in chromosomal disorders	Familial hypoplastic glomerulocystic kidney
Trisomies 13, 18, 21	
Oligomeganephronia	DYSGENETIC KIDNEYS
Usually sporadic	Autosomal recessive
Autosomal recessive	Congenital hypernephronic nephromegaly with tubular
Syndromal	dysgenesis
	Perlman syndrome
	ACQUIRED CYSTIC DISEASE

* Usually sporadic.
† Occasionally recessive or dominant.
‡ PUV have been reported in siblings.
§ Some kindreds with recessive, others with dominant inheritance.
‖ Dominant inheritance has been reported.

infection. Reasons for removal have included infection, injury and the possibility of malignant transformation. However, most cases are monitored by US and spontaneous resolution often occurs without compli-cations [36–38]. The preliminary results of a prospective study [38] are summarized in Table 11.6. The possibility of malignant degeneration has been the most compelling reason to consider nephrectomy [38]. However, this is an extremely rare outcome because only three cases of malignancy associated with multicystic kidney have been reported in the past 25 years [38]. It has been estimated that 8000 multicystic kidneys would need to be removed to prevent one tumour, and that 20 000 nephrectomies would need to be done to save one life [38].

Renal dysplasia

Abnormal parenchymal development or acquired insults can cause unilateral and/or bilateral small kidneys (Table 11.7). The usual types of congenitally small kidneys

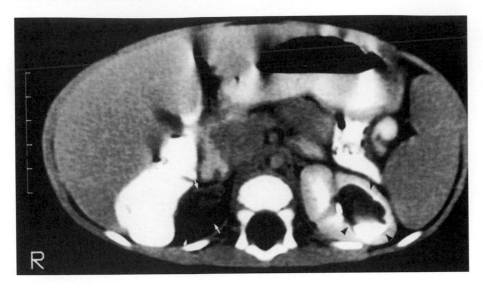

Fig. 11.1 Multicystic kidney disease (MKD) and hydrocalyx. A contrast computed tomography scan shows nonfunctioning MKD on the right (arrows) and contrast stasis in a large dilated obstructed calyx (hydrocalyx) (arrowheads) in the left kidney.

Table 11.5 Associations of congenital hepatic fibrosis (CHF). From [25].

CHF and polycystic kidneys
  Autosomal recessive polycystic kidneys
  Autosomal dominant polycystic kidney

CHF and hereditary tubulointerstitial nephritis
  Juvenile nephronophthisis (Boichis syndrome)
  Juvenile nephronophthisis with tapetoretinal degeneration
  Biedl–Bardet syndrome
  CHF, cystic kidneys, colobomas and encephalopathy
  Asphyxiating thoracic chondrodystrophy (Jeune syndrome)

CHF and hereditary renal dysplasias
  Meckel syndrome
  Chondrodysplasia syndromes
  Renal–hepatic–pancreatic cystic dysplasia (Ivemark syndrome)
  Zellweger syndrome

Table 11.6 Multicystic kidney registry: preliminary findings. Modified from [38].

Establishment of multicystic kidney registry	1986
Number of patients registered	441
Prenatal diagnosis by ultrasound	288
Presentation with flank mass	80
Male : female ratio	250 : 191
Left : right kidney ratio	233 : 198
Abnormal contralateral kidney	19%
Vesicoureteric reflux (VCU done in 65 patients)	43%
Nephrectomy	181
Usual age at nephrectomy (months)	7–12
Pathological confirmation of multicystic kidney	175
Pelviureteric junction obstruction	6
Follow-up of patients not operated on:	
Urinary tract infection	12
Minimal hypertension (unrelated to MKD)	4
Malignancy	0/260
Cumulative rate of radiological undetectability of MKD	
By year 1	18%
By year 2	31%
By year 5	54%

MKD, multicystic kidney disease; VCU, vesicoureteric reflux.

are simple hypoplasia and renal dysplasia. Another congenital form, oligomeganephronic hypoplasia, is less common.

In simple renal hypoplasia there is a quantitative deficiency of renal parenchyma with normal renal architecture, reduced numbers of reniculi and decreased numbers and sizes of nephrons [39]. Renal dysplasia is a qualitative deficiency that results from altered metanephric differentiation. Characteristic features are primitive ducts, poorly differentiated nephrons, rudimentary medullary development and metaplastic cartilage [29,39]. Oligomeganephronic kidneys are small and have decreased numbers of nephrons which are hypertrophied [40,41]. Oligomeganephronia can be sporadic or familial, isolated or syndromal. There is early onset of polyuria, dehydration, anaemia and severe growth retardation.

Table 11.7 Causes of small kidneys.

Inherited or congenital
  Renal hypoplasia
  Renal dysplasia
  Oligomeganephronic hypoplasia

Acquired
  Renal venous thromboses
  Renovascular accidents
  Pyelonephritis
  Vesicoureteric reflux
  Chronic glomerulonephritis
  Renal artery stenosis

Causes of dysplasia include autosomal recessive inheritance [42], autosomal dominant inheritance [43], multifactorial modes of inheritance [44], a mutation on chromosome 8q [45], chromosomal disorders [46], obstructive uropathy [29] and exposure to teratogens.

Isolated adysplasia/dysplasia

The incidence of bilateral renal dysplasia at birth is 0.15 per 1000 [47]. The mode of transmission is not well defined in all cases and may differ among kindreds, but includes

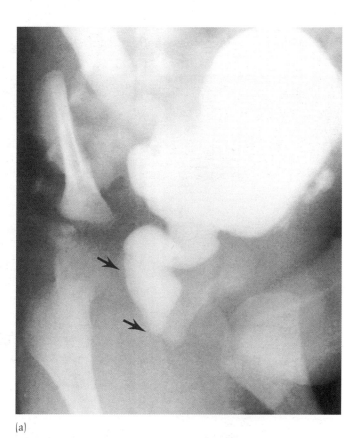

(a)

Fig. 11.2 (a) Obstructive cystic dysplasia (posterior urethral valves). Voiding cystourethrography shows dilated posterior urethra and valves (arrows). (b) US (same infant) shows large echogenic kidney with multiple cortical/medullary cysts.

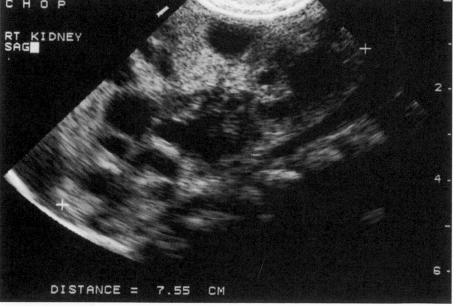

(b)

autosomal dominant inheritance with reduced penetrance [47] or multifactorial inheritance [48]. Parents and siblings may be normal or have unilateral dysplasia, unilateral agenesis or bilateral dysplasia [43]. There are no renal phenotypic differences between sporadic and familial dysplasia. Sporadic dysplasia may be caused by a new mutation or inheritance of the gene(s) from a non-manifesting parent. Apparently normal relatives should be screened by renal US if genetic counselling is requested. The empirical risk of bilateral renal adysplasia for future siblings is 3.5% and the recurrence risk increases if two siblings are affected. Prenatal diagnosis by US is possible if there is oligohydramnios. It is important to note that this may not be feasible before 20 weeks' gestation.

Clinical features of renal dysplasia depend on the severity of the renal disorder. The neonate may appear

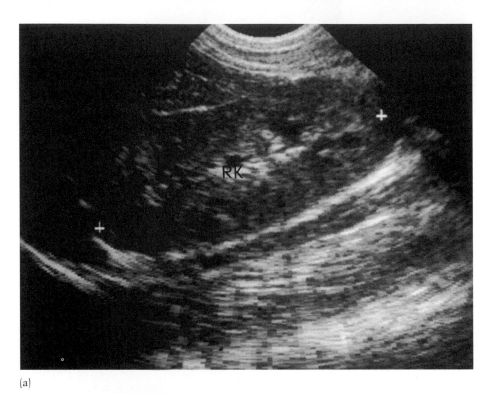

(a)

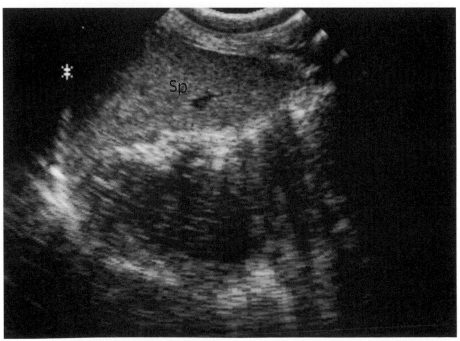

(b)

Fig. 11.3 Ectodermal dysplasia–ectrodactyly–cleft lip syndrome. (a,b) Solitary kidney. US shows normal compensatory hypertrophy (RK). Sp, spleen.

normal or, if bilateral dysplasia is present, may have features of the oligohydramnios sequence. There may be massive renal salt wasting, failure to thrive and dehydration. Unilateral dysplasia with a normal contralateral kidney rarely causes clinical disease and most of these cases are found by chance. Children with isolated bilateral dysplasia may come to attention because of urinary tract infection or progressive renal insufficiency. There is no specific treatment for the dysplasia.

Adysplasia/dysplasia in conjunction with obstructive uropathy

In patients with prune belly syndrome and those with posterior urethral valves, survival initially depends on the severity of pulmonary hypoplasia, and subsequently on the severity of renal dysplasia. The kidneys may be minimally affected or there may be severe dysplasia with or without cysts (Fig. 11.2).

Adysplasia/dysplasia in syndromes with multiple congenital abnormalities

Branchio-oto-renal syndrome (BOR)

The incidence is estimated at 1:40000. Inheritance is autosomal dominant with high penetrance and variable expression (see Table 11.1). The gene for the branchio-oto-renal (BOR) syndrome has been linked to chromosome 8q [45]. Manifestations include pre-auricular pits, branchial clefts, sensorineural deafness, lachrymal duct atresia and a spectrum of renal involvement. The kidneys may be normal, or there can be unilateral dysplasia, renal agenesis and/or reflux [2,49]. The risk of severe renal dysplasia is estimated to be 6% [49]. Renal function may be normal or severely reduced. Prognosis depends on the severity of the kidney abnormality.

Acrorenal syndromes

EEC syndrome. Inheritance is autosomal dominant, penetrance and expression are variable, and all patients and first-degree relatives should be evaluated for genitourinary abnormalities [50] (Fig. 11.3).

VACTERL. (VATER) VACTERL is a constellation of defects of *v*ertebral anomalies, *a*nal atresia, *c*ongenital heart disease, *t*racheo-oesophageal fistula, *r*enal abnormalities and radial *l*imb abnormality. VACTERL is usually sporadic.

Townes–Brock REAR syndrome. Urogenital anomalies include unilateral hypoplasia, posterior valves and meatal stenosis. Inheritance is autosomal dominant with variable expression [51].

Fanconi pancytopenia syndrome. This has non-renal and renal features that overlap with VACTERL [52] and radial adysplasia syndromes. Microcephaly and chromosomal breaks differentiate these patients from those with VACTERL. The inheritance is autosomal recessive.

Autosomal recessive skeletal dysplasias

These may be associated with a variety of renal abnormalities [53] (Table 11.8).

Polycystic kidneys

Autosomal recessive polycystic kidney disease

Inheritance is autosomal recessive, parents are unaffected and there is often variable expression within a sibship [53]. The gene for autosomal recessive PKD has been localized to chromosome 6p21-cen by linkage analysis in 16 families [56] (Table 11.9). There is no evidence for genetic heterogeneity among the different clinical phenotypes [56]. The prevalence is estimated at 1:10000 to 1:40000.

Autosomal recessive PKD may be diagnosed after 24 weeks' gestation by sonographic demonstration of hyperechoic kidneys, oligohydramnios, an apparently absent bladder and enlarged kidneys [57–59]. Renal involvement is more evident than hepatic involvement when presentation is in the neonate, and liver disease is more prominent in older children [60]. Neonates with severe renal involvement *in utero* may have the oligohydramnios sequence with varying degrees of respiratory and renal involvement. In infancy, hypertension is often severe and hyponatremia is often a problem [60].

Imaging studies

The kidneys are large. Cysts are not typically seen on excretory urography and there is delayed excretion of contrast. The nephrogram often has a mottled or streaky appearance from pooling of contrast medium in dilated collecting ducts. The renal sonographic appearance in the neonate with a history of oligohydramnios is that of large kidneys with markedly increased echogenicity. There is no corticomedullary differentiation and there is loss of the central echo complex. Sonographically resolvable cysts are rare and, in the neonate, are seen with much less frequency than in autosomal dominant PKD (Fig. 11.4). However, the kidneys may be similar in appearance in either entity and therefore renal US does not always distinguish autosomal recessive PKD from autosomal dominant PKD or from transient nephromegaly [61]. US can demonstrate a 'coarse', echogenic liver (Fig. 11.5) in most cases and dilated biliary radicals in some patients (Fig. 11.6).

Table 11.8 Autosomal recessive syndromes with renal cysts and/or dysplasia. Modified from [53].

	Phenotype	Renal involvement	CHF	Prognosis	Prenatal diagnosis
Chondrodysplasia punctata	Rhizomelic dwarfism, stippled epiphyses; joint contractures, characteristic face	Microcysts	No	Lethal in infancy	Amniotic fluid amniocytes
Chondroectodermal dysplasia	Acromelic dwarfism, cone-shaped epiphyses, polydactyly, hypoplastic nails, dysplastic teeth, congenital heart disease	Agenesis, tubular microcysts, megaureter, TIN	Yes	Death in childhood	Ultrasound
Short rib syndromes	Dwarfism, short ribs, polydactyly, visceral abnormalities	Agenesis, hypoplasia, cystic dysplasia	Yes	Lethal in infancy	Ultrasound, fetoscopy
Type I (Majewski syndrome)	Short tibia, arhinencephalia				
Type II (Saldino–Noonan syndrome)	Metaphyseal/pelvic dysplasia	Tubular microcysts, interstitial nephritis	Yes		
Type III (Naumoff syndrome)	Shortening of skull base	Tubular microcysts, interstitial nephritis	Yes		
Jeune asphyxiating thoracic dystrophy syndrome	Respiratory distress, dysostoses, short ribs; narrow, long thoracic cage; small pelvis; trident acetabular margins; short, thick 2nd and 3rd phalanges; cone-shaped epiphyses; handle-bar clavicle; mesomelic shortening of limbs	Renal cystic diseases	Yes	Survivors develop metaphyseal dystrophy dysplasia with post-natal short-limbed dwarfism	Ultrasound by 18 weeks
Acrodysplasia with retinitis pigmentosa (Saldino–Mainzer syndrome)	Cone-shaped epiphyses, retinitis pigmentosa, cerebellar ataxia	Tubular microcysts, interstitial nephritis	?	Renal failure in childhood	
Marden–Walker syndrome	Blepharophimosis, contractures, hypotonia, kyphoscoliosis, cleft palate	Microcysts	No	Failure to thrive	
Roberts syndrome	Hypomelia, craniofacial dysmorphism, clitoral/penile enlargement, congenital heart disease	Cystic dysplasia, fused kidneys	Yes	Lethal in infancy or childhood	Ultrasound
Brachymesomelia renal syndrome	Brachymesomelia, craniofacial anomalies, congenital heart disease	Glomerular cysts	No	Lethal in infancy	
Acrocephalopoly syndactyly dysplasia	Organomegaly, craniosynostosis, polysyndactyly	Renal enlargement, tubular and glomerular cysts	Yes	Lethal in infancy	
Fraser syndrome	Cryptophthalmos, cutaneous syndactyly, abnormal genitalia	Renal adysplasia or dysplasia; many major, minor anomalies. Renal cystic dysplasia, renal agenesis, thickening of muscular layer and fibrosis of bladder are reported		Most patients die in the newborn period	Ultrasound by 18–19 weeks
Fitch–Fryns syndrome	Distal limb hypoplasia, cleft palate/lip, genital anomalies	Cystic dysplasia, double ureters	No	Lethal in infancy	Ultrasound by 20 weeks

continued

Table 11.8 *Continued.*

	Phenotype	Renal involvement	CHF	Prognosis	Prenatal diagnosis
Meckel syndrome	Postaxial polydactyly, microphthalmia, encephalocele, ambiguous genitalia	Cystic kidneys	Yes	Usually lethal in infancy	Ultrasound
Goldston syndrome	Dandy–Walker malformation, autosomal recessive	Cystic kidneys	Yes	Lethal in infancy	Ultrasound, increased fetoprotein
Renal–hepatic–pancreatic dysplasia (RHPD)	Fibrosis of the liver and pancreas	Cystic kidneys	Yes	Neonatal death by respiratory failure in most cases	
Glutaric aciduria type II (multiple acyl dehydrogenase deficiencies)	Prematurity, hypotonia, hepatomegaly, craniofacial anomalies, rocker bottom feet, anterior abdominal wall defects, external genital anomalies, sweaty feet odour, brain heterotopias	Renal cystic dysplasia, nephromegaly		Death in days to months. No treatment for biochemical abnormalities	Enzyme assay in amniocytes and/or elevated glutaric acid in amniotic fluid. Ultrasound
Zellweger cerebro–hepato–renal syndrome	Similar to glutaric aciduria type II; nystagmus, cataracts, pigmentary retinopathy, optic disc pallor, brain heterotopias, abnormal gyri, absent corpus callosum, micronodular cirrhosis, stippled epiphyses of patella, acetabulum; abnormal peroxisomal enzymes	Cortical renal cysts	Yes	Most die in 6 months; some with milder form survive into adolescence with retardation, deafness and seizures	Enzyme assays in amniocytes or chorionic villus cells
Carbohydrate-deficient glycoprotein syndrome [54]	Olivopontocerebellar atrophy, retinitis pigmentosa, testicular atrophy, hypothyroidism, immune deficiency	Multiple microcysts	Yes	May live to 10 years	

CHF, congenital hepatic fibrosis (biliary dysgenesis); TIN, tubular interstitial nephritis.

Table 11.9 Chromosome loci of renal cystic and dysplastic diseases.

	Chromosome loci
Autosomal dominant diseases	
PKD1	16p13
PKD2	4q13-q23
Tuberosclerosis	16p
von Hippel–Lindau syndrome	3p25-p26
Branchio-oto-renal syndrome	8q
Autosomal recessive diseases	
Autosomal recessive PKD	6p21-cen
Juvenile nephronophthisis	2q11.1-2q21.1
Biedl–Bardet syndrome	8q12.11

Pathology

The kidneys are large, spongy and reniform (Fig. 11.7). Dilated collecting ducts are perpendicular to the surface of the kidney (Fig. 11.8). There is no dysplasia. Portal areas of the liver are expanded by increased numbers of dilated bile ductules surrounded by fibrous tissue (Fig. 11.9). Dilated ductules may become cystic and liver cells are normal. Pancreatic ductules may be dilated and may also be surrounded by fibrous tissue.

Treatment

Frusemide can correct hyponatraemia and reduce hypertension. The hypertension often responds to an angiotensin-converting enzyme inhibitor [62]. Bilateral nephrectomies have been advocated for neonates whose massive kidney enlargement restricts diaphragmatic excursion and prevents weaning from a ventilator [63].

Outcome

Many affected neonates die from respiratory and/or renal failure. Seventy-five per cent of the patients who survive the first year can survive beyond the age of 15 years [62] and patients can survive into the third decade. Portal hypertension with bleeding oesophageal varices can be a life-threatening problem. Renal and/or liver transplantations have been performed successfully.

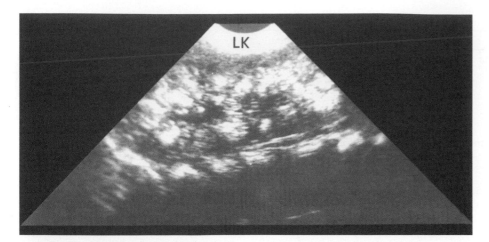

Fig. 11.4 Autosomal recessive PKD. US of the left kidney (LK) shows a large kidney with markedly echogenic pyramids due to renal tubular ectasia.

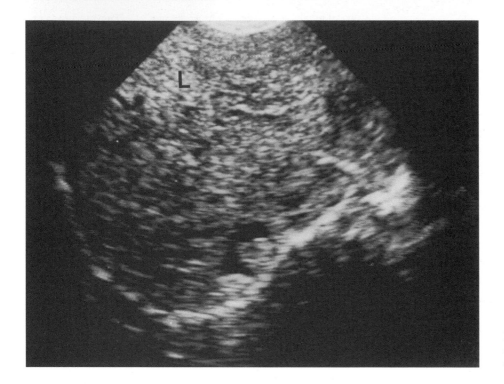

Fig. 11.5 Autosomal recessive PKD. In congenital hepatic fibrosis US shows a coarse, echogenic liver (L).

Autosomal dominant polycystic kidney disease

This is the second most common autosomal dominant mutation in humans. The incidence in liveborns is 1–3 in 100 000 and the estimated prevalence in the population is between 1:200 and 1:1000. The mutation rate is 6.5×10 [64]. PKD may not be detected for years and may be diagnosed by US, by genetic probes, or it may be found unexpectedly at postmortem. PKD can present in infants [65–67] and children [68–73] with abdominal distension, unilateral or bilateral abdominal masses, haematuria, lumbar pain, urinary tract infection, hypertension or a ruptured berry aneurysm. Gross haematuria may follow blunt trauma to the abdomen [71]. Blood pressure, liver size

and serum creatinine concentrations are usually normal in the first decade of life [72,73]. In some patients only one kidney may be affected initially [71]. Diagnosis of PKD in a child has led to its diagnosis in an apparently normal parent or in one with unexplained hypertension.

Reduced renal blood flow, renin system activation and increased body sodium precede the clinical manifestations of autosomal dominant PKD, and end-stage renal failure is a common consequence of autosomal dominant PKD [74]. The differential diagnosis includes autosomal recessive PKD and the PKD that can occur in association with the tuberosclerosis complex [13,15] (Fig. 11.10), von Hippel–Lindau disease [16], Hajdu–Cheney syndrome [19,20] and oro–facial–digital syndrome type I [18]. PKD may coseg-

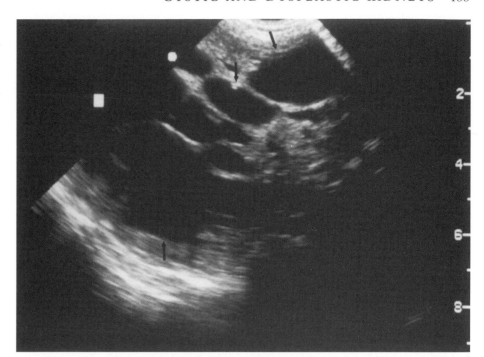

Fig. 11.6 Autosomal recessive PKD. US in this infant shows larger, anechoic tubular structures (arrows). These represent non-obstructive, dilated intrahepatic biliary ducts.

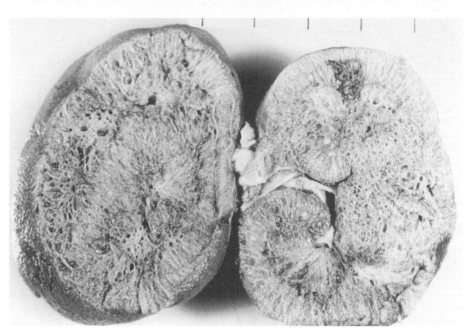

Fig. 11.7 Autosomal recessive PKD. Cut section of a kidney showing a spongy appearance.

regate with an overlap connective tissue disorder [12] (see Table 11.3).

Imaging studies

In PKD, intravenous urography can reveal normal kidneys, or unilateral or bilateral involvement. Kidneys may be normal in size or enormously enlarged and the appearance can be lobular. Non-opacified cysts stretch and distort calyces and produce smooth or irregular indentations. The parenchyma contains numerous cysts of various sizes. US

[75,76] is more sensitive than intravenous urography for detecting cysts (Fig. 11.11). The kidneys are usually enlarged in affected persons over the age of 18 years. There are usually equal numbers of cysts in each kidney and the cysts tend to be of similar sizes. Cysts may also be detected in the liver, pancreas and spleen.

Pathology

By the time the kidneys are examined pathologically they are enlarged and have numerous cysts on the external

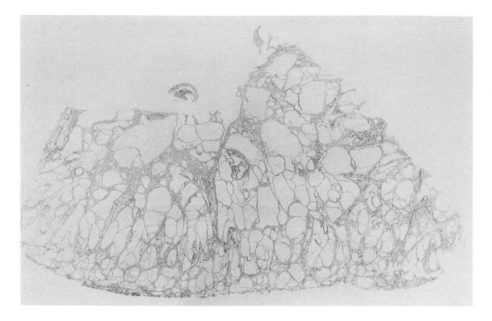

Fig. 11.8 Autosomal recessive PKD. Low-power microscopy section showing numerous dilated tubules with few glomeruli (×20).

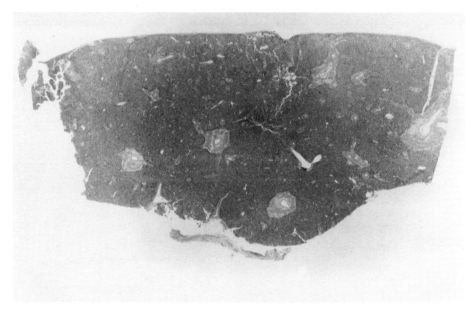

Fig. 11.9 Autosomal recessive PKD. Low-power microscopy of a section of liver. The portal tracts are expanded, there is bile duct proliferation and periportal fibrosis (×20).

surface [77] (Fig. 11.12). Cysts are randomly distributed throughout the parenchyma and involve any segment of the nephron. The lining epithelium may be similar to that of the segment of tubule from which the cyst arose. Cysts vary in size and may contain pale fluid or blood. The cyst epithelium is able to secrete and reabsorb actively [5]. Basement membranes are thick and the cysts are surrounded by interstitial fibrosis. Epithelial hyperplasia, with small polyps or adenomas, accompanies the formation of the cysts [78]. Cyst formation may be the result of epithelial hyperplasia with sequestration of fluid delivered to the cyst by transepithelial secretion and, in cysts that communicate with the tubule, by glomerular filtration. There may be an increased prevalence of renal neoplasia in adults with PKD [78].

Genetics

Inheritance is autosomal dominant and therefore each offspring has a 50% chance of inheriting the gene. Penetrance is almost 100% but expression varies within and between kindreds in age at presentation, severity of involvement and frequency of associated abnormalities. In about 85% of families there is linkage with a gene, PKD1, on the short arm of chromosome 16 (16p13.3) [7,8]. Many different mutations occur in this gene; there is a tendency for each family to have its own mutation which gives rise to PKD1 [79]. Among the remaining 5% of families linkage has been established between autosomal dominant PKD (PKD2) and chromosome 4q13–q23 [9,10]. These patients have the same clinical

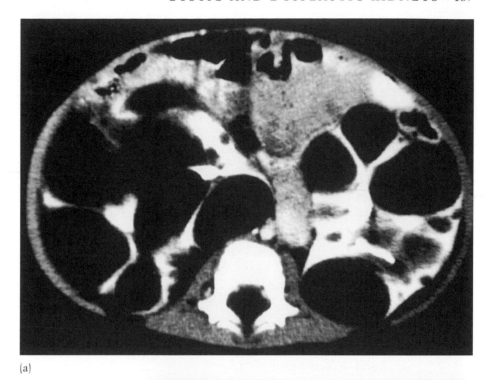

(a)

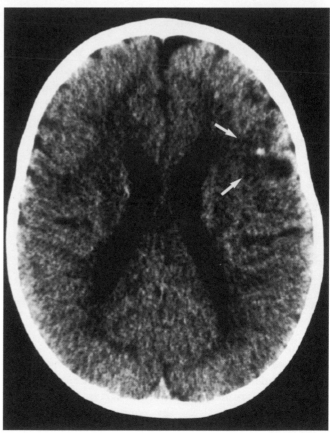

(b)

Fig. 11.10 Tuberosclerosis. (a) Polycystic kidneys. A contrast computed tomography (CT) scan shows massive renal enlargement with multiple cysts. (b) Central nervous system involvement. A cranial CT scan in the same patient shows a subcortical tuber (arrows) with calcification.

phenotypes as PKD1. There is evidence of a third locus for PKD [11].

Tests for the presymptomatic diagnosis of PKD are done for genetic counselling purposes. Prediction by DNA complements ultrasonography for detection and is not age dependent. The gene status of the affected person has to be

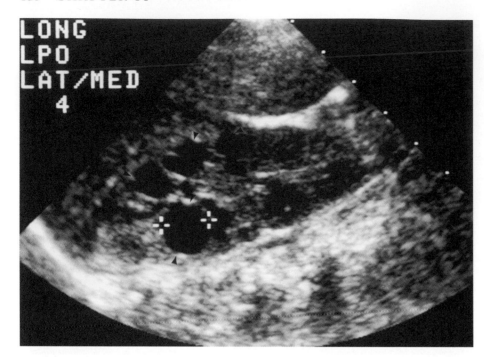

Fig. 11.11 Autosomal dominant PKD. US in a pre-school child shows a large kidney with multiple cortical and medullary cysts (arrows).

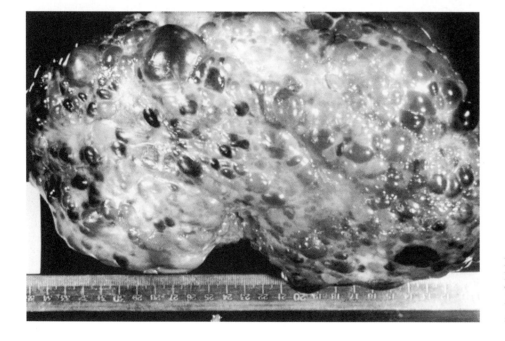

Fig. 11.12 Autosomal dominant PKD. Nephrectomy specimen from an adult. The kidney is enormously enlarged and there are numerous cysts on the surface.

determined first. Sonographic diagnostic criteria for PKD1 are summarized in Table 11.10. Although early identification of asymptomatic individuals may provide a rational approach to treatment of urinary infection and hypertension, there is no treatment that alters the course in asymptomatic individuals. Therefore, investigation of children at risk is not routinely done except to confirm manifestations of the disease or at the insistence of a parent. The frequency of serious complications in children with PKD is very low and therefore a decision whether to be tested can be deferred [81].

Treatment

Stimulation of the renin–angiotensin–aldosterone system, possibly by renal ischaemia caused by expansion of cysts, contributes to the development of hypertension in PKD [82]. Control of hypertension, restriction of dietary protein and control of renal infection in individuals who have not developed renal insufficiency has not improved outcome [83,84]. However, it is important to treat hypertension and it has been suggested that angiotensin-converting enzyme

Table 11.10 Sonographic diagnostic criteria for PKD1 by age group (assessed on basis of DNA linkage studies). Modified from [80].

| Criteria | Age | | | | | | | |
| | 20 years | | 30 years | | 40 years | | 50 years | |
	PPV (%)	NPV (%)	PPV (%)	NPV (%)	PPV (%)	NPV (%)	PPV (%)	NPV (%)
>1 cyst	100	96.6	97.7	100	96.9	100	77.2	100
>2 cysts (one/both kidneys)	100	96.6	99.2	100	98.9	100	95.6	100
>2 cysts in one kidney, >1 cyst in the other	100	90.5	99.2	100	98.9	100	98.2	100
>2 cysts each kidney	100	87.7	100	100	100	100	100	100
>4 cysts each kidney	100	85.1	100	89.9	100	100	100	100

NPV, negative predictive value; PPV, positive predictive value.

inhibition may be of particular value in the treatment for this purpose [85].

Not all antibiotics penetrate optimally into the cysts. Antibiotics that are able to enter the cysts include ciprofloxacin, norfloxacin, chloramphenicol, trimethoprim, clindamycin, doxycycline, erythromycin, metronidazole and tetracycline [64]. Severe, refractory abdominal and flank pain can be treated successfully, albeit temporarily, by surgical decompression [86]. Uninephrectomy, in adults, has almost no effect on the rate of progression to end-stage renal failure [87]. Nephrectomy is rarely indicated prior to renal transplantation and the disorder does not recur in the allograft.

Outcome

Most neonates or infants who presented with PKD used to die from respiratory failure or sepsis [66,67] but the prognosis has improved. Sedman et al. noted that only three patients progressed to end-stage renal failure at 3, 15 and 39 years out of 154 asymptomatic children from 83 families with PKD [72]; the first two were diagnosed in the first year of life [72]. In a study by Fick et al., six patients diagnosed in utero, and five in the first year of life, were followed for 3–15 years; two had end-stage renal disease, eight had normal or near normal renal function, four developed a reduced renal concentrating ability and nine were hypertensive [73]. In a third study, none of seven patients diagnosed in childhood developed chronic renal failure before the age of 20 years, but three became hypertensive by the age of 15 years [71].

More recent studies on the prognosis in adults reveal more cause for optimism [88,89] than earlier studies [68,69]. An individual diagnosed presymptomatically by US can be advised that the chance of developing end-stage renal failure before the age of 40 years is 2%; before 50 years 22%; and by 73 years 53% [88]. Uninephrectomy for uncontrolled urinary tract infection, calculi, trauma or haemorrhage has no effect on the rate of progression to end-stage renal failure in adults with PKD [87]. Intracranial aneurysms rarely rupture prior to the age of 21 years. Screening for aneurysms should focus on patients with a prior episode of rupture and on those with a family history of an aneurysm [90].

Glomerulocystic kidneys

The term glomerulocystic is descriptive and does not signify quantity. Bernstein [91] uses the term glomerulocystic kidneys to encompass the entire group of heterogeneous conditions, and reserves the term glomerulocystic kidney disease for non-syndromal cases (Table 11.11). The kidneys may be large or small and the liver is normal. Most cases are sporadic but autosomal dominant inheritance has been reported [92]. The cysts are often subcapsular and may contain more than one glomeruloid structure. The sonographic appearance of glomerulocystic kidney disease in infants can resemble autosomal recessive PKD [93].

Familial juvenile nephronophthisis

Nephronophthisis is an autosomal recessive disorder with linkage to chromosome 2 [94,95]. Polydipsia, polyuria, renal salt wasting, anaemia and growth failure begin in the first decade and end-stage renal failure occurs in most patients by 13 years. Cysts develop at the corticomedullary junction. Initially there are peritubular lymphohistiocytic

Table 11.11 Classification of glomerulocystic kidneys. Modified from [91].

Glomerulocystic kidney disease (GCKD)
  Dominant GCKD in older patients
  Sporadic non-syndromal GCKD
  Familial (dominant) hypoplastic GCKD

GCKD in autosomal dominant PKD in infants

Glomerulocystic kidneys in heritable malformation syndromes
  Tuberosclerosis
  Oro–facial–digital, type 1 syndrome
  Brachymesomelia renal syndrome
  Trisomy 13
  Short rib polydactyly syndrome
  Jeune asphyxiating thoracic dystrophy syndrome
  Zellweger cerebro–hepato–renal syndrome
  Familial nephronophthisis

Glomerular cysts in dysplastic kidneys
  Diffuse cystic dysplasia
  Renal–hepatic–pancreatic dysplasia

Acquired glomerular cysts
  Indomethacin-induced fetopathy
  In utero exposure to phenacetin

---

infiltrates and later there is chronic tubulointerstitial disease with sclerosis, dilated tubules and thick, split tubular basement membranes.

Nephronophthisis is also associated with other syndromes that have congenital hepatic fibrosis [96], cone-shaped epiphyses, cerebellar ataxia [97] and retinitis pigmentosa [98]. Medullary cystic kidney disease, which is similar to nephronophthisis, presents in young adults, progresses rapidly to end-stage renal failure, and is inherited in an autosomal dominant mode. Nephronophtisis and medullary cystic kidney disease must be differentiated from medullary sponge kidney.

Medullary sponge kidney

Medullary sponge kidney is a relatively benign, sporadic condition. Clinical features include urinary tract infection, haematuria and renal calculi. Medullary sponge kidneys can be confused with renal tubular ectasia, a phenotypic expression of autosomal recessive PKD presenting in childhood or adolescence.

Dysgenetic kidneys

Congenital hypernephronic nephromegaly with tubular dysgenesis

In this disorder there is late-onset oligohydramnios after 24 weeks [99]. The kidneys are large and do not function [100] and the calvarium is underdeveloped. US shows that the kidneys are enlarged symmetrically, there is no evidence of cysts or obstruction, and the corticomedullary junction is poorly defined. Histological studies show an apparent increase in the number of glomeruli and immature tubules without proximal convolutions [99]. Inheritance is autosomal recessive. Prenatal diagnosis is not possible before 20 weeks and death occurs in the neonatal period.

Perlman syndrome

This is characterized by polyhydramnios, macrosomia,

Table 11.12 Renal abnormalities reported after *in utero* exposure to toxins.

Toxin	Abnormality	Reference
Angiotensin-converting enzyme inhibitors	Fetal hypotension, anuria, oligohydramnios, growth restriction, pulmonary hypoplasia, renal tubular dysplasia and abnormal calvaria	Pryde *et al.* [102]
Anticonvulsants	Urogenital anomalies found occasionally after exposure to valproic acid and other anticonvulsants	Ardinger *et al.* [103]
Cocaine	Maternal cocaine use may cause genitourinary abnormalities	Chasnoff *et al.* [104]
Indomethacin	May cause renal dysgenesis after prolonged high doses	Restaino *et al.* [105]
Lead	Incriminated as a possible cause of the VACTERL association	Levine & Muenke [106]
Phenacetin and salicylate	Glomerulocystic disease reported in one infant	Krous *et al.* [107]
Warfarin	Unilateral renal agenesis and ectopia reported in three infants	Hall [108]

bilateral nephromegaly with nephroblastomatosis, visceromegaly, cryptorchidism, diaphragmatic hernia, interrupted aortic arch, hypospadias and polysplenia [101].

Teratogens and renal abnormalities

Associations between teratogens and renal abnormalities (Table 11.12) are speculative. In most reported cases there is no convincing proof of cause and effect. However, exposure to teratogens should be considered in all cases of cystic and dysplastic kidneys [102-108].

References

1 Kaplan BS, Kaplan P, Ruchelli E. Hereditary and congenital malformations of the kidneys in the neonatal period. *Perinat Clin North Am* 1992;**19**:197–211.
2 Fitch N, Srolovitz H. Severe renal dysgenesis produced by a dominant gene. *Am J Dis Child* 1976;**130**:1356–7.
3 Kaplan BS, Kaplan P. Chronic renal disease in the neonate. In: Spitzer A, ed. *Intensive Care of the Fetus and Neonate*. Mosby-Year Book, 1996;1070–8.
4 Kissane JM. Renal cysts in pediatric patients. A classification and overview. *Pediatr Nephrol* 1990;**4**:69–77.
5 Gardner KD Jr. Pathogenesis of human cystic renal disease. *Ann Rev Med* 1988;**39**:185–91.
6 Kaplan BS, Kaplan P, Rosenberg HK, Lamothe E, Rosenblatt DS. Polycystic kidney disease. *J Pediatr* 1989;**115**:867–880.
7 Reeders ST, Breuning MH, Corney G *et al.* Two genetic markers closely linked to adult polycystic kidney disease on chromosome 16. *Br Med J* 1986;**292**:851–3.
8 Reeders ST, Keith T, Green P *et al.* Regional localization of the autosomal dominant polycystic kidney disease locus. *Genomics* 1988;**3**:150–5.
9 Kimberling WJ, Kumar S, Gabow PA, Connolly CJ, Somlo S. Autosomal dominant polycystic kidney disease: localization of the second gene to chromosome 4q13-q23. *Genomics* 1993;**18**:467–72.
10 Peters DJM, Spruit L, Saris JJ *et al.* Chromosome 4 localization of a second gene for autosomal dominant polycystic kidney disease. *Nature Genet* 1993;**5**:359–62.
11 Daoust MC, Reynolds DM, Bichet DG, Somlo S. Evidence for a third genetic locus for autosomal dominant polycystic kidney disease. Genomics. 1995;**25**:733–6.
12 Somlo S, Rutecki G, Giuffra LA *et al.* A kindred exhibiting cosegregation of an overlap connective tissue disorder and the chromosome 16 linked form of autosomal dominant polycystic kidney disease. *J Am Soc Nephrol* 1993;**4**:1371–8.
13 Bernstein J. Renal cystic disease in the tuberous sclerosis complex. *Pediatr Nephrol* 1993;**7**:490–5.
14 European Chromosome 16 Tuberose Sclerosis Consortium (ECTSC). Identification and characterization of the tuberous sclerosis gene on chromosome 16. *Cell* 1993;**75**:1305–15.
15 Kandt RS, Haines JL, Smith M, Northrup H *et al.* Linkage of an important gene locus for tuberose sclerosis to a chromosome 16 marker for polycystic kidney disease. *Nature Genet* 1992;**2**:37–41.
16 Lamiell JM, Stor RA, Hsia YE. von Hippel–Lindau disease simulating polycystic kidney disease. *Urology* 1980;**15**:287–90.

17 Latif F, Tory K, Gnarra J *et al.* Identification of the Hippel–Lindau disease tumor suppressor gene. *Science* 1993;**260**: 1317–20.
18 Salinas CF, Pai GS, Vera CL *et al.* Variability in expression of the orofaciodigital syndrome type I (OFD I) in black females: six cases. *Am J Med Genet* 1991;**38**:574–82.
19 Kaplan P, Ramos F, Zackai EH, Bellah RD, Kaplan BS. Cystic kidney disease in Hajdu–Cheney syndrome. *Am J Med Genet* 1995;**56**:25–30.
20 Rosenmann E, Penchas S, Cohen T, Aviad I. Sporadic idiopathic acro-osteolysis with cranio-skeletal dysplasia, polycystic kidneys and glomerulonephritis. *Pediatr Radiol* 1977;**6**:116-20.
21 Osathanondh V, Potter EL. Pathogenesis of polycystic kidneys. Type I due to hyperplasia of interstitial portions of collecting tubules. *Arch Pathol Lab Med* 1964;**77**:466–78.
22 Blyth H, Ockenden BG. Polycystic disease of the kidneys and liver presenting in childhood. *J Med Genet* 1971;**8**:257–84.
23 Bernstein J. Hepatic involvement in hereditary renal syndromes. In: Gilbert EF, Opitz JM, eds. *Genetic Aspects of Developmental Pathology*. Birth Defects Original Article Series No. 23. New York: March of Dimes Birth Defects Foundation, 1987:115–30.
24 Cobben JM, Breuning MH, Schoots C *et al.* Congenital hepatic fibrosis in autosomal-dominant polycystic kidney disease. *Kidney Int* 1990;**38**:880–5.
25 Kaplan BS, Kaplan P. Autosomal recessive polycystic kidney disease. In: Spitzer A, Avner ED, eds. *Inheritance of Kidney and Urinary Tract Diseases*. Boston: Kluwer Academic Press, 1990:265–76.
26 Pavenello RdeCM, Eigier A, Otto PA. Relationship between Mayer–Rokitansky–Kuster (MRK) anomaly and hereditary renal adysplasia (HRA). *Am J Med Genet* 1988;**29**:845–9.
27 Tarry WF, Duckett JW, Stephens FD. The Mayer–Rokitansky syndrome: pathogenesis, classification and management. *J Urol* 1986;**136**:648–52.
28 McHugh K, Stringer D, Hebert D, Babiak CA. Simple renal cysts in children: diagnosis and follow-up with US. *Radiology* 1991;**178**:383–5.
29 Bernstein J. The multicystic kidney and hereditary renal adysplasia. *Am J Kidney Dis* 1991;**17**:495–6.
30 Buchta RM, Viseskul C, Gilbert EF, Sarto GE, Opitz JM. Familial bilateral renal agenesis and hereditary renal adysplasia. *Eur J Pediatr* 1973;**115**:111–29.
31 Greene LF, Feinzaig W, Dahlin DC. Multicystic dysplasia of the kidney: with special reference to the contralateral kidney. *J Urol* 1971;**105**:482–7.
32 Atiyeh B, Husmann D, Baum M. Contralateral renal abnormalities in multicystic-dysplastic kidney disease. *J Pediatr* 1992;**121**:65–7.
33 Kelalis PP, Malek RS. Infundibular stenosis. *J Urol* 1981; **125**:568–71.
34 Uhlenhuth E, Amin M, Harty JI, Howerton LW. Infundibulopelvic dysgenesis: a spectrum of obstructive renal disease. *Urology* 1990;**35**:334-7.
35 Gordon AC, Thomas DFM, Arthur RJ, Irving HC. Multicystic dysplastic kidney: is nephrectomy still appropriate? *J Urol* 1988;**140**:1231–4.
36 Hartman GE, Smolik LM, Shochat SJ. The dilemma of the multicystic dysplastic kidney. *Am J Dis Child* 1986; **140**:925–8.

37 Stanisic TH. Review of 'The dilemma of the multicystic dysplastic kidney'. *Am J Dis Child* 1986;**140**:865.

38 Wacksman J, Phipps L. Report of the multicystic kidney registry: preliminary findings. *J Urology* 1993;**150**:1870–2.

39 Bernstein J. Developmental abnormalities of the renal parenchyma—renal hypoplasia and dysplasia. *Pathol Ann* 1968;**3**:213–47.

40 Royer P, Habib RN, Mathieu H, Broyer M. *Pediatric Nephrology*. Philadelphia: WB Saunders, 1974.

41 Moerman P, Fryns J-P, Vandenberghe K, Devlieger H, Lauweryns JM. The syndrome of diaphragmatic hernia, abnormal face and distal limb anomalies (Fryns syndrome): further delineation of this multiple congenital anomaly (MCA) syndrome. *Am J Med Genet* 1988;**31**:805–14.

42 Cole BR, Kaufman RL, McAlister WH, Kissane JM. Bilateral renal dysplasia in three siblings. Report of a survivor. *Clin Nephrol* 1976;**5**:83–7.

43 Kaplan BS, Milner LS, Jequier S, Kaplan P, De Chadarevian J-P. Autosomal dominant inheritance of small kidneys. *Am J Med Genet* 1989;**32**:120–6.

44 Holmes LB. Prevalence, phenotypic heterogeneity and familial aspects of bilateral renal agenesis/dysgenesis. In: Spitzer A, Avner ED, eds. *Genetics of Kidney Disorders*. Boston: Kluwer Academic Press, 1990; 1–11.

45 Kumar S, Kimberling WJ, Kenyon JB *et al.* Autosomal dominant branchio-oto-renal syndrome—localization of a disease gene to chromosome 8q by linkage in a Dutch family. *Hum Mol Genet* 1992;**1**:491–5.

46 Van Allen MI. Urinary tract. In: Stevenson RE, Hall JG, Goodman RM, eds. *Human Malformations and Related Anomalies*, Vol. 2. Oxford: Oxford University Press, 1993: 501–50.

47 McPherson E, Carey J, Kramer A *et al.* Dominantly inherited renal adysplasia. *Am J Med Genet* 1987;**26**:863–72.

48 Buchta RM, Viseskul C, Gilbert EF *et al.* Familial bilateral renal agenesis and hereditary renal adysplasia. *Z Kinderheilk* 1973;**115**:111–29.

49 Fraser FC, Sproule JR, Halal F. Frequency of the branchio-oto-renal syndrome in children with profound hearing loss. *Am J Med Genet* 1980;**7**:341–9.

50 Rollnick BR, Hoo JJ. Genitourinary anomalies are a component manifestation in the ectodermal dysplasia, ectrodactyly, cleft lip/palate (EEC) syndrome. *Am J Med Genet* 1988;**29**:131–6.

51 Kurnit DM, Steele MW, Pinsky L, Dibbins A. Autosomal dominant transmission of a syndrome of anal, ear, renal and radial congenital malformations. *J Pediatr* 1978;**93**: 270–3.

52 Glanz A, Fraser FC. Spectrum of anomalies in Fanconi anemia. *J Med Genet* 1982;**19**:412–16.

53 Torres VE. Genetics of renal cystic diseases. In: Spitzer A, Avner ED, eds. *Inheritance of Kidney and Urinary Tract Diseases*. Boston: Kluwer Academic, 1990:175-219.

54 Strom EH, Stromme P, Westvik J, Pedersen SJ. Renal cysts in the carbohydrate-deficient glycoprotein syndrome. *Pediatr Nephrol* 1993;**7**:253–5.

55 Kaplan BS, Kaplan P, de Chadarevian J-P *et al.* Variable expression within a family of autosomal recessive polycystic kidney disease and congenital hepatic fibrosis. *Am J Med Genet* 1988;**29**:639–47.

56 Zerres K, Mucher G, Bachner L *et al.* Mapping of the gene for

57 Romero R, Cullen M, Jeanty P *et al.* The diagnosis of congenital renal anomalies with ultrasound. II. Infantile polycystic kidney disease. *Am J Obstet Gynecol* 1984;**150**: 259–262.

58 Luthy DA, Hirsch JH. Infantile polycystic kidney disease: observations from attempts at prenatal diagnosis. *Am J Med Genet* 1985;**20**:505–517.

59 Townsend RR, Goldstein RB, Filly RA *et al.* Sonographic identification of autosomal recessive polycystic kidney disease associated with increased maternal serum/amniotic fluid alpha-fetoprotein. *Obstet Gynecol* 1988;**71**:1008–1012.

60 Lieberman E, Salinas-Madrigal L, Gwinn JL *et al.* Infantile polcystic disease of the kidneys and liver: clinical, pathological and radiological correlations and comparison with congenital hepatic fibrosis. *Medicine* 1971;**50**:277–318.

61 Stapleton FB, Hilton S, Wilcox J. Transient nephromegaly simulating infantile polycystic disease of the kidneys. *Pediatrics* 1981;**67**:554–9.

62 Kaplan BS, Fay J, Shah V, Dillon MJ, Barratt TM. Autosomal recessive polycystic kidney disease. *Pediatr Nephrol* 1989; **3**:43–9.

63 Sumfest JM, Burns MW, Mitchell ME. Aggressive surgical and medical management of autosomal recessive polycystic kidney disease. *Urology* 1993;**42**:309–12.

64 Grantham JJ, Gabow PA. Polycystic kidney disease. In: Schrier RW, Gottschalk CW, eds. *Diseases of the Kidney*. Boston: Little, Brown, 1988:583–615.

65 Ross DG, Travers H. Infantile presentation of adult-type polycystic kidney disease in a large kindred. *J Pediatr* 1975; **87**:760–3.

66 Proesmans W, Van Damme B, Casaer P, Marchal G. Autosomal dominant polycystic kidney disease in the neonatal period: association with a cerebral arteriovenous malformation. *Pediatrics* 1982;**70**:971–5.

67 Freycon M-T, Boyer C, Lauras B, Annino R, Freycon F. Reins polykystiques a transmission dominante chez un nourrisson. *Pediatrie* 1982;**38**:287–94.

68 Dalgaard OZ. Bilateral polycystic kidney disease of the kidneys. *Act Med Scand* 1957;**158**(Suppl. 328):1–255.

69 Dalgard OZ. Polycystic disease of the kidneys. In: Strauss MB, Welt LG, eds. *Diseases of the Kidney*, 2nd edn. Boston: Little, Brown, 1971:1223–58.

70 Gabow PA, Ikle DW, Holmes JH. Polycystic kidney disease: prospective analysis of non-azotemic patients and family members. *Ann Intern Med* 1984;**101**:238–47.

71 Kaplan BS, Rabin I, Nogrady MB, Drummond KN. Autosomal dominant polycystic kidney disease in children. *J Pediatr* 1977;**90**:782–3.

72 Sedman A, Bell P, Manco-Johnson M, Schrier R *et al.* Autosomal dominant polycystic kidney disease in childhood: a longitudinal study. *Kidney Int* 1987;**31**:1000-5.

73 Fick GM, Johnson AM, Strain JD *et al.* Characteristics of very early onset autosomal dominant polycystic kidney disease. *J Am Soc Nephrol* 1993;**3**:1863–70.

74 Harrap SB, Davies DL, Macnicol AM *et al.* Renal, cardiovascular and hormonal characteristics of young adults with autosomal dominant polycystic kidney disease. *Kidney Int* 1991;**40**:501–8.

75 Rosenfield AT, Lipson MH, Wolf B *et al.* Ultrasonography and

nephrotomography in the presymptomatic diagnosis of dominantly inherited (adult-onset) polycystic kidney disease. *Radiology* 1980;**135**:423–7.

76 Striker GE, Striker LJ. Renal cysts in polycystic kidney disease. *Am J Nephrol* 1986;**6**:161–4.

77 Grantham JJ, Geiser JL, Evan AP. Cyst formation and growth in autosomal dominant polycystic kidney disease. *Kidney Int* 1987;**31**:1145–52.

78 Bernstein J, Evan AP, Gardner KD Jr. Epithelial hyperplasia in human polycystic kidney diseases. Its role in pathogenesis and risk of neoplasia. *Am J Pathol* 1987;**129**:92–101.

79 Peral B, Ward CJ, San Millan JL *et al*. Evidence of linkage disequilibrium in the Spanish polycystic kidney disease 1 population. *Am J Hum Genet* 1994;**54**:899–908.

80 Ravine D, Gibson RN, Walker RG *et al*. Evaluation of ultrasonographic diagnostic criteria for autosomal dominant polycystic kidney disease 1. *Lancet* 1994;**343**:824–7.

81 Ravine D, Walker RG, Gibson RN *et al*. Treatable complications in undiagnosed cases of autosomal dominant polycystic kidney disease. *Lancet* 1991;**337**:127–9.

82 Chapman AB, Johnson A, Gabow PA, Schrier RW. The renin–angiotensin–aldosterone system and autosomal dominant polycystic kidney disease. *N Engl J Med* 1990;**323**:1091–6.

83 Klahr S, Beck G, Breyer J *et al*. Dietary protein restriction and reduced blood pressure goal in adults with polycystic kidney disease (APKD) [Abstract]. *J Am Soc Nephrol* 1993;**4**:263.

84 Sklar AH, Caruana RJ, Lammers JE *et al*. Renal infections in autosomal dominant polycystic kidney disease. *Am J Kidney Dis* 1987;**10**:81–8.

85 Watson ML, Macnicol AM, Allan PL, Wright AF. Effects of angiotensin converting enzyme inhibition in adult polycystic kidney disease. *Kidney Int* 1992;**41**:206–10.

86 Elzinga LW, Barry JM, Bennett WM. Surgery in the management of autosomal dominant polycystic kidney disease. *Am J Kidney Dis* 1992;**19**:89–92.

87 Zeir M, Gebeth S, Gonzalo A *et al*. The effect of uninephrectomy on progression of renal failure in autosomal dominant polycystic kidney disease. *J Am Soc Nephrol* 1992;**3**:1119–23.

88 Bear JC, McManamon P, Morgan J *et al*. Age at clinical onset and at ultrasonographic detection of adult polycystic kidney disease: data for genetic counselling. *Am J Med Genet* 1984;**18**:45-53.

89 Churchill DN, Bear JC, Morgan J *et al*. Prognosis of adult onset polycystic kidney disease re-evaluated. *Kidney Int* 1984;**26**:190–3.

90 Chauveau D, Pirson Y, Verellen-Dumoulin C *et al*. Intracranial aneurysms in autosomal dominant polycystic kidney disease. *Kidney Int* 1994;**45**:1140–6.

91 Bernstein J. Glomerulocystic kidney disease—nosological considerations. *Pediatr Nephrol* 1993;**7**:464-70.

92 Kaplan BS, Pincott J, Gordon I, Barratt TM. Autosomal dominant hypoplastic glomerulocystic kidney disease. *Am J Med Genet* 1989;**34**:569–73.

93 Fitch SJ, Stapleton FB. Ultrasonographic features of glomerulocystic disease in infancy: similarity to infantile polycystic kidney disease. *Pediatr Radiol* 1986;**16**:400–2.

94 Antignac C, Arduy CH, Beckmann JS *et al*. A gene for familial juvenile nephronophthisis (recessive medullary cystic disease) links to chromosome 2p. *Nature Genet* 1993;**3**:342–5.

95 Hildebrandt F, Singh-Sawhney I, Schnieders B *et al*. Mapping of a gene for familial juvenile nephronophthisis: refining the map and defining flanking markers on chromosome 2. *Am J Hum Genet* 1993;**53**:1256–61.

96 Boichis H, Passwell J, David R *et al*. Congenital hepatic fibrosis and nephronophthisis. *Q J Med* 1973;**165**:221–33.

97 Mainzer F, Saldino R, Ozonoff MB, Minagi H. Familial nephropathy associated with retinitis pigmentosa, cerebellar ataxia, and skeletal abnormalities. *Am J Med* 1970;**49**:556–62.

98 Proesmans W, Van Damme B, Macken J. Nephronophthisis and tapetoretinal degeneration associated with liver fibrosis. *Clin Nephrol* 1975;**3**:160–4.

99 Swinford AE, Bernstein J, Toriello HV *et al*. Renal tubular dysgenesis: delayed onset of polyhydramnios. *Am J Med Genet* 1989;**32**:127–32.

100 Allanson JE, Pantzar JT, MacLeod PM. Possible new autosomal recessive syndrome with unusual renal histopathological changes. *Am J Med Genet* 1983;**16**:57–60.

101 Greenberg F, Copeland K, Gresik MV. Expanding the spectrum of the Perlman syndrome. *Am J Med Genet* 1988;**29**:773–6.

102 Pryde PG, Sedman AB, Nugent CE, Barr M Jr. Angiotensin-converting enzyme inhibitor fetopathy. *J Am Soc Nephrol* 1993;**3**:1575–82.

103 Ardinger HH, Atkin JF, Blackstone RD *et al*. Verification of the fetal valproate syndrome phenotype. *Am J Med Genet* 1988;**29**:171–85.

104 Chasnoff IJ, Chisum GM, Kaplan WE. Maternal cocaine use and genitourinary tract malformations. *Teratology* 1988;**37**:201–4.

105 Restaino I, Kaplan BS, Kaplan P *et al*. Renal dysgenesis in a monozygotic twin. Association with *in utero* exposure to indomethacin. *Am J Med Genet* 1991;**39**:252–7.

106 Levine F, Muenke M. VACTERL association with high prenatal lead exposure. *Pediatrics* 1991;**87**:390–2.

107 Krous HF, Richie JP, Sellers B. Glomerulocystic kidney. A hypothesis of origin and pathogenesis. *Arch Pathol Lab Med* 1977;**101**:462–3.

108 Hall BD. Warfarin embryopathy and urinary tract anomalies: possible new association. *Am J Med Genet* 1989;**34**:292–3.

12   Anomalies of Renal Position and Fusion and Pelviureteric Junction Obstruction

A.M.K.Rickwood and J.V.Harney

Anomalies of renal position and fusion

Of themselves these anomalies seldom amount to more than anatomical curiosities and, as such, tend to pass unnoticed except when complicated by urinary infection or obstruction, or when associated with sundry congenital anomalies of the genitourinary tracts or with certain genetic conditions or congenital malformations of other systems. The latter include tracheo-oesophageal fistula [1], anal imperforation [2,3], vertebral anomalies [4,5], cardiac malformations [6], cloacal exstrophy [7] and myelomeningocele [8].

Embryology

During the fourth week of gestation the ureteric bud develops from the mesonephric duct close to its conjunction with the cloaca. With cephalad growth, the bud comes to adjoin the nephrogenic cord of the intermediate mesoderm which later forms the metanephros. After further cephalad migration, the ureteric bud branches successively to form the major and minor calyces and the distal collecting tubules [9]. Simultaneously, the metanephric cap differentiates from the intermediate mesoderm to surround this developing collecting system. Further upward migration of the kidney occurs from a combination of true migration and differential lumbar growth and at each stage in its ascent the organ successively gains its blood supply from adjacent major vessels. The process is completed, during the seventh to eighth week of gestation, by axial rotation of the kidney through 90°.

Most anomalies of position and fusion are explicable by disturbances in the timing or extent of this sequence of events.

Inferior ectopia

The various degrees of this anomaly, affecting the left kidney a little more often than the right but equally distributed between the sexes, occur from some measure of failure of migration (pelvic, iliac or abdominal kidney). In autopsy series the condition is found in 1:500 [10] to 1:1200 [11] individuals. Occasionally the kidney is solitary [12].

The pelvic kidney, which is the commonest type, lies inferior to the aortic bifurcation, opposite the sacral concavity; the iliac kidney lies at the level of the sacral promontary, anterior to the iliac vessels, and the abdominal kidney lies above the iliac crest opposite the second or third lumbar vertebra. Their vasculature is derived locally, with the renal artery arising from the distal aorta, from the common or external iliacs or from the inferior mesenteric artery. Multiple arteries are common. Their axes of rotation vary from transverse to vertical and, because renal rotation represents a late stage in migration, the renal pelvis usually faces anteriorly. The adrenal gland, developing quite independently, is always normally sited.

Fetal lobulation often persists and the organ's configuration may be further distorted by compression from surrounding structures, factors which may cause bizarre appearances on imaging studies. With intravenous urography (IVU), tomographic views may help delineate the organ from adjacent bony structures, whilst accurate views of pelvic or iliac kidneys by radionuclide scintigraphy require anterior placement of the gamma camera.

Associated anomalies of the genital tract are recorded in 15–45% of cases [6,12]; in females these take the form of a unicornuate, bicornuate or rudimentary uterus and, in males, testicular maldescent, urethral duplication or hypospadias.

Pelvic kidney is particularly associated with primary vesicoureteric reflux (Fig. 12.1) and occasionally with pelviureteric junction (PUJ) obstruction [13]. Even in the absence of these complications, the organ may exhibit a degree of hypoplasia.

Superior ectopia

Upward migration of the kidney beyond the eighth week of

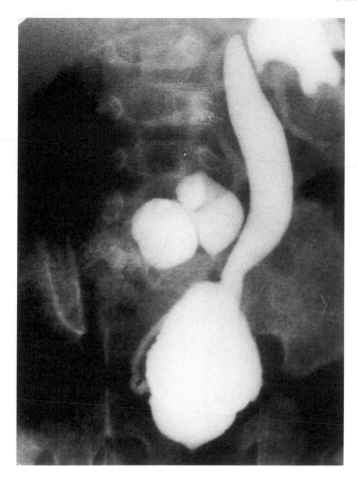

Fig. 12.1 Pelvic kidney. Cystography demonstrates bilateral ureteric reflux, on the left to an orthotopic kidney and on the right to a pelvic kidney.

gestation is prevented by development of the diaphragm, and superior ectopia presumably results from accelerated migration or from delayed closure of the diaphragm [14]. In the extreme, and rarest, form the kidney lies entirely within the thoracic cavity (Fig. 12.2). The renal vessels arise from the aorta and vena cava above their normal sites and whilst the adrenal gland may be carried upwards by the kidney more often it lies at its normal level.

This rare condition (1 : 13 000 individuals in an autopsy series [10]) tends to be discovered incidentally by chest radiography and, unusually among anomalies of position and fusion, has no urinary or non-urinary associations.

Anomalies of rotation

Partial or complete failure of the final phase of migration, axial rotation of the kidney, leaves the renal pelvis facing anteriorly and the calyces posteriorly. Less often, excessive rotation positions the pelvis posteriorly and, rarer still, the kidney may rotate ventrolaterally so that the renal pelvis faces outward from the midline. In any event, the renal vessels wind around the long axis of the kidney in a manner predictable from the extent of the malrotation.

In an autopsy series, rotational anomalies were found in approximately 1 : 2000 individuals [15]. As with superior ectopia, they have no urinary or non-urinary associations and are of clinical significance only in that they may be confused, on imaging studies, with extrinsic compression of the kidney, its collecting system or the renal pelvis.

Crossed renal ectopia

Classification of these anomalies, according to McDonald and McClellan [16], is illustrated in Fig. 12.3. In the

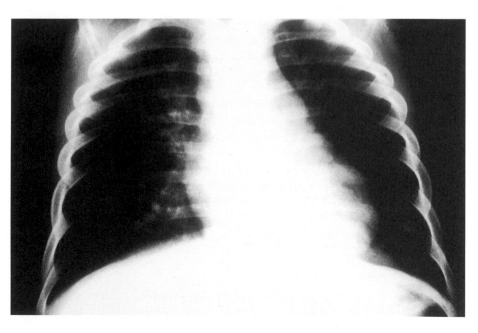

Fig. 12.2 Thoracic kidney. A routine chest X-ray incidentally reveals the soft tissue outline of a thoracic kidney emerging to the left of the cardiac shadow.

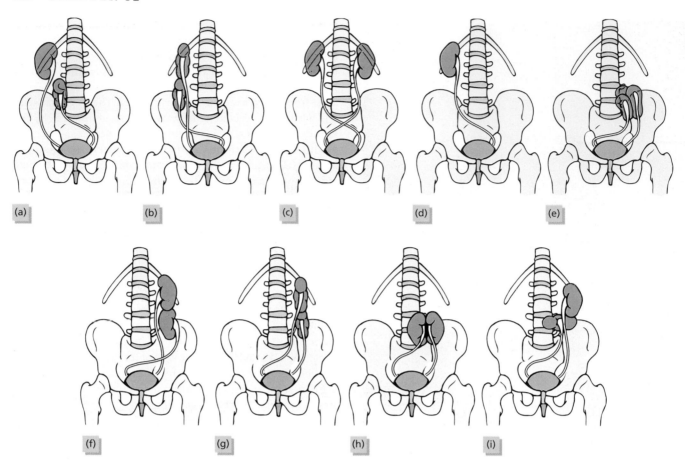

Fig. 12.3 Crossed Renal Ectopia (McDonald S. McCellan [16].
(a) Unilateral inferior ectopia without fusion. (b) Unilateral fusion
with inferior ectopia. (c) Unilateral fusion with pelvic ectopia and
malrotation. (d) Sigmoid kidney with inferior ectopia.

(e) Unilateral fusion with superior ectopia. (f) Bilateral ectopia.
(g) Solitary unilateral ectopia. (h) Unilateral fusion with pelvic
ectopia. (i) Unilateral fusion with inferior ectopia and
malrotation.

commonest form, unilateral fused kidney with inferior
ectopia, the upper pole of the ectopic organ is fused with
the lower pole of the orthotopic kidney and, because both
fail to undergo rotation, their pelvises face anteriorly [17]
(Fig. 12.4). With sigmoid kidney, the second commonest
form, the anomaly is similar except in that, because there
is normal rotation of both organs, the pelvis of the crossed
kidney faces laterally and that of the orthotopic kidney
medially [17] (Fig. 12.5). Solitary crossed ectopia and
bilateral crossed ectopia are extremely rare [16].

The blood supply of such kidneys is variable and
unpredictable. Primary vesicoureteric reflux is prevalent in
all varieties of crossed ectopia [18] and presumably
accounts for the appreciable incidence of pyelonephritis
and urolithiasis found in adult patients [17].

Horseshoe kidney

Here, fusion of the kidneys across the midline almost
always involves the lower renal poles and the isthmus may
consist of a fibrous band or, more often, of functioning
renal tissue. In adult autopsy series the anomaly is found in
approximately 1:400 individuals [16]. The proportion is
greater in paediatric series due to association with certain
lethal congenital anomalies [19]. Fusion of the lower renal
poles is believed to occur during the fourth week of
gestation when the metanephric masses most closely
approximate.

The presence of the isthmus prevents final upward renal
migration beyond the origin of the inferior mesenteric
artery. The kidneys not only lie a little caudally but
rotation is also prevented so that the renal pelvises face
anteriorly and the calyces posteriorly. The lowermost
calyces typically face the midline and the vertical axes of
the kidneys run inferomedially towards the isthmus. Their
blood supply is variable and multiple renal arteries are
common.

Ureteric duplication occurs in some 10% of cases [20]
and vesicoureteric reflux is demonstrable in more than half
[20]. In approximately 30% of patients there is PUJ

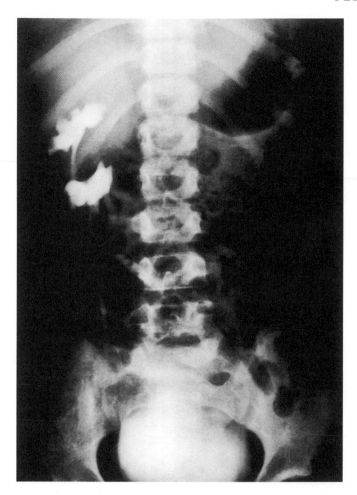

Fig. 12.4 Unilateral fused kidney with inferior ectopia. IVU showing left to right cross-fused ectopia; both renal pelves face anteriorly.

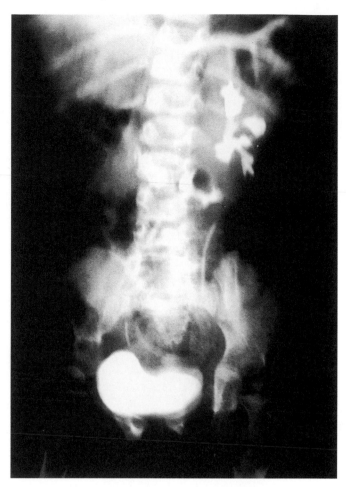

Fig. 12.5 Sigmoid kidney. IVU showing right to left cross-fused ectopia; calyces of the orthotopic left kidney face outwards and the solitary visible calyx of the ectopic right kidney medially.

obstruction [21] (Fig. 12.6); this is sometimes bilateral. Remoter genitourinary associations include a 4% incidence of testicular maldescent and hypospadias in males and a 7% incidence of bicornuate uterus or septate vagina in females [20].

Horseshoe kidney exists in 21% [22] of patients with trisomy 18 and 7% of those with Turner syndrome [20,23]. All varieties of renal tumour have been described in horseshoe kidney ·and in particular the anomaly carries a sevenfold increase in risk of nephroblastoma [24]. An inherited chromosomal deletion exists predisposing affected individuals to aniridia, mental retardation, horseshoe kidney and nephroblastoma [25].

Pelviureteric junction obstruction

The PUJ is far the commonest site of urinary obstruction in children and is also a quite frequent site of obstruction in adults of all ages. The obstruction may be caused by some intraluminal lesion, by a functional abnormality of the proximal ureter (intrinsic obstruction), by external compression, usually by an aberrant renal vessel (extrinsic obstruction) or may be secondary to some other urinary tract abnormality, usually vesicoureteric reflux (secondary obstruction).

Intrinsic obstruction, accounting for upwards of 90% of cases, is more common in males than females and affects the left kidney more often than the right [26]. Bilateral involvement occurs in approximately 15% of cases [27]. Occasionally there is a familial predisposition, with inheritance as an autosomal dominant trait [28] with incomplete penetration [29], due to an abnormality at the 6p locus [30].

Patients with intrinsic PUJ obstruction are more likely to have various congenital abnormalities than the population at large. Non-urological associations include congenital heart disease, tracheo-oesophageal fistula [1], anal imperforation [3] and vertebral anomalies [4]. Within

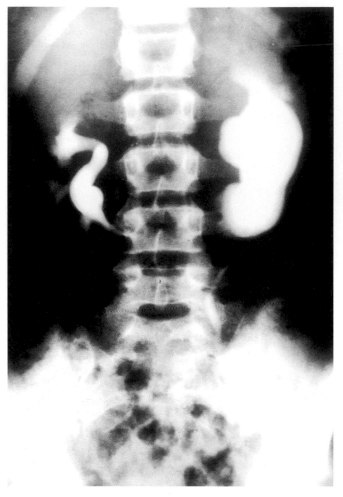

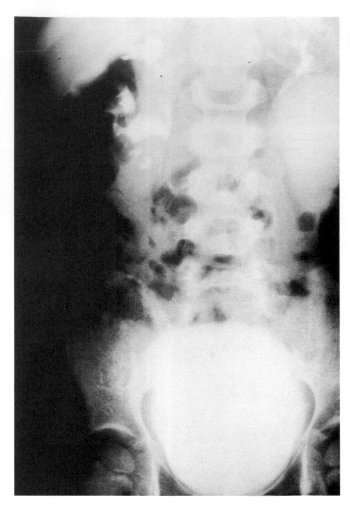

Fig. 12.6 Horseshoe kidney. On IVU the lowermost calyces of both kidneys face inwards towards the isthmus and pelviureteric junction obstruction affects the left kidney.

Fig. 12.7 Pelviuretric obstruction in the lower pole of a duplex kidney. The IVU shows duplicated drainage systems bilaterally with hydronephrosis due to pelviureteric junction obstruction affecting the left lower moiety.

the urinary tracts, the condition may coexist with most anomalies of position and fusion or may occur in the lower moiety of a duplicated upper renal tract (Fig. 12.7). Occasionally the contralateral kidney is absent or exhibits congenital hypoplasia or dysplasia, including multicystic dysplasia [31]. Primary vesicoureteric reflux, ipsilaterally or contralaterally, has been described in as many as 40% of cases [32].

Pathology

Intraluminal obstruction

True intraluminal obstruction is exceptional and most recorded examples have been due to fibro-endothelial polyps [33,34] (Fig. 12.8). In infants, obstruction has been ascribed to ureteric mucosal folds, supposedly causing a flap-valve effect [35]. Such folds, which represent a normal stage in

fetal development, are seldom, if ever, truly obstructive and, in time, resolve to leave a ureter of normal configuration [36].

Intrinsic obstruction

The pelviureteric junction is typically non-dependent and usually the renal pelvises and proximal ureter are united by flimsy adhesions. These phenomena are not themselves the cause of the obstruction which persists after pelviure-terolysis. Characteristically there is a persistent narrow aperistaltic segment of ureter, 2–10 mm long, immediately below the PUJ.

The nature of the functional obstruction within this segment is undetermined. The ureter initially develops as a solid cord, with subsequent canalization, and partial failure of the latter process has been invoked as a cause [37].

Extrinsic obstruction

An aberrant lower polar renal artery exists in some 35% of patients with PUJ obstruction [46]. It is necessary to distinguish incidental occurrence of such a vessel in the presence of intrinsic obstruction from the much rarer entity of true extrinsic obstruction where mobilization of the vessel from the PUJ results in clear and immediate relief of the obstruction [47]. Such obstruction is practically never seen before the age of 5 years.

Secondary obstruction

This may be suspected in patients with vesicoureteric reflux (primary or secondary) where the pelvicalyceal dilatation is disproportionately greater than the degree of reflux [32] (Fig. 12.9). Such 'obstruction' is apparent rather

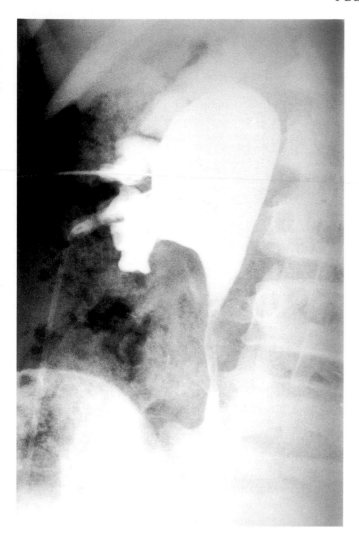

Fig. 12.8 Intraluminal pelviureteric junction obstruction. Antegrade pyelogram showing obstruction due to a fibroendothelial polyp within the proximal ureter.

Various histological changes have been described within the narrowed segment, including neuronal dysplasia (R. van Weltzen, personal communication), increase in the usual collagen–muscle ratio and thickening of the lamina propria [38–41], but it is uncertain whether these appearances are primary or secondary. Vector analysis of the orientation of the muscle fibres within the segment has demonstrated a persistent fetal circular arrangement rather than the predominantly longitudinal pattern of older children and adults [42].

The long established view that hydronephrosis due to intrinsic PUJ obstruction is both congenital and permanent requires qualification. Children presenting clinically with the complaint usually have no hydronephrosis fetally [43], whilst among those diagnosed prenatally, improvement or resolution of the hydronephrosis occurs in some 30% of cases [44,45].

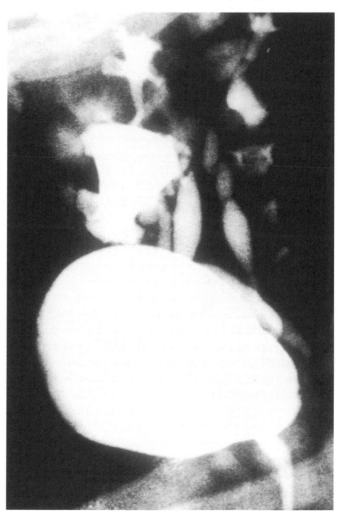

Fig. 12.9 Secondary pelviureteric junction obstruction. Cystography demonstrates bilateral vesicoureteric reflux. The right upper renal tract is duplicated and the dilatation of the lower polar pelvicalyceal system is disproportionately greater than the severity of the reflux.

than real and the hydronephrosis, which may develop only during voiding, disappears once the reflux resolves or has been surgically corrected. This should be distinguished from a conjunction of true intrinsic obstruction with incidental reflux and the issue may be determined by dynamic isotope renography, with the bladder catheterized, or by antegrade pressure–perfusion studies (Whitaker test [48]).

Pelviureteric junction obstruction and renal function

Most affected kidneys function normally, or almost so, regardless of the degree of hydronephrosis, the form of obstructive curve (type II vs IIIb) on renography, or whether the condition was presented clinically [49] or was detected prenatally [45,50–52]. Severe functional impairment (<20% differential) exists in less than 10% of cases. Functional impairment may sometimes be due to primary hypoplasia or dysplasia, rather than acquired obstructive uropathy, and this may be suspected when the affected kidney is small and the contralateral organ exhibits compensatory hypertrophy [53].

The characteristic symptom of PUJ obstruction, episodic loin pain, suggests that the obstruction is at least of variable severity if not frankly intermittent. Intrapelvic pressures are almost always normal in patients asymptomatic at the time of the examination [26]; limited material indicates that they become appreciably elevated during episodes of loin pain (A.M.K. Rickwood, unpublished data).

Although periodic or sustained increases in intrarenal pressure almost certainly initiate the process of renal impairment, this does not proceed by pressure atrophy but rather the pressure changes trigger a sequence of pathophysiological events leading to intrarenal vascular changes which ultimately become irreversible [54,55].

Experience thus far of patients diagnosed prenatally and managed expectantly indicates that PUJ obstruction does not inevitably, or even commonly, lead to impaired renal function [45,49,50] and that the risk of this event is not predictable from dynamic renography [45,56] or the Whitaker test [57] but may be increased in the presence of massive hydronephrosis [56]. Moreover, function impaired neonatally may improve spontaneously during the first few months of life [53]. To what extent these observations are applicable to older patients presenting clinically is yet to be determined.

Complications

Renal calculi

In children, PUJ obstruction is the commonest anatomical cause of renal calculi [58] and, in paediatric series of PUJ obstruction, approximately 3% of cases develop this complication [26].

As a rule there are three to five discrete stones, typically 5–8 mm in diameter, and in most cases there is a history of urinary infection, usually with *Proteus vulgaris*. Metabolic investigation is seldom rewarded and stone recurrence is exceptional provided the obstruction has been relieved.

Hypertension

In a few individuals there is moderate and often fluctuant hypertension which resolves following pyeloplasty. Less often there is more sustained and severe hypertension [59], typically in cases where function of the affected kidney is severely impaired, and this may persist even after nephrectomy, presumably as a result of secondary damage to the contralateral organ.

Clinical presentation

Prenatal diagnosis

Approximately one-third of neonates with significant fetal hydronephrosis prove to have anatomical appearances of PUJ obstruction [60,61]. They do not differ from patients presenting clinically in terms of sex distribution or lateralization of the lesion. Quite often the hydronephrosis manifests only during the final 10 weeks of gestation. It does not seem that the gestational age at which the hydronephrosis becomes detectable relates to risk of renal impairment except where gross hydronephrosis has developed by 20 weeks' gestation (D.F.M. Thomas, personal communication).

Approximately one-fifth of cases do not have obstruction using the criteria of dynamic diuresis renography [44] and here renal function is almost always normal and spontaneous resolution of the hydronephrosis is common [44,61].

Apart from the occasional case with global renal failure associated with bilateral disease or a solitary functioning kidney, there are no symptoms neonatally, and rarely subsequently, and the relevant physical sign, renomegaly, is found in less than 20% of cases [50].

Presentation during infancy

In the very young, PUJ obstruction may be discovered during the course of routine assessment of some other anomaly (e.g. imperforate anus). Presentation clinically is most commonly with urinary infection. Other occasional presenting features include a renal mass, haematuria, failure to thrive and persistent vomiting.

Presentation in older children and adults

Some 60% of patients present with episodic loin pain which is typically severe, prolonged for several hours and often accompanied by vomiting. Fever is absent, as are other features of urinary infection. In adult males episodes are commonly precipitated by beer drinking. In time symptoms tend to become more frequent and more extended. Occasionally an episode does not resolve and anuria may ensue if there is bilateral involvement or a solitary functioning kidney.

In some younger children the pain is located periumbilically and it may be difficult to decide whether this is ascribable to the renal lesion or whether the problem is one of non-specific abdominal pain of childhood with incidental hydronephrosis. Prolonged episodes of pain accompanied by vomiting point to the former.

Some 15% of older children, and a rather smaller proportion of adults, present with symptoms of upper urinary tract infection (fever, loin pain), with or without accompanying lower tract symptoms. Frank pyonephrosis is rare and usually supervenes in kidneys with pre-existing functional impairment.

In almost a quarter of childhood cases the lesion is detected quite incidentally (an IVU obtained during cardiac catheterization, an isotope bone scan for some orthopaedic complaint, etc.) or presents with symptoms which are either irrelevant (nocturnal or diurnal enuresis, lower urinary tract infection) or are precipitated rather than spontaneous (post-traumatic haematuria).

Investigation

Investigation aims to determine the anatomy of the lesion, the renal function and whether the hydronephrosis is, or is not, obstructive. In children these aims are largely satisfied by a combination of ultrasonography (Fig. 12.10), dynamic diuresis renography (Fig. 12.11) and a plain abdominal X-ray (to exclude calculi). Intravenous renography or retrograde pyelography are indicated where the anatomy is in doubt or where PUJ obstruction is associated with anomalies of position or fusion or with duplication of the upper renal tract [62]. Their role otherwise seems essentially one of personal preference.

Although vesicoureteric reflux may accompany PUJ obstruction [32], cystography can reasonably be restricted to those patients presenting with urinary infection or who have an element of distal ureteric dilatation detected by ultrasound or IVU.

Definition of 'obstruction' by the criteria of dynamic diuresis renography is dependent upon several variables (see Chapter 6) and, in particular, this examination is apt to be misleading in the presence of massive hydronephrosis or materially impaired renal function [63,64]. The Whitaker test [48] represents an alternative means of determining 'obstruction' in these circumstances, although in both cases it is almost always positive. An alternative view of the role of the Whitaker test is that it is restrictable to a few patients in whom the clinical picture is equivocal and the findings on renography are similarly equivocal or, occasionally, negative.

In a few patients with PUJ obstruction, hydronephrosis is absent except during episodes of loin pain [65,66]. Sometimes the phenomenon is precipitated during dynamic renography by the injection of a diuretic. Otherwise the diagnosis can be confirmed only by imaging during an attack of pain.

Very occasionally, PUJ obstruction and primary ureterovesical junction obstruction coexist ipsilaterally. As a rule they are diagnosed, and treated, sequentially (i.e. ureterovesical junction obstruction becomes evident only following relief of PUJ obstruction or vice versa). Sometimes the conjunction is suspected at the outset when typical appearances of PUJ obstruction are associated with a degree of non-refluxing distal ureteric dilatation and the diagnosis can be confirmed by combined antegrade pyelography and pressure–perfusion studies. Usually it is better to treat the distal obstruction first.

Management

General

Formerly, typical anatomical appearances of PUJ obstruction, usually as displayed by IVU, were considered sufficient justification in themselves for surgical intervention. Considerations which have led to a more conservative approach are the realization that the hydronephrosis is not always obstructive, the demonstration, by radionuclide studies, that renal function is usually better preserved than suggested by IVU [67] and the appreciation, from experience with cases diagnosed prenatally, that the natural history of the complaint is rather more benign than once supposed.

Patients presenting clinically

Clear indications for active intervention are:
1 relevant symptoms;
2 impaired renal function — the exact level of impairment is debatable although <40% differential with unilateral lesions represents a general concensus;
3 complications in the form of calculi or hypertension.

In as many as 20% of children, though a smaller proportion of adults, none of these considerations apply. Their number includes a few with bilateral involvement. Whether they require surgery, or whether expectant management is more appropriate, remains an open question.

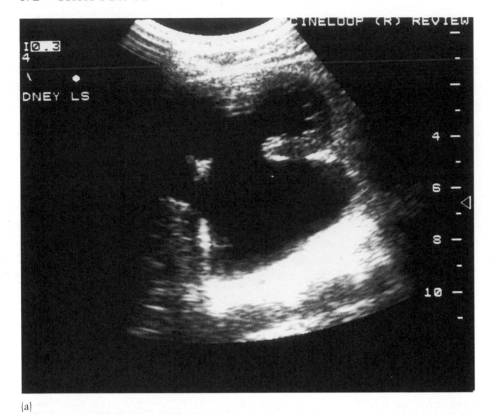

(a)

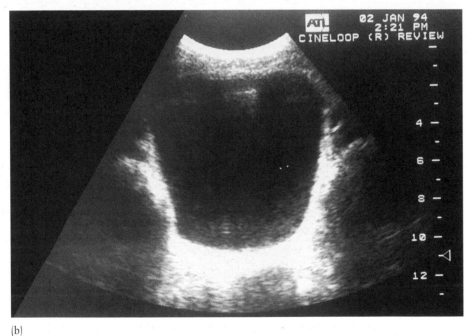

(b)

Fig. 12.10 Pelviureteric junction obstruction. On ultrasonography, there is marked pelvicalyceal dilatation affecting the left kidney with attenuation of the context (top): ultrasonography of the full bladder (bottom) reveals no sign of ureteric dilatation distally.

Whilst active management normally comprises surgical relief of the obstruction, an exception exists in unilateral cases, where function of the kidney is severely compromised (<20% differential). Despite sporadic reports of remarkable recovery following pyeloplasty [49,68], the usual outcome in this circumstance is a kidney which still functions poorly, albeit a little less so than preoperatively. Sometimes function declines further, despite technically satisfactory surgery, presumably due to advanced vascular changes intrarenally [69]. The prospects for functional recovery are better predicted by static than by dynamic radionuclide scintigraphy [70] and are less hopeful when

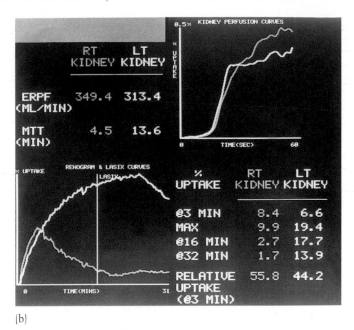

(b)

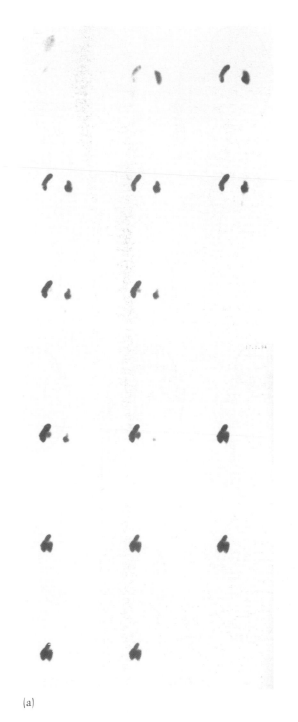

(a)

Fig. 12.11 Pelviureteric junction obstruction. On [^{99m}Tc] MAG$_3$ renography images (a) there is retention of isotope within the left pelvicalyceal system with none seen entering the ureter. The renographic curves (b) confirm an obstructive picture on the left with minimal elimination of isotope following administration of Lasix. Function of the left kidney is a little impaired both on 3 minutes uptake of isotope and ERPF.

the affected kidney is small and the contralateral organ exhibits compensatory hypertrophy [53]. In doubtful cases, the issue may be clarified by establishing percutaneous nephrostomy drainage and reassessing function 4–6 weeks later. Nephrectomy is usually advisable where function remains poor [71].

Emergency intervention may be indicated for patients with persistent loin pain, pyonephrosis or global renal impairment. Although emergency pyeloplasty is feasible in the absence of urinary infection, these situations are usually better handled by percutaneous nephrostomy drainage followed by definitive surgery once anatomy and renal function have been established.

Patients diagnosed antenatally

Very few of these patients require intervention because of symptoms and accumulating experience indicates that most can be managed expectantly [45,50,52,53,71].

Except for the occasional neonate with global renal

impairment, the initial assessment of function and obstruction, by dynamic diuresis renography, is best deferred for 1–2 months [44,53,72]. Hitherto, early elective pyeloplasty has been advocated where function is materially, though not severely, impaired (20–40% differential with unilateral involvement) [45,50,71], but recent reports, showing spontaneous functional improvement during infancy [53,73], suggest that further renographic reassessment at 3–6 months of age should be undertaken before recommending pyeloplasty. Management of severe functional impairment follows the lines described in the previous section.

Various regimens of surveillance have been described for expectantly managed cases, the authors' being to undertake ultrasonography at 4-monthly intervals during the first 2 years of life, and 6–12 monthly thereafter, and to repeat renography at 2-yearly intervals. Earlier renographic reassessment, at 1 year of age, is undertaken in those with gross hydronephrosis or with function bordering on 40% differential; renography is also re-performed whenever ultrasound examination shows increasing hydronephrosis. It should be noted, however, that deteriorating function is not necessarily accompanied by an increase in hydronephrosis [45,71]. Urinary infections are rare in these patients [45] so that there is no compelling indication for routine cystography or for antibiotic prophylaxis.

Experience to date shows that declining renal function is uncommon [43,74] and, in one controlled trial, the levels of renal function at 2 years of age did not differ significantly between those undergoing early pyeloplasty and those managed expectantly [71].

Surgery

Pyeloplasty

Open pyeloplasty remains the usual means of correcting PUJ obstruction. The techniques employed (Fig. 12.12) comprise Y-V plasty of the PUJ (Foley [75]), flap pyeloureteroplasty (Culp and de Weerd [76] and Scardino and Prince [77]) and dismembered pyeloureterostomy (Anderson–Hynes [78]). These procedures all aim to bypass, or excise, the functionally obstructed proximal ureteric segment and to provide dependent pelviureteric drainage. The Anderson–Hynes procedure is the most widely favoured and is applicable to almost all anatomical variations of PUJ obstruction.

The approach to the kidney [79] (anterior, transperitoneal or extraperitoneal (best restricted to young children) approaches, standard loin incision, posterior lumbotomy) is one of personal preference, as also is the choice of absorbable suture material (catgut or synthetic) and placement of the suture line (interrupted or continuous). As a rule, with the Anderson–Hynes procedure, the

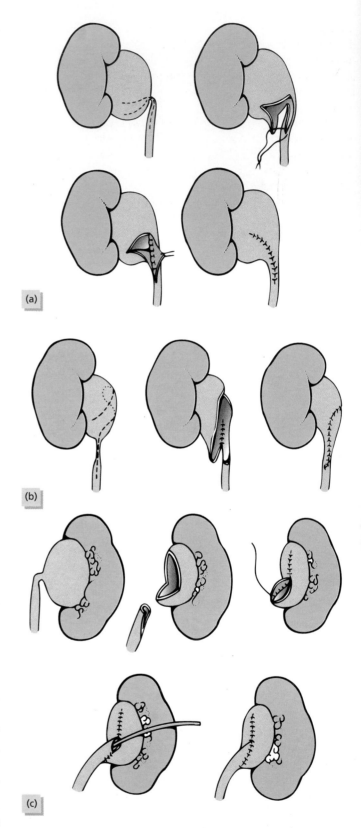

Fig. 12.12 Operative correction of pelviureteric junction obstruction. (a) Y-V plasty (Foley [75]); (b) Pelviureteroplasty (Culp [76]); (c) Dismembered pyeloureterostomy (Anderson–Hynes [78]).

pelviureteric anastomosis should be at least 2 cm in length. It may be impracticable to excise the entire narrowed ureteric segment where this is exceptionally long; in this circumstance it should be ensured that the apex of the anastomosis extends appreciably into ureter of normal calibre.

Drainage postoperatively [80,81] may comprise purely extra-anastomotic drainage, nephrostomy plus transanastomotic splint (4–6 F) or a double-J pyelovesical stent. Except in infants or in cases in some way complicated, extra-anastomotic drainage is usually the preferred means [80,81], with the drain removed some 24 h after any urinary leakage has ceased. Transanastomotic splints are removed 7–10 days postoperatively; the nephrostomy is clamped simultaneously and removed 24 h later provided there is no evidence of ongoing obstruction. A double-J stent should not be employed in a male child without first ascertaining that the urethra can accommodate the instrument necessary for its removal from the bladder.

Early complications of pyeloplasty are uncommon and usually comprise prolonged urinary leakage where extra-anastomotic drainage has been employed or delayed drainage of the anastomosis where a nephrectomy plus ureteric splint have been utilized. Persistence of either complication beyond 14 days postoperatively can often be rectified by retrograde passage of a ureteric catheter (3–6 F). More persistent anastomotic failure is manageable by retrograde balloon dilatation [82] or, rarely, by reoperation [83]. Neither procedure is advisable before 1 month postoperatively and in the interim the kidney can be drained, if necessary, by a percutaneous nephrostomy.

As a rule, investigations following pyeloplasty should be deferred until at least 1 month postoperatively and normally for at least 3 months. Appreciable lessening of hydronephrosis on ultrasonography or the appearance of free pyeloureteric flow on IVU are clear indications of a technically satisfactory outcome, but absence of these features does not necessarily indicate persistent obstruction. Here the issue is usually determinable by dynamic radionuclide renography [84], although in the presence of massive hydronephrosis or materially impaired renal function a Whitaker test may be necessary to confirm or exclude residual obstruction. In cases where renal function was impaired postoperatively and where early postoperative investigations indicate a technically satisfactory outcome, reassessment of function can reasonably be deferred for 2 years or so because functional recovery beyond that time is seldom more than slight.

The technical results of pyeloplasty are satisfactory in upwards of 90% of cases [26,49,80,85]. Persistent obstruction is rare and late restenosis of the pelviureteric junction is virtually unknown.

Nephropexy

In the presence of true extrinsic obstruction by an aberrant lower polar renal artery, mobilization of the vessel and its fixation at a higher level on the renal pelvis gives a satisfactory result. Most surgeons, however, prefer pyeloplasty in this situation; in this event the vessel should be transposed behind the anastomosis.

Ureterocalycostomy

This procedure, whereby the spatulated ureter is anastomosed to the lowermost renal calyx [86], plays little if any part in primary treatment but may be considered for salvage of a failed pyeloplasty where there is gross hydrocalycosis and the renal pelvis is, for some reason, unusable.

Minimally invasive surgery

Retrograde balloon dilatation of the PUJ has been successfully employed both as a primary treatment and for salvage of a failed pyeloplasty [82].

Endopyelotomy [87], involving a cold-knife incision of the stenotic ureteric segment using an endoscope passed via a nephrostomy tract, represents an alternative minimally invasive procedure. Satisfactory results have been reported in both adults and children [88]. Lack of success does not preclude subsequent pyeloplasty, though it may render the procedure more difficult than usual [89].

Both forms of treatment require 6–8 weeks' splintage with a double-J stent to prevent restenosis. The role of these procedures in the treatment of PUJ obstruction has yet to be defined, nor is it known whether early satisfactory results will be maintained long term.

References

1 Atwell JD, Beard RC. Congenital anomalies of the upper urinary tract associated with esophageal atresia and tracheo-esophageal fistula. *J Pediatr Surg* 1974;**9**:825.

2 Belman AB, King LR. Urinary tract anomalies associated with imperforate anus. *J Urol* 1972;**108**:823.

3 Singh MP, Haddadin A, Zachary RB, Pilling DW. Renal tract disease in imperforate anus. *J Pediatr Surg* 1974;**9**:157.

4 Uehling DT, Gilbert E, Chesney R. Urologic implications of the VATER association. *J Urol* 1983;**129**:352.

5 Strubbe EH, Lemmens JA, Thijn CJ, Willemsen WN, van Toor BS. Spinal abnormalities and the atypical form of Mayer–Rokitansky–Kuster–Hauser syndrome. *Skeletal Radiol* 1993; **22**:459.

6 Malek RS, Kelalis PP, Burke EC. Ectopic kidney in children and frequency of association with other malformations. *Mayo Clin Proc* 1971;**46**:461.

7 Soper RT, Kilger K. Vesicointestinal fissure. *J Urol* 1964;**92**:490.

8 Wilcock AR, Emery JL. Deformities of the renal tract in

children with myelomeningocele and hydrocephalus compared with those children showing no such nervous system deformities. *Br J Urol* 1970;**42**:152.

9 Osathanondh V, Potter H. Development of human kidney as shown by microdissection. *Arch Pathol* 1963;**76**:271.

10 Campbell WF. Renal ectopia. *J Urol* 1930;**240**:187.

11 Thompson GJ, Pace JM. Ectopic kidney: a review of 97 cases. *Surg Gynecol Obstet* 1937;935.

12 Downs RA, Lane JW, Burns E. Solitary pelvic kidney: its clinical implications. *Urology* 1973;**1**:51.

13 Kramer SA, Kelalis PP. Ureteropelvic junction obstruction in children with renal ectopy. *J Urol (Paris)* 1984;**5**:331.

14 N'Guessan G, Stephens FD, Pick J. Congenital superior ectopic (thoracic) kidney. *Urology* 1984;**24**:219.

15 Campbell WF. Anomalies of the kidney. In: *Urology*, 3rd edn. Philadelphia: WB Saunders, 1970:1416.

16 McDonald JH, McClellan DS. Crossed renal ectopia. *Am J Surg* 1957;**93**:995.

17 Abeshouse BS, Bhisitkul I. Crossed renal ectopia with and without fusion. *Urol Int* 1959;**9**:63.

18 Kelalis PP, Malek RS, Segura JW. Observations on renal ectopia and fusion in children. *J Urol* 1972;**108**:333.

19 Segura JW, Kelalis PP, Burke EC. Horseshoe kidney in children. *J Urol* 1972;**108**:333.

20 Boatman DL, Koln CP, Flocks RH. Congenital anomalies associated with horseshoe kidney. *J Urol* 1971;**113**:147.

21 Whitehouse GH. Some urographic aspects of the horseshoe kidney anomaly; review of 59 cases. *Clin Radiol* 1975;**26**:107.

22 Dollman A, Jaeger W. Uberzahliges Chromosomenfragment bet einam oligophrenen kind mit multiplen Entwicklungstorungen. *Monatsschr Kinderheilkd* 1968;**116**:144.

23 Bishop PMF, Lessof MH, Palini PE. Turner's syndrome and allied conditions. *Mem Soc Endocrinol* 1960;**7**:162.

24 Mesrobian HJ, Kelalis PP, Habrovsky E *et al.* Wilms tumour in horseshoe kidney: a report from the national Wilms tumour study group. *J Urol* 1985;**133**:1002.

25 Fantes JA, Bickmore WA, Fletcher JM *et al.* Submicroscopic deletions at the WARG locus revealed by non-radioactive *in situ* hybridisation. *Am J Hum Genet* 1992;**51**:1286.

26 Johnston JH, Evans JP, Glassberg KI, Shapiro SR. Pelvic hydronephrosis in children: a review of 219 personal cases. *J Urol* 1977;**117**:97.

27 Frering V, Sabatier E, Takvorian P, Dodat H. Improved prognosis and treatment of hydronephrosis due to ureteropelvic junction obstruction syndrome in children. *Prog Urol* 1991;**1**:1000.

28 Atwell JD. Familial pelviuretric junction obstruction and its association with duplex pelvicalyceal system and vesicouretric reflux. A family study. *Br J Urol* 1985;**57**:365.

29 Cohen B, Goldman SM, Kopilnick M *et al.* Uretropelvic junction obstruction: its occurrence in 3 members of a single family. *J Urol* 1978;**120**:361.

30 Izquierdo, Porteous M, Paramo PG, Connor JM. Evidence for genetic heterogeneity in hereditary hydronephrosis caused by pelviureteric obstruction, with one locus assigned to chromosome 6 p. *Hum Genet* 1992;**89**:557.

31 Williams DI, Karlaftis CM. Hydronephrosis due to pelviureteric obstruction in the newborn. *Br J Urol* 1966;**38**:138.

32 Lebowitz RI, Blickmanan JG. The co-existence of ureteropelvic junction obstruction and reflux. *Am J Roentgenol* 1983;**140**:231.

33 Gup A. Benign mesodermal polyp in childhood. *J Urol* 1975;**114**:610.

34 Williams PR, Fegetter J, Miller RA, Wickham JEA. The diagnosis and management of benign fibrous ureteric polyps. *Br J Urol* 1980;**52**:253.

35 Maizels M, Stephens FD. Valves of the ureter as a cause of primary obstruction of the ureter: anatomic, embryological and clinical aspects. *J Urol* 1980;**123**:742.

36 Leiter J. Persistent fetal ureter. *J Urol* 1979;**122**:251.

37 Ruano-Gil D, Coca-Pereras A, Tajedo-Maten A. Obstruction and normal re-canalization of the ureter in the human embryo: its relation to congenital ureteric obstruction. *Eur Urol* 1975;**1**:287.

38 Notley RG. The structural basis for normal and abnormal ureteric mobility. *Ann R Coll Surg Engl* 1971;**49**:248.

39 Murneghan JF. Mechanisms of congenital hydronephrosis with reference to factors influencing surgical treatment. *Ann R Coll Surg Engl* 1958;**23**:25.

40 Hanna MK, Jeffs RD, Sturgess JM, Barkin M. Ureteral structure and ultrastructure. Part II. Congenital ureteropelvic junction obstruction and primary obstructive megaureter. *J Urol* 1976;**116**:725.

41 Gosling JA, Dixon JS. Functional obstruction of the ureter and renal pelvis: a histological and electron microscopic study. *Br J Urol* 1978;**50**:145.

42 Kaneto H, Orikasa S, Chiba T, Takahasi T. Three-D muscular arrangement at the ureteropelvic junction and its changes in congenital hydronephrosis: a stereo morphometric study. *J Urol* 1991;**146**:909.

43 Rickwood AMK, Harney J, Jones MO, Oak S. Limitations of fetal ultrasonography in the detection of pelviureteric junction obstruction. *Br J Urol* 1995;**75**:529.

44 Arnold AJ, Rickwood AMK. Natural history of pelviureteric obstruction detected by prenatal sonography. *Br J Urol* 1990;**65**:91.

45 Freedman ER, Rickwood AMK. Prenatally diagnosed pelviureteric junction obstruction: a benign condition? *J Pediatr Surg* 1994;**29**:769.

46 Nixon HH. Hydronephrosis in children: a clinical study of seventy eight cases with special reference to the role of aberrant renal vessels and the results of conservative operations. *Br J Surg* 1953;**40**:601.

47 Stephens FD. Ureterovascular hydronephrosis and the aberrant renal vessels. *J Urol* 1982;**117**:984.

48 Whitaker RH. The Whitaker test. *Urol Clin North Am* 1979;**6**:529.

49 O'Reilly PH. Functional outcome of pyeloplasty for ureteropelvic junction obstruction. Prospective study in 30 consecutive cases. *J Urol* 1989;**142**:273.

50 Madden NP, Thomas DF, Gordon AC *et al.* Antenatally discovered pelviureteric junction obstruction. Is non-operation safe? *Br J Urol* 1991;**67**:96.

51 Najmaldin AS, Burge DM, Atwell JD. Outcome of antenatally diagnosed pelviureteric junction hydronephrosis. *Br J Urol* 1991;**67**:96.

52 Cartwright PC, Duckett JW, Keating MA *et al.* Managing apparent ureteropelvic junction obstruction in the newborn. *J Urol* 1992;**148**:1224.

53 Koff SA, Campbell R. Nonoperative management of unilateral neonatal hydronephrosis. *J Urol* 1992;**148**:525.

54 Yarger WE, Schocken DD, Harris RH. Obstructive nephropathy

in the rat: possible roles for the renin–angiotensin system, prostaglandins and thromboxanes in postobstructive renal function. *J Clin Invest* 1980;**65**:400.

55 Leahy AL, Ryan PC, McEntee GM *et al.* Renal injury and recovery in partial ureteric obstruction. *J Urol* 1989;**142**:199.

56 Josephson S, Dhillon HK, Ransley PG. Post-natal management of antenatally detected bilateral hydronephrosis. *Urol Int* 1993;**51**:79.

57 Gill B, Levitt S, Kogan S *et al.* The dilated urinary tract in children. Prospective analysis with correlation of radiological, isotope, pressure perfusion and surgical findings. *Br J Urol* 1988;**61**:413.

58 Diamond DA. Clinical patterns of paediatric urolithiasis. *Br J Urol* 1991;**68**:195.

59 Grossman IC, Cromie WJ, Wein AJ, Duckett JW. Renal hypertension secondary to ureteropelvic junction obstruction. *Urology* 1981;**17**:69.

60 Turnock RR, Shawis R. Management of fetal urinary tract anomalies detected by prenatal ultrasonography. *Arch Dis Child* 1984;**53**:962.

61 Homsy YL, Saad F, Laberge I *et al.* Transitional hydronephrosis of the newborn and infant. *J Urol* 1990;**144**:579.

62 Cockrell SN, Hendren WH. The importance of visualising the ureter before performing a pyeloplasty. *J Urol* 1990;**65**:91.

63 Koff SA, McDowell G, Byard M. Diuretic radionuclide assessment of obstruction in the infant: guidelines for successful management. *J Urol* 1988;**140**:1167.

64 Chung S, Majd M, Rushton HG, Belman AB. Diuretic renography in the evaluation of neonatal hydronephrosis: is it reliable? *J Urol* 1993;**150**:765.

65 Hoffer FA, Lebowitz RI. Intermittent hydronephrosis: a unique feature of ureteropelvic junction obstruction caused by a crossing vessel. *Radiology* 1985;**156**:655.

66 Hortsman WG, Davey MD. Intermittent hydronephrosis as cause for a false-negative pressure–flow study. *Cardiovasc Intervent Radiol* 1991;**14**:185.

67 Lupton EW, Testa HJ. The obstructive diuresis renogram: an appraisal of the significance. *J Urol* 1992;**147**:981.

68 Bassiouny IE. Salvage pyeloplasty in nonvisualising hydronephrotic kidney secondary to ureteropelvic junction obstruction. *J Urol* 1992;**148**:685.

69 Grapin C, Chartier-Kastler E, Audry G *et al.* Failures observed after repair of the pelviureteric junction in children based on a series of thirteen cases. *Ann Pediatr (Paris)* 1990;**37**:26.

70 O'Flynn KJ, Gough DC, Gupta S *et al.* Prediction of recovery in antenatally diagnosed hydronephrosis. *Br J Urol* 1993;**71**:478.

71 Ransley PG, Dhillon HK, Gordon I *et al.* The postnatal management of hydronephrosis diagnosed by prenatal ultrasound. *J Urol* 1990;**144**:584.

72 Dector SW, Gibbons MD. The fate of infant kidneys with fetal hydronephrosis but initially normal ultrasound. *J Urol* 1989;**140**:1305.

73 Gordon I, Dhillon HK, Peters AM. Antenatal diagnosis of renal pelvic dilatation—the natural history of conservative management. *Pediatr Radiol* 1991;**21**:272.

74 Gordon I, Dhillon HK, Gatanash H, Peters AM. Antenatal diagnosis of pelvic hydronephrosis: assessment of renal function and drainage as a guide to management. *J Nucl Med* 1991;**32**:1649.

75 Foley FEB. A new plastic operation for stricture of the ureteropelvic junction: a report of 20 patients. *J Urol* 1937;**38**:643.

76 Culp OS, de Weerd JH. A pelvic flap operation for certain types of ureteropelvic obstruction: preliminary report. *Proc Staff Mat Mayo Clin* 1951;**26**:483.

77 Scardino PL, Prince CL. Vertical flap ureteropelvioplasty: preliminary report. *South Med J* 1953;**46**:325.

78 Anderson JC, Hynes W. Retrocaval ureter: a case diagnosed preoperatively and treated successfully by a plastic operation. *Br J Urol* 1949;**21**:209.

79 Sheldon CA, Duckett JW, Snyder HM. Evolution in the management of infant pyeloplasty. *J Pediatr Surg* 1992;**27**:501.

80 Rickwood AMK, Phadke D. Pyeloplasty in infants and children with particular reference to the method of drainage postoperatively. *Br J Urol* 1978;**50**:227.

81 Wollin M, Duffy PG, Diamond DA *et al.* Priorities in urinary diversion following pyeloplasty. *J Urol* 1989;**142**:576.

82 McClinton S, Steyn H, Hussey JR. Retrograde balloon dilatation for pelviureteric junction obstruction. *Br J Urol* 1993;**71**:152.

83 Bratt CG, Nilsson S. Late results after surgical correction of pyeloplasty failure in idiopathic hydronephrosis. *J Urol* 1984;**132**:231.

84 O'Flynn KJ, Gough DC, Gupta S *et al.* Prediction of recovery in antenatally diagnosed hydronephrosis. *Br J Urol* 1993;**71**:478.

85 Vihma Y, Perkkulainen KV. Pelviureteric junction obstruction in children. *Z Kinderchir* 1983;**38**:43.

86 Ross JH, Streem SB, Novick AC, Kay R, Montic J. Ureterocalycostomy for reconstruction of complicated pelviureteric junction obstruction. *Br J Urol* 1990;**65**:322.

87 Ramsey JWA, Miller RA, Kellett MJ *et al.* Percutaneous pyelolysis: indications, complications and results. *Br J Urol* 1984;**56**:586.

88 Tan HL, Najmaldin A, Webb DR. Endopyelotomy for pelviureteric junction obstruction in children. *Eur Urol* 1993;**24**:84.

89 Motola JA, Fried R, Badiani GH, Smith AD. Failed endopyelotomy: implications for future surgery on the ureteropelvic junction. *J Urol* 1993;**150**:821.

13   Congenital Abnormalities of the Ureter
J.D.Frank and H.McC.Snyder III

Embryology of the ureteric bud

Normal embryology

In order to have a better understanding of the ureteric anomalies to be presented, it is useful to be familiar with the embryology of the ureteric bud and the role that the developing ureteric bud has in determining renal differentiation from the metanephric ridge. During normal development (Fig. 13.1) the ureter begins development near the end of the fourth week of embryonic life as a bud growing from the mesonephric (wolffian) duct. The bud rapidly grows toward, and penetrates, the ridge of metanephric blastema. At 5 weeks the beginning of a renal pelvis can be seen. During subsequent renal differentiation the ureteric bud will give rise to the entire collecting system of the kidney: ureter, renal pelvis, calyces, papillary ducts and collecting tubules.

The proximal end of the ureteric bud joins the mesonephric duct at the dorsomedial aspect of the elbow where the mesonephric duct bends forward and medially to join the ventral aspect of the cloaca. The mesonephric duct will be progressively absorbed into the central segment of the cloaca that is destined to become the urogenital sinus. By the eighth week of development the common stem of the mesonephric duct has been absorbed into the urogenital sinus and the ureter and mesonephric duct have achieved independent entry points into the urogenital sinus. The ureteric bud is initially below and medial to the mesonephric duct and they are quite close together. With further development, the ureteric orifice moves in a cephalad and lateral direction while the mesonephric duct (later to become the vas deferens) moves downwards and medially to reach its ultimate position in the posterior urethra at the verumontanum. As a result of this movement the mesonephric duct, and thus eventually the vas, comes to cross over the ureter ventrally. By the 12th week of development, the final location of the ureteric orifice and mesonephric duct have been achieved.

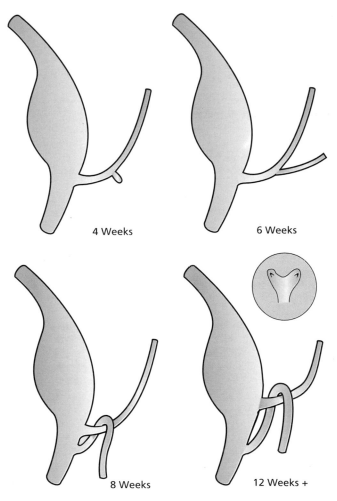

Fig. 13.1 Normal embryology of the ureteric bud from the mesonephric duct.

The initial point where the distal mesonephric duct joins the urogenital sinus appears to indicate the eventual location of the bladder neck. As the common stem of the mesonephric duct below the ureteric bud is incorporated into the expanding urogenital sinus, it forms the tissue of

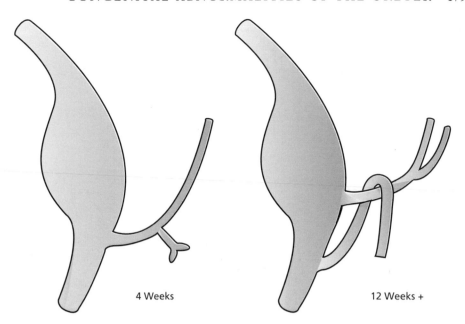

Fig. 13.2 Bifid ureteric bud leading to incomplete duplication of the ureter.

4 Weeks

12 Weeks +

the trigone. The final position of the ejaculatory duct (the end of the vas) and the ureteric orifice are usually approximately equidistant from the opening of the bladder neck.

Abnormal embryology

With this outline of normal embryology in mind, the process by which the pathological states to be discussed in this chapter arise, as well as some covered elsewhere in this volume, can be proposed. They are best understood as anomalies of origin or division of the ureteric bud.

If the bud takes origin at a normal site but bifurcates shortly after its origin, an incomplete duplication of the ureter will result (Fig. 13.2). If division occurs at the end of the period during which the ureter is growing into the metanephric blastema (the fifth week), then only a bifid pelvis will result. Bifurcation before that period will lead to varying degrees of ureteric duplication with fusion to form a single ureter entering the bladder.

Primary vesicoureteric reflux would be expected if the ureteric bud took its origin at a position lower than normal on the mesonephric duct (Fig. 13.3). In this situation, as the ureter is incorporated into the urogenital sinus, it would be carried more cranially and laterally than usual during the standard period of ureteric migration. It would be further from its normal position on the trigone and might be expected to be less well supported. The result would be just what is generally found in primary reflux: a laterally ectopic orifice with a short submucosal tunnel.

If the ureteric bud were to arise only slightly higher than normal on the mesonephric duct, then a mild degree of ureteric ectopia in the direction of the bladder neck might

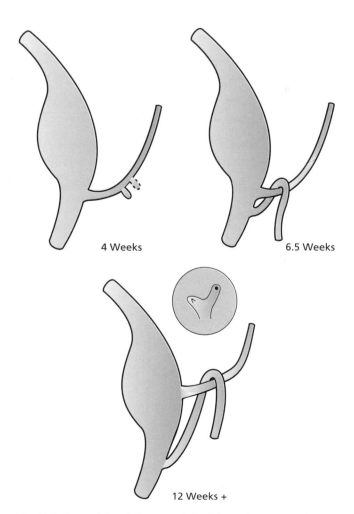

4 Weeks

6.5 Weeks

12 Weeks +

Fig. 13.3 Low origin of the ureteric bud from the mesonephric duct leading to a laterally ectopic ureteric orifice and vesicoureteric reflux.

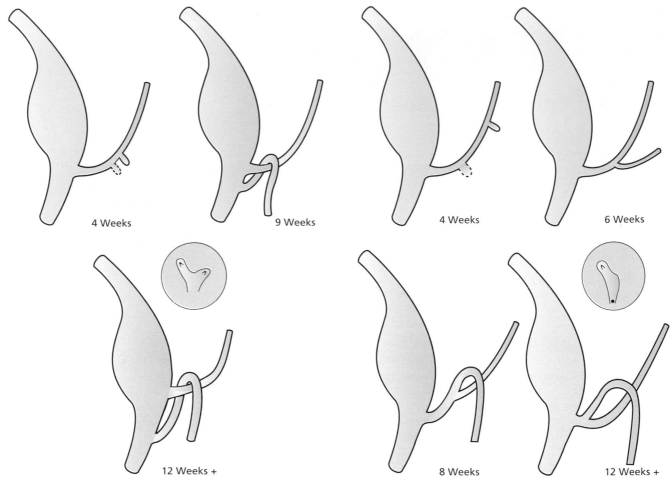

4 Weeks   9 Weeks

12 Weeks +

4 Weeks   6 Weeks

8 Weeks   12 Weeks +

Fig. 13.4 High origin of the ureteric bud from the mesonephric duct leading to a mild degree of ureteric ectopia toward the bladder neck, but with the ureter still on the trigone.

Fig. 13.5 Very high origin of the ureteric bud from the mesonephric duct leading to a ectopic ureter which maintains contact with the mesonephric remnants (vas, epididymis or seminal vesicle).

be expected (Fig. 13.4). While this might not be patho-logical, if the bud were to take a very high point of origin from the mesonephric duct (Fig. 13.5), it might end by joining the urethra or, in the male, maintain a connection with the mesonephric remnants (vas, epididymis or seminal vesicle). In the female, the high bud may end in the urethra or in a more distal remnant of the mesonephric duct — Gartner's duct. Gartner's duct runs from the broad ligament of the uterus along the lateral wall of the vagina as far as the hymen. A very high ureteric bud might end anywhere along this structure and, with secondary rupture of the duct, result in a vaginal communication. This explains the major sites for ectopic ureters in the male and female. The major difference between the two sexes lies in the fact that in the male the sites of ectopic termination all lie above the level of the external urethral sphincter so that urinary incontinence is not seen. Conversely, in the female, as an ectopic ureter may be below the sphincter, constant dribbling in-continence may be produced.

If there are two ureteric buds both originating from the normal site on the mesonephric duct (Fig. 13.6), a complete duplication of the ureter may result without any pathological sequelae. However, if there are two buds with one in a normal location and one in a low position (Fig. 13.7, see p. 182), then one would expect to see complete duplication with reflux into the ureter which was carried most superiorly and laterally during development — the lower pole one. And, indeed, this is what is most commonly found clinically. If there are two ureteric buds taking origin from the mesonephric duct, with one in a normal location and one in a high location (Fig. 13.8, see p. 182), then the second ureter to be incorporated into the developing bladder can be expected to end more distal and medial than normal. Hence, it is the upper pole ureter which ends ectopically. This, then, is the embryological explanation of the Meyer–Weigert law: with complete ureteric duplication, it is the medial and distal ureter which serves the upper pole of the kidney [1,2].

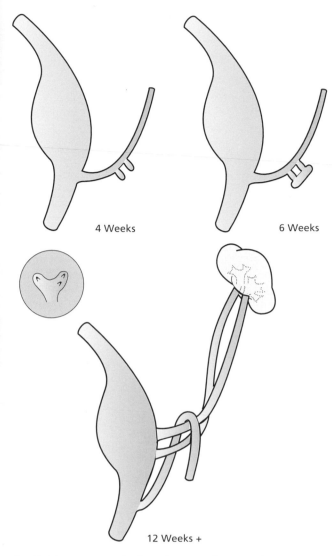

4 Weeks

6 Weeks

12 Weeks +

Fig. 13.6 Two ureteric buds at the normal site on the mesonephric duct leading to the complete duplication of the ureter without pathological sequelae.

A discussion of the caudal embryology of the ureter would be incomplete without a discussion of the aetiology of ureteroceles. Ureteroceles are cystic dilatations of the terminal segment of the ureter. While they may be associated with single ureters, most commonly they are found at the distal end of the ureter draining the upper pole collecting system in total ureteric duplication. Chwalla [3] postulated an obstructive aetiology for this anomaly. He pointed out that there exists in the embryo a two-cell-layer ureteric membrane which is present at the time of the origin of the ureteric bud from the mesonephric duct. This membrane, he reasoned, must break down or be completely reabsorbed to leave an unobstructed meatal opening. Persistence of the membrane would produce a ureteric obstruction. This theory fits nicely with the ureteroceles

which are found to have a stenotic orifice and are associated with hypertrophy of the ureter, suggesting obstruction. However, as Stephens [4] and others have pointed out, there are ureteroceles with large orifices and some which are associated with a blind-ending ureter, making obstruction unlikely as the complete explanation.

Stephens [5] and Tanagho [6,7] have postulated that the distal ureter may be acted on by the same driving force that leads to the expansion of the urogenital sinus to form the bladder. However, if this were an explanation for all ureteroceles, then any ectopic ureteric orifice should be associated with a ureterocele, which is not the case. To try to resolve this, Tanagho has postulated an additional factor [6,7]. There may be a delay in the establishment of the lumen of the ureteric bud with that of the mesonephric duct. This delay, in turn, may be the triggering factor that leads to ureteric expansion (Fig. 13.9, see p. 183). It is clear that no one explanation adequately covers all ureteroceles.

Relation of the ureteric bud position to renal morphology

It has long been recognized that ectopic ureters and ureters associated with ureteroceles frequently drain renal tissue which is hypoplastic or dysplastic and often non-functional. Mackie and Stephens [8] have postulated that this finding may also be related to an anomalous origin of the ureteric bud from the mesonephric duct (Fig. 13.10, see p. 183). This theory postulates that the metanephric ridge contains blastema with varying potential for the induction of normal renal tissue. A central zone which would correspond to the area normally reached by a ureteric bud taking origin in a normal location on the mesonephric duct has the potential for developing normal renal parenchyma. On either side of this zone, the potential of the metanephric blastema to form normal renal tissue is less. Accordingly, when a ureteric bud arises above or below the normal point of origin, it may grow to induce renal tissue with an increased likelihood of dysplasia or hypoplasia. This theory seems to hold best for upper pole ureters seen in complete duplication. Less commonly, some laterally ectopic ureteric orifices associated with reflux are also found to be associated with primarily abnormal renal tissue. This theory is an attractive way to explain the abnormal renal morphology which may be associated with a ureteric orifice away from the normal site on the trigone. It is possible that when normal renal tissue is found associated with ectopic orifices or ureteroceles, this may result from growth of the ureteric bud, which is not perfectly straight, to reach the metanephric blastema. Thus, occasionally, when the ureteric bud does arise at an abnormal site it may still reach metanephric blastema with good potential.

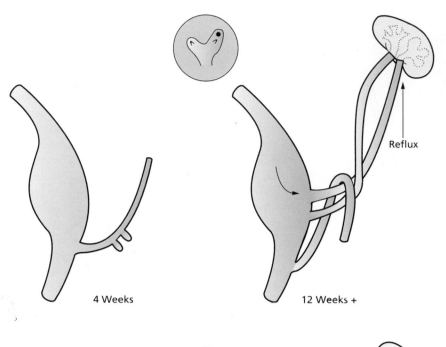

Fig. 13.7 Two ureteric buds, one normal and one low on the mesonephric duct, leading to complete ureteric duplication with lower pole vesicoureteric reflux.

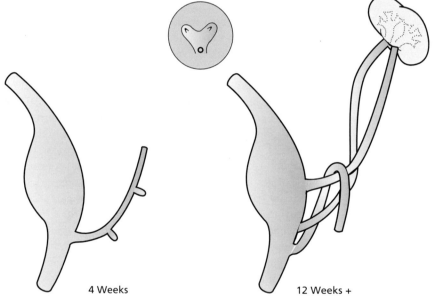

Fig. 13.8 Two ureteric buds, one normal and one high on the mesonephric duct, leading to complete ureteric duplication with an ectopic upper pole ureter.

Ureteric duplication

Ureteric duplication constitutes the most common ureteric anomaly. Frequently, it is an incidental finding not associated with any pathology. With urinary infection, however, there is an increased incidence of ureteric duplication, as will be described. Upper urinary tract stasis with obstruction or reflux is more common in duplication and provides the explanation for this finding. The incidence of ureteric duplication appears to be approximately 1:125 or 0.8% [9,10]. Unilateral duplication is approximately six times more frequent than bilateral. The right and left sides are affected equally.

An examination of the genetics of duplication suggests that this anomaly may be determined by an autosomal dominant trait with incomplete penetrance [11]. With an index child with ureteric duplication in a family, the likelihood of another sibling with a duplication rises from the expected 1:125 to 1:8 or 9 [12,13].

Other anomalies of the urinary tract have an increased incidence in patients with ureteric duplication. The most common is renal hypoplasia or dysplasia, probably reflecting the abnormal metanephric blastema induced by an anomalously located ureteric bud. In a radiographic review of duplications [14], an increased incidence of radiographic renal anomalies was also found. Twenty-nine

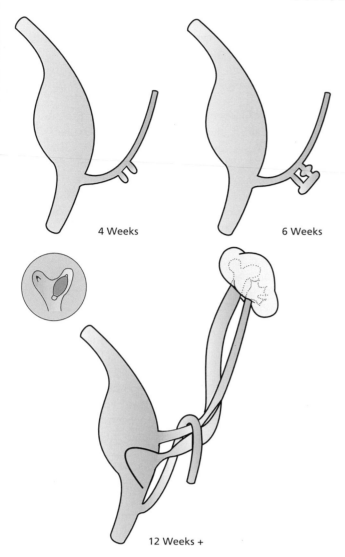

Fig. 13.9 Two ureteric buds with delay in establishment of the lumen of the upper ureteric bud leading to development of an upper pole ureterocele.

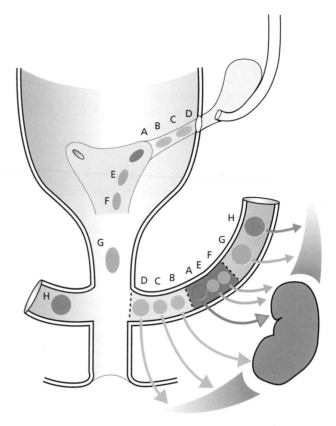

Fig. 13.10 Stephens' theory that an abnormal origin of the ureteric bud from the mesonephric duct leads to the induction of mesonephric blastema with limited potential for the formation of normal renal tissue. This composite diagram shows how a ureteric bud with a near-normal origin (A, E, F) from the mesonephric duct will induce kidney from the main mass of metanephric blastema and will form a good kidney associated with a ureteric orifice on the trigone. Ureteric buds with an abnormal origin will induce blastema with limited potential and will be associated with an ectopic ureteric orifice.

per cent of duplex units exhibited scarring, hydronephrosis or both. This is not surprising, based on the embryological discussion given above. Likewise, one would expect an increased incidence of childhood urinary tract infections with duplications because of the associated reflux or obstruction that is seen. Indeed, this has been the reported experience [9,15].

Incomplete ureteric duplication

Y ureter

Incomplete ureteric duplication is presumably due to bifurcation of the ureteric bud above its junction with the mesonephric duct. The level of bifurcation will determine

the degree of duplication seen. Of incomplete duplications, roughly 25% are found to divide in the distal third of the ureter, 50% in the middle third and 25% in the upper third of the ureter. In many instances, ureteric duplication is merely an incidental finding and not associated with any clinical problem. However, with a Y junction in the ureter, it is possible for a peristaltic wave to arrive at the junction and then be passed in a retrograde fashion up the other side of the Y. This back and forth movement of urine has been called a 'yo-yo' movement and can lead to stasis and ureteric dilatation. Uncommonly, there is associated infection or flank discomfort.

The diagnosis is usually evident on intravenous urography (IVU) using fluoroscopic observation or on a mercapto acetyl triglycine (MAG_3) renogram. A micturating cystourethrogram (MCU) is important to rule out dilatation due to vesicoureteric reflux.

In the rare case warranting surgical treatment, the operative procedure depends upon the level of the duplication. If the duplication is very low, it may be possible to carry out a reimplantation of the ureters with separate ureteric orifices in the bladder. For higher duplications, a high ureteropyelostomy or uretero-ureterostomy with excision of most of the extra duplicated ureter serves to eliminate the problem.

Blind-ending duplication

Very rarely, a ureteric duplication is present with a blind-ending ureter [16,17]. Although the ureteric bud appears to have bifurcated, only one limb succeeds in inducing the development of associated renal parenchyma. In some reported series, ureteric diverticula may be confused with this entity. Most are duplications of the mid or distal ureter. Women are three times as likely to exhibit this anomaly and it is seen most frequently on the right side.

The occasional patient who develops symptoms generally does so in the third or fourth decade. Flank pain with infection or calculi is most frequently observed. The diagnosis may require a retrograde ureterogram as the blind duplication may not fill on IVU. Treatment consists of surgical excision of the duplication.

Inverted Y

This constitutes the most rare anomaly of ureteric branching. Presumably, two separate ureteric buds arise from the mesonephric duct but fuse prior to inducing renal differentiation. Almost all reported patients have been female [18]. One limb may be ectopic and produce incontinence. Treatment of this rare anomaly is directed at correcting any problem caused by the ectopic limb. This generally involves its resection.

Complete ureteric duplication and vesicoureteric reflux

In kidneys with complete ureteric duplication, vesi-coureteric reflux is the most common cause of acquired disease. Reflux generally occurs into the lower segment of the kidney drained by a ureter which had an abnormally caudal origin from the mesonephric duct, resulting in a lateral ureteric orifice with a shortened submucosal course which permits reflux. By contrast, the upper pole ureter, because its orifice lies medial and distal (Meyer–Weigert law [1,2]), has a longer submucosal course and is only rarely subject to reflux. Occasionally, reflux will be seen into both upper and lower pole orifices. In this situation, cystoscopy usually reveals that both orifices lie side by side in a laterally ectopic position. This presumably arises because both ureteric buds have taken origin close by one another

and in a position caudal to normal on the mesonephric duct. Reflux into the upper pole ureter may also occur if its orifice is ectopic at the bladder neck or urethra, and the ureter reaches this point separately without trigonal support with complete duplication and vesicoureteric reflux.

Urinary tract infection is the most frequent presentation of the child with duplication and reflux. Occasional neonates will be diagnosed on prenatal ultrasound examination. The diagnosis is established by an MCU showing reflux into the lower pole collecting system and an IVU showing duplication of the renal collecting system. An ultrasound will often diagnose a duplex system but it is unusual for the reflux to be diagnosed. A MAG$_3$ scan is useful for looking at differential function of the upper and lower poles, and an indirect radionuclide cystogram can be performed and the reflux diagnosed. We still prefer to confirm the reflux with a contrast study in order to define the anatomy and to rule out any other associated anomalies.

Management of the refluxing duplicated ureter depends upon the amount of function in the lower pole seen on a dimercapto succinic acid (DMSA) or MAG$_3$ isotope scan. Low grades of reflux with reasonable function may resolve spontaneously with linear growth of the child accompanied by lengthening of the submucosal tunnel of the ureter. Low-dose antibiotic prophylaxis and intermittent radio-logical monitoring are all that are required. Higher grades of reflux are often associated with poor function and may benefit from surgical intervention. Poor function of the lower pole (less than 10% of individual renal function) is best treated by a lower pole heminephroureterectomy. Removing the lower pole of the kidney is not easy because the calyces erode into the upper pole of the kidney so that the upper moiety sits like an inverted egg-cup on an egg. The ureter should be taken as low down as possible before the ureters join in a common sheath. The refluxing stump should be ligated. If there is reasonable function of the lower pole a double-barrelled reimplantation of the ureters may be performed. Both ureters should be mobilized together and reimplanted in the common sheath.

Ureteric triplication

One of the rarest anomalies of the upper urinary tract is ureteric triplication (Fig. 13.11). The embryological explanation for this anomaly is the presence of three buds arising from the mesonephric duct. Early fusion of the ducts could account for the partial triplications that have been seen. Most cases are trifid ureters with all three ureters draining through a single orifice. In a review of 61 cases, Perkins et al. [19] found that the left side was affected most commonly and that the problem was seen most frequently in females. Symptoms may be infection,

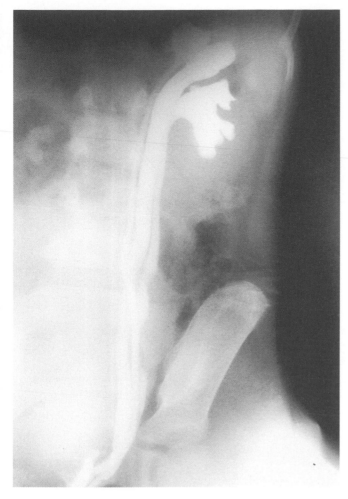

Fig. 13.11 A retrograde ureterogram showing ureteric triplication.

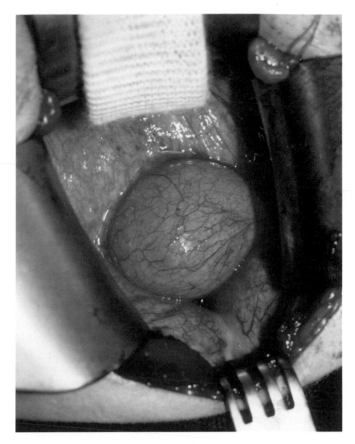

Fig. 13.12 A large intravesical ureterocele.

incontinence or pain [20]. Surgical treatment, when required, must be individualized.

Ureterocele

A ureterocele may be defined as a cystic dilatation of the intravesical submucosal ureter. Most frequently, it is associated with the upper pole ureter of a kidney with complete ureteric duplication. Ureteroceles are much more common in girls than boys. Rarely, a ureterocele may be associated with a blind-ending ureter. The embryology of ureteroceles has been much debated (see above) and it is evident that no one explanation accounts for all ureteroceles. Characteristically, the wall of the ureterocele demonstrates attenuated muscle and collagen. Ureteroceles may vary in size from small ones which may be difficult to visualize to those which are so large as to fill virtually the entire bladder (Fig. 13.12). The orifice of the ureterocele may be located intra- or extravesically and may be stenotic, normal in size or even patulous in a minority of cases.

The first effort at classification of ureteroceles was by Ericsson [21]. He defined simple ureteroceles as those contained entirely within the bladder. These are more common with a single system as opposed to a duplex system and are termed intravesical as opposed to ectopic. Ectopic ureteroceles are defined as ureteroceles which extend to the bladder neck or posterior urethra. This classification continues to be widely used today. Stephens [4] provided a classification which furthers our understanding of the pathological anatomy of ureteroceles. He divided ureteroceles into four categories.

1 *Stenotic ureteroceles* (approximately 40%) have a small ureteric orifice and the ureterocele is usually located entirely in the bladder, corresponding to Ericsson's simple ureterocele. The degree of stenosis of the ureteric orifice varies from pin-point, with the ureterocele being tensely distended at all times, to larger ones which result in the ureterocele being visible only as a peristaltic wave prepares to eject a stream of urine from the meatus. Pathological examination reveals that the wall of a stenotic ureterocele tends to exhibit more musculature than other varieties of ureterocele. It is in a predominantly longitudinal orientation.

2 *Sphincteric ureteroceles* (approximately 40%) are defined

as those with an orifice located within the confines of the internal sphincter. They constitute a type of ectopic ureterocele. The meatus of the ureterocele may be normal in size or even large. Obstruction to drainage is secondary to incorporation of the meatus within the internal sphincter, thus drainage of the ureterocele takes place during voiding. This variety of ureterocele may be subject to reflux. Pathological examination reveals that the walls of sphincteric and sphincterostenotic ureteroceles exhibit deficient musculature which is oriented in a more helical than longitudinal pattern.

3 *Sphincterostenotic ureteroceles* (approximately 5%) exhibit a stenotic meatus located ectopically at the level of the internal sphincter. This is another variant of the ectopic ureterocele. They tend to be larger and tense. During micturition, instead of emptying as the sphincteric ones do, they may ball-valve into the bladder outlet, producing urethral obstruction or, in the female, may prolapse through the urethral meatus.

4 *Caecoureteroceles*. Stephens has defined another type of ureterocele which he calls the caecoureterocele [5]. In this type, the meatus of the ureterocele is located in the bladder, but a tongue of the ureterocele extends down the urethra submucosally (Fig. 13.13). This tongue-like projection may lead to a mucosal flap capable of obstructing the urethra if great care is not taken at the time of ureterocele excision.

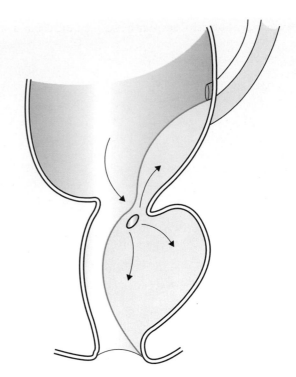

Fig. 13.13 Caecoureterocele—a ureterocele with a tongue-like projection extending down the urethra submucosally.

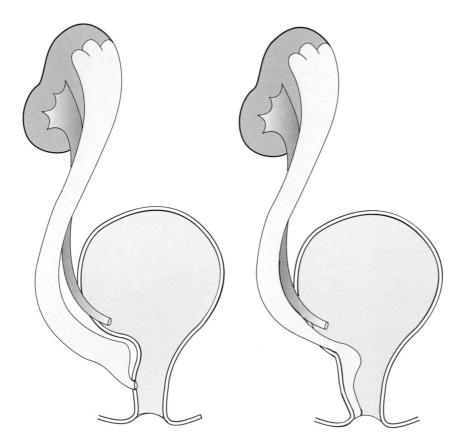

Fig. 13.14 Pseudoureterocele—the dilated terminal end of a ectopic ureter elevating the trigone to give the appearance of a ureterocele.

An apparent ureterocele may be seen on ultrasound or on cystoscopy which is in fact the dilated end of an ectopic ureter elevating the trigone. This has been termed a pseudoureterocele [22] (Fig. 13.14).

The classification of ureteroceles has changed slightly and we now refer to the ureteroceles as intravesical or ectopic in accordance with the definition of the American Academy of Pediatrics section of urology [23] rather than as ectopic or orthotopic.

The incidence of ureteroceles was reported by Campbell [24] to be 1:4000 autopsies in children. It seems likely that small ureteroceles were being missed. Uson et al. [25] reported an incidence of 1:500 autopsies. Ureteroceles are more common in Caucasians and are rare in Blacks. Females are reported to be affected four to seven times as commonly as males. Some series demonstrate a left-sided predominance; 10–15% are bilateral. Duplication of the ureter is present in 75% of patients with ureteroceles. Ectopic ureteroceles, as opposed to simple ones, make up 60–80% of most cases [4,21,26]. Single system ectopic ureteroceles are rare and are seen usually in males. Associated urological anomalies are common. When the ureterocele is associated with ipsilateral ureteral duplication, there is a 30–50% likelihood of contralateral duplication. Renal anomalies, especially fusions and ectopia, are common. When the ureterocele arises from the upper pole in a duplication, renal dysplasia of that moiety is frequent.

Presentation

Infection was one of the most common presentations for a child with a ureterocele. Often this is in the first few months of life with a picture of Gram-negative sepsis. Infants may fail to thrive or have gastrointestinal symptoms. Rarely a neonate will present with a prolapsed ureterocele (Fig. 13.15). Prenatal diagnosis as a result of routine maternal ultrasound has become more frequent in the past 10 years. In the report by Blyth et al. [27] of 115 children with a ureterocele, 20 patients presented with a urinary infection and 19 were antenatally diagnosed. Lee et al. [28] recently reported on the experience of prenatally diagnosed duplex systems from Liverpool. Of 39 patients, 15 had a ureterocele, 15 ureteric ectopia, six lower pole reflux, two a pelviureteric junction stenosis of the lower pole and one yo-yo reflux in association with an incomplete duplex. Occasionally, an infant will be found to have a palpable abdominal mass which may represent the bladder or a dilated renal drainage system. Prolapse of the ureterocele may lead to bladder outlet obstruction. This constitutes the most common cause of urethral obstruction in little girls. Usually, obstruction is produced by tense non-compressible ureteroceles which are the ones which tend to be large. Most ureteroceles do not produce

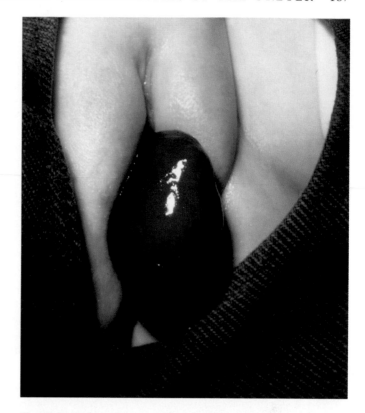

Fig. 13.15 Prolapsed ureterocele in a neonate.

obstruction because they are compressible during voiding. Haematuria from trauma to the dilated associated drainage system or from the presence of a stone secondary to stasis is another presentation. Flank or abdominal pain is more common with intravesical than with ectopic ureteroceles. Incontinence may be a presenting symptom as well. Most commonly this is secondary to bladder infection. However, if the ureterocele is large with an intraurethral extension, there may rarely be an abnormal and lax internal sphincter that may permit incontinence even after surgical treatment of the ureterocele [29].

The diagnosis of a ureterocele either pre- or postnatally is most commonly made using an ultrasound examination of the kidneys and bladder (Fig. 13.16a). This will detect the hydronephrotic upper moiety of a duplex kidney or the hydronephrosis of the whole kidney in a single system ureterocele. The dilated ureter running behind the bladder and the intravesical ureterocele can usually be visualized [30,31]. On occasions when the kidney is severely hydronephrotic it may be difficult to differentiate between a single system and duplex system ureterocele.

The IVU remains useful in diagnosis. If function in the associated kidney is good, there will be the typical 'cobra head' deformity produced by opacified urine in the ureterocele surrounded by a radiolucent halo produced by the wall of the ureterocele (Fig. 13.17, see p. 189). This type of picture is most common with intravesical ureteroceles.

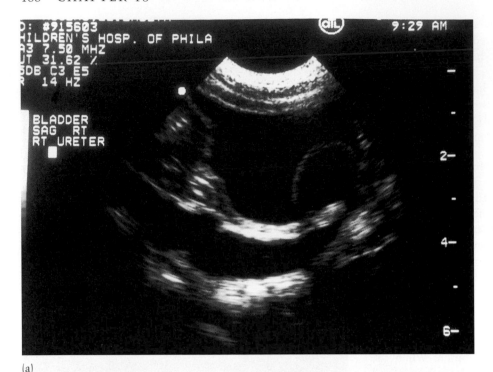

(a)

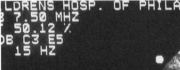

(b)

Fig. 13.16 (a) Intravesical ureterocele seen on ultrasound with a dilated ureter behind the bladder before puncture. (b) Appearance of the ureterocele after puncture. The ureterocele has collapsed and the dilated ureter is no longer seen behind the bladder.

Most ectopic ureteroceles are associated with a poor or non-functioning renal moiety and the degree of associated hydroureteronephrosis is greater. Because of poor function, the radiographic signs are primarily negative ones reflecting the effect of the dilated non-functioning segment on the functioning lower pole unit. Typically, the kidney appears to have too few calyces and the long upper pole infundibulum will be missing. Hydronephrosis of the upper pole will push the lower pole downwards and laterally, producing the characteristic 'drooping lily' sign (Fig. 13.18).

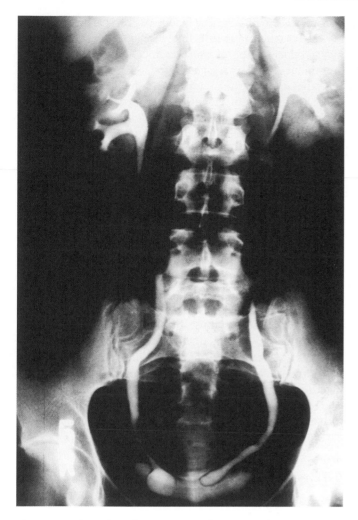

Fig. 13.17 Bilateral single system simple ureteroceles. IVU showing the typical 'cobra head' deformity of the distal ureter associated with small single system ureteroceles.

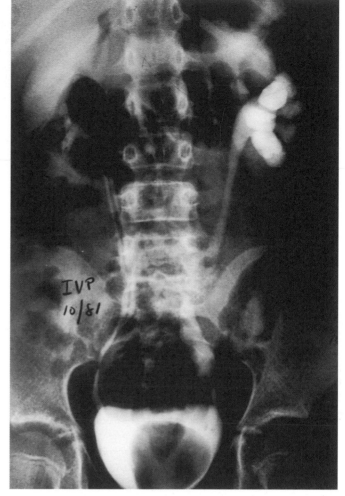

Fig. 13.18 Left ureteric duplication with an associated ureterocele shown as a filling defect in the bladder.

The hydroureter may displace the lower pole ureter laterally and the lower pole ureter may be tortuous as it is intertwined with the upper pole one. In the bladder, there is typically a negative shadow reflecting the ureterocele (see Fig. 13.18). This may vary from a large, tense, rounded shadow filling much of the bladder to a poorly defined irregularity along the floor of the bladder. It is best to examine early and post-void films in the urogram series for the ureterocele, because once the bladder is filled with opaque medium, the ureterocele may be obscured.

The MCU is an essential part of ureterocele evaluation. When the ureterocele is associated with the upper pole of a duplication, reflux to the lower pole occurs in about 50% of cases. These tend to be compressible ureteroceles with poor support for the submucosal course of the lower pole ureter. In 10–15% of ureteroceles, there is reflux into the ureterocele itself. This is usually a wide-mouthed ureterocele (often sphincteric), a caecoureterocele or a ruptured ureterocele. In approximately 25% of cases there is contralateral reflux [32]. The typical radiographic sign of the rare ruptured ureterocele is the filling of an irregular cavity beyond the bladder outline with an edge which forms a filling defect within the bladder shadow. Another variable of ureteroceles which can be determined from the MCU is the degree of detrusor backing. If this is poor and the ureterocele prolapses through the detrusor during voiding, the radiographic picture may mimic that of a bladder diverticulum (Fig. 13.19). Interestingly, after decompression of the ureterocele, the detrusor backing may appear to improve substantially. Tense ureteroceles may obstruct the ipsilateral lower pole ureter or contralateral ureter and may ball-valve into the bladder neck, producing bladder outlet obstruction. Thus, the radiographic findings with ureteroceles may constitute some of the most challenging tasks of interpretation in paediatric urology. Not only may the ureterocele be associated with ipsilateral

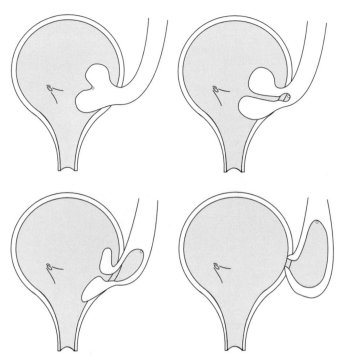

Fig. 13.19 Illustration of how prolapse of a ureterocele through the ureteric hiatus may mimic a bladder diverticulum.

and contralateral duplication, but obstruction or reflux of any of the renal moieties may also be present. Radionuclide examination of the kidneys is an essential investigation particularly in duplex kidneys with a ureterocele. A DMSA or MAG$_3$ scan is probably most accurate in determining the differential function of the upper and lower moieties of the duplex kidney. This in turn will influence the decision as to which type of treatment should be undertaken, although the upper pole usually provides only one-third of the kidney's function [14] and thus function is not a major issue in choosing therapy.

Findings at cystoscopy are quite variable and may be confusing. There may be a small ureterocele which is most evident as it fills with a peristaltic wave before ejecting a fine stream of urine from its meatus. The ureterocele may be so large as to make identification of its orifice and other ureteric orifices in the bladder impossible. With bilateral obstruction it may be difficult to ascertain from which side the ureterocele has its origin. In this situation, it may be useful to inject the ureterocele with contrast medium and obtain a radiograph. This is most easily accomplished by wedging a small needle into the end of a fine ureteric catheter and puncturing the ureterocele under direct vision at cystoscopy. Injection can also be carried out by passing a spinal needle through the lower abdominal wall into the bladder and into the ureterocele again under direct vision. In order to avoid missing a compressible ureterocele that may appear as a minor mucosal fold on the bladder floor, it

is important to observe the bladder when it is nearly empty as well as when it is full. Likewise, massage of the flank may produce filling of the ureterocele and make it more prominent. Flank massage may also produce a jet of pus from the orifice of the ureterocele in the frequently infected cases, permitting the identification of the meatus. When detrusor backing of the ureterocele is poor and the ureterocele prolapses through the detrusor, the cystoscopic picture may be confused with that of a bladder diverticulum. The diagnosis will be made if the bladder is emptied and the flank massaged, permitting the ureterocele to appear again within the bladder. Because of the frequent occurrence of contralateral duplication with ureteroceles, every effort should be made to assess the contralateral anatomy carefully at cystoscopy. This may save considerable embarrassment at the time of surgery.

Management

A number of factors must be taken into account when considering the treatment of ureteroceles. These are the patient's age; the amount of functioning renal parenchyma; the intravesical or ectopic position of the ureterocele; whether it is associated with a single or duplex system; the degree of ipsilateral ureteric dilatation; the presence of ipsilateral or contralateral reflux and the degree of detrusor backing of the ureterocele.

Intravesical ureteroceles

Intravesical ureteroceles tend to be associated with single ureters, better upper tract function and less hydro-ureteronephrosis; it is therefore appropriate to discuss their therapy separately from that of the ectopic ureterocele. It must be emphasized, though, that there are broad areas of overlap. It is interesting to read this chapter in the previous edition of this book: 'The endoscopic incision of a ureterocele in children is usually followed by reflux and a secondary operation has generally been required.' Blyth *et al.* [27] reported 81% of single system ureteroceles were intravesical as opposed to 40% of duplex system ureteroceles.

The current recommended approach for the primary treatment of an intravesical ureterocele whether presenting due to an antenatal diagnosis or as a result of sepsis is endoscopic incision. The technique of incision is important (Fig. 13.20a). It is essential that the incised opening into the ureterocele is located within the bladder when the bladder is empty to ensure that there is adequate drainage. The opening into the ureterocele is made using a 3 F Bug-bee electrode with the point of puncture into the ureterocele just above the base. The direction of incision should be parallel to the floor of the bladder taking care to avoid incising below the lumen, which is easier than it would

Fig. 13.20 Technique for incision of a ureterocele. (a) With an intravesical ureterocele a 3 F Bug-bee electrode is punctured low on the anterior wall to preserve a flap valve of decompressed ureterocele. (b) With an ectopic ureterocele it is necessary to drain the urethral segment without leaving an occluding distal lip. This can be achieved by a longitudinal incision extending from the distal extent of the ureterocele through the bladder neck sufficiently proximal to ensure that bladder neck closure does not occlude opening (1); alternatively, by puncturing the urethral and intravesical segments of the ureterocele satisfactory drainage is achieved (2).

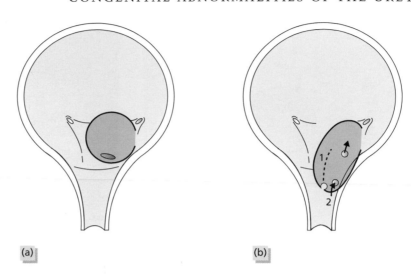

(a) (b)

seem. The opening created by a 3 F Bug-bee is more than adequate to decompress the ureterocele (see Fig. 13.16).

In the series by Blyth *et al.* [27], 25 of 27 ureteroceles were satisfactorily decompressed and reflux was present in only two of 27 patients at 6 months follow-up. Secondary procedures were only needed in two patients. Both of these were in duplex systems and were due to failure to decompress the upper pole in one patient and a bladder outlet obstruction in the other. Single system intravesical ureteroceles are therefore usually treated successfully using endoscopic Bug-bee puncture without morbidity or the necessity of a secondary procedure.

Other surgical options include nephrectomy for poor or non-function [33]. Persistent reflux with infection will require a ureterocelectomy and reimplantation of the ureter. Occasionally, the ureteric calibre may be so large that a tapered reimplantation may be necessary. Poor detrusor backing, if present, must be repaired. It is usually possible to separate the inner lining of the ureterocele and save a part of the side wall. The detrusor is then brought together to repair the defect. If the defect is large and the detrusor very thin it can be brought together plicating the muscle and creating a repair like the keel of a ship. The mucosa is then closed over the top. When the excision of the ureterocele involves the bladder neck, often in intravesical ureteroceles and always in extravesical ones, this 'keeling' repair of the bladder neck is essential to maintain the functional integrity of the bladder neck. It is essential that any dilatation of the bladder neck caused by the ureterocele or its excision is repaired by successive stitches everting ('keeling') the bladder neck detrusor until a normal bladder neck ring is reconstructed [34]. A transtrigonal method of reimplantation enables the reimplantation to be done away from the area of the ureterocele excision and detrusor reconstruction. A small asymptomatic minimally obstructive ureterocele may be observed.

Ectopic (extravesical) ureteroceles

There are a number of different treatment options for ectopic ureteroceles (Fig. 13.21). There has been a move to being more conservative in recent years. The traditional approach to an ectopic ureterocele was to carry out a ureterocele excision, reconstruction of the detrusor and reimplantation of the ipsilateral lower pole ureter and contralateral ureter if necessary. Through a separate flank incision a partial upper pole nephroureterectomy was performed [35]. The procedure could be staged by bringing the upper pole ureter out as a temporary cutaneous ureterostomy. Whether done in a single stage or as a two-stage procedure, this operative undertaking was a considerable technical challenge and led to a closer examination of alternative methods of treatment.

As the upper pole unit of an ectopic ureterocele associated with duplication is rarely of sufficient quality to warrant salvage, an approach based on its primary removal with decompression of the ureterocele and a staged approach to surgery at the bladder level was tried in some centres [36–38]. This approach avoided surgery on the ureterocele until it had had a chance to shrink down in size following decompression. It was felt that this would simplify bladder surgery or possibly eliminate the need for an operation at the bladder level. Following decompression of the ureterocele, it was also noted that frequently ipsilateral and contralateral reflux or obstruction would subside. Even cases where the ureterocele appears to have poor backing are observed on occasion to reconstitute the bladder wall after ureterocele decompression. The ureterocele usually collapses so well that it is hard to see subsequently by MCU.

Currently, persistent ipsilateral lower pole reflux is the most common indication for excision of the ureterocele and reimplantation of the lower pole ureter. While some series [36,37] have reported as low as a 25–30% need for

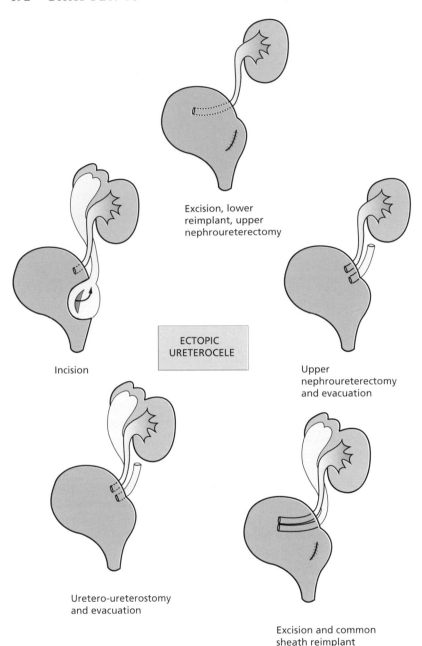

Excision, lower
reimplant, upper
nephroureterectomy

Incision

ECTOPIC
URETEROCELE

Upper
nephroureterectomy
and evacuation

Uretero-ureterostomy
and evacuation

Excision and common
sheath reimplant

Fig. 13.21 Surgical options for ectopic ureteroceles.

eventual ureterocele excision, a review of ureteroceles at the Children's Hospital of Philadelphia [38] revealed that ipsilateral lower pole reflux which persisted for more than 2 years after ureterocele decompression usually failed to resolve spontaneously. In that series, if all persistent ipsilateral lower pole reflux came to surgery, it would raise the incidence of a needed secondary operation at the bladder level to 50%. There are occasional other cases where reflux into the ureterocele and upper ureteric stump leads to sufficient problems with infection or post-micturition dribbling to warrant surgery. When dealing with a caecoureterocele this surgery is often difficult and may even lead to complications if attempts are made to excise all the ureterocele from above. The majority of the ureterocele should be excised from above and the defect closed, but a distal lip may be left behind. This can then be better dealt with from below. At the end of the surgical procedure the urethra is visualized from below and a hook passed up the urethra to catch the distal lip of the ureterocele which can then be incised with diathermy. All in all, however, it is becoming increasingly evident that the staged approach to the treatment of ectopic ureteroceles will lead to the avoidance of a secondary bladder procedure in a great many children.

When the upper pole unit associated with an ectopic ureterocele exhibits function [39], indicating that moiety warrants salvage (less than 10% of cases), a high uretero-ureterostomy or ureteropyelostomy may be undertaken but it is only appropriate if there is an extrarenal pelvis or dilated lower pole ureter. The decompressed ureterocele can be managed as mentioned above. The alternative method of salvaging the upper pole by excision of the ureterocele and common sheath reimplant of both the upper and lower pole ureter is usually technically difficult because of the size of the obstructed upper pole ureter.

In recent years, as endoscopic treatment has gained favour, some have advocated a primary endoscopic incision of the ureterocele and a 'waiting period' to see if the upper pole will regain some function [40]. The recent paper by Blyth et al. [27] indicates that endoscopic incision of an extravesical ureterocele has a limited part to play in the management of this abnormality and that a secondary surgical procedure is more likely to be required than for an intravesical ureterocele. Incision of an ectopic ureterocele was the definitive treatment in only 50% of patients with persistent reflux—the usual indication for subsequent surgery. The secondary surgical procedure required usually consisted of a partial nephrectomy with ureterocelectomy, excision of the ureterocele and reimplantation of the lower pole ureter or a ureterocele excision and duplex system reimplantation. Thus, while endoscopic incision of ectopic ureteroceles still has an important role in ureterocele management, there will be a significant number of children who will require subsequent open surgery.

In the neonate, the ureterocele can be punctured as a minor procedure decompressing an obstructed system and lowering the risk of sepsis. If further surgery is required it can be deferred until the child is 1 year of age when bladder surgery can be more successfully undertaken. In the older child, incision is most successful for intravesical ureteroceles or ureteroceles associated with a single system. In the toilet-trained child, especially if there is no associated reflux, a primary upper pole partial nephrectomy (avoiding the need for bladder surgery in the majority of patients) will minimize the surgical discomfort of the child which is created when ureterocele excision and bladder neck reconstruction is needed. While the endoscopic treatment of ureteroceles continues to evolve it is clear that it has a greater role than previously thought.

Occasionally, one will begin an operation for what appears to be primary vesicoureteral reflux into a single system and, at mobilization of the ureter, find a second small ureter running to a small non-obstructed ureterocele [41]. Treatment by common sheath reimplantation is usually successful without the need for later removal of the poorly functioning upper pole renal moiety.

Occasionally, an ectopic ureterocele will be associated with such a severe degree of ipsilateral lower pole obstruction or reflux that the lower pole has very poor function. In this situation a primary nephroureterectomy may be justified as decompression of the ureterocele and/or preservation of the lower pole rarely, if ever, results in improved function. Fortunately, this situation is rare.

There are several technical points in the performance of an upper pole partial nephrectomy undertaken to decompress a ureterocele that need to be mentioned. In children, complete renal mobilization to facilitate surgery on the upper pole is generally possible through a relatively short transverse flank incision just below the tip of the 12th rib. The vasculature to the upper pole is often variable and anomalous. During renal mobilization, care should be taken to identify the quite small vessels which may run directly into the upper pole. By tracing them toward the parenchyma before their division, one can be safely assured of not damaging the blood supply to the lower pole. The ureter to the upper pole usually courses posterior to the renal vessels; however, it should be remembered that occasionally an aberrant vessel will be behind the ureter. Having clearly identified the ureter to the upper pole, it may be divided and the upper end put on gentle traction to guide dissection of the upper pole parenchyma to be removed. If the capsule is not too adherent from previous inflammation, it is useful to strip this back to be used later in closure. The critical ingredient in the upper pole partial nephrectomy is the removal of the complete upper pole collecting system. The parenchymal incision is made just on the upper pole side of the line of demarcation with the lower pole. Resection of the usually hypoplastic or dysplastic upper pole is not usually associated with a significant blood loss. The distal end of the upper pole ureter is then dissected down to below the level of the iliac vessels. The ureter is often significantly dilated and tortuous. It may appear to wrap around the small lower pole ureter. In order to avoid damage to the lower pole ureter, dissection should be kept immediately upon the wall of the upper pole ureter. Below the iliac vessels, the upper and lower pole ureters begin to share a common muscular sheath. No effort need be made to remove this portion of the upper pole ureter. If there is no reflux into the ureterocele, the lower end is irrigated and then left open. If the ureterocele refluxes, the ureter should be ligated. In this situation, there is an increased likelihood that a subsequent bladder operation to remove the ureterocele and ureteric stump will be required. A small Penrose drain is left to the area of the ureteric stump, as well as to the area of the removed renal parenchyma.

Ectopic ureter

An ectopic ureter is defined as one which does not open at its normal location on the corner of the trigone. The embryological explanation for this anomaly is found in the high origin of the ureteric bud from the mesonephric duct with delayed or no separation from the duct. The orifice of

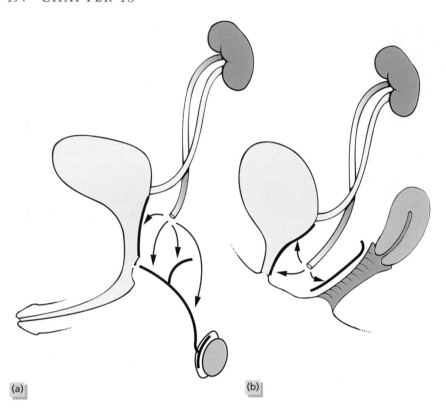

Fig. 13.22 (a) Ureteric ectopia in a male. The possible sites of ectopic ureter are above the external sphincter. (b) Ureteric ectopia in a female. An ectopic ureter may be located beyond the continence mechanism and may produce incontinence.

the ectopic ureter may be found at any of a number of possible sites in a male or female (Fig. 13.22). This leads to different clinical presentations in the male and female, as will be considered below. The exact incidence of ectopic ureter is uncertain, because many mildly ectopic ureters cause no symptoms. Campbell [9] reported 10 ectopic ureters in 19076 autopsies in children, or an incidence of 1:1900 children. In 80% of these cases, the ectopic orifice was associated with the upper pole ureter of a kidney with duplication of its drainage system. In females this percentage is even higher than 80%, as in males it is much more common for an ectopic ureter to drain a single system [42]. Ectopic ureters are much more common in females with a series reporting two to 12 female cases for each male [43]. Ten to 20% of ectopic ureters are bilateral. When a single system is ectopic on one side, the contralateral system may be duplicated in up to 80% of cases [44].

The anomaly most commonly seen with the ectopic ureter is hypoplasia or dysplasia of the associated renal tissue. This is not surprising considering the embryological discussion above. The most ectopic ureteric orifices are associated with the most abnormal renal parenchyma. Rognon *et al.* [45] reported 10 males with ureters emptying into the seminal tracts and in all cases the renal parenchyma failed to visualize at urography [45]. While a single ectopic ureter will rarely result in weakness of the bladder neck, this is a much more common problem with

bilateral single ectopic ureters, as will be discussed separately below.

Ectopic ureter in the female

The primary difference between males and females lies in the fact that ectopic ureters in the latter can come to lie distal to the continence mechanism of the bladder neck and external sphincter and, accordingly, may be associated with incontinence (see Fig. 13.22). About one-third of ectopic ureters are located either at the level of the bladder neck or slightly more distal in the urethra at the level of the external sphincter. The more proximal the orifice, the less continence will be a problem, but obstruction of the ectopic ureter as it traverses the musculature of the bladder neck will be more frequent. These high ectopic ureters drain only during micturition when the sphincters are open. Reflux into the ureter is frequent in the higher placed ectopic orifices, producing the paradoxical finding of both obstruction and reflux. Lower ureters traversing the level of the external sphincter can less commonly be demonstrated to reflux. The most frequent site of ureteric ectopia in the female is the vaginal vestibule, with approximately one-third of ectopic orifices being found in this area (Fig. 13.23). This is the site of the terminal end of Gartner's duct—the mesonephric duct remnant in the female. Approximately 25% of ectopic ureters in females will enter the vagina.

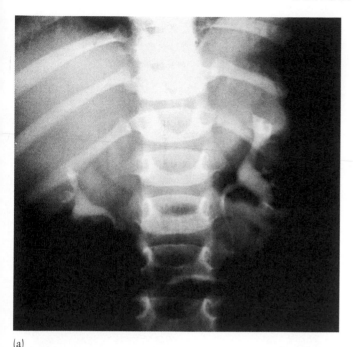

(a)

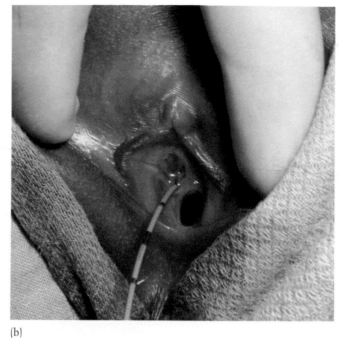

(b)

Fig. 13.23 Ectopic ureter in the vaginal vestibule in a female who presented with constant dribbling incontinence as well as normal voiding. (a) IVU shows right duplication with minimal upper pole function and down and out displacement of the lower pole — 'drooping lily' sign. (b) Ureteric catheter in ectopic ureter.

Rarer cases of ectopic ureters can be found at the level of the cervix or even the uterus. These vaginal, cervical and uterine cases presumable represent rupture of Gartner's duct into the ureterovaginal canal along their common wall.

Although today there is a rising incidence of ectopic ureters detected by antenatal maternal ultrasound, about one-half of females with ectopic ureters present with a classic history of continuous dribbling incontinence, in spite of what appears to be a normal voiding pattern [44–46]. If the associated ureter is very dilated, the child may be continent when recumbent and may present with daytime wetting only. A persistent foul-smelling vaginal discharge is another common presentation. If the orifice of the ectopic ureter is quite high and associated with significant obstruction or reflux, urinary tract infection is frequent. In the infant, obstruction may be severe enough to cause presentation with an abdominal mass formed by the dilated obstructed drainage system. Interestingly, there have been females with ectopic ureters at the level of the vestibule or distal urethra without incontinence. Presumably this is due to obstruction of the ureter as it traverses the sphincteric musculature with emptying only during voiding. This type of case may subsequently develop

incontinence after puberty or childbirth [47,48] and may be confused with stress-type urinary incontinence.

The diagnosis of an ectopic ureter in the female is often problematical. There is frequently non-visualization of the renal element. With duplications of the drainage system, there may be inference of the upper pole system by radiographic changes of the lower pole. Duplication with bilateral ectopic ureters is possible and the radiographic findings may be subtle (Fig. 13.24). If the ureter is single, the diagnosis may be even more difficult. The problem is compounded by the fact that the kidneys associated with ectopic single ureters may themselves be ectopic or even crossed and fused. Renal function may be so poor as to preclude visualization by either IVU or renal scanning. Ultrasound may be particularly useful in this situation. The ureters are usually dilated and can be traced behind the bladder. There are cases, however, where exploratory surgery, picking up the ureter first just above the bladder, will be required. Having found the ureter, it can be traced upward to its associated renal moiety.

As the function of renal tissue associated with ectopic ureters is frequently poor, the administration of indigo carmine or methylene blue intravenously in order to try to demonstrate the distal ureteric orifice is rarely successful. In order to ascertain that a suspected case of incontinence is truly due to an ectopic ureter, it is useful to fill the bladder with indigo carmine or methylene blue-stained saline via a Foley catheter and then observe the perineum closely. The continued slow drip of clear urine strongly suggests the presence of an ectopic ureteric orifice. Meticulous scrutiny of the area immediately around the

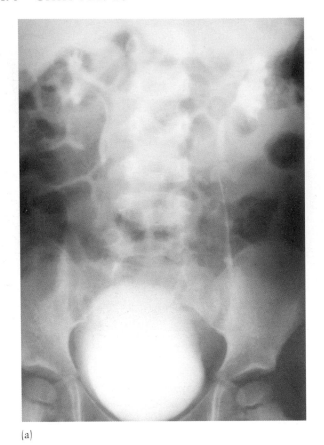

(a)

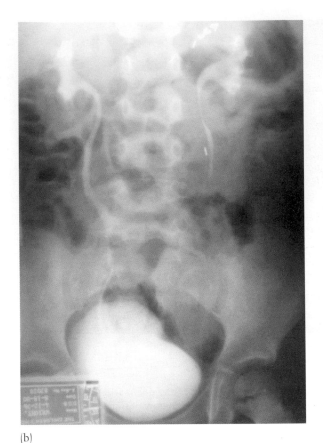

(b)

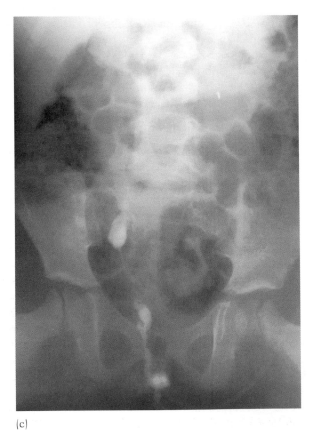

(c)

Fig. 13.24 Bilateral ectopic ureters in a female who presented with constant incontinence as well as normal voiding. (a) Initial IVU shows down and out displacement of the left kidney and lateral displacement of the ureter suggesting duplication with an ectopic ureter. The right kidney was not felt to be duplicated. Left upper pole partial nephrectomy did not correct the incontinence. (b) Follow-up IVU shows vertical access to the right kidney and mild tortuousity of the right ureter suggesting duplication with a second ectopic ureter. (c) Retrograde ureterogram of a vestibular ectopic right ureteric orifice confirms suspicion of bilateral duplication with ectopia by showing the upper pole ureter. The child was cured of incontinence by right upper pole partial nephrectomy.

urethral meatus and the distal vagina will frequently reveal a tiny dimple which can be probed and then subsequently retrogradely injected to demonstrate the ectopic ureter. Deeper in the vagina, the ectopic orifice may be found by vaginoscopy with the cystoscope.

Management

The surgical treatment of an ectopic ureter in the female depends on the quality of the associated renal parenchyma. In single system ureteric ectopia, nephroureterectomy is most commonly required. However, there are cases where function is adequate to justify a ureterovesical reimplantation of the ureter. When dealing with an ectopic ureter associated with the upper pole of a duplicated renal unit, a partial nephrectomy is the usual procedure. If function is good, a ureteropyelostomy or ureteroureterostomy to the lower pole drainage system may be justified.

In either single or duplex systems, the entire distal ureter need not always be removed. If the ectopic ureteral stump joins the bladder neck it may fill like a diverticulum during voiding and cause either post-void dribbling or serve as a reservoir for infection. Thus primary excision of such an ectopic stump should be considered. By maintaining dissection immediately on the wall of the ureter and using a catheter in the urethra the junction can be identified and sutured without any injury to the bladder neck. Only very rarely is a transtrigonal approach needed. If the troublesome ureteric stump is not very dilated its lining may be endoscopically cauterized with the bug-bee electrode leading to obliteration of the lumen. Ectopic ureteral stumps to the introitus or vagina rarely cause later problems and no primary treatment of them is recommended. Occasionally a vaginally ectopic ureter associated with a Gartner's duct cyst may become infected producing a purulent vaginal discharge. In such cases, marsupialization of the cyst into the vagina is usually effective in correcting the problem.

Ectopic ureter in the male

In the male, the orifice of an ectopic ureter may come to lie anywhere along the ectopic pathway that extends to the verumontanum and encompasses the mesonephric duct derivatives (epididymis, seminal vesicles and vas deferens) (see Fig. 13.22a). The most common location of the ectopic orifice is in the posterior urethra where approximately half the ectopic ureters in males will be found [43] (Fig. 13.25). About one-third of ectopic ureters enter the seminal vesicle [49,50]. The other possible locations are seen more rarely. The drainage of ectopic ureters into the male genital tract accounts for the association of epididymitis with ectopic ureters. This is the reason the prepubertal male with epididymitis should be investigated for an ectopic ureter.

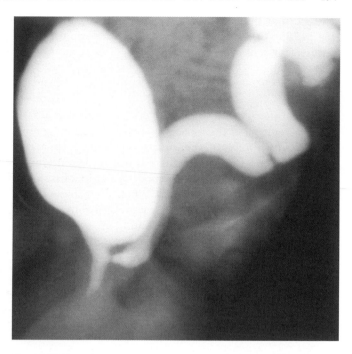

Fig. 13.25 Ectopic ureter to a posterior urethra in a male who presented as an infant with sepsis. A voiding cystourethrogram shows vesicoureteric reflux into a single ectopic ureter entering the posterior urethra from a solitary left kidney.

Interestingly, in some males, symptoms do not arise until the onset of sexual activity. There may then be seen prostatitis, seminal vesiculitis, epididymitis or a seminal vesicle cyst with infection which may produce pain on bowel motions or on rectal examination. Ectopic ureters which enter the posterior urethra do not produce incontinence because they are above the external sphincter, but may lead to symptoms of urgency and frequency from the constant drip of urine into the posterior urethra.

The diagnosis of an ectopic ureter in the male requires a high index of suspicion. An ectopic ureter entering the genital tract is often single and drains a non-functioning renal element [45,51]. Ultrasound may assist in locating the responsible renal element. When the ectopic ureter is from the upper pole of a duplicated renal drainage system, then the indirect signs of hydroureteronephrosis which have been described above will again apply. The most difficult diagnostic problems arise in duplicated kidneys with a tiny upper pole draining into a small minimally obstructed ectopic ureter. The diagnosis may be suggested by finding contralateral duplication. In MCU, only an approximately 15% of ectopic ureters in males show reflux [44]. As in the female, ectopic ureters at the level of the sphincters may exhibit the paradox of both obstruction and reflux.

At cystoscopy and examination under anaesthesia it may be possible to feel a mass in the area of the seminal vesicle or see elevation of the floor of the bladder in that area, which can at times mimic the appearance of a ureterocele (see p. 185). In the instance of a single ureteric ectopia, a hemitrigone will be noted.

Management

The treatment of ectopic ureters in males generally involves removal of the associated poorly functioning renal tissue. Only rarely is the function adequate to justify reimplantation of the ureter in a single ectopic ureter, or diversion to the lower pole pelvis or ureter in a case of an ectopic ureter with duplication. When the ectopic ureter enters the male genital ducts they are generally rendered unfit for the passage of sperm, and, in order to avoid recurrent epididymitis, it is wise to ligate the vas. This is less likely to endanger the contralateral genital ducts than an effort to remove all of the distal ureter or seminal vesicle cyst, if one is present. An occasional large seminal vesical cyst with reflux will need excision and this is best accomplished transtrigonally.

Bilateral single ectopic ureter

Bilateral single ectopic ureters continue to be a very rare entity with less than 50 reported in the literature. Because the bladder neck and trigonal musculature appear to be derived from the tissue of the common stem of the mesonephric duct below the point of origin of the ureteric bud, if the bud is very caudal in its origin there will be little or no formation of the bladder neck and trigone. Thus, characteristically with bilateral single ectopic ureters at the level of the urethra or more distal, there will be a poorly developed small bladder with absent trigone and poorly formed bladder neck. Females present with incontinence and are usually found to have the ectopic ureters located in the distal urethra. In general, they have poorer bladders and worse associated renal anomalies than males [52,53]. Males also present with incontinence. Enough urine may enter the bladder to permit some voiding to take place. As a result, the bladder in males is often slightly larger than in females.

It should be emphasized that this situation is seen only when bilateral single ectopic ureters are very distal in their location. Patients with bilateral single ectopic ureters ending at the bladder neck level may present with infection and upper urinary tract dilatation from obstruction or reflux, but have a better prognosis with respect to continence and bladder function.

The diagnosis may be possible by IVU and MCU. Often, however, the kidneys exhibit poor function and while the MCU may demonstrate a small bladder with no evidence of a bladder neck, it will not show the ureters if they are further down the ectopic pathway than the urethra. Ultrasound examination may be very useful. At cystoscopy,

a poorly defined funnel-shaped bladder neck associated with a small bladder is seen. Most often, the ureteric orifices in the male are observed in the distal bladder neck. In the female they may be occasionally difficult to locate.

Treatment of the incontinent child with bilateral single ectopic ureters constitutes a major surgical challenge. If there is adequate bladder capacity, reimplantation of the ureters and a Young–Dees–Leadbetter-type reconstruction of the bladder outlet may be possible [54–56]. If the bladder is not sufficient for this, it may be possible to construct a long detrusor tube of the entire bladder, as has been suggested by Arap [57], and augment this by a sigmoid cystoplasty with antirefluxing ureteric anastomoses to the colon segment. If a Young–Dees–Leadbetter bladder neck reconstruction does not work and the patient continues to be incontinent after bladder neck reconstruction and augmentation a Mitrofanoff [58] procedure with division of the urethra and the use of a catheterizable non-refluxing appendix may be required.

Non-refluxing primary obstructive megaureter

We are all agreed that megaureter means big ureter, but whether it is obstructed or not is an endless source of disagreement. The classification by Smith et al. [59] in 1977 has helped to define the problem of the megaureter (Table 13.1).

Pathophysiology

There is no single explanation for the pathophysiology of a non-refluxing megaureter. Light and electron microscopic studies offer differing suggestions as to the cause of the ureteric abnormality [60–62]. What is agreed is that the distal ureter just prior to its insertion into the bladder is relatively narrow and fails to allow normal bolus propagation to occur (Fig. 13.26). That segment of ureter, therefore, must be excised and the dilated proximal ureter reimplanted with or without a manoeuvre to diminish the ureteric calibre.

Table 13.1 International classification of megaureter.

	Primary	Secondary
Obstructed	Intrinsic ureteral obstruction	To urethral obstruction or extrinsic lesions
Reflux	Reflux is only abnormality	Associated with bladder outlet obstruction or neurogenic bladder
Non-refluxing, non-obstructed	Idiopathic ureteral dilatation	To polyuria (diabetes insipidus) or infection (?)

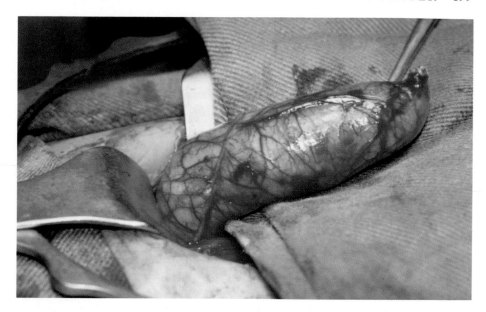

Fig. 13.26 A divided obstructive megaureter showing a grossly dilated ureter with a narrow terminal segment.

Presentation

The presentation of patients with megaureters has changed dramatically in the last 15 years. Before this, patients presented with the classic symptoms of a urinary infection due to urinary stasis and not infrequently the formation of a stone. There is a male:female preponderance of 5:1 with a higher incidence of involvement on the left side. Before the advent of antenatal maternal ultrasound nearly one-third of patients presented in the first year of life [63]. In 1992 Rickwood et al. [64] published a series of 38 patients with non-refluxing megaureters detected antenatally. A number of other reports have been published recently and will be discussed later (see p. 202).

Diagnosis

The investigations for prenatally diagnosed megaureters are similar to those for patients presenting with symptoms. An ultrasound examination is the initial investigation when the dilated ureter will be seen running behind the bladder and the degree of hydronephrosis associated with the megaureter can be assessed. The hydronephrotic kidney is in fact the first abnormality to be picked up on the antenatal ultrasound. Postnatally, a further ultrasound is undertaken on the second day of life to confirm the diagnosis. An MCU must be performed to exclude posterior urethral valves and/or reflux. There are a few patients who demonstrate both reflux and obstruction. They usually present postnatally with a urinary infection and suffer recurrent urinary infections in spite of antibiotic prophylaxis [65]. They require ureteric reimplantation. The cystogram in these patients is diagnostic because the contrast that refluxes into the ureter is very dilute as opposed to the contrast in the bladder. This occurs because of the dilution of the contrast by the column of urine trapped within the dilated ureter above the obstructive segment of ureter.

For those patients diagnosed antenatally, providing the patient has two kidneys, a normal cystogram and is otherwise well, further investigations are deferred until after the period of transitional nephrology at about 6 weeks of age. A dynamic isotope scan is then carried out using either [^{99m}Tc] diethylenetriamine penta-acetic acid (DTPA) or MAG$_3$. Individual kidney glomerular filtration rates (GFRs) can be calculated [66] and individual percentage kidney function can be assessed. The criteria for making the diagnosis of obstruction are based upon those defined by O'Reilly [67] in 1978. The Philadelphia group [66] has suggested that if renal function is normal based on the extraction factor and/or equal to the contralateral non-dilated renal unit, the dilatation seen does not represent a functionally significant obstructive uropathy. This non-operative approach has seen no deterioration in function or development of obstructive symptoms. An IVU is still used in many centres and we find that with an equivocal renogram the calyceal morphology, in particular the presence of calyceal crescents (Fig. 13.27a), is helpful in trying to establish the diagnosis of an obstructive megaureter.

There will remain a 'grey area' where the decision as to whether the kidneys are obstructed or not remains difficult. In this small group of patients the antegrade pressure–perfusion study or Whitaker test may be helpful [68] but modern imaging techniques, especially radio-isotopes, make this rarely necessary. In patients in whom

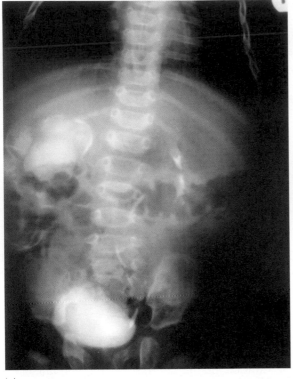

(a)

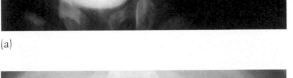

(b)

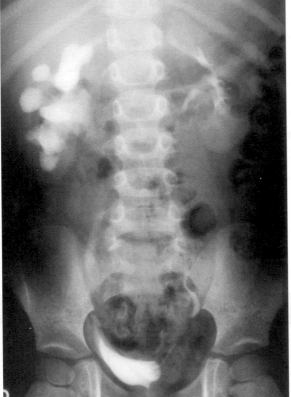

(c)

Fig. 13.27 Right obstructive megaureter in a 5-month-old baby who presented with a severe urinary tract infection. (a) IVU showing calyceal crescents in the right kidney and normal left kidney. (b) Grossly dilated right megaureter. (c) Follow-up urogram showing improvement following remodelling and reimplantation of the right ureter in association with a psoas hitch.

all the other tests are equivocal, the Whitaker pressure may also not be diagnostic. The presence of a negative test with a pressure below 16 cmH$_2$O at an appropriate perfusion rate would seem to exclude obstruction.

Management

Preliminary drainage

Rarely, a patient may present with a pyonephrosis secondary to an obstructed megaureter. There may or may not be an associated stone at the lower end of the ureter. An ultrasound will be diagnostic in this situation and, if the patient is sick and pyrexial, a percutaneous nephrostomy catheter should be inserted to drain the pus. A functional assessment of the kidney can be undertaken after 2–4 weeks and the decision then taken as to whether to proceed

to a nephrectomy or a ureteric reimplantation depending upon the function of that kidney. If the ureter is very large a low end ureterostomy can be performed, particularly in a sick infant, allowing the ureter to decompress before carrying out a reimplantation a few months later.

Non-operative management

Prenatal diagnosis makes the decision as to which patient requires an operation more difficult because these patients are asymptomatic, whereas the older child will present with significant urinary symptoms to make a decision easier. Management of a prenatally diagnosed obstructive uropathy, whether it is at the pelviureteric junction or the ureterovesical junction should initially be non-operative (Fig. 13.28). The paper by Koff and Campbell [69] showed how well patients do with conservative management of an

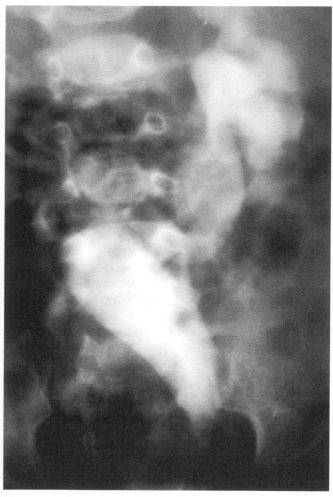

(a)

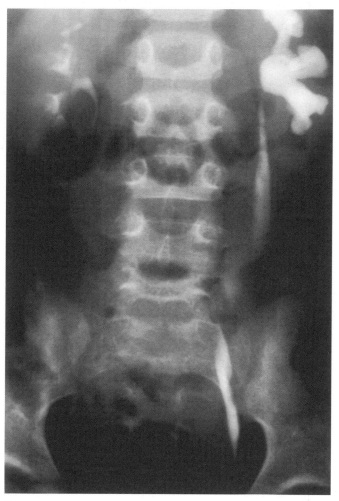

(b)

Fig. 13.28 Left megaureter non-operative management. (a) Initial urogram showing the left megaureter. The abnormality was first detected on a prenatal maternal ultrasound scan. An isotope scan showed good function of the left kidney. The baby was managed non-operatively. (b) A follow-up urogram 5 years later showing the left ureter and kidney returning to normal without surgical intervention.

apparent pelviureteric junction obstruction. Recently the paper by Baskin et al. [70] reported on 25 patients conservatively managed out of a total of 35 neonates with primary obstructed megaureters. Of these 25 patients, 17 were antenatally diagnosed and were followed-up for 7.5 years. One patient was lost to follow-up but all the other 16 patients had renal scans that showed the expected increase in GFR. No patient developed stones, pain or pylonephritis. The group from Great Ormond Street [71] reporting on 67 megaureters followed-up for 3.1 years found that 34% resolved spontaneously, 49% persisted and only 17% required a reimplantation. The reasons for reimplantation were break-through infections in three patients and deteriorating renal function in eight. Interestingly enough there was no difference prognostically between those megaureters diagnosed prenatally and those detected postnatally. They did, however, find a correlation between ureteric size and prognosis. The majority of megaureters less than 6 mm in diameter resolved while 50% of those greater than 10 mm underwent surgery. Sixty per cent of those patients with poor drainage on the [^{99m}Tc] DTPA scan required surgery although it must be emphasized that the very capacious nature of the ureter in these cases makes the diuretic phase of the renal scan the least reliable.

The absolute indications therefore for surgery are:
1 deteriorating renal function on a renal isotope scan;
2 recurrent symptomatic urinary infections in spite of chemoprophylaxis;
3 pyonephrosis or stones;
4 intermittent pain.
Relative indications are failure to drain on an isotope scan, using Lasix with moderate renal function, and urinary infection when chemoprophylaxis has been stopped.

Surgery

The operation required depends to an extent upon the age of the patient and therefore the bladder capacity and the width of the ureter. The aim of surgery is to excise the distal obstructive ureteral segment to produce an unobstructive ureter which does not reflux, as safely as possible. The surgical options as follows.

Mild to moderate dilatation

1 Reimplantation of the ureter using the Ahmed [72], Politano–Leadbetter [73] or Cohen [74] techniques.
2 Ureteral folding and reimplantation — Kalicinski technique [75].
3 Plication and reimplantation — Starr technique [76].

Grossly dilated ureters (unilateral)

1 Hendren remodel and reimplantation technique [77,78].

2 Psoas hitch with reimplantation ± Hendren remodel (see Fig. 13.27).

Grossly dilated ureters (bilateral)

Transuretero-ureterostomy, psoas hitch and long remodel reimplantation.

Moderately dilated ureters may not require any remodelling. This is unusual because the majority of these patients do not come to surgery, but, if they do, a Cohen [74] reimplantation or the modification described by Ahmed [72] may be used, always excising the narrowed aperistaltic segment. One is trying to achieve a ratio of reimplantation tunnel to ureteric diameter of 4–5:1 to achieve reflux prevention. The more dilated ureter requires the Starr [76] or Kalicinski [75] folding techniques which avoid having to excise part of the ureter with the associated risk to the blood supply or the risk of a urinary leak postoperatively. For the very wide ureters, however, this technique leaves a large sausage-shaped mass to be reimplanted submucosally which is unsatisfactory. For these larger ureters some form of excisional tapering technique is required. This has been well described by Hendren [77], but the important features are that the ureter should not be narrowed too much and the blood supply must not be jeopardized. There is nothing worse than trying to salvage a ureter which has been previously reimplanted and has then stenosed from ischaemia. It is always better to err on the side of leaving the ureter slightly too wide and risk reflux than narrow the ureter too much and risk stenosis. For the very wide ureter it is safest to reimplant it into a bladder which has been hitched on the psoas muscle so that a long tunnel can be obtained leaving a relatively wide ureteric diameter. In the patient with bilateral gross obstructive megaureters, a transuretero-ureterostomy with a psoas hitch and single ureteric reimplantation is a useful technique to avoid major complications [78]. The length of ureter that requires remodelling need only be slightly longer than the length of ureter required to be placed in the submucosal tunnel. Almost never do both the upper and lower ureter require remodelling, as described originally by Hendren [78]. It is always best to remodel and reimplant the lower ureter first because the vast majority of kidneys and upper ureters will improve once the obstruction has been relieved.

Any patient who has a ureteric tailoring should have the ureter stented and a bladder catheter left in situ for 8–9 days.

Follow-up

The patient should remain on antibiotic prophylaxis until a follow-up cystogram at 3–6 months after surgery demonstrates no reflux. The upper tracts can be followed using ultrasound and/or isotope renal scans. If at 3 months everything appears satisfactory antibiotics can be stopped and the patient followed with an intermittent ultrasound.

References

1 Meyer R. Anatomie und Entwicklungsgeschickte der Ureterverdoppelung. *Virchows Arch [A]* 1907;**187**:408–34.

2 Weigert C. Ueber einige Bildungsfehler der Ureteren. *Virchows Arch [A]* 1877;**70**:490–501.

3 Chwalla R. The process of formation of cystic dilatations of the vesical end of the ureter and of diverticula at the ureteral ostium. *Urol Cutan Rev* 1927;**31**:499–504.

4 Stephens FD. *Congenital Malformations of the Rectum, Anus and Genitourinary Tracts*. London: E & S Livingstone, 1963:178–95.

5 Stephens FD. Caecoureterocele and concepts on the embryology and aetiology of ureteroceles. *Aust NZ J Surg* 1971;**40**:239–47.

6 Tanagho EA. Embryologic basis for lower ureteral anomalies: a hypothesis. *Urology* 1976;**7**:451–64.

7 Tanagho EA. Ureteroceles: embryogenesis, pathologenesis and management. *JCE Urol* 1979;**18**:13–37.

8 Mackie GG, Stephens FD. Duplex kidneys: a correlation of renal dysplasia with position of the ureteral orifice. *J Urol* 1975;**114**:274–80.

9 Campbell MF. Anomalies of the ureter. In: Campbell MF, Harrison JH eds. *Urology*, 3rd edn. Philadelphia: Saunders Co. 1970:1487–1542.

10 Nation EF. Duplication of the kidney and ureter: a statistical study of 230 new cases. *J Urol* 1944;**51**:456–65.

11 Cohen N, Berant M. Duplications of the renal collecting system in the hereditary osteo-onychodysplasis syndrome. *J Pediatr* 1976;**89**:261–3.

12 Whitaker J, Danks DM. A study of the inheritance of duplication of the kidneys and ureters. *J Urol* 1966;**95**:176–8.

13 Atwell JD, Cook PL, Howell CJ et al. Familial incidence of bifid and double ureters. *Arch Dis Child* 1974;**49**:390–3.

14 Privett JTJ, Jeans WD, Roylands J. The incidence and importance of renal duplication. *Clin Radiol* 1976;**27**:521–30.

15 Kretschmer HL. Hydronephrosis in infancy and childhood: clinical data and a report of 101 cases. *Surg Gynaecol Obstet* 1937;**64**:634–45.

16 Albers DD, Geyer JR, Barnes SD. Clinical significance of blind-ending branch of bifid ureter: report of 3 additional cases. *J Urol* 1971;**105**:634–7.

17 Schultze R. Der Blind endende Doppelureter. *Z Urol Nephrol* 1967;**4**:271–89.

18 Klauber GT, Reid EC. Inverted Y reduplication of the ureter. *J Urol* 1972;**107**:362–4.

19 Perkins PJ, Kroovand RL, Evans AT. Ureteral triplication. *Radiology* 1973;**108**:533–8.

20 Livaditis A, Maurseth K, Skog PA. Unilateral triplication of the ureter and renal pelvis: report of a case. *Acta Chir Scand* 1964;**127**:181–4.

21 Ericsson NO. Ectopic ureterocele in infants and children. *Acta Chir Scand Suppl* 1954;**197**:1–93.

22 Gill B. Ureteric ectopy in children. *Br J Urol* 1980;**52**:257–61.

23 Glassberg KI, Braren V, Duckett JW et al. Suggested termino-logy for duplex systems, ectopic ureters and ureteroceles. *J Urol* 1984;**132**:1153–4.

24 Campbell M. Ureterocele: a study of 94 instances in 80 infants and children. *Surg Gynecol Obstet* 1951;**93**:705–8.

25 Uson AC, Lattimer JK, Melicow MM. Ureteroceles in infants and children: a report based on 44 cases. *Pediatrics* 1961;**27**:971–83.

26 Mandell J, Colodny AH, Lebowitz R, Bauer SB, Retik AB. Ureteroceles in infants and children. *J Urol* 1980;**123**:921–6.

27 Blyth B, Passerini-Glazel G, Camuffo C, Snyder HM III, Duckett J. Endoscopic incision of ureteroceles: intravesical versus ectopic. *J Urol* 1993;**149**:556–60.

28 Lee LD, Rickwood AMK, Williams MPL, Anderson PAM. Experience with duplex system anomalies detected by prenatal ultrasonography. *J Urol* 1993;**149**:808–10.

29 Leadbetter GW Jr. Ectopic ureterocele as a cause of urinary incontinence. *J Urol* 1970;**103**:222–6.

30 Athey PA, Carpenter RJ, Hadlock FP, Hedrick TD. Ultrasonic demonstration of ectopic ureterocele. *Pediatrics* 1983;**71**:568–71.

31 Summer TE, Crowe JE, Resnick MI. Diagnosis of ectopic ureterocele using ultrasound. *Urology* 1980;**15**:82–5.

32 Sen S, Beasley SW, Ahmed S, Durham Smith E. Renal function and vesicoureteric reflux in children with ureteroceles. *Pediatr Surg Int* 1992;**7**:192–4.

33 Snyder HM, Johnston JH. Orthotopic ureteroceles in children. *J Urol* 1978;**119**:543–6.

34 Stephens DF. Congenital malformations of the urinary tract. *Praeger Sci* 1983;**200**–5.

35 Hendren WH, Monfort GK. Surgical correction of ureteroceles in childhood. *J Pediatr Surg* 1971;**6**:235–44.

36 King LR, Kozlowski JM, Schacht MJ. Ureteroceles in children: simplified and successful approach to management. *J Am Med Assoc* 1983;**249**:1461–5.

37 Cendron J, Melin Y, Valayer J. Simplified treatment of ectopic ureteroceles in 35 children. *Eur Urol* 1981;**7**:321–3.

38 Caldamone A, Snyder HM, Duckett JW. Ureteroceles in children: follow up management with upper tract approach. *J Urol* 1984;**131**:1130–2.

39 Prewett JTL, Jeans WD, Roylance J. The incidence and importance of renal duplication. *Clin Pediatr* 1976;**27**:521.

40 Tank ES Jr. Unroofing of ureteroceles. *Soc Pediatr Urol Newsl* 1980;**4**:30.

41 Bauer SB, Retik AB. The non-obstructive ectopic ureterocele. *J Urol* 1978;**119**:804–7.

42 Schulman CC. The single ectopic ureter. *Eur Urol* 1976;**2**:64–9.

43 Ellerker AG. The extravesical ectopic ureter. *Br J Surg* 1958;**45**:64–9.

44 Malek RS, Kelalis PP, Stickler GB, Burke EC. Observations on ureteral ectopy in children. *J Urol* 1972;**107**:308–13.

45 Rognon L, Brueziere J, Soret JY et al. Abouchement ectopique de l'uretere dans le tractus seminal: a propos de 10 cas. *Chirurgie* 1973;**99**:741–8.

46 Schulman CC. Les implantations ectopiques de l'uretere. *Acta Urol Belg* 1972;**40**:201–478.

47 Davis DM. Urethral ectopic ureter in the female without incontinence. *J Urol* 1930;**23**:463–76.

48 Childlow JH, Utz DC. Ureteral ectopia in vestibule of vagina with urinary continence. *South Med J* 1970;**63**:423–5.

49 Gordon HL, Kessler R. Ectopic ureter entering the seminal

vesicle associated with renal dysplasia. *J Urol* 1972;**108**: 389–91.

50 Seitzman DM, Patton JF. Ureteral ectopia: combined ureteral and vas deferens anomaly. *J Urol* 1960;**84**:604–8.

51 Cendron J, Bonhomme C. Uretere a terminasion ectopique extravesicale chez des sujets de sexe masculin (a propos de 10 cas). *J Urol Nephrol* 1968;**74**:31–50.

52 Williams DI, Lightwood RG. Bilateral single ectopic ureters. *Br J Urol* 1972;**44**:267–72.

53 Cox CE, Hutch JA. Bilateral single ectopic ureter: a report of 2 cases and review of the literature. *J Urol* 1966;**95**: 493–7.

54 Young HH. An operation for the cure of incontinence associated with epispadias. *J Urol* 1922;**7**:1–32.

55 Dees JE. Congenital epispadias with incontinence. *J Urol* 1949;**62**:513–22.

56 Leadbetter GW. Surgical correction of total urinary incontinence. *J Urol* 1964;**91**:261–6.

57 Arap S, Giron AM, Goes GM. Initial results of the complete reconstruction of bladder exstrophy. *Urol Clin North Am* 1980;**7**:477–91.

58 Mitrofanoff P. Cystostomie continente trans-appendiculaire dans le traitement des cessies neurologiques. *Chir Pediatr* 1980;**21**:297–305.

59 Smith ED, Cussen LJ, Glenn J *et al.* Report of working party to establish an international nomenclature for the large ureter. *Birth Defects* 1977;**13**:3–8.

60 Marnaghan GF. Experimental investigation of the dynamics of the normal and dilated ureter. *Br J Urol* 1957;**29**:403–9.

61 MacKinnon KJ, Foote JW, Wiggleworth FW, Blennerhassett JB. Pathology of adynamic distal ureteral seqment. *J Urol* 1970;**103**:134–7.

62 Notley RG. The musculature of the human ureter. *Br J Urol* 1970;**42**:724–7.

63 Williams DI, Hulme-Moir I. Primary obstructive megaureter. *Br J Urol* 1970;**42**:140–3.

64 Rickwood AMK, Lee JD, Williams MPL, Anderson PAM. Natural history of obstructed and pseudo-obstructed megaureters detected by prenatal ultrasonography. *Br J Urol* 1992;**70**:322–5.

65 Whitaker RH, Flower CRR. Ureters that show both reflux and obstruction. *Br J Urol* 1979;**51**:471–4.

66 Keating MA, Escala J, Snyder HMcC III, Heyman S, Duckett JW. Changing concepts in management of primary obstructive megaureter. *J Urol* 1989;**142**(2):636–40.

67 O'Reilly PH, Tester HJ, Lawson RS, Farrar DJ, Charlton-Edwards E. Diuresis renography in equivocal urinary tract obstruction. *Br J Urol* 1978;**50**:76–80.

68 Whitaker RH. The Whitaker test. *Urol Clin North Am* 1979;**6**:529–39.

69 Koff SA, Campbell K. Non operative management of unilateral neonatal hydronephrosis. *J Urol* 1992;**148**:525–31.

70 Baskin LS, Zderic S, Snyder H, Duckett JW. Primary dilated megaureter. Long term follow up [Abstract]. In: *American Academy of Paediatrics Annual Meeting*, 1993:69–70.

71 Liu A, Dillon HK, Young CK, Duffy PG, Ransley PG. Prognosis and management of primary megaureters detected in the newborn period [Abstract]. *American Academy of Paediatrics Annual Meeting*, 1993:67–8.

72 Ahmed S. Transverse advancement ureteral reimplantation: pullthrough alternative in megaureter. *J Urol* 1980;**123**: 218–20.

73 Politano VA, Leadbetter WF. An operative technique for the correction of vericoureteral reflux. *J Urol* 1958;**79**: 932–41.

74 Cohen SJ. Ureterozystoneostomie: ein neue antiveflux technik. *Urologie* 1975;**6**:1–6.

75 Kalicinski ZH, Sansy K, Kitarbinska B, Joszt W. Surgery of megaureters — modification of Hendren's operation. *J Pediatr Surg* 1977;**12**:183–8.

76 Starr A. Ureteral plication. A new concept in ureteral tailoring for megaureter. *Invest Urol* 1979;**17**:153.

77 Hendren WH. Operative repair of megaureter in children. *J Urol* 1969;**101**:491–5.

78 Hendren WH. Reoperative ureteral reimplantation. Management of the difficult case. *J Pediatr Surg* 1980;**15**:770–86.

14 Congenital Disorders of the Bladder and the Urethra

P.D.E.Mouriquand

Epispadias, bladder exstrophy and cloacal exstrophy

Definition and embryology

Epispadias, bladder exstrophy and cloacal exstrophy are developmental abnormalities of increasing severity, resulting from the interruption of the caudal delimitation of the embryo. The delimitation is the processus allowing the 3D rolling-up of the embryonic layers (ectoderm, mesoderm, entoderm), leading to the tubularization of the embryo (germinal disc) [1] (Figs 14.1 and 14.2). This phenomenon, which occurs during the first 2 months of gestation, is both transversal and longitudinal. It allows the formation and the anterior junction of the two pelvic bones, the cavitation of the pelvic organs, the partitioning of the pelvic cavity and separate connections to the pelvic floor of the anorectal, uterovaginal and vesicourethral conduits.

The cloacal membrane is a bilaminar layer (ectoderm and entoderm) situated at the caudal end of the germinal disc, which occupies the infra-umbilical abdominal wall. Mesenchymal ingrowth [2] between the ectodermal and entodermal layers results in formation of the lower abdominal muscles and the pelvic bones [3]. During the development of the urorectal septum the cloacal membrane undergoes a reverse rotation so that the ectodermal surface is no longer directed towards the developing anterior abdominal wall but gradually comes to face caudally and slightly posteriorly. This change facilitates the partitioning of the cloaca and it is brought about mainly by the development of the infra-umbilical portion of the anterior abdominal wall, and by the retrogression of the tail. The mesoderm that passes round the cloacal membrane to the caudal attachment of the umbilical cord undergoes further proliferation and growth so forming a surface elevation, the

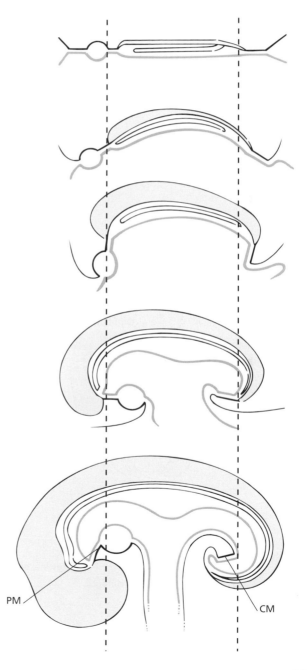

Fig. 14.1 Kinetic of the process of longitudinal delimitation of the human embryo [1]. CM, cloacal membrane; PM, pharyngeal membrane.

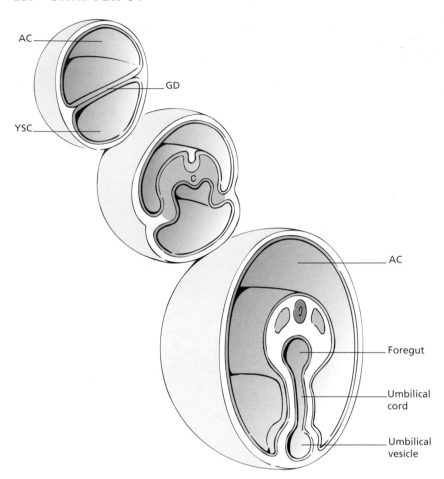

Fig. 14.2 Kinetic of the process of transversal delimitation of the human embryo [1]. AC, amniotic cavity; GD, germinal disc; YSC, yolk sac cavity.

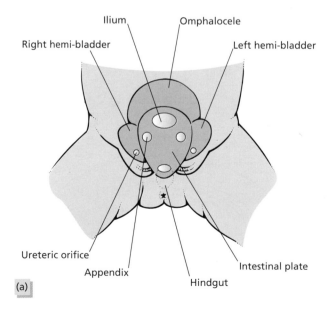

(a)

Fig. 14.3 Cloacal exstrophy [5].

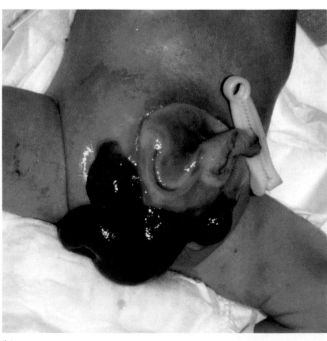

(b)

genital tubercle. The further growth of this part of the abdominal wall progressively separates the attachment of the umbilical cord from the genital tubercle [4]. When the caudal delimitation is aborted, the mesenchymal ingrowth between the ectodermal and entodermal layers fails to progress and the overstretched cloacal membrane becomes fragile and subject to a premature rupture leading to exstrophy (or non-cavitation) of the pelvic organs. Delimitation progresses from the cephalic to the caudal extremity, and from the dorsum to the ventrum of the embryo.

When the caudal delimitation halts at an early stage of gestation (cloacal exstrophy) (Fig. 14.3), all pelvic organs appear as contiguous and often duplicated plates. When it occurs later, the bowel tract is formed, the anus brought out to the pelvic floor although antepositioned, and both

the bladder and the urethra are exstrophied (bladder exstrophy) (Fig. 14.4), and when it occurs at the end of the processus of delimitation, only the urethra is exstrophied (epispadias) (Fig. 14.5a,b). This 'zip down' processus explains the progressive closure of the pelvis and the cavitation of the pelvic organs from the back to the front of the embryo and from the top to the bottom.

It appears that the middle period of the cloacal delimitation is more vulnerable than the early and late stages. This would explain why bladder exstrophy (60% of the patients born with these abnormalities) [6] is more frequent than cloacal exstrophy (10%) and epispadias (30%). Other theories explaining the cause of these abnormalities have been published. Patton and Barry [7] and Ambrose and O'Brien [8] have postulated an abnormal caudal development of the genital hillocks with fusion in

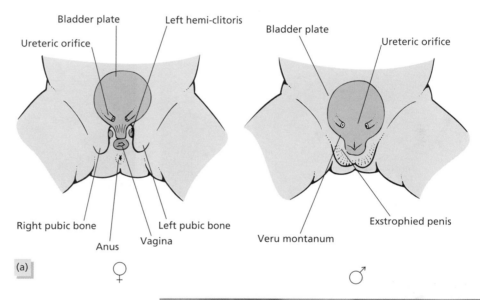

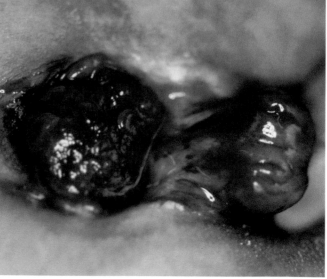

Fig. 14.4 Bladder exstrophy [5].

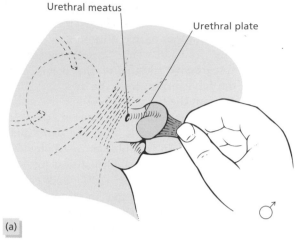

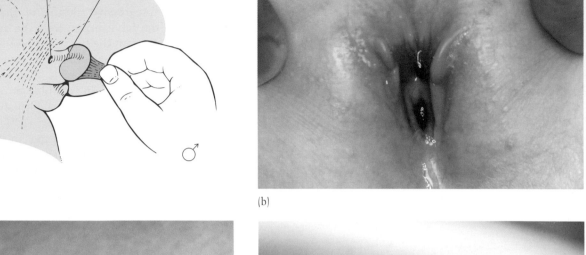

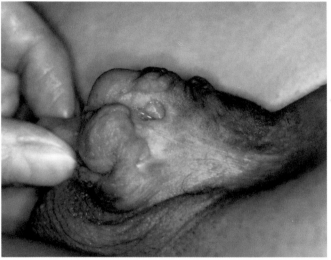

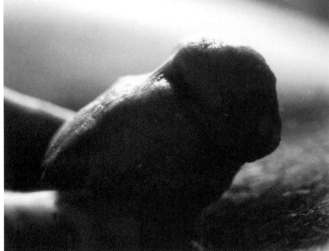

Fig. 14.5 (a) Epispasdiac penis [5]. (b) Female epispadias. (c) Cripple male epispadias. (d) Dorsal aspect of the penis after 40 mg of papaverine (same patient as (c)).

the midline below rather than above the cloacal membrane. Thomalla *et al.* [9] raised the possibility of a local infarction of the cloacal membrane. Mildenberger *et al.* [10] have suggested that there is an abnormal caudal insertion of the body stalk (mesoderm). The common association of cloacal exstrophy with vertebral (48–80%) [11,12] and neurological anomalies (29–75%) [11,13,14] suggests that these complex abnormalities may arise at an even earlier stage of embryogenesis and could represent some sort of failed duplication of the caudal extremity of the embryo.

Incidence and inheritance

The incidence of bladder exstrophy is between 1:10 000 [15] and 1:50 000 [16,17]. A 5:1 to 6:1 ratio of male:female exstrophy births is reported [18,19]. The incidence of epispadias is 1:117 000 births [20] with a 5:1 ratio of male:female epispadias. The incidence of cloacal exstrophy is 1:250 000 live births [13]. The risk of recurrence of bladder exstrophy in a given family is approximately 1:100 [18]. Shapiro *et al.* [21] determined that the risk of bladder exstrophy in the offspring of individuals with bladder exstrophy and epispadias is 1:70 live births, a 500-fold greater incidence than in the general population.

Anatomy (Figs 14.3–14.5a,b)

Pelvic wall anomalies

The non-closure of the pelvic ring is one of the main characteristics of these abnormalities. The outward rotation, the horizontalization and lateral displacement of the innominate bones and the pubic rami explain the large pubic gap, the divergence of the rectus muscles on each side of the vesical plate, the increased distance between the hips, the waddling gait and the outward rotation of the lower limbs. The triangular defect caused by the premature rupture of the abnormal cloacal membrane is occupied by an open bladder. In cases of cloacal exstrophy, the exstrophied caecum sits between the two hemibladders and an omphalocele is commonly associated. The fascial defect is limited inferiorly by the intersymphyseal band, which represents the divergent urogenital diaphragm. Inguinal hernias are very frequent (65%), especially in male patients in whom the risk of strangulation is greater than in girls [22]. The perineum is short, broad and tilted anteriorly. The puborectal sling is spread open anteriorly explaining the frequent anal prolapse seen when the child strains.

Urinary defects

The vesical plate is usually smooth at birth and the two ureteric orifices are usually easily identified as small nipples. If the bladder is not closed soon after birth or if it is not covered and humidified properly (using clingfilm and damp swabs), the mucosal surface changes quickly and becomes metaplasic, inflamed or infected, with pseudo-polyps and ulcers. This is one of the reasons why early bladder closure has often been advocated. After a few days, the characteristics of the bladder wall change quite dramatically [23] and the bladder becomes fibrotic and inelastic, and functional closure may become difficult or impossible. The size of the bladder plate varies a lot but is never normal and can be as small as the trigonal surface making bladder closure almost impossible without augmentation.

Islets of ectopic bowel mucosa are often found in bladder biopsies. It seems that the function and the presence of muscarinic cholinergic receptors are normal in exstrophic bladders after closure [24]. In cases of cloacal exstrophy, the bladder is split into two parts, each of them receiving the corresponding ureter. The two hemibladders are separated by an intestinal plate which represents the exstrophic caecum. The orifices of the terminal ileum, rudimentary hindgut and a single (or paired) appendix are apparent on the surface of the everted caecum. The hindgut (or tailgut) is blind-ending, and the ileum may be prolapsed. The autonomic innervation to the hemibladders and corporal bodies arises from a pelvic plexus on the anterior surface of the rectum and also from a sacral pelvic plexus [25].

The upper tract is usually normal although multiple associated anomalies have been described, especially in cloacal exstrophy, such as pelvic kidneys (23–31%) [11,26], renal agenesis (11–33%) [26,27], and dilated pelvis and ureters (33%) [27]. Multicystic dysplastic kidneys, horseshoe kidneys, abnormal aorta and iliac arteries [28] and fusion anomalies are seen less frequently. Ectopic ureters draining into the vasa in the male and into the uterus, vagina or fallopian tubes in the female, are also reported [13]. Ureteric reflux is almost constant and distal ureteric dilatation due to meatal obstruction is occasionally noticed [3]. The epispadiac urethra is represented by a short and wide mucosal strip extending from the bladder to the dorsal aspect of the glans or to the vaginal orifice. The sphincteric structures, although poorly developed, can be identified near the site of the bladder neck [5].

Genital defects

In the male

The epispadiac penis appears foreshortened because of the wide separation of the corporal insertions [29,30]. The displacement of each hemipelvis leads to a malrotation of each corpus, explaining the dorsal curvature of the erected penis (Fig. 14.5c,d). The flaccid epispadiac penis cannot dangle. The erection mechanisms are preserved but sexual intercourse is rendered impossible by the size and shape of the erected penis. The dorsum of the penis is covered by the urethral plate which is wide and tethered on to the underlying corpora. The hooded foreskin is only represented ventrally, although a complete foreskin may be seen in epispadiac penis. The corpus spongiosum is vestigial and sits under the urethral plate between the two corpora cavernosum.

In the exstrophic penis, the dorsal neurovascular pedicle is replaced by two neurovascular bundles which run on the external aspect of each corpus, witness of their malrotation [31]. No vascular anastomosis exists between the epispadiac corpora. The verumontanum and the seminal tracts are normal [32], provided they are not injured iatrogenically. Retrograde ejaculation may occur following bladder closure, because the proximal sphincteric mechanisms are in essence defective. The prostatic glands are only represented behind the proximal urethral plate. The testicles are normal although frequently located near the pubic tubercles, above the corresponding scrotum which usually appears wide. Duplicated urethra and penis have been reported [33].

In cases of cloacal exstrophy, the phallus is separated into the right and left halves with the adjacent labium or scrotal half. In isolated epispadias, two forms of increasing severity may be distinguished: (i) the distal epispadias where continence is preserved but where a dorsal chordee is almost always present, requiring a complete penile reconstruction (Fig. 14.9, p. 216–18); and (ii) the proximal epispadias where incontinence is constant, implying a complete penile reconstruction and a bladder neck reconstruction (Fig. 14.11, p. 220).

In the female

The clitoris is bifid. The urethral plate and the vagina are short. The vaginal orifice is often stenotic and displaced anteriorly. A hairless area separates the two hemimons pubis. The labia are divergent. The uterus, fallopian tubes and ovaries are normal except for occasional uterine duplication. The defective pelvic floor may predispose mature females to uterine prolapse development. Uterine prolapses are less frequent when osteotomy and closure of the anterior defect are performed early in life [3].

Anorectal defects

The anal sphincter mechanism is anteriorly displaced. The divergent levator ani and puborectalis muscles and the distorted anatomy of the external sphincter contribute to varying degrees of anal incontinence and rectal prolapse. Prolapse virtually always disappears after bladder closure [3].

Exstrophy variants

A spectrum of anomalies has been described [34] under the term 'split symphysis variants'. These variants are 10 times rarer than the classic bladder exstrophy [5] and more frequent in female babies.

Pseudoexstrophy is characterized by isolated parietal anomalies with a normal urinary tract [6]. In the superior vesical fissure variant, only the upper part of the bladder is exstrophied; the lower part of the bladder, the bladder neck and the urethra are intact.

The inferior vesical fissure variant, 'duplicate exstrophy' (where a small subumbilical vesical plate is found near a normal lower urinary tract) [2,35,36], exstrophy of a duplicated bladder [5,34,37–40] and the ectopic duplicated bladder are other variants of 'failed' exstrophy.

The variants of cloacal exstrophy are even more complex [41–43] and an attempt to classify them has been proposed by Manzoni and others [11,44,45].

Diagnosis

Antenatal diagnosis

Ultrasound showing the absence of bladder filling, along with a low-set umbilicus, are highly suggestive of bladder exstrophy [46–48]. However, bilateral ectopic ureters could provide very similar ultrasonic images. Langer *et al.* [49] published one case of cloacal exstrophy in which a prenatal diagnosis was made at 17 weeks, prior to rupture of the cloacal membrane seen at 26 weeks. No reports of the biochemistry of the amniotic fluid in these patients have been published to date.

Postnatal diagnosis

This is obvious and should lead to the immediate transfer of the child to a paediatric urological unit.

Management

Management at birth

When the umbilical cord is divided, heavy clamps that can scrape and scuff the exposed normal transitional epithelium should be avoided. Sutures should be used to tie the cord, and the stump prevented from lying on the bladder. The bladder plate should be covered by wet swabs and the baby should be wrapped with clingfilm which will avoid drying and excoriation of the bladder surface. Stimulation of the bladder by foreign material causes detrusor contraction, pain, tenesmus and unnecessary straining that can promote rectal prolapse [50]. A complete clinical examination of the child is required to define the anatomical defects. An ultrasound scan defines whether or not upper urinary tract anomalies and myelomeningoceles are associated.

A staged surgical reconstruction of these abnormalities has been advocated by most paediatric urologists [51,52]. The first stage is the closure of the exstrophied bladder, the second is the bladder neck reconstruction and the third is the epispadias repair. The schedule and order of these three steps vary with the surgeon but it is commonly accepted that bladder closure should be performed soon after birth to avoid mucosal damage of the bladder. The reconstruction of the bladder neck is performed, by some, between 3 and 5 years of age, followed 1 year later by the urethroplasty. Other paediatric urologists prefer to perform the urethral and penile reconstruction prior to the bladder neck reconstruction, to increase the bladder outlet resistance and let the bladder capacity increase before repairing the bladder neck. In older children, these steps can be combined.

Bladder closure and pelvic osteotomy

The primary objective in closure of the bladder exstrophy, in the hours following birth, is to convert the exstrophy to a complete epispadias with incontinence while preserving renal function. Concomitant pelvic osteotomy is performed by most surgeons for three main reasons.
1 Reapproximation of the symphysis diminishes the tension on the abdominal closure and eliminates the need for fascial flaps.
2 Placement of the urethra within the pelvic ring reduces the excessive urethrovesical angle.
3 Reapproximation of the urogenital diaphragm and approximation of the levator ani may aid in eventual urinary control [53,54].

The majority of patients referred to the Johns Hopkins Hospital following partial or complete dehiscence have not undergone a prior osteotomy [55]. However, bladder closure is possible without pelvic osteotomy during the first 24 h of life and, for some urologists, during the first 72 h of life [3]. Everyone would agree that from the orthopaedic viewpoint,

pelvic osteotomies are not necessary in exstrophy patients.

There are four main types of osteotomy.

1 The posterior bilateral iliac osteotomy [56,57] (Fig. 14.6a) does not provide a very good mobility of the pubis, it may result in occasional delayed or malunion of the ilium, and, most importantly, it involves the need to turn the patient

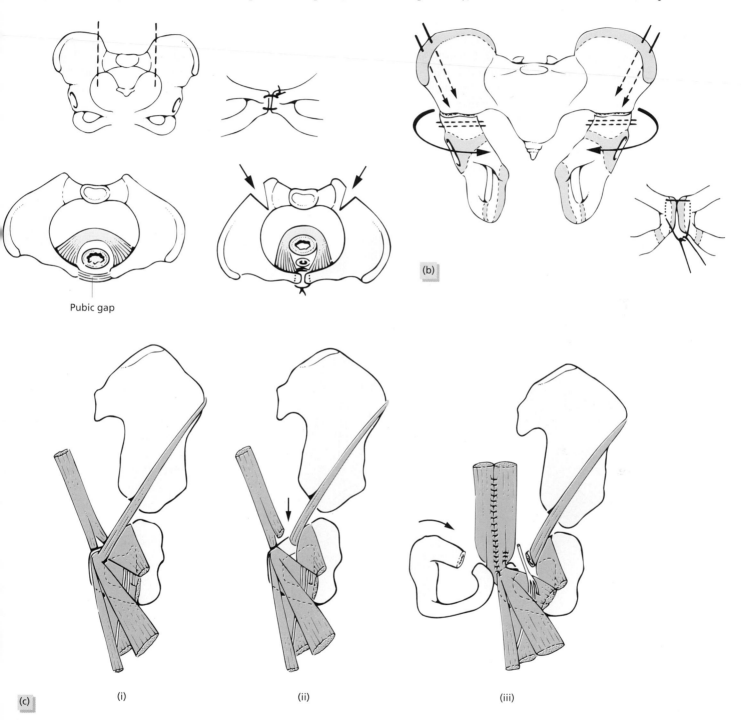

Pubic gap

(b)

(c)   (i)   (ii)   (iii)

Fig. 14.6 (a) Posterior bilateral iliac osteotomy [5]. (b) Bilateral transverse innominate osteotomy [60]. (c) Anterior pelvic osteotomy of the superior ramus of the pubic bone [61].

intraoperatively from the prone to the supine position [3].

2 The bilateral transverse innominate osteotomy [58–60], (Fig. 14.6b) offers a better mobility of the two bones, but still requires the change of position of the child during the procedure.

3 The anterior pelvic osteotomy of the superior ramus of the pubic bone [61–63] (Fig. 14.6c).

4 Anterior diagonal mid-innominate osteotomy [64,65], recently described, seems to offer an excellent mobilization of the bones, without extra incisions. It can be performed after bladder closure and is less time consuming.

Bladder closure (Fig. 14.7) starts by dissecting the peritoneum off the bladder plate whilst preserving the vascular pedicles. The edge of the rectus fascia is a reliable landmark which leads to the pubic insertion of the remnants of the urogenital diaphragm. Some paediatric urologists divide the urethral plate distally to the verumontanum, allowing the proximal urethra, prostate and bladder neck to separate from the corpora cavernosa. These structures are then moved downward behind the symphysis, allowing the relocation of the bladder deeper in the pelvis. After lengthening of the penis, the gap between the posterior urethra and the penile urethra is bridged by two paraexstrophic skin flaps [66]. Paraexstrophic flaps can be used in girls [5,67] for lengthening the urethra. Other paediatric urologists do not divide the urethral plate and do not use paraexstrophic flaps, in order to avoid the interposition of cutaneous tissues between the proximal urethra (and the genital ducts behind it) and the penile urethra which may cause late problems of stricture after epispadias reconstruction [68]. It is also uncertain whether or not the division of the urethral plate gives any extra length to the exstrophic penis.

Reconstruction of the umbilicus has cosmetic and functional value. Its greatest use may lie in concealment of a continent catheterizable stoma [69–71].

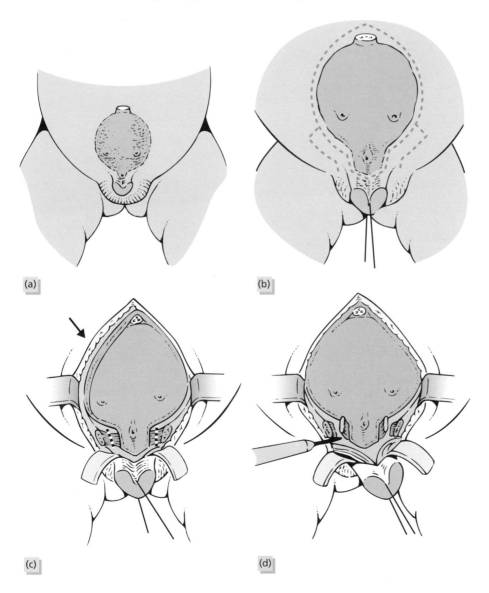

Fig. 14.7 Bladder closure: the traditional technique [5]. (a) The exstrophied bladder after excision of the umbilical cord. (b) Classic incision following the bladder plate and delineation of the paraexstrophic flaps. (c) The dissection follows the medial edge of each rectus fascia and the peritoneum is dissected off the bladder plate (arrow). (d) Division of the interpubic band of fibrous tissue.

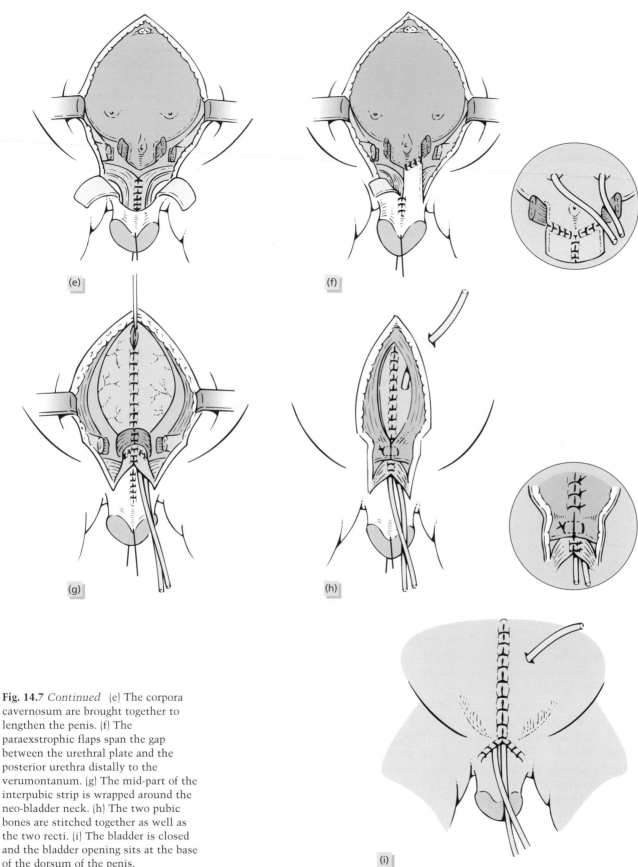

Fig. 14.7 *Continued* (e) The corpora cavernosum are brought together to lengthen the penis. (f) The paraexstrophic flaps span the gap between the urethral plate and the posterior urethra distally to the verumontanum. (g) The mid-part of the interpubic strip is wrapped around the neo-bladder neck. (h) The two pubic bones are stitched together as well as the two recti. (i) The bladder is closed and the bladder opening sits at the base of the dorsum of the penis.

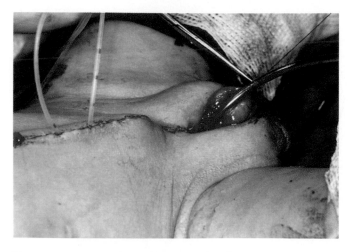

Fig. 14.7 *Continued* (j) Bladder exstrophy closure.

After bladder closure, both pelvises are kept together either with a Bryant traction (Fig. 14.8a), an external fixator [57] (Fig. 14.8b) or plaster keeping both limbs internally rotated (Fig. 14.8c) for 4–8 weeks. Some surgeons do not use any fixation [72]. The gap between the two pubic bones reappears in almost all cases within 2 years after osteotomy. This does not really matter because the pelvic osteotomy does not have any orthopaedic purpose but helps considerably in the bladder closure and in the relocation of the lower urinary tract into the pelvic cavity. A new technique of bladder exstrophy closure using rectus abdominis muscle has been recently reported in patients with a very poor bladder plate [73]. In any case, a close and regular urological and orthopaedic follow-up is required until the next step.

Epispadias repair

In the male

This step aims at correcting the dorsal chordee, reconstructing the epispadiac urethra and lengthening the penis. Although many procedures have been described over the years [74–76], the technique of Cantwell–Ransley [77] is currently accepted by most paediatric urologists as the most reliable [3,78,79] (Fig. 14.9). The urethral plate is fully dissected off the corpora cavernosum from the urethral opening down to the glans. Both corpora bodies are dissected free of adhesion to the pubic rami for 1–2 cm. The neurovascular bundles are elevated from the bodies of the corpora and retracted. The urethral plate is then tubularized over a 10 F silastic catheter. Both corpora are derotated to correct the chordee and a cavernocavernostomy is carried out to maintain the derotation, lengthen the corpora and to keep the reconstructed urethra

on the ventral side of the penis. A glanuloplasty is performed, allowing the ventral relocation of the urethral meatus and a cosmetically satisfactory glans with a low rate of fistula formation [80]. The penile skin cover is achieved by a redistribution of the ventral skin.

A midline division of the glans is advocated by Mitchell [81], allowing the complete separation of the two hemipenises and subsequently an easier reconstruction of the whole penis. Other techniques using a reverse Duckett procedure have been reported [82,83].

In the female (Fig. 14.10)

The urethral plate is dissected and tubularized which increases the bladder outlet resistance. The triangular hairless area separating both major labia and the hemiclitoris is excised. Two lateral flaps of fat tissue are brought medially to fill the gap separating the two hemimons. The hemiclitoris are sutured together and the clitoridal hood is reconstituted. Subsequent surgery to improve genital cosmesis is often indicated when the child approaches puberty, to rotate hair-bearing skin into the mons area [84].

Bladder neck reconstruction and surgery of incontinence

This is the most critical stage of exstrophic reconstruction because none of the techniques available provides fully satisfactory results.

The Young–Dees–Leadbetter procedure

The Young–Dees–Leadbetter procedure [20,85,86] (Fig. 14.11) remains the most commonly used operation to make these children dry. It is usually performed around the age of 3 years old when the bladder capacity is over 60 ml [87]. Performing epispadias repair prior to bladder neck reconstruction allows a significant increase of the bladder capacity [88]. An additional increase of bladder outlet resistance can be obtained by combining this technique with the Marshall–Marchetti–Kranz [89] bladder neck suspension. The principle is to lengthen the urethra endovesically and to overlap it with two triangular flaps of trigone. This increases the bladder outlet resistance and should balance the endovesical pressure enough to keep the child dry but not so much as to allow transurethral bladder emptying. A transtrigonal ureteric mobilization is required not only to correct the reflux but also to move the ureters away from the bladder neck so that sufficient trigonal tissue is available for bladder neck reconstruction [90]. Intraoperative urethral pressure profilometry is used to approximate a continence length of 3.5 cm and urethral closure pressure of 60–90 ml water when the bladder is distended with 50 ml of saline [91,92].

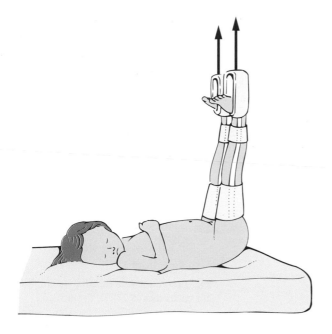

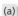

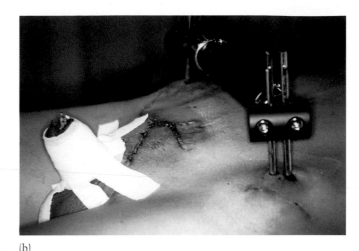

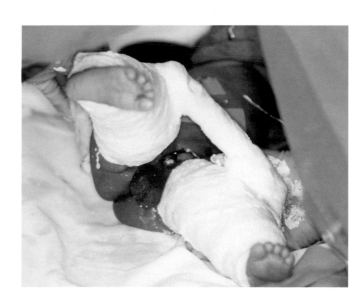

Fig. 14.8 (a) The Bryant traction [5]. (b) Hoffman external fixator. (c) Internal rotation of both inferior limbs.

Other techniques of bladder neck reconstruction

Several variants of the Young–Dees–Leadbetter technique have been described [93–96], as well as several associated procedures, such as bladder augmentation, appendicovesicostomy and artificial urinary sphincter [97,98], which are often used after failed bladder neck reconstruction.

Surgery of cloacal exstrophy

The same therapeutic principles can be applied for cloacal exstrophy. However, several additional problems need to be considered at the time of closure.

1 *Bladder closure.* The bowel can be either separated from the hemibladders or integrated in the bladder closure if the bowel length is sufficient. An ileostomy or short colostomy is performed and the two hemibladders are rejoined as two side-by-side exstrophic hemibladders to close the defect [11]. Secondary bladder reconstruction is often required using stomach or ileum [99,100]. A continent conduit [101–103] offers a second access to the reconstructed bladder, which can be very useful.

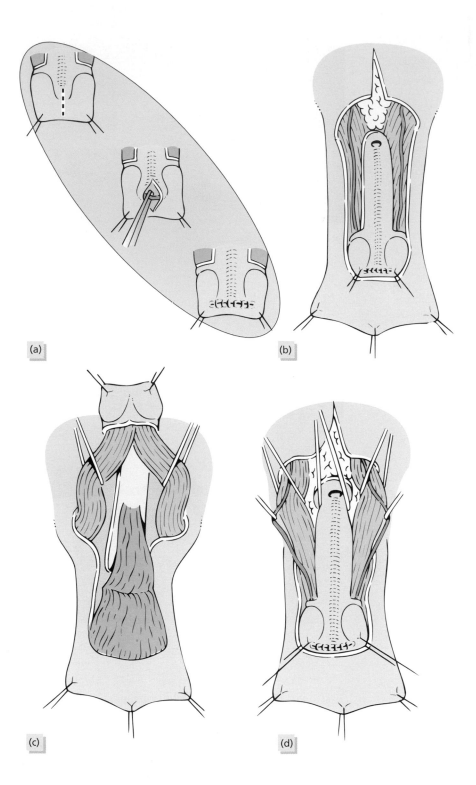

Fig. 14.9 Cantwell–Ransley technique for epispadias [5,77]. (a) Preliminary glanuloplasty (IPGAM procedure) which makes a great difference to the final cosmetic appearance by displacing the terminal urethral meatus ventrally. (b) The incision begins in the midline above the urethral opening and is extended far enough upwards to provide good access to the proximal corpora for mobilization. It continues down on each side of the urethral plate (backed by the corpus spongiosum) and sweeps ventrally around the coronal sulcus separating the prepuce and ventral skin from the corpora. (c) Dissection of the urethral plate commences on the ventral surface, preserving a pedicle to the dartos. Alternate dorsal and ventral dissection is continued until the urethral plate is completely free from the corpora. Dissection then continues backwards to separate adhesion of the prostate and interpubic bar from the convex dorsal surface of the corpora. The urethral plate from the urethral opening to the glans should be completely free of corporal attachment at completion. (d) Dissection of neurovascular bundles and the corpora cavernosum. The neurovascular bundles are sweeping laterally and ventrally at the midpoint of the corpora. Artificial erection at this stage will show dorsal angulation of the corpora at this point.

2 *Associated anomalies.* These are common [13], involving the central nervous system (spina bifida, myelomeningocele), the urinary tract (pelvic kidney, renal agenesis), the müllerian remnants (duplicated uterus and vagina), the skeletal system (vertebral and limb deformities), the gastrointestinal tract (omphalocele, malrotation, duplication, short gut syndrome) and the cardiovascular and pulmonary systems.

3 *Gender reassignment* to female is often required when the two hemipenises are too small.

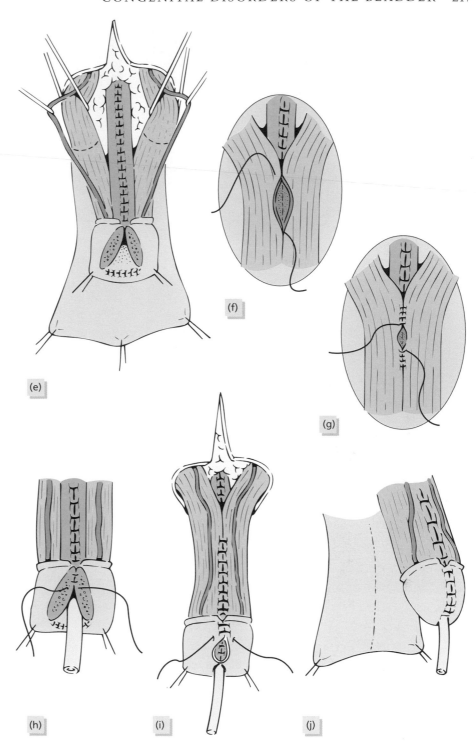

Fig. 14.9 *Continued* (e) Tubularization of the urethral plate over a 10 F silastic urethral stent or catheter. (f–j) Glanuloplasty, derotation of the corpora and cavernocavernostomy. Cavernocavernostomy and corporal rotation are performed to correct the dorsal chordee and approximate the corpora on the dorsal aspect of the urethra.

The failed exstrophy

Dehiscence of the bladder closure is mainly due to an excess of tension of the abdominal wall, local infection or bladder prolapse. Reclosure with or without repeated osteotomy, associated with bladder augmentation and a continent conduit, allows dryness and preservation of the upper tract in most cases. Spontaneous transurethral micturitions are nevertheless unlikely after repeated reconstruction [46,68].

Options after a failed bladder neck reconstruction are:
1 repeated bladder neck reconstruction [94,104], associated with or without a bladder augmentation and a continent conduit;

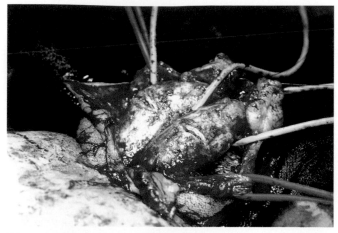

(k)

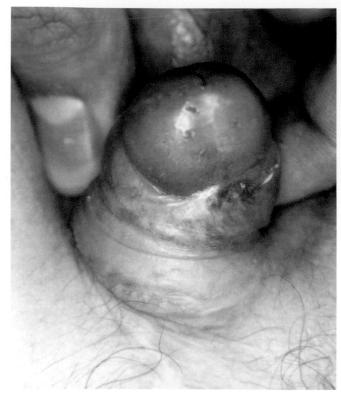

(l)

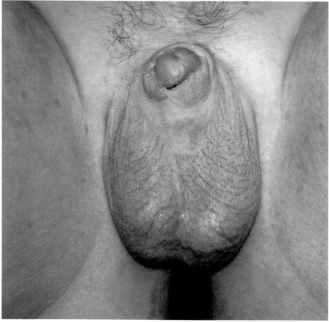

(m)

Fig. 14.9 *Continued* (k) Dorsal view of the penis showing the dissection of the epispadiac penis. The blue slings are placed around the corpora cavernosum. The red slings are placed around the neurovascular bundles. Note the two dorsal transversal incisions on the corpora which will allow their derotation and the cavernocavernostomy. (l,m) Long-term results of the Cantwell–Ransley procedure.

2 bladder outlet resistance can also be increased by injecting silicone particles (Macroplasty®) around the Young–Dees tube;

3 an artificial urinary sphincter can be inserted around the bladder neck [105–107];

4 urinary diversion is only considered by most paediatric urologists when all the other options have failed.

The failed epispadias reconstruction is less common since the technique of Cantwell–Ransley [77] has been used by most paediatric urologists. However, urethral fistulas and strictures, especially when the paraexstrophic flaps have been used, require repeated urethroplasty, sometimes using a free graft of buccal mucosa [108]. Epispadias treated a long time ago or operated for on several occasions often require a full reconstruction associated, in some cases, with an osteotomy.

Urinary diversions

Urinary diversions (ureterosigmoidostomies, ileal conduit and ureterostomies) were the only treatment of these anomalies until 1950. Diversions are still used in some rare cases when the bladder plate is severely damaged and not usable for a primary closure. Undiversion can be subsequently considered to improve the quality of life of these patients.

Ureterosigmoidostomy has fallen out of favour as a means to manage bladder exstrophy largely because of

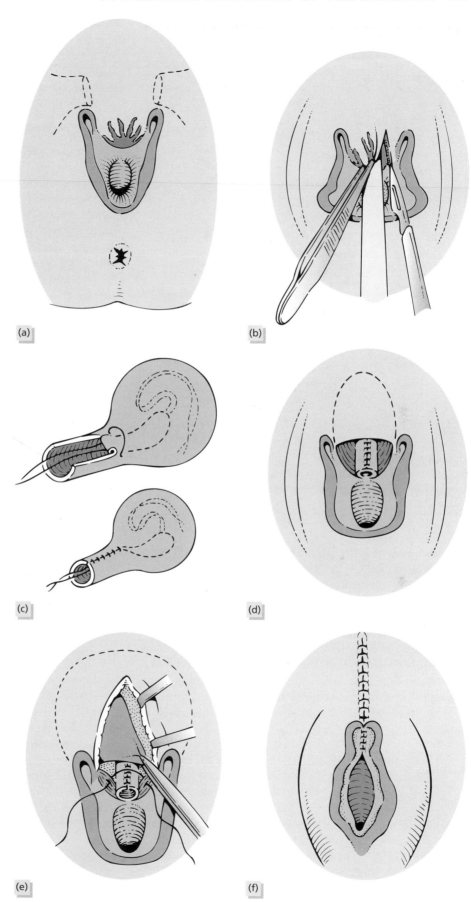

Fig. 14.10 Female epispadias [5].
(a) Female epispadias. (b) Hendren technique excising the roof of the urethra. (c) Urethroplasty. (d) Excision of a triangular area of hairless skin which separates the two major labia and the two hemiclitoris. (e) Two lateral flaps of fat tissue are brought medially to fill the gap separating the two hemimons. (f) Suture of the two hemiclitoris and clitoridal hood.

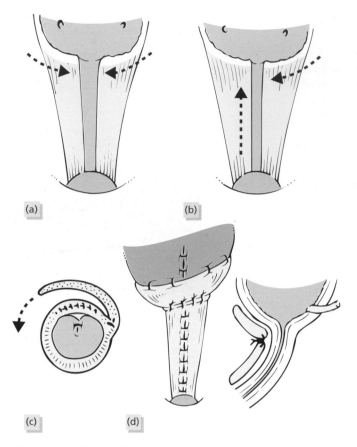

Fig. 14.11 Bladder neck reconstruction [5]. (a) The classic incision line of the Young–Dees–Leadbetter technique. (b–d) The Mollard modification. Note the urethrocervical angulation achieved by this technique.

its association with significant upper urinary tract deterioration [109,110], metabolic acidosis and, more recently, the recognition of an increasing incidence of colonic neoplasia [94,111–115]. Rectal leakage [116], recurrent urinary tract infections [110], delayed continence and absence of transurethral voiding are some other drawbacks of ureterosigmoidostomy [94]. However, Stöckle *et al.* [117] reports that the success rate of ureterosigmoidostomy on continence and social adaptation is much higher (97.4%) than the staged reconstruction. Continent urinary reservoir may be an alternative in this group of patients [118].

Results

Bladder closure

Bladder closure is much safer today. Mollard *et al.* [119] report a success rate of 92% (46/50) in patients followed from 1963 to 1985. The failure rate in 207 patients followed from 1945 to 1985 by Connor *et al.* was 31% [120].

Oesterling and Jeffs [121] reported the causes of failed bladder closure in 31 patients (out of 144) followed from 1975 to 1985 and concluded that the successful initial bladder closure is essential for the result of the bladder neck reconstruction.

Bladder emptying and continence

The various paediatric urologists involved in this type of surgery do not have the same criteria of success when evaluating bladder emptying and continence. For some [87,94], regular and complete transurethral emptying should be achievable without using intermittent catheterization when the adequate balance is found between the detrusor activity and the bladder outlet resistance. For others, the exstrophic bladder does not behave normally [97,122] and transurethral micturitions, although possible, are not particularly encouraged and intermittent catheterization seems to be a safer way to empty the bladder. For Mollard *et al.* [94], continence and transurethral voiding were achieved in 69% of 73 children (girls 77%, boys 63%). For Hollowell and Ransley [97], 57/68 patients were dry and void or used clean intermittent catheterization, but 11 (20%) did not have a satisfactory outcome of the continence procedure. For Merguerian *et al.* [123], 61% of 37 patients had a satisfactory continence. Bladder capacity, high urethral continence length and high urethral closing pressure are the main determinants of success. For Connor *et al.* [120], 82% of 207 patients had an acceptable urinary continence. For Gearhart and Jeffs [124], 74% (55 patients) were dry for at least 3 h, 16% between 1 and 3 h, and 8% were wet.

Sexual implications

After successful epispadias repair, the penis, although straight, remains short. This does not seem to be a major obstacle to sexual intercourse. However, fertility seems to be seriously affected by the various procedures performed on the posterior urethra. Only three of 68 men [125] and four of 72 men [126] had successfully fathered children. Six of 26 and seven of 27 women with bladder exstrophy in these respective series successfully bore offspring. A survey of 2500 exstrophy and epispadias patients identified 38 males who had fathered children and 131 female who had borne offspring [24]. It seems that patients who underwent a ureterosigmoidostomy have better semen analyses than patients who underwent a stage reconstruction (iatrogenic injury of the verumontanum during bladder closure) [3]. In exstrophy the vagina lies parallel to the pelvic floor when the girl is standing and the introitus is seen on the lower abdominal wall rather than in the perineum. Episiotomy is required in 34% and formal vaginoplasty in 23% of the cases [127].

Carcinomas

There are around 80 cases of adenocarcinoma reported in exstrophy patients [128]. Mesrobian *et al.* [110] found eight carcinomas in their series of 108 bladder exstrophies. These colonic carcinomas are developed from the intestinal islets of mucosa which sit on the bladder mucosa. It is also likely that exstrophy patients with augmented bladders are at risk of developing carcinomas during adulthood.

Posterior urethral valves and other congenital anomalies of the urethra

Definition and embryology

Congenital lesions of the human urethra occur during the first 4 months of pregnancy and involve several embryological structures. The urogenital sinus (UGS), the urogenital membrane (which is the anterior part of the cloacal membrane), the distal part of the wolffian system and the glanular ectodermal plug are the four protagonists of urethral construction [129–133]. Subsequently to the division of the cloaca (the confluence between the distal part of the bowel and the allantois) at 6 weeks, the UGS becomes a distinctive entity which presents two parts located above and below the insertion of the two wolffian ducts on its posterior wall (Fig. 14.12). The urological zone is located above the wolffian ducts and the genital zone is located below them. During weeks 7 and 8, the posterior wall of the UGS enlarges and absorbs the distal part of the ureteric buds, whereas the distal part of each wolffian duct reaches the posterior part of the urethra. The two ureteric orifices and the opening of the two wolffian ducts delineate the trigone, which is a wolffian structure.

The genital zone of the UGS is also subdivided in two segments; (i) the pelvic segment, which is vertical; and (ii) the phallic segment, which is horizontal. The posterior urethra located above the verumontanum derives from the urological zone of the UGS, and the posterior urethra located below the verumontanum is the superior part of the genital zone of the UGS. The construction of the posterior urethra (prostatic urethra) occurs during the third month. The distal part of the pelvic segment of the UGS becomes the membranous urethra. At week 11 (Fig. 14.13), the genital tubercle in the male becomes elongated and will form the future penis. The horizontal segment of the genital zone of the UGS constitutes the urogenital plate which lies under the genital tubercle. At the end of the third month, the genital folds bordering the urogenital plate merge, giving the urogenital plate a tubular shape. It is the

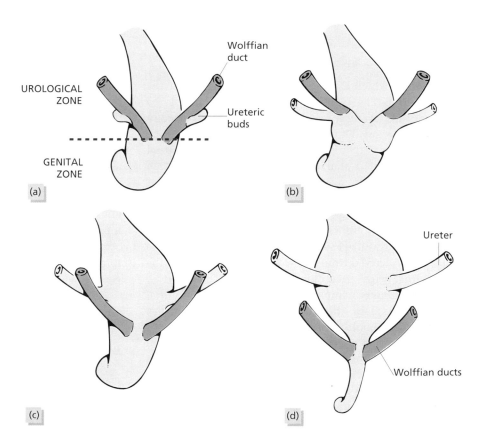

Fig. 14.12 Embryological evolution of the UGS [129] between 5 and 8 weeks' gestation.

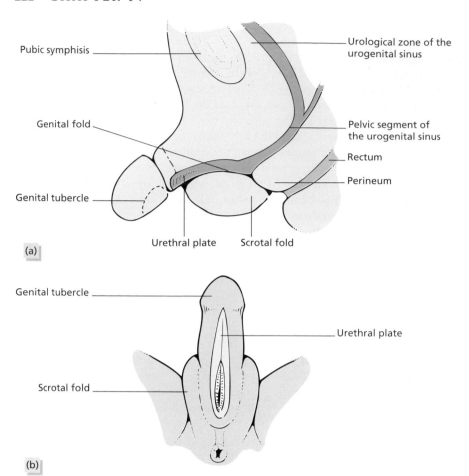

Pubic symphisis

Urological zone of the urogenital sinus

Genital fold

Pelvic segment of the urogenital sinus

Rectum

Perineum

Genital tubercle

Urethral plate   Scrotal fold

(a)

Genital tubercle

Urethral plate

Scrotal fold

(b)

Fig. 14.13 Genitalia of an 11-week-old fetus—the closure of the urogenital plate (urethral plate) [129].

penile urethra which stops before reaching the end of the genital tubercle (Fig. 14.14a,b). The urogenital plate is the precursor of the urethral plate which is commonly used in hypospadias surgery. During the fourth month (Fig. 14.14c), two epithelial buds penetrate the distal end of the genital tubercle: one forms a plain cord of cells in the glans which becomes secondarily a tubular structure (the glanular urethra); the second one is circular and will cleave the prepuce from the glans.

This sequence of embryological events is not universally accepted and Chwalla [134] believed that the trigone of the bladder is not derived from the wolffian duct and that it is of entodermal origin from cloacal remains.

The extraordinary complexity and length of the urethral construction explain the numerous occasions of faulty development. It should be stressed that the most vulnerable parts of the urinary tract are located at the junction between two (or more) different embryological structures (Fig. 14.14d). The calycotubular junction, the pyeloureteric junction, the ureterovesical junction and the vesicourethral junction are the four most vulnerable parts of the urinary tract and all represent complex crossroads between two

or more embryological structures. The anatomical construction of the urethra is closely linked to the physiology of the fetal urethra. The myogenesis of the urethra is a slow phenomenon which is not achieved before the last trimester of pregnancy. The urethral musculature is a complex apparatus and is possibly represented by two separate muscular systems [135,136]. Its histological connections with the bladder and trigonal musculature do not occur before 26 weeks of pregnancy. This late development of the muscular system and its late connections with other embryological structures raise the question of the function of the fetal urethra during the first trimester of gestation (see p. 224).

Congenital lesions of the posterior urethra

Posterior urethral valves

Definition and incidence

A posterior urethral valve (PUV) is a congenital submontanal membrane obstructing the posterior urethra

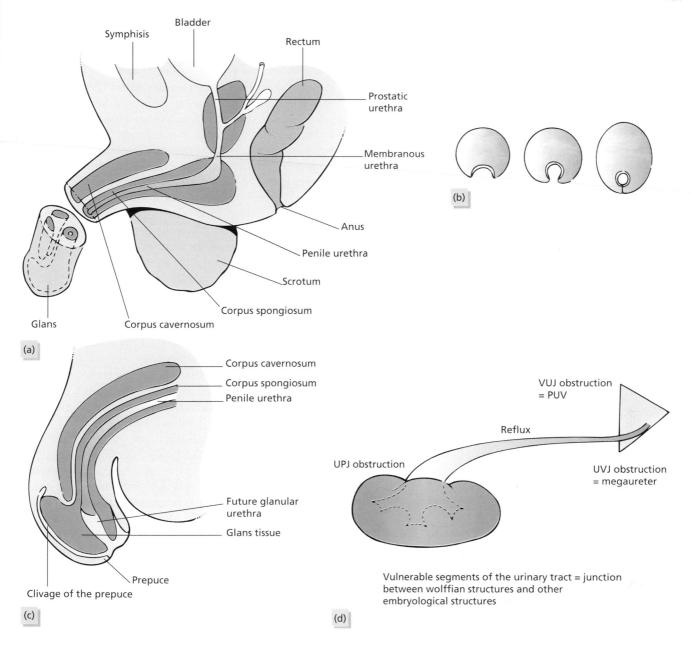

Fig. 14.14 (a,b) The penis at 4 months' gestation [129]. (c) Embryology of the glanular urethra at 4 months. (d) Vulnerable segments of the urinary tract.

more or less severely. It is rarely described in females [137–139], although it is the most common cause of lower urinary obstruction in male children. Late diagnosis of PUV during adulthood is not uncommon [140].

PUVs are related to the faulty development of either the urogenital membrane (type III of the Young classification) or the wolffian system (type I of the Young classification). It is therefore most likely that two different anatomical congenital disorders are grouped under the same generic term.*

The first description of such a disorder was done by Morgagni [141] in the eighteenth century and then by Langenbeck [142] in 1802, Budd [143] in 1840, Pickard [144] in 1855, Tolmatschew [145] in 1870 and Knox and Sprunt [146] in 1912. In 1919 Young et al. [147] published the first classification which distinguished three anatomical types (Fig. 14.15a). Subsequent studies done by Robertson and Hayes [148], Bazy [149] and Stephens [150] show that two main types should be considered. A type I valve of the

---

* It is not certain that these two embryopathies lead to the same urological damage. It is actually difficult radiologically and endoscopically to distinguish these two types of PUV. Both types have the same treatment.

Young classification is the most common and is due to the anterior fusion of the urethrovaginal folds (wolffian structures) (Fig. 14.15a). A type III valve of the Young classification is probably due to the persistence of the urogenital membrane (Fig. 14.15c). A type I valve would appear around 7 weeks of pregnancy and type III around 11 weeks.

The exact timing of these embryological events is not known. However, the Young classification is probably inaccurate because the techniques used for postmortem dissection [151] and the insertion of instruments or catheters into the urethra often convert a type III to a type I valve. Therefore, it is possible that there is only one type of valve which can be described as follows. The membrane is usually attached posteriorly immediately below the level of the verumontanum, with a pin-hole meatus posteriorly, adjacent to the verumontanum. The anterior anchorage of the membrane can be very distal and can go through the external sphincter.

Paramedian parallel reinforcements and distal ballooning are also common features of this congenital obstruction [148,151]. Stephens also describes a type IV valve [150] where the obstructive agent is formed in the anterior instead of the posterior urethral wall and lies below the level of, and is unrelated to, the verumontanum or inferior crest of the urethra.

The probable incidence of PUV is 1:5000 to 1:8000 in boys [152], but these figures should be interpreted cautiously, considering the small size of the series published.

Pathophysiology

PUV obstruction of the urinary tract. It is remarkable that antenatal ultrasound scans of PUV patients rarely show dilatation of the posterior urethra before 20 weeks' pregnancy although the valve appears between 7 and 11 weeks of pregnancy. At 25 weeks of pregnancy, more than a half of the nephronic construction is achieved (Fig. 14.16) and the muscular walls of the excretory tract remain very immature. Histological connections between the bladder and the posterior urethra do not occur before 26 weeks of pregnancy [131]. How and where does the dialysate flow between 9 weeks (first mature nephron) and 26 weeks (histological connections between bladder and posterior urethra) of pregnancy? Does this dialysate flow down to the bladder through a very immature excretory system? Or does it partially filtrate or suffuse through the fetal membranes to reach the amniotic cavity at the early stages of the urinary tract construction?

As the fetus grows, the excretory tract becomes permeable [153,154] and drives the dialysate from the fetal kidney to the bladder. This could explain transitory dilatations of the fetal urinary tract which are currently observed during the first part of pregnancy. Is the fetal urethra a physiological conduit, allowing bladder emptying between 9 and 26 weeks' pregnancy?

If dilatation of the urinary tract does not occur in early stages of gestation in most fetuses with PUV, could it mean that the urethra is not in use because it is immature? The urachus may represent a transitory physiological conduit between 9 and 26 weeks of pregnancy. This hypothesis is supported by the fact that a fetus with prune belly syndrome usually presents with early dilatation of the urinary tract (12–15 weeks' pregnancy) and the urachus is often abnormal (although patent) or absent. Dissection of human fetuses (Fig. 14.17) shows that the urachus is rarely a patent conduit after 22 weeks of pregnancy and actually connects the dome of the bladder to placental structures and not to the amniotic cavity.

Anatomical consequences of PUV on the urinary tract [155]. Anatomical effects of PUV on the urinary tract are mainly represented by the dilatation and elongation of the posterior urethra, the thickening of the bladder neck which can be widely open or very narrow and the thickening of the detrusor, [156] which is often trabeculated. The posterior lip of the bladder neck can become prominent, creating another potential outlet obstruction. Subsequent vesicoureteric reflux is often noticed, with a marked dilatation of the upper tract and renal deterioration. Thickness of the bladder wall can cause a secondary obstruction at the level of the ureterovesical junction and indeed opening of the bladder enclosure (by doing a vesicostomy or by augmenting the bladder) often relieves ureterovesical obstruction. Primary or secondary renal dysplasia and hypoplasia have been discussed in association with fetal urinary tract obstruction and, especially, PUV [157,158]. The timing of the onset of obstruction determines the type of renal damage: early obstruction seems to generate dysplasia, whereas late obstruction seems to generate mainly dilatation of the excretory system [159].

Some associated lesions of the urinary tract, such as vesicoureteric reflux (22–70% of patients with PUV) [152], bladder diverticula and urine extravasation (with or without ascites) can provide a pressure 'pop-off' mechanism which minimizes the renal consequences of PUV [160–163]. However, some authors [164] did not notice any beneficial effect of unilateral reflux in 114 boys with PUV assessed in Great Ormond Street Hospital.

Bladder failure. Hyperplasia, hypertrophy of bladder muscle and collagen are commonly associated with bladder outlet obstruction and especially PUV. Smooth muscle is infiltrated with increased amounts of type III collagen and elastin [165] which results in a loss of compliance and the development of a small capacity, high pressure bladder.

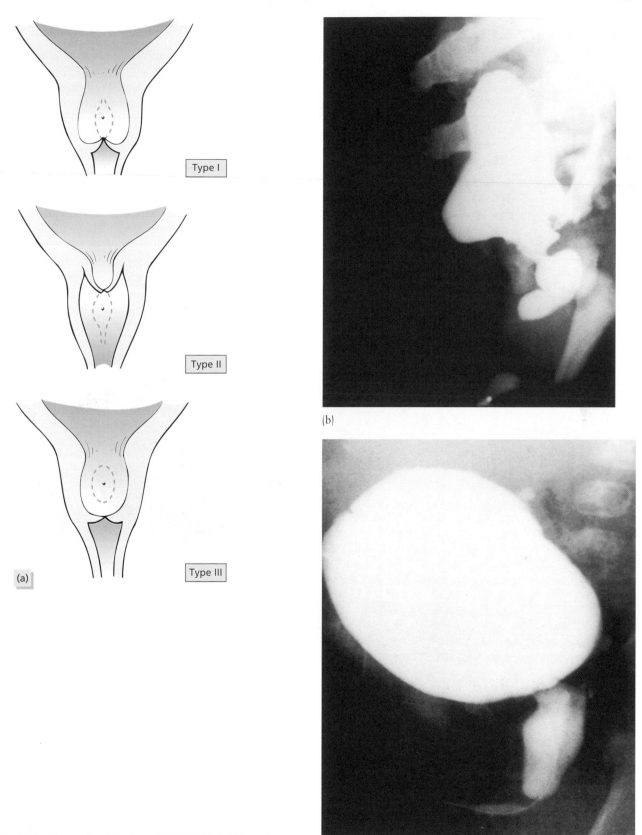

Fig. 14.15 (a) The Young classification of PUV [147]. (b) Note the prominent posterior lip of the bladder neck. (c) Valve type III.

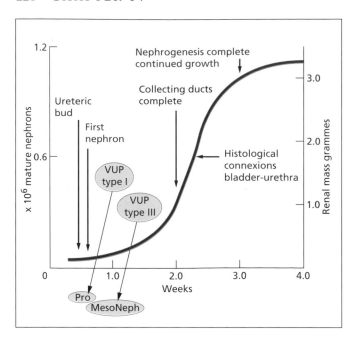

Fig. 14.16 Fetal renal development.

Changes in neurotransmitter receptor concentrations may be responsible for hyperreflexia [166–168]. These changes may be partially or completely reversed after treatment of the valve.

Urodynamic changes and PUV are the direct consequences of anatomical deterioration of the urinary tract, although they are not constant. Variable urodynamic bladder profiles have been reported in boys with PUV and it is sometimes difficult to know if these urodynamic disorders are related to the congenital disorder or its treatment. There is no doubt that some incontinence is related to damage of the external sphincter during endourethral manoeuvres [169]. It is also true that several urodynamic profiles are classically described in patients with bladder outlet obstruction [170]: myogenic failure, hyperreflexia, bladder hypertonia and non-compliant bladder [171–173]. Significant overlap may be seen between these categories. Incontinence may also be the consequence of renal damage and particularly the tubular failure to concentrate urine (polyuria), implying that large volumes

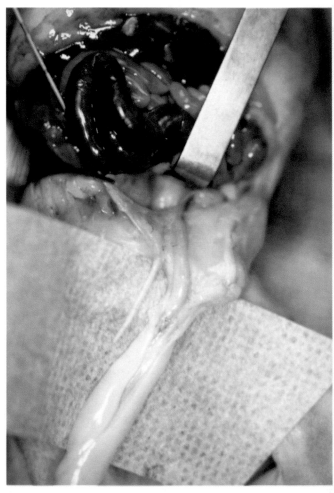

(a)

(b)

Fig. 14.17 (a) Dissection of the urachus in (a) a 20-week-old human fetus, and (b) a 22-week-old human fetus.

of urine flood the bladder which does not have the urodynamic capacity to hold such volumes [174]. Incontinence was found in 33% of the patients followed at Great Ormond Street by D.I. Williams and P.G. Ransley (114 boys followed between 1966 and 1975) [164] and in 22% of 77 patients followed by P. Mollard (unpublished data). Parkhouse reported that only 4% of the children without incontinence under the age of 5 years developed renal failure, whereas 46% of the children with incontinence under the age of 5 years did develop renal failure [164]. Similar statements were also reported by Connor and Burbige in 1990 [175]. This would support the hypothesis that renal failure and bladder failure are closely linked.

Renal function and PUV. When and how can PUV affect renal function? Normal fetal renal function is most likely low considering the blood pressure in the fetal renal artery (fetal blood circulation) which implies a low glomerular filtration; and the very slow maturation of the excretory system associated with high excretory pressure which also implies a limited tubular function. Most of the fetal

dialysis is therefore supported by the placenta and the fetal membranes which represent a huge surface of exchange, and by the mother who represents the system of reference (Fig. 14.18a,b). Two facts illustrate the secondary role of the kidney *in utero*: (i) anephric children have normal blood electrolytes at birth; and (ii) neonates have the same creatinaemia as their mothers.* Renal dysplasia is often associated with PUV and explains why *in utero* bladder shunts inserted quite early during pregnancy in fetuses with PUV have not proven to be efficient in improving function [176]. Renal failure is a common complication of PUV and is recorded in 40–50% of the cases at the time of the diagnosis [177,178]. Long-term outcome for renal function is poor with one-third of patients with PUV dying of renal failure [164]. Amazingly, children with PUV represent a small number of those requiring paediatric renal

---

* It would be interesting to follow creatinaemia of newborns whose mothers have chronic renal failure. However, fertility of these women is rather low which explains the small number of data published.

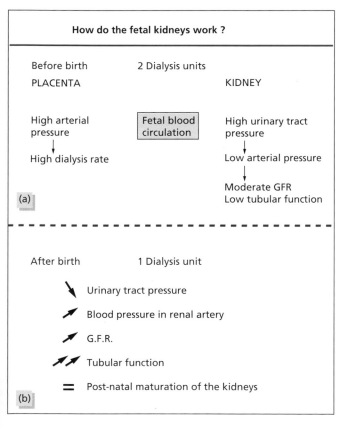

(a)

(b)

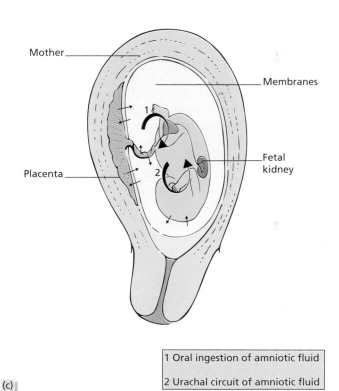

(c)

1 Oral ingestion of amniotic fluid

2 Urachal circuit of amniotic fluid

Fig. 14.18 Fetal dialysis. (a) Fetal blood circulation and dialysis. (b) Dialysis in the newborn. (c) Physiological model of fetal dialysis showing the circulation of amniotic fluid through two closed circuits of dialysis: the orodigestive circuit and the vesicoplacental circuit.

transplantation (4.6% for Reinberg et al. [179] and 1% for Uehling [180]).

Sexual consequences. Woodhouse et al. [181] reported that nine out of 21 men treated in infancy for PUV had slow or dry ejaculation. Retrograde ejaculation is rare (1:21) and semen counts were within the fertile range.

Diagnosis

Antenatal diagnosis of PUV. Antenatal ultrasound is nowadays able to pick up most of the anomalies of cavitary systems. Cavities containing fluids are easily measurable with ultrasound scanning and most obstruction of the fluid circulation, or any lack or excess of fluid, are seen on ultrasound. Dilatation of the urinary tract related to PUV can be detected from 18 weeks' gestation but is often found after 25 weeks. Unfortunately, interpretation of abnormal ultrasound scans is often difficult because dilatation does not always mean obstruction and transient in utero obstructions can be either physiological (see above) or pathological [182]. PUV will be suspected in a fetus with bilateral dilatation of the upper urinary tract thick-walled bladder, associated or not with renal dysplasia and oligohydramnios. Oligohydramnios is usually noticed during the second part of pregnancy when most of the amniotic fluid is conveyed through the fetal urinary tract. As mentioned before, it is doubtful that the dialysate* goes through the fetal urethra during the first part of pregnancy. However, this needs to be proven.

Antenatal ultrasound can also pick up structural anomalies such as the echo-anatomy of the kidneys [187–191] and it seems that the absence of corticomedullary differentiation is more common in children renal failure and vesicoureteric reflux [192]. Another aspect of antenatal diagnosis of PUV is extravasation of urine. As mentioned above, fetal urinary ascites is a quite favourable predictive

* The fetal kidney probably works poorly considering the low blood pressure (fetal blood circulation; see Fig. 14.18a) [183] in the fetal renal artery and the slow maturation of the urinary tract. It is reported that fetal glomerular function and fetal tubular function increase markedly at the end of pregnancy [184,185], and even hyperfiltration could occur in utero in damaged kidneys, leading to glomerular sclerosis [186]. This statement remains questionable and it seems more likely that the glomerular filtration rate does not change a lot but more dialysate goes through the urinary tract which has matured significantly during the second part of gestation. The amniotic fluid, which is mainly represented by the fetal dialysate, goes through the fetal digestive tract and the fetal urinary tract (see Fig. 14.18c), creating two closed circuits of dialysis. If the urinary tract is bilaterally obstructed (PUV), one closed circuit is defective and oligohydramnios progressively appears during the second part of gestation.

factor of renal function [163,193]. Children with antenatal diagnosis of PUV seem to have a worse renal prognosis than those with later diagnosis, and earlier diagnosis and treatment does not improve the clinical prognosis [194].

The idea of predicting the renal function by measuring electrolytes in fetal urine came in the early 1980s [195,196]. Following these criteria, a good predicted renal function is made in a fetus with dilated urinary tract but moderately decreased amniotic fluid volumes at the time of presentation, normal to echogenic renal parenchyma, fetal urine sodium < 100 mEq/ml, fetal urine chloride < 90 mEq/ml, fetal urine osmolarity < 210 mosmol and fetal urine output > 2 ml/h. Iothalamate excretion failed to differentiate good from poor function [185]. Oligohydramnios, cortical cysts and higher urinary levels of sodium, chloride or osmolarity suggest irreversible renal dysplasia. For some, these criteria, however, fail to detect severe renal damage in many cases [176,197]. For others [198], fetal urine electrolyte levels and ultrasonographic images appear helpful in predicting residual fetal renal function and neonatal outcome, and prenatal decompression may prevent the development of fetal pulmonary hypoplasia. Other parameters such as β-microglobulin do not seem to have more predictive value.

It is surprising that most studies are focused on the fetal kidney, which is probably of secondary importance in the overall fetal dialysis (see footnote on p. 228 and Fig. 14.18). The placenta and the fetal membranes have an essential role in fetal dialysis, at least during the first part of pregnancy, and it would seem more appropriate to find a marker of placental clearance. The fetal kidneys, like the fetal lung, start working on their own when the blood circulation suddenly changes at birth.

Clinical features:
1 In the newborn, symptoms of severe metabolic disorders related to renal failure (hyperchloraemic acidosis, anaemia), respiratory failure (spontaneous pneumothorax or pneumomediastinum) and urinary tract infection (septicaemia, meningitis) imply urgent measures of resuscitation. Palpation of the kidney(s) and the bladder is usually easy. Azotaemia, hyponatraemia, hyperkalaemia, dehydration, haematuria and acidosis are commonly noticed. The features of Potter's syndrome may be seen in newborns with PUV. These include intrauterine growth deficiency, pulmonary hypoplasia, limb-positioning defects (e.g. talipes equinovarus) and the characteristic Potter facies [152,194–197].
2 In infants and young children, urinary symptoms are more common (dysuria, haematuria, urinary tract infection) sometimes accompanied by rectal prolapse. Renal failure may be present.
3 In older children, urinary incontinence, urinary urgencies and dysuria are variable.

Investigations:

1 *Ultrasound scan* of the urinary tract is the first investigation to do. It shows the dilatation of the upper urinary tract, the possible abnormal echogenicity of the renal parenchyma, the thick bladder wall (Fig. 14.19) associated or not with bladder diverticula, and the dilated posterior urethra. Perineal ultrasound, with a 7.5 MHz probe, marks a progression in the detection of urethral anomalies. With miniaturization of the ultrasound probes, transrectal scans may be a promising investigation.

2 *Micturating cystogram* remains the investigation of reference to detect PUV and its associated anomalies. Insertion of a transurethral catheter can damage the anatomy of the valve and some paediatric urologists prefer to perform suprapubic micturating cystograms. Distinction between type I and type III valves (if they exist) [151] has actually no practical interest because treatment is identical (Fig. 14.20).

3 *Isotope studies* are essential to assess the renal consequences of PUV and its associated lesions [203,204]. Intravenous urograms (IVUs) are no longer of much interest because of the development of ultrasound scans and isotope studies. IVUs are often poor because of the high plasma creatinine and the subsequent poor secretion of contrast medium by the kidneys. However, IVUs can be normal in nearly 25% of cases [205,206].

4 *Urodynamic studies* (see p. 226) are of no interest in the diagnosis of PUV but are useful in the treatment and follow-up of the associated anomalies and complications, mainly urinary incontinence.

Management

Antenatal treatment. Antenatal treatment is rarely indicated but justified for some when biological criteria (see p. 228) and oligohydramnios are getting worse in a fetus with

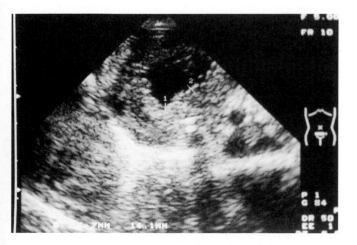

Fig. 14.19 Ultrasound of a thick-walled bladder in a newborn with PUV.

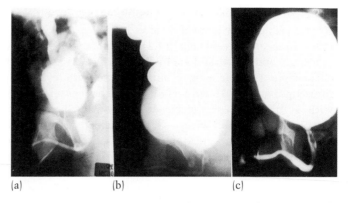

Fig. 14.20 Micturating cystogram of a patient with posterior urethral valves. (a) Prior to endoscopic resection. (b) A minute after resection on the operating table. (c) A month later.

bilateral dilatation of the upper urinary tract. Insertion of a double-J stent between the fetal bladder or the dilated kidneys and the amniotic cavity, under ultrasound guidance, allows decompression of the urinary tract, possible preservation or development of the fetal kidney and possible maturation of the fetal lungs by restoration of an adequate volume of amniotic fluid. These antenatal diversions are usually done quite late in pregnancy and, once again, the benefit of such interventions in children with PUV has not been demonstrated yet.

Postnatal treatment. After birth, three main principles should be respected: it is first essential to resuscitate the child when necessary, make urine drainage free and destroy the valve.

1 Resuscitation implies hydration, electrolyte replacement and antibiotics and should be done in a neonatal intensive care unit.

2 Urine drainage can be achieved either by inserting a transurethral feeding tube or a suprapubic catheter. A transurethral catheter left a few days before the destruction of the valve helps the insertion of the resectoscope in neonates. It is a simple option which may damage the valve (does it matter?) and does not always allow complete drainage of the upper tract because of the thickness of the bladder wall and its poor compliance. In these cases, surgical vesicostomy is a reasonable option [207] which entirely modifies the muscular status of the bladder and often relieves ureterovesical obstruction.

If the child is severely sick and infected, drainage of the upper tract may be the best option (ureterostomy or percutaneous nephrostomy). Ureterostomies (terminal or loop ureterostomy) have less indications nowadays because they often damage the ureter, do not always provide a good drainage and are often difficult to close [208]. A significant post-obstructive diuresis may occur following these diversions and implies a careful follow-up of the electrolyte balance.

3 Destruction of the valve is possible when resuscitation is achieved, usually a few days after birth.

Retrograde endoscopy (Fig. 14.21) is the most common procedure and was first done by Randall in 1921 [209]. The endoscopic treatment uses either a neonate cystoure-throscope (7, 9 or 10 F with a built-in 0° channel telescope), with a high-frequency electrode (3 F; or Bug-bee) or an infant resectoscope with a hooked electrode. Several techniques are widespread using a hooked electrode, or a Bug-bee electrode (metallic mandrin of a No. 3 ureteric catheter). For some [206,208] it is technically safer to use the knee of the hooked electrode and push it gently on the upper commissure of the valve (12 o'clock position) toward the bladder. A 12 o'clock cut is usually sufficient but other cuts can be done at 8 o'clock and 2 o'clock. It is probably more dangerous to hook the valve and withdraw the hooked electrode because the anterior anchorage of the membrane can be very distal and can go through the external sphincter [151]. It is therefore most likely that some incontinence can be due to the endoscopic treatment [169].

Laser can be used to destroy the valve [210–212]. The neodymium yttrium aluminium garnet (YAG) laser beam is transmitted by advancing a 600 μm bare fibre through the side channel of a No. 8 cystourethroscope. The valve is vaporized advancing centrifugally and small marginal fins can be left to undergo spontaneous shrinkage.

Percutaneous antegrade valve ablation [213,214] is another endoscopic approach of the valve which avoids urethral instrumentation and possible urethral strictures. This technique implies the percutaneous placement of a 12 F suprapubic cystocatheter and uses a 9.5 F resectoscope with a 90° hooked electrode. The primary advantage of this technique is its applicability to the premature or low birth weight infant, or to the infant with a small-calibre urethra that would not accommodate the smallest paediatric endoscope.

The valve can be hooked blindly and destroyed in the newborn without anaesthetic. Sir David Innes Williams (1973) [177] had this original idea which was subsequently developed by R.H. Whitaker (1986) [215]. The principle is that the sterile, lubricated hook is passed up the urethra in the neonate without anaesthetic, in the X-ray department, immediately after the valve has been demonstrated by micturition cystourethrography (MCU). It is expected that only the valve can engage in the hook. The bare metal used as a diathermy electrode is limited to the small area inside the hook. The rest of the instrument, including the outside of the tip of the hook, is insulated.

Fogarty balloon catheter ablation of PUV was also the idea of Sir David Innes Williams. A No. 4 Fogarty balloon catheter is placed into the bladder which has been filled beforehand with some contrast medium. The balloon is inflated with approximately 0.75 cm³ saline. With gentle withdrawal, the operator visualizes valve engagement by the balloon. Sharp withdrawal of the catheter ruptures the obstructing anterior membrane without injuring the sphincter. The procedure may be repeated immediately if appropriate. Urethral extravasation of contrast material is common and, therefore, postoperative catheter drainage is recommended [216,217]. Whichever endoscopic technique is chosen, an X-ray control on the operating table is advisable.

A perineal urethrotomy approach of PUV is certainly not recommended nowadays in western countries but still has indications when endoscopic and radiological equipment are not available [218]. There are no longer any indications for an open anterior approach of PUV [149].

Postoperative period and treatment of associated anomalies. Post-obstructive diuresis with concomitant losses in sodium and potassium with acidosis and the risk of urinary tract infection after urethral instrumentation, imply a strict follow-up of these patients. Some authors

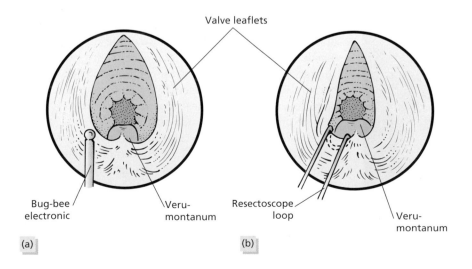

Valve leaflets

Bug-bee electronic

Veru-montanum

(a)

Resectoscope loop

Veru-montanum

(b)

Fig. 14.21 Endoscopic views of valve resection. (a) Bug-bee destruction of the valve. (b) Hooking of the valve.

leave a bladder catheter after fulguration of the PUV, while others do not. It actually depends on the overall condition of the patient. In most cases, there is a progressive improvement of the bladder and the upper tract after complete destruction of the PUV, although it takes years for the dilatation to come down [178,219].

Vesicoureteric reflux disappears in most cases if the kidney keeps a reasonable function [220]. If the kidney is destroyed, a nephroureterectomy is indicated. However, vesicoureteric reflux may act as a 'pop-off' valve and may have a protective effect by reducing intravesical pressure. Urodynamic studies are therefore required before considering a nephroureterectomy or a ureteric reimplantation in a patient with PUV. Ureteric reimplantation in a trabeculated bladder is often difficult and unsuccessful, and associated with a poor prognosis with regard to recovery of renal function [168]. However, antireflux surgery does not apparently affect outcome [168]. Endoscopic treatments of reflux may be safer in this particular indication.

Surgery of the bladder neck should be always avoided [208] because it is unnecessary and dangerous (incontinence, retrograde ejaculation). True secondary bladder neck obstruction is rarely found [221,222].

Persistent dilatation of the upper tract without reflux is often related to a degree of obstruction at the ureterovesical junction. This obstruction may be intermittent or permanent, i.e. it may exist only when the bladder is full.

Pressure–perfusion studies [223] are often unreliable [224,225] in detecting obstruction of the upper tract. Intermittent catheterization could be a reasonable option in these children, but practically it is a poorly accepted procedure in children with normal urethral sensitivity. Bladder augmentation [226] has rare indications but, like vesicostomy, changes the muscular behaviour of the bladder, improves its capacity and compliance and often relieves ureterovesical obstruction (without reimplanting the ureters). The child may have difficulties in emptying his or her bladder completely after augmentation and intermittent catheterization may be required. Early valve destruction with concomitant ureteric reimplantation and tapering [227,228] is considered by many as an excessive and dangerous procedure [177,205,208,220,229].

Incontinence is reported to be between 14 and 38% [230,231] after treatment of PUV. The incontinence tends to improve with puberty, presumably as a result of further prostatic development. Treatment of incontinence will not be considered in this chapter. The association of bad outcome with incontinence points to continuing bladder dysfunction as a major determinant of long-term outcome for renal function [168]. Even if major progress has been achieved in early diagnosis and early treatment of PUV, mortality, renal failure and persistent incontinence remain major problems and it does not seem that antenatal treatment has changed the prognosis of this severe and common congenital anomaly of the posterior urethra. The type of primary surgical treatment (fulguration, vesicostomy, high urinary diversion) does not seem to influence progression of renal failure or body growth in children with PUV. Regardless of the surgical or medical treatment, which can greatly influence mortality, renal failure developed in almost 50% of the children with PUV [232]. Four factors have been identified as being associated with poor long-term outcome: (i) presentation before the age of 1 year; (ii) bilateral vesicoureteric reflux; (iii) proteinuria; or (iv) day-time incontinence at the age of 5 years old [168].

Other congenital lesions of the posterior urethra

Polyps

Congenital posterior urethral polyps are benign growths arising from the verumontanum and are almost invariably found in young boys. Only 50 cases were reported by 1982 [233]. The main clinical signs are dysuria, sudden stoppage of micturition (clapper), haematuria and occasionally infection [234–236]. Diagnosis is made with MCU (the appearance of the polyp can change with the position of the child) and urethroscopy (Fig. 14.22). Upper tract dilatation is noted in 20% of the patients, reflux in 8% and bladder diverticula in 8% [233]. Endoscopic treatment allows a complete excision of the tumour which has a fibrovascular stalk covered with transitional epithelium [235]. In children the stalk is attached to the proximal verumontanum which is different to the adult male where polyps are composed of prostatic-type glands located distally to the verumontanum [237]. No recurrence has been described in the paediatric population.

Cysts

Cysts of the posterior urethra are either müllerian duct* cysts or utricular cysts. They can be associated with hypospadias or prune belly syndrome [238]. Symptoms are mainly represented by dysuria, urogenital infection (epididymitis), haematuria and haemospermia [239,240]. Rectal examination often reveals a midline cystic structure at the base of the prostate [152]. Diagnosis is made with ultrasound, MCU and urethroscopy. Treatment is not necessary in small and well-drained cysts. Aspiration of the cyst does not always give good long-term results, as well as causing transurethral endoscopic unroofing of the cyst; open surgery is then required. Suprapubic transvesical, perineal or posterior [241] approaches have been described.

---

* Müllerian ducts regress under the influence of müllerian-inhibiting factor produced by the fetal testis, leaving the prostatic utricle as a vestige. The utricle is a short, blind-ending pouch located on the verumontanum [152].

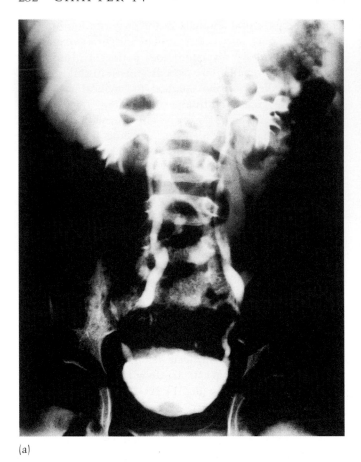

(a)

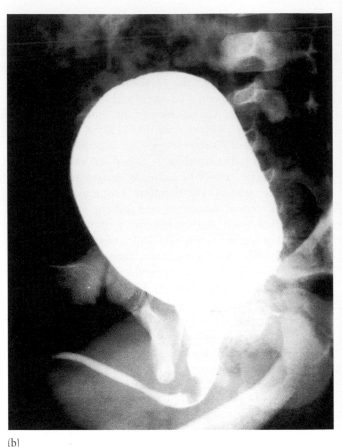

(b)

Fig. 14.22 Polyp of the posterior urethra. (a) IVU: note the defect in the bladder. (b) MCU: note the defect in the posterior urethra (same patient).

Urethral diverticula in females are common [242], acquired lesions probably related to the infection of Skene glands [243–245] which will not be developed here.

Duplications of the urethra

In the male

By 1986, only 150 cases had been reported [246,247]. Several classifications have been reported but Effmann's classification (Fig. 14.23) seems to be adopted by many authors. Type I is a blind incomplete urethral duplication; type IIA is a complete duplication with two meatuses (type IIA1: two non-communicating urethras arising independently from the bladder; and type IIA2: a second channel arising from the first and coursing independently to a second meatus); type IIB is a complete patent urethral duplication with one meatus (two urethras arising from the bladder or posterior urethra and uniting to form a common distal channel); and type III is a urethral duplication as a

component of partial or complete caudal duplication. Type I is the most common and type III the least common.

Some variations are reported, such as collateral urethral duplication in the frontal plane [248] and trifurcation of the urethra [249]. Williams and Kenawi [250] and Woodhouse and Williams [251] describe urethral duplications in a frontal plane (complete or abortive) and in a sagittal plane (epispadias, hypospadias, Y duplication and spindle duplication) and posterior urethral duplication. Stenosis at the urethral junction (obstruction) is possible and one urethra can be located outside the sphincteric muscular structures (incontinence).

Embryology of these lesions is totally confusing and is possibly related to some aberrations of cloacal septations [150]. Troyer [132] lists a large number of embryological hypotheses, none of which has been demonstrated. A partial failure or an irregularity of the ingrowth of the lateral mesoderm between the ectodermal and endodermal layers of the cloacal membrane in the midline can account for the forms with a dorsal epispadiac channel. On the other hand, canalization of the urethral plate readily explains distal hypospadiac duplications but does not explain the more complete hypospadiac form that involves a perineal or pre-anal opening. These last cases probably are secondary to defective urorectal fold development [252].

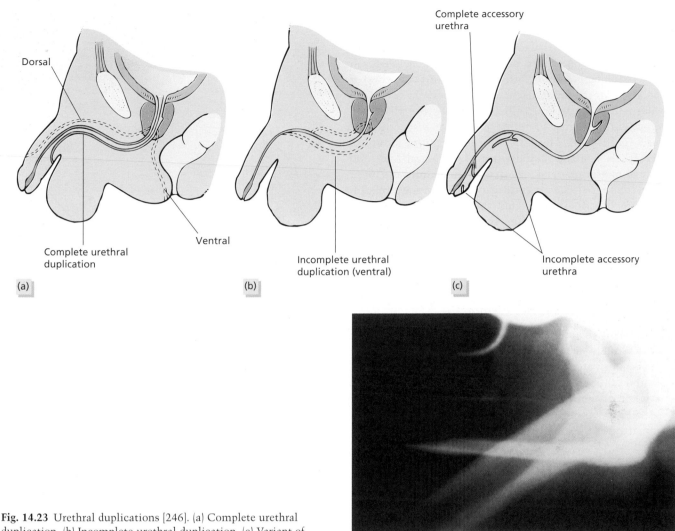

Fig. 14.23 Urethral duplications [246]. (a) Complete urethral duplication. (b) Incomplete urethral duplication. (c) Variant of accessory urethra. (d) Complete duplication of the penile urethra.

Patients with urethral duplication can be asymptomatic or can present with a double stream, urinary incontinence, urinary tract infections or outflow obstruction. Physical examination usually will reveal two meatuses and nothing else. Other anomalies of the genitalia can be noticed (ambiguity, epispadias, chordee). MCU and a retrograde urethrogram will allow the anatomical type to be defined. Associated urological anomalies are possible, such as duplication of the bladder, duplication of external genitalia [253,254], dilatation of the upper tract, renal agenesis, PUV, etc. Treatment is not always necessary if the patient is totally asymptomatic. If not, endoscopic treatment or open surgery is required — excision of an epispadiac urethra; partial urethrotomy; urethrourethrostomy; marsupialization and urethroplasty; electrofulguration of a perineal urethra [255–257], etc.

In the female

Urethral duplication in females is a very rare congenital anomaly. Three main types can be distinguished [208].
1 Urethral duplication associated with bladder duplication.
2 Urethral duplication with a single bladder [258,259].
3 Urethral duplication with a phallic urethra (female pseudohermaphrodism), associated with anomalies of the genitalia.

These three types could be related to an abnormal development of the müllerian ducts [260,261]. A clitoridoplasty and perineoplasty are required [262].

Congenital anomalies of the anterior urethra

Megalourethra

Originally described by Nesbitt [263], the megalourethra is

a rare condition (45 cases reported by 1986) [264,265] which may be associated with severe, sometimes lethal, urological anomalies (e.g. the triad syndrome) [266]. The megalourethra is not related to a urethral obstruction but to an atresia of the corpus spongiosum (scaphoid megaurethra) or to an arrest in the embryogenesis of the corpora cavernosa (fusiform megalourethra) [150,267,268]. Rather than two distinct entities, megalourethra represents a spectrum of defects (Fig. 14.24). Megalourethra results from failure of differentiation of the mesoderm in the urethral folds and failure of migration of spongy tissue formed from the inner genital folds [267]. Treatment depends a lot on the situation of the upper urinary tract and the associated anomalies [269]. Supravesical diversion is the suggested primary treatment if the upper tract is grossly dilated [266]. A reduction urethroplasty then can be performed at a later date.

Diverticulum of the anterior urethra

This anomaly is a minor expression of megalourethra. The diverticulum is saccular and due to a local deficiency of the corpus spongiosum [270]. Another explanation for congenital urethral diverticulum is that it may arise from cystic dilatation of normal or accessory urethral glands that eventually communicate with the urethra [270–273]. Two different types of urethral diverticula have been described, both of which are uncommon [274]: (i) a narrow-necked type with a small sac, which does not cause obstruction but is associated with stasis and calculus formation; and (ii) a wide-necked type that often has a much larger sac. This latter type of diverticulum presents with obstruction due to the distal lip of the ostium, which is said to act as a flap valve and is pushed up against the dorsal wall of the urethra on attempted micturition. Endoscopic treatment or open surgery is required.

Anterior urethral valves

The nosological distinction between anterior valves and urethral diverticula is vague. However, urethral valves have been described all along the entire course of the anterior urethra. Most anterior valves occur between the penoscrotal junction and the midbulbar urethra, with those between the midbulbar urethra and distal urethra being less common [275]. They appear as a filmy, ventrally based cusp of tissue, but can be like a diaphragm perforated in its centre. No clear embryological origin has been reported, although they could be aborted urethral duplications [276]. Symptoms, diagnosis and treatment are similar to symptoms encountered in diverticulum of the urethra. Valves in the fossa navicularis* [277] have been described as well as valves at different places along the urethra [278].

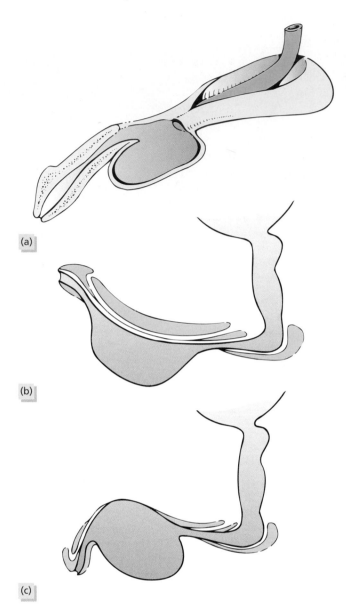

Fig. 14.24 Megalourethra. (a) Saccular diverticulum. (b) Scaphoid and (c) fusiform types of megalourethra.

Polyps of the anterior urethra

Polyps of the anterior urethra are very rare lesions [279,280] which may cause urethral symptoms. Treatment is endoscopic.

---

* The lacuna magna or the sinus of Guérin is a dorsal diverticulum in the roof of the fossa navicularis and is present in approximately 30% of boys as either a small pit or a sinus up to 4–6 mm long. It is not an obstructive structure but it can be stretched during micturition and can occasionally bleed [270].

Cowper syringoceles

Cowper's main glands are paired and lie posterolateral to the membranous urethra and caudal to the external urethral sphincter. The two ducts run a submucosal course along the back of the urethra to open into the floor of the bulbus urethra through two minute side-by-side orifices [150,270]. Two accessory glands are located in the depth of the corpus spongiosum of the bulb. Abnormal opening of the ducts into the urethra could be the cause of the obstruction [281]. The gland itself will form a cyst which sticks out into the urethral lumen (Fig. 14.25). Spontaneous opening of the gland into the urethra is possible and leaves the ducts wide open. These cysts are usually asymptomatic although they can obstruct the urethral lumen with severe (sometimes lethal) repercussion on the urinary tract [282–284]. Urethral symptoms are more common. Perineal tumour is rare [285]. Diagnosis is made with perineal ultrasound, transrectal ultrasound, urethrogram (there may be a reflux of contrast medium into the ruptured gland) and urethroscopy (blue bulge). Differential diagnosis with a false passage, venous reflux, urethral diverticulum or urethral duplication can be difficult [208]. Treatment is endoscopic.

Cysts of the Littré glands

These glands are located mainly in the bulbous and distal penile urethra. Their ducts may become ectatic and may be opacified. Recurrent painless bleeding after micturition or haematuria are the main symptoms of these lesions, which can be treated by endoscopic fulguration [270].

Skene duct cysts

These are rare cystic masses located just around the female urethral meatus (0.04% of female births for Nam Hyuk and Sang Youn [286] and (2/year for Mollard [208]). The cause of ductal obstruction is not known and several glands can be involved [287]. The cyst usually measures 1 cm but can be bigger [288]. Histology shows a transitional or squamous epithelium [289,290]. Differential diagnosis with Gartner cysts, urethral prolapse, prolapsed ectopic ureterocele and imperforate hymen can be difficult. Symptoms seem to be rare. Although spontaneous rupture is possible, treatment is usually required (excision, marsupialization or simple needle aspiration).

Urethral prolapse

A urethral prolapse is a bright red or cyanotic oedematous lump which can become infected, ulcerated or necrotic and which occurs in approximately 1:3000 children.

The aetiology is unknown and symptoms are characterized by painless vaginal bleeding and, rarely, by

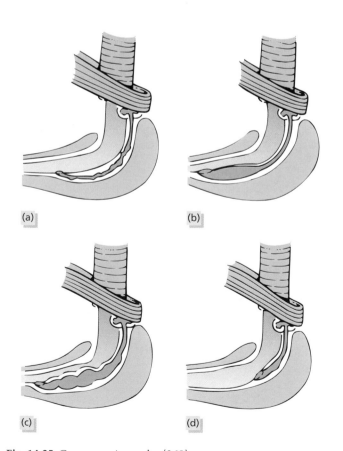

(a)　　　(b)

(c)　　　(d)

Fig. 14.25 Cowper syringoceles [269].

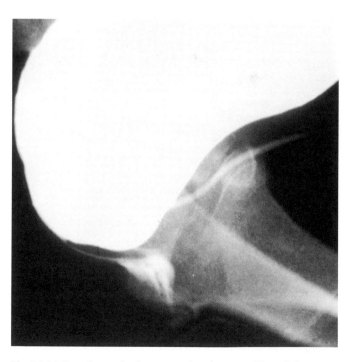

Fig. 14.26 Female urethral atresia related to a wolffian defect.

micturitional disturbances [291]. Examination is essential and shows that urine comes from the middle of the everted mass, which is confirmed by catheterization of the bladder. Differential diagnoses include urethral or vaginal neoplasia, urethral caruncle, condyloma and prolapsing ureterocele. Surgery (excision of the prolapsed mucosa) appears to be the best option [291–294], although some authors recommend conservative treatment [294]. Complications of surgical treatment are rare although urethral stenosis, urinary incontinence, acute urinary retention, vaginal bleeding and recurrence of prolapse have been reported [291,296–298].

Agenesia and congenital strictures of the urethra

These are extremely rare and may not exist [299]. Total agenesia is lethal and has been reported in 28 cases by

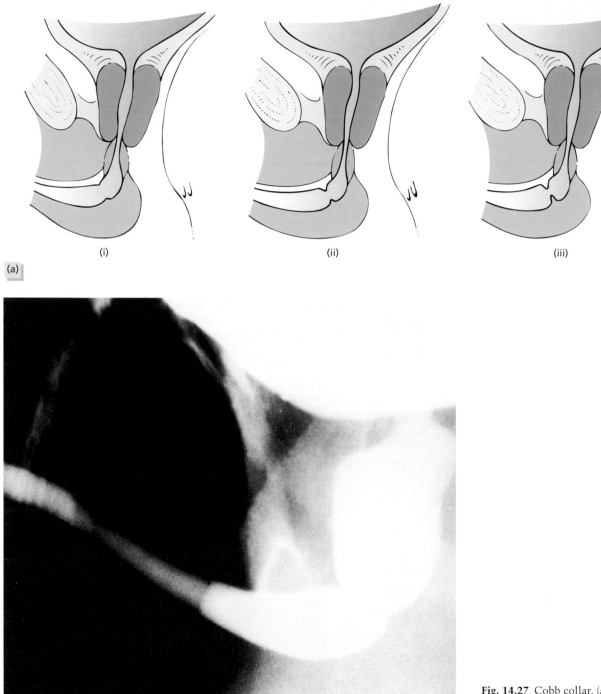

Fig. 14.27 Cobb collar. (a) Classification of Cobb collar [318]. (b) Urethrogram of a child with Cobb collar.

Palmer and Russi [300]. This malformation is incompatible with normal renal development [152,301]. Nearly all examples of urethral atresia in girls have occurred in stillbirths in which the bladder was also atretic. Children who survive all had a fistula between the urinary tract and the vagina or the rectum and dysplastic kidneys [302–303] (Fig. 14.26). Partial congenital atresia has been described in children of both sexes with a high imperforate anus.

It is reported that congenital stricture may exist at the junction between the bulbar and the membranous urethras [272,304,305]. Family cases have been published [306,307]. However, most of these cases have been diagnosed during adulthood and it is therefore not certain that they are congenital strictures.

Urethrocutaneous fistulas

Most urethrocutaneous fistulas are actually urethral duplications. However, Mollard [208] reports that Williams and himself each encountered one case.

Congenital meatal stenosis

Congenital meatal stenosis is rare in males [308], even in males with hypospadias. They are exceedingly rare in females [309], although they are possible when associated with other anomalies (anorectal imperforation, female hypospadias). A distal urethral ring has been found at the junction between the two portions of the urethra (the UGS and müllerian portion) [310–312] and may be stenotic in some cases, causing micturating problems in girls. This concept of a distal urethral ring made urethral dilatation in girls a fashionable treatment for girls with recurrent urinary symptoms [311] but no longer has any support nowadays. Graham et al. [313] and Averous et al. [314] have shown that the urethral calibre is normal during urinary tract infections.

Urethral haemangiomas

Urethra haemangiomas are rare and benign lesions that cause significant haemorrhagic morbidity. Although benign in nature, these lesions tend to recur unless completely eradicated [315,316]. Urethrorrhagia and haematuria are the main symptoms. Total urethral excision seems to be avoidable although urethral marsupialization is sometimes required to have a full control of the lesion [316].

Congenital stricture of the proximal urethral bulb (Cobb collar or Moormann ring)

In 1968, Cobb et al. [304] published 52 cases of bulb urethral stricture, among which 26 patients were under 16 years of age. In 1972, Moormann [317] described a similar

finding in 38 males. Three different anatomical types are reported [318]: (i) a simple ridge of tissue (Cobb collar I); (ii) a definite stricture in the area described (Cobb collar II); or (iii) a very tight pin-hole opening (Cobb collar III) (Fig. 14.27). Failure of complete dissolution of the urogenital membrane at the junction of the cloaca and genital groove has been suggested. However, Cranston et al. [318] believe that Cobb collar is the result of a narrowing at the level of the urogenital ostium, i.e. the opening of the pelvic part into the phallic part of the UGS [318,319]. It is usually a radiological or endoscopic finding but chronic retention and bilateral hydronephrosis have been described [319].

References

1 David G, Haegel P. La délimitation. In: Tuchmann-Duplessis H, ed. *Embryologie*. Paris: Ed. Masson, 1971:46–53.

2 Muecke EC. The role of the cloacal membrane in exstrophy: the first successful experimental study. *J Urol* 1964;**92**:659.

3 Gearhart JP. Bladder and urachal abnormalities: the exstrophy–epispadias complex. In: Kelalis PP, King LR, Belman AB, eds. *Clinical Pediatric Urology*. Philadelphia: WB Saunders, 1992:579–619.

4 Hamilton WJ. Cleavage and formation of germ layers. In: Hamilton WJ, Boyd JD, Mossman HW, eds. *Human Embryology*, 2nd edn. Cambridge: Heffer, 1959:57–8.

5 Mollard P, Mouriquand P, Joubert P. L'exstrophie vésicale et ses variantes. In: *Encyclopédie Médico-Chirurgicale*. Éditions Techniques *Paris:* 1988;**41180**:1–14.

6 Marshall VF, Muecke EC. Variations in exstroply of the bladder. *J Urol* 1962;**88**:766–96.

7 Patton BM, Barry A. The genesis of exstrophy of the bladder and epispadias. *Am J Anat* 1952;**90**:35.

8 Ambrose SS, O'Brien DP. Surgical embryology of the exstrophy–epispadias complex. *Surg Clin North Am* 1974; **54**:1379.

9 Thomalla JV, Rudolph RA, Rink RC, Mitchell ME. Induction of cloacal exstrophy in chick embryo using the CO_2 laser. *J Urol* 1985;**134**:991–5.

10 Mildenberger H, Kluth D, Dziuba M. Embryology of bladder exstrophy. *J Pediatr Surg* 1988;**23**:166–70.

11 Hurwitz RS, Manzoni GAM, Ransley PG, Stephens FD. Cloacal exstrophy: a report of 34 cases. *J Urol* 1987;**138**: 1060–4.

12 Spencer R. Exstrophia splanknica. *Surgery* 1965;**57**:751–66.

13 Diamond DA. Cloacal exstrophy: associated anomalies. *Dialog Pediatr Urol* 1990;**13**:6–8.

14 Brito CG, Mitchell ME, Rink RC. Cloacal exstrophy: reconstruction for urinary continence. 58th Annual Meeting of the American Academy of Pediatrics. Abstract No. 54. Chicago: American Academy of Pediatrics, 1989;76–7.

15 Rickman PP. Vesicointestinal fissure. *Arch Dis Child* 1960;**35**:967.

16 Higgins CC. Exstrophy of the bladder: report of 158 cases. *Am Surg* 1962;**28**:99–102.

17 Lattimer JK, Smith MJV. Exstrophy closure; a follow-up on 70 cases. *J Urol* 1966;**95**:356–9.

18 Ives E, Coffey R, Carter CO. A family study of bladder exstrophy. *J Med Genet* 1980;**17**:139–41.

19 Lancaster PAL. Epidemiology of bladder exstrophy; a

communication from the International Clearinghouse for Birth Defects monitoring systems. *Teratology* 1987;**36**:221.

20 Dees JE. Congenital epispadias with incontinence. *J Urol* 1949;**62**:513–22.

21 Shapiro E, Lepor H, Jeffs RD. The inheritance of classical bladder exstrophy. *J Urol* 1984;**132**:308.

22 Stringer MD, Duffy PG, Ransley PG. Inguinal hernias associated with bladder exstrophy. *Br J Urol* 1994;**73**:308–9.

23 Culp DA. The histology of exstrophied bladder. *J Urol* 1964;**91**:538–48.

24 Shapiro E, Jeffs RD, Gearhart JP, Lepor H. Muscarinic cholinergic receptors in bladder exstrophy: insights into surgical management. *J Urol* 1985;**134**:309.

25 Schlegel PN, Gearhart JP. Neuroanatomy of the pelvis in an infant with cloacal exstrophy: a detailed microdissection with histology. *J Urol* 1989;**141**:583.

26 Soper RT, Kilger K. Vesicointestinal fissure. *J Urol* 1964;**92**:490–501.

27 Howell C, Caldamone A, Snyder H. Optimal management of cloacal exstrophy. *J Pediatr Surg* 1983;**18**:365–9.

28 Dykes EH, Oesch I, Ransley PG, Hendren WH. Abnormal aorta and iliac arteries in children with urogenital abnormalities. *J Pediatr Surg* 1993;**28**:696–700.

29 Woodhouse CRJ. The management of erectile deformity in adults with exstrophy and epispadias. *J Urol* 1986;**135**:932.

30 Kelley J, Eraklis AJ. A procedure for lengthening the phallus in boys with exstrophy of the bladder. *J Pediatr Surg* 1971;**6**:645–9.

31 Hurwitz RS, Woodhouse CRJ, Ransley PGR. The anatomical course of the neurovascular bundles in epispadias. *J Urol* 1986;**136**:68–70.

32 Hanna MK, Williams DI. Genital function in males with vesical exstrophy and epispadias. *Br J Urol* 1972;**44**:169–174.

33 Schultze KA, Pfister RR, Ransley PG. Urethral duplication and complete bladder exstrophy. *J Urol* 1985;**133**:276–8.

34 Williams DI, Jolly HR. Long-term results of transplantation of the ureters for ectopia vesicae. *Great Ormond St J* 1952;**3**:9–13.

35 Arap S, Giron AN. Duplicated exstrophy: report of three cases. *Eur Urol* 1986;**12**:451.

36 Sheldon CA, McLorie GA, Khoury A, Churchill BM. Duplicate bladder exstrophy: a new variant of clinical and embryological significance. *J Urol* 1990;**144**:334–6.

37 Kogan SJ, Hankin LG, Levitt SB. Total duplicate exstrophic bladder and urethra. Variation of incomplete bladder exstrophy. *Urology* 1976;**8**:55–7.

38 Turner-Warwick R, Ransley PG, Bloom DA, Williams DI. Variants of the exstrophy complex. *Urol Clin North Am* 1978;**5**:127.

39 Weiss RE, Garden RJ, Cohen EL, Stone NN. Covered exstrophy with sequestered colonic remnant. *J Urol* 1993;**149**:185–7.

40 Mahdavi R. Covered exstrophy and visceral sequestration with complete double bladder. *J Urol* 1994;**151**:455–6.

41 Hendren WH. Urological aspects of cloacal malformations. *J Urol* 1988;**140**:1207–13.

42 Allen TD, Husmann DA. Cloacal anomalies and other urorectal septal defects in female patients: a spectrum of anatomical abnormalities. *J Urol* 1991;**145**:1034–9.

43 Cerniglia FR, Roth DR, Gonzales ET. Covered exstrophy and visceral sequestration in a male newborn: case report. *J Urol* 1989;**141**:903–4.

44 Manzoni GA, Ransley PG, Hurwitz RS. Cloacal exstrophy and cloacal exstrophy variants: a proposed system of classification. *J Urol* 1987;**138**:1065–8.

45 Ransley PG, Manzoni GA, Hurwitz RS. Management of the bowel in cloacal exstrophy. *Dialog Pediatr Urol* 1990;**13**:2–3.

46 Gearhart JP, Jeffs RD. Augmentation cystoplasty in the failed exstrophy reconstruction. *J Urol* 1988;**139**:790–3.

47 Mirk M, Calisti A, Feleni A. Prenatal sonographic diagnosis of bladder exstrophy. *J Ultrasound Med* 1986;**5**:291.

48 Verco PW, Khor BH, Barbary J, Enthoven C. Ectopic vesicae *in utero*. *Australas Radiol* 1986;**30**:117.

49 Langer JC, Brennan B, Lappalainen RE *et al*. Cloacal exstrophy: prenatal diagnosis before rupture of the cloacal membrane. *J Pediatr Surg* 1992;**27**:1352–5.

50 Jeffs RD. Exstrophy and cloacal exstrophy. *Urol Clin North Am* 1978;**5**:127–39.

51 Cendron J. La reconstruction vésicale. *Ann Chir Infant* 1971;**12**:371.

52 Jeffs RD, Charrios R, Many M, Juransz AR. Primary closure of the exstrophied bladder. In: Scott R, ed. *Current Controversies in Urologic Management*. Philadelphia: WB Saunders, 1972:235.

53 Gearhart JP, Jeffs RD. Bladder exstrophy: increase in capacity following epispadias repair. *J Urol* 1989;**142**:525–6.

54 Jeffs RD, Guice SL, Oesch I. The factors in successful exstrophy closure. *J Urol* 1982;**127**:974.

55 Gearhart JP, Jeffs RD. Complications of exstrophy and epispadias repair. In: Smith RB, Ehrlich RM, eds. *Complications of Urologic Surgery*, 2nd edn. Philadelphia: WB Saunders, 1990:569.

56 Schultz WG. Plastic repair of exstrophy of the bladder combined with bilateral osteotomy of the ilia. *J Urol* 1958;**79**:453–8.

57 Bérard J, Bugman P, Mollard P. Faut-il fixer les ostéotomies pelviennes réalisées dans le cadre de l'exstrophie vésicale [Lecture]. Presented to the Meeting of the Société Française de Chirurgie Pédiatrique, Marseille, 1988.

58 Gokcora IH, Yazar T. Bilateral transverse iliac osteotomy in the correction of neonatal bladder exstrophy. *Int Surg* 1989;**74**:123.

59 Montagnani CA. Functional reconstruction of exstrophied bladder: timing and technique. Follow-up of 39 cases. *Kinderchirurgie* 1988;**43**:322.

60 Sponseller PD, Gearhart JP, Jeffs RD. Anterior innominate osteotomies for failure or late closure of bladder exstrophy. *J Urol* 1991;**146**:137–40.

61 Frey P, Cohen SJ. Blasenekstrophie — anteriore osteotomie des beckens — eine neue operative technik zur erleichterung der stabilisierung des beckens und des abdominalverschlusses. *Kinderchirurgie* 1988;**43**:171–3.

62 Frey P, Cohen SJ. Anterior pelvic osteotomy. A new operative technique facilitating primary bladder exstrophy closure. *Br J Urol* 1989;**64**:641–3.

63 Perovic S, Brdar R, Scepanovic D. Bladder exstrophy and anterior pelvic osteotomy. *Br J Urol* 1992;**70**:678–82.

64 McKenna PH, Khoury AE, McLorie GA, Churchill BM, Wedge JH. Anterior diagonal mid-innominate osteotomy. *Dialog Pediatr Urol* 1993;**16**:5–6.

65 McKenna PH, Khoury AE, McLorie GA *et al*. Iliac osteotomy:

a model to compare the options in bladder and cloacal exstrophy reconstruction. *J Urol* 1994;**151**:182–7.

66 Duckett JW. Epispadias. *Urol Clin North Am* 1978;**74**:729–37.

67 Spindel MR, Winslow BH, Jordan GH. The use of paraexstrophy flaps for urethral reconstruction in neonatal girls with classical exstrophy. *J Urol* 1988; **140**:574–6.

68 Gearhart JP, Peppas DS, Jeffs RD. Complications of paraexstrophy skin flaps in the reconstruction of classical bladder exstrophy. *J Urol* 1993;**150**:627–30.

69 Sumfest JM, Mitchell ME. Reconstruction of the umbilicus in exstrophy. *J Urol* 1994;**151**:453–4.

70 Hanna MK. Reconstruction of umbilicus during functional closure of bladder exstrophy. *Urology* 1986;**27**:340.

71 Hanna MK, Ansong K. Reconstruction of umbilicus in bladder exstrophy. *Urology* 1984;**24**:324.

72 Allen TD, Husmann DA, Bucholz RW. Exstrophy of the bladder: primary closure after iliac osteotomies without external or intenal fixation. *J Urol* 1992;**147**:438–40.

73 Büyükünal SNC. Interim report in humans of a previously described technique in an animal model: closure of bladder exstrophy with rectus abdominis muscle flap – II. *J Urol* 1994;**152**:706–9.

74 Cantwell FV. Operative treatment of epispadias by transplantation of the urethra. *Ann Surg* 1895;**22**:689.

75 Young HH. An operation for cure of incontinence associated with epispadias. *J Urol* 1922;**7**:1.

76 Gross RE, Cresson SL. Treatment of epispadias: a report of 18 cases. *J Urol* 1952;**68**:477–88.

77 Ransley PG, Duffy PG, Wolin M. Bladder exstrophy closure and epispadias repair. In: Dudley H, Caryer D, Russel RCG, eds. *Operative Surgery*. London: Butterworth, 1988:620–32.

78 Borzi PA, Thomas DFM. Cantwell–Ransley epispadias repair in male epispadias and bladder exstrophy. *J Urol* 1994;**151**:457–9.

79 Perovic S, Scepanovic D, Sremcevic D, Vukadinovic V. Epispadias surgery – Belgrade experience. *Br J Urol* 1992;**70**:674–7.

80 Diamond DA, Ransley PG. Improved glanuloplasty in epispadias repair: technical aspects. *J Urol* 1994;**152**:1243–5.

81 Mitchell ME, Bägli DJ. Complete penile disassembly for epispadias repair: the Mitchell technique. *J Urol* 1995;**155**:300–4.

82 Duckett JW. The island flap technique for hypospadias repair. *Urol Clin North Am* 1981;**8**:503–11.

83 Monfort G, Morisson-Lacombe G, Guys JM, Coquet M. Transverse island flap and double flap procedure in the treatment of congenital epispadias in 32 patients. *J Urol* 1987;**138**:1069–71.

84 Kramer SA, Jackson IT. Bilateral rhomboid flaps for reconstruction of external genitalia in epispadias exstrophy. *Plast Reconstr Surg* 1986;**77**:621–31.

85 Young HH. Exstrophy of the bladder: first case in which normal bladder and urinary control have been obtained by plastic operations. *Surg Gynecol Obstet* 1942;**74**:729–37.

86 Leadbetter GW. Surgical correction of total urinary incontinence. *J Urol* 1964;**91**:261–6.

87 Jeffs RD. Exstrophy, epispadias and cloacal and urogenital sinus abnormalities. *Pediatr Clin North Am* 1987;**34**:1233–57.

88 Gearhart JP. Bladder neck reconstruction in complete epispadias. *Dialog Pediatr Urol* 1987;**10**:2–3.

89 Marshall VT, Marchetti AA, Krantz KE. The correction of stress incontinence by simple vesico-urethral suspension. *Surg Gynecol Obstet* 1949;**88**:509–18.

90 Canning DA, Gearhart JP, Peppas DS, Jeffs RD. The cephalotrigonal reimplant in bladder neck reconstruction for patients with exstrophy or epispadias. *J Urol* 1993;**150**:156–8.

91 Lepor H, Jeffs RD. Primary bladder closure and bladder neck reconstruction in classical bladder exstrophy. *J Urol* 1983;**130**:1142–5.

92 Gearhart JP, Williams KA, Jeffs RD. Intraoperative urethral pressure profilometry as an adjunct to bladder neck reconstruction. *J Urol* 1986;**136**:1055–6.

93 Mollard P. Bladder reconstruction in exstrophy. *J Urol* 1980;**124**:525–9.

94 Mollard P, Mouriquand PDE, Buttin X. Urinary continence after reconstruction of classical bladder exstrophy (73 cases). *Br J Urol* 1994;**73**:298–302.

95 Jones JA, Mitchell ME, Rink, RC. Improved results using a modification of the Young–Dees–Leadbetter bladder neck repair. *Br J Urol* 1993;**71**:555–61.

96 Koff SA. A technique for bladder neck reconstruction in exstrophy: the cinch. *J Urol* 1990;**144**:546–9.

97 Hollowell JG, Ransley PG. Surgical management of incontinence in bladder exstrophy. *Br J Urol* 1991;**68**:543–8.

98 Longaker MT, Harrison MR, Langer JC, Crombleholme TM. Appendicovesicostomy: a new technique for bladder diversion during reconstruction of cloacal exstrophy. *J Pediatr Surg* 1989;**24**:639–41.

99 Burbige KA, Libby C. Enterovesical cystoplasty for bladder closure in bladder exstrophy. *J Urol* 1987;**137**:948–50.

100 Mitchell ME, Brito CG, Rink RC. Cloacal exstrophy reconstruction for urinary continence. *J Urol* 1990;**144**:554–8.

101 Mitrofanoff P. Cystostomie continent trans-appendiculaire dans le traitement des vessies neurologiques. *Chir Pediatr* 1980;**21**:297.

102 Benchekroun A, Essakalli N, Faik M. Continent urostomy with hydraulic ileal valve in 136 patients: 13 years of experience. *J Urol* 1989;**142**:46–51.

103 Hendren WH. Ileal nipple for continence in cloacal exstrophy. *J Urol* 1992;**148**:372–9.

104 Gearhart JP, Jeffs RD. Management of the failed bladder exstrophy closure. *J Urol* 1991;**146**:610–12.

105 Decter RM, Roth DR, Fishman IJ *et al.* Use of the AS800 device in exstrophy and epispadias. *J Urol* 1988;**140**:1202–3.

106 Ransley PG. Artificial urinary sphincter in the treatment of incontinence in patients with exstrophy and epispadias [Lecture]. Presented to the first meeting of the British Association of Paediatric Urologists, Cambridge. 1992.

107 Ransley PG. Management of cloacal exstrophy. *Dialog Pediatr Urol* 1990;**13**:2–3.

108 Etker S, Mouriquand PDE, Manzoni GA, Duffy PG, Ransley PG. Buccal graft mucosa and hypospadias repair [Poster presentation]. Presented to the American Academy of Pediatrics, Dallas, 1994.

109 Husmann DA, McLorie GA, Churchill BM. A comparison of renal function in the exstrophy patient treated with staged reconstruction versus urinary diversion. *J Urol* 1988;**140**:1204–6.

110 Mesrobian HG, Kelalis PP, Kramer SA. Long-term follow-up

of 103 patients with bladder exstrophy. *J Urol* 1988;**139**: 719–22.

111 Hensle TW. Editorial comment. *J Urol* 1990;**143**:774.

112 Eraklis AJ, Folkman MJ. Adenocarcinoma at the site of ureterosigmoidostomies for exstrophy of the bladder. *J Pediatr Surg* 1979;**13**:730.

113 Warren RB, Warner TFCS, Hafez GR. Late development of colonic adenocarcinoma 49 years after ureterosigmoidostomy for exstrophy of the bladder. *J Urol* 1980;**124**:550.

114 Zabbo A, Kay R. Ureterosigmoidostomy and bladder exstrophy: a long-term follow-up. *J Urol* 1986;**136**:396–7.

115 Woodhouse CRJ, Strachan JR. Malignancy in exstrophy patients [Abstract No. 61]. Presented to the meeting of the British Association of Urological Surgeons, Scarborough, 1990.

116 Purcell MH, Duckro PN, Schultz K, Gregory JG. Follow-up of ureterosigmoidostomy diversion for bladder exstrophy — behavioral biofeedback as an alternative treatment for fecal–urinary incontinence: a case report. *J Urol* 1987;**137**:945–7.

117 Stöckle M, Becht E, Voges G, Riedmiller H, Hohenfellner R. Ureterosigmoidostomy; an outdated approach to bladder exstrophy? *J Urol* 1990;**143**:770–5.

118 Bassiouny IE. Continent urinary reservoir in exstrophy/epispadias complex. *Br J Urol* 1992;**70**: 558–62.

119 Mollard P, Basset T, Deseubis M, Bringeon G. Résultats de la reconstruction vésicale et urétrale pour exstrophie. *Chir Pediatr* 1986;**27**:27–32.

120 Connor JP, Hensle TW, Lattimer JK, Burbige KA. Long-term followup of 207 patients with bladder exstrophy; an evolution in treatment. *J Urol* 1989;**142**:793–6.

121 Oesterling JE, Jeffs RD. The importance of a successful initial bladder closure in the surgical management of classical bladder exstrophy: analysis of 144 patients treated at the John Hopkins Hospital between 1975 and 1985. *J Urol* 1987;**137**: 258–62.

122 Hollowell JG, Hill PD, Duffy PG, Ransley PG. Evaluation and treatment of incontinence after bladder neck reconstruction in exstrophy and epispadias. *Br J Urol* 1993; **71**:743–9.

123 Merguerian PA, McLorie GA, McMullin ND *et al.* Continence in bladder exstrophy: determinants of success. *J Urol* 1991;**145**:350–2.

124 Gearhart JP, Jeffs RD. Exstrophy of the bladder, epispadias, and other bladder anomalies. In: Walsh PC, Retik AB, Starney TA, Vaughan ED Jr, eds. *Campbell's Urology*, Vol. 2, 6th edn. Philadelphia: WB Saunders, 1992:1772.

125 Bennett AH. Exstrophy of the bladder treated by ureterosigmoidostomies. *Urology* 1973;**2**:165.

126 Woodhouse CRJ, Ransley PG, Williams DI. The patient with exstrophy in adult life. *Br J Urol* 1983; **55**:632.

127 Woodhouse CRJ. The sexual and reproductive consequences of congenital genitourinary anomalies. *J Urol* 1994;**152**: 645–51.

128 Nielsen K, Nielsen KK. Adenocarcinoma in exstrophy bladder: the last case in Scandinavia? A case report and review of literature. *J Urol* 1983;**130**:1180–2.

129 Tuchmann-Duplessis H. *Embryologie du Sinus Uro-Génital in Embryologic-Organogenèse.* Paris: Ed. Masson, 1970: 66–87.

130 Gonzales J, Gonzales M, Mary JY. Size and weight study of human kidney growth velocity during the last three months of pregnancy. *Eur Urol* 1980;**6**:37–44.

131 Gonzales J. Relation structure et fonction dans le développement de l'appareil urinaire du foetus. *J Urol (Paris)* 1985;**91**: 108–117.

132 Troyer JR. Embryology of the urethra. *Dialog Pediatr Urol* 1987;**10**:2–4.

133 Altemus AR, Hutchins GM. Development of the human anterior urethra. *J Urol* 1991;**146**:1085–93.

134 Chwalla R. Ueber die Entwicklung der Harnblase und der Primären Harnröhre des Menschen mit Besonderer Berücksichtigung der Art und Weise, in der sich die Ureteren von der Urnierengängen Treunen, nebst Bemerkungen über die Entwicklung der Müllerschen Gänge und des Mastdarms. *Z Anat Entwicklungs* 1927;**83**:615–733.

135 Droës JTPM. Observations on the musculature of the urinary bladder and the urethra in the human fetus. *Br J Urol* 1974;**46**:179–85.

136 Brockis JG. The development of the trigone of the bladder with a report of a case of ectopic ureter. *Br J Urol* 1952;**24**: 192–200.

137 Bakker NJ. Valves in female urethra. *Urol Int* 1958;**6**:187.

138 Nesbit RM, McDonald HP, Busby S. Obstructive valves in the female urethra. *J Urol* 1964;**91**:79.

139 Stevens WE. Congenital obstruction of female urethra. *J Am Med Assoc* 1936;**106**:89.

140 Marsden RTH. Posterior urethral valves in adults. *Br J Urol* 1969;**41**:586–91.

141 Morgagni JB. *Adversaria Anatomica Omnia*, Part 1, Article 10. Padua: J. Cominus, 1719:5.

142 Langenbeck B. Mémoire sur la lithotomie. Cited by Campbeu MF. In: *Pediatric Urology*. Philadelphia: WB Saunders, 1937.

143 Budd G. Case of extraordinary dilatation of the kidneys, ureters and bladder. *Lancet* 1840;**1**:767.

144 Pickard. Cited by Campbell MF. In: *Pediatric Urology*. Philadelphia: WB Saunders, 1937.

145 Tolmatschew N. Ein Fau Scmilunaren Klappen der Harnröhre und von Vergrösserter Vesicula Prostatica. *Arch Pathol Anat* 1870;**49**:348.

146 Knox JHM, Sprunt TP. Congenital obstruction of the posterior urethra: report of a case in a boy aged five years. *Am J Dis Child* 1912;**4**:137.

147 Young HH, Frontz WA, Baldwin JC. Congenital obstructions of the posterior urethra. *J Urol* 1919;**3**: 289.

148 Robertson WB, Hayes JA. Congenital diaphragmatic obstruction of the male posterior urethra. *Br J Urol* 1969; **41**:592.

149 Bazy P. Rétrécissement congénital de l'urèthre chez l'homme. *Presse Med* 1903;**11**:215.

150 Stephens FD. Congenital intrinsic lesions of the posteror urethra. In: Stephens FD, ed. *Congenital Malformations of the Urinary Tract*. New York: Praeger, 1983:95–125.

151 Dewan PA, Zappala SM, Ransley PG, Duffy PG. Endoscopic reappraisal of the morphology of congenital obstruction of the posterior urethra. *Br J Urol* 1992;**70**:439–44.

152 Kaplan GW, Scherz HL. Infravesical obstruction. In: Kelalis PP, ed. *Clinical Pediatric Urology*, 3rd edn. Philadelphia: WB Saunders, 1992:821–64.

153 Ruano-Gil D, Coca-Payeras A, Tejedo-Mateu A. Obstruction and normal recanalization of the ureter in the human embryo: its relation to congenital ureteric obstruction. *Eur Urol* 1975;**1**:287–93.

154 Alcaraz A, Vinaixa F, Tejedo-Mateu A *et al.* Obstruction and

recanalization of the ureter during embryonic development. *J Urol* 1991;**145**:410–16.

155 Duckett JW, Snow BW. Disorders of the urethra and penis. In: Walsh PC, Gittes RF, Perlmutter AD, eds. *Campbell's Urology*, 5th edn. Philadelphia: WB Saunders, 1986:2000

156 Workman SJ, Kogan BA. Fetal bladder histology in posterior urethral valves and the prune belly syndrome. *J Urol* 1990;**144**:337–9.

157 Henneberry MO, Stephens FD. Renal hypoplasia and dysplasia in infants with posterior urethral valves. *J Urol* 1980;**123**:912–15.

158 Bellinger MF, Comstock CH, Grosso D, Zaino R. Fetal posterior urethral valves and renal dysplasia at 15 weeks gestational age. *J Urol* 1983;**128**:1238–9.

159 Beck AD. The effect of intra-uterine urinary obstruction upon the development of the fetal kidney. *J Urol* 1971;**105**:784.

160 Rittenberg MH, Hulbert WC, Snyder HM, Duckett JW. Protective factors in posterior urethral valves. *J Urol* 1988;**140**:993–6.

161 Greenfield SP, Hensle TW, Berdon WE, Geringer AM. Urinary extravasation in the newborn male with posterior urethral valves. *J Pediatr Surg* 1982;**17**:751–6.

162 Burbige KA, Hensle TW. Posterior urethral valves in the newborn: treatment and functional results. *J Pediatr Surg* 1987;**22**:165.

163 Symonds DA, Driscoll SG. Massive fetal ascites, urethral atresia and cytomegalic inclusion disease. *Am J Dis Child* 1974;**127**:895–7.

164 Parkhouse HF, Barratt TM, Dillon HS *et al.* Long-term outcome of boys with posterior urethral valves. *Br J Urol* 1988;**62**:59.

165 Ewalt DH, Howard PS, Blyth B. Is lamina propria matrix responsible for normal bladder compliance. *J Urol* 1992; **148**:544–9.

166 Elbadawi A, Meyer S, Malkowicz SB. Effects of short-term partial bladder obstruction on the rabbit detrusor: an ultrastructural study. *Neurourol Urodyn* 1989;**8**:89–93.

167 Kato K, Wein AJ, Kitada S. The functional effect of mild outlet obstruction on the rabbit urinary bladder. *J Urol* 1988;**140**:880–4.

168 Speakman MJ, Brading AF, Gilpin CJ. Bladder outflow obstruction: a cause of denervation supersensitivity. *J Urol* 1987;**138**:1461–6.

169 Nijman RJM, Scholtmeijer RJ. Complications of transurethral electro-incision of posterior urethral valves. *Br J Urol* 1991;**67**:324–6.

170 Husmann D, McConnell JD. The bladder's response to outlet obstruction. *Dialog Pediatr Urol* 1989;**12**:2–8.

171 Campaiola JM, Perlmutter AD, Steinhardt GF. Noncompliant bladder resulting from posterior urethral valves. *J Urol* 1985;**134**:708–10.

172 Lortat-Jacob S, Dietrich JC, Nihoul-Fékété C. Séquelles vésicales des valves de l'urèthre postérieur. Etude urodynamique de 14 cas. Implications thérapeutiques [Lecture]. Presented to the Congrès de Chirurgie Pédiatrique, Paris, 1990.

173 Peters GA, Bolkier M, Bauer SB *et al.* The urodynamic consequences of posterior urethral valves. *J Urol* 1990;**144**: 122–6.

174 Dinneen MD, Duffy PG, Barratt TM, Ransley PG. Persistent polyuria after valve ablation. *Br J Urol* 1994;**74**:785–9.

175 Connor JP, Burbige KA. Long-term urinary incontinence and renal function in neonates with posterior urethral valves. *J Urol* 1990;**144**:1209–11.

176 Sholder AJ, Maizels M, Depp R *et al.* Caution in antenatal intervention. *J Urol* 1988;**139**:1026–9.

177 Williams DI, Whitaker RH, Barratt TM, Keeton JE. Urethral valves. *Br J Urol* 1973;**45**:200.

178 Scott JES. Management of congenital posterior urethral valves. *Br J Urol* 1985;**57**:71.

179 Reinberg Y, Gonzales R, Fryd D, Mauer SM, Najarian JS. The outcome of renal transplantation in children with posterior urethral valves. *J Urol* 1988;**140**:1491–3.

180 Uehling DT. Posterior urethral valves: functional classification. *Urology* 1980;**15**:27.

181 Woodhouse CRJ, Reilly JM, Bahadur G. Sexual function and fertility in patients treated for posterior urethral valves. *J Urol* 1989;**142**:586–8.

182 Mouriquand P, Mollard P, Ransley PG. Dilemmes soulevés par le diagnostic anténatal des uropathies obstructives et leurs traitements. *Pediatrie* 1989;**44**: 357–63.

183 Amiel-Tison G, Lebrun F, Larroche JC. Circulation foetale et pourcentages de saturation de l'hémoglobine. In: *Médicine Néonatale. Encyclopédie Médico-Chirurgicale. Obstétrique.* Paris: 1979;**5114L30**:1

184 Arant BS. Clinical evaluation of neonatal renal function. *Dialog Pediatr Urol* 1987;**10**:2–4.

185 Bellinger MF. Evaluation of fetal renal function. *Dialog Pediatr Urol* 1987;**10**:4–5.

186 Moore ES. Glomerular hyperfiltration *in utero. Dialog Pediatr Urol* 1987;**10**:5–7.

187 Glazer GM, Filly RA, Callen PW. The varied sonographic appearance of the urinary tract in the fetus and newborn with urethral obstruction. *Radiology* 1982;**144**:563–8.

188 Grisoni ER, Gauderer MWL, Wolfson RN, Izant RJ, Cleveland JR. Antenatal ultrasonography: the experience in a high risk perinatal center. *J Pediatr Surg* 1986;**21**:358–61.

189 Gauderer MWL, Jassani MN, Izant RJ. Ultrasonographic antenatal diagnosis: will it change the spectrum of neonatal surgery? *J Pediatr Surg* 1984;**19**:404–7.

190 Bowie JD, Rosenberg EC, Andreotti RF, Fields SI. The changing sonographic appearance of fetal kidneys during pregnancy. *J Ultrasound Med* 1983;**2**:505–7.

191 Lawson TL, Foley WD, Berland LL, Clark KE. Ultrasonic evaluation of fetal kidneys. *Radiology* 1981;**138**:153–6.

192 Hulbert WC, Kotlus Rosenberg H, Cartwright PC, Duckett JW, Snyder HW. The predictive value of ultrasonography in evaluation of infants with posterior urethral valves. *J Urol* 1992;**148**:122–4.

193 Adzick NS, Harrison MR, Flake AW, Laberge JM. Development of a fetal renal function test using endogenous creatinine clearance. *J Pediatr Surg* 1985;**20**:602.

194 Reinberg Y, De Castano I, Gonzales R. Prognosis for patients with prenatally diagnosed posterior urethral valves. *J Urol* 1992;**148**:125–6.

195 Harrison MR, Golbus MS, Filly RA *et al.* Management of the fetus with congenital hydronephrosis. *J Pediatr Surg* 1982;**17**: 728.

196 Glick PL, Harrison MR, Golbus MS. Management of the fetus with congenital hydronephrosis. II. Prognosis criteria and selection for treatment. *J Pediatr Surg* 1985;**20**:276–87.

197 Elder JS, O'Grady PJ, Ashmead G, Duckett JW, Philipson E.

Evaluation of fetal renal function: unreliability of fetal urinary electrolytes. *J Urol* 1990;**144**:574–8.

198 Crombleholme TM, Harrison MR, Golbus MS *et al.* Fetal intervention in obstructive uropathy: prognostic indicators and efficacy of intervention. *Am J Obstet Gynecol* 1990; **162**:1239–44.

199 Potter EL. Bilateral renal agenesis. *J Pediatr* 1946;**29**:68.

200 Potter EL. Facial characteristics of infants with bilateral renal agenesis. *Am J Obstet Gynecol* 1946;**51**:885.

201 Potter EL. Oligohydramnios: further comments. *J Pediatr* 1974;**84**:931–2.

202 Symchych PS, Winchester P. Animal model: amniotic fluid deficiency and fetal lung growth in the rat. *Am J Pathol* 1978;**90**:779–82.

203 Van Der Vis Melsen MJE, Baert RJM, Rajnherc JR *et al.* Scintigraphic assessment of lower urinary tract function in children with and without outflow tract obstruction. *Br J Urol* 1989;**64**:263–9.

204 Groshar D, Embdon OM, Sazbon A, Koritny ES, Frenkel A. Radionuclide assessment of bladder outlet obstruction: a noninvasive (1-step) method for measurement of voiding time, urinary flow rates and residual urine. *J Urol* 1988;**139**: 266–9.

205 Williams DI, Eckstein HB. Obstructive valves in the posterior urethra. *J Urol* 1965;**93**:236.

206 Mollard P, Sarkissian S, Tostain J. Traitement des lésions du haut-appareil en amont des valves de l'urèthre postérieur (65 cas). *Chir Pediatr* 1981;**22**:411–15.

207 Rushton HG, Parrott TS, Woodard JR, McClellan W. The role of vesicostomy in the management of anterior urethral valves in neonates and infants. *J Urol* 1987;**138**:107–9.

208 Mollard P. In: Mollard P, ed. *Précis d'Urologie de l'Enfant.* Paris: Ed. Masson, 1984:264–94.

209 Randall A. Congenital valves of the posterior urethra. *Ann Surg* 1921;**73**:477.

210 Ehrlich RM, Shanberg A, Fine RN. Neomydium YAG lascr ablation of posterior urethral valves. *J Urol* 1987;**138**:959–62.

211 Ehrlich RM, Shanberg A. Neomydium YAG laser ablation of posterior urethral valves. *Dialog Pediatr Urol* 1988;**11**:4–5.

212 Biewald W, Schier F. Laser treatment of posterior urethral valves in neonates. *Br J Urol* 1992;**69**:425–7.

213 Zaontz MR, Gibbons MD. An antegrade technique for ablation of posterior urethral valves. *J Urol* 1984;**132**:982.

214 Datta NS. Percutaneous transvesical antegrade ablation of posterior urethral valves. *Urology* 1987;**30**: 561–4.

215 Whitaker RH, Sherwood T. An improved hook for destroying posterior urethral valves. *J Urol* 1986;**135**:531–2.

216 Diamond DA, Ransley PG. Fogarty balloon catheter ablation of neonatal posterior urethral valves. *J Urol* 1987;**137**: 1209–11.

217 Kalicinski HZH. Foley's balloon procedure in posterior urethral valve. *Dialog Pediatr Urol* 1988;**11**:7.

218 Garg SK, Lawrie JH. The perineal urethrotomy approach to posterior urethral valves. *J Urol* 1983;**130**: 1146–9.

219 Gonzales ET Jr. Posterior urethral valves and bladder neck obstruction. *Urol Clin North Am* 1978;**5**:57.

220 Johnston JH. Vesicoureteral reflux with urethral valves. *Br J Urol* 1979;**51**:100.

221 Bauer SA, Dieppa RA, Labib KK, Retik AB. The bladder in boys with posterior urethral valves. *J Urol* 1979;**121**: 769.

222 McGuire EJ, Weiss RM. Secondary bladder neck obstruction in patients with urethral valves. *Urology* 1975;**5**:756.

223 Whitaker RH. The ureter in posterior urethral valves. *J Urol* 1973;**45**:395.

224 Dhillon HK, Gordon I, Ransley PG, Duffy PG. The antegrade pressure perfusion study in infants with prenatally diagnosed hydronephrosis [Lecture]. Presented to the 59th Annual Meeting of the Boston, (Section of Urology), American Academy of Pediatrics, 1990.

225 Dhillon HK, Duffy PG, Gordon I, Ransley PG. A randomised clinical trial in infants with prenatally diagnosed unilateral hydronephrosis [Lecture]. Presented to the 61st Annual Meeting of the American Academy of Pediatrics, (Section of Urology), San Francisco, 1992.

226 Glassberg KL, Schneider M, Haller J. Observations of persistently dilated ureter after posterior urethral valve ablation. *Urology* 1982;**20**:20.

227 Hendren WH. Posterior urethral valves in boys: a broad clinical spectrum. *J Urol* 1971;**106**:298.

228 Monfort G, Morisson-Lacombe G, Bensoussan A, Carcassonne M. Les valvules de l'urètre postérieur chez le garçon. *Ann Chir Infant* 1976;**17**:15.

229 Cukier J. Compte-rendu de l'Assemblé Internationale d'Urologie Pédiatrique. Pinchurst 1980. *J Urol (Paris)* 1981; **87**:97.

230 Johnston JH, Kulatilake AE. The sequelae of posterior urethral valves. *Br J Urol* 1971;**43**:743.

231 Cass AS, Stephens FD. Posterior urethral valves: diagnosis and management. *J Urol* 1974;**112**:519.

232 Reinberg Y, De Castano I, Gonzales R. Influence of initial therapy on progression of renal failure and body growth in children with posterior urethral valves. *J Urol* 1992;**148**: 532–3.

233 Kimche D, Lash D. Congenital polyp of the posterior urethra. *J Urol* 1982;**127**:134.

234 Cendron J, Melin Y, Baviera D, Alaoui-Drai A. Polypes de l'urètre postérieur. A propos de 6 cas. *Chir Pediatr* 1985; **26**:356–61.

235 Foster RS, Garrett RA. Congenital posterior urethral polyp. *J Urol* 1986;**136**:670–2.

236 Dodat H, Paulhac JB, Macabeo V, Bouvier R. Tumeurs bénignes de l'urètre postérieur chez l'enfant. A propos d'un cas exceptionnel de rhabdomyome de type foetal. *J Urol (Paris)* 1987;**93**:43–6.

237 Goldstein AMB, Bragin SD, Terry R, Yoell JH. Prostatic urethral polyps in adults: histopathologic variations and clinical manifestations. *J Urol* 1981;**126**:129.

238 Devine PC, Kessel HC. Surgical correction of urethral prolapse. *J Urol* 1980;**123**:856.

239 Schuhrke TD, Kaplan GW. Prostatic utricle cysts (müllerian duct cysts). *J Urol* 1978;**119**:765.

240 Van Poppel H, Verreecken R, Degetter P, Verduyn H. Hemosperm owing to utricular cyst: embryological summary and surgical review. *J Urol* 1983;**129**:608.

241 Kaplan KW, Piconi J. Müllerian duct and terminal vesical cyst. *Birth Defects* 1977;**13**:241.

242 Sholem SL, Weschler M, Roberts M. Management of the urethral diverticulum in women: a modified operative technique. *J Urol* 1974;**112**:485–6.

243 Cukier J, Foix E, Vacant J. Les poches sous-uréthrales chez la femme adulte. *J Urol Nephrol* 1976;**3**:161–72.

244 Davis BL, Robinson DG. Diverticula of the female urethra: essay of 120 cases. *J Urol* 1970;**104**:850–3.

245 Benoit G, Boccon-Gibod L, Steg A. Les poches sous-urétrales sont-elles une affection bénigne? *Ann Urol* 1983;**17**:151–2.

246 Effmann EL, Lebowitz RL, Colodny AH. Duplication of the urethra. *Radiology* 1976;**119**:179.

247 Kossow JH, Morales PA. Duplication of the bladder and the urethra and associated anomalies. *Urology* 1973;**1**:71.

248 Kennedy HA, Steidle CP, Mitchell ME, Rink RC. Collateral urethral duplication in the frontal plane: a spectrum of cases. *J Urol* 1988;**139**:332–4.

249 Gülerçe Z, Nazli O, Killi R, Girgin C, Erhan O. Trifurcation of the urethra: a case report. *J Urol* 1992;**148**:403–4.

250 Williams DI, Kenawi MM. Urethral duplications in the male. *Eur Urol* 1975;**1**:209.

251 Woodhouse CRJ, Williams DI. Duplications of the lower urinary tract in children. *Br J Urol* 1979;**51**:481.

252 Psihramis KE, Colodny AH, Lebowitz RL, Retik AB, Bauer SB. Complete patent duplication of the urethra. *J Urol* 1986;**136**:63–7.

253 Kapoor R, Saha MM. Complete duplication of the bladder, urethra and external genitalia in a neonate. A case report. *J Urol* 1987;**137**:1243–4.

254 Sharma SK, Kapoor R, Kumar A, Mandal AK. Incomplete epispadiac urethral duplication with dorsal penile curvature. *J Urol* 1987;**138**:585–6.

255 Holst S, Peterson NE. Fulguration–ablation of atypical accessory urethra. *J Urol* 1988;**140**:347–8.

256 Rabinovitch HH. Urethral duplication. *Dialog Pediatr Urol* 1987;**10**:7–8.

257 Ortolano V, Nasrallah PF. Urethral duplication. *J Urol* 1986;**136**:909.

258 De Nicola RR, McCartney RC. Urethral duplication in female child treated with sclerotic solution. *J Urol* 1949;**61**:1065.

259 Boissonnat P. Two cases of complete double functional urethra with a single bladder. *Br J Urol* 1961;**33**:453.

260 Bellinger MF, Duckett JW. Accessory phallic urethra in the female patient. *J Urol* 1982;**127**:1159.

261 Sotolongo JR, Gribetz ME, Saphir RL, Begun GR. Female phallic urethra and persistent cloaca. *J Urol* 1983;**130**:1186–7.

262 Bonney WW, Young HH, Levin D, Goodwin WE. Complete duplication of the urethra with vaginal stenosis. *J Urol* 1975;**113**:132.

263 Nesbitt TE. Congenital megalourethra. *J Urol* 1955; **73**:839.

264 Appel RA, Kaplan GW, Brock WA, Streit D. Megalourethra. *J Urol* 1986;**135**:747–51.

265 Kester RR, Mooppan UMM, Ohm HK, Kim H. Congenital megalourethra. *J Urol* 1990;**143**:1213–15.

266 Mortensen PHG, Johnson HW, Coleman GU *et al.* Megalourethra. *J Urol* 1985;**134**:358–61.

267 Dorairajan T. Defects of spongy tissue and congenital diverticula of the penile urethra. *Aust N Z J Surg* 1963;**32**: 209.

268 Lockart JL, Reeve HR, Krueger RP, Glenn JF, Henry HH. Megalourethra. *Urology* 1978;**12**:58.

269 Locke JR, Noe HN. Megalourethra: surgical technique for correction of an unusual variant. *J Urol* 1987;**138**:110–11.

270 Cook WA, Stephens FD. Congenital lesions of the anterior urethra. Developmental anomalies and their management. In: King LR, ed. *Problems in Urology*, Vol. 2. Philadelphia: Lippincott, 1988:81–6.

271 Ortlip SA, Gonzales R, Williams RD. Diverticula of the male urethra. *J Urol* 1980;**114**:350.

272 Firlit CF. Urethral abnormalities. *Urol Clin North Am* 1978;**5**:31.

273 Bissada NK, Hanash KA. Obstructive urethral diverticula in children. *Urology* 1982;**30**:281–3.

274 Baker AR, Neoptomelos JP, Wood KF. Congenital anterior urethral diverticulum: a rare cause of lower urinary tract obstruction in childhood. *J Urol* 1985;**134**: 751–2.

275 Kusuda L, Das S. Anterior urethral valves. *Scand J Urol Nephrol* 1989;**23**:231.

276 Williams DI, Retik AB. Congenital valves and diverticula of the anterior urethra. *Br J Urol* 1969;**41**:228.

277 Scherz HC, Kaplan GW, Packer MG. Anterior urethral valves in the fossa navicularis in children. *J Urol* 1987;**138**:1211.

278 Graham SD, Krueger RP, Glenn JF. Anterior urethral diverticulum associated with posterior urethral valves. *J Urol* 1982;**128**:376.

279 Foster RS, Weigel JW, Mantr FA. Anterior urethral polyps. *J Urol* 1980;**124**:145.

280 Moriya K, Kobayakawa H, Yasumoto R. Anterior urethral polyps. *Br J Urol* 1988;**62**:183.

281 Cook FE, Shaw JL. Cystic anomalies of the ducts of Cowper's gland. *J Urol* 1961;**85**:659.

282 Weinberger MA. Urethral cysts arising in Cowper's gland ducts. Etiology, pathogenesis and clinico-pathologic aspects. *J Urol* 1961;**85**:818.

283 Abrams HJ, Joshi DP, Neier CR. Intra uterine urinary retention and electrolyte imbalance secondary to Cowper's gland cyst. *J Urol* 1966;**95**:565.

284 Howell G, Lisansky ET, Scott E. Congenital cysts of the urethra in a three-week old male infant causing pyonephrosis and death. *Bull Med Maryland* 1942;**26**:241.

285 Brock WA, Kaplan GW. Lesions of Cowper's glands in children. *J Urol* 1979;**122**:121.

286 Nan Hyuk L, Sang Youn K. Skene's duct cysts in female newborns. *J Pediatr Surg* 1992;**27**:15–17.

287 Gottesman JE, Sparkuhl A. Bilateral Skene's duct cysts. *J Pediatr* 1979;**94**:945–6.

288 Blaivas JG, Pais VM, Retik AB. Paraurethral cyst in female neonate. *Urology* 1976;**7**:504–7.

289 Cohen HJ, Klein MD, Laver MB. Cysts of the vagina in the newborn infant. *Am J Dis Child* 1957;**94**:322–4.

290 Bartone FF. Abnormalities of the urethra, penis, and scrotum. In: Welch KJ, Randolph JG, O'Neil J, eds. *Pediatric Surgery*. Chicago: Year Book, 1986:1314–26.

291 Mitre A, Nahas W, Gilbert A *et al.* Urethral prolapse in girls: familial case. *J Urol* 1987;**137**:115.

292 Klaus H, Stein RT. Urethral Prolapse in young girls. *Pediatrics* 1973;**52**:645.

293 Devine CJ Jr, Gonzales-Serva L, Stecker JF Jr. Utricular configuration in hypospadias and intersex. *J Urol* 1980; **123**:407.

294 Lowe FC, Hill GS, Jeffs RD, Brendler CB. Urethral prolapse in children: insights into etiology and management. *J Urol* 1986; **135**:100–3.

295 Richardson DA, Hajj SN, Herbst AL. Medical treatment of urethral prolapse in children. *Obstet Gynecol* 1982;**59**:69.

296 Turner RW. Urethral prolapse in female children. *Urology* 1973;**2**:530.

297 Akpo EC, Aguessy-Ahyi B, Padonou N *et al.* Le prolapsus

muqueux urétral de l'enfant au CHU de cotonou. A propos de 13 observations. *J Urol (Paris)* 1983;**89**:351.

298 Capraro VJ, Bayonet-Rivera NP, Magoss I. Vulvur tumor in children due to prolapse of urethral mucosa. *Am J Obstet Gynecol* 1970;**108**:572.

299 Harshman MW, Cromie WJ, Wein AJ. Urethral stricture disease in children. *J Urol* 1981;**126**:650.

300 Palmer JM, Russi MF. Persistent urogenital sinus with absence of the bladder and urethra. *J Urol* 1969; **102**:590.

301 Aaronson IA, Cremin BJ. Lower urinary tract obstruction. In: *Clinical Paediatric Uroradiology*. Edinburgh: Churchill Livingstone, 1984:210–32.

302 Valiki BF. Agenesis of the bladder: a case report. *J Urol* 1973; **109**:510–11.

303 Knight H, Phillips N, Mouriquand PDE. Female hypospadias a case report *J Pediatr Surg* 1995;**30**:1738–40.

304 Cobb BG, Wolf SA, Ansell JS. Congenital stricture of the proximal urethral bulbe. *J Urol* 1968;**99**:629.

305 Kelalis PP. Anterior urethra. In: Kelalis PP, King LR, Belman AB, eds. *Clinical Pediatric Urology.* Philadelphia: WB Saunders, 1976:328–41.

306 Michon J. Rétrécissement 'familial' de l'urètre. *J Urol Nephrol (Paris)* 1978;**84**:107.

307 Redman JF, Fraiser LP. Apparent congenital anterior urethral strictures in brothers. *J Urol* 1979;**122**:707.

308 Allen JS, Summers JL, Wickerson JE. Meatal calibration in newborn boys. *J Urol* 1972;**107**:498.

309 Bueschen AJ, Royal SA. Urethral meatal stenosis in a girl causing severe hydronephrosis. *J Urol* 1986;**136**:1302–3.

310 Lyon RP, Smith DR. Distal urethral stenosis. *J Urol* 1963; **89**:414.

311 Lyon RP, Tanagho EA. Distal urethral stenosis in little girls. *J Urol* 1965;**93**:379.

312 Lyon RP. Distal urethral stenosis. In: Johnston JH, Goodwin WE, eds. *Reviews in Pediatric Urology.* Amsterdam: Excerpta Medica, 1974.

313 Graham JB, King LR, Kropp KA, Uehling DT. Significance of distal urethral narrowing in young girls. *J Urol* 1967;**97**: 1045.

314 Averous M, Guiter J, Grasset D. Les sténoses urétrales de la fillette: mythe ou réalité. *J Urol (Paris)* 1981;**87**:67.

315 Manuel EJ, Seery WH, Cole AT. Capillary hemangioma of the male urethra: case report with literature review. *J Urol* 1977;**117**:804.

316 Steinhardt G, Perlmutter A. Urethral hemangioma. *J Urol* 1987;**137**:116–17.

317 Moormann JG. Congenital bulbar urethral stenosis as a cause of disease of the urogenital junction. *Urologe* 1972;**11**: 157–60.

318 Cranston D, Davies AH, Smith JC. Cobb's collar — a forgotten entity. *Br J Urol* 1990;**66**:294–6.

319 Glenister JW. A correlation of the normal and abnormal development of the penile urethra and of the infra umbilical abdominal wall. *Br J Urol* 1958;**30**:117–26.

15 Congenital Anomalies of the Testis and Scrotum

J.Spencer Barthold and J.F.Redman

Introduction

Congenital anomalies of the testis and surrounding structures are significant because of their frequency, the risk of bilateral effect despite unilateral disease and the long interval between treatment and determination of prognosis. These characteristics apply particularly to cryptorchidism, varicocele and testicular torsion and, consequently, the optimal management of these disorders remains controversial.

Cryptorchidism

Aetiology and pathophysiology

Cryptorchidism, meaning 'hidden testis', encompasses a range of disorders including anorchia, testicular ectopy and truly undescended testes. Anorchia is most commonly due to prenatal demise of a previously formed testis due to torsion or vascular accident, since blind-ending spermatic vessels and vas with calcification and haemosiderin deposition are often present and ipsilateral müllerian ductal structures are absent [1,2]. Testicular ectopy is presumably due to abnormal migration of the gubernaculum or obstruction of the normal pathway to descent [3]. Ectopic testes in the superficial inguinal pouch (anterior to the rectus sheath) are common; while perineal, penile and penopubic ectopy is rare [4,5]. A true undescended testis occurs as an isolated anomaly (which may be hereditary) or in association with intersex disorders, deficiencies in the synthesis or action of testicular hormones, or congenital malformation syndromes [6,7]. The frequent association of gonadotropin or androgen insufficiency with undescended testes suggests that androgens are required for normal testicular descent. Abnormalities of the synthesis or action of müllerian-inhibiting substance (MIS) (or anti-müllerian hormone) are also associated with cryptorchidism, due to failure of direct MIS stimulation of testicular descent or mechanical blockade of descent by persistent müllerian duct structures

[8,9]. Patients with genital ambiguity or hypospadias in addition to cryptorchidism are found to have intersex disorders in 53 and 27% of cases, respectively [10].

The population of patients with isolated cryptorchidism appears to be heterogeneous. Some patients have abnormalities which suggest that forme fruste hypogonadotropic hypogonadism is present [11–13] (Table 15.1). The aetiology of these hormonal and developmental anomalies is unknown. Although androgen production at puberty is unimpaired in cryptorchid males, early postnatal hormone deficiency may contribute to subnormal testicular exocrine function in adulthood [12].

Many clinical and experimental data suggest that one or more testicular hormones stimulate testicular descent. Androgens appear to be required for descent of human (see above), rodent [14,15] and porcine [16] testes, although experimental evidence suggests that other hormones and/or factors may be important [8,17]. Conclusive evidence of a direct role for MIS is lacking to date [9]. Other factors which may or may not be regulated by androgens, such as epidermal growth factor, calcitonin gene-related peptide (CGRP) or as yet unidentified testicular substances, may also participate in testicular descent (8,18–20]. Although the embryology of human descent has been more fully elucidated in recent years, the exact role of hormonal and mechanical factors in this process remains poorly understood. It is known that the testis forms in the presence of the SRY gene (sex-determining region, Y

Table 15.1 Data supporting an underlying endocrinopathy in boys with isolated cryptorchidism.

Reduced postnatal surge in serum testosterone and luteinizing hormone
Atrophy of neonatal Leydig cells
Delayed or absent germ cell maturation
Bilateral histological abnormalities and impaired semen quality in unilateral disease
Epididymal anomalies
Increased risk of tumour in contralateral descended testes

chromosome) [21] and remains adjacent to the future inguinal canal until the 24th week of gestation [3,22,23]. The testis and epididymis are anchored distally by the gubernaculum, a jelly-like mesenchymal structure which rarely extends beyond the external ring [3,23]. Prior to descent, the spermatic cord elongates, the gubernaculum begins to swell and a peritoneal evagination (the processus vaginalis), accompanied by the cremaster muscle, migrates distally within the peripheral gubernaculum [3]. The remarkable increase in gubernacular bulk is due to an increase in extracellular matrix material and uptake of water, and causes dilatation of the inguinal canal, presumably to allow the passage of the testis [3]. Testicular descent usually occurs between 24 and 28 weeks' gestation; the testis and gubernaculum (which is unattached distally) rapidly traverse the canal together. Subsequent gubernacular regression and movement of the testis to a dependent scrotal position occur gradually [23].

There are a number of hypotheses of hormonal–mechanical interaction during testicular descent in humans, but none are proven and some are not supported by embryological data [23]. Traction by the gubernaculum or cremaster cannot occur since these structures do not have a distal point of attachment during descent. Some investigators report that the gubernaculum attaches solely to the epididymis and postulate that normal epididymal descent is necessary for testicular descent [24]. However, gubernacular swelling and distal migration of the processus vaginalis appear to be the most critical events in epididymotesticular descent, and identification of the factor(s) which controls these processes is critical. The gubernacula of pigs and dogs is similar to humans; in these species gubernacular swelling is testis dependent, but not necessarily androgen dependent [17]. In rodents, gubernacular anatomy is somewhat different in that swelling of the mesenchyme is subtle and the processus vaginalis is comprised of cremasteric muscle [17]. Formation of the rat cremasteric sac appears to require innervation of the cremaster muscle by the genitofemoral nerve (GFN) and release of CGRP by GFN fibres; processes which may or may not be androgen dependent [8,25]. Confirmation of a role for the GFN in mammals with a peritoneal processus vaginalis must await further studies.

Incidence and classification

A classic report by Scorer reported an incidence of isolated cryptorchidism of 4.3% at birth (21% in premature males), 1% at 3 months and 0.8% at 1 year of age [26]. Recently, a higher incidence of cryptorchidism in infancy was noted in one series (rates of 4.9% at birth and 1.55% at age 3 months) [27] but not in another (rates of 3.7% at birth, 1.1% at age 3 months and 1.0% at age 1 year) [28]. The likelihood of spontaneous descent is greatest in premature and/or low birth weight infants and decreases significantly after the age of 3 months.

Although an increased incidence of cryptorchidism has not been confirmed, a marked increase in the rate of orchidopexy has been reported in recent years [29,30]. The possible causes of these increasing rates include misdiagnosis of retractile testes as undescended testes and 'ascent' of testes previously noted to be descended. The former may be more likely as testicular retractility to the scrotal neck or above occurs in 65% of boys aged 6 months to 11 years [31]. Retractile testes are defined as testes which reside extrascrotally, but can be manipulated into a dependent scrotal position at least temporarily [32]. Differentiation of retractile testes from truly undescended testes may occasionally be difficult but is best achieved by examination of the patient in a supine position with the hips externally rotated and abducted and the knees flexed or in a squatting position [32,33]. Ascent of the testis appears to be uncommon [34–36]. Possible causes of apparent or real testicular ascent include relative spermatic cord shortening with age, an associated hernia or a testis in the superficial inguinal pouch which can be manipulated into the scrotum during infancy but becomes less mobile with age [33–36]. Testes may ascend in patients with a history of retractility or of previous spontaneous descent in infancy [27,32,35]. Because difficulties may be encountered in differentiating retractile from truly undescended testes, and some retractile testes may ascend, it is advisable to reexamine boys with retractile testes periodically until puberty [32].

True undescended testes may initially be classified as palpable or non-palpable [33,37]. The exact position is best determined by both physical examination and surgical findings since interobserver variation based solely on an examination may be marked [38]. Palpable testes may be subclassified as ectopic or located along the normal path of descent. Iatrogenic cryptorchid testes are those which are undescended after previous inguinal surgery. Non-palpable testes comprise approximately 20% of cryptorchid testes and are extra-abdominal, intra-abdominal or absent [39]. Canalicular testes may not be palpable due to atrophy or associated obesity. Testicular absence due to agenesis is extremely rare, while absence due to presumed torsion (blind-ending vessels and vas, 'vanishing' testis) comprises 20–40% of cases of non-palpable testis [7]. Contralateral testicular hypertrophy is suggestive of, but not diagnostic of, monorchia [40,41].

Management

The finding of histological abnormalities in cryptorchid testes by the age of 1 year and the reduced likelihood of spontaneous descent after the age of 3 months has prompted recent recommendations for treatment at or soon after 1 year of age [7]. Optimal treatment remains controversial.

Palpable testes

Options for the management of palpable testes include surgery or hormonal therapy with human chorionic gonadotropin (hCG), luteinizing hormone-releasing hormone (LHRH) or both. Specific indications for surgery include ectopic testes, iatrogenic cryptorchidism or clinical hernia. Placement of palpable testes in a scrotal position is successful in the majority of cases (94% in one large series [42]). If adequate spermatic vessel length is in question, and particularly if a long-looping vas is present, dissection between the vas and vessels should be avoided and Fowler–Stephens orchidopexy (spermatic vessel transection) should be considered. Retroperitoneal or transperitoneal mobilization of the spermatic vessels may achieve adequate spermatic vessel length for orchidopexy without vessel transection. If the length of the vessels remains inadequate, options include microvascular or staged orchidopexy or orchiectomy. The benefits of primary surgical treatment of undescended testes include the repair of a frequently associated hernia, assessment of epididymal configuration and a high success rate. Testicular biopsy at the time of orchidopexy has been recommended for determination of the number of spermatogonia per tubule (S:T ratio) and assessment of potential fertility prognosis [43]. Biopsy is safe in adults [44], but its effect on the long-term function of the infant testis is not known. If performed, injury to subcapsular vessels is least likely at the medial and lateral aspects of the upper pole [45].

The benefits of primary hormonal therapy include avoidance or facilitation of surgery and a low risk. However, success rates for hormonal therapy are variable and not as good as those reported for surgery (Table 15.2). Because classification of testicular position is often variable [38], placebo-controlled trials are most reliable, yet many report poor results. Older patients, those with more caudally situated testes or retractile testes, or those with testes documented to be scrotal at birth tend to respond more favourably to hormonal therapy [46,47,51]. However,

Table 15.2 Results of hormonal therapy for cryptorchidism [46–53].

Treatment	Success rate (%)	
	Controlled studies	Uncontrolled studies
LHRH	8–38	13–78
hCG	6–23	25–55
LHRH and hCG	–	38–67
Buserelin	26	–

hCG, human chorionic gonadotropin; LHRH, luteinizing hormone-releasing hormone.

recurrent cryptorchidism may occur in up to 70% of patients after long-term follow-up [52]. Buserelin, an LHRH analogue, may stimulate descent of prescrotal testes when used in dosages low enough to prevent pituitary down-regulation (10–20 µg daily or every other day) [53]. In addition, buserelin has been recommended for stimulation of germ cell maturation in patients with a low S:T ratio (≤0.1) [54]. Short-term studies confirm improvement in the mean S:T ratio of buserelin-treated testes, but the long-term impact on fertility is not known.

Non-palpable testes

Non-palpable testes respond poorly to hormonal therapy and surgery is indicated in most cases. However, if neither testis is palpable, anorchia can be reliably diagnosed and surgical exploration avoided if there is both an elevation of serum gonadotrophins (particularly follicle-stimulating hormone, FSH) and an absence of any rise in serum testosterone in response to hCG stimulation [55]. Exceptions include post-pubertal males with secondary testicular failure characterized by elevated serum gonadotrophins and an absent response to hCG and anorchid boys aged 3–9 years, in whom FSH and LH may be normal (but gonadotrophin response to LHRH stimulation is exaggerated) [56]. As imaging studies are not reliable for localization of non-palpable testes [57], laparoscopy may be particularly useful in patients with suspected anorchia but equivocal hormonal studies or after a previous 'negative' inguinal exploration for a non-palpable testis. In addition, laparoscopy may be helpful for localization and even primary treatment of intra-abdominal testes [58–63]. Even in young infants, the procedure is usually technically successful and safe. Non-palpability of the testis and cord structures is confirmed after induction of anaesthesia, prior to laparoscopy. If intra-abdominal blind-ending vessels are visualized, no further surgery is needed unless placement of a testicular prosthesis is planned. If the vas and vessels exit the internal ring and the processus vaginalis is not patent, an intracanalicular testicular remnant is usually present, whereas an open processus vaginalis is associated with a viable testis in most cases [61–63]. Excision of extra-abdominal blind-ending vessels and vas is indicated as microscopic tubules are present in 5–13% of cases examined [2,59,61,62]. Contralateral scrotal orchidopexy has been advocated in patients with monorchia, yet the risk of torsion of the remaining testis appears to be minimal [64]. If no spermatic vessels are found laparoscopically, laparotomy is necessary to confirm testicular agenesis [61].

Results of surgery

A recent meta-analysis by Docimo summarizes the results of surgery for cryptorchidism [65]. In this review, a successful result was defined as a scrotal position and lack of atrophy of the testis. The results of this study are summarized in Table 15.3. Analysis of these data suggests that surgical success is significantly less for proximally-located testes, that staged Fowler–Stephens orchidopexy may not be superior to the original Fowler–Stephens technique and that microvascular autotransplantation may be superior to other orchidopexy techniques for intraabdominal testes. The fact that more than 25% of orchidopexies for abdominal testes are considered failures underscores the lack of an optimal procedure in these cases. Although a testis emerging from the internal ring may be amenable to standard orchidopexy, postoperative testicular position may be suboptimal in many cases [42]. High rates of atrophy were noted in one series of staged orchidopexy after long-term follow-up, suggesting that this approach may be more hazardous because of potential injury to both the vas and vessels [66]. The use of microvascular orchidopexy is limited by the requirement for technical expertise and possible increased difficulty and risk of testicular atrophy in young infants [67–69]. Laparoscopy is being used for both diagnosis and therapy of high undescended testes, but insufficient data are available to support its routine use. Laparoscopic clip placement in two-stage Fowler-Stephens orchidopexy [70], laparoscopic orchiectomy [60,71] and laparoscopy-assisted orchidopexy [72,73] have all been used in selected cases. The latter procedure is performed by mobilization of the spermatic vessels, creation of a new medially placed 'inguinal ring' and scrotal pouch orchidopexy without inguinal exploration or spermatic vessel transection.

Prognosis

Untreated cryptorchidism results in progressive deterioration in spermatogenesis within the affected testis. However, the degree to which this effect is reversed by the

Table 15.3 Results of orchidopexy. Data from [65].

	No. of cases reviewed	Success (%)
Testicular position		
Abdominal	842	74
Peeping	294	82
Canalicular	681	87
Distal	674	93
Type of orchidopexy		
Inguinal	1566	89
Transabdominal	80	81
Fowler–Stephens	321	67
Staged Fowler–Stephens	56	77
Two-stage	248	73
Microvascular	86	84

various forms of treatment is unclear. Mean sperm density is reduced in men with a history of unilateral or bilateral cryptorchidism but is more severe in the latter group (Table 15.4). The type and timing of treatment have not been shown conclusively to influence fertility, as estimated by semen analysis, in most studies [74]. Despite a significant incidence of depressed sperm density in previously cryptorchid men, remarkably good paternity data have been reported (see Table 15.4). Although proof of paternity cannot be obtained for ethical reasons, impregnation is clearly possible even for some patients with severe oligospermia, and may be a better measure of fertility than sperm density alone [76].

Malignant transformation of germ cells is more likely in cryptorchid men; a risk factor of 4.7-fold was recently reported as compared to 40–50-fold in older studies [77]. Approximately 15–20% of tumours occur in a contralateral descended testis. The tumours in scrotal testes after previous orchidopexy are usually non-seminomatous (50–71%), while those arising in abdominal testes are most frequently seminomas (60–87%) [78–80]. Giwercman and associates found carcinoma *in situ* (CIS) in 1.7–3% of testes of men with a history of cryptorchidism and have estimated that the risk of subsequent transformation of CIS to invasive carcinoma is at least 50% [81]. Consequently, these authors recommend biopsy of all previously cryptorchid testes in adults, followed by unilateral orchiectomy with contralateral biopsy if CIS is diagnosed, and radiation therapy if CIS is present in the remaining testis.

Other testicular anomalies

Polyorchidism (supernumerary testis) is extremely rare and postulated to result from transverse division of the genital ridge [82–84]. The left side is usually affected and the patient most commonly presents with a scrotal mass. The supernumerary testis may share an epididymis and vas or vas only with its ipsilateral mate; less frequently it lacks both epididymal and vasal attachments. Associated problems include cryptorchidism (15–50%), hernia (20–30%), torsion (13%) or tumour (1–5%). Exploration is indicated for diagnosis or treatment of the associated abnormalities.

Transverse testicular ectopia is also rare and is defined as two ipsilateral testes with absence of a contralateral testis

Table 15.4 Fertility in cryptorchidism. Data from [74–76].

	Unilateral (%)	Bilateral (%)
Oligospermia	31	31
Azoospermia	14	42
Oligospermia or azoospermia	43	75
Paternity	71–92	43–62

[85]. Characteristically, both testes have an accompanying epididymis and vas and a hernia is present. The condition may be isolated or associated with persistent müllerian duct syndrome [9,86]. In the absence of retained müllerian ducts, some authors recommend contralateral exploration to rule out polyorchidism [85]. Transverse orchidopexy is recommended with partial excision of müllerian ductal structures (if present) as needed; however, radical excision is avoided to prevent vasal injury [9,86].

Epididymal anomalies

The most common cause of epididymal maldevelopment is cryptorchidism [87–93]. Abnormalities of the cystic fibrosis gene may also cause epididymal and vasal anomalies (see below). Severe epididymal anomalies associated with cryptorchidism include agenesis (0–2%), atresia (0–14%), absent fusion of the caput and testis (0–7%) and complete epididymal separation (0–11%). Abnormalities of 'ductal suspension' are less well defined and variably observed; these include widening of the mesentery between the testis and epididymis (7–15%) and epididymal elongation and/or looping (14–79%). A normal epididymis is reportedly present in 97% of boys with descended testes (those explored for hydrocele, hernia, torsion or varicocele) but a narrow mesentery between the testis and epididymis was usually present [94]. However, epididymal anomalies appear to be more common in association with patency of the processus vaginalis irrespective of testicular position [93] (Table 15.5). These data suggest that normal epididymal development is not required for testicular descent, and that epididymal development and closure of the processus vaginalis may both be androgen dependent.

Vasal anomalies

Congenital absence of the vas deferens is due to wolffian duct agenesis and typically includes absence of the body and tail of the epididymis [95]. This anomaly is found in

Table 15.5 Association of epididymal anomalies with patency of the processus vaginalis (PV).

	Incidence of epididymal anomalies (%)		
	Patent PV	Non-patent PV	Reference
Cryptorchid testes	78	38	Mininberg & Schlossberg [88]
	75	20	Heath et al [89]
	65	6	Hazebroek et al. [92]
	71	16	Elder [93]
Scrotal testes	50	10	Elder [93]

70–90% of males with cystic fibrosis [96]. Otherwise healthy males with bilateral vasal agenesis frequently have mutations in the cystic fibrosis gene and therefore have a primary genital form of cystic fibrosis [97]. Paternity may be attempted by epididymal sperm aspiration and in vitro fertilization [98]. Unilateral vasal agenesis is frequently associated with agenesis (79%) or anomalies (12%) of the ipsilateral kidney and contralateral renal anomalies (10%) [99]. Accessory vas deferens-like structures may be found in 1–4% of hernia sacs examined microscopically and are embryonic remnants rather than cases of true vasal duplication [100,101]. They may be differentiated from normal vasa by their small diameter (0.2–0.3 mm vs 1–1.5 mm normal vasal diameter) and the absence of muscle. Ectopic insertion of the vas into the ureter or bladder (persistent common mesonephric duct) is extremely rare and may be associated with anorectal and ureteral anomalies or renal agenesis [102].

Varicocele

Aetiology

Varicocele is defined as ectasia of the internal spermatic venous system or pampiniform plexus. Dilatation is restricted to the left side in 78–93% of patients, presumably due to asymmetrical development of the spermatic venous drainage [103]. Venographic studies of patients with varicocele suggest that the cause of this anomaly is retrograde flow in the internal spermatic venous system due to incompetent valves, renal venous anastomoses (persistent intercardinal veins) and/or renal vein stenosis [104].

Incidence and classification

Varicocele is rare before the age of 10 years and the incidence plateaus by age 14 [105]. The incidence in both adolescents and adults is approximately 16% [106]. The patient is examined in the upright position and the varicocele is classified as: (i) type I: small and palpable during the Valsalva manoeuvre; (ii) type II: moderate and palpable without the Valsalva manoeuvre; and (iii) type III: large and visible as well as palpable. Grade II or III varicoceles comprise less than half of those identified in adolescent screening studies but comprise the vast majority of those recognized clinically [106]. Clinical varicoceles are usually asymptomatic, although occasional boys may note a mass or complain of pain.

Natural history and management

Although the incidence of varicocele in the male population does not change after puberty, several observations suggest that varicocele is a progressive lesion that adversely affects both testes. Internal spermatic vein dilatation in animals increases intratesticular bloodflow and temperature bilaterally via a yet unexplained mechanism [107]. Similar changes may occur in human testes, with impairment of fertility in a proportion of affected males [108]. Of men presenting with infertility, 19–41% have varicoceles [103] as opposed to 17% in a population of fertile males [109]. After varicocelectomy, improvement in sperm quality and successful paternity occur in 66 and 43% of infertile males, respectively [103]. While many men with varicoceles are fertile [103,109], some may have subclinical impairment in semen quality [110]. The likelihood of testicular impairment and infertility appears to be progressive as older men with varicoceles are more likely to be infertile [111]. Varicoceles were reported to be more common in men with secondary infertility (69–81%) than those with primary infertility (35–50%) [112,113] but more recent data have not confirmed this observation [114].

Testicular growth failure (hypotrophy), abnormal testicular histology, impaired semen quality and abnormalities of the hypothalamic–pituitary–gonadal axis have been observed in some adolescents with varicoceles [115–118]. However, no specific parameter has been shown to be predictive of subsequent fertility. The left testis was reported to be significantly smaller than the right testis in as many as 77% of adolescents with a left varicocele [115]. Both ipsilateral (72%) and contralateral (26%) hypotrophy were reported in a study which compared testicular size to population norms [116]. Ultrasound may be more accurate than calipers or orchiometers for testicular volume measurement [119].

Varicocelectomy is followed by testicular catch-up growth in more than two-thirds of adolescents, while progressive hypotrophy occurs in untreated boys [116,120,121]. However, many men with a varicocele and small left testis are normospermic and/or fertile and enlargement of adult testes after varicocelectomy does not correlate with fertility prognosis [122–124]. Semen analysis data in adolescents with varicoceles are limited, but a prospective, controlled study showed no significant difference in sperm

density between patients and age-matched controls [121]. Moreover, increases in sperm concentration and testicular size in response to varicocelectomy were not consistently correlated with each other [121]. Similarly, exaggerated gonadotrophin responsiveness to gonadotrophin-releasing hormone (GnRH) was present in 31% of adolescents with varicoceles but did not correlate with testicular hypotrophy [118]. In adults with varicoceles and oligospermia, semen parameters improve after varicocelectomy only if gonadotrophin hyperresponsiveness is present preoperatively and normalizes postoperatively [125]. Therefore, it is postulated that endocrine testing may identify adolescents at risk for infertility better than testicular volume measurements [118]. Some authors recommend that varicocelectomy should be performed in any adolescent with a grade II or III varicocele, or 5–13% of all adolescent males [106]. Others recommend varicocelectomy only in adolescents with significant left testicular hypotrophy, defined as a reduction in relative testicular size of 10–20% or 2–3 cm^3 [119, 126–128]. Some data suggest that bilateral hypotrophy and gonadotrophin hyperresponsiveness to GnRH may be more significant prognostic parameters [118]. Future longitudinal, controlled studies are needed to resolve these issues.

Varicocelectomy techniques in adolescents are similar to those used in adults, yet recurrence rates tend to be higher [103,106,126,127,129–140] (Table 15.6). Intraoperative venography has been advocated for the identification of persistent venous collaterals which may cause recurrence, but false-negative findings and technical problems may be encountered and recurrence rates may be as high as 6–9% despite its use [141,142]. Recently, the retroperitoneal approach with spermatic artery transection (Palomo technique) has been advocated for adolescents because of its universal success without testicular atrophy [126,127]. While some authors strongly discourage spermatic artery transection because of potential adverse effects on spermatogenesis [137], arterial transection did not prevent the recovery of spermatogenesis or fertility in a randomized study in adults [143]. Hydrocele formation, due to transection of the lymphatics, requires repair in approximately

Procedure	Adolescents (%)		Adults (%)	
	Recurrence	Hydrocele	Recurrence	Hydrocele
Non-artery sparing*	0–15	0–3	0	7
Artery sparing				
Standard*	11–52	0–3	0.1–28	0–3
Microscopic	–	–	0.6	0
Percutaneous†	6–21	0	5	0
Laparoscopic	–	–	0–14	0

Table 15.6 Results of varicocelectomy. Data from [103,106,125,126,128–139].

*Retroperitoneal or inguinal.
†Technical success rate is 73–90%.

one-third of cases [106,127,133–135] and can be minimized by use of the laparoscope or operating microscope.

Spermatic cord (testicular) torsion

Torsion of the spermatic cord may be extravaginal, proximal to the attachment of the tunica vaginalis to the cord, or intravaginal, distal to the tunical attachment. Extravaginal torsion occurs almost exclusively in the perinatal period, prior to fixation of the tunica vaginalis within the scrotum. Intravaginal torsion occurs at any age and is due to an abnormally high attachment of the tunica vaginalis to the spermatic cord and lack of posterior fixation of the epididymis and testis, which results in marked testicular mobility or the 'bell-clapper' deformity (Fig. 15.1j). The incidence of torsion prior to the age of 25 years has been estimated to be 1 : 160 males [144]. In an autopsy series, the bell-clapper deformity was associated with 12% of scrotal testes examined [145]. Clearly, therefore, not all males with bell-clapper testes develop testicular torsion. The proximate cause of torsion in a susceptible individual is not known.

Extravaginal torsion

In a recent review of the literature, the majority of reported cases of perinatal torsion occurred prenatally (72%), while the remainder occurred in the neonatal period [146]. Approximately 20% of cases were bilateral and 80% of these were synchronous. Characteristically, the patient with *in utero* torsion presents with painless scrotal discoloration and a firm testis but minimal oedema or inflammatory reaction. In contrast, postnatal torsion in neonates occurs acutely, after a previously negative scrotal examination, and is more frequently associated with inflammation [147]. The differential diagnosis of perinatal torsion includes hernia, hydrocele, haematocele, meconium peritonitis, epididymitis, appendiceal torsion and tumour. Salvage of testes after perinatal torsion is highly unlikely; therefore, emergent exploration is not indicated. However, prompt exploration via an inguinal approach has been recommended to confirm the diagnosis and exclude the possibility of tumour or other inguinal or testicular pathology [146,147]. Postnatal torsion should be managed emergently; it is occasionally intravaginal. Contralateral testicular fixation after extravaginal torsion is controversial, but proponents argue that the risk of asynchronous torsion and subsequent anorchia, albeit low, warrants this approach [146,147].

Intravaginal torsion

Although intravaginal torsion of the spermatic cord may occur at any age, a peak incidence is seen at puberty, between 13 and 15 years [144,148]. Symptoms typically begin acutely, and most commonly include scrotal and/or abdominal pain and vomiting. Inguinal pain, urinary symptoms or a history of recent trauma or exercise may also be present. One-third to one-half of patients report previous bouts of pain. Elevation of the testis and a palpable

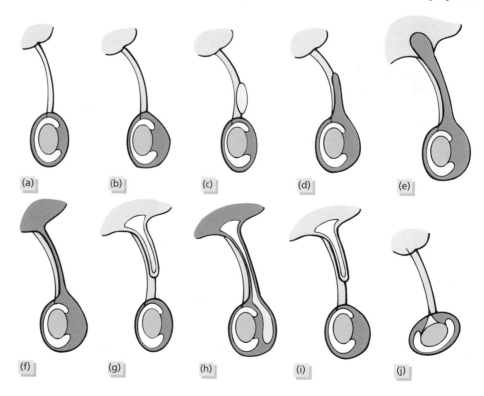

Fig. 15.1 Congenital anomalies of development of the processus and/or tunica vaginalis. (a) Normal anatomy; (b) scrotal hydrocele; (c) hydrocele of the cord; (d) inguinoscrotal hydrocele; (e) abdominoscrotal hydrocele; (f) communicating hydrocele; (g) inguinal hernia; (h) scrotal hernia; (i) inguinal hernia and scrotal hydrocele; (j) bell-clapper deformity.

supratesticular mass (the twisted spermatic cord) may be noted on examination. Approximately 25% of infants and children presenting with acute scrotal symptoms have testicular torsion [148,149]. The most common alternative diagnoses are torsion of a testicular appendage, epididymitis and hernia. Useful physical findings which strongly support a diagnosis other than torsion include the presence of a cremasteric reflex [148] and the ability to distinguish the testis from the epididymis by palpation [150].

Immediate surgical exploration in cases of suspected torsion is indicated, particularly when symptoms have been present for 6–12 h or less. Manual detorsion may be attempted by external rotation [151] and bilateral scrotal orchidopexy performed urgently if detorsion is successful. Colour Doppler ultrasound imaging has been recommended to evaluate intratesticular bloodflow in all patients with acute scrotal pain because it is highly accurate and more expeditious than nuclear testicular scanning [149]. However, false-negative studies have been reported, and findings may be particularly misleading in very young patients or in cases of partial or recurrent torsion [150,152,153]. In cases of subacute torsion, grey scale ultrasonography may be confusing [154]. As no presently available test can infallibly diagnose torsion, imaging studies should probably be reserved for confirmation of normal blood flow when pathology other than torsion is suspected. If the history is suggestive of intermittent torsion, and particularly if a horizontal lie of the testis is noted on examination of the patient in the standing position, elective bilateral scrotal orchidopexy should be performed [155].

The risk of subsequent testicular atrophy after torsion increases with its severity and duration. The incidence of non-viability rises after 6 h of torsion, but occasional testes may survive despite 12–24 h of torsion [144,156]. Subsequent fertility potential appears to be impaired in some men with a history of unilateral torsion, but the aetiology of this effect is controversial. Contralateral abnormalities of spermatogenesis and reduced semen quality are reported in more than half of patients with unilateral torsion, suggesting that a pre-existing congenital testicular anomaly may be present [157]. However, other data suggest an inverse correlation between duration of torsion and semen quality, with poor outcome after prolonged torsion even if orchiectomy is performed [158,159]. The mechanism of the time-related injury to the contralateral testis is not known, but proof of an immunogenic mechanism in humans is lacking [157,159]. Interestingly, the effect of prepubertal torsion on subsequent fertility appears to be minimal [160].

Hernia/hydrocele

The spectrum of abnormalities of the processus and tunica vaginalis is shown in Fig. 15.1. The processus vaginalis normally closes around birth; failure of closure may allow transinguinal passage of the abdominal contents (a hernia) or peritoneal fluid (a communicating hydrocele). Partial closure may result in a scrotal, inguinoscrotal, abdominoscrotal or cord hydrocele, and combinations of hernia and hydrocele may occur. The appropriate diagnosis is usually made by history and inguinoscrotal examination with transillumination. Although both a scrotal hernia and hydrocele may transilluminate, the former is usually partially or completely reducible and associated with asymmetrical widening of the external ring. Ultrasound may occasionally be useful for confirmation of the cystic nature of a hydrocele of the cord or evaluation of the testis if a tumour is suspected.

Treatment may be delayed in newborns with hydrocele as closure of the processus vaginalis and resorption of hydrocele fluid frequently occurs in the first year of life. Persistent hydroceles in older children or those which fluctuate in size should be treated surgically via an inguinal approach to allow high ligation of an associated patent processus vaginalis. Abdominoscrotal hydroceles, although rare, pose a special problem in management. It is recommended that the intra-abdominal portion of the sac be completely excised, via a preperitoneal approach if necessary, with ligation of the processus vaginalis [161]. Hernias should be repaired soon after diagnosis, particularly in infants, because as many as one-third of patients in this age group may suffer incarceration prior to elective repair [162,163]. Incarceration is most likely in the first year of life, and is associated with a higher risk of postoperative complications. The reported rate of testicular atrophy after incarceration varies from 2 to 15%, but is lowest after successful reduction prior to operative repair [164]. After manual reduction of an incarcerated hernia, repair should be performed within 24–48 h [162]. Contralateral inguinal exploration is often recommended because of reports of a high incidence of contralateral patency of the processus vaginalis observed at surgery or laparoscopically [165]. However, longitudinal studies show that the incidence of subsequent contralateral clinical hernias is as low as 6% after unilateral herniorrhaphy in childhood [166] and 10% after unilateral herniorrhaphy in the first year of life [167]. The majority of contralateral hernias appear within 2 years of the initial surgery. Consequently, these authors discourage routine contralateral exploration, with the exception of patients with a history of prematurity or increased intra-abdominal pressure (e.g. in the presence of a ventriculoperitoneal shunt) [166].

Scrotal anomalies

The more common scrotal anomalies include penoscrotal

transposition and bifid scrotum. Penoscrotal transposition in the absence of other genital anomalies is very rare, it may be partial or complete (prepenile scrotum) [168] and it may be associated with anomalies of the vertebrae, urinary or gastrointestinal tract, or the caudal regression syndrome [169]. The aetiology is thought be a disturbance in the caudal migration of the labioscrotal swellings. Bifid scrotum has been reported to occur in 5% of patients with hypospadias [170]. Repair of penoscrotal transposition or bifid scrotum may be performed by excision of the angle of rugal skin cranial to the penile base [171] or via an 'M' incision with development of rotational flaps [170,172]. These techniques do not use circumferential penile incisions which may interfere with the penile vascular supply. Urethroplasty may be performed simultaneously or in two stages.

More unusual scrotal anomalies include scrotal ectopia and accessory scrotum [173,174]. The unilateral ectopic scrotum (also called unilateral penoscrotal transposition) contains the ipsilateral testis and is associated with anomalies of the penis and kidney. The aetiology is presumed to be abnormal caudal migration of one labioscrotal swelling. Surgical repair consists of rotation of the ectopic scrotum as a flap with suture to the contralateral hemiscrotum and orchidopexy [173]. In contrast, the accessory scrotum does not contain a testis, and is frequently associated with a perineal lipoma [174]. It is therefore hypothesized that the lipoma disrupts the continuity of the labioscrotal swelling during embryogenesis. Anorectal and other malformations are more common in patients without an associated perineal lipoma. Treatment consists of local excision.

Anatomical approach to inguinal surgery

The inguinal canal and underlying retroperitoneum are best approached via an incision which begins just craniolateral to the pubic tubercle, lies directly over the canal and follows the Langer lines. Except in infants, this corresponds to a position inferior to the lowest inguinal crease. Careful attention to anatomical detail facilitates the dissection, which is enhanced by the use of spring retractors [175,176]. Full access to the spermatic cord is obtained by exposing the external oblique caudally and medially until the cord is seen to emerge from the aponeurosis (Fig. 15.2). Extending the incision in the aponeurosis through the external ring and caudally into the contiguous external spermatic fascia fully exposes the cord and aids in delivery of the testis into the inguinal canal if needed.

If the surgeon approaches the canal by incision of the cremasteric fascia, rather than by separation of the ventral cremasteric fibres, superior exposure of the spermatic cord and inguinal floor is obtained. This is achieved by sweeping the cremasteric muscle and fascia cranially away from the dorsal aspect of the caudal leaf of the incised external oblique aponeurosis, until the external spermatic vessels which parallel the inguinal canal can be seen through the thin cremasteric fascia. Placement of a spring retractor between the arc of the cremaster and the inner aspect of the caudal leaf of the external oblique aponeurosis clearly displays the cremasteric fascia and vessels (Fig. 15.3). An incision in the fascia overlying the vessels is carried inferomedially along the cord as far as the proximal scrotum if possible. This manoeuvre also facilitates the

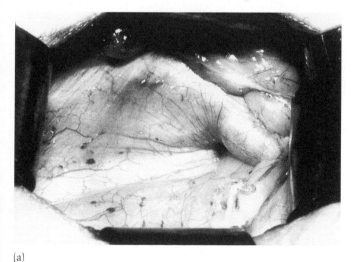

(a)

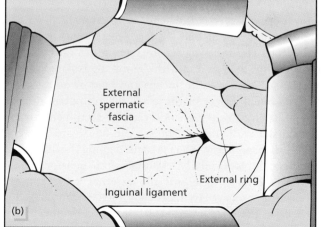

(b)

Fig. 15.2 (a) Intraoperative photograph and (b) line drawing showing the actual appearance of the external ring and external spermatic fascia covering the spermatic cord structures. (Reproduced from [175] with permission.)

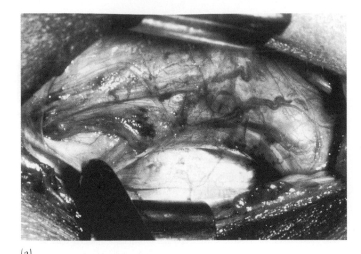

(a)

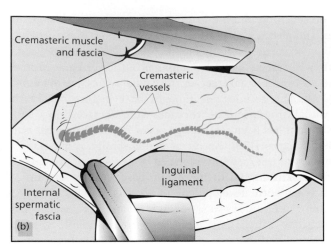

Fig. 15.3 (a) Intraoperative photograph and (b) line drawing showing incision of the cremasteric muscle and fascia parallel to their attachment to the inguinal ligament. (Reproduced from [175] with permission.)

delivery of the testis into the canal. The cremasteric fascial incision can be carried laterally along the inguinal ligament into the insertion of the cremasteric and internal oblique muscles to provide wide access to the internal ring and the retroperitoneum if necessary. Since the cremasteric vessels and genital branch of the genitofemoral nerve lie in the leaves of the cremasteric fascia, the innermost leaf of the fascia must be incised to allow free retraction of these structures inferiorly. The cremasteric muscle and fascia can then be retracted superiorly to expose and isolate the cord.

Surgical treatment of the spermatic cord

With the exposure of the cord as previously described, exposure of a hernia sac or varicocele is easily accomplished and the testis or accompanying scrotal hydrocele can be easily delivered into the groin. To isolate a hernia sac, the sac is grasped in forceps and held by an assistant. On the caudal aspect of the cord, the retroperitoneal fat which accompanies the cord can be seen beneath the internal spermatic fascia. The sac can be isolated intact if the internal spermatic fascia is incised along this line of fat. A varicocele is similarly exposed after incision of the internal spermatic fascia. If the external spermatic and cremasteric fascia overlying the cord have been incised to the neck of the scrotum, the testis and/or a hydrocele may be delivered into the inguinal canal. The internal spermatic fascia proximally and the cremasteric fascia distally are grasped and countertraction is applied, resulting in evagination of the cremasteric muscle and fascia and visualization of the tunica vaginalis covered by internal spermatic fascia (Fig. 15.4). Large hydroceles may not

negotiate the neck of the cremasteric fascia, but partial exposure allows aspiration of fluid and subsequent delivery into the groin. Following windowing of the hydrocele, sharp downward traction of the invaginated scrotum draws the testis into its normal position, thereby preventing iatrogenic cryptorchidism. Low undescended testes may also be delivered by evagination of the cremasteric muscle and fascia.

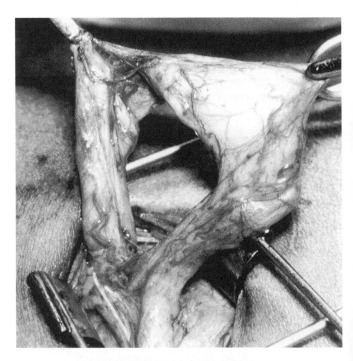

Fig. 15.4 Testis and cord structures completely invested in internal spermatic fascia which has been freed by countertraction from the cremasteric fascia. The left forceps holds the distal aspect of the evaginated cremasteric muscle and fascia and the right forceps holds the internal spermatic fascia overlying testis. Note the bridging cremasteric vessels (left) and the clean plane of dissection. (Redrawn from [175] with permission.)

Surgical treatment of the retroperitoneum through an inguinal approach

The internal inguinal ring may be opened widely by incising the internal spermatic fascia circumferentially as the cord emerges from the body wall [177] (Fig. 15.5). The inguinal floor may be incised medially if necessary. Repair of the floor is easily accomplished because the transversalis fascia cranially (transversus abdominus arch) and the thickening of the transversalis fascia which parallels the inguinal ligament (the iliopubic tract) can be clearly distinguished [178]. In addition, the internal ring may be enlarged laterally by detaching the internal oblique muscle from the inguinal ligament. Alternatively, the retroperitoneum may be exposed via a LaRoque incision in the external oblique aponeurosis 4–5 cm craniolateral to the inguinal canal with splitting of the internal oblique and transversus abdominis muscles in the direction of their fibres [179,180].

An anatomical concept which is useful in the surgical approach to the retroperitoneum is the 'secondary internal ring', a membranous thickening of the intermediate stratum of retroperitoneal connective tissue just proximal to the internal ring [181,182]. The cord may be transposed medially during orchidopexy by incision of this membranous layer and subsequent mobilization of the spermatic vessels and vas from the peritoneum. Similarly, passage of the cord under the inferior epigastric vessels is facilitated by dissecting the membranous fascial layer from the fat surrounding the vessels. To identify blind-ending vessels and vas within the retroperitoneum requires the deliberate incision of the membranous layer along the anticipated course of these structures, as merely separating the retroperitoneal connective tissue from the transversalis fascia will usually be inadequate.

Specific orchidopexy techniques

The principles of successful orchidopexy include atraumatic placement of the testis in a dependent scrotal position without tension. The testis is adequately mobilized, and a scrotal pouch is created via a transverse incision in the upper scrotum. Dissection between the dartos and external spermatic fascia is simple and effective; the more difficult dissection between the dartos and skin is not required [183]. The testis is brought through an opening in the external spermatic fascia, which is then closed to prevent testicular retraction but with care to avoid compromise of the cord. Secure fixation of the testis in the pouch can be achieved without potentially deleterious transparenchymal sutures if the tunica vaginalis is completely everted [184]. This concept is also valid for orchidopexy after testicular torsion as scrotal fixation may be inadequate if the tunica vaginalis is not everted, even if permanent transparenchymal sutures are used [184].

Operations for orchidopexy after previous inguinal surgery can be arduous [185]. The operation is facilitated if the spermatic cord can be identified first in a virginal site. In most cases the retroperitoneum is inviolate; therefore, if the lateral aspects of the cremasteric arch and medial aspect of the adjacent internal oblique muscle are freed from the inguinal ligament, the cord may be identified in the retroperitoneum and then dissected distally from its fibrotic surroundings.

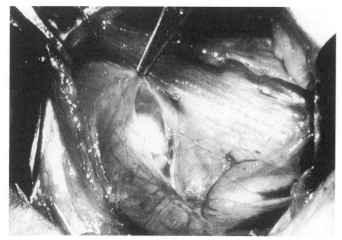

(a)

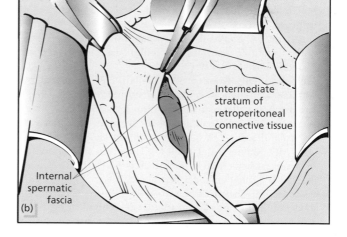

(b)

Fig. 15.5 (a) Intraoperative photograph and (b) line drawing showing an incision in the transversalis fascia as it becomes the internal spermatic fascia in surgical exposure of the internal ring. (Reproduced from [175] with permission.)

References

1 Kogan SJ, Gill B, Bennett B et al. Human monorchism: a clinicopathological study of unilateral absent testes in 65 boys. J Urol 1986;135:758–61.

2 Turek PJ, Ewalt DH, Snyder HM et al. The absent cryptorchid testis: surgical findings and their implications for diagnosis and etiology. J Urol 1994;151:718–21.

3 Backhouse KM. Embryology of testicular descent and maldescent. Urol Clin North Am 1982;9:315–25.

4 Redman JF. Observations on course of cremasteric muscle in perineal testes with commentary on gubernaculum. Urology 1993;41:462–5.

5 Redman JF, Golladay ES. Penopubic and penile testicular ectopia. South Med J 1991;84:535–6.

6 Rajfer J. Congenital anomalies of the testis. In: Walsh PC, Retik AB, Stamey TA, Vaughan ED Jr, eds. Campbell's Urology. Philadelphia: WB Saunders, 1992:1543–54.

7 Kogan S. Cryptorchidism. In: Kelalis PP, King LR, Belman AB, eds. Clinical Pediatric Urology; Philadelphia: WB Saunders, 1992:1050–83.

8 Hutson JM, Terada M, Zhou B, Paxton G. Factors in testis descent and causes of cryptorchidism. Curr Opin Urol 1993;3:465–9.

9 Josso N, Cate L, Picard JY et al. Anti-Mullerian hormone: the Jost factor. Recent Prog Horm Res 1993;48:1–59.

10 Rajfer J, Walsh PC. The incidence of intersexuality in patients with hypospadias and cryptorchidism. J Urol 1976;116: 769–70.

11 Job JC, Toublanc JE, Chaussain JL et al. The pituitary–gonadal axis in cryptorchid infants and children. Eur J Pediatr 1987;146:2–5.

12 Hadziselimovic F, Thommen L, Girard J, Herzog B. The significance of postnatal gonadotropin surge for testicular development in normal and cryptorchid testes. J Urol 1986;136:274–6.

13 Huff DS, Hadziselimovic F, Snyder HM, Blyth B, Duckett JW. Early postnatal testicular maldevelopment in cryptorchidism. J Urol 1991;146:624–6.

14 Spencer JR, Torrado T, Sanchez RS, Vaughan ED Jr, Imperato-McGinley J. Effects of flutamide and finasteride on rat testicular descent. Endocrinology 1991;129:741–8.

15 Husmann DA, McPhaul MJ. Time-specific androgen blockade with flutamide inhibits testicular descent in the rat. Endocrinology 1991;129:1409–16.

16 McMahon DR, Kramer SA, Tindall DJ, Husmann DA. Antiandrogen induced cryptorchidism in the pig is related to failed gubernacular regression. J Urol 1994;151:275A.

17 Wensing CJG, Colenbrander B. Normal and abnormal testicular descent. Oxf Rev Reprod Biol 1986;8:130–64.

18 Cain MD, Kramer SA, Tindall DJ, Husmann DA. Alterations in maternal epidermal growth factor (EGF) affect testicular descent and epididymal development. Urology 1994;43:375–8.

19 Fentener JM, Zoelen EJJ, Ursem PFJ, Wensing CJG. In vitro model of the first phase of testicular descent: identification of a low molecular weight factor from fetal testis involved in proliferation of gubernaculum testis cells and distinct from specified polypeptide growth factors and fetal gonadal hormones. Endocrinology 1988;123:2868–77.

20 Visser J, Heyns CF. Demonstration of a 26 KD protein in testicular extracts inducing proliferation of gubernaculum cells during testicular descent in the pig fetus. J Urol 1994;151:328A.

21 McElreavey K, Vilain E, Cotinot C, Payen E, Fellous M. Control of sex determination in animals. Eur J Biochem 1993;218:769–83.

22 Arey LB. The Genital System. In: Developmental Anatomy. Philadelphia: WB Saunders, 1974:315–34.

23 Heyns CF. The gubernaculum during testicular descent in the human fetus. J Anat 1987;153:93–112.

24 Hadziselimovic F, Herzog B. The development and descent of the epididymis. Eur J Pediatr 1993;152:6–9.

25 Van der Schoot P. Androgens in relation to prenatal development and postnatal inversion of the gubernaculum in rats. J Reprod Fert 1992;95:145–58.

26 Scorer CG. The descent of the testis. Arch Dis Child 1964;39:605–9.

27 John Radcliffe Hospital Cryptorchidism Study Group. Cryptorchidism: a prospective study of 7500 consecutive male births, 1984–8. Arch Dis Child 1992;67:892–9.

28 Berkowitz GS, Lapinski RH, Dolgin SE et al. Prevalence and natural history of cryptorchidism. Pediatrics 1993;92:44–9.

29 Chilvers C, Pike MC, Forman D, Fogelman K, Wadsworth MEJ. Apparent doubling of frequency of undescended testis in England and Wales in 1962–81. Lancet 2 1984:330–2.

30 Fenton EJM, Woodward AA, Hudson IL, Marschner I. The ascending testis. Pediatr Surg Int 2 1990;5:6–9.

31 Farrington GH. The position and retractility of the normal testis in childhood with reference to the diagnosis and treatment of cryptorchidism. J Pediatr Surg 1968;3:53–9.

32 Wyllie GG. The retractile testis. Med J Aust 1984;140:403–5.

33 Kaplan GW. Nomenclature of cryptorchidism. Eur J Pediatr 1993;152:17–19.

34 Atwell JD. Ascent of the testis: fact or fiction. Br J Urol 1985;57:474–7.

35 Belman BA. Acquired undescended (ascended) testis: effects of human chorionic gonadotropin. J Urol 1988;140:1189–98.

36 Robertson JFR, Azmy AF, Cochran W. Assent to ascent of the testis. Br J Urol 1988;61:146–7.

37 Whitaker RH. Undescended testis—the need for a standard classification. Br J Urol 1992;70:1–6.

38 Olsen LH. Inter-observer variation in assessment of undescended testis. Br J Urol 1989;64:644–8.

39 Levitt SB, Kogan SJ, Engel RM et al. The impalpable testis: a rational approach to management. J Urol 1978;120:515–20.

40 Koff SA. Does compensatory testicular enlargement predict monorchism? J Urol 1991;146:632–3.

41 Huff DS, Snyder HM III, Hadziselimovic F, Blyth B, Duckett JW. An absent testis is associated with contralateral testicular hypertrophy. J Urol 1992;148:627–8.

42 Saw KC, Eardley I, Dennis MJS, Whitaker RH. Surgical outcome of orchiopexy. I. Previously unoperated testes. Br J Urol 1992;70:90–4.

43 Hadziselimovic F, Hecker E, Herzog B. The value of testicular biopsy in cryptorchidism. Urol Res 1984;12:171–4.

44 Hjort T, Linnet L, Skaakebaek NE. Testicular biopsy: indications and complications. Eur J Pediatr 1982;138:23–5.

45 Jarow JP. Intratesticular arterial anatomy. J Androl 1990;11: 255–9.

46 De Muinck Keizer-Schrama SMPF, Hazebroek FWJ. Hormonal treatment of cryptorchidism: role of the pituitary gonadal axis. Semin Urol 1988;6:84–95.

47 Rajfer J, Handelsman DJ, Swerdloff RS et al. Hormonal therapy of cryptorchidism. A randomized, double-blind study comparing human chorionic gonadotropin and gonadotropin-releasing hormone. N Engl J Med 1986;314:466–70.

48 Christiansen P, Muller J, Buhl S et al. Hormonal treatment of cryptorchidism—hCG or GnRH—a multicentre study. Acta Paediatr 1992;81:605–8.

49 Olsen LH, Genster HG, Mosegaard A et al. Management of the non-descended testis: doubtful value of luteinizing-hormone-releasing-hormone (LHRH). A double-blind, placebo-controlled multicentre study. Int J Androl 1992;15:135–43.

50 Lala R, Matarazzo P, Chiabotto P et al. Combined therapy with LHRH and HCG in cryptorchid infants. Eur J Pediatr 1993;152:S31–3.

51 Karpe B. Prognosis of hormonal treatment of undescended testis related to testicular position at birth. Pediatr Surg Int 1991;6:221–2.

52 Waldschmidt J, Doede T, Vygen I. The results of 9 years of experience with a combined treatment with LH-RH and HCG for cryptorchidism. Eur J Pediatr 1993;152:S34–6.

53 Bica DG, Hadziselimovic F. The behavior of epididymis, processus vaginalis and testicular descent in cryptorchid boys treated with buserelin. Eur J Pediatr 1993;152:S38–42.

54 Hadziselimovic F, Herzog B, Hocht B et al. Screening for cryptorchid boys risking sterility and results of long-term buserelin treatment after successful orchiopexy. Eur J Pediatr 1987;146:S59–62.

55 Levitt SB, Kogan SJ, Schneider KM et al. Endocrine tests in phenotypic children with bilateral impalpable testes can reliably predict 'congenital' anorchism. Urology 1978;11: 11–17.

56 Lustig RH, Conte FA, Kogan BA, Grumbach MM. Ontogeny of gonadotropin secretion in congenital anorchism: sexual dimorphism versus syndrome of gonadal dysgenesis and diagnostic considerations. J Urol 1987;138:587–91.

57 Hrebinko RL, Bellinger MF. The limited role of imaging techniques in managing children with undescended testes. J Urol 1993;150:458–60.

58 Diamond DA, Caldamone AA. The value of laparoscopy for 106 impalpable testes relative to clinical presentation. J Urol 1992;148:632–4.

59 Plotzker ED, Rushton HG, Belman AB, Skoog SJ. Laparoscopy for nonpalpable testes in childhood: is inguinal exploration also necessary when vas and vessels exit the inguinal ring? J Urol 1992;148:635–8.

60 Poenaru D, Homsy YL, Peloquin F, Andze GO. Laparoscopic management of the impalpable abdominal testis. Urology 1993;42:574–9.

61 Moore RG, Peters CA, Bauer SB, Mandell J, Retik AB. Laparoscopic evaluation of the nonpalpable testis: a prospective assessment of accuracy. J. Urol 1994;151:728–31.

62 Tennenbaum SY, Lerner SE, McAleer IM et al. Preoperative laparoscopic localization of the nonpalpable testis: a critical analysis of a 10-year experience. J Urol 1994;151:732–4.

63 Elder JS. Laparoscopy for inpalpable testes: significance of the patent processus vaginalis. J Urol 1994;152:776–8.

64 Lamesch A. L'anorchidie unilaterale ou monorchidie. Chirurgie 1992;118:328–33.

65 Docimo SG. The results of surgical therapy for cryptorchidism: a literature review and analysis. J Urol 1995;154: 1148–52.

66 Corbally MT, Quinn FJ, Guiney EJ. The effect of two-stage orchiopexy on testicular growth. Brit J Urol 1993;72:376–8.

67 Hazebroek FWJ, Molenaar JC. The management of the impalpable testis by surgery alone. J Urol 1992;148:629–31.

68 Bianchi A. Management of the impalpable testis. The role of microvascular orchidopexy. Pediatr Surg Int 1990;5:48–53.

69 Kogan SJ, Houman BZ, Reda EF, Levitt SB. Orchiopexy of the high undescended testis by division of the spermatic vessels: A critical review of 38 selected transections. J Urol 1989; 141:1416–19.

70 Elder JS. Two-stage Fowler-Stephens orchiopexy in the management of intra-abdominal testes. J Urol 1992;148: 1239–41.

71 Thomas MD, Mercer LC, Saltzstein EC. Laparoscopic orchiectomy for unilateral intra-abdominal testis. J Urol 1992;148:1251–3.

72 Jordan GH, Robey EL, Winslow BH. Laparoendoscopic surgical management of the abdominal/transinguinal undescended testicle. J Endourol 1992;6:159–63.

73 Bogaert BA, Kogan BA, Mevorach RA. Therapeutic laparoscopy for intra-abdominal testes. Urology 1993;42: 182–8.

74 Chilvers C, Dudley NE, Gough MH, Jackson MB, Pike MC. Undescended testis: the effect of treatment on subsequent risk of subfertility and malignancy. J Pediatr Surg 1986;8: 691–6.

75 Lee PA. Fertility in cryptorchidism. Does treatment make a difference? Endocrinol Metab Clin N Am 1993;22:479–90.

76 Lee PA, Bellinger MF, Songer NJ et al. An epidemiologic study of paternity after cryptorchidism: initial results. Eur J Pediatr 1993;152:S25–7.

77 Giwercman A, Grindsted J, Hansen B, Jensen O, Skakkebaek NE. Testicular cancer risk in boys with maldescended testis: a cohort study. J Urol 1987;138:1214–16.

78 Batata MA, Whitmore WF, Chu FCH et al. Cryptorchidism and testicular cancer. J Urol 1980;124:382–7.

79 Halme A, Kellokumpu-Lehtinen P, Lehtonen T, Teppo L. Morphology of testicular germ cell tumours in treated and untreated cryptorchidism. Br J Urol 1989;64:78–83.

80 Jones BJ, Thornhill JA, O'Donnell B et al. Influence of prior orchiopexy on stage and prognosis of testicular cancer. Eur Urol 1991;19:201–3.

81 Giwercman A, Bruun E, Frimodt-Moller C, Skakkebaek NE. Prevalence of carcinoma in situ and other histopathological abnormalities in testes of men with a history of cryptorchidism. J Urol 1989;142:998–1002.

82 Thum G. Polyorchidism: case report and review of literature. J Urol 1991;145:370–2.

83 Merida MG, Miguelez C, Galiano E, Lopez Perez GA. Polyorchidism: an exceptional case of three homolateral testes. Eur Urol 1992;21:338–9.

84 Kale N, Basaklar AN. Polyorchidism. J Pediatr Surg 1991;12: 1432–4.

85 Dogruyol H, Ozcan M, Balkan E. Two rare genital abnormalities: crossed testicular and scrototesticular ectopia. Br J Urol 1992;70:201–3.

86 Martin EL, Bennett AH, Cromie WJ. Persistent Müllerian duct syndrome with transverse testicular ectopia and spermatogenesis. J Urol 1992;147:1615–17.

87 Marshall FF, Shermeta DW. Epididymal abnormalities associated with undescended testis. J Urol 1979;121:341–3.

88 Mininberg DT, Schlossberg S. The role of the epididymis in testicular descent. *J Urol* 1983;**129**:1207–8.

89 Heath AL, Man DWK, Eckstein HB. Epididymal abnormalities associated with maldescent of the testis. *J Pediatr Surg* 1984;**19**:47–9.

90 Gill B, Kogan S, Starr S, Reda E, Levitt S. Significance of epididymal and ductal anomalies associated with testicular maldescent. *J Urol* 1989;**142**:556–8.

91 Koff WJ, Scaletscky R. Malformations of the epididymis in undescended testis. *J Urol* 1990;**143**:340–3.

92 Hazebroek FWJ, de Muinck Keizer-Schrama SMPF, van Maarschalkerweerd M, Visser HKA, Molenaar JC. Why luteinizing-hormone-releasing-hormone nasal spray will not replace orchiopexy in the treatment of boys with undescended testes. *J Pediatr Surg* 1987;**22**:177–82.

93 Elder JS. Epididymal anomalies associated with hydrocele/ hernia and cryptorchidism: implications regarding testicular descent. *J Urol* 1992;**148**:624–6.

94 Turek PJ, Ewalt DH, Snyder HM III, Duckett JW. Normal epididymal anatomy in boys. *J Urol* 1994;**151**:726–7.

95 Charny CW, Gillenwater JY. Congenital absence of the vas deferens. *J Urol* 1965;**93**:399–401.

96 Hcaton ND, Pryor JP. Vasa aplasia and cystic fibrosis. *Br J Urol* 1990;**66**:538–40.

97 Anguiano A, Oates RD, Amos JA *et al.* Congenital bilateral absence of the vas deferens. A primary genital form of cystic fibrosis. *J Am Med Assoc* 1992;**267**:1794–7.

98 Mathieu C, Guerin J-F, Cognat M *et al.* Motility and fertilizing capacity of epididymal human spermatozoa in normal and pathological cases. *Fertil Steril* 1992;**57**: 871–6.

99 Donohue RE, Fauver HE. Unilateral absence of the vas deferens. A useful clinical sign. *J Am Med Assoc* 1989;**261**: 1180–2.

100 Gill B, Favale D, Kogan SJ *et al.* Significance of accessory ductal structures in hernia sacs. *J Urol* 1992;**148**:697–8.

101 Popek EJ. Embryonal remnants in inguinal hernia sacs. *Human Pathol* 1990;**21**:339–49.

102 Nesbitt JA II, King LR. Ectopia of the vas deferens. *J Pediatr Surg* 1990;**25**:335–8.

103 Pryor JL, Howards SS. Varicocele. *Urol Clin N Am* 1987;**14**:499–513.

104 Braedel HU, Steffens J, Ziegler M, Polsky MS, Platt ML. A possible ontogenic etiology for idiopathic left varicocele. *J Urol* 1994;**151**:62–6.

105 Oster J. Varicocele in children and adolescents. An investigation of the incidence among Danish school children. *Scand J Urol Nephrol* 1971;**5**:27–32.

106 Steeno OP. Varicocele in the adolescent. In: Zorgniotti AW, ed. *Temperature and Environmental Effects on the Testis.* New York: Plenum Press, 1991:295–321.

107 Turner TT, Lopez TJ. Testicular blood flow in peripubertal and older rats with unilateral experimental varicocele and investigation into the mechanism of the bilateral response to the unilateral lesion. *J Urol* 1990;**144**:1018–21.

108 Goldstein M, Eid J-F. Elevation of intratesticular and scrotal skin surface temperature in men with varicocele. *J Urol* 1989;**142**:743–5.

109 Kursh ED. What is the incidence of varicocele in a fertile population? *Fertil Steril* 1987;**48**:510–11.

110 Nagao RR, Plymate SR, Berger RE, Perin EB, Paulsen CA. Comparison of gonadal function between fertile and infertile men with varicocele. *Fertil Steril* 1986;**46**:930–3.

111 Russell JK. Varicocele, age, and fertility. *Lancet* 1957;**2**:222.

112 Gorelick JI, Goldstein M. Loss of fertility in men with varicocele. *Fertil Steril* 1993;**59**:613–16.

113 Witt MA, Lipshultz LI. Varicocele: a progressive or static lesion? *Urology* 1993;**42**:541–3.

114 Jarow JP, Coburn M, Sigman M. Incidence of varicoceles in men with primary and secondary infertility. *Urology* 1996; **47**:73–6.

115 Lyon RP, Marshall S, Scott MP. Varicocele in childhood and adolescence: implication in adulthood infertility? *Urology* 1982;**19**:641–4.

116 Okuyama A, Nakamura M, Namiki M *et al.* Surgical repair of varicocele at puberty: preventive treatment for fertility improvement. *J Urol* 1988;**139**:562–4.

117 Hadziselimovic F, Herzog B, Liebundgut B, Jenny P, Buser M. Testicular and vascular changes in children and adults with varicocele. *J Urol* 1989;**142**:583–5.

118 Kass EJ, Freitas JE, Salisz JA, Steinert BW. Pituitary gonadal dysfunction in adolescents with varicocele. *Urology* 1993; **42**:179–81.

119 Costabile RA, Skoog S, Radowich M. Testicular volume assessment in the adolescent with a varicocele. *J Urol* 1992;**147**:1348–50.

120 Kass EJ, Belman AB. Reversal of testicular growth failure by varicocele ligation. *J Urol* 1987;**137**:475–6.

121 Laven JSE, Haans LCF, Mali WPTM *et al.* Effects of varicocele treatment in adolescents: a randomized study. *Fertil Steril* 1992;**58**:756–62.

122 Lipshultz LI, Corriere JN. Progressive testicular atrophy in the varicocele patient. *J Urol* 1977;**117**:175–6.

123 Pinto KJ, Kroovand RL, Jarow JP. Varicocele related testicular atrophy and its predictive effect upon fertility. *J Urol* 1994;**152**:788–90.

124 Gentile DP, Cockett ATK. The effect of varicocelectomy on testicular volume in 89 infertile adult males with varicoceles. *Fertil Steril* 1992;**58**:209–11.

125 Hudson RW. The endocrinology of varicoceles. *Fertil Steril* 1988;**49**:199–208.

126 Kass EJ, Marcol B. Results of varicocele surgery in adolescents: a comparison of techniques. *J Urol* 1992;**148**:694–6.

127 Parrott TS, Hewatt L. Ligation of the testicular artery and vein in adolescent varicocele. *J Urol* 1994;**152**:791–3.

128 Belman AB. Editorial comment. *J Urol* 1994;**152**:793.

129 Gorenstein A, Katz S, Schiller M. Varicocele in children: 'To treat or not to treat'—venographic and manometric studies. *J Pediatr Surg* 1986;**12**:1046–50.

130 Thon WF, Gall H, Danz B, Bahren W, Sigmund G. Percutaneous sclerotherapy of idiopathic varicocele in childhood: a preliminary report. *J Urol* 1989;**141**:913–15.

131 Reyes BL, Trerotola SO, Venbrux AC *et al.* Percutaneous embolotherapy of adolescent varicocele: results and long-term follow-up. *J Vasc Interven Radiol* 1994;**5**:131–4.

132 Sayfan J, Adam YG, Soffer Y. A new entity in varicocele subfertility: the 'cremasteric reflux'. *Fertil Steril* 1980;**33**: 88–90.

133 Szabo R, Kessler R. Hydrocele following internal spermatic vein ligation: a retrospective study and review of the literature. *J Urol* 1984;**132**:924–5.

134 Ross LS, Ruppman N. Varicocele vein ligation in 565 patients

under local anesthesia: a long-term review of technique, results and complications in light of proposed management by laparoscopy. *J Urol* 1993;**149**:1361–3.

135 Dubin L, Amelar RD. Varicocelectomy: 986 cases in a twelve-year study. *Urology* 1977;**10**:446–9.

136 Homonnai ZT, Fainman N, Engelhard Y *et al.* Varicocelectomy and male fertility: comparison of semen quality and recurrence of varicocele following varicocelectomy by two techniques. *Int J Androl* 1980;**3**:447–58.

137 Goldstein M, Gilbert BR, Dicker AP, Dwosh J, Gnecco C. Microsurgical inguinal varicocelectomy with delivery of the testis: an artery and lymphatic sparing technique. *J Urol* 1992;**148**:1808–11.

138 Donovan JF, Winfield HN. Laparoscopic varix ligation. *J Urol* 1992;**147**:77–81.

139 Jarow JP, Assimos DG, Pittaway DE. Effectiveness of laparoscopic varicocelectomy. *Urology* 1993;**42**:544–7.

140 Ralph DJ, Timoney AG, Parker C, Pryor JP. Laparoscopic varicocele ligation. *Br J Urol* 1993;**72**:230–3.

141 Gill B, Kogan SJ, Maldonado J, Reda E, Levitt SB. Significance of intraoperative venographic patterns on the postoperative recurrence and surgical incision placement of pediatric varicoceles. *J Urol* 1990;**144**:502–5.

142 Hart RR, Rushton HG, Belman AB. Intraoperative spermatic venography during varicocele surgery in adolescents. *J Urol* 1992;**148**:1514–16.

143 Matsuda T, Horii Y, Yoshida O. Should the testicular artery be preserved at varicocelectomy? *J Urol* 1993;**149**:1357–60.

144 Williamson RCN. Torsion of the testis and allied conditions. *Br J Surg* 1976;**63**:465–76.

145 Caesar RE, Kaplan GW. Incidence of the bell-clapper deformity in an autopsy series. *Urology* 1994;**44**:114–16.

146 Das S, Singer A. Controversies of perinatal torsion of the spermatic cord: a review, survey and recommendations. *J Urol* 1990;**143**:231–3.

147 Brandt MT, Sheldon CA, Wacksman J, Matthews P. Prenatal testicular torsion: principles of management. *J Urol* 1992;**147**:670–2.

148 Rabinowitz R. The importance of the cremasteric reflex in acute scrotal swelling in children. *J Urol* 1984;**132**:89–90.

149 Kass EJ, Stone KT, Cacciarelli AA, Mitchell B. Do all children with an acute scrotum require exploration? *J Urol* 1993;**150**:667–9.

150 Steinhardt GF, Boyarsky S, Mackey R. Testicular torsion: pitfalls of color Doppler sonography. *J Urol* 1993;**150**:461–2.

151 Cattolica EV. Preoperative manual detorsion of the torsed spermatic cord. *J Urol* 1985;**133**:803–5.

152 Patriquin HB, Yazbeck S, Trinh B *et al.* Testicular torsion in infants and children: diagnosis with doppler sonography. *Radiology* 1993;**188**:781–5.

153 Ingram S, Hollman AS, Azmy A. Testicular torsion: missed diagnosis on colour Doppler sonography. *Pediatr Radiol* 1993;**23**:483–4.

154 Pryor JL, Watson LR, Day DL *et al.* Scrotal ultrasound for evaluation of subacute testicular torsion: sonographic findings and adverse clinical implications. *J Urol* 1994;**151**:693–7.

155 Schulsinger D, Glassberg K, Strashun A. Intermittent torsion: association with horizontal lie of the testicle. *J Urol* 1991;**145**:1053–5.

156 Donahue RE, Utley WLF. Torsion of spermatic cord. *Urology* 1978;**11**:33–6.

157 Anderson JB, Williamson RCN. Fertility after torsion of the spermatic cord. *Br J Urol* 1990;**65**:225–30.

158 Fisch H, Laor E, Reid RE, Tolia BM, Freed SZ. Gonadal dysfunction after testicular torsion: luteinizing hormone and follicle-stimulating hormone response to gonadotropin releasing hormone. *J Urol* 1988;**139**:961–4.

159 Anderson MJ, Dunn JK, Lipshultz LI, Coburn M. Semen quality and endocrine parameters after acute testicular torsion. *J Urol* 1992;**147**:1545–50.

160 Puri P, Barton D, O'Donnell B. Prepubertal testicular torsion: subsequent fertility. *J Pediatr Surg* 1985;**20**:598–601.

161 Luks FI, Yazbeck S, Homsy Y, Collin PP. The abdominoscrotal hydrocele. *Eur J Pediatr Surg* 1993;**3**:176–8.

162 Stephens BJ, Rice WT, Koucky CJ, Gruenberg JC. Optimal timing of elective indirect inguinal hernia repair in healthy children: clinical considerations for improved outcome. *World J Surg* 1992;**16**:952–7.

163 Stylianos S, Jacir NN, Harris BH. Incarceration of inguinal hernia in infants prior to elective repair. *J Pediatr Surg* 1993;**28**:582–3.

164 Puri P, Guiney EJ, O'Donnell B. Inguinal hernia in infants: the fate of the testis following incarceration. *J Pediatr Surg* 1984;**19**:44–6.

165 Holcomb GW III. Laparoscopic evaluation for a contralateral inguinal hernia or a nonpalpable testis. *Pediatr Ann* 1993;**22**:678–84.

166 Given JP, Rubin SZ. Occurrence of contralateral inguinal hernia following unilateral repair in a pediatric hospital. *J Pediatr Surg* 1989;**24**:963–5.

167 Surana R, Puri P. Is contralateral exploration necessary in infants with unilateral inguinal hernia? *J Pediatr Surg* 1993;**28**:1026–7.

168 Cohen-Addad N, Zarafu IW, Banna MK. Complete penoscrotal transposition. *Urology* 1985;**26**:149.

169 Hemal AK, Khanna S, Sharma SK. Incomplete penoscrotal transposition associated with hemivertebrae. *Aust N Z J Surg* 1991;**61**:233–5.

170 Redman JF. The surgical correction of incomplete scrotal transposition associated with hypospadias. *J Urol* 1983;**129**:565–7.

171 Ehrlich RM, Scardino PT. Surgical correction of scrotal transposition and perineal hypospadias. *J Pediatr Surg* 1982;**17**:75–7.

172 Mori Y, Ikoma F. Surgical correction of incomplete penoscrotal transposition associated with hypospadias. *J Pediatr Surg* 1986;**21**:46–8.

173 Lamm DL, Kaplan GW. Accessory and ectopic scrota. *Urology* 1977;**9**:149–53.

174 Sule JD, Skoog SJ, Tank ES. Perineal lipoma and the accessory labioscrotal fold: an etiological relationship. *J Urol* 1994;**151**:475–7.

175 Redman JF. Applied anatomy of the groin. Part I (basic anatomy). *Am Urol Assoc Update Ser* 1989;**8**:65–71.

176 Redman JF. Applied anatomy of the groin. Part II (applied anatomy). *Am Urol Assoc Update Ser* 1989;**8**:74–9.

177 Griffith CA. The Marcy repair revisited. *Surg Clin North Am* 1984;**64**:215–27.

178 Clark JU, Hashimoto EI. Utilization of Henle's ligament, iliopubic tract, aponeurosis transversus abdominis and

Cooper's ligament in inguinal herniorrhaphy. *Surg Gynecol Obstet* 1946;**82**:480–4.

179 LaRoque GP. The intra-abdominal method of removing inguinal and femoral hernia. *Arch Surg* 1932;**24**:189–203.

180 Redman JF. A retroperitoneal approach to orchiopexy. *J Urol* 1972;**108**:107–8.

181 Fowler R. The applied surgical anatomy of the peritoneal fascia of the groin and the 'secondary internal ring'. *Aust N Z J Surg* 1975;**45**:8–14.

182 Redman JF. Anatomy of the retroperitoneal connective tissue. *J Urol* 1983;**130**:45–50.

183 Redman JF. A simplified technique for scrotal pouch orchiopexy. *Urol Clin North Am* 1990;**17**:9–12.

184 Rodriguez LE, Kaplan GW. An experimental study of methods to produce intrascrotal testicular fixation. *J Urol* 1988; **139**: 565–7.

185 Redman JF. Reoperative orchiopexy: approach through the cremasteric fascia. *Dialog Pediatr Urol* 1993;**16**:5–7.

Vesical Dysfunction in Children
S.L.Schulman and J.D.van Gool

Functional incontinence

Functional incontinence due to bladder–sphincter dysfunction is an entity assigned to children with urinary incontinence when organic causes (i.e. anatomical and neurogenic) have been excluded. Unfortunately, there is confusion because of the misuse of medical terminology and an inability to define strictly the subsets of functional incontinence: urge syndrome and dysfunctional voiding. For the purposes of this chapter we define enuresis as normal voiding at an inappropriate time when urinary control is expected. Enuresis differs from incontinence, which is a failure of voluntary control of bladder and/or urethral muscle activity, with constant or frequent involuntary passage of urine. Hence, enuretic children usually empty their bladders and incontinent ones simply leak.

The complex of dysfunctional voiding and recurrent urinary tract infection (UTI) is an established clinical entity seen in school-age children, especially in girls. Among 7-year-old Swedish school children the prevalence of this condition is 8.4% in girls and 1.7% in boys [1]. In this study the mutual association of dysfunctional voiding and UTI, already known from retrospective clinical studies [2–5], was documented epidemiologically. Text-books and editorials treat the two parts of the complex separately [6,7] leading to separate treatment of the individual UTI and the primary symptom of dysfunctional voiding, wetting. Equally confusing is the improper treatment of children with nocturnal enuresis with behaviour modification and pharmacotherapy when, in fact, some of these children have symptoms suggestive of urge incontinence or dysfunctional voiding. There is evidence that dysfunctional voiding is associated with vesicoureteral reflux (VUR) [8,9], hence potentially reflux nephropathy, as well as a social stigma. School-age children consider wetting in school the third worst stress following the death of a parent and going blind [3].

Physiology and maturation of normal voiding

Bladder storage and emptying involve several complex processes and depend on an intact nervous system including the cerebral cortex, midbrain, spinal cord and peripheral nerves. The somatic and autonomic nervous systems (sympathetic and parasympathetic) are both responsible for effective lower urinary tract function. The somatic component innervates the external sphincter. The parasympathetic branch of the autonomic nervous system is primarily responsible for bladder emptying. The preganglionic nerves arise from the sacral area of the spinal cord (S2–4) and synapse close to the bladder. The major neurotransmitter is acetylcholine and its receptors are located throughout the bladder fundus and at the posterior urethra. Stimulation causes a detrusor contraction. The sympathetic branch of the autonomic nervous system arises from the thoracolumbar area of the spinal cord (T10–12,L1) with ganglia near the cord and function to facilitate the storage/filling phase of micturition. Noradrenaline is the primary neurotransmitter. Alpha-receptors, primarily located in the bladder neck and posterior urethra, respond to stimulation by contracting, thereby increasing resistance. Beta-receptors, primarily located at the bladder fundus, respond to stimulation by relaxing the detrusor muscle.

The micturition reflex pathways involve afferent nerves carrying impulses secondary to bladder distension reaching the sacral spinal cord. Spinal tract neurones carry impulses to the brainstem. The cortex communicates with the brainstem either permitting or inhibiting micturition. When normal voiding occurs there is both contraction of the detrusor and relaxation of the sphincter. Interruption of the higher pathways still allows reflex detrusor contraction but in an uncoordinated fashion with improper relaxation of the sphincter causing dyssynergia. More detail can be found in a contemporary text [10].

Maturation of these pathways allow the child to progress toward toilet training. The infants' bladder serves as a reservoir with intermittent and coordinated emptying.

Eventually the child develops an appreciation of bladder distension, and voiding is inhibited by consciously contracting the sphincter during a detrusor contraction until he or she is able to reach the toilet. Further maturation involves cortical inhibition of the contractions allowing the child more time to wait before 'needing' to void. Ultimately, by the age of 4–5 years the child can voluntarily choose to void prior to any sensation of bladder fullness [Fig. 16.1].

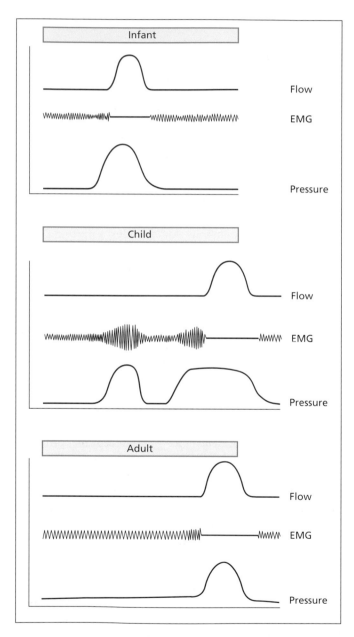

Fig. 16.1 Before volitional control is attained the sphincter relaxes as the bladder contracts. During the toilet-training period the child attempts to suppress the detrusor contraction by tightening the external sphincter. Eventually this process becomes automatic on a subconscious level [88].

Clinical characteristics of dysfunctional voiding

Urge syndrome and urge incontinence

These are characterized by frequent attacks of an imperative urge to void, countered by hold manoeuvres such as squatting [11,12]. Urge incontinence, when present, usually peaks in the afternoon, and consists of small quantities of urine loss. Many children do not express their urine loss, choosing instead to use techniques to camouflage their wetting. Parents of these children know the location of every toilet outside the home. Urge incontinence may have a nocturnal component, again in the form of slight loss of urine, which may or may not wake up the child. The symptoms and signs are caused by uninhibitable detrusor contractions countered by voluntary contraction of the pelvic floor. The functional capacity of the bladder is small for the child's age. Micturition is normal with complete relaxation of the pelvic floor in many cases, although some children may prematurely contract their sphincter resulting in incomplete emptying. This habit of inhibiting urge with voluntary pelvic floor contraction leads to postponement of defaecation leading to constipation and faecal soiling [11,13], not to be confused with the encopresis of children with behavioural problems.

Dysfunctional voiding

Staccato voiding is often termed dyssynergic voiding, in analogy to the true detrusor–sphincter dyssynergia in neuropathic bladder–sphincter dysfunction, and is sometimes combined with urge syndrome. This peculiar voiding pattern is caused by periodic bursts of pelvic floor activity during voiding resulting in peaks of bladder pressure coinciding with dips in urine flow rate. Flow time is prolonged and often incomplete increasing the child's risk of developing UTI.

Fractionated, incomplete voiding is characterized by infrequent voiding with micturition occurring in several small fractions. This is usually associated with incomplete bladder emptying, and thus post-void residuals. The bladder is large for age secondary to a hypoactive bladder and urge is easily inhibited. Micturition occurs in fractions secondary to unsustained bladder contractions with abdominal pressure necessary to shorten the flow time. The flow rate is highly irregular, due to reflex activity of the pelvic floor muscles, triggered by increases in abdominal pressure. Ostensibly, wetting in this form of dysfunctional voiding is secondary to overflow incontinence.

Other forms

The lazy bladder syndrome [14] is the net result of

longstanding fractionated and incomplete voiding. Abdominal pressure is the primary driving force for voiding and detrusor contractions are virtually absent. These children void infrequently and leave large post-void residuals subjecting them to an increased risk of developing UTI. This should not be confused with pure diurnal enuresis, an entity associated with normal, albeit infrequent, voiding usually seen in boys who simple delay emptying until it becomes too late.

The Hinman syndrome (non-neurogenic neurogenic bladder), first elaborated by Hinman [15], may represent one end of the natural history of dysfunctional voiding, characterized first by detrusor overactivity followed by bladder–sphincter dyssynergia and ultimately lazy bladder syndrome. Radiographs show thick trabeculated bladder walls, VUR and reflux nephropathy. Initially, severe psychological disturbance was postulated as the aetiology in these patients and hypnotherapy was recommended. Surgical treatment prior to correcting this imbalance is discouraged [16].

History and physical examination

A complete history and physical examination are essential to help identify children with neurogenic bladders as well as to distinguish between classifications of enuresis and the different forms of functional incontinence. Daytime wetting is usually the hallmark of dysfunctional voiding. The wetting is usually in small amounts, causing damp spots on the underwear. The wetting is most prevalent in the late afternoon because, during school, children are most anxious about remaining dry. Children with advanced stages of dysfunctional voiding will wet as well, but tend to skip early morning voiding. The nocturnal component usually involves losses of small amounts of urine with some children awakening. This is in contrast to nocturnal enuresis where voiding is complete and unnoticed until the morning.

Voiding frequency should be charted by the child for at least 2 weeks in a diary. Children with urge syndrome usually void at least seven times a day, those with infrequent voiding empty only one to three times a day and may strain or use manual pressure to assist in complete emptying. A staccato flow is a reliable sign of sphincter overactivity during voiding.

Sudden and imperative sensations of urge, numerous times a day, are characteristic of urge syndrome. Most children with urge syndrome have adopted typical hold manoeuvres to prevent wetting with each contraction. Despite this they are not successful and dampen their underwear. Children with lazy bladder syndrome never demonstrate urge. Finally, children with classic diurnal enuresis deny urge and ignore uncontrolled voiding.

Other features include obtaining a history of recurrent UTI which points to dysfunctional voiding associated with incomplete bladder emptying as the aetiology [2,3,17,18]. Incontinence in conjunction with stress may be seen in children with urge syndrome when increasing abdominal pressure provokes a detrusor contraction, as opposed to pure stress incontinence caused by structural incompetence of the ureteral closure mechanism. Likewise, incontinence associated with laughing may, in some cases, represent children with urge syndrome with detrusor instability exacerbated by increased abdominal pressure; this is in contrast to true giggle micturition which is defined as sudden, involuntary, uncontrollable and complete emptying of the bladder upon giggling in otherwise normal children [19]. Finally, constipation is associated with dysfunctional voiding [13].

The physical examination should focus on findings that might lead one to suspect an occult neuropathic bladder. These include lipomeningocele, sacral dimple, café-au-lait spots, lipoma and a hairy tuft at the sacrum. An absent or asymmetrical gluteal cleft suggests sacral agenesis. The neurological examination includes careful attention to the lower extremity including tone, strength, sensation and reflexes. Anal tone and the child's gait should be assessed.

Urodynamics

We and others [20] believe that urodynamic studies, by showing the interaction between detrusor and sphincter activity, are an essential adjunct to the diagnosis and therapy of children with functional incontinence in most patients because they help reveal the pathophysiological patterns behind the signs and symptoms of the condition.

Careful review of the literature supports the idea that most urodynamic patterns fit into two categories of bladder–sphincter overactivity [18,21]. One category is characterized by strong uninhibited detrusor contractions early in the filling phase, countered by voluntary pelvic floor activity giving rise to frequency, urgency, hold manoeuvres and urge incontinence with essentially normal voiding parameters. The other is characterized by incomplete relaxation (or frank overactivity) of striated pelvic floor muscles during actual voiding causing a staccato or fractionated flow associated with incomplete emptying despite a normal filling phase. One should note that the clinical patterns – urge syndrome and dysfunctional voiding (staccato or fractionated pattern), to which may be added the lazy bladder syndrome – may not be the distinct entities they seem and probably represent different stages in the natural history of non-neurogenic bladder–sphincter dyssynergia in children [22].

Radiological findings

All children with daytime wetting should have an

ultrasound of the kidneys and bladder to exclude anatomical abnormalities responsible for incontinence. In addition a voiding cystourethrogram (VCU) is performed those children with UTI. Not surprisingly, children with dysfunctional voiding will show, on VCU, ultrasound and intravenous urography, the abnormalities that are characteristic for the paediatric population with recurrent UTI, such as VUR and reflux nephropathy, with the prevalence known from studies on recurrent UTI in school-age children [2,5,23].

Some patients demonstrate a peculiar anomaly found at VCU; the so-called spinning-top configuration of the urethra. Seen during filling or voiding, whenever a girl or boy with urge syndrome tries to inhibit an imperative urge by contracting the pelvic floor, the force of the detrusor contraction will dilate the proximal urethra down to the closed external sphincter [24,25].

The detrusor muscle contracting against a tightly closed urethra generates high pressures explaining the variability in grade of VUR in children with urge syndrome and recurrent UTI [5]. Traditionally, VUR is graded on the appearance of the refluxing urinary tract on one or more static images, taken during filling and micturition. Elevated bladder pressures will momentarily dilate a refluxing urinary tract making VUR a dynamic event difficult to grade consistently on a static VCU [22,26,27]. As a consequence, the incidence of reflux nephropathy in children with dysfunctional voiding and recurrent UTI does not show the expected correlation with the grade of VUR [22].

Management

Only a proportion of children with functional incontinence will become free of symptoms with traditional methods of treatment (i.e. careful explanation of the problem, voiding instructions and control of recurrent UTI). Children may remain incontinent despite treatment under the auspices of a urotherapist in a structurally organized out-patient programme [28]. The primary treatment modalities we provide include antibiotic prophylaxis, anticholinergics and biofeedback with psychological counselling when indicated.

Long-term chemoprophylaxis has a definite place in the management of children with recurrent UTI and functional incontinence [29]. If recurrences can be avoided for a period of at least 6 months, signs and symptoms may diminish appreciably breaking the dysuria–tentative (dysfunctional) voiding–UTI cycle.

Children with urge syndrome respond to therapy with anticholinergic drugs aimed specifically at reducing the number of overactive detrusor contractions and restoring the reduced functional bladder capacity. This has, in some cases, reduced the degree of VUR [30,31]. However, results are often unpredictable and not long lasting. The best results with anticholinergic treatment are obtained in combination with a well-organized traditional treatment programme, and one might postulate that the general measures of the programme itself are more essential to success than the anticholinergic medication.

Children with urge syndrome must learn how to recognize the first sensations of urge and how to suppress these sensations by normal central inhibition, instead of emergency procedures such as urethral compression. Children with dysfunctional voiding must learn to void with a relaxed pelvic floor. A programme aimed at retraining the child to remain continent and empty effectively is the best approach, assuming the child has sufficient cognitive ability to understand what they are being taught and provided that an element of feedback can be incorporated into the retraining process [18]. Biofeedback, a term coined by Miller [32], is defined as the use of modern instrumentation to give a person better moment-to-moment information about a specific physiological process that is under the control of the central nervous system, but which is not clearly or accurately perceived. Urodynamic signals such as urine flow rate, pelvic floor electromyogram (EMG) or detrusor pressure are perfectly suited for biofeedback [18,28,33–36]. The success rate of such programmes, estimated to be as great as 70% in uncontrolled studies, underlies the importance of the physiological concept behind the clinical complex of bladder–sphincter dyssynergia and recurrent UTI.

Other forms of therapy have been suggested for the child with daytime wetting. Severing the filum terminale has been recommended by some [37], especially in the presence of spina bifida occulta, but has been discouraged by others [38]. Neuromodulation and acupuncture have also been advocated, although the mechanisms leading to successful treatment have yet to be elucidated [39,40]. Schneider et al. [41] taught the Kegel exercise to children with voiding dysfunction and found considerable improvement in the incidence of incontinence.

Neuropathic bladder–sphincter dysfunction

The entities associated with a neuropathic bladder in children include myelodysplasia, spinal dysraphism (which includes lipomeningocele, diastomyelia, dermoid cysts associated with tethering of the filum terminale) and sacral agenesis. This chapter will deal with the most common cause of neurogenic bladder dysfunction, myelomeningocele which is seen in 1–3 : 1000 live births, the greatest incidence in the world being in Wales. Myelomeningoceles account for over 90% of myelodysplastic newborns [42] and most commonly affects the lumbar and sacral spinal levels. The clinical expression of myelomeningocele ranges from prenatal hydrocephalus and Arnold–Chiari malformation (seen in approximately 85% of children) to syringomyelia with secondary tethering of the spinal cord. Unfortunately, renal failure secondary to neuropathic bladder–sphincter dysfunction is still seen in adolescents, making evaluation as early as the newborn period [43] vital to maximize renal function.

The initial approach to children with myelomeningoceles involved correcting the incontinence [44] and was associated with significant morbidity and mortality from obstructive uropathy and reflux nephropathy. In myelomeningocele, functional obstruction of the bladder outlet by detrusor–sphincter dyssynergia is responsible for upper urinary tract dilatation and high-pressure VUR. The dilatation and reflux increase with the age of the child and should not be considered in the realm of associated primary renal malformations [45]. Incomplete bladder emptying increases the risk of UTI, which makes the functional obstruction of the bladder outlet in myelomeningocele equivalent to an anatomical obstruction.

The lower urinary tract (detrusor, bladder neck and external sphincter) normally works in a coordinated fashion. The mutually exclusive functions of storage and emptying are controlled and coordinated at different levels of the central nervous system, converging at the sacral micturition centre which is structurally abnormal in almost every child with myelomeningocele. Thus, proper diagnosis and effective therapy can only be instituted based on an assessment of all of the components of the lower urinary tract [46,47].

Urodynamic studies in children with myelomeningoceles, by combining the registration of bladder pressure, rectal pressure, pelvic floor EMG and urine flow rate, produce pertinent evidence about the activity of both the detrusor muscle and the urethral sphincter mechanism during bladder filling and emptying. These studies should be performed in the newborn period to assess the child's risk of further deterioration [43,48–51].

Classification of detrusor and sphincter function

Overactivity of the sphincter mechanism throughout filling and emptying indicates functional obstruction. Conversely, inactivity of the sphincter represents incontinence. One can add the effect of the detrusor to these clinically relevant categories, such that detrusor overactivity implies a small bladder capacity and detrusor inactivity a large bladder capacity. Thus children with myelomeningoceles can fall into four discrete categories of bladder–sphincter dysfunction. Table 16.1 provides the distribution of the four main patterns of bladder–sphincter dysfunction that were determined by the urodynamic assessment of a cohort of 188 children with myelomeningoceles followed from birth with serial urodynamic, uroradiological and neurological studies [48]. A total of 473 urodynamic studies were performed over a 16-year period (1976–92), with each child averaging 2.5 studies.

In most cases a reciprocal relationship was seen between detrusor and sphincter activity, implying that the detrusor and sphincter display the same type of neurological lesion. There was also a consistency between the four categories of detrusor–sphincter function with repeat urodynamic studies demonstrating similar findings [43,48]. Changes usually occur in a single urodynamic parameter, such as bladder compliance and capacity, voiding pressure and urine flow rate. However, real changes in the urodynamic pattern can also occur. These are usually secondary to changes in the neurological lesion itself, such as secondary tethering of the spinal cord, or to the late expression of associated lesions such as hydromyelia or syringomyelia [43,52,53]. The changes in urodynamic patterns, commonly seen in children with 'minor' lesions and normal urodynamics [53,54] who develop secondary tethering of the spinal cord, will consist of the development of detrusor–sphincter dyssynergia or of a decrease in activity of the detrusor or sphincter muscles. Although specific categories can be elicited on urodynamic studies and their interpretation has become the basis of classification of neuropathic bladder–sphincter dysfunction, interpreting urodynamic data alone may be insufficient. A VCU should be performed with the urodynamic study, with video urodynamics as the ideal choice [55].

Pelvic floor inactivity

Incontinence is the main problem in the two categories of neurogenic bladder–sphincter dysfunction with inactivity

Table 16.1 Distribution of four patterns of neuropathic bladder-sphincter dysfunction in 188 children with myelomeningocele.

	Detrusor inactive	Detrusor overactive	Detrusor normal	Total
Inactive sphincter	44(43)	20(20)	–	63(64)
Overactive sphincter	28(26)	83(85)	–	111(111)
Normal sphincter	–	–	14(13)	14(13)
Total	71(70)	103(105)	14(13)	188(188)

Number in parentheses donote distribution at onset with six children showing a definite change in pattern.

of the urethral sphincter, with functional bladder capacity based on the activity of the detrusor. Extremely low values are seen in detrusor overactivity with low to normal values in detrusor inactivity. It is difficult to achieve continence without surgically increasing the outflow resistance of the bladder neck and urethra.

The therapy of choice for the child with a combination of sphincter and detrusor inactivity is clean intermittent self-catheterization (CIC) [56]; despite low bladder capacity, CIC will reduce the degree of incontinence to a socially acceptable level. This in turn increases the patient's independence, especially when the child is able to catheterize him or herself [57]. If bladder capacity is sufficient and a greater degree of bladder neck competence is necessary, surgical procedures such as colposuspension [58] or artificial sphincter implantation [59] are indicated, once the child has mastered the technique for CIC.

The combination of urethral sphincter inactivity and detrusor overactivity requires an increase in bladder capacity prior to success with CIC. This can be achieved by pharmacological or neurosurgical denervation of the bladder [60,61], or by bladder augmentation [55,62] with the primary goal being conversion of the bladder from a low compliance, low capacity system to an inactive reservoir. It is essential that the child and the parents are facile at CIC prior to resorting to augmentation. Techniques have been developed that provide both a high compliance reservoir and easy access for catheterization, such as an appendicovesicostomy [63,64].

UTI and VUR rarely cause problems in a patient with inactivity of the urethral sphincter, as the reflux is usually low grade with a high rate of spontaneous resolution as long as there is complete emptying of the bladder. With bladder emptying through manual expression (Credé method), recurrent UTI may be a problem. Manual expression is a tempting alternative to CIC in children with inactivity of the pelvic floor, but is unsatisfactory because of its tendency to displace caudally and kink the urethra. One should be aware that UTI in children with myelomeningoceles may be difficult to diagnose because of the absence of obvious signs such as dysuria or frequency causing considerable delay in the treatment of these children [65].

Pelvic floor overactivity

Functional infravesical obstruction, due to detrusor–sphincter dyssynergia, is the primary problem in children with myelomeningoceles and pelvic floor overactivity regardless of the pattern of detrusor activity. When combined with detrusor inactivity, urinary retention will develop with overflow incontinence and high bladder pressures at the end of the filling phase. CIC provides both an opportunity to prevent damage secondary to obstruction

and allows the child to regain continence as the bladder capacity in these children is generally high. Once again, attempts to empty with manual expression or Valsalva manoeuvres will increase emptying pressures and result in incomplete emptying.

When both the detrusor and urethral sphincter are overactive, obstructive uropathy may ensue secondary to increased pressures during emptying. The bladder capacity may not always be small as the neurological lesion may be incomplete in both the detrusor muscle and the urethral sphincter. Bladder–sphincter dysfunction may remain compensated, at the price of detrusor hypertrophy, high bladder pressures and a small functional capacity. Decompensation and obstructive uropathy are heralded by increased bladder capacity and residual urine that can appear as continence along with a high rate of UTI [66]. Treatment with CIC alone will not effectively treat incontinence, nor will it prevent obstructive uropathy associated with elevated detrusor pressures. Thus pharmacological conversion of the overactive bladder to an inactive reservoir with the use of anticholinergic medications is necessary in conjunction with CIC. Oxybutynin, an anticholinergic medication with a high rate of success in bladder–sphincter dysfunction, is usually prescribed at a dosage of 0.3–0.4 mg/kg/day divided into three or four doses. The common side effects seen with this class of drug can be minimized by instilling the drug, dissolved in water, directly into the bladder after emptying by CIC [67].

There is evidence that this pattern of bladder–sphincter dysfunction will result in a small, poorly compliant bladder with continuously elevated pressures, both during filling and emptying, with structural changes in the bladder consisting of collagen deposition [68]. Thus, in some cases, surgical conversion of the poorly compliant bladder through the use of augmentation will be necessary to protect the upper tracts and gain sufficient functional capacity for continence. Early reports describing selective sacral rhizotomy in children with this form of neuropathic bladder–sphincter dysfunction have shown promising results, possibly obviating the need for augmentation or diversion [61].

Incomplete bladder emptying is to be expected in children with overactivity of the pelvic floor musculature. The resultant residual urine is likely to become infected if CIC is not introduced. Despite the fear that CIC may contaminate the bladder, studies have shown fewer infections in children treated this way [57]. Also, patient compliance with prophylaxis may improve with the concomitant improvement in incontinence. The combination of high bladder pressures and VUR permits transmission of the elevated pressures directly to the upper urinary tract where the pressure-dependent phenomenon of intrarenal reflux can initiate renal scarring, particularly in young children. Early detection and treatment of functional obstruction are crucial to prevent the progressive scarring of reflux nephropathy.

Conclusion

The urodynamic patterns in infants and children with myelomeningoceles provide a neuropathological basis for classification of their bladder–sphincter dysfunction. The classes are clinically relevant since they are defined by the two most important urological problems: incontinence and obstruction. In this respect, sphincter activity is clinically more important; however, detrusor activity will have long-term sequelae such as hypertrophy and abnormal collagen composition that will render the bladder useless as a reservoir. In individual patients, the urodynamic parameters serve to grade the clinical problems and to monitor medical and surgical interventions. Without urodynamics, in is impossible to tailor therapy to the patient. This may create troublesome social, psychological, financial and emotional implications [69].

Urodynamics is also the only diagnostic technique that can detect functional obstruction before it manifests itself as obstructive uropathy or reflux nephropathy. Serial urodynamic observations are needed to follow the evolution of detrusor–sphincter dyssynergia, with the recognition of either compensated bladder function or frank functional obstruction. Static imaging techniques such as cystography do not meet this objective and should be considered complementary to urodynamic studies. A combination of imaging and urodynamic techniques offers the best method for investigation of the lower urinary tract in children with myelomeningoceles [55].

Primary nocturnal enuresis

Primary nocturnal enuresis is a heterogenous condition that affects between 5 and 8% of children aged 7 years, with a spontaneous resolution rate of 15% per year [70,71]. Because the vast majority of cases do resolve spontaneously, some physicians choose to ignore the problem. Although enuresis does not cause physical harm to children it can cause emotional disturbances and poor self-esteem. Some parents feel as though they have failed and often both the children and their parents choose to keep enuresis a family secret [72].

Aetiology

After excluding structural and neurogenic causes, systemic diseases and functional incontinence — usually after obtaining a thorough history and physical examination — there is no single aetiology to explain enuresis in every child. Clearly genetics plays an important part as 40% of offspring will be enuretic if one parent has the condition and 70% will be enuretic if both parents are affected [73,74]. Some investigators have found small functional bladder capacities in children with nocturnal enuresis created by the development of detrusor contractions during sleep [75]. These children may fall into our category of urge syndrome, especially when symptoms are associated with daytime frequency, urgency and wetting. Others feel that children with nocturnal enuresis are unusually heavy sleepers, although sleep studies have failed to show a clear difference between children with enuresis and children who can remain dry. In addition, most children able to remain dry at night do so without awakening, suggesting more than a dyssomnia as the aetiology.

A deficiency of antidiuretic hormone, first reported by Nørgaard and Rittig [76,77], has been used to explain enuresis, especially in young adolescents. Thus, these children are prone to produce more urine than their functional bladder capacity will allow at night. This theory is inconsistent when one considers that approximately half of children with diseases causing resistance to antidiuretic hormone, such as sickle cell disease, can remain dry at night [78,79].

Evaluation

Little more than a complete history and physical examination is necessary when evaluating children with nocturnal enuresis. Careful attention to daytime voiding behaviour is important to exclude bladder–sphincter dysfunction. Children with a history of UTI should be evaluated with imaging studies. Constipation can cause enuresis and should be treated. The physical examination should include emphasis on normal growth and blood pressure to exclude chronic renal failure, and a neurological examination to exclude an occult neuropathic bladder. A urinalysis should be performed to look for proteinuria, haematuria and normal concentrating ability. Imaging studies are not necessary if history, physical examination and urinalysis are normal.

Therapy

The treatment for nocturnal enuresis should be directed in a manner that is age appropriate and is either behavioural or pharmacological. Usually it is best for younger children to have a motivationally based programme, with medications used in older children and adolescents. Many studies have shown improvement in nocturnal enuresis when medication is used, compared to placebos, but few, if any, compare one therapy to another.

Behavioural therapy in the form of self-awakening can be used by having the child pretend that his or her bladder is full and trying to awaken the child. Others recommend self-hypnosis with the post-hypnotic suggestion that the child will use the bathroom at night [80]. Dry bed training involves the parents more and teaches the child to self-awaken by going through a series of programmed awakenings over several days until the child becomes independent. A high cure rate (92%) has been reported with a relapse rate of 20% [81].

Enuresis alarms are very popular and, if the family and child are motivated, can be quite successful (approximately 70%) [71]. Most commercially available alarms are easy to use, free of risk, inexpensive and relatively comfortable. Their disadvantages include the time commitment necessary until they can be discontinued. They are not very helpful if the alarm is triggered several times per night because of decreased bladder capacity or polyuria.

Three medications are currently available for treatment of nocturnal enuresis; oxybutynin, imipramine and desmopressin acetate (DDAVP). Oxybutynin may be useful for the nocturnal component in children with urge syndrome, but has not been proven beneficial in children with primary isolated nocturnal enuresis [82]. Imipramine has been used extensively for nocturnal enuresis and seems to exert both an anticholinergic effect aimed at increasing bladder capacity and a central effect that decreases the amount of time spent in rapid-eye-movement sleep [83]. Imipramine when taken in a dose of 50–75 mg at bedtime had a positive effect in 10–60% of patients, with some children relapsing after withdrawal [84]. Imipramine can cause nausea, anxiety and malaise with some children experiencing personality changes, cardiac arrhythmias or sleep disorders. It must be kept out of the reach of small children because of its potentially lethal effects when taken at inappropriately high doses.

In 1985, Nørgaard et al. suggested that a component of nocturnal enuresis may be caused by a deficiency of the normal surge of antidiuretic hormone usually seen in children able to remain dry at night [76]. Hence DDAVP, at a dose of 20–40 μg/night intranasally, would appear to be useful because it would reduce a child's urine output such that he or she could remain dry prior to needing to void. DDAVP seems to be more effective in children where there is a family history of nocturnal enuresis (91% success rate) as compared to where a family history was not observed (7%) [85]. Moffatt evaluated 18 randomized controlled trials and determined that DDAVP produces complete dryness in only a minority of patients for a short period of time and suggested that an enuresis alarm should be primary therapy [86]. Water intoxication has been observed extremely infrequently with more common side effects including nasal stuffiness, epistaxis and mild abdominal pain. DDAVP is recently available in an oral formulation with comparable results to intranasal dosing [87].

It is essential that one recognizes that isolated primary nocturnal enuresis should not be confused with the other forms of wetting described above. Children who do not respond to conventional therapy may have diurnal enuresis, which is a complex behavioural problem, urge syndrome or dysfunctional voiding.

References

1 Hellström A, Hanson E, Hannson S, Hjälmås K, Jodal U. Association between urinary symptoms at 7 years old and previous urinary tract infection. Arch Dis Child 1991;66:232–4.
2 Gool JD van, Tanagho EA. External sphincter activity and recurrent urinary tract infections in girls. Urology 1977; 10:348–53.
3 Meadow SR. Day wetting. Pediatr Nephrol 1990;4:178–84.
4 Snodgrass W. Relationship of voiding dysfunction to urinary tract infection and vesicoureteral reflux in children. Urology 1991;38:341–4.
5 Gool JD van, Hjälmås K, Tamminen-Möbius T, Olbing H. Historical clues to the complex of dysfunctional voiding and vesicoureteral reflux. J Urol 1992;148:1699–702.
6 Editorial. Diurnal enuresis. Lancet 1987;2:314–15.
7 Marcovitch H. Treating bed wetting. Br Med J 1993;306:536.
8 Seruca H. Vesicoureteral reflux and voiding dysfunction: a prospective study. J Urol 1989;142:494–8.
9 Steele BT, De Maria J. A new perspective on the natural history of vesicoureteral reflux. Pediatr 1992;90:30–2.
10 Van Arsdalen K, Wein AJ. Physiology of micturition and continence. In: Krane RJ, Sirorsky MB, eds. Clinical Neuro-Urology. Boston: Little, Brown, 1991:25–82.
11 Vincent SA. Postural control of urinary incontinence—the curtsey sign. Lancet 1966;2:631–2.
12 Gool JD van, Jonge GA de. Urge syndrome and urge incontinence. Arch Dis Child 1989;64:1629–34.
13 O'Regan S, Yazback S, Hamberger B, Schick E. Constipation—a commonly unrecognized cause of enuresis. Am J Dis Child 1986;140:260–1.
14 Luca FG, Swenson O, Fisher JH, Loutfi AH. The dysfunctional 'lazy' bladder syndrome in children. Arch Dis Child 1962; 37:117–20.
15 Hinman F Jr. Urinary tract damage in children who wet. Pediatr 1974;54:143–50.
16 Hinman F Jr. Noneurogenic neurogenic bladder (the Hinman syndrome)—15 years later. J Urol 1986;136:769–77.
17 Koff SA. Bladder–sphincter dysfunction in childhood. Urology 1982;19:457–61.
18 Gool JD van, Kuijten RH, Donckerwolcke RA, Messer AP, Vijverberg MAW. Bladder–sphincter dysfunction, urinary infection and vesicoureteral reflux—with special reference to cognitive bladder training. Contrib Nephrol 1984;39:190–210.
19 Cooper CE. Giggle micturition. In: Kolvin I, MacKeith RC, Meadow SR, eds. Bladder Control and Enuresis. London: Heinemann, 1973:61–3.
20 Weerasinghe N, Malone PS. The value of videourodynamics in the investigation of neurologically normal children who wet. Br J Urol 1993;71:539–42.
21 Mayo ME, Burns MW. Urodynamic studies in children who wet. Br J Urol 1990;65:641–5.
22 Gool JD van, Vijverberg MAW, Jong TPVM de. Functional daytime incontinence—clinical and urodynamic assessment. Scand J Urol Nephrol Suppl 1992;141:58–69.
23 Allen TD. Vesicoureteral reflux as a manifestation of

dysfunctional voiding. In: Hodson CJ, Kincaid-Smith P, eds. *Reflux Nephropathy*. New York: Masson Publications, 1979: 171–80.

24 Saxton HM, Borzyskowski M, Mundy AR, Vivian GC. Spinning top urethra: not a normal varient. *Radiol* 1988;**168**:147–50.

25 Saxton HM, Borzyskowski M, Robinson LB. Nonobstructive posterior urethral widening (spinning top urethra) in boys with bladder instability. *Radiol* 1992;**182**:81–5.

26 Borzyskowski M, Mundy AR. Videourodynamic assessment of diurnal urinary incontinence. *Arch Dis Child* 1987;**62**:128–31.

27 Nielson JB, Djurhuus JC, Jörgenson TM. Lower urinary tract dysfunction in vesicoureteral reflux. *Urol Int* 1984;**39**:29–31.

28 Hellström A, Hjälmås K, Jodal U. Rehabilitation of the dysfunctional bladder in children: method and 3-year followup. *J Urol* 1984;**138**:847–9.

29 Smellie JM, Grünberg RN, Bantock HM, Prescod N. Prophylactic co-trimoxazole and trimethoprim in the management of urinary tract infection in children. *Pediatr Nephrol* 1988;**2**:12.

30 Homsey YL, Nsouli I, Hamburger B, Laberge I, Schick E. Effects of oxybutynin on vesicoureteral reflux in children. *J Urol* 1985;**134**:1168–71.

31 Scholtmeijer RH, Mastrigt R van. The effect of oxyphenonium bromide and oxybutynin hydrochloride on detrusor contractility and reflux in children with vesicoureteral reflux and detrusor instability. *J Urol* 1991;**146**:660–2.

32 Miller NE. Learning of visceral and glandular responses. *Science* 1969;**163**:434–7.

33 Wear JB, Wear RB, Cleeland C. Biofeedback in urology using urodynamics: preliminary observations. *J Urol* 1979;**121**:464–8.

34 Sugar EC, Firlit CF. Urodynamic feedback: new therapeutic approach for childhood incontinence/infection (vesical voluntary sphincter dyssynergia). *J Urol* 1982;**128**:1253–8.

35 Jerkins GR, Noe HN, Vaugn WR, Roberts E. Biofeedback training for children with bladder sphincter incoordination. *J Urol* 1987;**138**:1113–15.

36 Kjölseth D, Knudsen LM, Madsen B, Nørgaard JP, Djurhuus JC. Urodynamic biofeedback training for children with bladder–sphincter dyscoordination during voiding. *Neurourol Urodyn* 1993;**12**:211–21.

37 Khoury AE, Hendrick EB, McLorie GA, Kulkarni A, Churchill BM. Occult spinal dysraphism: clinical and urodynamic outcome after division of the filum terminale. *J Urol* 1990;**144**:426–9.

38 Kondo A, Gotoh M, Kato K et al. Treatment of persistent enuresis. Results of severing a tight filum terminale. *Br J Urol* 1988;**62**:42–5.

39 Minni B, Capozza N, Creti G et al. Bladder instability and enuresis treated by acupuncture and electro-therapeutics: early urodynamic observations. *Acupunct Electrother Res* 1990; **15**:19–25.

40 Tanagho EA. Neuromodulation on the management of voiding dysfunction in children. *J Urol* 1992;**148**:655–7.

41 Schneider MS, King LR, Surwit RS. Kegel exercises and childhood incontinence: a new role for an old treatment. *J Pediatr* 1994;**124**:91–2.

42 Bauer SB, Labib KB, Dieppa RA et al. Urodynamic evaluation in a boy with myelodysplasia and incontinence. *Urology* 1977;**10**:354–62.

43 Bauer SB, Hallet M, Khoshbin S et al. The predictive value of urodynamic evaluation in the newborn with myelodysplasia. *J Am Med Assoc* 1984;**152**:650–1.

44 Lie HR, Lagergren J, Rasmussen F et al. Bowel and bladder control of children with myelomeningocele—a Nordic study. *Dev Med Child Neurol* 1991;**33**:1053–61.

45 Hunt GM, Whitaker RH. The pattern of congenital renal anomalies associated with neural tube defects. *Dev Med Child Neurol* 1987;**29**:91–5.

46 Wein AJ. Classification of neurogenic voiding dysfunction. *J Urol* 1981;**125**:605–10.

47 Hald T, Bradley WE. *The Urinary Bladder—Neurology and Urodynamics*. Baltimore: Williams and Wilkins, 1982:56–61.

48 Gool JD van. Interpretation of urodynamic assessment: activity patterns of detrusor and striated urethral muscles. *Spina Bifida and Neurogenic Bladder Dysfunction — a Urodynamic Study*. Utrecht: Impress, 1986:129–38.

49 McGuire EJ, Woodside JR, Burden TA et al. Prognostic value of urodynamic testing in myelodysplastic patients. *J Urol* 1981;**126**:205–9.

50 Sidi AA, Dykstra DD, Gonzalez R. The value of urodynamic testing in the management of myelodysplastic neonates with myelodysplasia: a prospective study. *J Urol* 1986;**135**:90–3.

51 Perez LM, Khoury J, Webster GD. The value of urodynamic studies in infants less than 1 year old with congenital spinal dysraphism. *J Urol* 1992;**148**:584–7.

52 Spindel MR, Bauer SB, Dyro FM et al. The changing neurologic lesion in myelodysplasia. *J Am Med Assoc* 1987;**258**:1630–2.

53 Toet M, Gool JD van, Witkamp TH, Wieringen H van. Spina bifida aperta and the tethered cord syndrome. *Eur J Pediatr Surg* 1991;1(Suppl.):48–9.

54 Dator DP, Hatchett L, Dyro FM, Shefner JM, Bauer SB. Urodynamic dysfunction in walking myelodysplastic children. *J Urol* 1992;**148**:362–5.

55 Borzyskowski M, Mundy AR. The management of the neuropathic bladder in childhood. *Pediatr Nephrol* 1988;**2**: 56–66.

56 Withycombe J, Whitaker RH, Hunt G. Intermittent catheterisation in the management of children with neuropathic bladder. *Lancet* 1978;**2**:981–3.

57 Gool JD van, Jong TPVM de, Boemers ThM. Einfluβ des intermittierender Katheterismus auf Harnwegsinfekte und Inkontinenz bei Kindern mit Spina bifida. *Monatsschr Kinderheilkd* 1991;**139**:592–6.

58 McGuire E, Wang C-C, Usitalo H et al. Modified pubovaginal sling in girls with myelodysplasia. *J Urol* 1986;**135**:94–6.

59 Light JK. The artificial urinary sphincter in children. *Urol Clin North Am* 1985;**12**:103–10.

60 Amark P, Nergardh A. Influence of adrenergic agonists and antagonists on urethral pressure, bladder pressure and detrusor hyperactivity in children with myelodysplasia. *Acta Pediatr Scand* 1991;**80**:824–32.

61 Franco I, Storrs B, Firlit CF et al. Selective sacral rhizotomy in children with high pressure neurogenic bladder: preliminary results. *J Urol* 1992;**148**:648–50.

62 Kass EJ, Koff SA. Bladder augmentation in the pediatric neurogenic bladder. *J Urol* 1983;**129**:552–5.

63 Duckett JW, Snyder HM. Continent urinary diversion: variations on the Mitrofanoff principle. *J Urol* 1986;**136**:58–62.

64 Kock NG, Nilson AE, Nilsson LO, Norlén LJ, Philipson BM. Urinary diversion via a continent ileal reservoir: clinical results in 12 patients. *J Urol* 1982;**128**:469–75.

65 Smellie JM. Management of urinary tract infections. In: Borzyskowski M, Mundy AR, eds. *Neuropathic Bladder in Childhood*. Oxford: Oxford University Press, 1990:59–71.

66 Gool JD van, Kuijten RH, Donckerwolke RAMG, Kramer PP. Detrusor–sphincter dyssynergia in children with myelomeningocele — a prospective study. *Z Kinderchir* 1982;**37**: 148–51.

67 Greenfield SP, Fera M. The use of intravesical oxybutynin chloride in children with neurogenic bladder. *J Urol* 1991; **146**:532–4.

68 Ghoniem GM, Bloom DA, McGuire EJ, Stewart KL. Bladder compliance in meningomyelocele children. *J Urol* 1989;**141**: 1404–6.

69 Bloom DA, Ritchey ML. The high cost of continence. *Dialog Pediatr Urol* 1992;**15**:3–4.

70 Fergusson DM, Horwood LT, Sannon FT. Factors related to the age of attainment of nocturnal bladder control: an 8-year longitudinal study. *Pediatr* 1986;**78**:884–90.

71 Forsythe WI, Redmond A. Enuresis and spontaneous cure rate: study of 1129 enuretics. *Arch Dis Child* 1974;**49**:259–69.

72 Foxman B, Valdez RB, Brook RH. Childhood enuresis: prevalence, perceived impact and prescribed treatments. *Pediatr* 1986;**77**:482–7.

73 Bakwin H. The genetics of enuresis. In: Kolvin I, MacKeith RC, Meadow SR, eds. *Bladder Control and Enuresis.* Philadelphia: JB Lipincott, 1973:73–8.

74 Hallgren B. Nocturnal enuresis in twins. *Acta Psychol Neurol Scand* 1960;**35**:73.

75 Starfield B. Functional bladder capacity in enuretic and non-enuretic children. *J Pediatr* 1967;**70**:777–81.

76 Nørgaard JP, Pederson EB, Djurhuus JC. Diurnal antidiuretic levels in enuretics. *J Urol* 1985;**134**:1029–31.

77 Rittig S, Knugdson UB, Nørgaard JP, Pederson EB, Djurhuus JC. Abnormal diurnal rhythm of plasma vasopressin and urinary output in patients with enuresis. *Am J Physiol* 1989;**256**: F664–71.

78 Akinyanju O, Agbato O, Ogunmekan AO, Okoye JU. Enuresis in sickle cell disease, I: prevalence studies. *J Trop Pediatr* 1976;**35**:24–6.

79 Readett DR, Morris JS, Serjeant GR. Nocturnal enuresis in sickle cell haemoglobinopathies. *Arch Dis Child* 1990;**65**: 290–3.

80 Olness K. The use of self-hypnosis on the treatment of childhood nocturnal enuresis: a report of forty patients. *Clin Pediatr* 1975;**14**:273.

81 Azrin NH, Thienes PM. Rapid elimination of enuresis by intensive learning without a conditioning apparatus. *Behav Res Ther* 1978;**9**:342.

82 Lovering JS, Tallett SE, McKendry JBJ. Oxybutynin efficacy in the treatment of primary enuresis. *Pediatr* 1988; **81**:104.

83 Kales A, Kales JD, Jacobson A, *et al.* Effects of imipramine on enuretic frequency and sleep stages. *Pediatr* 1977;**60**:431.

84 Kolvin I, Taunch J, Currah J *et al.* Enuresis: a descriptive analysis and a controlled trial. *Dev Med Child Neurol* 1972;**14**:715.

85 Hogg RJ, Husmann D. The role of family history in predicting response to desmopressin in nocturnal enuresis. *J Urol* 1993;**150**:444–5.

86 Moffatt MEK, Harlos S, Kirshen AJ, Burd L. Desmopressin acetate and nocturnal enuresis: how much do we know? *Pediatr* 1993;**92**:420–5.

87 Matthiesen TB, Rittig S, Djurjuus JC, Nørgaard JP. A dose titration and an open 6-week efficacy and safety study of desmopressin tablets in the management of nocturnal enuresis. *J Urol* 1994;**151**:460–3.

88 Siroky RJ, Krane MB. Clinical Neuro-Urology 2e Little-Brown, Lippincott-Raven. 1991:399.

17 Childhood Urinary Tract Infection and Vesicoureteric Reflux

L.M.Dairiki Shortliffe

Introduction

Urinary tract infections (UTIs) in children often serve as markers for urinary tract abnormalities that may need correction or that may subject a child to a risk of renal damage from infection. For this reason it is important to identify children at risk for urinary infection and those at risk for further renal damage from infection. This chapter will concentrate on factors that lead to bacteriuria and renal damage in children and their management.

Urinary tract infections

Natural history in children

From screening studies for UTI it has been documented that in the first few months of life boys have more frequent bacteriuria than girls. During this period about 2.7% of boys and 0.7% girls are bacteriuric [1,2]. Uncircumcised boys, moreover, have an increased rate of infections over circumcised boys. While after the first 6–12 months the incidence of infections falls to below 1% in both circumcised and uncircumcised boys, it increases to 1–3% in girls during school years [3–5].

Approximately 30–40% of these children have urinary obstruction and vesicoureteric reflux (VUR). A certain group of these children are, furthermore, susceptible to recurrent urinary infections. Winberg found that the risk of recurrent infection during the year after an infection is directly proportional to the number of previous infections (i.e. the more infections a child has, the more likely they are to get another). If there has been one earlier infection the risk is greater than 25% of getting another infection in the next year, if there have been two earlier infections the risk is greater than 50%, and after three infections the risk is almost 75% [6]. There is, therefore, a group of children who can be identified to be at high risk of getting subsequent infections. Why these children are at high risk of infection is not totally clear, but there are both bacterial and host factors. While many children have little morbidity from the recurrent infections, save bladder irritative symptoms, a certain group with anatomical abnormalities such as obstruction or VUR may risk renal damage from future infections. The future history of these children depends upon these risk factors.

Associated bacteria

The most common bacteria infecting the urinary tract is *Escherichia coli*, but other Enterobacteriaceae and enterococci may also cause urinary infection. Various bacterial traits that may cause virulence for the urinary tract have been identified. Particular bacterial cell wall O antigens identified by serotyping (e.g. O1, O2, O4, O6, O7, O75) [6,7], mannose-resistant haemagglutination, bacterial fimbriae [8,9] and other properties have been implicated. In 1981 Väisänen and associates [9] and Källenius and associates [8] reported that the two best markers for pyelonephritogenic *E. coli* were mannose-resistant haemagglutination and P blood group-specific adhesins (p fimbriae or p pili). Of 32 strains of *E. coli* found to cause pyelonephritis in children, 91% (29/32) had mannose-resistant haemagglutination characteristics and 81% had p fimbriae [9]. Källenius found, moreover, that 94% of *E. coli* causing pyelonephritis had p fimbriae, but only 19% of *E. coli* causing cystitis or 14% involved with asymptomatic bacteriuria had it [8].

Childhood risk factors

Previous studies in both children and adults show that increased periurethral bacterial colonization is associated with increased risk for recurrent bacteriuria [8,10–12]. In newborn children the periurethral area is massively colonized with aerobic bacteria (especially *E. coli*, enterococci and staphylococci) [10], but this colonization disappears during the first year of life and after about 5 years of age is found only in children who get recurrent UTIs.

In neonatal boys who are circumcised, however, the

periurethral area (prepuce) is significantly less colonized by bacteria than in uncircumcised boys [10,13,14], and this finding has been used to rationalize why uncircumcised boys have a higher incidence of urinary infections in the first few months of life than circumcised boys. In both circumcised and uncircumcised boys, after 6 months of age the increased periurethral colonization dramatically decreases and the incidence of infections decreases as well.

Age is also a variable with regard to the incidence of bacteriuria. The incidence of bacteriuria in babies under a year old is higher than at any other time during childhood. In older adults, moreover, the incidence of urinary infection appears to rise about 1% for every decade. While the increased incidence of UTIs in neonates is usually attributed to the immature and compromised immune system and increased bacterial colonization, the reasons for the slow increase of bacteria during adult years is unclear. It has been reported that children with recurrent UTIs may have lower urinary concentrations of secretory immunoglobulin A (IgA) in their urine than children without infections [15], suggesting some immunological differences may affect risk.

Another factor affecting this increased bacterial colonization appears to be the presence of bacterial receptors on the epithelial cells. When p fimbriae were identified as a virulence factor, it was found that glycolipids characterizing the P blood group system found on host uroepithelial cells may serve as receptors for bacteria. As a result, children with a P blood group phenotype were examined for evidence of recurrent infections as they might have a special increased susceptibility for urinary infection [16]. While 97% (35/36) of girls with recurrent pyelonephritis with minimal (international reflux grade 1) or no reflux had the P1 blood group phenotype, 84% of girls with reflux (international reflux grades II–V) had the P1 blood group phenotype, and 75% of those without history of infection had it. There was no significant difference in the rate of infections between girls with reflux and infections and those without infections, thus suggesting that in children with reflux the VUR is a more important risk factor for pyelonephritis than having receptors for the bacterial fimbriae.

Since the urothelial surface antigens have been found to influence susceptibility to UTI, several other blood group antigens have been implicated. Adult women with Lewis non-secretor blood phenotypes (Le(a–b–) and Le (a+b–)) have three times the risk of recurrent urinary infection than women with a Le(a–b+) phenotype, and uroepithelial cells from non-secretor women have more receptors than secretor women [17]. Similarly, it appears that children with anatomical abnormalities and a non-secretor phenotype may be more susceptible to urinary infections than secretors [18]. This work suggests that non-secretor

status may allow an exposure of structures that serve as bacterial receptors leading to increased bacterial adherence.

Primary vesicoureteric reflux

Under normal conditions urine does not reflux from the bladder to the ureter. When VUR occurs, bladder urine may pass retrogradely into the ureter, renal pelvis and calyces. Often the refluxing ureteric orifice is in a more lateral position and has a shorter intramural tunnel [19]. While the appearance of reflux may be associated with unusually high bladder pressures as in neurogenic bladders [20], in children with reflux the condition is usually thought to be present from birth but may be affected by dynamics of the immature bladder [21].

In asymptomatic children the incidence of reflux varies from 0.4 to 1.8% [22] with the incidence decreasing with age. In multiple studies following both animals and children in whom reflux was identified, it has been found that the reflux may disappear spontaneously depending upon its extent and severity [23–26]. Presumably this spontaneous disappearance relates to changes that occur during bladder maturation involving both anatomical and dynamic changes.

While reflux is unusual in normal asymptomatic children, reflux is the most common anatomical abnormality found in children who are evaluated for UTI. Epidemiological studies in bacteriuric children have shown that 21–57% have reflux [7,27–29]. In children found to have reflux after evaluation of a urinary infection, the reflux may also resolve spontaneously. It has been calculated that when reflux resolves spontaneously the rate of resolution is about 30–35% each year [30].

Of great importance are studies that have shown that 8–45% of siblings of children with reflux have reflux themselves [31–33]. The specific genetics of the trait are unknown, but this high familial incidence has led some to recommend screening young siblings of children with urinary infections for reflux.

Bladder dynamics and vesicoureteric reflux

While abnormal bladder dynamics have been associated with causing VUR in individuals with neurogenic bladders, abnormal bladder dynamics in children with reflux have been identified more recently. Urodynamic testing in neurologically normal children with recurrent infections and reflux has also shown abnormal cystometry and voiding patterns [21,34–41]. In 1979, Koff and associates proposed that increased intravesical pressures resulting from voluntary urethral sphincteric contraction during involuntary uninhibited bladder contractions may contribute to the initiation or persistence of VUR in neurologically normal children [21]. They and others found that anticholinergic treatment of uninhibited bladder contractions associated with reflux may increase rates of reflux resolution.

Complications of vesicoureteric reflux and urinary tract infections

Reflux nephropathy

Most focal renal scarring is related to a combination of VUR and bacteriuria. To differentiate this kind of scarring from that of other renal injuries, this has been termed reflux nephropathy. In general the greater the degree of reflux, the greater the incidence of renal scarring and impaired renal growth [42,43]. Reflux nephropathy is diagnosed radiologically by calyceal deformity and renal parenchymal thinning over localized or multiple calyces. A small shrunken irregular kidney may be the result of VUR and infections, but may be confused with congenitally small, dysplastic, poorly or non-functioning kidneys. This distinction may be difficult and sometimes impossible to make radiologically, because it is a histological diagnosis. Although these gross lesions are easily detected radiologically, more subtle changes related to infection, such as cortical pitting, mild global renal shrinkage or poor growth, or reflux nephropathy changes related to histology alone [44] will not be detected by radiological tests, but may cause significant alteration in renal function.

A number of studies have shown that about 17% of childen who are bacteriuric on a screening urine culture have renal scarring [5,28,29]. While further examination revealed that these children may not have been totally asymptomatic, the childen did not go to a physician for symptoms related to urinary infections. Thus, asymptomatic or 'covert' infections may at times be associated with renal scarring.

If a child is found to have radiological changes associated with reflux nephropathy and is then evaluated for VUR, about 60% still have reflux present [5,28,29], and it is possible that it may have already resolved in others.

If radiological evaluation is prompted by infection, often the kidney is already scarred. It has been hypothesized that these scars result from neonatal or early childhood infections during a period when the kidney is more susceptible to scarring. While the kidneys in children under 5 years appear to be particularly susceptible, several studies have documented that new or progressive scarring may occur after the age of 5 years, but occurs rarely after the age of 10 years [42,45,46]. At least two studies have recorded significant rates of renal scarring between the ages of 5 and 10 years, and one documented that 38% (14/37) of children who developed new scarring had a previously normal intravenous urogram (IVU) [45,46]. Almost all the episodes

of new or progressive scarring were associated with symptomatic or persistent infections and persistent reflux. In an adult with a normal urinary tract, however, focal renal cortical scarring from infection is extremely rare. Rarely papillary and calyceal distortion or generalized renal shrinkage may occur after acute non-obstructive pyelonephritis [47].

Multiple factors appear to affect whether a renal scar will form following reflux and infection. First, Rolleston and associates found that foci of renal scarring were associated with areas of intrarenal reflux (pyelotubular backflow) of contrast on voiding cystourethrography (VCU) in children under the age of 4 years [48]. Animal studies confirmed that certain 'compound' calyces found at the renal poles allowed intrarenal reflux, and renal scarring occurred when both reflux and bacteriuria were present [49,50]. Experimentally, renal scarring with reflux alone could be created only if there were abnormally high bladder pressures [51,52]. Other experimental work in rats has shown that bacteriuria alone without reflux may cause abnormally elevated renal pelvic pressures [53].

Secondly, when bacterial access to the kidney from the bladder occurs, the bacteria stimulate both humoral and cellular immune responses that mediate fibrosis and scarring. In experimental rat models of pyelonephritis, maximal renal suppuration and exudation occur 3–5 days after infection; this is followed by collagen infiltration, scarring and loss of renal mass [54–59]. This process can be ameliorated if antimicrobial treatment is started within the first few days of infection [54,56,58,59]. Other studies have shown that the inflammatory release of enzymes, superoxide and oxygen radicals causes renal tubular damage; inhibition of the superoxide production may, therefore, decrease damage [60].

Two consequences of reflux nephropathy are renal-associated hypertension and renal failure. While the incidence of childhood hypertension depends upon age and sex, renal hypertension is the most common cause [61]. Children with reflux nephropathy, who are normotensive, have at least a 10–20% risk of future hypertension [62,63] with its complications and associated renal deterioration. When Wallace and associates examined normotensive children who had renal scarring and ureteric reimplantation to correct the reflux, 17% became hypertensive over 10 years [63]. When Smellie and Normand followed 83 children with reflux nephropathy, 13% (11) were hypertensive initially, six with malignant hypertension, and another 19% (14) became hypertensive over the next 4–20 years. Similarly, in Sweden, Jacobson and associates found that 23% (7/30) of children with non-obstructive focal renal scarring developed hypertension after 27 years (none had hypertension initially) and 10% developed end-stage renal disease [64]. In both studies, however, hypertension occurred independently of the degree or extent of scarring in one or both kidneys, thus no prediction of risk can be made related to renal damage. More recently, however, data suggest that specific genetic variants may have increased risk for renal scarring.

Renal dysfunction and reflux nephropathy

Glomerular lesions and progressive proteinuria have been found in patients who have reflux nephropathy [65,66]. Significant proteinuria (greater than 1 g/24 h) has been found in patients with VUR and progressive deterioration in renal function [66]. When radiologically normal, unscarred kidneys, found contralateral to a kidney with unilateral reflux nephropathy, are biopsied glomerular sclerosis and histological findings associated with reflux nephropathy have been found [44,65,67,68]. This suggests that radiological demonstration of renal scarring or shrinkage is gross, and more extensive signs of reflux nephropathy may be occurring at the histological level. The reasons for progressive renal damage once reflux has ceased, however, are unclear. Two theories have emerged: one proposes that progressive renal damage occurs from hyperfiltration of the remaining nephrons and the other proposes that progressive immunological damage to the kidney occurs. The latter hypothesizes that a chronic inflammatory response develops as part of an autoimmune phenomenon related to reflux damage.

Diagnosis and management of urinary tract infections

Initial infection

Clinical and experimental data show that rapid diagnosis and treatment with antimicrobial agents is the most effective means of preventing renal damage. Treatment varies depending upon the age and severity of symptoms of the child. The neonate or child who is so ill that he or she is unable to take fluids, or who has a highly resistant organism, or who is immune compromised will require broad-spectrum parenteral antimicrobial agents (e.g. aminoglycoside and ampicillin) until bacterial sensitivities are obtained and will allow the selection of a drug with a more narrow spectrum. Although the exact length of treatment is controversial, pyelonephritis in the neonate or immune compromised child is usually treated with 7–10 days of parenteral antimicrobial agents, with oral agents continued until a total of 10–14 days of treatment are attained. At that point prophylactic antimicrobial agents are started. In the older child who is seriously ill and requires initial parenteral antimicrobial agents, treatment should be continued until the child is afebrile for 48 h and an oral agent to which the organism is sensitive can be selected. This is continued for a total of 10–14 days of

treatment and followed with maintenance on prophylactic agents until radiological evaluation is complete. In a child who is a few years or older, who does not appear severely systemically ill and has a clinical cystitis, many oral broad-spectrum antimicrobial agents will probably cure the infection in a course of 3–5 days [69–72]. Whichever course of treatment is chosen, the child should be placed on antimicrobial treatment until full radiological evaluation is performed.

Radiological evaluation

Children who have a documented first UTI should receive a full radiological evaluation allowing visualization of both the upper and lower urinary tract. These studies can be performed when convenient after the urine is sterile and the bladder irritative symptoms are gone. A renal and bladder ultrasound should be performed acutely if the child is acutely ill when diagnosed, has new azotaemia, has a poor response to appropriate antimicrobials after 3 or so days, has an unusual organism (tuberculosis or urea-splitting organisms such as *Proteus*) or has a known congenital urinary tract abnormality. Certain investigators advocate a radiological study such as a dimercapto succinic acid (DMSA) nuclear scan that will show renal inflammation and determine if the infection is upper or lower tract; however, in most instances this kind of information will probably not change the acute management. In specific cases, for instance when a seriously ill infant has a poor urinary specimen (i.e. bagged specimen) taken and it cannot be determined if a urinary infection is present or not, this kind of information may be useful to determine further evaluation and management plans.

A VCU may be performed as soon as the urine is sterile and bladder irritability has disappeared. This means that the study may be performed within a few days to weeks of the initiation of treatment, as convenient. The urine must be sterile when the VCU is performed to prevent forcing infected urine into the collecting systems during the study should reflux be present. For the study to be reliable, however, the bladder must be filled adequately so that bladder irritability is absent. Studies have shown that reflux is not caused by urinary infection or associated inflammation [73]; however, even if it were associated with inflammation this information would be useful for management.

In most situations, the most useful upper tract imaging study is ultrasound and the bladder should be included in the study [74–78]. While IVU may be performed in many situations, the IVU may not disclose poorly or non-functioning systems, especially in the neonate, as well as ultrasound. On the other hand, ultrasound may be less likely to show the details of renal scarring or collecting system duplication.

If VUR has been detected on VCU and surveillance on prophylactic antimicrobial agents is planned, an IVU with select tomograms or a [99mTc] DMSA scan may document baseline renal scarring that is not apparent on ultrasound [77,79,80]. Renal growth measurements obtained after the initial renal imaging studies must be interpreted cautiously, because initial renal size may be overestimated from the acute inflammation and scars may take several months to years to become completely apparent [42,79–81]. After initial radiological studies have already diagnosed reflux or if screening for reflux is required, a nuclear VCU may be useful to assess the presence of reflux with lower radiation exposure. The nuclear VCU will not allow detailed evaluation of the urethra, bladder wall or filling defects, or clear definition of reflux grade, however. In situations in which reflux is suspected (from frequent episodes of pyelonephritis) but has not been otherwise documented with routine VCU, the nuclear VCU may be more sensitive at disclosing reflux as scanning is performed during the entire study.

Other anatomical abnormalities and obstruction demonstrated by radiological studies may require other evaluation specific to their diagnosis before definitive management. These situations need to be evaluated and treated individually.

Reflux and bacteriuria

Management of VUR should minimize renal bacteriuria to prevent risk of renal damage. This can usually be accomplished by daily antimicrobial treatment to maintain a sterile urine or by surgical prevention of the reflux. VUR may, in many instances, resolve depending upon its extent and degree, in situations with low or moderate reflux, therefore, antimicrobial prophylaxis and surveillance (if practical) may be worthwhile. During this treatment the urine should be cultured at various intervals, and the urinary tract should be re-evaluated for persistence of reflux or new scarring annually. If no clinical infections have occurred and the child is older re-examinations may be delayed for longer intervals.

Low-dose prophylactic antimicrobial agents are useful to maintain a child with VUR free from infections. Ideally the agent should achieve high urinary concentrations with low systemic drug concentrations, cause no change or minimal change to the faecal flora, be well tolerated by a child, and be of low cost. As urinary concentrations of the drug should be much greater than systemic concentrations, antimicrobial resistance in gut organisms should not occur and these organisms should continue to be susceptible to the prophylactic agent.

Several antimicrobial agents have been documented to be useful in preventing recurrent urinary infections in children. Nitrofurantoin, at doses of 1.2–2.4 mg/kg each

evening [82], produces high urinary concentrations with very low serum levels when a child has normal renal function. When renal function is reduced to less than half of the normal level, the efficacy of the nitrofurantoin, which is based in part on renal-concentrating ability, may be reduced. The drug is also contraindicated in children with glucose-6-phosphate dehydrogenase (G6PD) deficiencies because it may cause haemolysis as an oxidizing agent. The G6PD deficiency may be seen in about 10% of US Blacks, and some Sardinians, non-Ashkenazi Jews, Greeks, Eti-Turks and Thais [83].

Cephalexin has been studied as a prophylactic agent primarily in adults. While faecal resistance developed in patients taking full-dose cephalexin (500 mg qid), adults taking a low dose (one-quarter to one-eighth of the full dose, 250–125 mg/day) did not appear to develop resistance in the faecal organisms and there was a good prophylactic effect of the drug. As this drug has no specific contraindications except for specific allergic reactions, it may be useful in infants.

A successful combination drug that has been studied as a prophylactic agent is trimethoprim-sulphamethoxazole at a dose of approximately 2 mg/kg of the trimethoprim portion [84,85]. As the combination includes a sulphonamide, it may compete for bilirubin-binding sites on albumin in neonates and probably should not be prescribed during an infant's first few months of life when hyperbilirubinaema may be of concern.

Although most studies have been performed in adult women, trimethoprim (approximately 2 mg/kg once nightly) has been found to be as effective as trimethoprim-sulphamethoxazole and nitrofurantoin in preventing recurrent urinary infections [86], and may be useful in individuals who are allergic to sulphur-containing drugs.

While nalidixic acid was used to treat children before the production of more powerful quinolones, the newer quinolones (norfloxacin, cinoxacin) have been contraindicated in prepubertal children because of studies in immature animals that claimed cartilage erosion and arthropathy occurred. Other studies have been unable to document specific problems in paediatric patients related to quinolone usage, but the drug is still not recommended for routine use [87].

Surgical correction of reflux may be required when reflux is grade 4–5, the child has had breakthrough infections while on appropriate antimicrobial prophylaxis, new or significant progression of renal scarring is observed, long-term antimicrobial prophylaxis is impossible for social or medical reasons, reflux fails to improve or resolve after multiple years of appropriate surveillance, or open bladder surgery to correct other anomalities is required. Renal scarring from pyelonephritis may not be apparent on ultrasound within the first few months after the infection; therefore, it is important that renal scarring that appears while a child is on prophylaxis and clinically well should not be interpreted as new scarring.

Recurrent urinary infections unassociated with reflux

When radiological evaluation reveals a normal urinary tract, there are no currently available routine tests that can predict those children at risk of recurrent urinary infections. When the history reveals a well-documented history of recurrent infections urinary prophylaxis with antimicrobial agents may be worthwhile as epidemiological data show that the risk of recurrent infections increases dramatically with each recurring infection. Prophylaxis may be continued for periods of 3–6 months with withdrawal of the drugs after these periods to see if susceptibility remains high. The natural history has shown that patients with high susceptibility will often have periods of months to years of remission from infection.

Whether so-called asymptomatic bacteriuria is actually asymptomatic is debatable. In most instances, with further questioning, signs and symptoms of urinary infection or incontinence are elicited even though they may not be the primary reason for the patient seeking attention [5,88]. For this reason it has been recommended that these infections be called 'covert' [5]. While about 30% of schoolgirls will clear these infections spontaneously without treatment [89,90], the majority will get reinfected or remain persistently infected [5,90,91]. In addition, there is some suggestion that treatment of asymptomatic bacteriuria by antimicrobial selection may lead to later colonization with a more virulent bacteria that will cause symptomatic cystitis or pyelonephritis [92,93]. Therefore, in refractory cases of recurrent covert infection follow-up without further treatment might be considered.

Urinary tract infections and voiding dysfunction

In the child with documented infections and reflux, who continues to have symptoms of voiding dysfunction even when the urine has been kept free from infection, treatment of the voiding problems using anticholinergic agents such as oxybutynin may be helpful in both improving reflux and decreasing the frequency of urinary infections. Several investigators have shown that treatment of such children with both antimicrobial prophylaxis and anticholinergic agents may cause more rapid than expected resolution or improvement of the reflux [21,94–96]. In children with recurrent infections unassociated with reflux and incontinence from voiding dysfunction, some have shown that bladder rehabilitation involving timed voiding or biofeedback, or the use of anticholinergics, may decrease the frequency of urinary infections and improve continence [21,28,37,39].

Summary

The diagnosis of UTIs in children is important because these infections may be markers for identifying children at risk of further renal damage from infection. While most children with VUR will have this risk of future renal infection diminished by antimicrobial prophylaxis or surgical correction of the problem, there may be confounding problems that may increase the risk of infection if not that of renal damage. Most children with frequent UTIs appear to have a biological predisposition for these infections and, as such, these children need to be warned that future bacteriuria may occur even if their reflux ceases whether spontaneously or surgically. In addition, children with any signs of reflux nephropathy should be followed for future hypertension and proteinuria. Children with associated incontinence or voiding problems may need additional evaluation and treatment. While familial screening may not be routine at present, families in whom a member has been identified as having VUR, should be warned of the familial nature of the problem and that early identification of VUR and UTI in young family members is important.

References

1 Fasth A, Bjure J, Hellström M, Jacobsson B, Jodal U. Autoantibodies to Tamm–Horsfall glycoprotein in children with renal damage associated with urinary tract infections. *Acta Paediatr Scand* 1980;**69**:709–15.

2 Wettergren B, Fasth A, Jacobsson B, Jodal U, Lincoln K. UTI during the first year of life in a Göteborg area 1977–79. *Pediatr Res* 1980;**14**:981.

3 Asscher AW. Urinary tract infection: the value of early diagnosis. *Kidney Int* 1975;**7**:63–7.

4 Bailey RR. Vesicoureteric reflux in healthy infants and children. In: Hodson J, Kincaid-Smith P, ed. *Reflux Nephropathy*. New York: Ed. Masson, 1979:59.

5 Savage DCL. Natural history of covert bacteriuria in schoolgirls. *Kidney Int Suppl* 1975;**8**:90–5.

6 Winberg J, Anderson HJ, Bergström T *et al.* Epidemiology of symptomatic urinary tract infection in childhood. *Acta Paediatr Scand Suppl* 1974;**252**:1–20.

7 Kunin CM, Deutscher R, Paquin A. Urinary tract infection in school children: an epidemiologic, clinical and laboratory study. *Medicine* 1964;**43**:91–130.

8 Källenius G, Möllby R, Svenson SB *et al.* Occurrence of P-fimbriated *Escherichia coli* in urinary tract infections. *Lancet* 1981;**2**:1369–72.

9 Väisänen V, Elo J, Tallgren LG *et al.* Mannose-resistant haemagglutination and P antigen recognition are characteristic of *Escherichia coli* causing primary pyelonephritis. *Lancet* 1981;**2**:1366–9.

10 Bollgren I, Winberg J. The periurethral aerobic bacterial flora in healthy boys and girls. *Acta Paediatr Scand* 1976;**65**:74–80.

11 Bollgren I, Winberg J. The periurethral aerobic flora in girls highly susceptible to urinary infections. *Acta Paediatr Scand* 1976;**65**:81–7.

12 Stamey TA, Sexton CC. The role of vaginal colonization with Enterobacteriaceae in recurrent urinary infections. *J Urol* 1975;**113**:214–17.

13 Fussell EN, Kaack MB, Cherry R, Roberts JA. Adherence of bacteria to human foreskins. *J Urol* 1988;**140**:997–1001.

14 Wiswell TE, Miller GM, Gelston HM, Jones SK, Clemmings AF. Effect of circumcision status on periurethral bacterial flora during the first year of life. *J Pediatr* 1988;**113**(3):442–6.

15 Fliedner M, Mehls O, Rauterberg E-W, Ritz E. Urinary sIgA in children with urinary tract infection. *J Pediatr* 1986;**109**:416–21.

16 Lomberg H, Hanson LÅ, Jacobsson B *et al*. Correlation of P blood group, vesicoureteral reflux, and bacterial attachment in patients with recurrent pyelonephritis. *N Engl J Med* 1983;**308**:1189–92.

17 Sheinfeld J, Schaeffer AJ, Cordon-Cardo C, Rogatko A, Fair WR. Association of the Lewis blood-group phenotype with recurrent urinary tract infections in women. *N Engl J Med* 1989;**320**(12):773–7.

18 Sheinfeld J, Cordon-Cardo C, Fair W, Wartinger D, Rabinowitz R. Association of type 1 blood group antigens (BGA) with urinary tract infections in children with genitourinary structural abnormalities. *J Urol* 1990;**143**(4):189A.

19 Stephens FD. Correlation of ureteral orifice position with renal morphology. *Trans Am Assoc Genitourin Surg* 1977;**68**:53–5.

20 Hutch JA. Vesico-ureteral reflux in the paraplegic: cause and correction. *J Urol* 1952;**68**(2):457–67.

21 Koff SA, Lapides J, Piazza DH. Association of urinary tract infection and reflux with uninhibited bladder contractions and voluntary sphincteric obstruction. *J Urol* 1979;**122**:373–6.

22 Bailey RR. A overview of reflux nephropathy. In: Hodson JJ, Kincaid-Smith P, eds. *Reflux Nephropathy*. New York: Ed. Masson, 1979:3–13.

23 Lenaghan D, Cussen LJ. Vesicoureteral reflux in pups. *Invest Urol* 1968;**5**:449–61.

24 Lenaghan D, Whitaker JG, Jensen F, Stephens FD. The natural history of reflux and long-term effects of reflux on the kidney. *J Urol* 1976;**115**:728–30.

25 Edwards D, Norman ICS, Prescod N, Smellie JM. Disappearance of vesicoureteric reflux during long-term prophylaxis of urinary tract infection in children. *Br Med J* 1977;**2**:285–8.

26 Roberts JA. Studies of vesicoureteral reflux: a review of work in a primate model. *South Med J* 1978;**71**:28–30.

27 Abbott GD. Neonatal bacteriuria: a prospective study in 1460 infants. *Br Med J* 1972;**1**:267.

28 Asscher AW, McLachlan MSF, Verrier-Jones R *et al*. Screening for asymptomatic urinary-tract infection in schoolgirls. *Lancet* 1973;**2**:1.

29 Newcastle Asymptomatic Bacteriuria Research Group. Asymptomatic bacteriuria in schoolchildren in Newcastle upon Tyne. *Arch Dis Child* 1975;**50**:90.

30 Skoog SJ, Belman AB, Majd M. A nonsurgical approach to the management of primary vesicoureteral reflux. *J Urol* 1987;**138**:941–6.

31 Noe HN. The role of dysfunctional voiding in failure or complication of ureteral reimplantation for primary reflux. *J Urol* 1985;**134**:1172–5.

32 Noe H. The long-term results of prospective sibling reflux screening. *J Urol* 1992;**148**:1739–42.

33 Van den Abbeele AD, Treves ST, Lebowitz RL *et al*. Vesicoureteral reflux in asymptomatic siblings of patients with known reflux: radionuclide cystography. *Pediatrics* 1987;**79**(1):147–53.

34 Hansson S, Hjälmås K, Jodal U, Sixt R. Lower urinary tract dysfunction in girls with untreated asymptomatic or covert bacteriuria. *J Urol* 1990;**143**:333–5.

35 Kass EJ, Diokno AC, Montealegre A. Enuresis: principles of management and result of treatment. *J Urol* 1979;**121**:794–6.

36 Koff SA. Bladder–sphincter dysfunction in childhood. *Urology* 1982;**19**(5):457–61.

37 Passerini-Glazel G, Cisternino A, Camuffo MC *et al*. Video-urodynamic studies of minor voiding dysfunctions in children: an overview of 13 years' experience. *Scand J Urol Nephrol Suppl* 1992;**141**:70–84.

38 Qvist N, Kristensen ES, Nielsen KK *et al*. Detrusor instability in children with recurrent urinary tract infection and/or enuresis. *Urol Int* 1986;**41**:196–8.

39 van Gool JD, Vijverberg MAW, de Jong TPVM. Functional daytime incontinence: clinical and urodynamic assessment. *Scand J Urol Nephrol Suppl* 1992;**141**:58–69.

40 Bauer SB, Retik AB, Colodny AH *et al*. The unstable bladder of childhood. *Urol Clin North Am* 1980;**7**(2):321–36.

41 Kondo A, Kobayashi M, Otani T, Takita T, Mitsuya H. Children with unstable bladder: clinical and urodynamic observation. *J Urol* 1983;**129**:88–91.

42 Filly R, Friedland GW, Govan DE, Fair WR. Development and progression of clubbing and scarring in children with recurrent urinary tract infections. *Pediatr Radiol* 1974;**113**:145–53.

43 Smellie JM, Edwards D, Normand ICS, Prescod N. Effect of vesicoureteric reflux on renal growth in children with urinary tract infection. *Arch Dis Child* 1981;**56**:593–600.

44 Kincaid-Smith P. Reflux nephropathy without overt radiological lesions. In: Bailey R, ed. *Second CJ Hodson Symposium on Reflux Nephropathy*. Christchurch, New Zealand: Christchurch School of Medicine, 1991:19–22.

45 Berg U. Long-term followup of renal morphology and function in children with recurrent pyelonephritis. *J Urol* 1992;**148**:1715–20.

46 Smellie JM, Ransley PG, Norman ICS, Prescod N, Edwards D. Development of new renal scars: a collaborative study. *Br Med J* 1985;**290**:1957–60.

47 Davidson AJ, Talner LB. Late sequelae of adult-onset acute bacterial nephritis. *Radiology* 1978;**127**:367–71.

48 Rolleston GL, Maling TMJ, Hodson CJ. Intrarenal reflux and the scarred kidney. *Arch Dis Child* 1974;**49**:531–9.

49 Ransley PG, Risdon RA. Renal papillae and intrarenal reflux in the pig. *Lancet* 1974;**2**:1114.

50 Ransley PG, Risdon RA. Reflux and renal scarring. *Br J Radiol Suppl* 1978;**51**:1–35.

51 Hodson J, Maling TMJ, McManamon PJ, Lewis MG. Reflux nephropathy. *Kidney Int Suppl* 1975;**8**:50–8.

52 Ransley PG, Risdon RA, Godley ML. High pressure sterile vesicoureteral reflux and renal scarring: an experimental study in the pig and minipig. In: Hodson CJ, Heptinstall RH, Winberg J, eds. *Reflux Nephropathy Update: 1983*. New York: Karger, 1984:320–43.

53 Issa M, Shortliffe L. Effect of bacteriuria on bladder and renal pelvic pressures in the rat. *J Urol* 1992;**148**:559–63.

54 Glauser MP, Lyons JM, Braude AI. Prevention of chronic experimental pyelonephritis by suppression of acute suppuration. *J Clin Invest* 1978;**61**:403.

55 Miller TE, Stewart E, North JDK. Immunobacteriological aspects of pyelonephritis. *Contrib Nephrol* 1979;**16**:11–15.

56 Miller T, Phillips S. Pyelonephritis: the relationship between infection, renal scarring, and antimicrobial therapy. *Kidney Int* 1981;**19**:654–62.

57 Roberts JA, Domingue GJ, Martin LN *et al.* Immunology of pyelonephritis in the primate model: live versus heat-killed bacteria. *Kidney Int* 1981;**19**:297–305.

58 Shimamura T. Mechanisms of renal tissue destruction in an experimental acute pyelonephritis. *Exp Mol Pathol* 1981;**34**: 34–42.

59 Slotki IN, Asscher AW. Prevention of scarring in experimental pyelonephritis in the rat by early antibiotic therapy. *Nephron* 1982;**30**:262.

60 Roberts JA, Roth JK, Domingue GJ. Immunology of pyelonephritis in the primate model. V. Effect of superoxide dismutase. *J Urol* 1982;**128**:1394–400.

61 Dillon MJ. Recent advances in evaluation and management of childhood hypertension. *Eur J Pediatr* 1979;**132**:133–9.

62 Holland NH, Kotchen T, Bhathena D. Hypertension in children with chronic pyelonephritis. *Kidney Int Suppl* 1975;**8**:243–51.

63 Wallace DMA, Rothwell DL, Williams DI. The long-term follow-up of surgically treated vesicoureteric reflux. *Br J Urol* 1978;**50**:479–84.

64 Jacobson SH, Eklöf O, Eriksson CG *et al.* Development of hypertension and uraemia after pyelonephritis in childhood: 27 year follow up. *Br Med J* 1989;**299**:703–6.

65 Kincaid-Smith P. Glomerular lesions in atrophic pyelonephritis and reflux nephropathy. *Kidney Int Suppl* 1975;**8**:81–3.

66 Torres VE, Velosa JA, Holley KE *et al.* The progression of vesicoureteral reflux nephropathy. *Ann Int Med* 1980; **92**:776–84.

67 Bailey RR, Swainson CPL, Burry AF. Glomerular lesions in the 'normal' kidney in patients with unilateral reflux nephropathy. In: Hodson CJ, Heptinstall RH, Winberg J, eds. *Reflux Nephropathy Update: 1983.* New York: Karger, 1984:126–31.

68 Kincaid-Smith PS. Diffuse parenchymal lesions in reflux nephropathy and the possibility of making a renal biopsy diagnosis in reflux nephropathy. In: Hodson CJ, Heptinstall RH, Winberg J, eds. *Reflux Nephropathy Update: 1983.* New York: Karger, 1984:111–15.

69 Copenhagen Study Group of Urinary Tract Infections in Children. Short-term treatment of acute urinary tract infection in girls. *Scand J Infect Dis* 1991;**23**:213–20.

70 Jójárt G. Comparison of 3-day versus 14-day treatment of lower urinary tract infection in children. *Int Urol Nephrol* 1991;**23**(2):129–34.

71 Lohr JA, Hayden GF, Kesler RW *et al.* Three-day therapy of lower urinary tract infections with nitrofurantoin macrocrystals: a randomized clinical trial. *Pediatrics* 1981;**99**(6): 980–3.

72 Madrigal G, Odio CM, Mohs E, Guevara J, McCracken GH. Single dose antibiotic therapy is not as effective as conventional regimens for management of acute urinary tract infections in children. *Pediatr Infect Dis J* 1988;**7**(5):316–19.

73 Lebowitz R. The detection of vesicoureteral reflux in the child. *Invest Radiol* 1986;**21**(7):519–31.

74 Alon U, Pery M, Davidai G, Berant M. Ultrasonography in the radiologic evaluation of children with urinary tract infection. *Pediatrics* 1986;**78**(1):58–64.

75 Alon U, Berant M, Pery M. Intravenous pyelography in children with urinary tract infection and vesicoureteral reflux. *Pediatrics* 1989;**83**(3):332–6.

76 Honkinen O, Ruuskanen O, Rikalainen H, Mäkinen E, Välimäki I. Ultrasonography as a screening procedure in children with urinary tract infection. *Pediatr Infect Dis J* 1986;**5**(6):633–5.

77 Lindsell D, Moncrieff M. Comparison of ultrasound examination and intravenous urography after a urinary tract infection. *Arch Dis Child* 1986;**61**:81–2.

78 Macpherson RI, Gordon L. Vesicoureteric reflux: radiologic aspects. *Semin Urol* 1986;**4**(2):89–98.

79 Conway JJ. The role of scintigraphy in urinary tract infection. *Semin Nucl Med* 1988;**18**(4):308–19.

80 Gordon I. Use of Tc-99m DMSA and Tc-99m DTPA in reflux. *Semin Urol* 1986;**4**(2):99–108.

81 Johansson B, Troell S, Berg U. Urographic renal size in acute pyelonephritis in childhood. *Acta Radiol* 1988;**29**:155–8.

82 Lohr JA, Nunley DH, Howards SS, Ford RF. Prevention of recurrent urinary tract infections in girls. *Pediatrics* 1977;**59**(4):562–5.

83 Thompson RB. *A Short Textbook of Haematology.* Philadelphia: JB Lippincott, 1969.

84 Grüneberg RN, Smellie JM, Leaky A *et al.* Long-term low-dose cotrimoxazole in prophylaxis of childhood urinary tract infection: bacteriological aspects. *Br Med J* 1976;**2**(2):206.

85 Stamey TA, Condy M, Mihara G. Prophylactic efficacy of nitrofurantoin macrocrystals and trimethoprim-sulfamethoxazole in urinary infections. *N Engl J Med* 1977;**296**: 780–3.

86 Stamm WE, Counts GW, Wagner KF *et al.* Antimicrobial prophylaxis of recurrent urinary tract infections. *Ann Intern Med* 1980;**92**:770–5.

87 Schaad UB. Use of quinolones in pediatrics. *Eur J Clin Microbiol Infect Dis* 1991;**10**(4):355–60.

88 Kunin CM, Zacha E, Paquin A. Urinary-tract infections in schoolchildren: I. Prevalence of bacteriuria and associated urologic findings. *N Engl J Med* 1962;**266**:1287–96.

89 Lindberg U, Claesson I, Hanson LÅ, Jodal U. Asymptomatic bacteriuria in schoolgirls: VIII. Clinical course during a 3-year follow-up. *J Pediatr* 1978;**92**(2):194–9.

90 Verrier-Jones ER, Meller ST, McLachlan MSF *et al.* Treatment of bacteriuria in schoolgirls. *Kidney Int Suppl* 1975;**4**:85–9.

91 Jodal U. The natural history of bacteriuria in childhood. *Infec Dis Clin North Am* 1987;**1**(4):713–29.

92 Hansson S, Caugant D, Jodal USEC. Untreated asymptomatic bacteriuria in girls: I. Stability of urinary isolates. *Br Med J* 1989;**298**:853–5.

93 Hansson S, Jodal U, Lincoln K, Svanborg-Edén C. Untreated asymptomatic bacteriuria in girls: II. Effect of phenoxymethylpenicillin and erythromycin given for intercurrent infections. *Br Med J* 1989;**298**:856–9.

94 Homsy YL. Vesicoureteric reflux: the urodynamic dimension. *Dialog Pediatr Urol* 1983;**6**:2–7.

95 Homsy YL, Nsouli I, Hamburger B, Laberge I, Schick E. Effects of oxybutynin on vesicoureteral reflux in children. *J Urol* 1985;**134**:1168–71.

96 Koff SA, Murtagh D. The uninhibited bladder in children: effect of treatment on vesicoureteral reflux resolution. In: Hodson CJ, Heptinstall RH, Winberg J, eds. *Reflux Nephropathy Update: 1983.* New York: Karger, 1984:211–20.

18　Intersex Disorders

G. Passerini Glazel and F. Aragona

Sexual differentiation: notes of embryology

Before 7 weeks of life the fetus is phenotypically indifferent, with both female and male embryos sharing common primordia. At the seventh week of gestation sexual differentiation starts as shown in Fig. 18.1: the presence of the testis-determining factor (TDF) on the short arm of the Y chromosome (H-Y antigen) provides the signal for testicular development and the primitive gonad differentiates into Sertoli cells and steroid-producing Leydig cells. The absence of the Y chromosome results in the differentiation of the gonad into an ovary, occurring around 80 days. It is important to stress that the development of phenotypic sex is governed by the action of or absence of testicular secretions [1–3]. When testicular secretions are present a male phenotype is induced, whereas female differentiation is not dependent on the presence of an ovary and therefore does not require secretions from the embryonic gonad.

The two types of secretions of the fetal testis involved in male development are müllerian-inhibiting factor (MIF) and androgens [4]. MIF is a peptide hormone, secreted by Sertoli cells of the fetal testis, that acts to induce regression of the paramesonephric (müllerian) ducts. However, normal testicular differentiation can still occur with isolated defects in MIF biosynthesis. The second substance secreted by the fetal testis is testosterone [5], produced by Leydig cells under the influence of placental (maternal) human chorionic gonadotropin (hCG). Testosterone acts both within the fetal testis, where it has a role in promoting maturation of the spermatogonia, and beyond the testis, where its paracrine and endocrine actions play an essential part in the development of the male phenotype. Under the influence of testosterone, the mesonephric duct differentiates into the epididymis, the vas deferens, the ejaculatory ducts and the seminal vesicles. In the absence of testosterone, the mesonephric duct involutes; and in the absence of MIF, the paramesonephric duct develops into the oviduct, uterus, cervix and upper portion of the vagina [6].

The response of both the urogenital sinus and external genitalia to androgen requires the conversion of testosterone to dihydrotestosterone (DHT) by the enzyme 5α-reductase. DHT binds directly to specific high-affinity receptor proteins; the hormone–receptor complex induces an increase in transcription of specific mRNA inducing, as the final effect, male phenotypic differentiation and, in particular, virilization of the external genitalia and the male urethra.

Virilization is completed by the 12th week: the penis is fully formed in all its components, even if by this time it is the same size as the clitoris. In the remaining two trimesters of pregnancy a 10-fold increase in penile size occurs, under the influence of fetal testosterone, whose production is in turn regulated by the secretion of fetal pituitary luteinizing hormone (LH).

In the absence of MIF, the paramesonephric ducts persist and develop into the ovarian tubes, uterus and upper portion of the vagina; in the absence of testosterone the wolffian ducts regress and the urogenital sinus and the external genitalia develop into bladder, urethra, the lower portion of the vagina and clitoris.

It is therefore evident that the testis is the main organ responsible for sexual differentiation; its secretions inhibit müllerian ducts, stimulate wolffian derivatives and masculinize external genitalia. Normal masculinization is a complex phenomenon that requires:
1 normal sex chromosomes;
2 normal testicular development;
3 normal testosterone biosynthesis;
4 normal testosterone to DHT conversion;
5 normal receptor sensitivity in the target organs.

Testicular absence will induce feminization of the genitalia, while anomalies of normal testicular development can produce genital ambiguity in subjects with a male XY karyotype.

Classification of intersexuality

There is no uniformly accepted classification of sexual

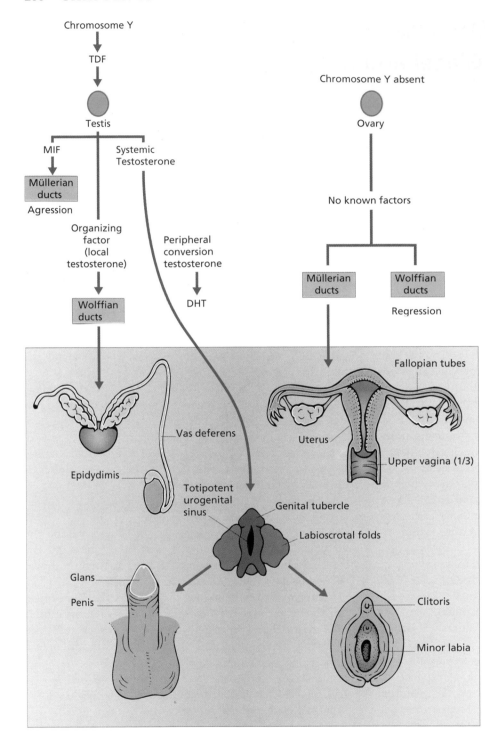

Chromosome Y

TDF

Testis

MIF

Müllerian ducts

Agression

Systemic Testosterone

Organizing factor (local testosterone)

Wolffian ducts

Peripheral conversion testosterone

DHT

Chromosome Y absent

Ovary

No known factors

Müllerian ducts

Wolffian ducts

Regression

Vas deferens

Epidydimis

Totipotent urogenital sinus

Genital tubercle

Labioscrotal folds

Glans

Penis

Fallopian tubes

Uterus

Upper vagina (1/3)

Clitoris

Minor labia

Fig. 18.1 Normal sexual differentiation.

differentiation disorders. The most widely accepted classification is based on the histology of the gonad present, with subclassification according to the aetiology, as proposed by Allen [7]. By this gonadal classification there are five major categories.

1 Ovary only (female pseudohermaphrodite).

2 Testis only (male pseudohermaphrodite).

3 Ovary plus testis (true hermaphrodite).

4 Testis plus streak (mixed gonadal dysgenesis).

5 Streak plus streak (pure gonadal dysgenesis).

The usual features of the classic intersex states are detailed in Table 18.1.

The presentation of children with ambiguous genitalia occurs typically in the neonate; a different group presents

Table 18.1 The usual characteristics of the classic intersex states. From [7] with permission.

Diagnosis	Karyotype	Gonad	Internal ducts	External ducts	Pubertal change	Fertility	Gonadal malignancy	Sex assignment	Comment
Female									
Pseudohermaphrodite									
3β-ol-dehydrogenase deficiency	XX	Ovary	Müllerian	Mildly ambiguous	Feminization (if treated)	Yes (if treated)	No	Female	Severe salt wasting
11β-hydroxylase deficiency	XX	Ovary	Müllerian	Ambiguous	Feminization (if treated)	Yes (if treated)	No	Female	Hypertension
21-hydroxylase deficiency	XX	Ovary	Müllerian	Ambiguous	Feminization (if treated)	Yes (if treated)	No	Female	Frequent salt wasting
Secondary to maternal androgens	XX	Ovary	Müllerian	Ambiguous	Feminization	Yes	No	Female	
True hermaphrodite	XX,XY, XX/XY,etc.	Ovary and testis	Müllerian and wolffian	Ambiguous	Tendency to virilization; gynaecomastia	No	Rare*	Variable	
Male									
Pseudohermaphrodite									
Herni uteri inguinalis	XY	Testis	Müllerian and wolffian	Cryptorchid male	Virilization	Rare	Rare*	Male	
20α-hydroxylase deficiency	XY	Testis	Wolffian	Female	Unknown	No	No*	Female	Severe salt wasting
3β-ol-dehydrogenase deficiency	XY	Testis	Wolffian	Hypospadiac male	Partial virilization with gynaecomastia	No	No*	Usually male	Severe salt wasting
17α-hydroxylase deficiency	XY	Testis	Wolffian	Female	Usually eunuchoid	No	No*	Female	Hypertension
17,20-desmolase deficiency	XY	Testis	Wolffian	Ambiguous	Unknown	No	No*	Uncertain	
17-ketosteroid reductase deficiency	XY	Testis	Wolffian	Female	Partial virilization with gynaecomastia	No	No*	Female	
Lubs syndrome	XY	Testis	Wolffian	Ambiguous (feminization)	Feminization	No	No*	Female	Elevated testosterone and LH levels
Gilbert–Dreyfus syndrome	XY	Testis	Wolffian	Ambiguous	Partial virilization with gynaecomastia	No	No*	Variable	Elevated testosterone and LH levels

Continued on p. 282

Table 18.1 *Continued.*

Diagnosis	Karyotype	Gonad	Internal ducts	External ducts	Pubertal change	Fertility	Gonadal malignancy	Sex assignment	Comment
Reifenstein syndrome	XY	Testis	Wolffian	Hypospadiac male	Virilization with gynaecomastia	No	No*	Usually male	Elevated testosterone and LH levels
Testicular feminization syndrome	XY	Testis	Wolffian	Female	Feminization	No	Yes	Female	Elevated testosterone and LH levels
Pseudovaginal perineoscrotal hypospadias	XY	Testis	Wolffian	Female	Virilization	No	No*	Female	
Dysgenetic testes	XO/XY, etc.	Testis	Wolffian and müllerian	Ambiguous	Virilization	No	Yes	Variable	
	XXY, XX, etc.	Testis	Wolffian	Variable	Partial virilization	No	No	Variable	
Mixed gonadal dysgenesis	XO/XY, etc.	Testis and streak	Wolffian and müllerian	Ambiguous	Usually virilization	No	Yes	Variable	
Gonadal dysgenesis									
Turner syndrome	XO, etc.	Streak	Immature müllerian	Female	Eunuchoid	No†	Usually no	Female	Webbed neck, shield chest, etc.
Pure gonadal dysgenesis									
XX type	XX	Streak	Immature müllerian	Female	Eunuchoid	No	Usually no	Female	
XY type	XY	Streak	Immature müllerian	Female	Eunuchoid	No	Yes	Female	

*All patients with cryptorchid testes have an increased incidence of gonadal malignancy.
†One exception.
LH, luteinizing hormone.

later in life with a functional failure of the assigned gender role. In this chapter, presentation in the neonate is, therefore, considered separately from that in later life.

Clinical presentation

Ambiguous genitalia in the neonatal period

Female pseudohermaphrodites

This is the most important group because they constitute 60–70% of all intersex cases presenting in the neonatal period. All patients have a 46,XX karyotype, are TDF gene negative and have exclusively ovarian tissue. The müllerian system develops into fallopian tubes, the uterus and the upper portion of the vagina, and the wolffian system regresses. Clinically, the virilization of the external genitalia varies from minimal clitoral enlargement to almost complete masculinization (Fig. 18.2). At birth there is usually hypertrophy of the clitoris with severe chordee, a variable degree of labioscrotal fold fusion and even a glandular urethra in the more masculinized cases. In the affected female, the labioscrotal folds are bulbous and rugated, giving the general appearance of a male with bilateral cryptorchidism and hypospadias.

Female pseudohermaphrodites can be divided into two groups: (i) those fetuses in whom abnormal masculinization occurs from the presence of inappropriate androgens; and (ii) those affected by a non-steroidal mechanism (Table 18.2).

Cases resulting from abnormal androgens constitute the majority of female pseudohermaphrodites. Masculinization is limited to the external genitalia and clitoral hypertrophy if the androgenic stimulus is received after 12 weeks of gestation. If the stimulus is received earlier, clitoral hypertrophy still occurs, plus retention of the urogenital sinus and labioscrotal fusion. These patients must be correctly diagnosed because they should be raised as females. The prognosis of these patients when raised as females is excellent for pubertal development and the attainment of normal female characteristics, sexual activity and reproductive capability. Abnormal androgens may be the result of fetal biosynthetic anomalies (in the majority) or from a maternal source of androgens, either endogenous or exogenous. Fortunately, these cases of maternal androgen origin are now very rare. Congenital adrenal hyperplasia (CAH) makes up the majority of these cases of female pseudohermaphrodites [8]. There are six types

Table 18.2 Aetiology of female pseudohermaphroditism.

Inappropriate androgens
Congenital adrenal hyperplasia (CAH)
21α-hydroxylase (21-OH) deficiency
11β-hydroxylase (11-OH) deficiency
3-hydroxysteroid dehydrogenase (3-HSD) deficiency

Non-steroidal causes
Maternal tumours
Iatrogenic fetal virilization
Idiopathic forms

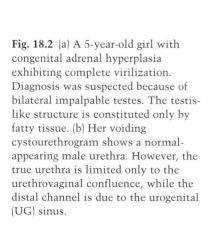

Fig. 18.2 (a) A 5-year-old girl with congenital adrenal hyperplasia exhibiting complete virilization. Diagnosis was suspected because of bilateral impalpable testes. The testis-like structure is constituted only by fatty tissue. (b) Her voiding cystourethrogram shows a normal-appearing male urethra. However, the true urethra is limited only to the urethrovaginal confluence, while the distal channel is due to the urogenital (UG) sinus.

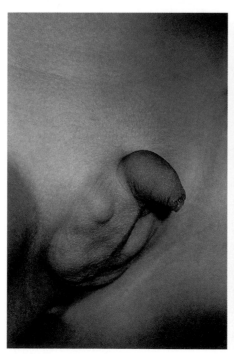

(a)

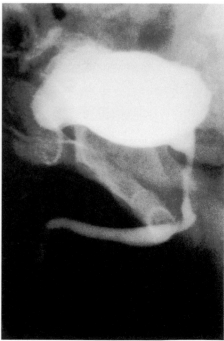

(b)

of adrenogenital syndromes [9] but only types I–IV are virilizing and cause female pseudohermaphroditism (Fig. 18.3).

In type I there is a deficit of 21-hydroxylase (21-OH), localized in the zona fasciculata of the adrenal cortex, that results in increased production of 17-hydroxyprogesterone (17-OHP) and a block in cortisol production. The overproduction of androgens resulting from the block causes the inappropriate masculinizing effect on the urogenital sinus and external genitalia.

In type II CAH, the 21-OH deficiency involves the zona granulosa as well and, in addition to the virilizing effect, there is a deficiency of biologically active mineralocor-

ticoid. The latter results in an electrolyte imbalance with salt and water loss, usually requiring treatment.

In type III CAH, the enzymatic block occurs at the 11-OH level and two important proximal metabolites, 17-OHP and androgen, accumulate. In addition, there is an accumulation of a biologically active and very potent mineralocorticoid, deoxycorticosterone. In affected children, the electrolyte imbalance with hypokalaemic acidosis, hypervolaemia and secondary hypertension can be life threatening if left untreated.

Type IV CAH is the only enzyme deficiency that causes CAH and ambiguity in both males and females. The enzymatic block occurs more proximally at the 3β-OH-

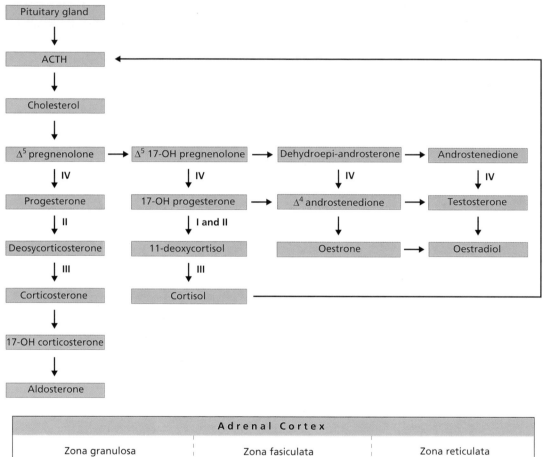

Fig. 18.3 Steroidal biosynthetic pathways in the adrenal glands. I–IV correspond to the enzyme deficiencies that are responsible for CAH: I, II, deficiency of 21-OH; III, deficiency of 11β-OH; IV, deficiency of 3β-hydroxysteroid dehydrogenase. ACTH, adrenocorticotrophic hormone; OH, hydroxylase.

dehydrogenase level. It is the rarest of the four forms of CAH and, because it is associated with the greatest degree of salt wasting, survival is rare. The principal androgen that accumulates proximal to the block is dehydroepiandrosterone (DHEA), a weak androgen, and thus the degree of virilization encountered in affected females is usually not as severe as seen in other types of CAH. Most patients have separate urethral and vaginal orifices. The hormonal deficiencies found are in cortisol and mineralocorticoids, with excess adrenocorticotrophic hormone (ACTH) and severe hyponatraemia.

All patients with types I–IV CAH require cortisol replacement. Hydrocortisone sodium succinate (50 mg/m²) should be given as a bolus, and another 50–100 mg/m² should be added to the infusion of parenteral fluid over the next 24 h [9]. Regular monitoring of serum electrolytes and blood pressure measurements are essential to avoid the potential catastrophe of shock or hypokalaemic acidosis and hypertension that may occur in most children with female pseudohermaphroditism and mineralocorticoid deficiency or excess, respectively. If profound hypotension and hyperkalaemia are present, 1–2 mg of deoxycorticosterone acetate should be given intramuscularly over 12–14 h. If the patient is in shock, 20 ml/kg of saline must be given in the first hours of therapy.

Male pseudohermaphrodites

This group comprises patients presenting in the neonatal period with genital ambiguity who have a 46,XY karyotype, exclusively testicular tissue and who develop their wolffian system while the müllerian system regresses. External genitalia exhibit a variable degree of feminization depending on the severity of enzymatic deficit.

The many aetiologies of male pseudohermaphroditism are listed in Table 18.3. All of them cause genital ambiguity because of a defect in the synthesis of steroid hormones or, more frequently, as a consequence of the failure of the target organ to respond to circulating testosterone. There are five types of enzymatic defects that result in male pseudohermaphroditism and ambiguous genitalia in the

Table 18.3 Aetiology of male pseudohermaphroditism.

Adrenal steroidogenesis deficiency (congenital adrenal hyperplasia)
 20,22-desmolase deficiency
 17α-hydroxylase (17-OH) deficiency
 3β-hydroxysteroid dehydrogenase (3β-HSD) deficiency

Sexual hormones synthesis deficiency
 17,20-desmolase deficiency
 17β-hydroxysteroid dehydrogenase (17β-HSD) deficiency

Leydig cell aplasia

5α-reductase deficiency (lack of conversion of testesterone into dihydrotestosterone)

Deficit of androgen receptors
 Complete androgen insensitivity (complete testicular feminization)
 Incomplete androgen insensitivity (incomplete testicular feminization)

Isolated müllerian-inhibiting factor (MIF) activity deficiency
 Müllerian duct persistance syndrome (hernia uteri inguinalis)

Idiopathic forms

neonate (Fig. 18.4). A deficiency in 20,22-desmolase, 17α-hydroxylase and 3β-ol-dehydrogenase interferes in the cascade production of cortisol and results in death in the majority of affected males. A few patients with the 3β-oldehydrogenase deficiency have survived into adulthood and have shown a mixture of partial virilization and gynaecomastia at puberty, but no fertility has been reported [10]. The virilization phenomena are caused by the accumulation of a weak androgen (DHEA) behind the enzyme block. The deficiency in 17,20-desmolase and 17β-ol-dehydrogenase involves only the synthesis of sexual hormones; it produces genital ambiguity with some virilization at the time of puberty, without interference in the synthesis of cortisol, no increase in the ACTH drive and no elevation of precursor steroids behind the block [10].

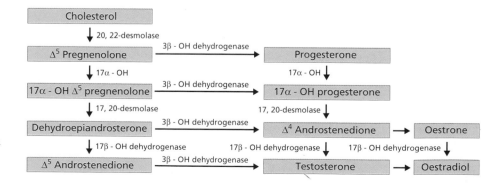

Fig. 18.4 Adrenal and/or testicular enzymatic deficiencies responsible for a reduced testosterone synthesis. OH, hydroxylase.

The inability of a target organ to respond to circulating testosterone is the result of androgen insensitivity, which can be complete or partial. Complete androgen-insensitivity syndromes (AISs) (or the Morris syndrome) are rare, occurring in one in 20 000 to one in 64 000 male births. The incomplete forms are even rarer, with an incidence one-tenth of the complete form. As the complete form does not present with ambiguity in the neonatal period, it is discussed later. Although incomplete forms of androgen insensitivity result in ambiguity in the neonatal period, because their pathophysiology is so closely related to the complete forms, they also are discussed later.

True hermaphrodites

These constitute 10% of the intersex pool [10]. A 46,XX karyotype is found in 57–80% of these patients [11]. The others have a 46,XY pattern (13%) [12] or a mosaic with 46,XX/XY (31%). True hermaphrodites have ovarian and testicular tissue present in the same individual. This may take the form of an ovary on one side and a testis on the other, or an individual may have both components in the same gonad — an ovotestis. According to van Niekerk [13] the following are the most frequent associations: an ovary and a testis (30%), an ovary and an ovotestis (30%), bilateral ovotestes (20%) an ovotestis and a testis (10%) and a unilateral ovotestis/other (10%).

Internal duct differentiation follows the appropriate ipsilateral gonad: a fallopian tube develops when an ovary is present and a vas deferens with the epididymis when a testis is present. When an ovotestis is present, the differentiation of the ducts is variable. A uterus is almost always present [14] although it may be hypoplastic or unicornuate [10]. Although the appearance of the external genitalia varies from feminine with slight clitoral prominence to full masculinization, a tendency to maleness with asymmetrically descended gonads and hypospadias predominates in 75% [14].

The changes at puberty are variable but generally correlate with the gonadal tissue present. It seems that at puberty almost one-half of true hermaphrodites will have normal menses [15] and as the reconstructive surgery for sex-assigned females gives by far the better result, it would appear logical to assign preferentially the true hermaphrodite to the female gender, especially the 46,XX karyotype individual. Assignment to the male gender exposes the individual to several reconstructive procedures with a sometimes poor functional and cosmetic result and, inevitably, primary hypogonadism because most testes are dysgenetic when adulthood is reached [11]. Gonadal malignancies have been reported; thus, all discordant and dysgenetic tissue should be removed after sex assignment. Three cases of true hermaphroditism and pregnancy have been reported in the literature [16–18]. These three cases constitute the only evidence that there might be a potential for fertility in true hermaphrodites. In at least two of the three, the karyotype was 46,XX. There is also a report of spermatogenesis in the testes of true hermaphrodites [15]. All these observations are indicative of the possible fertility potential in true hermaphrodites, but further studies are required.

Mixed gonadal dysgenesis

The gonads of these subjects are classically asymmetrical as there is testicular tissue on one side and a dysgenetic gonad (streak) on the other. A mosaic 46,XY/45,XO karyotype is found in most of these patients. The testis is composed of Sertoli and Leydig cells, but no germinal cells are present. The streak gonad appears similar to the ovarian stroma but without oocytes. The müllerian duct usually persists unilaterally or bilaterally; the testis is often provided with a fallopian tube rather than a vas deferens and an epididymis. The streak gonad is usually drained by a müllerian duct. A bicornuate or unicornuate uterus is generally present.

Malignancy will develop in about 15–25% of the streak gonads, usually in the form of gonadoblastomas, dysgerminomas or both [14]. Individuals with a 46,XY karyotype are at a much higher risk than those with a mosaic pattern. Individuals tend to virilize and have gynaecomastia at the time of puberty. No fertility has been reported so far and sex assignment should be individualized. The response of the phallus to androgenic stimulation should be assessed in borderline cases, but the female gender is usually preferred as the development of the phallus is usually inadequate for functional and cosmetic surgical results to be successful.

Patients assigned as female require gonadectomy, clitoroplasty and vaginoplasty. Those assigned to the male gender should most probably undergo removal of any dysgenetic gonadal tissue and repair of the usually severe hypospadias.

Non-ambiguous genitalia in the neonatal period

Female phenotype

Androgen-insensitivity syndromes

AISs represent the lack of response by the different target organs to androgen stimulation. They can be divided into two categories: (i) complete AIS (testicular feminization syndrome or Morris syndrome); and (ii) incomplete forms (Reifenstein syndrome).

In AIS, hormonal secretion occurred normally *in utero* but the urogenital sinus and external genitalia did not develop along the male line because of the lack of response of all target organs (including pubic and axillary hair, the larynx and the hypothalamic–pituitary axis) to the normally secreted androgen. The defect is thought to be localized at the level of the cytoplasmic androgen receptor of the 5α-reductase enzyme. Two major types of defects have been described: a receptor-negative form (AR–) and a receptor-positive form (AR+). In the AR– syndrome the specific intracellular androgen receptors are undetectable in all target organs, whereas in the AR+ variant there is a structural abnormality of the receptor [19]. These measurements are usually performed in fibroblast cultures from the genital skin, where the 5α-reductase enzyme is located that is deficient in AIS [20]. Clinically, the AR– type normally represents the complete form of the AIS whereas the AR+ type is probably responsible for the clinically incomplete forms.

Individuals affected by complete AIS present in the neonatal period as normal females. The syndrome has now been identified as an X-linked mutation that precludes the normal synthesis of the androgen receptors located in the cytosol [21]. The incidence varies from one in 20 000 to one in 64 000 male births. All patients have a 46,XY karyotype and have exclusively testicular tissue (seminiferous tubules with no spermatogenesis and increased numbers of Leydig cells). The internal ducts develop normally as wolffian ducts, and there is regression of all müllerian structures as MIF is normally secreted. They are phenotypically normal, tall and hairless females with non-ambiguous feminine external genitalia and symmetrically undescended gonads. They usually have a shallow vaginal cavity probably corresponding to a vast prostatic utricle (Fig. 18.5). At the time of puberty, normal breasts develop and axillary and pubic hair is absent or scanty. There is slight vulval hair development and amenorrhoea is the rule. Clinically, these patients usually present in the post-pubertal period for evaluation of primary amenorrhoea or, less often, during the pre-pubertal period because of inguinal hernias.

The gonads are at higher risk of malignancy because of cryptorchidism in this condition, and gonadectomy is recommended. The timing of gonadectomy must be individualized. Because the testes tumours that can occur rarely develop before puberty, surgical intervention is

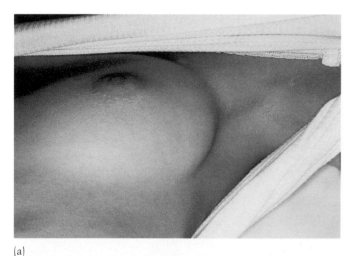

(a)

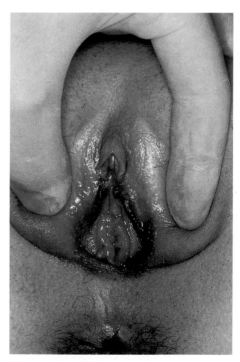

(b)

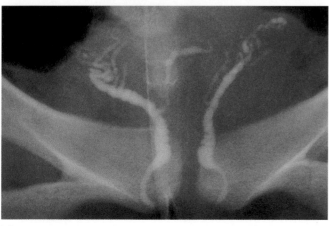

(c)

Fig. 18.5 (a) A well-developed breast and scanty axillary hair in a 17-year-old girl with the Morris syndrome (complete testicular feminization). (b) A normal looking clitoris and vulvar region in the same girl. The vaginal cavity — the embryological prostatic utricle — admits only the ungual phalanx. (c) Dye injection into both the vas deferens during orchiectomy visualizes long abnormal seminal vesicles whose endings surround the enlarged utricle (a tiny 'vagina').

indicated in the pre-pubertal period only if the presence of testes in the labia majora or in the inguinal region results in discomfort or hernia formation. Oestrogen therapy will be necessary for individuals who undergo pubertal gonadectomy to ensure normal growth and breast development. When castration is performed post-pubertally, oestrogen withdrawal symptoms are the rule and oestrogen supplements are necessary.

In contrast to the complete form, incomplete AIS forms cause ambiguity in the neonatal period. Their incidence is about one in 10 of the complete form; individuals have a 46,XY karyotype, have exclusively testicular tissue, their wolffian ducts develop normally (sometimes there is a hypoplastic or absent vas deferens) and there is regression of the müllerian structures. There is a lesser defect of virilization of the external genitalia consisting of partial fusion of the labioscrotal folds and some degree of clitoromegaly present at birth which is responsible for the ambiguity. The gonads are usually symmetrically undescended, and there is a short blind-ending vagina. At puberty some degree of virilization and feminization occurs, including the development of normal pubic hair and gynaecomastia (Fig. 18.6). Sex assignment should be individualized and made thoughtfully. The same considerations as in true hermaphrodites and mixed gonadal dysgenesis apply. The potential for fertility is usually considered non-existent. Because some virilization is expected at the time of puberty, in the sex-assigned female, gonadectomy should be performed during the pre-pubertal period. At puberty in the different forms of androgen insensitivity, despite very low affinity of the cytoplasmic receptors for testosterone, some virilization occurs, because testosterone is secreted in such excess; the voice deepens, the muscle mass increases and the phallus lengthens.

5α-Reductase deficiency

The deficiency in 5α-reductase is a rare syndrome originally described in humans in 1974 [22]. The phenotypic appearance is generally represented by a severe hypospadias (Fig. 18.7). The deficit is found in the genital sinus and hepatic tissues; the diagnosis in adults is made by measuring the ratio of testosterone to DHT, which is increased. However, in affected children past infancy, the basal plasma testosterone and DHT levels are too low for accurate determination of the testosterone:DHT ratio. This measurement can be done after hCG administration. Demonstration that the genital skin is unable to convert the testosterone to DHT in tissue culture is the ultimate test for diagnosis [14].

Male pseudohermaphrodites

The deficiency of 17α-hydroxylase and 17-keto-reductase in the synthesis of steroid hormones is a cause of male pseudohermaphroditism that is not associated with ambiguous genitalia in the neonatal period. These individuals have a 46,XY karyotype, normal testicular tissue with development of the wolffian ducts and

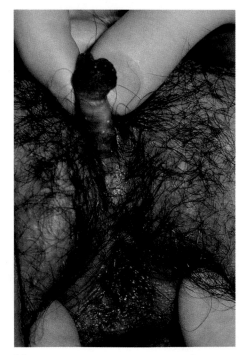

(a)

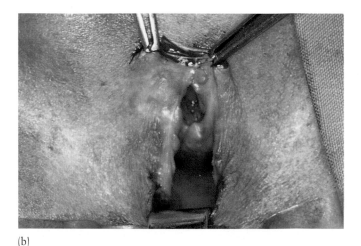

(b)

Fig. 18.6 (a) The tiny phallus of an 18-year-old with Reifenstein syndrome (incomplete testicular feminization) who previously underwent several operations for penile lenghtening. (b) After penile reconstruction with myocutaneous flaps and the closure of a perineal urethral fistula, a previously undetected, enlarged prostatic utricle is revealed.

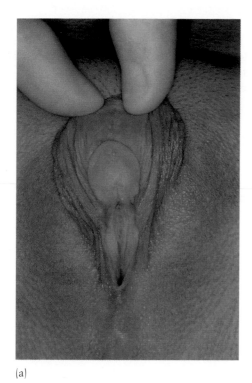

(a)

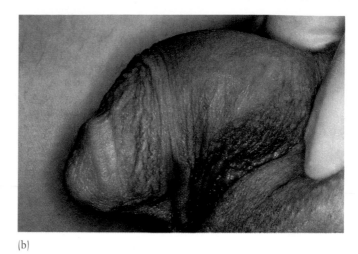

(b)

Fig. 18.7 A 7-year-old boy with 5α-reductase deficiency and severe hypospadias: (a) frontal view, and (b) lateral view.

regression of the müllerian structures. These subjects present later in life as amenorrhoeic phenotypic females.

Pure gonadal dysgenesis

These patients have variable karyotypes (45,XO; 46,XX; 46,XY), have bilateral undescended streak gonads with müllerian structures developed yet hypoplastic, while the wolffian ducts have regressed. There is no ambiguity in the neonatal period but usually the patients present later in life as phenotypic females with sexual infantilism. Dysgerminoma and gonadoblastoma are particularly frequent and present clinically with pelvic mass, signs of virilization or both. Bilateral gonadectomy is thus essential at the time of diagnosis for patients with a 46,XY karyotype.

Male phenotype

Klinefelter syndrome

The original description referred to a man with bilaterally small and firm testes, varying degrees of impaired sexual maturation, azoospermia, gynaecomastia and elevated levels of urinary gonadotrophins. The karyotype can be 47,XXY, 46,XX/47,XXY or even 48,XXXY or 49,XXXXY. The chromatin as well as the H-Y antigen are positive. These patients have symmetrically descended testes, which at birth have normal histology; however, in early infancy, there is a drastic loss of germ cells, followed by progressive tubular hyalinization during adolescence. They usually seek medical attention at puberty because of sexual infantilism or later in life for infertility, which occurs secondary to primary hypogonadism.

Hernia uteri inguinalis

The persistent müllerian duct syndrome (or hernia uteri inguinalis) is a rare syndrome resulting from an isolated deficiency of testicular MIF secretion or from peripheral insensitivity to MIF. Males affected are not ambiguous at birth and generally present later with symmetrically or asymmetrically undescended testes for orchidopexy or repair of inguinal hernias. They have a 46,XY karyotype and the gonadal tissue is exclusively testicular. Both wolffian and müllerian duct derivatives are present with a vas deferens and epididymis alongside an ipsilateral uterus, fallopian tube and the upper portion of a vagina.

Surgical removal of the müllerian structures is recommended [23], although the fertility potential of these patients can be compromised when surgery is attempted to salvage testicular tissue as the vas deferens is intimately related to the broad ligament and uterus. These adhesions make primary or staged orchidopexy a very difficult intervention.

XX male reversal

The majority of XX sex-reversal males contain fragments of

DNA from the short arm of the Y chromosome [24–26] in the distal end of the short arm of the X chromosome. They have a 46,XX karyotype but have exclusively testicular tissue with a normally developed wolffian system and regression of the müllerian ducts.

The external genitalia are not ambiguous at birth with a normal male phenotype. The testes are small and firm but bilaterally descended; later in life these patients develop gynaecomastia and hyalinization of the seminiferous tubules at puberty with incomplete pubarche. All these findings make this rare disorder very similar to the Klinefelter syndrome.

Diagnosis

Early and exact diagnosis is essential in patients with ambiguous genitalia because a late diagnosis can be responsible for behavioural disorders (due to late or wrong gender assignment) and some of the clinical and pathological entities which can be life threatening, such as fluid imbalance and gonadal neoplasias. Therefore, genital ambiguity can be considered a psychomedical emergency with two specific goals.
1 Accurate sex assignment.
2 Detection of the underlying endocrinopathies that may endanger the newborn, particularly the salt-losing variety.

Anamnesis

As the majority of conditions producing ambiguous genitalia are transmitted through a recessive autosomic mechanism, a similar anomaly is frequently found in the family. A maternal history of androgen exposure (either endogenous or exogenous) as well as a family history of neonatal death is a clue for a diagnosis of CAH. Moreover, it is important to look for maternal virilization (inadequate lactation, hirsutism, calvities, acne, clitoromegaly) which may indicate an androgen-producing neoplasia.

Physical examination

It is important to demonstrate whether or not the gonads are symmetrically or asymmetrically descended, because generally only testicular material fully descends (although ovotestes have been reported to descend completely into the bottom of the labioscrotal folds). Thus, if there are palpable inguinoscrotal gonads, the diagnosis of female pseudohermaphroditism and pure gonadal dysgenesis can be eliminated. On the other hand, the absence of palpable gonads in an apparently fully virilized infant should raise the possibility of a severely virilized female pseudohermaphrodite (see Fig. 18.2). Finally it is important to evaluate carefully the phallus and the urethral meatus to rule out a microphallus and/or hypospadias because the association of cryptorchidism and hypospadias is associated with intersex conditions in 53% of cases [27]. The measurement of phallic length and comparison with known nomograms [28] is important, especially in consideration for penile reconstruction.

Karyotype

The chromosomal sex is best determined by karyotyping and can be done within 48 h with activated T lymphocytes, but the regular 72 h lymphocyte culture is preferable. A reliable result can be achieved by microscopy without photography and banding at 3–4 days. A complete karyotype with banding and photography can be achieved in 6–7 days.

The usefulness of the buccal smear is limited in the neonatal assessment of sexual ambiguity because it is present in only 20% of infant female cells. For this reason it is practically abandoned nowadays.

Sonographic and radiological studies

Pelvic ultrasound and retrograde genitograms may detect the cervix and uterus, confirming müllerian duct structures. This rules out a diagnosis of male pseudohermaphroditism, except in those with hernia uteri inguinalis and or in those with dysgenetic gonads. Ultrasound cannot give any information about gonadal type. Therefore, gonadal sex evidence must be obtained through biopsies obtained by laparotomy or laparoscopy if other tests prove to be inconclusive [29].

Radiological evaluation of the vagina should also be obtained to evaluate its size and the level of its conjunction with the urogenital sinus. If a radio-opaque marker is placed on the perineal skin the radiological evaluation allows a better estimate of the level of the vaginal confluence because it is more objective and less invasive than an endoscopic evaluation. If vaginal filling is not obtained during a simple voiding cystourethrogram, retrograde filling of the urogenital sinus is performed in order to obtain vaginal visualization. Should this attempt also be negative, the authors prefer to obtain a vaginogram after introducing a catheter into the vagina during an endoscopic evaluation performed under the same anaesthetic used for the surgical correction. The authors believe that an adequate radiological evaluation of the level of vaginal confluence and vaginal size allows the most appropriate surgical approach to be determined.

Biochemical studies

As CAH female pseudohermaphrodites are the most common cause of genital ambiguity and require cortisone replacement, endocrine evaluation represents a diagnostic emergency in newborns with ambiguous genitalia. In order to prevent NA+ and Cl- losses and fatal dehydration, adrenal steroids must be evaluated within the first week of life even before the karyotype is known. The most common CAH syndrome, which is secondary to a 21α-hydroxylase deficit, is characterized by high 17-OHP (>2000 ng/dl) serum levels found in the first days of life. These levels can be rapidly evaluated by a radioimmunoassay test with no need to measure 17-ketosteroid or pregnanetriol urinary levels, as their evaluation is more difficult and slow and may be abnormally elevated in normal children in the first months of life. However, the determination of the plasma 17-OHP level should be delayed for 48 h after birth because earlier levels can reflect the presence of maternal progesterone.

The clinical presence of hypokalaemic alkalosis or hypertension may reflect underlying deficiencies of cortisol and mineralocorticoids or an excess of DOC, and requires urgent correction. Biochemical measurements of the various precursors can identify the exact enzymatic block in male and female pseudohermaphroditism (Table 18.4).

In the normal neonate, the testosterone:DHT ratio is 4.9 ± 2.8 and it remains almost unchanged after hCG stimulation because of a parallel increase of both testosterone and DHT. In 5α-reductase deficiency serum the testosterone:DHT ratio is elevated after hCG stimulation, while reduced 5α-reductase activity is detectable in vitro on genital skin fibroblasts [30]. In cases of AIS due to receptor deficiency, both testosterone and DHT increase after hCG stimulation but the genital skin fibroblast test shows an abnormal binding of androgens to their receptors [30].

Diagnostic algorithm in the newborn with ambiguous external genitalia

We can define ambiguous genitalia as any situation in which it is unclear whether a child is a male or a female.

The following conditions fit this definition:
1 hypospadias with bilateral impalpable testes;
2 hypospadias with unilateral impalpable testis;
3 micropenis with impalpable testes;
4 normal phallus with bilateral impalpable testes.

It is the authors' opinion that a micropenis and severe hypospadias with palpable testes should be regarded with caution because — although not true intersex — they could represent the consequence of a testosterone biosynthesis deficiency or partial testosterone insensitivity.

For a correct diagnosis in all these cases, the following diagnostic algorithms — mainly based on sex karyotype — should be followed.

Female karyotype (46,XX)

Genital ambiguity in patients with a 46,XX karyotype (Fig. 18.8) can be due to four possibilities.
1 Female pseudohermaphroditism (most frequent).
2 True hermaphroditism (rare) which exhibits a female karyotype in about 60% of cases.
3 Mixed gonadal dysgenesis (very rare).
4 Female embryo exposure to androgens or progestogens.

The presence or absence of palpable gonads and the 17-OHP levels are important in establishing the differential diagnosis. In cases of impalpable gonads and elevated 17-OHP serum levels, the diagnosis of female pseudohermaphroditism secondary to 21-OH deficiency can be established. Palpable gonads and normal 17-OHP serum levels are suggestive of true hermaphroditism (a biopsy will reveal the histological features of the gonads). If the gonads are impalpable and 17-OHP levels are normal, prenatal exposure to androgens or progestogens must be ruled out. Such exposure can occur because of pharmacological treatments or because of maternal virilizing tumours. Virilizing tumours can be suspected in cases of maternal hirsutism, clitoromegaly, acne, calvities or inadequate lactation. A gravid luteoma (a benign virilizing maternal

Table 18.4 The main endocrinological parameters for the diagnosis of congenital adrenal hyperplasia (CAH) in female patients and of adrenal and/or testicular steroidogenesis in male patients.

	Deficient enzyme	17-OHP	Androstanedione	DHEA	Testosterone
Male steroidogenesis deficiencies	20,22-desmolase	↓	↓	↓	↓
	17α-OH	↓	↓	↓	↓
	3β-OH dehydrogenase	N↑	N↓	↑↑	N
	17,20-desmolase	N↑	↓↓	N↑	↑
	17β-OH dehydrogenase	N	↑↑	N↑	N
Female CAH syndromes	21-OH	↑	↑	N↑	↑
	11β-OH	↑	↑	↑	↑
	3β-OH dehydrogenase	N↑	N↑	↑↑	N↓

↑, increased; ↑↑, much increased; ↓, decreased; ↓↓, much decreased; DHEA, dehydroepiandrosterone; N, normal; OH, hydroxylase; OHP, hydroxyprogesterone.

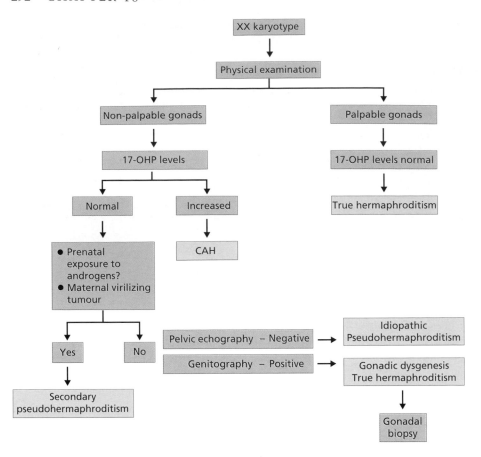

Fig. 18.8 Diagnostic algorithm in the newborn with ambiguous genitalia and a female karyotype. CAH, congenital adrenal aplasia; OHP, hydroxyprogesterone.

tumour) can, however, escape diagnosis if it is transient and if its androgen production is insufficient to produce maternal virilization.

If fetal exposure to androgens is excluded, pelvic ultrasound and, if indicated, genitography should be undertaken in order to differentiate between gonadal dysgenesis and true hermaphroditism with non-palpable gonads. In both cases gonadal biopsy provides the diagnosis. Idiopathic female pseudohermaphroditism must be considered if all tests are negative.

Male karyotype (46,XY)

An ambiguous phenotype with a male karyotype (Fig. 18.9) represents a more complex case than the same phenotype with a female karyotype. As a consequence the diagnostic approach is more complex. According to Migeon [31] the most common causes are represented by the following.

1 Male pseudohermaphroditism due to androgen insensitivity (50% of cases).

2 Pure gonadal dysgenesis (40% of cases).

3 Male pseudohermaphroditism due to several aetiologies such as testosterone biosynthesis deficiency, 5α-reductase deficiency, etc. (10% of cases).

If both gonads are palpable, male pseudohermaphroditism is the most likely aetiology. It can be related to testosterone biosynthesis or 5α-reductase deficiencies or to partial androgen insensitivity (the complete form has no ambiguous genitalia, which are totally feminized).

The diagnostic procedure starts with hCG stimulation if the child is more than three months old. An undetectable testosterone level can be related to a deficiency in its biosynthesis or, more rarely, to Leydig cell aplasia. The level of the biochemical blockage — therefore the enzymatic deficiency — can be evaluated by measuring the different testosterone precursors (see Table 18.4). A normal testosterone increase after hCG stimulation is related either to 5α-reductase deficiency or to partial androgen insensitivity. The testosterone : DHT ratio after hCG will allow the exact diagnosis: it is increased in cases of 5α-reductase deficiency while it is normal in cases of androgen receptor insensitivity. The diagnosis will be confirmed by evaluating the scrotal skin fibroblast enzymatic activity in cases of suspected 5α-reductase deficiency and by testing androgen receptor function in cases of androgen insensitivity. It must be stressed that a correct diagnosis is important because only patients with testosterone biosynthesis deficiency will adequately respond to testosterone administration at puberty.

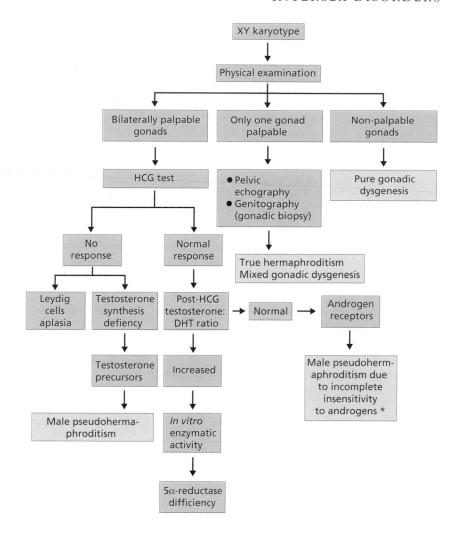

Fig. 18.9 Diagnostic algorithm in the newborn with ambiguous genitalia and a male karyotype. DHT, dihydrotestosterone; HCG, human chorionic gonadotrophin. * In the complete form (Morris syndrome) the external genitalia are not ambiguous.

If only one gonad is palpable the two possible diagnoses are: (i) true hermaphroditism (more likely, and exhibiting a 46,XY karyotype in 10% of cases); or (ii) mixed gonadal dysgenesis with a male karyotype. Pelvic ultrasound and/or genitography to detect müllerian derivatives and gonadal biopsy provide the correct diagnosis.

If no gonads are palpable, the most likely diagnosis is pure gonadal dysgenesis. Diagnosis must be confirmed by gonadal histology.

Mosaic karyotype

Two possibilities must be taken into consideration.
1 True hermaphroditism, which is associated with mosaicism in one-third of cases.
2 Gonadal dysgenesis — generally its mixed form is associated with mosaicism.

In both cases one gonad can be palpable but only in true hermaphroditism can they be palpated bilaterally. Gonadal biopsy is necessary to establish the diagnosis.

Guidelines for a sex assignment

Patients with genital ambiguity must be reared as males or females and this decision represents a true neonatal emergency. The decision must be taken after the correct diagnosis has been made in order to raise these patients in the gender in which they will best fit. There is no doubt that female pseudohermaphrodites should be raised as females. In other cases the decision must be taken after considering anatomical, psychological and oncological factors as discussed below.

1 *Phallic size.* Currently phallic size is still believed to be the most significant criterion in gender assignment in the newborn [28,32]. Although nomograms are available for penile length, it is not clearly defined what size of phallus is required to avoid male inadequacy [28]. Time–growth response to androgen stimulus can be a key factor in distinguishing borderline cases, although some claim — after rather questionable experimental and clinical observations — that early exposure to androgens accelerates the loss of androgen receptors [33,34].

2 *Fertility potential.* Except for female pseudoher-maphrodites and rare cases of true hermaphrodites, fertility potential is usually considered non-existent in mixed gonadal dysgenesis and uncertain in male pseudoher-maphroditism.

3 *Risk of gonadal malignancy.* Dysplastic and cryptorchid gonads have an increased risk of malignancy. Even though gonadoblastomas are not malignant, these tumours frequently contain dysgerminoma elements that can metastasize. The risk of neoplasia in streak gonads with an XY karyotype is much larger than is streak gonads with XX chromosomes.

4 *Patient or family wishes.* Family history, culture and preferences, particularly if based on prior experience, are of major importance. Parenteral wishes may even be very dominant in dictating one sex of rearing over another. This is most often based on longstanding cultural bias and may not be alterable by any medical advice.

The older child who presents with an originally assigned sex of rearing that is inappropriate represents one of the most complex situations in clinical surgery. Raising a female pseudohermaphrodite as a male is an example. Care, extensive psychiatric and endocrinological consultation and real communication with the family are of utmost importance.

Surgical treatment

Surgical treatment of patients with ambiguous genitalia can be classified as follows: (i) exploratory surgery for diagnostic purposes; (ii) excisional surgery of inappropriate tissues; and (iii) reconstructive surgery.

Exploratory surgery

As diagnosis and gender assignment represent a neonatal emergency in a child with ambiguous genitalia, exploratory surgery, if necessary, is usually carried out in the first days of life. Indications are represented by true hermaph-roditism, mixed gonadal dysgenesis and cases of male pseudohermaphroditism with unclear gender assignment. Although its safety in newborns has not been proved yet, laparoscopy may replace open surgery because it allows not only the inspection of internal ducts but also biopsies from the gonads can be obtained. It is important to stress that biopsies must be properly taken from the gonads, especially if an ovotestis is suspected. In some cases ovarian and testicular tissue can be separated and visualized at the gonadal surface; biopsies must be obtained from both regions. In other cases the two gonadal components are variously intertwined and biopsies must be taken at different surface appearances. In cases of suspected androgen insensitivity, genital skin biopsy for fibroblast culture is also useful.

Excisional surgery of inappropriate tissue

This should not be undertaken until a clear diagnosis and proper gender assignment have been done. It includes the following.

1 Removal of the gonadal tissue and its related duct, opposite to the chosen gender assignment in the case of ovotestes.

2 Removal of dysgenetic gonads for oncological reasons. Streak gonads can be removed precociously because they are not important for hormonal production. In cases of hormone-producing tissue, the authors prefer to delay its removal until around puberty to take advantage of its natural hormone production, which seems to be better than substitution therapy. However, others prefer earlier castration and subsequent substitution therapy. The risk of neoplasia is particularly high in streak gonads in the case of an XY karyotype. Malignancy will develop in 15–25% of streak gonads, usually gonadoblastomas, dysgerminomas or both [14]. In one large series of gonadoblastomas, 40% were in patients less than 15 years of age and 15% were in patients less than 10 years of age [35]. In cases of mixed gonadal dysgenesis, testes should be removed early if they cannot be relocated into the scrotum or if associated with ipsilateral müllerian duct structures because in these cases the risk of malignancy is about 50%.

3 Removal of müllerian structures in cases of MIF deficiency is debated because their dissection may injure the intimately related wolffian ducts.

4 Excision of redundant corpora cavernosa if a clitoris has to be reconstructed from an enlarged phallus.

5 Removal of excessive mammary tissue if gynaecomastia appears after puberty.

Reconstructive surgery

Masculinizing genitoplasty

In cases of masculinizing reconstruction it should be clear to the parents that this approach could be very difficult. Müllerian structures should also be removed in these patients. The easiest cases are represented by young children with hypospadias-like genitalia and corpora cavernosa of adequate size. A patient with a micropenis is more complicated because it is necessary to rely on the amount of phallic increase after testosterone or local DHT exposure.

The most difficult cases are represented by children or boys in whom a female gender assignment would be the better choice but who have already received a male assignment. Not much can be done in these cases apart from penile reconstruction with myocutaneous flaps. Unless severe psychological problems are forcing such a reconstruction, this is better performed after puberty.

Penile reconstruction with myocutaneous flaps before puberty has been performed in few cases (C.H. Horton, personal communication) but the follow-up is still too short to evaluate long-term results.

Feminizing genitoplasty

Feminizing genitoplasty has both cosmetic and functional aims. To provide a good cosmetic appearance, a redundant phallus must be reduced, the labia majora — that generally have a somewhat scrotal appearance — must be adjusted, the missing labia minora should be reconstructed and, finally, a vulval region should be created lined as much as possible with mucosa.

From a functional point of view the following goals should be obtained: a wide and supple, properly placed vaginal opening; a properly orientated and wide vagina; free menstrual drainage; and clitoral sensations.

From a surgical point of view, feminizing genitoplasty can be divided into two procedures: clitoroplasty and vaginoplasty. They can be performed at different ages or simultaneously. There is no controversy that clitoroplasty should be performed as early as possible. Indeed, there is general agreement that an enlarged phallus represents the main cause of parental confusion about the sex of their child. If this situation is maintained for too long it will produce major psychological problems for the child. Therefore, the age at which the authors prefer to perform this surgery is around 2 months.

In cases of favourable vaginal anatomy (a low vagina that can be easily opened to the perineum by a simple Fortunoff flap), vaginoplasty can be carried out at the same time as clitoroplasty. In more severe cases, when the vaginal entry is too high to make a Fortunoff flap possible (Fig. 18.10) most surgeons preferred an early clitoroplasty followed by a delayed vaginoplasty. Some surgeons used to perform a vaginoplasty at around 3–5 years of age [36] while others prefer to delay it until after puberty [37–39]. The reasons for a delayed vaginoplasty were mainly due to the tendency of most cases to stenose and to the subsequent need of periodic dilatations.

More recently, the authors published a technique [40] which enabled a clitoroplasty and vaginoplasty to be performed as a single stage procedure, even at an early age. With progressive experience the authors feel now that the exposure to maternal oestrogens produces a relatively larger and thicker vagina in the first few months of life than in later years. Also, with age, perineal structures deepen, vaginal walls become thinner and vaginal dissection can be more difficult. Subsequently, in CAH cases, an important increase in vaginal size occurs at the time of puberty due to the natural oestrogen production and vaginal dissection becomes easy again. Therefore, in the authors' experience the best timing for vaginoplasty in complex cases is either

the first few months of life (2–4 months) or soon after puberty. But it must be kept in mind that in some cases urethrovaginal confluence is responsible for urinary tract infections and correction of the malformation is the best way to prevent them [41].

Clitoroplasty

The earliest 'reconstructive' procedures for clitoral reduction were obtained simply by amputation (clitorectomy) [42] with unacceptable cosmetic and functional results. Clitoral recession was also suggested [43]: the corpora cavernosa were dissected out and anchored with interrupted sutures to the pubic bones. It is hard to say if this approach was really better then clitorectomy because

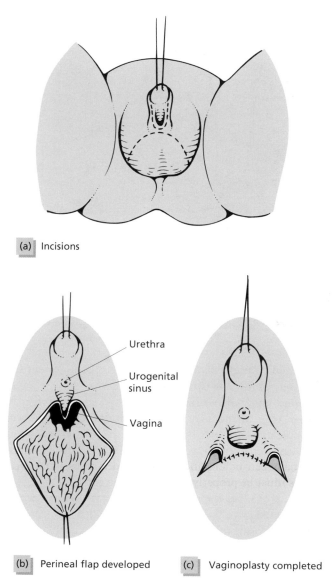

(a) Incisions

(b) Perineal flap developed

(c) Vaginoplasty completed

Urethra

Urogenital sinus

Vagina

Fig. 18.10 Vaginoplasty using a Fortunoff flap. Modified from Snyder *et al.* [36].

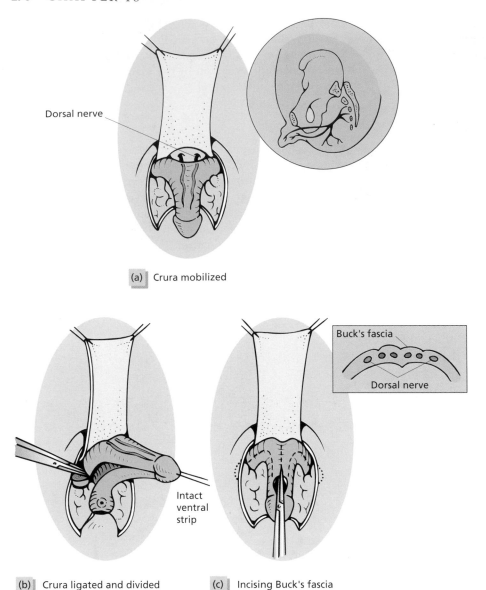

(a) Crura mobilized

(b) Crura ligated and divided

(c) Incising Buck's fascia

Fig. 18.11 Clitoroplasty by subtotal resection of the corpora: initial steps. Modified from Snyder *et al.* [36].

unreduced corpora engorged at the time of arousement and produced painful and excessive erection.

Spence and Allen in the USA [44] and Marberger in Europe [45] introduced almost simultaneously a true clitoroplasty with partial recession of the corpora and preservation of the neurovascular bundles to maintain glans sensations. The principles of both techniques were combined by Snyder *et al.* [36] (Figs 18.10–18.12). After dissecting out the dorsolateral skin, the corpora cavernosa are separated from the neurovascular bundles and from the ventral mucosal strip interposed between the glans and the urethral opening. The corpora are ligated and cut at the level of the crura proximally, and at the level of the balanic sulcus distally. The distal and proximal stumps of the corpora are then reanastomosed, thus performing a partial corporal amputation.

Kogan [46] suggested reducing the clitoris only by excising the erectile tissue (Fig. 18.13). After a lateral vertical incision is performed into the albuginea of the corpora cavernosa, the erectile tissue is progressively dissected out and extruded. Dissection is started, freeing completely the cavernous tissue from the distal end of the corpora and is extended proximally down to where desired. After a tie is passed around each cavernous tissue, the distal part is removed and the albuginea plicated.

All these techniques represented great improvements compared to clitorectomy or simple clitoral resection. However, some disadvantages were still present. Resection of the intermediate portion of the corpora cavernosa and reanastomosis of their distal stumps to the proximal portions can still leave a redundant clitoris. Simple resection of a good portion of the cavernous tissue is not as

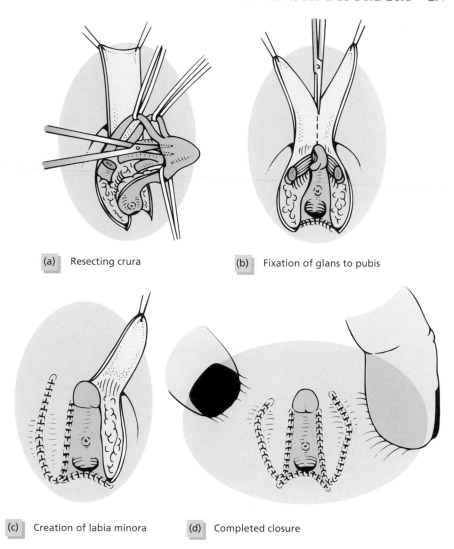

(a)   Resecting crura

(b)   Fixation of glans to pubis

(c)   Creation of labia minora

(d)   Completed closure

Fig. 18.12 Clitoroplasty by subtotal resection of the corpora completed. Modified from Snyder *et al.* [36].

easy as it may appear because of excessive bleeding during dissection. Preservation of the continuity of the mucosal strip running from the glans to the urethral meatus, as suggested by Snyder [36], is possible only in cases of moderate phallic size. With large phalluses, maintenance of this mucosal strip can result in mucosal redundancy.

Taking into account these considerations, the authors modified clitoral recession as shown in see Fig. 18.15f. The glans is degloved either by dissecting out the dorsolateral skin and the ventral mucosa separately (in a hypospadias-like phallus) or by a circumcising incision followed by skin retraction (in a fully virilized phallus). The corpora are freed mainly by dissecting them free from the neurovascular bundle dorsally, and from the mucosal covering (or from the urogenital sinus in severely virilized cases) ventrally. Most importantly the glans is dissected out from the tips of the corpora cavernosa. The whole procedure is easy to perform because all the dissecting planes are surprisingly easy to find. At the end of this part of the procedure the

glans is perfectly detached resulting in a cap-like structure, perfectly vascularized and innervated by well-connected neurovascular bundles. The corpora are then ligated and divided at the crus. The remainder of the glans is then tacked to the corporal stumps. Finally, the phallic skin is divided dorsally as with previous clitoroplasties in order to reconstruct the labia minora. Redundant ventral mucosa is removed in order to avoid unattractive plicatures.

Vaginoplasty

An exact anatomical evaluation of the urogenital sinus and of the level of branching of the urethrovaginal confluence is mandatory before surgery is planned (see p. 290). The technique for vaginoplasty should be selected on the basis of the distance between the vaginal entry and the perineal spot, where the vaginal opening will be placed. Some authors believe that the location of the so-called external urethral sphincter and its relationship with the vaginal

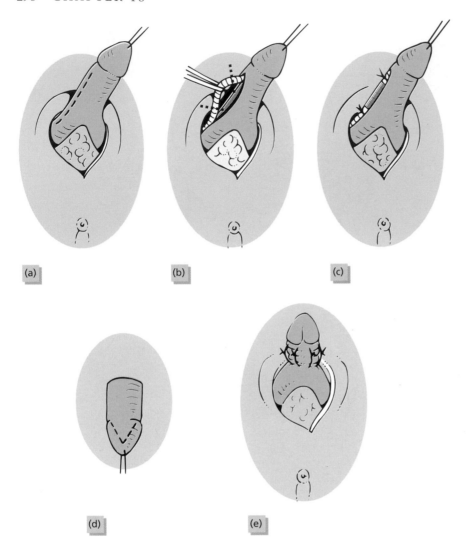

(a)   (b)   (c)

(d)   (e)

Fig. 18.13 Clitoroplasty by partial excision of erectile tissue. Modified from Kogan *et al.* [46].

entry is important for continence [47]. The authors are not concerned about the possible relationship between the vaginal entry and the external urethral sphincter because we have never been able to locate this functional structure, even during dissection of the highest vaginas. A careful dissection is probably the key to avoiding injury to the continence mechanism, which is mainly based on the bladder neck.

On the other hand it is extremely important to avoid connecting the vagina to the perineum by a simple procedure if it is too high to be treated in this way. This will end up with a single perineal opening and a female hypospadias. Such a situation is prone to producing recurrent urinary infections and, in the most severe cases, accumulation of stones within the vagina and severe local inflammation and discomfort has been described. Therefore, according to the anatomical situation, the following techniques can be adopted.

Simple cut back. This technique is represented by a

vertical incision from the single perineal opening down into the perineum where the posterior lip of the vaginal opening should be located. It must be stressed that this operation can be performed only in very rare cases resembling a vaginal fusion. The cases in which it can be employed do not require any investigations to outline the anatomy because the perineal opening is wide and the separate openings of the urethra and vagina are superficial and very easy to inspect. The thickness of the closing membrane is minimal.

Fortunoff flap. The Fortunoff flap [48] is developed from the labioscrotal or perineal skin starting with an inverted U- or V-shape incision whose apex is placed just at the level of the single perineal opening (see Fig. 18.10). The base of the flap should be placed where the posterior vaginal lip is desired. A thick flap is then developed taking care to follow the inferior (posterior) wall of the urogenital sinus. This wall is then incised vertically until the vaginal opening appears. At this point the incision is advanced more into

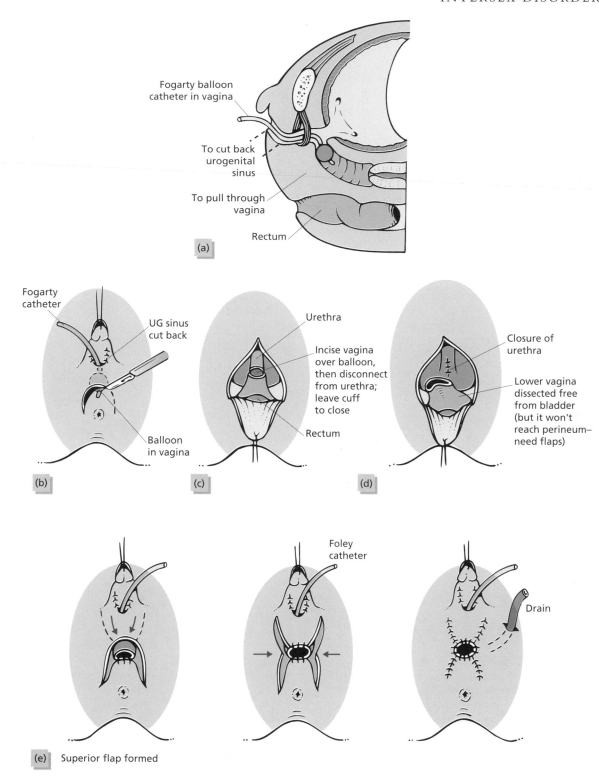

Fig. 18.14 Perineal pull-through vaginoplasty according to Hendrew-Crawford. (a) After degloving of the phallic shaft the Buck fascia and albuginea are ancised (dotted line). (b) (1) Excision of the erectile tissue from inside the tunica albuginea. (c) (2) & (2′) Proximal and distal ligation of the erectile tissue for haemostatic purpose. (3) The erectile tissue included within the haemostatic stitches is removed and most of the corpus cavernosum remains empty. (d) Wedge resection of the glans. (e) Shrinkage of the empty corpora by a few separate stitches. Modified from Hendren and Crawford [49].

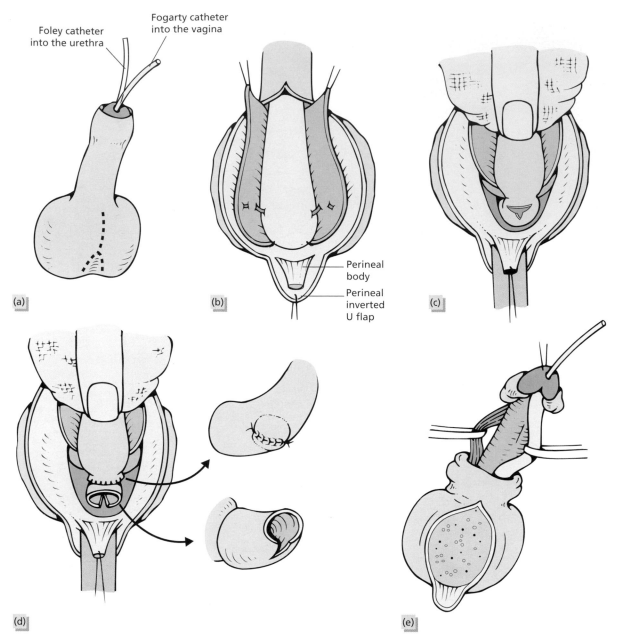

Fig. 18.15 Complete virilization in a girl with severe CAH syndrome. (a) A Fogarty catheter is placed into the vagina and a Foley catheter is placed into the urethra. The operation starts with an inverted Y incision at the level of the scrotum-like labioscrotal folds. (b) The bulbospongiosus muscles are incised on the midline. The perineal body is freed from its anterior connections and abated. (c) The bulbar segment of the urogenital sinus (UGS) is progressively exposed by freeing and displacing from it the superficial transversus perinei, the deep transversus perinei muscles and the prerectal fibres of the levator ani. This is a very important step because it will allow the surgeon to create a good space around the vagina. Inadequate dissection at this level can represent one of the reasons for subsequent vaginal stenosis. A wet sponge under the tip of the forefinger of the helping assistant retracts the bulbar portion of the UGS; this will help to superficialize the membranous portion and the urethrovaginal confluence. After the lower (posterior) wall of the vagina has been exposed and located with the help of the Fogarty catheter, a vertical incision is made near to the urethrovaginal confluence. The incision is stopped and completed with a transverse incision 5 mm away from the urethra. (d) By extending the transverse incision, the vagina is dissected free from its conjunction with the urethra. The inside view, obtained through the previous incision, will help the dissection which can be rather difficult around the distal end of the vagina due to the presence of fibrous tissue interposed between the vagina and urethra. The dissection must be continued until the vagina is completely freed from it and well mobilized. Care must be taken to leave an adequate length of vaginal stump to allow suturing. (e) A wet sponge is placed into the cavity and attention turned to the clitoroplasty. After a circular incision is made around the balanic sulcus, the phallic skin is retracted and dissection is made around

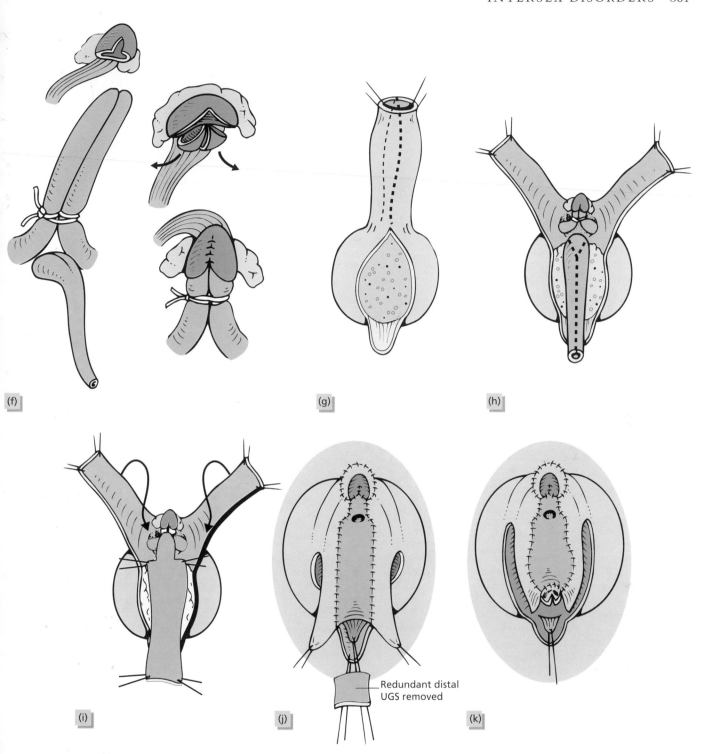

(f)   (g)   (h)

(i)   (j)   (k)

Redundant distal
UGS removed

Fig. 18.15 (*Continued*) the corpora in order to free the neurovascular bundles dorsally and the UGS ventrally. (f) The UGS is completely mobilized from the glans. Also, following the tips of the corpora cavernosa, a nice, almost avascular plane can be identified; this allows the corpora to be separated from the glans. The corpora are ligated where the clitoris will be located just above their conjunction. The distal part of the corpora is then removed by two oblique incisions on each corpus just above the haemostatic stitch. Glandular trimming is then performed.

As neurovascular structures move from the dorsal neurovascular bundles first laterally within the glans and then toward the tip of the glans, trimming is performed by removing triangular segments of tissue around the region of the previous 'urethral meatus'. The glans is then reconfigured with approaching stitches and adapted to the tip of the corporal stump. (g) The phallic skin is pulled up again and incised longitudinally, dorsally and ventrally. (h) The skin incisions develop two skin flaps. The UGS, which has been preserved intact, is now incised dorsally.

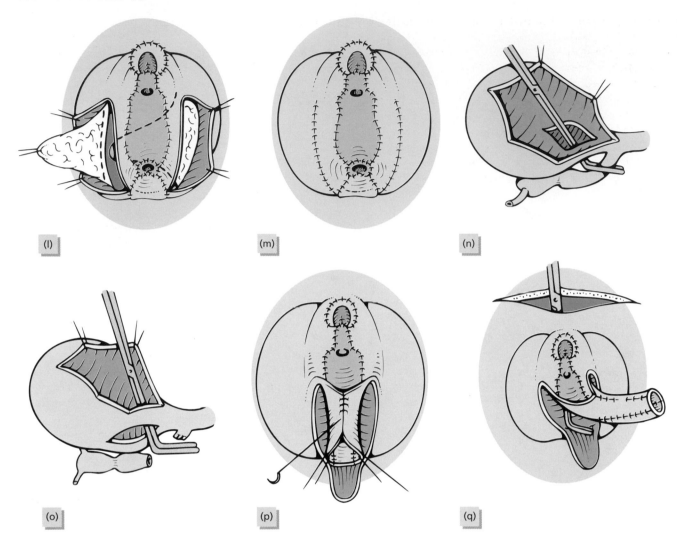

(l)

(m)

(n)

(o)

(p)

(q)

Fig. 18.15 (*Continued*) (f) The proximal end of the incision is performed in a V shape and terminated where the 'urethral' meatus is desired (dotted lines indicate the incision of the UGS). (i) The small V-shaped flap obtained from the dorsum of the UGS is rotated upwards and sutured to the reduced glans while the two lateral skin flaps are rotated downwards. (j) The two skin flaps are sutured around the glans and on each side of the divided UGS, thus obtaining a mucocutaneous rectangle. In case of redundancy, the distal end of the UGS is removed. (k) The distal end of the mucocutaneous rectangle is now inverted into the perineal opening and progressively sutured to the distal end of the vagina. A continuous mucous lining is present in the anterior wall of the vulvar and vaginal region, from the clitoris to the true vagina. (l) The initial Fortunoff-type skin flap is now rotated upwards and progressively sutured to the inferior (posterior) wall of the vagina and to the lateral wedges of the mucocutaneous rectangle. If the labioscrotal folds are too fatty they can be partially defatted. The fatty tissue of one side should be discarded, that of the opposite side is interposed between the UGS and urethra (above) and the reconstructed vagina below. This will help to produce a gentle curvature of the anterior vulvar region between the urethral and vaginal openings. This step is better performed before the suture of the mucocutaneous flap with the vagina is started. (m) Progressive suturing of the lateral edges of the mucocutaneous rectangle with the labioscrotal folds on each side will terminate the operation. (n) In cases of very high and small vagina difficult to dissect from the perineum, a transvesical approach is suggested. After the anterior bladder wall is opened, the trigone is incised from above the interureteric bar to the bladder neck. The vagina is easily visualized and sectioned. The incision is progressively carried out together with progressive suturing of the stump connected with the urethra. The holding stitch avoids the disappearance of the stump into the wound. (o) A right-angle clamp easily connects the perineal wound with the retrovesical space. (p) The mucocutaneous rectangle previously obtained by combining the splitted phallic skin and the opened UGS is progressively rolled into a tube. The skin and mucosa remain inside. (q) The tube is then pulled into the perineum. It will then be easily anastomosed to the vagina through the transtrigonal opening. After bladder closure the perineal wound is closed as in steps (l) and (m).

the posterior vaginal wall so that a wide vaginal opening is obtained. If the posterior wall of the urogenital sinus was not previously dissected sufficiently, further dissection can be accomplished. When the incision has been completely accomplished, the apex of the Fortunoff flap is sutured to the proximal end of the incision. The posterior wall of the distal vagina and the posterior vaginal lip are therefore reconstructed by the skin flap.

As previously stated, this procedure cannot be performed if the urogenital sinus below the urethrovaginal confluence is too long. The urethral meatus will remain too high and a female hypospadias will be produced. Secondly, a wide common perineal opening can produce unsatisfactory cosmetic and functional results. Discomfort during voiding due to severe urinary tract and local infection can be present and vaginal stones have been described.

Although possibly serious complications may occur if the indications for the procedure are wrong, the authors agree with others [47] that most patients with CAH, mixed gonadal dysgenesis and true hermaphrodites have an anatomical situation that will benefit from the Fortunoff flap. Therefore, this simple operation is probably the most utilized in intersex patients.

Pull-through procedure. This procedure, published in 1969 by Hendren and Crawford [49], was probably the one that solved most of the functional problems of high vaginal insertion (Fig. 18.14). In this technique vaginoplasty is performed as a separate procedure from clitoroplasty and the entire procedure is carried out through the perineum. After the child has been placed in the lithotomy position with good perineal exposure, cystoscopy is performed and a Fogarty catheter is placed into the vagina. The perineal skin is incised in order to develop four V- or U-shaped flaps that — after adequate mobilization — will be connected to the vagina at the end of the operation. Generally they can be obtained from labioscrotal folds and the final cosmetic appearance is acceptable. However, if the labioscrotal folds are diminished in size, most of the flaps can be obtained from flat perineal skin and the end result will be an isolated hole into the perineum with no mucosal lining.

After the vaginal dissection has been completed and the vaginal stump has been sutured, the vagina is connected to the perineum by anastomosing it to the previously obtained perineal skin flaps.

Hendren and Donahoe [50] noted the need for long-term vaginal dilatation with Hegar dilators. This observation, together with the need for some improvement in cosmetic results, urged others to improve this technique. However, it has the great merit of being the first good solution — and the only one available for 20 years after its publication — to solve a difficult surgical problem.

Combined clitoroplasty and vaginoplasty. Because of the suboptimal cosmetic and functional results of the Hendren and Crawford procedure, the authors recently presented a new one-stage clitorovaginoplasty [40] (Fig. 18.15) and a similar one was published in 1990 [51].

Vaginal enlargement. In some cases of male pseudohermaphroditism the 'vagina' (which actually is a prostatic utricle) can be either tiny — although the vulvar region looks normal — or absent. In cases of a small vagina, its opening is located in the normal position (see Fig. 18.5b). In these cases, progressive dilatations if started after puberty in well-motivated patients, can obtain excellent cosmetic and functional results without requiring surgery [52]. In our hands the procedure starts with plastic anal dilators maintained in place overnight, secured with plasters. As progressive dilatation is achieved, the size of dilator is increased until a phallic-size dilator can be easily inserted.

Total reconstruction for vaginal agenesis. In vaginal agenesis, the vagina must be completely reconstructed. There is no need for vaginal reconstruction in children and it should be undertaken after puberty. Skin grafts almost invariably result in vaginal contraction and stenosis. Moreover, the vagina will be completely dry. For these reasons skin grafts have been almost completely abandoned and replaced by bowel segments. Small bowel segments are fragile and easily traumatized during intercourse; transverse sigmoid and colon segments exhibit enough durability but produce excessive amounts of mucous which smells. According to R. Hohenfellner (personal communication, 1994) the caecum with some ascending colon seems to represent a good compromise between colon durability and reduced mucous production.

For cosmetic reasons and to avoid traumatic bleeding it is important to prevent intestinal mucosa prolapse from the perineum. Therefore, the perineal opening of the intestinal loop must be made well inside the perineum. If a vulval region is not evident, perineal skin flaps as in the Hendren–Crawford procedure will allow the bowel segment opening to be kept high enough to avoid its protrusion.

Conclusion

Intersex disorders represent a very demanding pathological entity from diagnostic, medical, surgical and psychological points of view. The establishment of the correct diagnosis represents a neonatal emergency both for psychological and medical reasons. It is important to keep in mind that a proper endocrinological treatment must be instituted promptly in the great majority of cases due to the prevalence of CAH, which can be life threatening if improperly treated. Also, the growth of these patients needs to be continuously monitored and therapeutic adjustments made when necessary. The surgical correction of the malformation requires experience and skill in order to select the proper technique, to perform it meticulously, to adapt, if necessary, details taken from different techniques for the best management of a single patient, to follow the patient long-term and be to ready to perform subsequent revisions of the initial operation if necessary. Early psychological support can be very important for the family, especially if obstetricians and neonatalogists did not exhibit a cautious approach. Also, psychological support can be very difficult and demanding in patients whose diagnosis and treatment were delayed. Therefore, the management of an intersex case can represent a difficult task that requires a team with special interest and experience in this particular field.

References

1 Jost A. The role of fetal hormones in prenatal development. *Harvey Lect* 1960;**55**:201–8.
2 Jost A. Hormonal factors in the sex differentiation of the mammalian fetus. *Proc R Soc Lond [Biol]* 1970;**259**:119–25.
3 Jost A. A new look at the mechanism controlling sex differentiation in mammals. *Johns Hopkins Med J* 1972;**130**: 38–53.
4 Jost A. Embryonic sexual differentiation (morphology, physiology, abnormalities). In: Jones HW, Scoot WW, eds. *Hermaphroditism, Genital Anomalies and Related Endocrine Disorders*. Baltimore: Williams and Wilkins, 1971:16–37.
5 Wilson JD, Siiteri PK. Developmental pattern of testosterone synthesis in the fetal gonad of the rabbit. *Endocrinology* 1973;**92**:1182–91.
6 Grumbach MM, Conte FA. Disorders of sex differentiation. In: Williams RH, ed. *Textbook of Endocrinology*. Philadelphia: WB Saunders, 1981:423–513.
7 Allen T. Disorder of sexual differentiation. In: Kelalis PP, King LR, Belman AB, eds. *Clinical Paediatric Urology*. Philadephia: WB Saunders, 1975:304–21.
8 Allen LE, Hardy BE, Churchill BM. The surgical management of enlarged clitoris. *J Urol* 1982;**128**:351–4.
9 Conte FA, Grumbach MM. Abnormalities of sexual differentiation. In: Smith DR, ed. *General Urology*. Los Altos: Lange Medical, 1984:574–97.
10 Allen T. Disorder of sexual differentiation. In: Kelalis PP, King LR, Belman AB, eds. *Clinical Pediatric Urology*, 2nd edn. Philadelphia: WB Saunders, 1985:904–21.
11 Lalau-Keraly J, Amice V, Chaussain JL *et al.* L'hermaphrodisme vrai. *Semin Hosp [Paris]* 1986;**62**:2375–9.
12 Luks FI, Hansborough F, Klotz DH, Kottmeier PK, Tolete-Velcek F. Early gender assignment in true hermaphroditism. *J Ped Surg* 1988;**23**:1122–6.
13 Van Niekerk WA. True hermaphroditism: an analytic review with a report of three new cases. *Am J Obstet Gynecol* 1976;**126**:890–907.
14 Lorge F, Wese FX, Sluysmans TH *et al.* L'ambiguité sexuelle: aspects urologiques. *Acta Urol Belg* 1989;**57**:647–62.
15 Van Niekerk WA. True hermaphroditism. *Pediatr Adolesc Endocrinol* 1981;**8**:80–5.

16 Mayou BG, Armon P, Linderbaum RH. Pregnancy and childbirth in true hermaphrodite following reconstructive surgery. *Br J Obstet Gynaecol* 1978;**85**:314–16.
17 Narita O, Manba S, Nakanishi T, Ishizuka H. Pregnancy and childbirth in a true hermaphrodite. *Obstet Gynecol* 1975;**45**:593–5.
18 Tegenkamp TR, Brazzel JW, Tegenkamp I *et al.* Pregnancy without benefit of reconstructive surgery in a bisexually active true hermaphrodite. *Am J Obstet Gynecol* 1979;**135**:427–8.
19 Brown TR, Maes M, Rothwell SW *et al.* Human complete androgen insensitivity with normal dihydrotestosterone receptor binding capacity in cultured genital skin fibroblasts: evidence for a qualitative abnormality of the receptor. *J Clin Endocrin Metab* 1982;**55**:61–8.
20 Hughes IA, Evans BAJ. The fibroblast as a model for androgen resistant states. *J Clin Endocrinol Metab* 1988;**28**:565–79.
21 Griffin JE, Wilson JD. The syndromes of androgen resistance. *N Engl J Med* 1980;**320**:198–209.
22 Imperato-McGinley J, Guerrero L, Gauthier T, Peterson RE. Steroid 5α-reductase deficiency in men: an inherited form of male pseudohcrmaphroditism. *Science* 1974;**186**:1213–15.
23 Beheshti M, Churchill BM, Hardy BE *et al.* Familial persistant Mullerian duct syndrome. *J Urol* 1984;**131**:968–9.
24 Magenis RE, Casanova M, Fellous M *et al.* Further cytological evidence for Xp-Yp translocation in XX males using *in situ* hybridization with Y-derived probe. *Hum Genet* 1987;**75**:228–33.
25 Page DC, de la Chapelle A. The parental origin of X chromosomes in XX males determined using restriction fragment length polymorphisms. *Am J Hum Genet* 1984;**36**:565–75.
26 Petit C, de la Chapelle A, Levilliers J *et al.* An abnormal terminal X-Y interchange accounts for most but not all cases of human XX maleness. *Cell* 1987;**49**:595–602.
27 Rajfer J, Walsh PC. The incidence of intersexuality in patients with hypospadias and cryptorchidism. *J Urol* 1976;**116**:769–70.
28 Beheshti M, Churchill BM, Hardy BE *et al.* Gender assignment in male pseudohermaphrodite children. *Urology* 1983; **22**:604–7.
29 Hughes IA, Davies PAD. Neonatal endocrine and metabolic emergencies. *Clin Endocrin Metab* 1980;**9**:583–604.
30 Sultan CH, Migeon CJ. La culture de fibroblastes: moyen d'étude des anomalies de l'action cellulaire des androgénes au cours du pseuhermaphroditisme male. *Ann Endocrinol [Paris]* 1980;**41**:305–10.
31 Migeon CJ. Male pseudohermaphroditism. *Ann Endocrinol [Paris]* 1980;**41**:311–43.
32 Perlmutter AD. Management of intersexuality. In: Harrison JH, Walsh PC, Gittes RF *et al. Campbell's Urology*, Vol. 2, 4th edn. Philadelphia: WB Saunders, 1979:1535–48.
33 Husmann DA, Cain MP. Microphallus: eventual phallic size is dependent on the timing of androgen administration. *J Urol* 1994;**152**:734–9.
34 McMahon DR, Kramer SA, Tindall DJ, Husmann DA. Micropenis: does early treatment with testosterone do more harm than good? Abstract no. 30. *Abstract Volume*. AAP Annual Meeting, Section on Urology, Dallas, Texas, 1994: 79–80.
35 Wilson JD, Walsh PC. Disorders of sexual differentiation. In: Harrison JH, Walsh PC, Gittes RF *et al.*, eds. *Campbell's*

Urology, Vol. 2, 4th edn. Philadelphia: WB Saunders, 1979: 1484–1532.

36 Snyder HM, Retik AB, Baner SB, Colodny AH. Feminizing genitoplasty: a synthesis. *J Urol* 1983;**129**:1024–6.

37 Mollard P. Chirurgie des États Intersexués. In: *Précis d'Urologie de l'Enfant*. Paris: Masson, 1984:377.

38 Sotiropulos A, Morishima A, Homsy Y, Lattimer JK. Long-term assessment of genital reconstruction in female pseudoher-maphrodites. *J Urol* 1976;**115**:599–605.

39 Wakefield AR. Intersex and related problems. *Surg Clin North Am* 1967;**47**:505–12.

40 Passerini-Glazel G. A new technique for vaginal reconstruction in severely masculinized female pseudohermaphrodites. *J Urol* 1989;**142**:565–68.

41 David M, Mollard P, Daudet M, Lauras B. L'ambiguité sexuelle dans le pseudohermaphroditisme feminin. *Pediatrie* 1972;**27**:871–89.

42 Gross RE, Randolph J, Crigler JF. Clitorectomy for sexual abnormalities: indications and technique. *Surgery* 1966;**59**:300.

43 Lattimer JK. Relocation and recession of the enlarged clitoris with preservation of the glans: an alternative to amputation. *J Urol* 1961;**86**:113–16.

44 Spence HM, Allen TD. Genital reconstruction in the female with the adrenogenital syndrome. *Br J Urol* 1973;**45**:126–30.

45 Marberger H. Hunterian Lecture. Presented to the Royal College of Surgeons, London, 1975.

46 Kogan SJ, Smey P, Levitt SB. Subtunical total reduction clitoroplasty: a safe modification of existing techniques. *J Urol* 1983;**130**:746–8.

47 Donahoe PK, Hendren WH. Perineal reconstruction in ambiguous genitalia infants raised as females. *Ann Surg* 1984;**200**:363–72.

48 Fortunoff S, Lattimer JK, Edson M. Vaginoplasty technique for female pseudohermaphrodites. *Surg Gynecol Obstet* 1964;**188**:545–8.

49 Hendren WH, Crawford JD. Adrenogenital syndrome: the anatomy of the anomaly and its repair. Some new concepts. *J Ped Surg* 1969;**4**:49–59.

50 Hendren WH, Donahoe PK. Correction of congenital abnormalities of the vagina and perineum. *J Pediatr Surg* 1980;**15**:751–63.

51 Gonzales R, Fernandes ET. Single-stage feminization genito-plasty. *J Urol* 1990;**143**:776–8.

52 Frank RT. The formation of an artificial vagina without opera-tion. *Am J Obstet Gynecol* 1938;**35**:1053–6.

19   Prune Belly Syndrome

P.C.Cartwright and B.W.Snow

Introduction

The characteristic wrinkled and lax abdominal wall makes the prune belly syndrome (PBS) readily recognized in the newborn (Fig. 19.1). It also provides the syndrome with its commonly used name. The true diagnosis of PBS relies upon three hallmark findings:

1 partial lack of abdominal wall musculature;
2 bilateral undescended testes;
3 dilated upper urinary tracts and bladder.

The syndrome has been given other names including: Eagle–Barrett syndrome [1], triad syndrome [2], abdominal muscular deficiency syndrome [3], mesenchymal dysplasia syndrome [4] and urethral obstruction/malformation complex [5]. Whatever name is applied, the syndrome broadly affects the urogenital tract and may have associated abnormalities of many other organ systems.

The descriptive term 'prune belly syndrome' was first coined by Sir William Osler in 1901 to describe patients with these characteristics [6]. As early as 1839, however, Frohlich [7] had described an affected infant and in 1895 the essential elements of this syndrome had been delineated in the autopsy series of Parker [8]. Eagle and Barrett later assembled the elements of the syndrome in a more modern context [1].

PBS occurs in between 1:30 000 and 1:40 000 live births [9,10]. With cryptorchidism as an essential element defining this syndrome, only males can express the full syndrome. There may, however, be occasional females (3% of total cases) exhibiting the abdominal wall and urinary tract portions of the syndrome [11]. As well, some boys may exhibit the typical urinary tract malformation without the abdominal wall deficiency or cryptorchidism. The term 'pseudo-PBS' has been applied to such patients [12]. These patients with partial characteristics of PBS are, in general, less severely affected. Anomalies present in pseudo-PBS should be managed just as in a patient with the complete syndrome.

The degree of urinary tract involvement varies, thus PBS exists in a broad spectrum which ranges from stillbirth or early neonatal death secondary to pulmonary hypoplasia or renal failure to very minimal involvement in children having an excellent prognosis without medical intervention. Severity of involvement may be formally characterized as category I, II or III (Table 19.1).

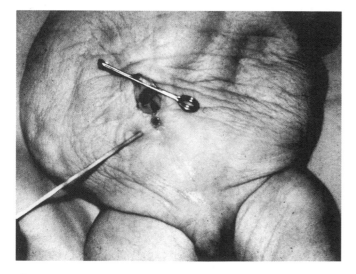

Fig. 19.1 Appearance of the abdominal wall in a newborn with PBS. The patient also has a patent urachus.

Table 19.1 Classification scheme for PBS. From [13] with permission.

Category classification	Distinguishing characteristics
I	Oligohydramnios, pulmonary hypoplasia or pneumothorax. May have urethral obstruction or patent urachus and club foot
II	Typical external features and uropathy of the full-blown syndrome but no immediate problem with survival. May have mild or unilateral renal dysplasia. May or may not develop urosepsis or gradual azotaemia
III	External features may be mild or incomplete. Uropathy is less severe and renal function stable

In the pre-antibiotic era, death from urosepsis or other complications occurred in as many as 50% of these patients in the first few years of life. Today, as many as 20% of newborns will die in the perinatal period as a consequence of pulmonary hypoplasia or other complications [14,15]. The increasing number of infants surviving with significant urinary tract dilatation has led to long-term management strategies which fall into two basic formats: early surgical reconstruction or sequential follow-up and observation with selective surgical intervention as indicated.

Embryogenesis

The fetal occurrences leading to the constellation of findings in PBS remain uncertain. Three lines of thought have emerged, each having strong and weak elements.
1 *Outlet obstruction*. This theory holds that transient urethral obstruction at a critical time in early fetal development could result in massive distension of the urinary tract with secondary underdevelopment of the abdominal wall and inguinal canals, poor descent of the testes and pulmonary hypoplasia (in severe cases) [5]. The obstruction could be due to delayed canalization of the junction between the anterior and posterior urethra or due to a 'functional valve' created by mucosal folding generated by a hypoplastic prostate. Recent fetal lamb projects support an obstructive aetiology but certainly other obstructive lesions do not cause PBS [16].
2 *Mesenchymal defect*. A noxious insult affecting thoracic somites in the first weeks of embryogenesis might result in: (i) poor development of the abdominal wall; (ii) disordered development of the ureteric and bladder wall with secondary dilatation; (iii) poor prostatic stroma; and (iv) a gubernaculum insensitive to hormonal stimulation [2]. This incorporates many features of PBS but fails to explain the male preponderance, and the better development that is usually seen of lateral abdominal muscles versus medial ones.
3 *Yolk sac abnormality*. Lateral fold overgrowth in the very young discoid embryo might retain abnormally large amounts of the yolk sac. This might explain the poorly developed abdominal wall and large bladder (retained allantois) in PBS, but not the ureteric dilatation or cryptorchidism [17].

Elements of prune belly syndrome

Abdominal wall

The typical PBS appearance results from deficient abdominal wall musculature. While affected infants have a similar appearance, the degree and location of abdominal wall involvement is highly variable. Musculature below the umbilicus is generally more severely affected than that above. Affected areas consist of skin, subcutaneous fat and a condensation of fibrous tissue with absent or sparse muscle fibres adherent to the peritoneum [18,19]. Segmental nerve and arterial supply to the abdominal wall appears normal [20,21]. The umbilicus is displaced superiorly as a result of contraction of the more normal upper rectus abdominis musculature. Intra-abdominal viscera can often be palpated easily through the abdominal wall and, in infants, intestinal peristalsis may be observed.

Problems that may arise from deficient abdominal wall musculature are:
1 difficulty going from supine to sitting position resulting in some infants rolling to use their arms for assistance [22];
2 chronic constipation [23];
3 poor cough with resultant trouble clearing pulmonary secretions and increased susceptibility to infection [24];
4 eventual poor body image [25,26].

Kidney

Hydronephrosis and renal dysplasia are the abnormalities typically associated with this syndrome. The range of severity is great, however, and some kidneys appear essentially normal [27]. Severely affected patients with urethral atresia or megaurethra and without a patent urachus will exhibit solid dysplastic kidneys as described by Potter and be stillborn [28]. In assessing autopsy specimens, Stephens commonly found both renal hypoplasia and dysplasia in PBS patients [17]. The degree of dysplasia may vary greatly even within the same patient, one side appearing normal while the other side is severely affected. Such abnormalities of renal embryogenesis are a major determinant of patient outcome. Stephens has theorized that dysplasia in PBS may be due to: (i) abnormal ureteric bud placement; (ii) deficiencies in the nephrogenic mesenchyme; (iii) abnormal acquisition of renal and ureteric vessels with resultant ischaemia; and (iv) early fetal bladder outlet obstruction [29].

The degree of hydronephrosis is, in general, less than the degree of hydroureter (Fig. 19.2). Calyces are often dilated and show narrow but unobstructed infundibula. Occasional true pelviureteric junction obstruction may be present [29]. Significant ureteric dilatation does not always predict poor renal parenchyma: it is, in fact, common to find more substantial renal parenchyma associated with the amount of ureteric dilatation than is expected in other diseases. There appears to be no correlation between the degree of abdominal wall deficit and the severity of renal abnormalities.

Ureter

A hallmark of PBS is hydroureter. The ureters are typically redundant, tortuous and dilated with the distal portion

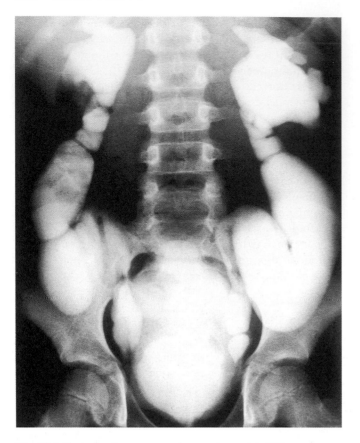

Fig. 19.2 Typical urinary system in a patient with PBS.

Bladder

The bladder in PBS is large, irregular and thick walled. A urachal pseudo-diverticulum is often present, but true trabeculations are unusual (Fig. 19.3). Examination of the thickened bladder wall reveals increased fibrocytes and collagen relative to smooth muscle [27]. Smooth muscle hypertrophy is generally not present but has been reported in fetuses with PBS [38]. Neurological innervation appears normal. Internally, the trigone is splayed with the ureteric orifices which are located laterally resulting in the high incidence of vesicoureteric reflux.

Urodynamic evaluation demonstrates normal voiding in some PBS patients despite grossly abnormal upper tracts and bladder [37,39]. Others will be noted to carry a significant post-void residual. Long-term follow-up of PBS patients in Toronto revealed three basic voiding patterns: (i) normal flow; (ii) prolonged, low-pressure voiding with slow flow; and (iii) intermittent flow. Patients with any of these patterns could demonstrate elevated residuals, and prior reduction cystoplasty appeared not to affect the post-void residual [40]. Those with elevated residual may have unbalanced voiding as described by Snyder *et al.* [41]. Patients must be clinically monitored for unbalanced bladder function manifested by incontinence, recurrent infections or worsening upper tracts. As a patient matures, various investigations have found that voiding patterns

more severely affected than the proximal portion [30,31] (see Fig. 19.2). True obstruction of these ureters is quite rare with only occasional cases of pelviureteric junction obstruction or a 'pleat valve' phenomenon in the distal ureter [32]. Vesicoureteric reflux occurs in over 70% of cases [33].

Histological evaluation of the ureter in PBS reveals architecture distinct from obstructed ureters of other causes. There is a marked decrease in smooth muscle with no definition of circular and longitudinal muscular layers [34]. Some portions of the ureter may be completely replaced by thick, hyaline substance that is largely acellular [35,36]. These changes occur along the entire ureter but are more pronounced distally [34,37]. In addition, the number of nerve plexuses appears to be decreased as does the number of thick and thin myofilaments [34,35].

With these histological abnormalities considered, it is not unexpected that, upon fluoroscopic evaluation, peristalsis is poor. The especially poor quality of the distal ureter makes it a poor choice for reconstructive procedures. The upper ureter, therefore, should be preserved if early diversion is required so that it will be available for future reconstructive efforts.

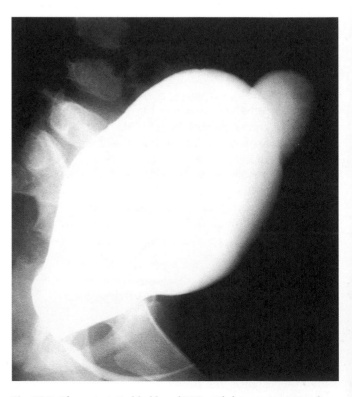

Fig. 19.3 Characteristic bladder of PBS with large capacity and urachal pseudodiverticulum.

may both improve [42] or worsen [13] making long-term follow-up necessary.

Prostate

Another radiographic hallmark of PBS is the appearance of the prostatic urethra. This is often roughly triangular with a widely separated bladder neck tapering at the level of the urogenital diaphragm, at which point the urethral calibre usually appears normal (Fig. 19.4). This may initially appear similar to the prostatic urethra in posterior urethral valve, but has more of a tapered funnel appearance rather than the abrupt calibre change of a valve. A small utricle is evident in some patients. There is uniform lack of development of the epithelial components of the prostate in PBS [37,43]. This prostatic hypoplasia contributes to later infertility [44].

Stephens [17] previously noted anterior folding of the prostatic urethral mucosa possibly working as a valve against outflow in some PBS patients. He termed this a type

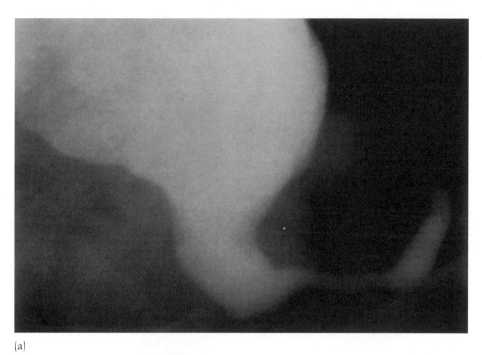

(a)

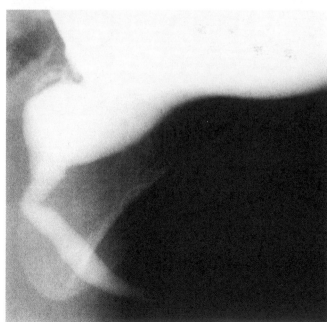

(b)

Fig. 19.4 The usual prostatic urethral dilatation in two patients with PBS.

IV posterior urethral valve and recommended an incision at the 12 o'clock position to relieve any symptoms associated with this. It is only occasionally a problem clinically.

Urethra

The anterior urethra in PBS patients is usually normal. There are, however, a number of reported anomalies of urethral development. Urethral atresia is occasionally present and is lethal unless associated with a patent urachus. A newborn autopsy series by Wigger and Blanc [27] showed seven out of 14 PBS patients had urethral atresia or severe stenosis. In surviving patients, a patent but diffusely narrowed urethra may be progressively dilated to a functional size as reported by Passerini-Glazel et al. [45].

Megaurethra has been associated with PBS [46,47] (Fig. 19.5). Patients with the fusiform variant of megaurethra suffer a high mortality rate, whereas those with scaphoid megaurethra fare better. Kroovand has suggested that minor urethral abnormalities occur in a relatively high percentage of PBS patients [48]. There is also an association of dorsal penile chordee with PBS.

Testis

Bilateral cryptorchidism is one of the three major findings of PBS. The testes are intra-abdominal and generally just inside the internal inguinal ring. Underdevelopment of the inguinal canal and gubernaculum may contribute to testicular non-descent in these patients [49]. As with all undescended testes, abnormalities of the epididymis are commonly recognized.

Reports concerning testicular histology have been varied. Nunn and Stephens found the testicular germinal elements of the fetus and newborn with PBS to be equivalent to normal [2]. Conversely, Orvis et al. reported Leydig cell hyperplasia and decreased spermatogonia counts [50]. Testes remaining in the abdomen for many years demonstrate findings of greatly diminished spermatogenesis, as in most undescended testes [51]. Woodhouse and Snyder found frequent azoospermia in adult PBS patients and testis biopsy results comparable to prolonged undescent of the testes in an otherwise normal man [52]. No man with PBS has fathered a child, although it is unknown if early orchiopexy might affect this.

Rare reports in the literature document the development of tumours in undescended testes in patients with PBS, but data are insufficient to compare the incidence versus standard undescended testes [53,54].

Orthopaedic anomalies

Musculoskeletal anomalies are the most common non-urogenital anomalies associated with PBS, affecting 50% of patients [55,56]. Many of the anomalies encountered are deformations caused by the limited intrauterine space associated with oligohydramnios. The milder manifestations of this include lateral knee and elbow dimpling and club foot (26%) (Fig. 19.6). More severe deformities such as arthrogryposis, lower limb hypoplasia, torticollis and congenital hip dislocation are also associated with the syndrome. Interestingly, some severe limb deformities in PBS have been theorized to occur secondary to vascular insult relating to compression of the external iliac artery by the enormously distended bladder and subsequent poor limb development [57]. Other anomalies represent true malformations and include pectus excavatum, pectus carinatum, hip dysplasia and various vertebral defects.

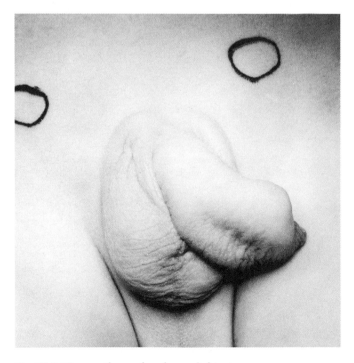

Fig. 19.5 Megaurethra and undescended testes.

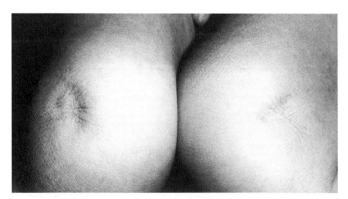

Fig. 19.6 Knee dimples commonly seen in patients with PBS.

Cardiac anomalies

Cardiac defects have been reported in 10% of patients with PBS. These include atrial and ventricular septal defects, tetralogy of Fallot and patent ductus arteriosus [58]. Urological abnormalities are seldom a pressing matter in the newborn and, as such, management of cardiac anomalies may dictate initial care of these patients.

Pulmonary anomalies

Severely affected patients with PBS may demonstrate pulmonary hypoplasia incompatible with life. These patients display splayed ribs, pectus deformities and weakened abdominal musculature, all of which impair respiratory activities. A number of other respiratory abnormalities have been observed including pneumothorax [59]. Recently, evaluation of 11 asymptomatic older boys with PBS was reported; nine had evidence of gas trapping and six demonstrated restrictive lung disease [60]. Such underlying pulmonary problems may be critically important during an anaesthetic or in the postoperative period.

Gastrointestinal anomalies

Intestinal malrotation is present in a significant number of PBS patients secondary to abnormal mesenteric attachments [61]. There also appears to be an increased incidence of distal bowel atresia or stenosis and persistent cloaca in PBS patients [62].

Management

Prenatal management

As the use of obstetric ultrasound has increased, larger numbers of patients with hydronephrosis are recognized, including those with PBS. Some or all of the typical features of PBS, including hydronephrosis, hydroureter, distended thick-walled bladder and lax abdominal wall, may be demonstrated with ultrasound [63–65].

Both antenatal intervention for vesicoamniotic shunting or elective termination of pregnancy have been suggested in fetuses demonstrating characteristics of PBS. Neither of these is generally warranted. It must be remembered that the diagnostic accuracy of ultrasound for PBS is only modest, being somewhere between 30 and 85% [66]. Thus, PBS may be confused sonographically with other conditions such as vesicoureteric reflux, posterior urethral valves or other causes of hydronephrosis. Even if PBS were correctly diagnosed *in utero*, the majority of these patients have dilated but unobstructed urinary tracts and will suffer minimal morbidity. Even in patients with clear obstruc-

tion, such as posterior valves, intervention is of unproven benefit. Thus, intervention or termination must be considered very cautiously. Occasionally, a massively distended fetal bladder will cause dystocia and sonographically guided bladder aspiration may be required [67].

Newborn management

Because of the typical abdominal wall laxity, the diagnosis of PBS is usually obvious at birth. Although the urologist is often notified immediately, there is rarely any urological emergency involved. Pulmonary considerations are usually foremost in the patient's management with the potential for respiratory failure due to pulmonary hypoplasia, pneumothorax or pneumomediastinum. A chest film shortly after birth is advisable. The presence of severe pulmonary hypoplasia, most commonly associated with antenatal oligohydramnios, may lead to progressive anoxia and early death.

After initial pulmonary assessment, cardiac evaluation is undertaken. Sonographic cardiac imaging is generally recommended. Finally, to complete the assessment, orthopaedic consultation should be sought to assess musculoskeletal development.

Initial urological evaluation involves sonography to assess renal length, renal parenchymal development and the degree of hydronephrosis and hydroureter present. Kidneys showing significant dysplasia or cystic change alert the clinician to follow closely for evidence of worsening renal function. Serum creatinine levels in the first 2 or 3 days of life reflects only maternal creatinine levels, but beyond this will reveal the newborn's renal function. Further urological evaluation will require urethral catheterization. This must always be approached cautiously since the introduction of bacteria into the bladder may result in clinically significant urinary infection which is difficult to clear. If the newborn is doing well clinically, we generally defer voiding cystourethrogram (VCU) and diuretic renogram until 2–4 weeks of age. The baby is placed on a prophylactic antibiotic and observed.

The diuretic renogram is achieved with a catheter in place. At the same visit, with only a single catheterization, the VCU is performed and the catheter is removed. A therapeutic dose of antibiotic is administered prior to, and following, this radiographic evaluation.

As discussed previously, PBS demonstrates a wide spectrum of involvement and is broadly categorized in Table 19.1. Category I patients are the most severely affected with pronounced renal dysplasia, pulmonary hypoplasia, or both. They may be stillborn with characteristic Potter facies or die shortly after birth from pulmonary or renal failure. Category II patients are intermediate in severity, showing mild to modest renal insufficiency but no pulmonary difficulties. These patients require the closest scrutiny to assure appropriate management in the first few years of life. Category III patients are mildly involved or show only partial features of the syndrome. They rarely require early intervention, but as with all PBS patients, they need long-term surveillance.

Long-term management

Overview

Four major approaches to the long-term management of the patient with PBS have emerged over the past few decades.

1 Early permanent urinary tract diversion.

2 Early high diversion (pyelostomy) with later urinary tract construction [20].

3 Complete urinary tract reconstruction as a newborn or young infant [29,68–70].

4 Observation with selective surgical intervention [33,71,72].

While some patients with PBS are so severely affected that early mortality is inevitable, others have such minor involvement that no urologist would see a need for urinary tract reconstruction. A large group of patients, however, falls in between, and there is ongoing controversy regarding the management of these patients.

Our approach is that of observation with selective surgical intervention. The urinary tract in these patients is, with rare exception, not obstructed. The significant dilatation is caused by deficient, smooth muscle in the renal pelvis, ureter and bladder. While these systems may become very dilated, there is often no elevation in storage pressures. While the gross anatomical abnormality is tempting to reconstruct, one must weigh this against the possibility of hastening a decrease in renal function due to an adverse surgical result or simply due to urinary tract infections from manipulation perioperatively. Unless a clear indication for surgical intervention, such as increasing creatinine or urinary tract infections, occurs we observe and sequentially follow-up these patients.

Others have advocated complete, extensive reconstruction of the urinary tract in the newborn patient [29,68,69]. This involves excision of the lower ureters, tapered reimplantation of the remaining upper ureter into the bladder, reduction cystoplasty and possibly concomitant orchiopexies and abdominal wall reconstruction (Fig. 19.7). Proponents of early reconstruction have more recently pushed their time of surgery back to possibly 6 or 12 months of age due to the high risk of pulmonary complications associated with newborn surgery in PBS patients [70]. In good outcomes, the urinary tract will have a less dilated appearance. Total early reconstruction attracts surgeons since it may reduce urinary stasis and resolve vesicoureteric reflux. Each of these problems may

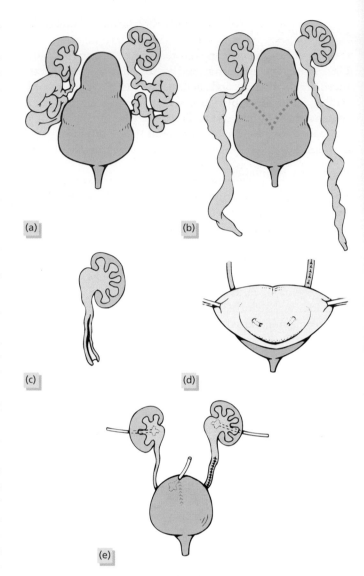

Fig. 19.7 Extensive urinary tract reconstruction: (a) initial appearance; (b) ureteric excision and reduction cystoplasty; (c, d) tapered ureteric reimplantation; (e) closure. (Reproduced from [13] with permission.)

cause declining renal function when associated with urinary tract infection. Woodard states in his experience that most group II patients managed non-operatively have an eventual indication for surgery such as urinary tract infection, increasing creatinine or increasing dilatation of the urinary tract [70]. Others have had the opposite experience with a majority of patients remaining free of infection with stable renal function [24]. Part of the dichotomy of management opinion is rooted in such differences in clinical experience.

Upper tracts

A minority of infants with PBS exhibit early problems with

rising creatinine levels or persistent urinary infection. Either of these may require prompt urinary diversion. In years past, diversion was commonly accomplished as an upper loop ureterostomy or pyelostomy. This may be required in particular, unusual cases but is deleterious and may render the upper ureter difficult to use in later reconstruction. An easier approach to early diversion, if required, is cutaneous vesicostomy. This is technically simple and allows for complete bladder decompression and, in the majority of cases, is adequate diversion.

The majority of PBS patients reflux into their massively dilated ureters (Fig. 19.8). In a stable, older patient, the need for ureteric reimplantation has been argued. While some believe that these ureters should be imbricated or tapered and reimplanted, we have not chosen this management approach unless recurring urinary infections are present. The abnormal cellular composition of these ureters results in poor peristalsis and makes the idea of tapering and reimplantation concerning. As well, the large dilated ureters may have some role in dissipation of voiding pressure and maintaining a 'balanced' system. Thus, a dilated but pressure-balanced ureteric system may be converted into an obstructed one. For patients who are infection free on prophylactic antibiotics, reports have

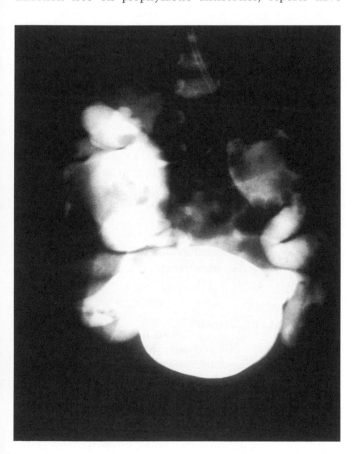

Fig. 19.8 Reflux into very tortuous and dilated ureters in a newborn with PBS.

documented preservation of renal function. In cases where reimplantation is required, the lower ureter is discarded, and the upper ureter is tailored and reimplanted with or without a psoas hitch.

Clinical awareness is required to diagnose the rare PBS patient with true ureteric obstruction which may occur at the pelviureteric or ureterovesical junctions. These patients need diagnostic evaluation using frusemide renography, renal scan with Lasix washout, or possibly a Whitaker antegrade infusion test. If obstruction is truly suspected, surgical repair is in order.

Bladder and urethra

As part of early extensive reconstruction, some surgeons have performed routine reduction cystoplasty because of the large bladder capacity and large pseudo-diverticulum often noted in these patients. Others have performed this as an isolated procedure in older children to improve bladder dynamics. Perlmutter [73] and Hanna [74] reported improved voiding in a small number of patients undergoing reduction cystoplasty. A similar idea of plicating rather than excising the dome of the bladder is reported by Williams and Parker [71]. Conversely, Duckett reported no improvement with this procedure [24]. Recently, Kinahan et al. from Toronto reported urodynamic evaluation of previously treated PBS patients and found no difference in voiding pattern or residual urine in those who had undergone previous reduction cystoplasty versus those who had not [40]. They concluded that there is no role for reduction cystoplasty in PBS.

Older patients with PBS may demonstrate elevated residuals after voiding. Such patients may have a type IV valve as described by Stephens. Cukier reported using a hot knife to incise the membranous urethra at the 12 o'clock position in these patients [75]. Snow and Duckett, as well, reported distinct voiding improvement following this procedure [24]. They noticed distinctly improved voiding and reduced residuals in the majority.

Urethral atresia associated with PBS is a fatal anomaly unless associated with a patent urachus to allow egress of urine. Those patients surviving may require a progressive urethral dilatation, as reported by Passerini-Glazel, in which sequentially larger catheters are used to dilate the urethral channel slowly to a functional size [45]. If this is not successful, standard urethroplasty techniques may be necessary. Megaurethra may also be associated with PBS and requires reconstruction of the dilated urethral segment [76].

Orchiopexy

The undescended testes of PBS must be addressed for reasons including: (i) maximizing all possible spermatogenesis; (ii) facilitating future examination of the testes; (iii) minimizing the risk of testicular loss from torsion; and (iv) minimizing the psychological impact of an empty scrotum. Though these testes function well hormonally, paternity is undocumented in PBS.

Testes in PBS are almost always in an intra-abdominal location on a broad mesorchium. The associated abdominal wall problem may result in an underdeveloped inguinal canal. Transinguinal orchiopexy in these patients is rarely feasible. Transabdominal orchiopexy has been reported to be highly successful when done in the first 6 months of life [77]. Others have found success common up to 2 years of age with the same transabdominal approach and extensive retroperitoneal mobilization but with preservation of the internal spermatic vessels [15]. These authors reported the ability to perform standard orchiopexy in 82% of patients less than 2 years old and in only 50% of those more than 2 years old. Our current approach is to perform orchiopexy at 12–18 months of age or sooner if other operative intervention is required.

Alternatives to standard orchiopexy in PBS patients include Fowler–Stephens orchiopexy, staged Fowler–Stephens orchiopexy and microvascular transplantation. Each has been applied to patients with PBS. Fowler–Stephens orchiopexy has resulted in approximately 75% successful placement of the testis into the scrotum [78]. Delayed performance of the Fowler–Stephens procedure following an initial ligation of the internal spermatic vessels offers a chance for the enhancement of collateral bloodflow to the testicle and a potentially a higher success rate [79]. Microvascular autotransplantation of the testicle has been applied successfully to patients with PBS [80]. Each procedure has its place in individualized management of these boys.

Abdominoplasty

Although laxity of the abdominal wall tends to improve over time, and wrinkling becomes less noticeable, the deformity remains significant and abdominoplasty is recommended in these patients. This results in a much improved truncal physique and offers an improved body image, something of enormous significance during childhood development. It also allows these patients to participate more freely in sports, wear normal trousers and not require an elastic abdominal binder. In addition, there is the potential for improvement of constipation and the ability to cough more effectively. Abdominoplasty is best performed in the first few years of life and may be performed along with urinary tract reconstruction or orchiopexies.

Randolph and associates in 1981 reported a long, transverse, smile-shaped lower abdominal incision as the optimal approach for reconstructing the PBS [25,81]. In their assessment, this excised the most abnormal segments of the abdominal wall while preserving neurological innervation [20]. The technique involves the excision of skin, abdominal musculature, fascia and peritoneum (Fig. 19.9). One later advantage is that the resulting scar is transverse and low enough to be covered by trousers or shorts.

Alternatively, a midline approach to reconstruction may be taken. In 1986, Ehrlich and colleagues reported a midline approach with vertical plication of the fascia and obtained favourable results in six patients [25]. More recently, the Monfort technique was described in which there is preservation of the umbilicus and a midline strip of abdominal wall fascia and muscle is maintained on the inferior and superior epigastric arteries [82,83]. Excess skin and fat are excised, and the lateral fascia is advanced from one side to the other over the midline fascial plate. This results in excellent cosmesis and is especially appropriate in the boy whose abdominal wall laxity is most pronounced laterally.

Atypical presentation

By definition, PBS involves the triad of abdominal musculature deficiency, dilated urinary tract and cryptorchidism. Some patients demonstrate incomplete PBS (pseudo-PBS). The majority of these patients show typical urinary tract features with either non-involved or minimally involved abdominal wall musculature or only a single undescended testis. Management of the urinary tract and undescended testes in these patients is identical to those with complete PBS.

Females have been reported with the typical abdominal wall and urinary tract findings [11]. A more recent series from Reinberg et al. found a high association of genital and anal anomalies in these patients [84]. Once again, the urinary tract is managed as in the standard patient with PBS.

Occasional patients will escape early diagnosis and come only to medical attention as adults. These patients may present with renal insufficiency, urinary infection or infertility [42,85,86].

Anaesthetic considerations

The patient with PBS presents anaesthetic and perioperative challenges. The deficient abdominal wall musculature appears to inhibit normal cough and predisposes to postoperative atelectasis and pneumonia. Henderson et al. [87] reported on 36 PBS patients undergoing 133 anaesthetic procedures. Eight pulmonary infections resulted which all responded to antibiotics and chest physiotherapy. They recommend postoperative chest physiotherapy in all PBS patients undergoing surgery. Deaths have been reported

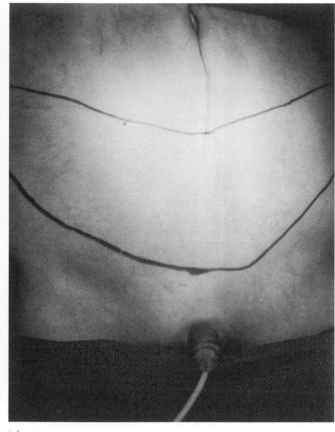

(a)

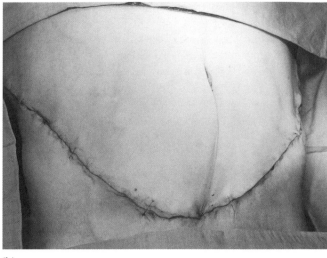

(b)

Fig. 19.9 (a) Before and (b) after abdominoplasty as described by Randolph [20,81].

secondary to pulmonary complications following newborn reconstruction [70]. In our experience, such problems have been most pronounced with abdominoplasty and may not be fully manifest until several days after surgery.

Renal transplantation

Progressive renal deterioration in PBS may result from intrinsic renal dysplasia or may be the result of obstruction or infection [88]. Renal transplantation may be required in some patients [88,89]. Prior to transplantation, these patients have generally undergone bilateral nephroureterectomy. Assessment of the bladder with VCU and urodynamics prior to considering transplantation is mandatory. A recent series reported eight patients with PBS who underwent renal transplantation [90]. The graft survival, quality of graft function and rate of death was no different than age-matched controls undergoing transplant with other disease entities.

Clinical experience

A review of reported clinical experience over the past decade gives some perspective on the management of patients with PBS.

Woodhouse and associates reported the cumulative experience with PBS at Great Ormand Street Hospital in 1982 [91]. Of 47 patients, there were five neonatal deaths, 13 patients undergoing high ureteral diversion relatively early for urinary tract infection or renal insufficiency, and 29 patients having no early intervention. In the patients with early high diversion, only a minority of later reconstructions (3/10) yielded a good result. The authors were impressed that the 29 patients with no early intervention did well overall, although 60% eventually underwent ureteric incision to relieve poor bladder emptying.

In 1986, Geary *et al.* in Toronto published their experience with 25 patients at the Sick Children's Hospital, although the status of urinary tract surgical intervention was not included [23]. There were three neonatal deaths and a high number of patients (75%) suffered significant morbidity from pulmonary, gastrointestinal and orthopaedic malformations. Long term, there was concern with diminished growth in one-third of the patients which was unrelated to their serum creatinine levels.

The experience at Baby's Hospital, New York City, was reported by Burbige and co-authors in 1987 [14]. Of 50 children with PBS, there was a 32% mortality rate. Of the survivors, roughly equal numbers underwent supravesical diversion with later reconstruction, early total reconstruction or initial observation. The groups did similarly in terms of eventual serum creatinine levels, and the group concluded that early reconstruction was as good as early diversion followed by later reconstruction, and that clinical judgement was required to individualize the management of each patient appropriately.

In 1989, Fallat and colleagues reported the experience at the Children's National Hospital in Washington, DC [15]. Of 20 patients, 15 underwent early total reconstruction. Orchiopexies and abdominoplasties went well while urinary tract reconstruction resulted in persistent reflux in 30% and ureteric obstruction in 40%.

In 1990, Adams and Hendren from Boston Children's Hospital reported 10% ureteric obstruction following ureteric reimplantation in PBS patients undergoing primary reconstruction and 40% in cases referred to them secondarily [92].

The Children's Hospital of Philadelphia data were reviewed by Snow and Duckett in 1991 [24]. Of 53 patients, there were four neonatal deaths and two later deaths secondary to renal failure. Twelve patients had been initially diverted and managed elsewhere, and 11 of them underwent subsequent undiversion. Of 21 patients managed completely at the Children's Hospital of Philadelphia, initial observation was pursued with nine eventually requiring vesicostomy, three requiring pyeloplasty and five undergoing ureteral reconstruction and reimplantation. Of the full group, nine have eventually required endoscopic ureteric incision. Eight of the nine showed improved voiding, lowered residuals and no incontinence following this procedure.

Conclusion

The PBS continues to be fascinating in the spectrum of manifestations seen. While immediate perinatal survival may be based on adequately developed lungs and kidneys, the long-term well being of the vast majority of PBS patients is largely dependent upon appropriate urological care. Of paramount importance is assuring no obstruction, adequate drainage and minimal infections of the urinary tract. The available data and our own clinical experience have led us to an approach of observation and follow-up with selective surgical intervention on an individual basis.

References

1 Eagle JF, Barrett GS. Congenital deficiency of abdominal musculature with associated genitourinary abnormalities. A syndrome: report of 9 cases. *Pediatrics* 1950;**6**:721–36.
2 Nunn IN, Stephens FD. The triad syndrome: a composite anomaly of the abdominal wall, urinary system and testes. *J Urol* 1961;**86**:782–94.
3 Pagon RA, Smith DW, Shepard TH. Urethral obstruction malformation complex: a cause of abdominal muscle deficiency and the 'prune belly.' *J Pediatr* 1979;**94**:900–6.
4 Welch K, Kearney GP. Abdominal musculature deficiency syndrome: prune belly. *J Urol* 1974;**111**:693–700.
5 Ives EJ. The abdominal muscle deficiency triad syndrome—experience with ten cases. *Birth Defects* 1974;**10**:127–37.
6 Osler WO. Absence of the abdominal muscles, with distended and hypertrophied urinary bladder. *Bull Johns Hopkins Hosp* 1901;**12**:331–2.
7 Frohlich F. Der Mangel der Muskeln, insbesondere der Seitenbauch muskeln. Dissertation, Wurzburg, Germany, 1839.
8 Parker RW. Case of an infant in whom some of the abdominal muscles were absent. *Trans Clin Soc Lond* 1895;**28**:201.
9 Garlinger P, Ott J. Prune belly syndrome: possible genetic implications. *Birth Defects* 1974;**10**:173–80.
10 Greskovich FJ, Hyberg LM. The prune belly syndrome: a review of its etiology, defects, treatment and prognosis. *J Urol* 1988;**140**:707–12.
11 Rabinowitz R, Schillinger JF. Prune belly syndrome in the female subject. *J Urol* 1977;**115**:454–6.
12 Duckett JW Jr. The prune belly syndrome. In: Kelalis PP, King LR, Belman AB, eds. *Clinical Pediatric Urology*. Philadelphia: WB Saunders, 1976:615–35.
13 Williams DI. Prune-belly syndrome. In: Harrison JH, Gittes RF, Perlmutter AD *et al.*, eds. *Campbell's Urology*, 4th edn. Philadelphia: WB Saunders, 1979:1743–55.
14 Burbige KA, Amodio J, Berdon WE *et al.* Prune belly syndrome: 35 years of experience. *J Urol* 1987;**137**:86–90.
15 Fallat MC, Skoog SJ, Belman AB *et al.* The prune belly syndrome: a comprehensive approach to management. *J Urol* 1989;**142**:802–5.
16 Gonzalez R, Reinberg Y, Burke B *et al.* Early bladder outlet obstruction in fetal lambs induces renal dysplasia and the prune-belly syndrome. *J Pediatr Surg* 1990;**25**(3):342–5.
17 Stephens FD. Triad (prune belly) syndrome. In: Stephens FD. *Congenital Malformations of the Urinary Tract*. New York: Praeger, 1983:485–511.
18 Afifi AK, Rebeiz JM, Adonia SJ *et al.* The myopathy of the prune belly syndrome. *J Neurol Sci* 1972;**15**:153–65.
19 Mininberg DT, Montoy F, Okada K *et al.* Subcellular muscle studies in the prune belly syndrome. *J Urol* 1973;**109**:524–6.
20 Randolph JG. Total surgical reconstruction for patients with abdominal muscular deficiency (prune belly) syndrome. *J Pediatr Surg* 1977;**12**:1033–43.
21 Stephens FD. *Congenital Malformations of the Urinary Tract*. New York: Praeger, 1983.
22 Duckett JW Jr. Prune belly syndrome. In: Welch KJ, Randolph JG, Ravith MM *et al.*, eds. *Pediatric Surgery*. Chicago: Year Book Medical, 1986:1193–203.
23 Geary DF, MacLusky IB, Churchill BM *et al.* A broader spectrum of abnormalities in the prune belly syndrome. *J Urol* 1986;**135**:324–6.
24 Snow BW, Duckett, JW. Prune belly syndrome. In: Gillenwater JY, Grayhack JT, Howards SS, Duckett JW eds. *Adult and Pediatric Urology*, Vol 2, 2nd edn. St Louis: Mosby Year Book, 1991:1921–38.
25 Ehrlich RM, Lesavoy MA, Fine RN. Total abdominal wall reconstruction in the prune belly syndrome. *J Urol* 1986; **136**:282–5.
26 Randolph JG, Cavett C, Eng G. Surgical correction and

rehabilitation for children with 'prune-belly' syndrome. *Ann Surg* 1981;**193**:757–62.

27 Wigger JH, Blanc WA. The prune belly syndrome. *Pathol Annu* 1977;**12**:17–39.

28 Potter EL. Abnormal development of the kidney. In Potter EL (ed). *Normal and Abnormal Development of the Kidney*. Chicago: Year Book Medical, 1972:154–220.

29 Woodard JR, Parrott TS. Reconstruction of the urinary tract in prune belly uropathy. *J Urol* 1978;**119**:824–30.

30 Berdon WE, Baker DH, Wigger HJ *et al*. The radiologic and pathologic spectrum of the prune belly syndrome. *Radiol Clin North Am* 1977;**25**:83–92.

31 Grossman H, Winchester PH, Waldbaum RS. Syndrome of congenital deficiency of abdominal wall musculature and associated genitourinary anomalies. *Prog Pediatr Radiol* 1970;**3**:327–43.

32 Maizels M, Stephens FD. Valves of the ureter as a cause of primary obstruction of the ureter: anatomic, embryologic and clinical aspects. *J Urol* 1980;**123**:742–7.

33 Duckett JW. The prune-belly syndrome. In: Kelalis PP, King LR, Belman AB eds. *Clinical Pediatric Urology*. Philadelphia: WB Saunders, 1976:615–35.

34 Palmer JM, Tesluk H. Ureteral pathology in the prune belly syndrome. *J Urol* 1974;**111**:701–7.

35 Hanna MK, Jeffs RD, Sturgess JM *et al*. Ureteral structure and ultrastructure: III. The congenitally dilated ureter (megaureter). *J Urol* 1977;**117**:24–7.

36 Ehrlich RM, Brown WJ. Ultrastructural anatomic observations of the ureter in the prune belly syndrome. *Birth Defects* 1977;**13**:101–3.

37 Nunn IN, Stephens FD. The triad syndrome: a composite anomaly of the abdominal wall, urinary system and testes. *J Urol* 1961;**86**:782–94.

38 Workman SJ, Kogan BA. Fetal bladder histology in posterior urethral valves and the prune belly syndrome. *J Urol* 1990;**144**:337–9.

39 Williams DI, Burkholder GV. The prune belly syndrome. *J Urol* 1967;**98**:244–51.

40 Kinahan TJ, Churchill BM, McLorie GA *et al*. The efficiency of bladder emptying in the prune belly syndrome. *J Urol* 1992;**148**:600–3.

41 Snyder HM, Harrison NW, Whitfield HM *et al*. Urodynamics in the prune belly syndrome. *Br J Urol* 1976;**48**:663–70.

42 Lee SM. Prune-belly syndrome in a 54 year old man. *J Am Med Assoc* 1977;**237**:2216–17.

43 DeKlerk DP, Scott WW. Prostatic maldevelopment in the prune belly syndrome: a defect in prostatic stromal epithelial interaction. *J Urol* 1978;**120**:341–4.

44 Hinman F. Alternatives to orchiopexy. *J Urol* 1980;**123**:548–51.

45 Passerini-Glazel G, Araguna F, Chiozza L *et al*. The PADUA (progressive augmentation by dilating the urethral anterior) procedure for the treatment of severe urethral hypoplasia. *J Urol* 1988;**140**:1247–9.

46 Sellers BB Jr, McNeal R, Smith RV *et al*. Congenital megalourethra associated with prune belly syndrome. *J Urol* 1976;**116**:814–15.

47 Shrom SH, Cromie WJ, Duckett JW. Megalourethra. *Urology* 1981;**17**:152–6.

48 Kroovand RL, Al-Ansari RM, Perlmutter AD. Urethral and genital malformations in prune belly syndrome. *J Urol* 1982;**127**:94–6.

49 Hadziselimovic F. *Cryptorchidism: Management and Implications*. New York: Springer Verlag, 1983.

50 Orvis BR, Bottles K, Kogan BA. Testicular histology in fetuses with prune belly syndrome and posterior urethral valves. *J Urol* 1988;**139**:335–7.

51 Uehling DT, Zadina SP, Gilbert E. Testicular histology in triad syndrome. *Urology* 1984;**23**:364–6.

52 Woodhouse CRJ, Snyder HM III. Testicular and sexual function in adults with prune belly syndrome. *J Urol* 1985;**133**:607–9.

53 Woodard JR, Trulock TS. Prune belly syndrome. In: Walsh PC, Retik AB, Stamey TA, Vaughn ED, eds. *Campbell's Urology*, 5th edn. Philadelphia: WB Saunders, 1986:2159–67.

54 Parra RO, Cummings JM, Palmer DC. Testicular seminoma in a long-term survivor of the prune belly syndrome. *Eur Urol* 1991;**19**:79–80.

55 Tuch BA, Smith TK. Prune belly syndrome: a report of twelve cases and review of the literature. *J Bone Joint Surg* [Am] 1978;**60**:109–11.

56 Loder RT, Guiboux JP, Bloom DA *et al*. Musculoskeletal aspects of prune-belly syndrome: description and pathogenesis. *Am J Dis Child* 1992;**146**:1224–9.

57 Perez-Aytes A, Graham JM, Hersh JH *et al*. Urethral obstruction sequence and lower limb deficiency: evidence for the vascular disruption hypothesis. *J Pediatr* 1993;**123**(3): 398–405.

58 Adebonojo FO. Dysplasia of the abdominal musculature with multiple congenital anomalies; prune belly or triad syndrome. *J Natl Med Assoc* 1973;**65**:327–33.

59 Weber ML, Rivard G, Perreault G. Prune belly syndrome associated with congenital cystic adenomatoid malformation of the lung. *Am J Dis Child* 1978;**132**:316–17.

60 Crompton CH, MacLusky IB, Geary DF. Respiratory function in the prune-belly syndrome. *Arch Dis Child* 1993;**68**:505–6.

61 Silverman FM, Huang N. Congenital absence of the abdominal muscle associated with malformation of the genitourinary and alimentary tracts: report of cases of review of literature. *Am J Dis Child* 1950;**80**:91–124.

62 Wright JR, Barth RF, Neff JC *et al*. Gastrointestinal malformations associated with prune belly syndrome: three cases and a review of the literature. *Pediatr Pathol* 1986;**5**: 421–48.

63 Bovicelli L, Rizzo N, Orsini LF *et al*. Prenatal diagnosis of the prune-belly syndrome. *Clin Genet* 1980;**18**:79–82.

64 Christopher CR, Spinelli A, Severt D. Ultrasonic diagnosis of prune-belly syndrome. *Obstet Gynecol* 1982;**59**:391.

65 Fisk NM, Dhillon HK, Ellis CE *et al*. Antenatal diagnosis of megalourethra in a fetus with the prune belly syndrome. *J Clin Ultrasound* 1990;**18**:124–8.

66 Elder JS. Intrauterine intervention for obstructive uropathy. *Kidney* 1990;**22**:19–24.

67 Gadziala NA, Kavade CY, Doherty FJ *et al*. Intrauterine decompression of megalocystis during the second trimester of pregnancy. *Am J Obstet Gynecol* 1982;**144**:355–6.

68 Hendren WH. Restoration of function in the severely decompensated ureter. In: Johnson JH, Scholtmeijer RJ, eds. *Problems in Paediatric Urology*. Amsterdam: Excerpta Medica, 1972:1–56.

69 Jeffs RD, Comisarow RH, Hanna MK. The early assessment for individualized treatment in the prune belly syndrome. *Birth Defects* 1977;**13**:97–9.

70 Woodard JR, Zucker I. Current management of the dilated

urinary tract in prune belly syndrome. *Urol Clin North Am* 1990;**17**:407–18.

71 Williams DI, Parker RM. The role of surgery in the prune belly syndrome. In: Johnston JH, Goodwin WF, eds. *Reviews of Paediatric Urology*. Amsterdam: Excerpta Medica, 1974: 315–31.

72 Woodhouse CR, Kellett MJ, Williams DI. Minimal surgical interference in prune belly syndrome. *Br J Urol* 1979;**57**:475.

73 Perlmutter AD. Reduction cystoplasty in prune belly syndrome. *J Urol* 1976;**116**:356–62.

74 Hanna MD. New concept in bladder remodeling. *Urology* 1982;**19**:6–12.

75 Cukier J. Resection of the urethra in the prune belly syndrome. *Birth Defects* 1977;**13**:95–6.

76 Appel RA, Kaplan GW, Brock WA *et al.* Megalourethra. *J Urol* 1986;**135**:747–51.

77 Woodard JR, Parrott TS. Orchiopexy in the prune belly syndrome. *Br J Urol* 1978;**50**:348–51.

78 Gibbons MD, Cromie WJ, Duckett JW. Management of the abdominal undescended testicle. *J Urol* 1979;**122**:76–9.

79 Ransley PG, Vordermark JS, Caldamone AA *et al.* Preliminary ligation of the gonadal vessels prior to orchidopexy for the intraabdominal testicle: a staged Fowler–Stephens procedure. *World J Urol* 1984;**2**:266–8.

80 Wacksman J, Dinner M, Staffon RA. Technique of testicular autotransplantation using a microvascular anastomosis. *Surg Gynecol Obstet* 1980;**150**:399–400.

81 Randolph JG, Cavett C, Eng G. Abdominal wall reconstruction in the prune belly syndrome. *J Pediatr Surg* 1981;**16**:960–4.

82 Monfort G, Guys JM, Bocciardi A *et al.* A novel technique for reconstruction of the abdominal wall in the prune belly syndrome. *J Urol* 1991;**146**:639–40.

83 Parrott TS, Woodard JR. The Monfort operation for abdominal wall reconstruction in the prune belly syndrome. *J Urol* 1992;**148**:688–90.

84 Reinberg Y, Shapiro E, Manivel JC *et al.* Prune belly syndrome in females: a triad of abdominal musculature deficiency and anomalies of the urinary and genital systems. *J Pediatr* 1991;**118**(3):395–8.

85 Culp DA, Flocks RH. Congenital absence of abdominal musculature. *J Iowa State Med Soc* 1954;**44**:155–9.

86 Kerbl K, Pauer W. Renal failure and uraemia leading to the diagnosis of prune belly syndrome in a 34-year old man. *Int Urol Nephrol* 1993;**25**(2):205–8.

87 Henderson AM, Vallis CJ, Sumner E. Anesthesia in the prune-belly syndrome: a review of 36 cases. *Anesthesia* 1987;**42**: 54–60.

88 Reinberg Y, Manivel JC, Pettinato G *et al.* Development of renal failure in children with the prune belly syndrome. *J Urol* 1991;**145**:1017–19.

89 Shenasky JH, Whelchel JD. Renal transplantation in prune belly syndrome. *J Urol* 1976;**115**:112–13.

90 Reinberg Y, Manivel JC, Fryd P *et al.* The outcome of renal transplantation in children with the prune belly syndrome. *J Urol* 1989;**142**:1541–2.

91 Woodhouse CRJ, Ransley PG, Williams DI. Prune belly syndrome—report of 47 cases. *Arch Dis Child* 1982;**57**:856–9.

92 Adams MC, Hendren WH. Reconstructive surgery in the prune belly syndrome [Abstract 73]. Presented to the American Academy of Pediatrics Meeting, Urology Section, 1990.

20 Hypospadiology

M.A.Keating and J.W.Duckett

Introduction

Hypospadias continues to challenge today's reconstructive urologists just as it has since the first contemporary repairs were reported by Thiersch and Duplay in the latter part of the nineteenth century [1]. Over 300 urethroplasties and their modifications have since been described and new additions continually appear in the literature (Table 20.1). This plethora of operations bears testimony to surgical ingenuity as well as a generalized dissatisfaction with many earlier repairs, where failures typically outnumbered successes. Fortunately, recent years have seen a continued improvement in the results of contemporary urethroplasties and a decline in morbidity. Nevertheless, clinicians who dabble with these anomalies are destined to repeat the errors of their predecessors. Surgeons who treat hypospadias must study the evolution of contemporary urethroplasties, understand the anatomical nuances of the anomaly and be able to offer a variety of solutions for its numerous variants. This body of knowledge comprises the art and science we now recognize as hypospadiology.

Significant changes have marked the field during the past two decades: optical magnification and microsurgical techniques are an important addition; outpatient surgery is done in nearly every case; most boys are operated on during the first year of life; preputial flaps are preferred over free grafts and one-stage procedures provide the standard for repair. Perhaps most importantly, better assessments of chordee and an improved understanding of the plasticity and resilience of the glans now allow us to project the neourethra beyond the coronal sulcus, where it was usually left by two-stage repairs. In the past, functional normality was the goal. In contrast, today's hypospadiologist strives to reconstruct a penis that is also normal cosmetically (Table 20.2). This new standard offers obvious benefits to afflicted boys when it can be achieved. It also sometimes blurs the indications for surgery for boys with distal hypospadias where function might not be affected if the anomaly were left uncorrected.

Preoperative management

Indications

Who needs surgery and when is it necessary to correct 'mild, glanular' or 'grade 1' hypospadias? These are common queries from parents and referring doctors, especially those trained in an earlier era when the results of urethroplasties were sometimes no better than the problems they were intended to correct. There is really no choice but to repair proximal hypospadias with chordee, otherwise the affected child will be obliged to sit to void and be unable to have children. However, it is impossible to predict which baby with distal hypospadias will return in later life with meatal stenosis, unappreciated chordee or the psychological burden of an altered body image.

Table 20.1. Highlights in management of hypospadias

Date	Clinician	Modification
200 AD	Heliodorus and Antyllus	First repair amputation of distal penis
1861	Bouisson	Attempted correction of chordee
1874	Duplay	Tubularization of previously transferred penile skin
1896	Hook	First vascularized preputial flap
1953	Denis Browne	'Buried strip' principle of epithelialization
1955	Devine and Horton	Free preputial graft urethroplasty
1970–2	Hodgson	Popularisation of vascularized cularizeo preputial flaps
1974	Gittes and McLaughlin	Saline artificial erection

Table 20.2. Goals of contemporary urethroplasty

1 Reposition neomeatus to tip of the penis
2 Creation of symmetric glans and penile shaft
3 Complete straightening of the penis
4 Construction of a hairless urethra with a uniform calibre
5 Normalization of voiding and erections

Fortunately, as a consequence of improved surgery, the benefits of contemporary urethroplasties now outweigh their risks in all but the most minor variants. Because hypospadias is much easier to manage in infancy than in adolescence or adulthood, we now correct virtually every variant encountered rather than risk dealing with their problems at a later age.

Preoperative evaluation

Misunderstanding and anxiety accompany the birth of a boy with hypospadias. Parents are told that their newborn son is abnormal, often by clinicians with very little understanding of the anomaly, its implications and the surgery necessary for its correction. In addition, guilt is commonplace, though the majority of hypospadias has no apparent underlying cause. To resolve these issues we have begun seeing affected infants at 1 or 2 months of age whenever possible. After examining the child, a frank discussion about the findings prepares the parents for future surgery and establishes a bond with the surgeon that is instrumental to a good working relationship. The complexity of any hypospadias should not be minimized or the possibility of secondary surgeries underestimated. Honesty and a commitment to finalization of the problem are critical to the surgeon's success outside the surgical suite where medicolegal issues can arise, especially if complications occur.

A thorough history is taken for every patient, paying special attention to prior genital surgery, including circumcision. The examination includes assessment of the size of the penis, position and calibre of its meatus, the presence of chordee and the quality of the prepuce and ventral shaft skin overlying the urethra. Though sometimes not as valid as the perioperative findings, these provide a basis for discussion of the different operations that might be used in repair. Checks are also made for other anomalies that commonly occur with hypospadias (Table 20.3) and may require correction. If cryptorchidism is

Table 20.3. Anomalies commonly associated with hypospadias

1 Torsion of the penis (50%)
2 Enlarged utricle—related to severity (30% with penoscrotal)
3 Penoscrotal transposition
4 Cryptorchidism—rule out intersex
5 Hernias (10%)

present, it may be the sign of an intersex state and warrants further investigation with a karyotype [2]. This association is more common with proximal hypospadias but can also occur with distal variants. Radiographical studies are not routinely obtained. The incidence of clinically significant upper tract anomalies associated with isolated hypospadias is no greater than that in the normal population, a finding explained by the asynchronous development of the urinary tract (early first trimester) and genitalia (third month gestation) [3]. Ultrasound of the abdomen is recommended, however, for the occasional child who also has anomalies of other organ systems (cardiac, anorectal, radial, etc.). These suggest a global insult in embryogenesis that also potentially affects the urinary tract. Finally, a more thorough evaluation is warranted in boys with a history of urinary tract infection.

Timing

Improvements in paediatric anaesthesia and microsurgical techniques have allowed a dramatic change in the timing of primary urethroplasties. We now prefer to correct most hypospadias between 6 and 12 months of life. Infants of this age are more easily managed, appear to have a higher pain threshold, are not yet toilet trained and are amnestic for their repairs later in development. In theory, genital awareness does not begin until 18 months of age [4]. As a consequence, we expect patients to benefit from early surgery; previously, hypospadias was operated on at a later age and patients experienced low self-esteem and other psychological drawbacks [5,6]. Fortunately, most infant penises are large enough that the same results can be achieved without increasing morbidity. Little benefit is gained by waiting because negligible penile growth occurs after infancy until adolescence. We occasionally give testosterone to infants with very small penises in anticipation of surgery but do not recommend it routinely [7]. Hormonal stimulation induces neovascularity and may increase the risk of bleeding. In addition, there are concerns that testosterone may down-regulate androgen receptors in infants and retard penile growth in later development.

Anatomical considerations

The decision to apply a particular urethroplasty is never made until the anatomical make-up of the hypospadias can be thoroughly appreciated at the time of surgery. Surgeons who opt to repair only 'simple' hypospadias or whose expertise is limited to one or perhaps two 'favourite' operations are not acting in their patients' best interest. Proximal hypospadias commonly hides behind the guise of a distal variant. This masquerade only becomes apparent when unrecognized chordee or deficiency of the corpus spongiosum are discovered at surgery. Suddenly, the well-intentioned yet simpler urethroplasty is no longer applicable (Fig. 20.1). To avoid this pitfall the hypospadiologist must have a number of solutions to the anatomical nuances that accompany these anomalies and ultimately dictate the options that might be used in their repair. Successful urethroplasty depends on thorough perioperative assessment and correction, when necessary, of the following.

Preputial and shaft skin

A classic hooded prepuce is found in most cases of hypospadias, though 1–2% of boys will have an intact prepuce. The latter classically occurs with megameatus variants. Dysgenetic ventral shaft skin is common, can make a major contribution to chordee and should be discarded. Its misalignment can form an abberant raphe that typically projects to the right. Fusion with the deficient investing layers of the underlying urethra is also common and separation of the two can be technically difficult. When a preputial flap urethroplasty is being considered, enough skin must be available to both construct the neourethra and cover the repair. This is rarely not the case.

Urethral plate

This relatively new term is used to describe the ventral shaft skin distal to the dystopic meatus. When composed of supple tissue, the urethral plate does not make the major contribution to chordee that we once supposed. The plate's quality, configuration and degree of extention into the glans have significant implications for technique selection (see p. 325). One or more tiny accessory urethras of variable depth are commonly found along its length. These are insignificant clinically and can be left undisturbed.

Meatus

The dystopic meatus occurs at any level and can take one of a number of different configurations. Glanular and subcoronal variants comprise the large majority (65–70%) when meatal position is assessed before the correction of chordee, but changes in position occur with correction of chordee (Fig. 20.2). Meatal stenosis is common, especially with distal hypospadias. At the other end of the spectrum are megameatus variants that have a widened distal urethra and meatus, a deeply splayed glans and intact prepuce [8]. A bougie à boule effectively gauges size and allows an assessment of the investing layers of the more proximal urethra that are sometimes deficient. In many patients with hypospadias a bridge or web of tissue is found at the level of the meatus that disrupts the plate. This can create turbulence in the neourethra, may increase the risk of fistula formation and should be corrected. A simple midline incision and its dorsal advancement effectively flatten the plate.

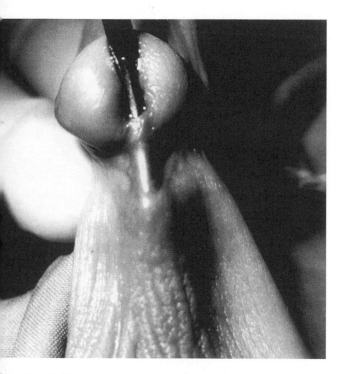

Fig. 20.1 Maldevelopment of the urethra and its investing layers with distal hypospadias. Urethral revision will cause reclassification as a more proximal variant.

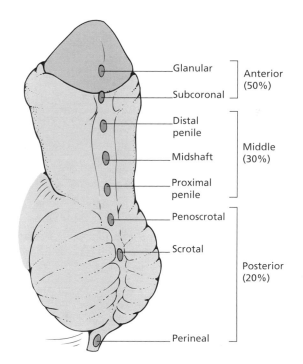

Fig. 20.2 Classification of hypospadias. Location of the meatus after correction of curvature provides the most practical classification for hypospadias.

Glans configuration

The end-on configuration of the hypospadiac glans is dictated by the width and distal projection of its urethral plate. The normal penis has a conical shape with its meatus positioned in the centre. A similar shape occurs with hypospadias having a narrow, minimally clefted plate with very little distal extension. Mobilization of glanular tissue around this type of plate is difficult and the lack of support for the neourethra can lead to breakdown with meatal retraction. In addition, these plates tend to be fibrotic and should be discarded rather than used in reconstruction. In contrast, variants with a glans that is flattened ventrally or is deeply clefted often have wider, healthier plates that extend near the end of the glans. Pinching the ventrum together mimics the normal configuration (Fig. 20.3). Differentiation of the two becomes important when preservation of the urethral plate is being considered. In the case of the former, the neourethra will fall short of the penile tip unless the plate is mobilized and advanced, allowing the neourethra to be recessed within the substance of the glans (see p. 328).

Chordee

Variable degrees of penile curvature, or chordee, can occur with hypospadias of any severity but the proximal variants are more uniformly affected. A number of different causes can contribute (Table 20.4). Superficial tethering from dysgenetic skin and dartos fascia and the yoking effect caused by the abnormal insertions of the hooded prepuce are by far the most common and can be solely responsible for significant degrees of curvature. Preoperative assessment, by placing the fingers at the base of the penis, can exaggerate their effect but may have little correlation with the presence of chordee by saline erection, especially after the shaft skin is taken down (see p. 324).

General principles

Tissue preparation and handling

The indications, if any, for preoperative antibiotics with urethroplasties remain open to debate. In pre-pubertal boys the perineal flora may be as innocuous as that on other parts of the body where surgical incisions are regarded as sterile and antibiotics not indicated. Nevertheless, many clinicians give a broad spectrum antibiotic, such as a cephalo-sporin, before surgery to theoretically maximize coverage. At the very least, post-pubertal males seem at greater risk for infection and benefit from this approach. Two or 3 days of antiseptic showers are also helpful for the older patient. In every case a thorough preoperative antibiotic preparation is necessary to eliminate local colonization. Special care is taken to separate any fusion of the prepuce and glans to remove the smegma beneath.

Table 20.4. Contributors to chordee

1 Skin tethering
2 Dysgenetic urethral plate
3 Pericorporal chordee—beneath/lateral to plate
4 Intrinsic corporal fibrosis/dysgenesis
5 Corporal disproportion

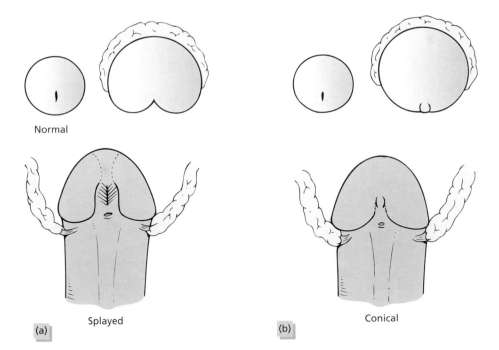

Normal

Splayed   Conical

(a)   (b)

Fig. 20.3 Glans configuration dictates the choice of urethroplasty. (a) A splayed glans projects the urethral plate to the glans tip. (b) A conical glans is an unsuitable candidate for plate-preserving techniques.

We suspect that many infections occur as a consequence of skin loss or haematoma rather than primary bacterial infections. To minimize these occurrences additional emphasis is placed on tissue-handling techniques and haemostasis. Optical magnification is used with every case. Tissues are gently manipulated with plastic surgical and ophthalmic instruments to lessen trauma and cautery is judiciously applied to individual vessels to limit its damage. Adrenaline (1 : 100 000) is invaluable to haemostasis and is injected along the lines of incision into the subcutaneous tissues and glans. A tourniquet rarely becomes necessary. Caudal or penile blocks help eliminate perioperative erections that initiate bleeding. They also lessen the requirement for general anaesthetic agents. Bleeding that occurs in the later stages of a case is often caused by a full bladder or lessening in the level of anaesthesia rather than a loss of the adrenaline's vasoconstrictive effect.

Skin takedown and coverage

The shaft skin of the penis is dissected to or below the penoscrotal junction in every case. The circumferential incision should be kept well below (7–10 mm) the coronal sulcus. This preserves the subcoronal skin and integrity of the corona when the ventral glans is ultimately reapproximated in the midline [9]. When taking down the dorsal skin, it is important to define the avascular plane between the Buck fascia and the overlying dartos fascia. The latter eventually becomes the vascular pedicle of any preputial flap that might become necessary in repair. At the completion of the case, skin coverage provides the final challenge. In some cases of distal hypospadias, the cylinder of penile skin can be reapproximated back to the glans. Redundant prepuce is then excised in a manner similar to circumcision. The more common alternative involves splitting the prepuce dorsally to the level of the coronal

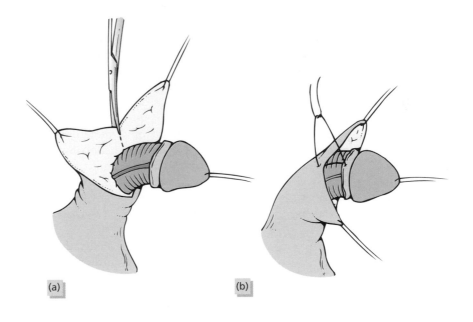
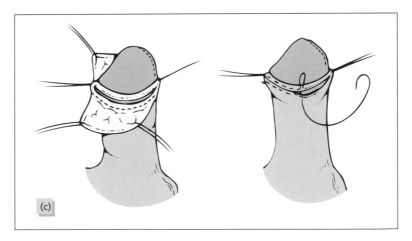

Fig. 20.4 The midline ventral skin closures possible after many urethroplasties. (a) Dorsal relaxing incision allows the transfer of lateral shaft skin. (b,c) After dorsal reapproximation and ventral realignment to cover any defect, excess prepuce is excised and the repair is completed.

sulcus. This permits rotational flaps to be transferred ventrally where a midline raphe can be created after excising the excess skin (Fig. 20.4). Byars flaps [10] and multiple Z-plasties occasionally become necessary but are cosmetically less pleasing and may increase the risks of skin loss and fistula formation.

Managing chordee

The ability to assess penile curvature, or chordee, using artificial saline erections has dramatically altered our perception of the problem and the techniques used to correct it [11]. We now realize that most chordee is caused by superficial tethering of the skin and its underlying dartos fascia. That which persists after their release is caused by either the urethral plate, corporal disproportion or intrinsic corporal maldevelopment. When the plate is soft and pliable, which is often the case, the corpora is usually the cause and removal of the plate will not effectively straighten the penis. Otherwise, the inelastic or fibrotic plate should be excised and traditional dissections of chordee completed along the corpora and into the glans itself.

Chordee that persists, whether the plate has been excised or not, can be corrected with dorsal plication sutures [12]. The tunica albuginea plication modification provides an effective solution to the problem. The Buck's fascia is elevated by lateral to medial dissections on either side of the midline (10 o'clock and 2 o'clock) to avoid damage to the neurovascular bundles. Transverse parallel incisions about 5 mm long and spaced 4–7 mm apart are made through the tunica albuginea opposite the point of greatest curvature (Fig. 20.5). Non-absorbable sutures (5/0 Prolene

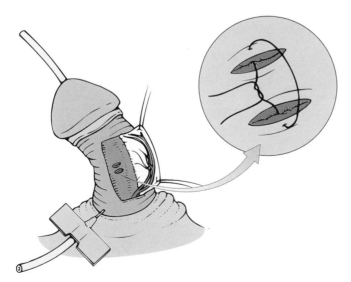

Fig. 20.5 Tunica albuginea plication. The neurovascular bundles are elevated with the Buck fascia. Non-absorbable sutures (insert) approximate the parallel incisions in the tunica albuginea.

in infants) reapproximate the tunica. As the technique relies on tissue approximation the long-term efficacy should be excellent. The early results (2.7 years follow-up) with this technique in nearly 200 boys have been encouraging [13]. Critics have exaggerated the penile length sacrificed by plications which, in actuality, amounts to less than 1 cm in all but the most severe cases. In cases of corporal disproportion this may actually be a corrective benefit. Dermal grafts are reserved for phalluses that are shorter and have more severe curvature [14,15]. Persistent glans tilt without ventral chordee is corrected by placing fine permanent sutures that hitch the dorsal glans to the corporal body, being careful to avoid the neurovascular bundles.

Preserving the urethral plate

Our understanding and management of this malpositioned, but not necessarily maldeveloped, tissue represents another dramatic departure of contemporary hypospadiology with its past. Historically, the urethral plate was routinely implicated as a major contributor to chordee. When preoperative curvature was present, the lines of incision of earlier urethroplasties would cross the plate so that dissections 'for chordee' could be done against the corporal bodies beneath. We now realize that this assumption is often incorrect. Instead, many cases of chordee are secondary to superficial tethering alone and receive little, if any, contribution from the urethral plate. This fact was underscored by a recent series from the Children's Hospital of Philadelphia where only a half of 374 patients with largely distal and midshaft hypospadias had chordee and less than one-third of these had curvature that persisted after releasing the shaft skin and dartos alone [16]. This realization expands the possibilities for application of the urethral plate and places additional emphasis on its preservation. It has also altered the approach to nearly every hypospadias where the initial incisions now keep the plate and its spongiosum intact and an initial artificial erection is done only after taking down the shaft skin.

Utilization of the urethral plate in urethroplasties is not novel. It is tubularized in the Duplay repair, kept intact with the Mathieu (flip-flap) repair and initially reconstructed in staged procedures [17]. In theory, the major advantage of constructing neourethras with plate is that they are composed of tissue with a portion of its vascularity intact. They are also easier to construct than the tubularized replacements that become necessary once the plate is excised. Despite these benefits not every hypospadias is a candidate for preservation of the plate. One major difficulty is positioning the neourethra to the tip of the penis when the glanular extension of the plate is inadequate. Another dilemma is posed by chordee that persists with the plate intact. In many instances it is difficult to tell whether the cause is deeper dysgenetic tissue, corporal disproportion or the plate itself.

Two modifications have been offered as potential solutions to these problems. Both preserve the technical simplicity of plate-based repairs yet potentially jeopardize vascularity by disrupting the tissue from its bed. The Barcat balanic groove technique completely detaches the plate and distal urethra from the glans [18]. This allows the glans to be split, deeper chordee to be excised and the neourethra advanced and more dorsally recessed within the substance of the glans to its tip. Historically, the major complication of urethral advancement techniques has been distal stenosis, yet this has not been cited as a problem with the Barcat technique. The cosmetic results and low complication rates of other recent series warrant its further consideration [19,20]. In the modifications described by Mollard and Perovich the distal plate is left attached to the glans. The remainder of its length is fully mobilized so that dissections for chordee can be done beneath. Though controversial, early reports of this approach are also encouraging [21,22].

Constructing the neourethra

We prefer to use preputial flaps whenever possible. Though the experience with free grafts in experienced hands has been commendable [23], it seems fundamentally sounder to use vascularized tissues whenever possible. The axial blood supply to the prepuce is predictable and with practice can be easily harvested with the dartos [24,25]. Concerns about compromising the overlying dorsal shaft skin are unfounded. Perimeatal-based flaps are effective, but should be applied judiciously. These flaps rely on vascularity that is sometimes deficient and may unpredictably supply the crucial hinge of the repair at the meatus.

Regardless of the type of urethroplasty used, multiple layers of tissue coverage help minimize the risks of fistula formation. Two layers are used to close the neourethra and the repair can be buttressed with additional coverage from the redundant pedicle [26]. Tunica vaginalis from an adjacent testis provides another option [27]. Finally, the normal calibre of a newborn male urethra is 8 F. Using this standard, neourethras are constructed to a calibre of 8–10 F in infants, 12 F in adolescents and at least 20 F in teenagers and adults. Appropriately sized red rubber catheters serve as a useful template during reconstruction.

Technique selection

Selecting a urethroplasty tailored to the individual's anatomy is probably the factor most crucial to optimizing results. Most hypospadias can be repaired by one of three repairs: (i) the meatal advancement and glanuloplasty (MAGPI) [28]; (ii) the onlay island flap (OIF) [29]; and (iii)

the tubularized transverse preputial island flap (TPIF) or Duckett procedure [30]. The incisions of each technique follow into the next in a logical sequence that allows them to address the evolving severity of some variants that can only be appreciated at surgery. In the case of distal hypospadias, for example, the investing layers of the distal urethra may be deficient or the mobility of the ventral urethra and glans insufficient to permit the tension-free tissue transfers required of the MAGPI. It then becomes a simple matter to outline the plate on to the glans and construct an onlay. But, in the same patient, if the plate is fibrotic and poorly developed or chordee is present, the TPIF can still be offered as an ideal solution. The exceptions to this triage are the megameatus hypospadias variants whose exaggerated urethral plate and distal urethra are best managed with a tubularization technique such as the pyramid procedure [8]. An algorithm for the primary repair of hypospadias, with its basis in the principles discussed above, is shown in Fig. 20.6 and discussed here.

Distal (glandular and coronal) hypospadias without chordee is usually an ideal candidate for the MAGPI

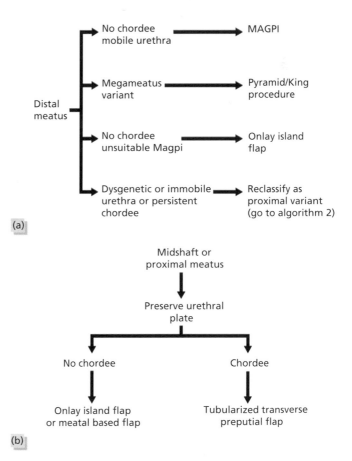

Fig. 20.6 (a) Algorithm for the repair of distal hypospadias. When chordee persists, reclassification is made to the more proximal variant. (b) Algorithm for the repair of midshaft and proximal hypospadias.

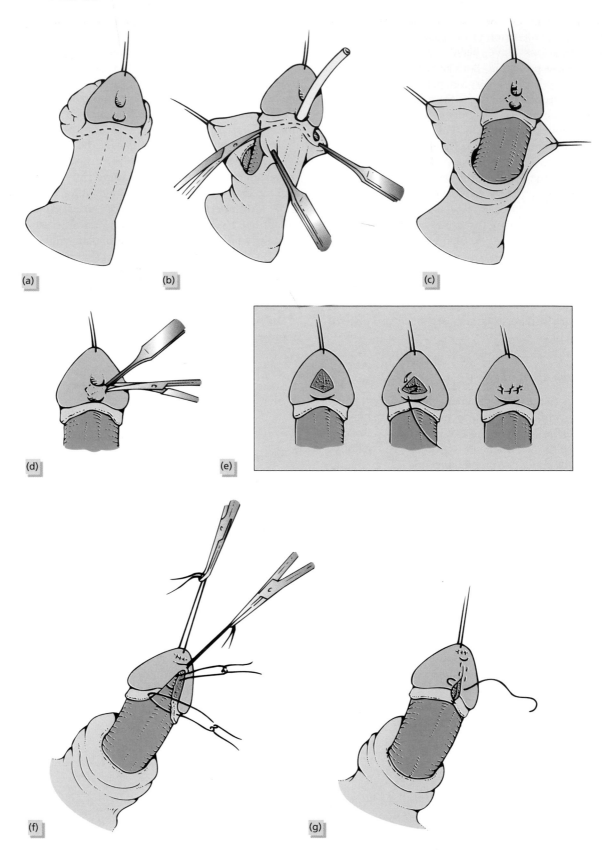

Fig. 20.7 The MAGPI repair. (a) Lines of incision. (b) Care is taken when addressing the ventral shaft skin, where fusion of the distal urethra and the overlying shaft skin often occur. (c–e) Wedge resection of the distal web and reapproximation completes the dorsal urethral advancement. (f,g) Traction completes the ventral urethral advancement as the glans is reapproximated around it.

technique. The simplicity of this procedure belies a subtle sequence of three tissue transfers required for its success. Mobility is required of the urethral plate, the ventral urethra and the glans, which is ultimately reapproximated around the advanced urethra. If urethral mobility is inadequate or the glans fish-mouthed or non-compliant, urethral retraction and glans breakdown become the inevitable consequence of tension [31]. If these are present an alternative technique such as the pyramid procedure or the OIF should be used. Any dissatisfaction with the MAGPI probably stems from its overapplication in unsuitable candidates. When properly deployed, the functional and cosmetic results are excellent. In one recent series, the MAGPI was used in over 1000 boys with a significant complication rate of only 1.2% [32].

Midshaft and proximal hypospadias without chordee or most distal variants not suitable for the MAGPI are ideal candidates for OIF urethroplasty. We sometimes still use perimeatal-based flaps in the occasional variant with a generous meatus and healthy ventral shaft skin. However, our preference for the OIF stems from its dependable vascular supply, adaptability to more proximal variants and the preservation of shaft skin that often enables a midline closure. In addition, the OIF has yielded slightly fewer complications than perimeatal-based flaps when applied to similar hypospadias (8 vs 10%) [33].

The best solution for proximal hypospadias with severe chordee remains the tubularized TPIF or Duckett procedure [30]. However, the decision to use the TPIF procedure is not made until other options are considered. We now begin nearly every repair with preservation of the urethral plate. If, after taking down the shaft skin and dartos, the penis is

straight and the tissues of the plate are healthy and well developed, the OIF rather than the more complex TPIF can be applied to even more proximal hypospadias. Advantages of the OIF over the TPIF include: (i) technical ease in constructing the neourethra; (ii) fixation of the neourethra by the plate, eliminating kinking and tortuosity; and (iii) avoiding circumferential anastomoses which makes stricture and stenosis less likely. In addition, significantly lower complication rates have been noted when compared to the TPIF (6 vs 15%) [16].

Preservation of the urethral plate by utilizing dorsal plication sutures for mid and proximal hypospadias with mild or moderate chordee remains controversial. When the plate is fibrotic it should be excised, more extensive dissections completed and the more technically demanding TPIF employed. However, if the plate is pliable and healthy it probably does not exert the bowstring effect once supposed and pericorporal dissections beneath it may not make a difference. The natural history of the unaltered urethral plate has not been defined but dorsal plications have become our preference for these variants. Problems are not apparent in early follow-up and the technical benefits of the simpler OIF appear to justify its use in this setting [34].

Primary techniques

The MAGPI procedure (Figs 20.7 and 20.8)

Incisions and dissection. A traction suture placed in the glans facilitates handling in this and other repairs. A circumferential incision is made approximately 5–7 mm

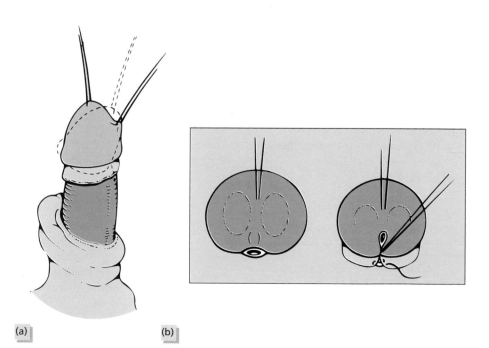

Fig. 20.8 An effective MAGPI procedure (a) eliminates glans tilt with its urethral advancement, and (b) allows a tension-free glans wrap of the urethra.

(a)

(b)

from the coronal edge which is carried proximal to the meatus and the shaft skin is taken down. Caution is required during the ventral part of this dissection; here the skin can be fused to deficient investing layers of urethra. It is helpful to define initially the better-developed tissue planes of the proximal shaft by bluntly spreading the scissors. The adherent tissues adjacent to the meatus can then be more easily appreciated and separated sharply by working distally. An 8 F feeding tube in the urethra is useful during this part of the dissection. Inadvertant urethrotomies can be repaired using fine inverting absorbable sutures. However, the risks of fistula formation increase markedly and, for more than the most minor urethrotomy, it is advisable to revise the injured urethra with an onlay flap of prepuce rather than attempt its repair.

Meatal advancement. A wedge of the dorsal meatal web is removed by making two cuts from its lateral edges that meet in the midline. This enlarges the meatus, flattens the urethral plate and eliminates 'dog ears'. The diamond-shaped defect in the plate that remains is closed transversely in the Heineke–Mikulicz fashion using 6/0 interrupted polyglycolic sutures, advancing the dorsal urethra. If the urethral plate is insufficiently mobile, the more forgiving glans tip must be pulled proximally to bridge the defect. This results in an unsightly depressed meatus. Urethral mobility can be tested using fine forceps and the MAGPI procedure should be deferred if mobility is suspect.

Glanuloplasty. Redundant remnants of the preputial insertions usually remain on either side of the glans wings after the skin incision. For cosmetic purposes, these are excised so that glans itself is approximated in the midline. Gentle traction on a stay suture or fine skin hook placed at the meatal lip completes the ventral urethral advancement. This allows the glans edges to rotate together creating a more anatomical conical shape. The glans is closed without tension in two layers over the advanced urethra. Deeper tissue is approximated with one or two 6/0 polyglycolic sutures. Fine interrupted chromic stitches reapproximate the skin. Extensive dissections beneath the lateral glans wings to access deeper tissues or achieve glanular mobility are unnecessary.

Penoplasty. A midline sleeve reapproximation of the shaft skin completes most repairs. Preservation of the prepuce is sometimes requested and is possible with the MAGPI.

OIF urethroplasty (Fig. 20.9)

Incisions and dissection. The urethral plate is kept intact by making two parallel incisions (width 5–7 mm) that extend from around the meatus to the tip of the glans. The subcoronal circumferential incision meets these at or proximal to the level of the meatus and the shaft skin is taken down. The glans wings are mobilized by defining the plane between the corporal bodies and glans cap, being careful not to undermine the plate.

Harvesting the flap. The urethra is revised by ventral spatulation and excision of any dysgenetic tissue back to healthy spongiosum. The length of the defect that must be bridged to the glans tip is measured. The combined width of the flap and plate should achieve that desired for the age of the patient. A flap of adequate size is isolated from the inner prepuce though exact sizing is unnecessary at this juncture. The flap is mobilized by developing its midline subcutaneous vascular pedicle to the base of the penis. Lateral dissections release the pedicle so that penile torsion does not occur after the flap is swung ventrally.

Urethroplasty and completion. After its ventral rotation, the onlay is approximated to one side of the urethral plate with a simple running suture that begins at the revised proximal meatus. Any excess flap is trimmed off. A running subcuticular stitch is used to close the flap's remaining side. Repairs can be tested by placing an 8 F feeding tube and injecting saline under gentle pressure after digitally occluding the proximal urethra. Redundant subcutaneous tissues of the pedicle are tacked to the corpora around the urethra to provide an additional layer of coverage. After reapproximating the glans wings in two layers, shaft skin coverage completes the repair.

The TPIF procedure (Fig. 20.10)

Incisions and dissection. Once the decision to perform the TPIF has been made, the urethral plate is divided. The corpora is cleared of any fibrous chordee and additional techniques (plications or dermal grafts) are completed. The now mobilized urethra is spatulated to healthy tissue and tacked back to the corpora at a more proximal level with interrupted sutures. This helps avoid kinking of the anastomosis. The length of the defect that must be bridged by the new urethra is measured.

Harvesting the flap. A transverse preputial flap of appropriate length and width is defined on the mucosal surface of the prepuce with tacking sutures. After its edges are incised, it is helpful to tubularize the flap over an appropriately sized red rubber catheter before completing its mobilization. An inverting locking suture approximates the epithelial edges. This is followed by a second layer that joins the overlying subcuticular tissue. Interrupted sutures are left at each end to allow for any tailoring in length that might become necessary. The completed neourethra is mobilized, using the catheter for traction, by developing its

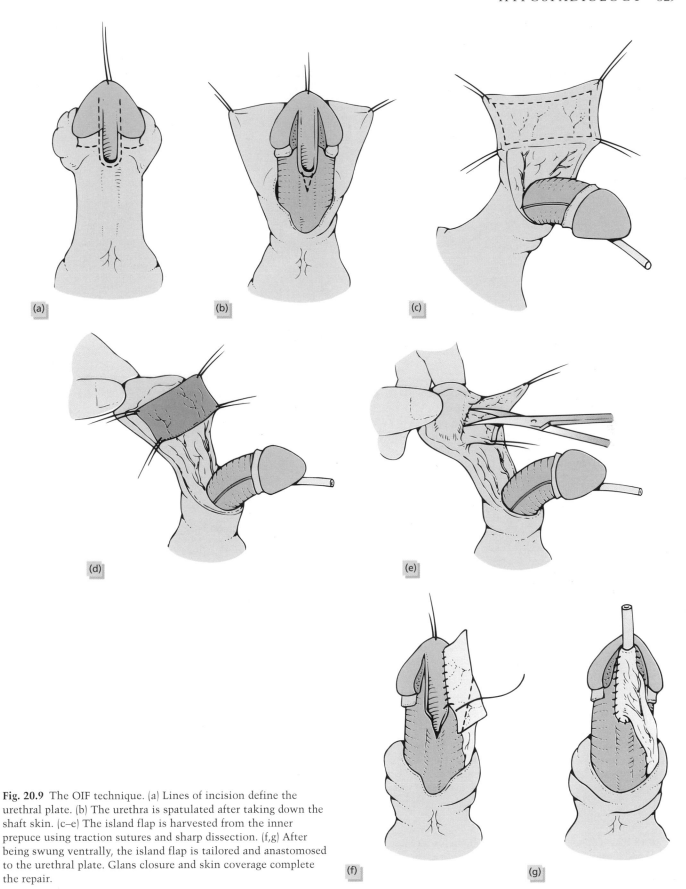

Fig. 20.9 The OIF technique. (a) Lines of incision define the urethral plate. (b) The urethra is spatulated after taking down the shaft skin. (c–e) The island flap is harvested from the inner prepuce using traction sutures and sharp dissection. (f,g) After being swung ventrally, the island flap is tailored and anastomosed to the urethral plate. Glans closure and skin coverage complete the repair.

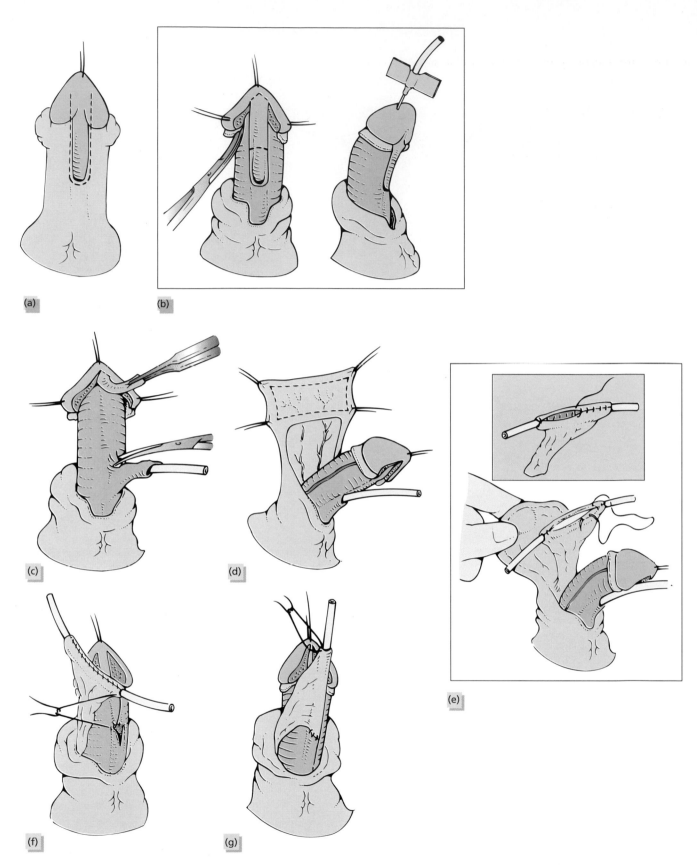

Fig. 20.10 The TPIF or Duckett repair. (a) Lines of incision outline and preserve the urethral plate. (b,c) Saline erection documents persistent curvature with the plate intact, requiring its excision (dotted lines) and urethral mobilization. (d) After correction of chordee, the inner preputial flap is outlined. Mobilization is done in a similar fashion to the OIF. (e) The flap is tubularized in two layers (insert). (f) The native urethra is tacked back to the corpora and spatulated before anastomosing the neourethra. (g) The preputial tube is matured without tension to the penile tip between widely splayed glans wings. A two-layer glans closure and skin coverage complete the repair.

midline subcutaneous pedicle to the base of the penis in a fashion similar to that of the OIF.

Completion. The neourethra is placed with its suture line against the corpora. The proximal anastomosis can be completed with either interrupted or running sutures. Redundant pedicle is fanned out to cover this area with a second layer. Distally, the neourethra is positioned between the glans wings where its meatus is matured with interrupted sutures. Ventral reapproximation of the glans is performed in two layers and skin coverage is completed using either the sleeve or Byars method. In occasional cases, the configuration of the glans warrants creation of a tunnel or channel. If so, removal of deeper spongiosal tissue is necessary so that a generous hiatus (18–20 F) for the neourethra is assured.

The pyramid procedure (Fig. 20.11)

The pyramid procedure was offered initially as a solution for the megameatus, intact prepuce (MIP) variant alone but its principles can be extended to any hypospadias having a

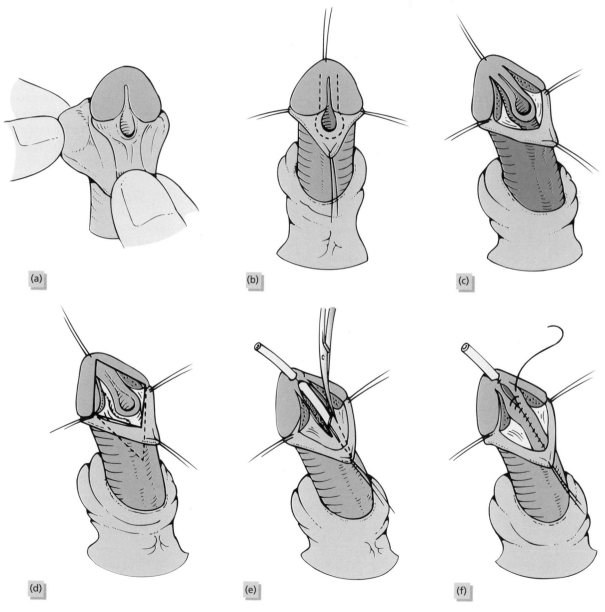

Fig. 20.11 The pyramid procedure. (a) A megameatus variant with a widely clefted glans and complete prepuce. (b) A tennis-racquet incision outlines the meatus and urethral plate. (c) Traction sutures define the base of the pyramid used for periurethral dissection and urethral mobilization. (d) The pyramid. (e) The widened distal urethral is tailored by removing a ventral wedge. (f) The proximal urethra is tubularized in continuity with the urethral plate. A two-layer glans closure and skin coverage complete the repair.

generously clefted glans [8]. The unusual configuration of the fish-mouthed meatus in MIP presents a formidable barrier to the glanuloplasty of the MAGPI, and its widened distal urethra and glans makes preparation of the urethral plate for an OIF or perimeatal-based flap difficult. In addition, the absence of chordee, in combination with an intact prepuce, causes the anomaly frequently to go unrecognized until after circumcision, removing much of the skin that might be used in reconstruction. The pyramid technique, a variant of the King repair which constructed a tubularized neourethra to the level of the sulcus [35], evolved from our experience with balanic epispadias whose findings mirror those of MIP. The 'pyramid' label describes its exposure, which allows for a simple and safe dissection of the megameatus and urethra in both the circumcised and uncircumcised child. Successful results with the pyramid or other similar procedures [36] rely upon on a generous plate and glans groove that can be mobilized and tubularized to an adequate size for the age of the patient. As with the MAGPI, caution must be exercised with selection. The plates of most distal hypospadias are not wide enough to be used with these types of repairs. As a consequence, their widespread application should probably be discouraged with concerns for long-term urethral calibre and patency.

Incisions and dissection. Four traction sutures define the megameatus and form the base of the pyramid. A tennis-racquet-shaped incision extends from the tip of the penis and is carried around the edges of the megameatus. This defines the urethral plate, which is kept wide (12–15 mm) and intact dorsally. Laterally, the edges of the glanular groove are deepened to mobilize the glans wings from the adjacent plate.

Urethroplasty. Proximally, the widened distal urethra is detached from the overlying shaft skin. Taking down the remainder of the shaft skin can be deferred unless chordee is present. The urethra is tailored in continuity with the plate by removing a wedge of ventral tissue as far proximally as necessary. Both are then tubularized over an appropriately sized catheter to form the neourethra.

Glanuloplasty and penoplasty. The glans wings are approximated in the midline in two layers and a sleeve approximation of the shaft skin completes the repair.

The perimeatal-based flap (Mathieu) procedure
(Fig 20.12)

Perimeatal-based flaps remain an option for the repair of distal hypospadias having a flattened ventral glans and healthy distal shaft skin overlying the urethra. Meatal stenosis is a relative contraindication to this repair. The correction of stenosis, which requires a dorsal meatotomy and advancement, can present technical difficulties when closing the two adjacent suture lines required of the urethroplasty.

Preparation of the plate and flap. The distance from the meatus to the tip of the penis determines the length of the flap. The plate is defined by making two parallel incisions 5–7 mm apart from the tip of the penis to the meatus. These incisions are extended down the penile shaft at the previously determined length and widened somewhat to create the flap. Less width should be taken from the plate to facilitate the subsequent glans wrap. The urethral plate is further defined and the glans wings are mobilized in a fashion similar to that used in the OIF.

Harvesting the flap. During mobilization of the flap, care is taken near its hinge at the meatus where the tissues are sometimes precariously thin. Traction sutures on the flap and a catheter in the urethra facilitate this dissection. The vascular subcutaneous tissues adjacent to the meatus that supply the flap should also be preserved.

Completion. The flap is 'flipped' distally to form the ventral neourethra. No tension should be present when suturing it to the distal extent of the plate. Running subcuticular sutures are used to close each side. A second layer of coverage can be harvested from the subcutaneous tissues of the dorsal skin. The glans is reconstructed in two layers and shaft coverage completes the repair. The Byars method may be required to cover the ventral skin defect left by the flap.

Postoperative management

Hypospadias, like so much other surgery, has seen significant alterations in its management as attempts at maximizing cost effectiveness are weighed against morbidity. Virtually every primary repair is now performed on an outpatient basis. Fortunately, an increase in complications has not resulted. Preoperative parental teaching and simplified dressings and methods of drainage have had a key role in this advancement.

Dressings

The dressing is instrumental in containing the penile bleeding and oedema which begin to subside 48–72 h after surgery. Subcutaneous wicks or vacuum tubes are rarely needed if the perioperative control of bleeding is adequate and the dressing effective. One option is to compress the penis against the lower abdomen with bio-occlusive dressing (Tegaderm) after placing it in a blanket of Telfa and gauze. This can be easily removed by the parents a few days

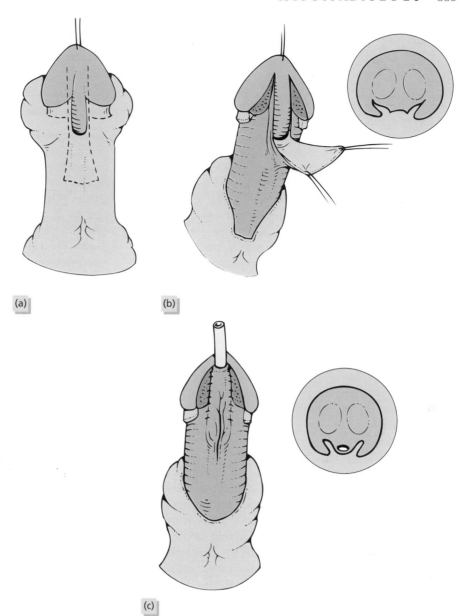

Fig. 20.12 The flip-flap (Mathieu) repair. (a) Lines of incision define the urethral plate and proximal flap that becomes the ventral neourethra. (b,c) The flap is mobilized distally and reanastomosed to the urethral plate. The glans wings (inserts) must be well mobilized in this and the OIF repair to enable tension-free anastomosis above the neourethra. Glans closure and skin coverage complete repair.

later. Another choice is a transparent, permeable dressing such as Opsite that applies direct compression to the penis without undue pressure. The repair is kept dry until 4 or 5 days after surgery when soaking in a warm bath is begun. This loosens the adhesive dressing and facilitates its removal at home.

Drains

We continue to divert every urethroplasty, with the exception of the MAGPI. A 6 F silastic tube (reinforced ventriculoperitoneal shunt tubing) is placed across the repair, lies proximal to the external sphincter and allows for continual urinary drainage. This soft tube, which is stitched to the glans with 5/0 polypropylene on a tapered needle, is well tolerated and has been very effective for younger children. Bladder spasms are usually not a problem. A suprapubic tube is used for older boys for whom nappies and open drainage are unacceptable. Urinary diversion is continued for 7–14 days, depending on the extensiveness of the repair and interval assessments of its healing. There has been a recent trend to doing away with urinary diversion for midshaft and distal hypospadias repairs by some clinicians. Our trials with this form of management have been unpleasant. Infants experience considerable discomfort with voiding and some return a few years later with fistulas that could only be appreciated once they were toilet training and watched voiding. Voiding through a reconstructed urethra, especially in the face of distal swelling, risks fistula formation [37].

Other

A broad spectrum antibiotic (sulphonamide or nitrofurantoin) is given as suppression for open urinary drainage and is continued a few days after the tube is removed to cover any residual infection or colonization. If bladder spasms are a problem opium suppositories, cut into thirds, provide immediate relief and oxybutynin can be used prophylactically. After the initial postoperative visit when the drainage tube and/or dressing is removed, additional evaluations are planned at 6 weeks and thereafter as needed. Calibration of the meatus and proximal anastomosis can be done using a bougie but actual dilatations are not routinely performed.

Complications

Acute complications

Minor problems during the early postoperative period are common. Fortunately, the penis is a forgiving organ and the majority require no more than supportive measures. Haematomas that become apparent after the dressing is removed usually organize and resolve but serial checks for infection should be done. When skin loss is noted, the defect typically fills in with granulation tissue. Grafts are unnecessary since healthy re-epithelialization with little scarring usually occurs. Multiple layers of underlying coverage assume additional importance to the neourethra in cases where skin viability is questionable. Infections are largely superficial and respond to local measures including warm soaks and topical antibiotics. Antibiotics are given to stem the local progression of the process but tissue debridment is rarely indicated.

The early appearance of a fistula is typically the most ominous problem encountered early after surgery. Acutely, fistulas become evident after discontinuing urinary diversion when leakage along a ventral incision is noted, usually at the site of the original meatus. The affected penis typically exhibits an impressive amount of induration and swelling during the early stages. The family should be reassured that the appearance of the penis will improve dramatically once the reaction subsides. Urinary drainage can be re-established but spontaneous closure rarely occurs. Proximal blow-outs of suture lines sometimes can occur and the meatus should be checked for stenosis or plugging with secretions. Distal obstruction is managed with periodic dilatation. Other than local care, the initial management of persistent complications usually entails patience alone. No corrective surgery should be attempted until penile induration and oedema have completely resolved and the surrounding tissues are healthy. Adequate healing usually occurs after 6 months but reoperations are sometimes deferred for up to 1 year in patients who have had multiple complications.

Surgical approach to persistent complications

Despite the improvements in management of hypospadias that have been described, complications still occur. Fistulas are the most common problem and rates of at least 5–10% can be expected in the best of hands for all but glanular repairs. Others complications include retraction of the meatus and glans breakdown, persistent chordee, urethral diverticula, strictures and loss of shaft skin [38]. Adherence to the principles outlined above should minimize these problems. Although management of individual entities goes beyond the scope of this discussion, the most challenging patients arrive with a combination of complications [39]. These unfortunate children have usually undergone a series of previous operations in an attempt to alleviate a cascade of compounded complications. Although we deplore the use of the term 'hypsopadias cripple' it is easy to see how the description became attached to their plight. Successful repair is contingent on a thorough evaluation of the individual components of the problem and use of the 'available resources'.

Whenever possible genital skin should be used to correct complex 're-do' hypospadias but the excess shaft skin that remains is often unhealthy or inadequate. Until recently, bladder mucosa was our preference for urethral replacement in these cases. However, bladder exhibits proliferative tendencies at its interface with the outside and the incidence of meatal problems (stenosis, ectropian, etc.) was excessive. As a consequence, free grafts of buccal mucosa have recently become our preference, though many of the technical modifications used with bladder mucosa still apply [40]. Because of its thick epithelium, buccal mucosa is easier to work with. In addition, the thinness of the tissue's dermis is, in theory, more conducive to revascularization. Finally, the harvest of buccal mucosa is less invasive than bladder and better tolerated by the patient [41,42]. Meatal prolapse has not been a problem.

Buccal mucosa graft (Fig. 20.13)

Preparing the graft bed. The best assessment of the different elements of the problem is done by making a subcoronal circumferential incision and taking down the penile shaft skin. When the skin is healthy it provides excellent coverage of the repair. The urethra is excised from the glans and shaft back to healthy tissue and chordee is corrected. When a dermal graft is necessary, a staged approach is recommended so that the buccal graft receives maximal vascularity at a later operation.

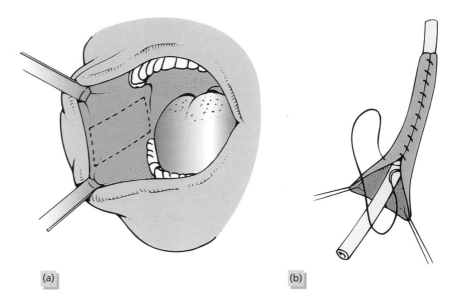

(a)   (b)

Fig. 20.13 Buccal mucosa graft. (a) The inner cheek mucosa is harvested, avoiding Stensen's duct, to make an appropriate urethral replacement for the age of the patient. (b) The neourethra is tubularized over a catheter template.

Harvesting the graft. After measuring the urethral deficit, a mucosal graft of appropriate length and width is taken from the inner cheek. Mucosa can also be taken from the inner lip but the graft width is limited. As two lip grafts are needed to create a tube this site is better suited to the harvest of onlays. Some allowance should be made for shrinkage (20%), which undoubtedly occurs. Care is taken to avoid damaging the deeper buccinator muscle or the Stensen's duct that lies opposite the third molar. Larger bleeders should be cauterized. The defect can be closed with chromic sutures but the wound also heals adequately by second intent.

Completion. Tubularization and urethral reanastomosis are performed in a manner similar to the TPIF. It may be helpful to recess the graft and eliminate any redundancy by initially maturing the meatus. The proximal anastomosis is then completed after pulling the neourethra proximally. Glanuloplasty and skin coverage by sleeve reapproximation complete the repair. A suprapubic tube is used for urinary diversion and a 6 or 8 F urethral stent is left across the graft, allowing secretions to drain. Patients are able to eat on the day following surgery. A cystourethrogram is performed 10 days after the procedure to assess healing before suprapubic drainage is discontinued. Daily meatal dilatations have helped minimize the incidence of stenosis.

Conclusions

The art and science of hypospadiology continue to evolve. There is currently no perfect operation that offers a solution to the spectrum of variants that comprise hypospadias. Surgical success depends on familiarity with a variety of contemporary techniques. Further advances are anticipated in the future for one of urology's most challenging and fascinating anomalies.

References

1 Horton CE, Devine CJ, Baran N. Pictoral history of hypospadias repair techniques. In: Horton CE, ed. *Plastic and Reconstructive Surgery of the Genital Area*. Boston: Little, Brown, 1973:237–48.

2 Rajfer J, Walsh PC. The incidence of intersexuality in patients with hypospadias and cryptorchidism. *J Urol* 1976;**116**: 769–70.

3 Cerasaro TS, Brock WA, Kaplan GW. Upper urinary tract anomalies associated with congenital hypospadias: is screening necessary? *J Urol* 1986;**135**:537–42.

4 Berg R, Berg G. Penile malformation, gender identity and sexual orientation. *Acta Psychiatr Scand* 1983;**68**: 154–66.

5 Berg G, Svensson J, Astrom G. Social and sexual adjustment of men operated for hypospadias during childhood: a controlled study. *J Urol* 1981;**125**:313–17.

6 Schultz JR, Klykylo WM, Wacksman JA. Timing of elective hypospadias repair in children. *Pediatrics* 1983;**71**:342–51.

7 Gearhart JP, Jeffs RD. The use of parenteral testosterone therapy in genital reconstructive surgery. *J Urol* 1987;**138**: 1077–8.

8 Duckett JW, Keating MA. Technical challenge of the megameatus intact prepuce (MIP) variant: the pyramid procedure. *J Urol* 1989;**141**:1407–8.

9 Firlit CF. The mucosal collar in hypospadias surgery. *J Urol* 1987;**137**:80–2.

10 Byars LT. Technique of consistently satisfactory repair of hypospadias. *Surg Gynecol Obstet* 1955;**100**:184–90.

11 Gittes RF, McLaughlin AP III. Injection techniques to induce penile erection. *Urology* 1974;**4**:473–4.

12 Nesbit RM. Operation for correction of distal penile curvature with and without hypospadias. *Trans Am Assoc Genitourin Surg* 1966;**58**:12–14.

13 Baskin LS, Duckett JW. Dorsal tunica albuginea plication for hypospadias curvature. *J Urol* 1994;**151**:1668–71.

14 Horton CE, Devine CJ. Peyronies' disease. *Plast Reconstr Surg* 1973;**52**:503.

15 Horton C, Gearhart JP, Jeffs RD. Dermal grafts for correction of severe chordee associated with hypospadias. *J Urol* 1993;**150**:452–5.

16 Baskin LS, Duckett JW, Ueoka K, Seibold J, Snyder HM. Changing concepts of hypospadias curvature lead to more onlay island flap procedures. *J Urol* 1994;**151**:191–6.

17 Mathieu JP. Traitment en un temps de l'hypospadias balanique et juxtabalanique. *J Chir* 1932;**39**:481–4.

18 Barcat J. Les hypospadias. III. Les urethroplasties, les resultats — les complications. *Ann Chir Infant* 1969;**10**:310.

19 Redman JF. The Barcat balanic groove technique for the repair of distal hypospadias. *J Urol* 1987;**137**:83–5.

20 Koff SA, Brinkman J, Ulrich J, Deighton D. Extensive mobilization of the urethral plate and urethra for repair of hypospadias: the modified Barcat technique. *J Urol* 1994;**151**:466–9.

21 Mollard P, Mouriquand P, Felfela T. Application of the onlay island flap urethroplasty to penile hypospadias with severe chordee. *Br J Urol* 1991;**68**:317–19.

22 Perovic S, Vukadinovic V. Onlay island flap urethroplasty for severe hypospadias: a variant of the technique. *J Urol* 1994;**151**:711–14.

23 Hendren WH, Horton CE Jr. Experience with 1-stage repair of hypospadias and chordee using free graft of prepuce. *J Urol* 1988;**140**:1259–64.

24 Duckett JW. Hypospadias. In: Walsh PC, Gittes RF, Permutter AD, Stamey TA, eds. *Campbell's Urology*, 5th edn. Philadelphia: WB Saunders, 1986:1969–99.

25 Hinman F Jr. The blood supply to preputial island flaps. *J Urol* 1991;**145**:1232–5.

26 Kass EJ, Bolong D. Single stage hypospadias reconstruction without fistula. *J Urol* 1990;**144**:520–2.

27 Snow B. Use of tunica vaginalis to prevent fistulas in hypospadias surgery. *J Urol* 1986;**136**:861–3.

28 Duckett JW. MAGPI (meatoplasty and glanuloplasty): a procedure for subcoronal hypospadias. *Urol Clin North Am* 1981;**8**:513–20.

29 Elder JS, Duckett JW, Snyder HM. Onlay island flap in the repair of mid and distal penile hypospadias without chordee. *J Urol* 1987;**138**:376–9.

30 Duckett JW. Transverse preputial island flap technique for repair of severe hypospadias. *Urol Clin North Am* 1980;**7**:423–31.

31 Gibbons MD, Gonzales ET Jr. The subcoronal meatus. *J Urol* 1983;**130**:739–42.

32 Duckett JW, Snyder HM III. Meatal advancement and glanuloplasty hypospadias repair after 1,000 cases: avoidance of meatal stenosis and regression. *J Urol* 1992;**147**:665–69.

33 Hollowell JG, Keating MA, Snyder HM, Duckett JW. Preservation of the urethral plate in hypospadias repair: extended applications and further experience with the onlay island flap urethroplasty. *J Urol* 1990;**143**:98–101.

34 Keating MA. Update, onlay island flap urethroplasty. *Dialog Pediatr Urol* 1990;**13**(10):1–8.

35 King LR. One-stage repair without skin graft based on a new principle: chordee is sometimes produced by skin alone. *J Urol* 1970;**103**:660–2.

36 Zaontz MR. The GAP (glans approximation procedure) for glanular/coronal hypospadias. *J Urol* 1989;**141**:359–61.

37 Buson H, Smiley D, Reinberg Y, Gonzalez R. Distal hypospadias without stents: is it better? *J Urol* 1994;**151**:1059–60.

38 Retik AB, Keating MA, Mandell J. Complications of hypospadias repair. *Urol Clin North Am* 1988;**15**:223–36.

39 Secrest CL, Jordan GH, Winslow BH *et al*. Repair of the complications of hypospadias surgery. *J Urol* 1993;**150**:1415–18.

40 Keating MA, Cartwright PC, Duckett JW. Bladder mucosa in urethral reconstructions. *J Urol* 1990;**144**:827–37.

41 Dessanti A, Rigamonti W, Merulla V *et al*. Autologous buccal mucosa for hypospadias repair: an initial report. *J Urol* 1992;**146**:1081–4.

42 Duckett JW. Successful hypospadias repair. *Contemp Urol* 1992;**4**:42–7.

21 Paediatric Urological Oncology

D. R. McMahon and S. A. Kramer

Wilms' tumour

Wilms' tumour is the most common malignant neoplasm of the urinary tract in children. It develops in approximately one child per 100 000, and more than 500 new cases occur annually in the United States [1]. Wilms' tumour presents in a bimodal fashion: sporadic unilateral cases occur with a peak incidence at 3.5 years and hereditary and bilateral cases occur at a mean patient age of 2.5 years [2]. There is no apparent sex predominance, but this tumour is more prone to develop in black children than in white children [3,4].

Genetics and markers

Recent advances in the molecular biology of Wilms' tumour have identified chromosomal abnormalities in some children [5]. Whereas the majority of patients with this tumour have a normal karyotype, an 11p abnormality is present in 30–50% of all patients with these tumours [6,7]. A specific constitutional chromosome abnormality has been identified in children with aniridia and Wilms' tumour. This abnormality, a deletion of band 13 on the short arm of chromosome 11 (11p13), is known as the WT1 gene [8,9]. The 11p13 chromosomal deletion may represent a mutation that results in loss of a tumour-suppressor function [6]. Deletion of 11p13 has been identified in specimens of nephroblastomatosis, in patients with bilateral Wilms' tumour, and in virtually all Wilms' tumours associated with the Denys–Drash syndrome [6,10]. However, an 11p13 deletion was present in only one of 20 sporadic Wilms' tumour specimens examined by Brown et al. [6].

A second Wilms' tumour gene (WT2) was initially identified in patients with the Beckwith–Wiedemann syndrome and has been mapped to chromosome 11p15 [5]. Knudson [11] and Yun et al. [12] reported that the IGF2 gene is located on 11p and proposed that production of this mitogen may be the common pathway that links both 11p13 and 11p15 abnormalities to the formation of Wilms' tumour. The loss of heterozygosity at the 16q locus in 20% of the specimens of Wilms' tumours examined supports the existence of a third Wilms' tumour gene [13,14].

The identification of reliable tumour markers would facilitate screening of high-risk individuals and would allow early detection of recurrent disease. A significant decrease in the level of the enzyme catalase has been used as a marker for an 11p13 deletion [15]. Unfortunately, children with sporadic aniridia may remain at risk for Wilms' tumour even in the absence of an 11p13 deletion [16]. The cellular oncogene n-myc is expressed at high levels in fetal renal tissue and Wilms' tumour but is quiescent in normal postnatal kidneys [17]. Activation of n-myc has been implicated in the genesis of a limited number of neoplasms arising from primitive precursor cells, including Wilms' tumour and neuroblastomas. Patients with Wilms' tumour may exhibit high levels of n-myc RNA expression from a single gene copy. However, in contrast to patients with neuroblastoma, there is usually no n-myc gene amplification at the DNA level [17]. Hyaluronic acid is a polysaccharide that is prominent in the embryonic kidney. Hyaluronic acid-stimulating activity is the measurement of a glycoprotein found in the fetal serum that stimulates the synthesis of hyaluronic acid. Of interest, increased levels of both hyaluronic acid and hyaluronic acid-stimulating activity have been reported in patients with Wilms' tumour [18,19]. Increased levels of erythropoietin and the prohormone, inactive renin, have also been identified in up to 67% of patients with Wilms' tumour [18,20] and neurone-specific enolase (a marker of neuroblastoma) was increased in five of 25 (20%) patients [18].

Associated conditions

Although most patients with Wilms' tumour have no associated congenital abnormalities, significant associations with congenital urinary tract defects, hemihypertrophy and sporadic aniridia have been well-documented [2,21] (Table 21.1). Genitourinary tract anomalies (renal

Table 21.1 Wilms' tumour (WT) and associated syndromes. Data from [4,11,16,22,23].

Syndrome	Incidence in general population	Incidence in WT patients (%)	Risk of WT (%)	Median age (years)
Sporadic aniridia	1:100 000	1–2.2	20	2.0
WAGR	–	<1	33	2.0
Denys–Drasch syndrome	Rare	<1	50	2.0
Hemihypertrophy	1:53 000	3	5	3.6
Beckwith–Wiedemann syndrome	1:53 000	2	10	2.2

WAGR, Wilms' tumour, aniridia, genitourinary tract anomalies and mental retardation.

hypoplasia, fusion anomalies, renal ectopy, duplication, hypospadias and cryptorchidism) are present in 4.5% of patients with Wilms' tumour [24]. This tumour occurs eight times more frequently in patients with horseshoe kidneys than in the general population [25]. The concurrence of Wilms' tumour, aniridia, genitourinary tract anomalies and mental retardation is well known by the acronym WAGR syndrome [2,5,16].

The frequency of aniridia in the general population is 1:50 000 to 1:100 000. The incidence of aniridia in patients with Wilms' tumour is increased to between 1.1% and 2.2% [16]. Wilms' tumour has been reported in between 18 [26] and 40% [27] of patients with sporadic aniridia (autosomal recessive). Conversely, in patients with 'familial aniridia' (autosomal dominant), only a single patient with Wilms' tumour has been documented [21]. Hemihypertrophy occurs in 3% of patients with Wilms' tumour. Similarly, patients with congenital hemihypertrophy have an increased risk for developing Wilms' tumour, adrenocortical neoplasms and hepatoblastoma [21].

Of the patients with the Beckwith–Wiedemann syndrome, 10% will be diagnosed to have Wilms' tumour, and those with hemihypertrophy are at particular risk of tumour formation [16]. Patients with the Beckwith–Wiedemann syndrome are also at an increased risk for rhabdomyosarcoma, adrenocortical carcinoma and hepatoblastoma [5,28].

Gonadal dysgenesis and male pseudohermaphroditism have been associated with Wilms' tumour [28,29]. Wilms' tumour can also occur with the nephrotic syndrome, glomerulonephritis and male pseudohermaphroditism in the Denys–Drasch syndrome [10,30,31]. An 11p13 deletion is invariably present in patients with this syndrome [6]. The WT1 gene (11p13) is highly expressed during normal development of both the metanephros and the urogenital ridge and, therefore, a mutation of this gene may be responsible for both the genital abnormalities and the development of Wilms' tumour [32,33].

The incidence of neurofibromatosis in patients with Wilms' tumour was reported to be approximately 30 times greater than expected [2,4]. In a review of 1482 patients with neurofibromatosis seen at the Mayo Clinic between 1950 and 1990, none acquired Wilms' tumour [34]. During this period, 194 patients with Wilms' tumour were also examined at the Mayo Clinic and none had neurofibromatosis. A recent review of data from the National Wilms' Tumor Study confirms that there is no increased risk of development of Wilms' tumour in patients with neurofibromatosis [21].

Recommendations for surveillance

Chromosomal analysis should be performed for patients with bilateral Wilms' tumour, Wilms' tumour–aniridia complex, Wilms' tumour and hemihypertrophy, Beckwith–Wiedemann syndrome, and Wilms' tumour and other associated congenital urological anomalies [15]. In addition, females with unexplained renal failure should be karyotyped to exclude male pseudohermaphroditism and the Denys–Drasch syndrome [21]. Routine chromosomal analysis is not warranted for otherwise healthy children with a normal family history and no other congenital abnormalities. Patients with aniridia, Denys–Drasch syndrome, hemihypertrophy and Beckwith–Wiedemann syndrome should undergo routine physical examination and renal ultrasonography at 3-monthly intervals for the first 7 years of life [19,35]. The limitations of screening for this rapidly growing tumour have been demonstrated by the National Wilms' Tumor Study. Screening for patients with aniridia identified only six of 20 (30%) of those in whom Wilms' tumour eventually developed [21].

Diagnosis

The main differential diagnosis lies in distinguishing Wilms' tumour from neuroblastoma; however, other considerations include clear cell sarcoma, rhabdoid tumour, congenital mesoblastic nephroma, cystic partially differentiated nephroblastoma, lymphoma, angiomyolipoma, solitary multilocular cyst and renal cell carcinoma [15,36]. Most patients with Wilms' tumour are thriving children who are seen because of an enlarging abdomen. An abdominal mass is palpable in 90% of these children and is usually detected by the parent or discovered by the paediatrician during routine physical examination. The tumour is usually smooth and firm to palpation, and large masses may extend across the midline. Vague abdominal pain is the second most frequent symptom and occurs in approximately 30% of children. The pain is often the result of capsular distention from acute haemorrhage into the neoplasm. Gross haematuria occurs rarely, but microscopic haematuria has been detected in 50% of patients at the time of diagnosis [15]. Hypertension is present in up to 60% of children and is secondary to either encroachment on the blood supply causing ischaemia or from renin secretion by the tumour itself [37].

The initial laboratory evaluation of any child with a retroperitoneal mass includes a complete blood cell count, urinalysis and culture, serum electrolyte determination, and renal function and liver function tests. Urinary catecholamines should be measured to rule out neuroblastoma. An abnormal serum level of creatinine suggests bilateral Wilms' tumour, solitary kidney or significant congenital or acquired disease. Bone marrow metastasis is rare in patients with Wilms' tumour, and bone marrow biopsy is not necessary if Wilms' tumour is the likely diagnosis.

During imaging of the abdomen of patients with suspected Wilms' tumour, it is imperative to note the anatomy and function of the contralateral kidney and to determine whether it contains any nephrogenic rests or frank tumours. It is important to determine the presence or absence of tumour within the renal vein or inferior vena cava and, if present, to note whether the thrombus extends into the right atrium [38]. Abdominal ultrasonography has supplanted excretory urography as the primary imaging technique for Wilms' tumour. This non-invasive procedure is the best method of detecting tumour extension into the renal vein or inferior vena cava [39]. Wilms' tumour extends into the renal vein in 11% [40] of patients and into the inferior vena cava in 6% [41]. The thrombus is usually floating in the lumen of the vessel, but invasion of the wall can occur. Tumour extends into the right atrium in 1% of patients. The routine evaluation of the inferior vena cava is important because 50% of patients with vena caval extension have no signs or symptoms at presentation [42,43].

Computed tomography (CT) is useful in differentiating cystic masses from solid masses and is superior to ultrasonography in demonstrating invasion of contiguous structures as well as in detecting an unsuspected contralateral Wilms' tumour. CT scans are useful for following the tumour's response to chemotherapy and for predicting the surgical resectability of the tumour. The most important limitation of CT is its inability to assess reliably the status of the lymph nodes [44].

The presence of bilateral Wilms' tumour alters the surgical approach significantly, so the status of the contralateral kidney must be determined before nephrectomy. Koo et al. [45] reviewed 48 consecutive children who underwent radiological and operative staging of Wilms' tumour. The imaging modalities used preoperatively included CT scanning, ultrasonography and magnetic resonance imaging (MRI). In five of the patients, the diagnosis of bilateral Wilms' tumour was made preoperatively and confirmed at operation. Radiological imaging of the other 43 patients showed unilateral Wilms' tumour only, without any contralateral abnormality. Operative exploration of the contralateral kidney in these 43 patients showed no evidence of Wilms' tumour. This report suggests that a CT scan alone may obviate contralateral renal exploration in selected patients.

Calcium deposits in the tumour are unusual, occurring in 5–10% of patients. When present, calcification is usually curvilinear and located peripherally. A non-functioning Wilms' tumour may occur in up to 10% of patients and is suggestive of extensive disease, including involvement of the renal pelvis or ureter or extension into the renal vein or inferior vena cava. Non-visualization of the kidney in a child with suspected Wilms' tumour should be evaluated by cystoscopy and retrograde pyelography [46–48].

Radiographic examination of the chest is essential because the thorax is the most common site for metastatic disease. Chest radiographs, preferably in four views, demonstrate the presence of pulmonary metastases with a lower false-positive error rate than do CT scans of the chest. In a series of 2500 patients enrolled in the National Wilms' Tumor Study III, only 32 (1%) had a negative finding on chest radiographs and positive findings on CT scan [44,49]. The National Wilms' Tumor Study data demonstrate that there is no worsening of prognosis in patients with negative findings on chest radiography and positive findings on CT when treated appropriately [49].

Pathology

Wilms' tumour originates from pleuripotential mesenchymal cells of the metanephrogenic blastema and has structural diversity, almost without parallel. The tumour is a triphasic embryonal renal neoplasm consisting of blastemal, stromal and epithelial cells. These cell types are mixed in complex and varied patterns. Some tumours are composed almost exclusively of sheets of primitive blastemal cells, whereas others may consist of a monomorphous population of highly differentiated tubular cells [50]. The majority of unilateral Wilms' tumours are unicentric; however, 7% of patients have a multicentric unilateral tumour [2,51]. There is no predilection for one side or the other, and the tumour may arise anywhere within the kidney.

Unfavourable histological variants have made up between 7 and 12% of patients in the National Wilms' Tumor Study [52,53]. Of interest, 39–52% of the deaths due to tumour occurred in this small group of patients [52]. The designation 'unfavourable histology' is now synonymous with 'anaplasia', or the presence of large hyperchromatic nuclei with multipolar mitotic figures. Anaplasia is present in 4.5% of Wilms' tumours [51].

Malignant rhabdoid tumour and clear cell sarcoma, previously considered unfavourable variants, are now classified as distinct pathological entities and not as Wilms' tumour variants. Clear cell sarcoma of the kidney, also referred to as bone metastasizing tumour of childhood, has a propensity to bone and brain metastases. The evaluation of these children should include bone scan, skeletal survey and MRI of the brain [54]. Rhabdoid tumour is characterized by cells that mimic rhabdomyoblasts; however, true muscle is not present. Brain metastases are common and MRI of the brain is indicated in the evaluation of these patients [55]. These tumours are discussed in detail elsewhere [15,52,54].

The tumour specimen must be examined carefully, because even focal anaplasia implies a poor prognosis [56]. Weeks *et al.* [57] identified four histological microsubstaging variables significantly associated with relapse.
1 Infiltration of tumour cells into the vessels or connective tissues of the renal sinus.
2 The presence of a granulation tissue in the perirenal soft tissue overlying the tumour (inflammatory pseudocapsule).
3 Extensive infiltration of the tumour capsule.
4 Tumour thrombi in the intrarenal vessels.

One or more of these features were present in all patients in the National Wilms' Tumor Study III who had relapse.

Portions of the tumour specimen should be placed in glutaraldehyde for electron microscopy and in tissue culture media for cytogenetic studies [58,59]. Flow cytometric analysis of specimens of Wilms' tumour has been used to correlate nuclear DNA ploidy patterns with tumour behaviour and response to treatment. In a review of 56 patients from the Mayo Clinic with Wilms' tumours, those with diploid and aneuploid patterns had a 100% 2-year survival [60]. In contrast, in those with a DNA tetraploid pattern, the 2-year survival was only 74%. Other medical centres have found that aneuploidy is associated with anaplasia and a high rate of relapse [61,62]. In a review of 32 tumours with favourable histological patterns, relapse occurred in four of five patients with aneuploid tumours but in only one of 27 with diploid tumours [63]. The refinement of flow cytometry, the application of fluorescent *in situ* hybridization and nuclear morphometry may help to further stratify patients into treatment groups [13,61–64].

Treatment

Surgical extirpation is still the cornerstone of therapy for all children with Wilms' tumour. The child is placed in the supine position and rotated slightly so that the involved side is up. A transverse transperitoneal incision and division of the ipsilateral rectus muscle afford adequate exposure. This incision allows for contralateral exploration, *en bloc* resection of the tumour and involved kidney and provides the least risk of tumour rupture during its removal from the abdominal cavity [65]. Invasion of the renal pelvis or ureter is an indication for nephroureterectomy. Meticulous surgical technique is mandatory because tumour spillage increases the stage of the tumour and exposes the patient to the morbidity associated with more aggressive therapies [66–68]. The current treatment protocol for the National Wilms' Tumor Study IV is shown in Table 21.2.

The presence or absence of lymph node metastases is of major importance in determining the appropriate regimen of chemotherapy and radiotherapy. The inability to determine the status of the lymph nodes preoperatively limits the clinicians' ability to treat each child with the regimen that will result in the best survival and the least long-term morbidity. Therefore, the National Wilms' Tumor Study protocol continues to recommend bilateral renal exploration with mobilization and palpation along with lymph node biopsy for accurate staging [19,44].

Aggressive and extended lymphadenectomy is not recommended and has not been associated with improved survival [70]. Complete tumour extirpation is desirable and *en bloc* resection of adjacent organs can be considered. It is noteworthy that tumour was present in only 17% of the adjacent organs removed in the patients in the National Wilms' Tumor Study III [67].

In a series of 36 children with advanced Wilms' tumour, Dykes *et al.* [71] performed percutaneous Trucut needle biopsy for diagnosis, followed by chemotherapy before definitive surgery. Nephrectomy was performed at a median of 14 weeks after chemotherapy. Tumour bulk was substantially decreased in 94% of patients. Concordance between the histological pattern of the tumour biopsy sample and the histological pattern at subsequent nephrectomy was 93%. Tumour seeding in the biopsy needle tract was not identified in any patient, but one child had a small peritoneal tumour nodule in the lateral abdominal wall which may have been related to the biopsy site. This nodule was completely excised at surgery, with no subsequent evidence of local recurrence. The authors' conclusion was that percutaneous biopsy was a safe

Table 21.2 National Wilms' Tumor Study IV protocol. From [69] with permission.

Disease	Initial therapy	Radiotherapy	Chemotherapy regimen
Stage I/favourable histology and stage I/anaplastic	Surgery	None	EE: actinomycin D plus vincristine (24 weeks) EE-4: pulsed, intensive actinomycin D plus vincristine (15 weeks)*
Stage II/favourable histology	Surgery	None	K: actinomycin D plus vincristine (22 and 65 weeks) K4: pulsed, intensive actinomycin D plus vincristine (24 and 60 weeks)*
Stage III/favourable histology	Surgery	1080 cGy	DD: actinomycin D, vincristine and doxorubicin (26 and 65 weeks) DD4: pulsed, intensive actinomycin D, vincristine and doxorubicin (24 and 52 weeks)*
High risk (clear cell sarcoma, all stages) and stage IV/favourable histology	Surgery	Yes†	DD: actinomycin D, vincristine and doxorubicin (26 and 65 weeks) DD4: pulsed, intensive actinomycin D, vincristine and doxorubicin (24 and 52 weeks)*

*Refer to latest National Wilms' Tumor Study protocol for dosage and length of treatment.
† Clear cell sarcoma patients receive 1080 cGy and stage IV/favourable histology cancer patients are given 1080 cGy if the primary tumour would qualify as stage III were there no metastases.

technique that allowed confirmation of diagnosis (with accurate histological classification in the majority of patients) before initiation of treatment. McLorie et al. [72] and Greenberg et al. [73] used similar approaches and were impressed that the tumours were more confined, less vascular and less friable after initial chemotherapy. There were no instances of needle track seeding or tumour rupture in either series [72,73].

The International Society of Pediatric Oncology (SIOP) protocols have used preoperative chemotherapy, without confirmatory biopsy, to reduce the frequency of tumour ruptures and to down-stage the tumours. However, it has been estimated that the radiographic diagnosis of Wilms' tumour without pathological confirmation is inaccurate in up to 5–10% of cases [74–76]. It is noteworthy that 1.5% of the patients who received chemotherapy in SIOP-6 had benign disease [77]. Operative tumour rupture occurred in 7% of SIOP-6 patients compared with 10% in the National Wilms' Tumor Study III. The 5-year survival rates in SIOP-6 for stage I, stage II and stage III tumours were 93, 86 and 75%, respectively [77]. An unusually large number of abdominal relapses occurred in patients with stage II tumour and disease-free nodes. Because of this increased rate of relapse, the current SIOP-9 protocol involves triple-agent chemotherapy.

Green et al. [78] and Green and Jaffe [79] showed that patients younger than 24 months with stage I tumours had an excellent prognosis and did not demonstrate improvement in disease-free survival after local radiation or systemic chemotherapy. In a recent prospective study of eight patients, Larsen et al. [80] confirmed that patients younger than 24 months at presentation who had small (less than 550 g of total kidney and tumour weight),

favourable histological patterns and stage I lesions had an excellent survival rate with surgery alone (100% overall survival and 88% disease-free survival). The application of microsubstaging criteria may allow improved stratification of patients [57]. In this subgroup of patients, adjuvant chemotherapy could be withheld, with the presumption that those who developed metastatic disease could be treated effectively by postoperative chemotherapy [78,79]. Hanna and Samowitz [81] suggested that partial nephrectomy should be considered in selected patients who have small polar tumours and favourable histological patterns. They reported four patients who underwent partial nephrectomy and postoperative chemotherapy with actinomycin D and vincristine. All four patients were alive without evidence of disease from 1 to 11 years post-operatively. McLorie et al. [72] have used preoperative chemotherapy to facilitate partial nephrectomy for both unilateral and bilateral Wilms' tumour.

Surgical complications were encountered in 20% of children in the National Wilms' Tumor Study III [82]. The factors that were most likely to be associated with the development of surgical complications were: (i) higher local tumour stage; (ii) intravascular tumour extension; and (iii) resection of other organs at the time of nephrectomy. The most frequent complications were small bowel obstruction (6.9%) and major intraoperative haemorrhage (5.9%). The overall survival of the patients with surgical complications was similar to that of patients without complications when matched for histological pattern and stage [82].

Significant morbidity and mortality are associated with the treatment of Wilms' tumour with caval extension. Primary excision of caval thrombi was associated with a 43% complication rate in the National Wilms' Tumor

Study III. Percutaneous biopsy and preoperative chemotherapy have been used to reduce the operative complications in this high-risk group [39]. In a series of 30 patients with caval or atrial extension of Wilms' tumour treated by primary cytoreductive chemotherapy, the thrombus markedly decreased in size in 11 patients and resolved completely in seven. Tumour embolization did not occur and the surgical complication rate was 25%; the most frequent complication was major haemorrhage, in 16% [41].

Staging and prognostic factors

The current staging system used by the National Wilms' Tumor Study is shown in Table 21.3.

A comprehensive statistical analysis of 1466 patients in the National Wilms' Tumor Study III who had favourable histology and non-metastatic disease was performed. This study demonstrated that lymph node involvement, age at diagnosis and tumour size (as measured by the weight of the excised specimen) were the most important determinants of outcome. Tumours dominated by blastemal cells were associated with a poor prognosis. Tumour size, tumour in the margin and capsular penetration were most significantly associated with abdominal recurrence. Intraoperative spillage of tumour is not an independent risk factor for relapse. However, meticulous surgical technique is mandatory because tumour spillage increases the stage of the tumour and exposes the patient to the morbidity of more aggressive therapy [83]. Lymph node involvement was associated most closely with pulmonary metastasis. Of the patients with a thrombus confined to the renal vein, 16.8% had tumour relapse in the lungs. In patients with tumour in

the inferior vena cava or right atrium, lung relapse developed in 6.9% [83]. In a review of 367 patients with recurrent disease from the National Wilms' Tumor Studies II and III, survival was greater than 40% if: (i) the relapse occurred only in the lung or in the abdomen if no abdominal radiation had been given; (ii) the initial tumour was stage I; (iii) only two-drug chemotherapy was given at presentation; or (iv) the tumour recurred later than 12 months after presentation [84,85].

Survival

The systematic design and evaluation of each National Wilms' Tumor Study have produced treatment refinements that have simultaneously improved survival and diminished morbidity. Results of National Wilms' Tumor Study III demonstrated that children with non-metastatic Wilms' tumour and favourable histological pattern had excellent prognoses. Survival rates at 4 years after diagnosis were 97% for those with stage I disease, 92% for those with stage II disease and 84% for those with stage III disease [86] (Table 21.4).

There is no statistically significant difference in survival between stage I tumours with favourable histology treated with 10 weeks or 6 months of actinomycin plus vincristine. In stage II or III tumours with favourable histology, survival is not improved by the addition of doxorubicin (Adriamycin). However, fewer intra-abdominal relapses occurred in stage III tumours treated with doxorubicin. In stage II tumours with favourable histology, survival was not improved with adjuvant radiation therapy. For stage III tumours with favourable histology, survival was not compromised by decreasing the radiation dose from 2000 cGy to 1000 cGy [86]. Diffuse anaplasia is associated with a 20–30% decreased survival rate compared with that of focal anaplasia [86].

Interestingly, involvement of the renal vein or inferior vena cava by tumour did not adversely affect the prognosis if treatment was appropriate [40,41]. The 3-year survival

Table 21.3 Staging system of the National Wilms' Tumor Study.

Stage I	Tumour limited to kidney, completely excised. Capsular surface intact; no tumour rupture. No residual tumour apparent beyond margins of resection
Stage II	Tumour extends beyond kidney but is completely excised. Regional extension of tumour; vessel infiltration; biopsy of tumour performed or local spillage of tumour confined to the flank. No residual tumour at or beyond the margins of excision
Stage III	Residual non-haematogenous tumour confined to the abdomen. Lymph node involvement of the hilus, periaortic chains or beyond; diffuse peritoneal contamination by tumour spillage or peritoneal implants of tumour; tumour extends beyond surgical margins either microscopically or macroscopically. Tumour not completely removable because of local infiltration into vital structures
Stage IV	Deposits beyond stage III, i.e. lung, liver, bone and brain
Stage V	Bilateral renal involvement at diagnosis

Table 21.4 Survival rates found in the National Wilms' Tumor Study III. Modified from [86] with permission.

	Four-year survival rate (%)
Favourable histology	
Stage I	97
Stage II	92
Stage III	84
Unfavourable histology	
Stage I*	87
Stages II–IV	55

* ADR, AMD, VCR, RT± cyclophosphamide.
ADR, doxorubicin (Adriamycin); AMD, dactinomycin; RT, radiation therapy; VCR, vincristine.

rates for patients with intracaval involvement were 88, 89 and 62% for stages I, II and III, respectively. The level of caval involvement had no effect on survival; all 16 children with intracardiac tumours and favourable histological features survived 3 or more years.

Although it is generally accepted that 2-year, disease-free survival after treatment is a measure of successful therapy, it is important to note that recurrence of Wilms' tumour beyond 2 years of treatment occurs in 1.5–4% of children. Clausen [87] reported on three patients who had recurrent Wilms' tumour at 9 years, 10 years and 11 years postoperatively.

Sequelae of therapy

Bone marrow toxicity and hepatic toxicity are the most frequent acute complications of treatment for Wilms' tumour. Bone marrow suppression occurs most commonly in the early months of treatment in patients undergoing both chemotherapy and radiation therapy. Acute toxicity in the liver, kidneys or lungs is rarely severe enough for chemotherapy to be discontinued.

Diastolic hypertension was noted in 7% of patients evaluated 5 years after nephrectomy [88]. Long-term follow-up evaluation of children with an acquired solitary kidney indicates that these patients are at risk of the development of proteinuria and chronic renal insufficiency. Argueso et al. [89] reviewed 152 patients who had an acquired solitary kidney, some of whom had Wilms' tumour, and who were followed up for a mean of 15 years postoperatively. Proteinuria developed in 17% of these patients and chronic renal insufficiency in 19%.

Reports from the National Wilms' Tumor Study on the late effects of therapy for Wilms' tumour indicate that the risk of a second malignancy is 1% at 10 years and may be as high as 8.5% at 20 years [90]. The predominant tumour types have included leukaemias, sarcomas and carcinomas [91]. Malignant neoplasms were more than twice as common in patients who had received radiation therapy than in those who had not received it, but the difference was not statistically significant. Radiation therapy has also been associated with the development of scoliosis, endocrine dysfunction, breast hypoplasia and pulmonary fibrosis [92–95]. However, improvements in the delivery of radiation therapy and decreases in both the intensity of treatment and the percentage of patients receiving radiation should decrease the morbidity encountered.

Bilateral disease

The incidence of synchronous bilateral Wilms' tumours ranges from 4.4 to 7.0%. Metachronous lesions occur in 1–1.9% of patients [2,96]. Synchronous bilateral Wilms' tumours usually have a favourable histological pattern and

behave in a less aggressive fashion than unilateral neoplasms. In a review of 145 patients with bilateral Wilms' tumours registered in the National Wilms' Tumor Studies II and III, unfavourable histological patterns were detected in 15 patients (10%) [97]. Of those 15 patients, discordant histological patterns (i.e. favourable on one side and unfavourable on the other side) occurred in six (40%). The unique characteristics of bilateral Wilms' tumours are depicted in Table 21.5.

The National Wilms' Tumor Study II recommended preservative rather than ablative surgery, because chemotherapy clearly has been shown to be effective in the treatment of bilateral disease. A transabdominal–transperitoneal incision is used and excisional biopsies are performed. The lymph nodes are sampled for accurate staging, and total nephrectomy should be avoided at this first operation. In patients with favourable histological patterns, chemotherapy is administered postoperatively, with the drug regimen and interval determined by the most advanced stage of disease according to the protocol of the National Wilms' Tumor Study IV (see Table 21.2). Imaging studies should be repeated at 3-monthly intervals, and objective response should be evident promptly. If there is no objective response or only minimal response (less than 50% decrease in tumour size, measured as the product of the two greatest diameters of the visible tumour), additional chemotherapy, i.e. ifosfamide and etoposide (VP16), can be initiated. Second-look procedures are undertaken with the intent of maximal conservation of renal parenchyma and consist of partial nephrectomy or excisional biopsy. If all the tumour can be removed without nephrectomy, chemotherapy is continued according to the stage of disease and radiation therapy is withheld. If nephrectomy seems inevitable at this time, definitive surgical treatment is deferred and repeat biopsy is advised. Chemotherapy is continued, and a third-look procedure is undertaken at an interval which should not exceed 6 months. The choices available at the time include the following: bilateral excisional biopsy, bilateral partial nephrectomy, bench surgery and nephrectomy with contralateral partial nephrectomy. Rarely, bilateral nephrectomy, dialysis and renal transplantation are required. Renal transplantation should be delayed for 1 year, if possible, because transplantation before that time is associated with a 62% recurrence rate and a 79% mortality

Table 21.5 Features unique to bilateral Wilms' tumours. From [69] with permission.

	Unilateral	Bilateral
Mean age (years)	3.5	2.5
Associated congenital anomalies (%)	8	60
Nephroblastomatosis (%)	44	100
Hypertension	Common	Rare

rate [98]. Unfortunately, this interval may be difficult to realize because of the hazards of prolonged dialysis in young children.

In a review of 185 patients with bilateral Wilms' tumour registered in the National Wilms' Tumor Studies II, III and IV, the overall survival was 83, 73 and 70% at 2, 5 and 10 years, respectively [96]. The important prognostic variables were unfavourable histological pattern, age at diagnosis and the most advanced stage of the individual tumours. No significant difference in survival was noted between patients undergoing initial surgical resection of the tumour and those undergoing initial tumour biopsy followed by chemotherapy and subsequent surgical resection [96,99]. Survival did not appear to be compromised by renal-sparing operations. The excellent survival rate may be the result of several factors, including the earlier age at which bilateral lesions occur, the high incidence of favourable histological patterns, the excellent response to chemotherapeutic agents and the different biological behaviour of bilateral tumours.

Nephrogenic rests

Nephroblastomatosis denotes a spectrum of histogenic abnormalities thought to be related to the pathogenesis of Wilms' tumour. Kidneys with nephroblastomatosis often have concomitant cystic and dysplastic areas of the renal cortex. The term nephrogenic rest has been suggested to replace the commonly used term of persistent nodular blastema. The term nephroblastomatosis should be restricted to the presence of multiple or diffuse nephrogenic rests [100]. Nephroblastomatosis occurs in three clinical settings: (i) in autopsy specimens; (ii) in association with Wilms' tumour; and (iii) as a primary diagnosis. In an autopsy series of infants less than 4 months old, nephroblastomatosis was found in one of 200–400 children. The majority of these lesions clearly regress before

becoming neoplastic [101]. Two major categories of nephrogenic rests have been identified: (i) perilobar nephrogenic rests; and (ii) intralobar nephrogenic rests (Table 21.6). The primary difference between perilobar and intralobar nephrogenic rests is the position of the rest within the renal lobe [100]. Nephroblastomatosis has been reported to occur in nearly 100% of kidneys with bilateral Wilms' tumour and in 23% of kidneys with unilateral Wilms' tumour [15]. It is likely that many of the cases of bilateral Wilms' tumour reported previously, especially those with favourable outcomes, were really examples of massive nephroblastomatosis.

Contrast-enhanced CT scanning is the most sensitive imaging method for detecting nephroblastomatosis [102], but false-negative results have been reported [103]. Nephroblastomatosis should be treated with chemotherapy according to the protocol of National Wilms' Tumor Study IV. Chemotherapy reduces the embryonal cell component of the nephrogenic rests and the lesions often regress, as seen on CT. The mature elements do not appear to be affected [100]. Nephrogenic rests that grow or become rounded warrant excision [101].

Genitourinary rhabdomyosarcoma in childhood

Rhabdomyosarcoma is the most common soft tissue sarcoma of childhood, accounting for 10–15% of all solid tumours in children. Of these tumours, 15–20% arise from the genitourinary tract [104]. Most patients present between 2 and 6 years of age; however, a second incidence peak occurs from 15 to 19 years of age [105]. Rhabdomyosarcoma of the urogenital tract occurs in approximately 0.7 cases per 1 million children annually. White children are affected more often than black children, and boys are affected more often than girls, in a ratio of 1.4 : 1 [105].

Table 21.6 Approximate prevalence of nephrogenic rests. From [100] with permission.

Population	Perilobar nephrogenic rests (%)	Intralobar nephrogenic rests (%)	Reference*
Infant autopsies	1	0.01†	[3]
Renal dysplasia	3.5	Unknown	[6]
Unilateral WT	25	15	[1]
Bilateral WT			[1]
(Synchronous)	74–79	34–41	
(Metachronous)	42	63–75	
BWS/HH/WT	70–77	47–56	[1]
Aniridia/WT	12–20	84–100	[1]
Drash/WT	11	78	[1]

* See Beckwith [100] reference list.
† Authors' unpublished observation (two cases with intralobar nephrogenic rests in 2000 infant autopsies).
BWS/HH, Beckwith–Wiedemann syndrome/hemihypertrophy; WT, Wilms' tumour.

Pathology

Rhabdomyosarcomas arise from undifferentiated mesenchyme that undergoes various degrees of differentiation into myxomatous tissue, fibrous tissue or striated muscle, [106]. The term sarcoma botryoides refers to a polypoid form of embryonal rhabdomyosarcoma that, grossly, appears as a cluster of grapes projecting into the vagina or bladder [106]. The three major histological subtypes are embryonal, alveolar and pleomorphic [104]. Microscopic examination shows embryonal histological features in 80% of patients with genitourinary rhabdomyosarcoma [104]. Unfavourable histological types include anaplastic rhabdomyosarcoma, monomorphous round cell rhabdomyosarcoma and alveolar tumours [107]. All other gross or cellular features are categorized as favourable [104,108,109].

Rhabdomyosarcomas are highly aggressive tumours with a propensity for early invasion of local structures. Both lymphatic metastases and haematogenous dissemination to the lungs, liver and bone have been noted in up to 20% of patients at presentation [104]. Flow cytometry has been studied as a means of discerning favourable from unfavourable tumours. Boyle et al. [108] examined 13 cases of rhabdomyosarcoma by flow cytometry and found that all were aneuploid tumours. All six cases treated after 1971 responded successfully to combination chemotherapy and surgery and were free of disease after a mean follow-up period of 75 months. Shapiro et al. [110] reported on 37 non-resectable tumours and found that the 10 diploid tumours had a 'uniformly poor prognosis'. In a review of 34 patients with clinical group III tumours from the Intergroup Rhabdomyosarcoma Study III, the 5-year progression-free survival was 91% for hyperdiploid tumours and 17% for diploid tumours [111]. Current investigations into the prognostic significance of cytogenetic abnormalities [112], P-glycoprotein expression [113,114] and the role of proto-oncogenes [115–117] may provide improved stratification of patients.

Diagnosis

Bladder rhabdomyosarcoma

Bladder lesions occur twice as often in boys as in girls, and most patients are younger than 5 years at the time of first presentation [105]. Rhabdomyosarcomas of the bladder usually originate in the submucosa and superficial layers of the trigone. Extension of tumour into the urethra, prostate, vulva and vagina occurs before lymphatic or haematogenous metastatic lesions develop [118]. Rhadomyosarcomas of the bladder often present in a botryoid form and may reach massive size before producing symptoms. The most common method of presentation is bladder outlet obstructive symptoms and, often, acute urinary retention. Occasionally, children have urinary tract infection or passage of tissue fragments through the urethra. Gross haematuria occurs infrequently and results from disruption of the overlying bladder mucosa. The tumour is often palpable as a suprapubic mass. Imaging of the upper tracts reveals hydroureteronephrosis in more than 50% of patients, and the cystogram shows the characteristic negative filling defects in the bladder. The radiographic evaluation should include ultrasonography of the abdomen; CT of the pelvis, abdomen and chest; and a bone survey or scan [104,118] (Fig. 21.1). More recently, MRI has been helpful in accurately staging the extent of pelvic tumours [119]. A definitive diagnosis is made at endoscopic evaluation when the typical polypoid, whitish growth can be removed for histological examination. Often, it is not possible to pass the cystoscope through the obstructed tortuous urethra; in those cases, a transperineal or transrectal biopsy is acceptable.

Prostatic rhabdomyosarcoma

The median age of patients with prostatic lesions is 3.5 years [118]. Prostatic rhabdomyosarcomas tend to be solid rather than botryoid. Continuous spread into the bladder often makes it difficult to distinguish histologically whether this tumour originates primarily in the prostate or in the bladder. The tumour infiltrates the bladder neck and posterior portion of the urethra and causes bladder outlet obstruction. Infiltration of the rectum by tumour may produce constipation as a presenting symptom. Unfortunately, the insidious onset of symptoms can result

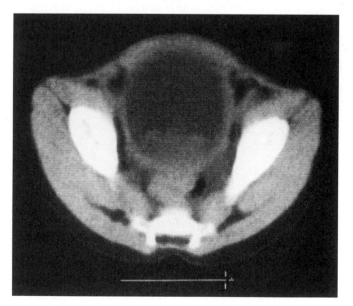

Fig. 21.1 CT scan of a pelvis showing marked soft tissue density, consistent with rhabdomyosarcoma, in the posterior portion of the bladder. (Reproduced from [15] with permission.)

in delayed diagnosis and treatment. Physical examination documents a distended bladder, and the tumour is easily palpable on rectal examination. Voiding cystourethrography shows elevation of the bladder base and distortion of the prostatic urethra. The diagnosis is confirmed by transurethral biopsy, if possible, or perineal or transrectal biopsy.

Pelvic rhabdomyosarcoma in females

Primary vaginal rhabdomyosarcoma is the most common tumour of the female genital tract in children [120]. Rhabdomyosarcomas of the vagina are invariably embryonal and usually appear when the patient is less than 2 years of age [104]. The tumour usually occurs on the anterior vaginal wall adjacent to the cervix, but it may arise from the distal portion of the vagina or from the labia. The tumour often extends through the vesicovaginal septum into the bladder and urethra. Because the rectovaginal septum acts as a barrier to posterior spread of tumour, the rectal wall is involved infrequently. Patients present with a prolapsing vaginal mass or bleeding; distant metastases are uncommon at initial presentation. The diagnosis of pelvic rhabdomyosarcoma in females is established by cystoscopy, vaginoscopy and biopsy. Uterine tumours usually develop in the second decade of life and are associated with a more ominous prognosis [104].

Staging

Clinical staging is based on the local extent of the tumour, the presence or absence of metastatic disease, and the microscopically verified completeness of surgical removal (Table 21.7).

Table 21.7 Staging of rhabdomyosarcoma. Modified from [121].

Group	Features
I	Localized disease, completely excised
IA	Confined to organ of origin
IB	Outside organ of origin; regional nodes not involved
II	Grossly excised tumour with microscopic residual disease
IIA	No evidence of gross residual tumour or regional node involvement
IIB	Completely excised tumour, no microscopic residual, regional nodes are positive or adjacent organ is involved
IIC	Regional nodes are positive with evidence of microscopic residual disease
III	Incomplete resection or biopsy with gross residual disease
IV	Distant metastases at presentation

Treatment — the Intergroup Rhabdomyosarcoma Studies

The Intergroup Rhabdomyosarcoma Study was established to provide a large number of patients for randomized trials. Intergroup Rhabdomyosarcoma Study I focused on complete surgical resection followed by postoperative radiotherapy and chemotherapy. The overall survival was 81%, with 70% of patients having no evidence of disease at 3 years [104,122]. The bladder was salvaged in 22% of patients [122]. Intergroup Rhabdomyosarcoma Study I documented that radiotherapy provided no benefit for group I patients and that doxorubicin (Adriamycin) did not improve the outcome for patients in group III or IV. The primary objective of Intergroup Rhabdomyosarcoma Study II was to improve on the survival rates of Intergroup Rhabdomyosarcoma Study I while preserving pelvic organs. In Intergroup Rhabdomyosarcoma Study II, initial radical surgery was replaced with primary chemotherapy, radiotherapy and conservative surgery [122,123]. Overall survival decreased to 70%, with only 52% of the patients without evidence of disease at 3 years. Also, bladder salvage was only 22% at 3 years [109,122,123]. Bladder salvage remained the focus in Intergroup Rhabdomyosarcoma Study III, and survival, excluding patients with group IV disease at diagnosis, was approximately 90%. Of the patients with group I, II or III disease, 60% were alive with a functional bladder at 3 years after diagnosis [124]. The treatment design for Intergroup Rhabdomyosarcoma Study IV is shown in Table 21.8. Alternatively, we have used vincristine, doxorubicin and cyclophosphamide, alternating this treatment with etoposide/ifosfamide for patients with bladder and prostatic rhabdomyosarcoma. Doxorubicin was not given during radiation therapy. This neoadjuvant chemotherapy regimen has been very effective and appears to facilitate local control in selected patients (C. Arndt, unpublished data).

The best prognostic indicators of survival are: (i) clinical stage; (ii) histological findings; and (iii) site of the primary tumour. In a review of 109 patients from the Intergroup Rhabdomyosarcoma Studies I and II, favourable outcomes were associated with tumours occurring between ages 1 and 5 years, non-prostate primary tumour, botryoid tumour and female sex [122]. LaQuaglia et al. [125] reviewed 25 patients at Memorial Sloan–Kettering and identified prostatic involvement as the most significant predictor of mortality. Local tissue invasion and distant metastases at diagnosis also predicted a poor outcome.

In females with pelvic rhabdomyosarcoma, anterior exenteration was the mainstay of therapy, but currently it is reserved for complicated recurrent disease (Table 21.9). When a hysterectomy is required for tumours of the proximal vagina, the ovaries should be preserved and repositioned to minimize the effects of radiation therapy. Fortunately, dilatation and curettage is adequate initial

Table 21.8 Intergroup Rhabdomyosarcoma Study IV treatment design. From [105] with permission.

Stage	Chemotherapy	Radiation
I*	Vincristine/actinomycin D/cyclophosphamide *or* vincristine/actinomycin D/ifosfamide	None
II	Vincristine/actinomycin D/cyclophosphamide *or* vincristine/actinomycin D/ifosfamide *or* vincristine/ifosfamide/etoposide	None
III	Vincristine/actinomycin D/cyclophosphamide *or* vincristine/actinomycin D/ifosfamide *or* vincristine/ifosfamide/etoposide	Conventional
IV†	Vincristine/melphalan *or* ifosfamide/etoposide *or* ifosfamide/Adriamycin } and vincristine actinomycin D/ cyclophosphamide	Conventional

* Excludes group 1 paratesticular patients who only received vincristine/actinomycin D.
† All stage IV patients receive VAC and one of the three 'new' drug pairs.

Table 21.9 Rhabdomyosarcoma of the female genital tract. Modified from [120].

Primary site	Total no. of patients	Total no. of living patients	No. of organs preserved		
			Bladder	Uterus	Ovary
Vagina	28	25	21	5	22
Uterus	10	6	6	4	6
Vulva	9	9	All	All	All

surgical therapy for the 60% of uterine tumours that are polypoid [120].

Paratesticular rhabdomyosarcoma

Paratesticular rhabdomyosarcoma accounts for about 75% of all genitourinary rhabdomyosarcomas. It is the most frequent spermatic cord tumour of childhood, accounting for 17% of malignant intrascrotal tumours [126,127]. This neoplasm usually is a unilateral, painless, firm and non-tender mass in the scrotum, lying superior to the testis.

Pathology

Paratesticular rhabdomyosarcomas arise from mesenchymal elements of the testicular or spermatic cord coverings and may originate in the testis itself, the epididymis or the testicular tunics [127]. Ninety-three to 97% of these tumours exhibit embryonal histological features [104,118].

Staging

Clinical staging is based on the local extent of the tumour, the presence or absence of metastatic disease, and the microscopically verified completeness of surgical removal

(see Table 21.7). A metastatic evaluation is performed, including CT scans of the abdomen and chest, because lymphatic spread is noted in up to 28% of patients [104]. A bone scan or skeletal survey is recommended in addition to a bone marrow aspirate or biopsy (or both) [118].

Therapy

Radical inguinal orchiectomy with early vascular occlusion at the level of the internal inguinal ring is still the first line of treatment. Trans-scrotal procedures should be avoided to prevent the likelihood of contamination. Intergroup Rhabdomyosarcoma Studies I, II and III advocated retroperitoneal lymphadenectomy for all patients with paratesticular rhabdomyosarcoma. The basis for this recommendation stems from a review of 20 children with paratesticular rhabdomyosarcoma [128]. Six of 15 patients (40%) undergoing retroperitoneal lymph node dissection (RPLND) had nodal involvement by tumour. The authors did not mention the clinical stage of disease in the 15 patients undergoing surgery, and it is unclear how many of those with stage I disease actually underwent node dissection. Raney *et al.* [129] concluded that 'a high incidence of retroperitoneal nodal involvement in para-testicular rhabdomyosarcoma supports the concept that radical orchiectomy should be followed by examination of the retroperitoneal nodes ...'. In a retrospective analysis of the Intergroup Rhabdomyosarcoma Study data, only three of 57 patients undergoing RPLND had pathologically positive nodes (unsuspected clinically and radiographically). Furthermore, in a retrospective series of 20 patients from Germany and 11 patients from Italy undergoing RPLND, no positive nodes were found in children with clinical stage I disease. Therefore, initial RPLND sampling was helpful in only three of 88 patients

(3%, Intergroup Rhabdomyosarcoma Study III, Germany and Italy) in determining the need for additional therapy [130]. All children received maintenance chemotherapy, and the 5-year survival rate for this combined group of patients was 92%.

In Intergroup Rhabdomyosarcoma Study IV, node dissection is not recommended in patients with localized, completely excised paratesticular rhabdomyosarcoma (clinical stage I) without clinical or radiographic evidence of lymph node involvement at diagnosis. Staging in these patients should be done carefully with thin-cut CT scans of the abdomen and pelvis. If these studies show no evidence of lymph node enlargement, retroperitoneal lymph node biopsy or sampling is not recommended, because the risk of lymph node involvement or nodal relapse is minimal.

Prognosis

Overall survival in the 95 patients entered in Intergroup Rhabdomyosarcoma Studies I and II with paratesticular rhabdomyosarcoma was 89% at 3 years and 80% at 5 years. The 3-year relapse-free survival was 93, 90 and 67% for stage I, II and III tumours, respectively [109]. LaQuaglia *et al.* [126] identified distant metastases at presentation and bulky retroperitoneal disease as the most reliable predictors of a fatal outcome. The spindle cell variant is associated with fewer metastases (16.3% vs 35.7%) and an improved 5-year survival of 95% when compared with the classic embryonal variant [121].

Testicular tumours in children

Testicular tumours are rare before puberty, constituting only 1% of all solid tumours in childhood [131]. The tumour occurs in approximately one in 1 million boys younger than 15 years [132]. The peak age for childhood testicular tumours is 2 years, and about 60% of patients are evaluated before that age. Although germ cell tumours account for about 95% of all testicular neoplasms, they represent only 60–75% of prepubertal testicular tumours [133] (Tables 21.10 and 21.11).

Diagnosis

Most children with testicular tumours are seen because of a non-tender, non-painful scrotal mass [134]. Physical examination reveals an enlarged, non-tender testicle that does not transilluminate. Fifteen to 20% of children have an associated hydrocele at presentation, and 7% of patients in the Prepubertal Testicular Tumor Registry were initially misdiagnosed as having a simple hydrocele [131]. In children with hormonally active tumours, scrotal examination may be unrevealing and the diagnosis is considered because of precocious puberty.

Table 21.10 The histology of testicular neoplasms according to the Prepubertal Testicular Tumor Registry. Modified from [131].

Histology	Number (%)
Yolk sac	207 (63)
Teratoma	46 (14)
Gonadal stromal tumour	15 (5)
Epidermoid cyst	6 (2)
Leydig cell	4 (1)
Sertoli cell	4 (1)
Gonadoblastoma	3 (1)
Juvenile granulosa cell	4 (1)
Other (rhabdomyosarcoma, leukaemia)	37 (11)
Unknown	1 (1)

Table 21.11 The histology of testis tumours in newborn infants. Modified from [131].

Histology	Number (%)
Yolk sac	6 (30)
Gonadal stromal tumour	6 (30)
Juvenile granulosa cell	2 (10)
Gonadoblastoma	2 (10)
Teratoma	1 (5)
Other	3 (15)

Imaging

Ultrasonography should be performed in the evaluation of a scrotal mass. Tumours concealed by a hydrocele are easily demonstrated by ultrasonography, and extratesticular tumours are readily differentiated from intratesticular lesions. The cystic appearance of a benign teratoma often allows preoperative discrimination from yolk sac carcinoma [135,136]. Abdominal CT scanning is extremely accurate in detecting metastatic disease and has replaced radionuclide liver scans and lymphangiography in the evaluation of patients with testicular tumours [132].

Markers

Tumour markers have proved to be extremely useful for staging and follow-up evaluation in patients with malignant testicular neoplasms. Alpha-fetoprotein is the primary fetal serum protein. In fetal life, it is produced by cells of the yolk sac, proximal gut and liver [137]. The level of α-fetoprotein is increased in 90% of patients with yolk sac tumours [131]. The interpretation of its levels in infants can be misleading, because the liver may produce α-fetoprotein until 2 years of age [132,137] (Fig. 21.2). The half-life of α-fetoprotein is approximately 5 days; therefore, serum levels should revert to normal (<10 ng/ml) within 25 days after orchiectomy [138]. The β-subunit of human chorionic gonadotrophin (β-hCG) is a glycoprotein that is synthesized by the normal syncytiotrophoblastic cells of

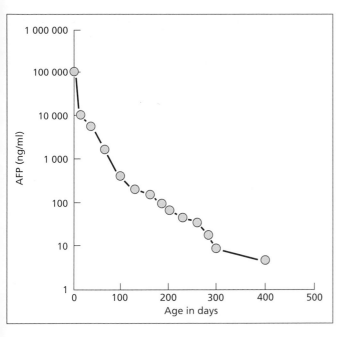

Fig. 21.2 Upper limits of normal α-fetoprotein (AFP) levels in infancy. (Redrawn from [137].)

the placenta and by specific tumours [138]. The half-life of β-hCG is approximately 24 h, so that this serum marker should normalize (<5 mIU/ml) within 5 days after all tumour has been excised. Approximately two-thirds of embryonal carcinomas and mixed teratomas secrete β-hCG [138].

Yolk sac carcinoma

Yolk sac tumour is the most common primary malignant testis tumour of germinal origin in children [131] (see Table

21.10). This tumour is a clinically and histologically distinct neoplasm of the testis that occurs primarily in children younger than 2 years [139]. Grossly, the tumour is firm, soft and yellow-white. It may have a diffuse microcystic pattern with areas of necrosis. Haemorrhage within the tumour is unusual but may occur. Histologically, the tumour has a characteristic 'organoid' pattern, with intermingling of epithelial and mesenchymal cells [134]. Yolk sac tumours have a pronounced variation in light microscopy appearance and may reveal a reticular pattern, a pseudopapillary pattern, a cystic or polyvesicular pattern, or a solid pattern [140]. Faintly eosinophilic spherical bodies are uniformly present in these tumours. A distinctive characteristic is the presence of perivascular Schiller–Duval bodies, structures that appear to be an attempt to form yolk sacs. Ultrastructural studies have demonstrated the presence of plasma proteins within the tumours [141–144]. Immunohistochemical staining may be of value in documenting the presence of various marker proteins within the tumour [140]. Although some authors have suggested that the specific proteins produced by the tumour may indicate differentiation of the neoplasm [141,145], we found no prognostic significance when rates of disease-free survival were compared [134].

Historically, children less than 1 year old have had a uniformly better prognosis than older children [131]. However, data from the Testicular Tumor Registry did not show a statistically significant difference in survival based on age. Metastases occurred in only 14% of the children younger than 2 years, but in 25% of those older than 2 years [131].

Radical inguinal orchiectomy at the level of the internal ring remains the first line of treatment. Haematogenous metastases to the lungs occur almost twice as frequently as do lymphatic metastases to the retroperitoneal nodes [131].

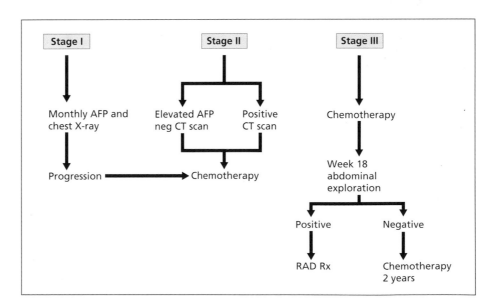

Fig. 21.3 Current recommendations for management after radical orchiectomy for yolk sac tumour. AFP, α-fetoprotein; chemotherapy, vinblastine, bleomycin, cisplatin and VP16; CT, computed tomography; RAD Rx, radiation therapy. (Redrawn from [146] with permission.)

Because of the low incidence of isolated retroperitoneal metastases, patients with localized disease as documented by normal radiographic studies and normal serum marker measurements should not be subjected to the potential morbidity of retroperitoneal lymphadenectomy (Fig. 21.3). Furthermore, adjuvant chemotherapy does not appear to improve survival of patients with stage I tumours [132]. Meticulous postoperative evaluation, including monthly determinations of serum α-fetoprotein, monthly chest radiographs and interval ultrasonographic or CT evaluations of the abdomen, is necessary if relapses are to be identified early. Children with advanced disease benefit significantly from the recently developed combination chemotherapeutic regimens. More than half of the patients with stage II or III disease were salvaged with vincristine, actinomycin D and cyclophosphamide (VAC) or cisplatin, vinblastine and bleomycin (PVB) chemotherapy [132,147].

Teratomas

Teratomas are germ cell tumours of infancy and early childhood, with a median age at presentation of 14 months [131]. These tumours usually appear as a painless testicular swelling and, because of their cystic component, often transilluminate. The tumour is derived from embryonic tissues and is composed of all three germ layers: ectoderm, mesoderm and endoderm. Grossly, the tumour is well encapsulated and contains multiple cysts of various sizes and consistency. Cartilage, muscle, fat, epidermal elements, glial tissue and bone are often present within the specimen. Haemorrhage and tumour necrosis are extremely rare. Approximately 15% of teratomas in children contain some poorly differentiated or malignant-appearing elements; however, the behaviour of these tumours has been universally benign [135]. In fact, metastasis from a testicular teratoma has not been reported in a prepubertal patient [136].

Radical inguinal orchiectomy is curative for stage I disease. However, interest in testis-sparing surgery for teratomas and other benign paediatric testis tumours is growing. Rushton and Belman [135] and Rushton et al. [136] have proposed that prepubertal patients who present without endocrine abnormalities, with normal α-fetoprotein levels and with well-circumscribed cystic lesions on ultrasonography may be safely treated with enucleation of the tumour. Frozen section evaluation of the specimen is required to support the diagnosis and to rule out the possibility of early pubertal changes within the testicle.

Gonadal stromal tumours

Gonadal stromal tumours are the most common non-germinal cell testicular tumours in children. These neoplasms are derived from a common mesenchymal stem cell that can give rise to pure Leydig cell tumours, pure Sertoli cell tumours, theca cell tumours, granulosa cell tumours or a combination of these [148].

Leydig cell tumours

Leydig cell tumours account for about 1% of childhood testicular neoplasms [131]. The peak incidence is at age 4–5 years. On the cut surface, the Leydig cell tumour is yellow to rusty brown, lobulated and spherical and often compresses the surrounding parenchyma. Reinke crystals, often found in adults, are generally absent in childhood tumours. These tumours can produce various hormones, including androgens (most commonly), oestrogens, progestins and corticosteroids. Sexual precocity is the usual presenting symptom [149]. The differential diagnoses in these children with testicular enlargement include Leydig cell tumour, Leydig cell hyperplasia, tumours of adrenal rest tissue and poorly controlled congenital adrenal hyperplasia [150].

From 10 to 15% of patients have gynaecomastia, which develops primarily because of an imbalance between circulating androgens and oestrogens. The feminization observed in patients with Leydig cell tumours is always superimposed on masculinization [149]. There have not been cases of malignancy associated with Leydig cell tumours in children [135]. Inguinal orchiectomy remains the treatment of choice; however, simple enucleation of the tumour has been reported and advocated [135].

Sertoli cell tumours

Children with Sertoli cell tumours usually present with an asymptomatic testicular mass. These tumours can secrete oestrogens or androgens, and gynaecomastia is present in up to 14% of boys [148]. Most Sertoli cell tumours are benign and metastasis has not been reported in children presenting before the age of 5 years [148]. The treatment of choice is inguinal orchiectomy, but retroperitoneal disease must be ruled out by CT or ultrasonographic studies.

Gonadoblastoma

Gonadoblastoma, an unusual tumour of the testis, may occur in patients with mixed gonadal dysgenesis. Although gonadoblastoma itself is a benign tumour, up to 60% of these tumours are associated with subsequent malignant germ cell tumours [148].

Epidermoid cysts

Epidermoid cysts of the testis account for 1–2% of testicular tumours in children. This tumour consists of stratified squamous epithelium with keratinization but without skin adnexal structures. These tumours are uniformly benign and either enucleation or orchiectomy is effective treatment [148].

References

1 Young JL Jr, Miller RW. Incidence of malignant tumors in US children. *J Pediatr* 1975;**86**:254–8.

2 Breslow NE, Beckwith JB. Epidemiological features of Wilms' tumor: results of the National Wilms' Tumor Study. *J Natl Cancer Inst* 1982;**68**:429–36.

3 Breslow NE, Langholz B. Childhood cancer incidence: geographical and temporal variations. *Int J Cancer* 1983;**32**:703–16.

4 Breslow N, Olshan A, Beckwith JB, Green DM. Epidemiology of Wilms' tumor. *Med Pediatr Oncol* 1993;**21**:172–81.

5 Koo HP, Hensle TW. Molecular biology of Wilms' tumor. *Urol Clin North Am* 1993;**20**:323–31.

6 Brown KW, Wilmore HP, Watson JE *et al.* Low frequency of mutations in the *WT1* coding region in Wilms' tumor. *Genes Chromo Cancer* 1993;**8**:74–9.

7 Wang-Wuu S, Soukup S, Bove K, Gotwals B, Lampkin B. Chromosome analysis of 31 Wilms' tumors. *Cancer Res* 1990;**50**:2786–93.

8 Riccardi VM, Sujansky E, Smith AC, Francke U. Chromosomal imbalance in the aniridia–Wilms' tumor association: 11p interstitial deletion. *Pediatrics* 1978;**61**: 604–10.

9 Francke U, Holmes LB, Atkins L, Riccardi VM. Aniridia–Wilms' tumor association: evidence for specific deletion of 11p13. *Cytogenet Cell Genet* 1979;**24**:185–92.

10 Coppes MJ, Huff V, Pelletier J. Denys–Drash syndrome: relating a clinical disorder to genetic alterations in the tumor suppressor gene *WT1. J Pediatr* 1993;**123**:673–8.

11 Knudson AG Jr. Introduction to the genetics of primary renal tumors in children. *Med Pediatr Oncol* 1993;**21**:193-8.

12 Yun K, Fidler AE, Eccles MR, Reeve AE. Insulin-like growth factor II and WT1 transcript localization in human fetal kidney and Wilms' tumor. *Cancer Res* 1993;**53**:5166–71.

13 Partin AW, Gearhart JP, Leonard MP *et al.* The use of nuclear morphometry to predict prognosis in pediatric urologic malignancies: a review. *Med Pediatr Oncol* 1993;**21**:222–9.

14 Newsham I, Cavenee W. Tumors and developmental anomalies associated with Wilms' tumor. *Med Pediatr Oncol* 1993;**21**:199–204.

15 Kramer SA, Kelalis PP. Pediatric urologic oncology. In: Gillenwater JY, Grayhack JT, Howards SS, Duckett JW, eds. *Adult and Pediatric Urology*, Vol. 2, 2nd edn. St Louis: Mosby Year Book, 1991:2245–87.

16 Clericuzio CL. Clinical phenotypes and Wilms' tumor. *Med Pediatr Oncol* 1993;**21**:182–7.

17 Brock WA, Rich MA. Implications of current tumor advances for the clinician. *Probl Urol* 1990;**4**:624–38.

18 Coppes MJ. Serum biological markers and paraneoplastic syndromes in Wilms' tumor. *Med Pediatr Oncol* 1993; **21**:213–21.

19 Anon. Summary and recommendations of the workshop held at the First International Conference on Molecular and Clinical Genetics of Childhood Renal Tumors, Albuquerque,

New Mexico, May 14–16, 1992. *Med Pediatr Oncol* 1993; **21**:233–6.

20 Johnston MA, Carachi R, Lindop GBM, Leckie B. Inactive renin levels in recurrent nephroblastoma. *J Pediatr Surg* 1991; **26**:613–14.

21 Miller RW, Fraumeni JF Jr, Manning MD. Association of Wilms' tumor with aniridia, hemihypertrophy and other congenital malformations. *N Engl J Med* 1964;**270**:922–7.

22 Green DM, Breslow NE, Beckwith JB, Norkool P. Screening of children with hemihypertrophy, aniridia, and Beckwith–Wiedemann syndrome in patients with Wilms' tumor: a report from the National Wilms' Tumor Study. *Med Pediatr Oncol* 1993;**21**:188–92.

23 Breslow N, Beckwith JB, Ciol M, Sharples K. Age distribution of Wilms' tumor: report from the National Wilms' Tumor Study. *Cancer Res* 1988;**48**:1653–7.

24 Pendergrass TW. Congenital anomalies in children with Wilms' tumor: a new survey. *Cancer* 1976;**37**:403–8.

25 Mesrobian H-GJ, Kelalis PP, Hrabovsky E *et al.* Wilms' tumor in horseshoe kidneys: a report from the National Wilms' Tumor Study. *J Urol* 1985;**133**:1002–3.

26 Freidman AL. Wilms' tumor detection in patients with sporadic aniridia: successful use of ultrasound. *Am J Dis Child* 1986;**140**:173–4.

27 Fraumeni JF Jr, Glass AG. Wilms' tumor and congenital aniridia. *J Am Med Assoc* 1968;**206**:825–8.

28 Beheshti M, Mancer JFK, Hardy BE, Churchill BM, Bailey JD. External genital abnormalities associated with Wilms' tumor. *Urology* 1984;**24**:130–3.

29 Rajfer J. Association between Wilms' tumor and gonadal dysgenesis. *J Urol* 1981;**125**:388–90.

30 Ringert RH, Pistor K. Nephroblastoma associated with mesangioproliferative glomerulonephritis. *Eur Urol* 1982;**8**: 125–6.

31 Spear GS, Hyde TP, Gruppo RA, Slusser R. Pseudohermaphrodism, glomerulonephritis with the nephrotic syndrome, and Wilms' tumor in infancy. *J Pediatr* 1971;**79**:677–81.

32 Kreidberg JA, Sariola H, Loring JM *et al.* WT-1 is required for early kidney development. *Cell* 1993;**74**:679–91.

33 Coppes MJ, Huff V, Pelletier J. Denys–Drash syndrome: relating a clinical disorder to genetic alterations in the tumor suppressor gene WT1. *J Pediatr* 1993;**123**:673–8.

34 Argueso L, Kramer SA. Indications for surveillance in patients at risk for Wilms' tumor. *Soc Pediatr Urol Newsl* 1991;**June**:45–7.

35 Palmer N, Evans AE. The association of aniridia and Wilms' tumor: methods of surveillance and diagnosis. *Med Pediatr Oncol* 1983;**11**:73–5.

36 Broecker B. Renal cell carcinoma in children. *Urology* 1991;**38**:54–6.

37 Ganguly A. Gribble J, Tune B, Kempson RL, Leutscher JA. Renin-secreting Wilms' tumor with severe hypertension: report of a case and brief review of renin-secreting tumors. *Ann Intern Med* 1973;**79**:835–7.

38 Cushing B, Slovis TL. Imaging of Wilms' tumor: what is important! *Urol Radiol* 1992;**14**:241–51.

39 Habib F, McLorie GA, McKenna PH, Khoury AE, Churchill BM. Effectiveness of preoperative chemotherapy in the treatment of Wilms' tumor with vena caval and intracardiac extension. *J Urol* 1993;**150**:933–5.

40 Ritchey ML, Othersen HB Jr, de Lorimier AA *et al.* Renal vein

involvement with nephroblastoma: a report of the National Wilms' Tumor Study-3. *Eur Urol* 1990;**17**:139–44.

41 Ritchey ML, Kelalis PP, Haase GM *et al.* Preoperative therapy for intracaval and atrial extension of Wilms' tumor. *Cancer* 1993;**71**:4104–10.

42 Clayman RV, Sheldon CA, Gonzales R. Wilms' tumor: an approach to vena caval intrusion. *Prog Pediatr Surg* 1982;**15**:285–305.

43 Nadas AS, Ellison RC. Cardiac tumors in infancy. *Am J Cardiol* 1968;**21**:363–6.

44 D'Angio GJ, Rosenberg H, Sharples K *et al.* Position paper; imaging methods for primary renal tumors of childhood: costs versus benefits. *Med Pediatr Oncol* 1993;**21**:205–12.

45 Koo AS, Koyle MA, Hurwitz RS *et al.* The necessity of contralateral surgical exploration in Wilms' tumor with modern noninvasive imaging technique: a reassessment. *J Urol* 1990;**144**:416–17.

46 Stevens PS, Eckstein HB. Ureteral metastasis from Wilms' tumor. *J Urol* 1976;**115**:467–8.

47 Cremin BJ. Non-function in nephroblastoma (Wilms' tumour): a report on the excretory urography of nine cases. *Clin Radiol* 1979;**30**:197–201.

48 Canty TG, Nagaraj HS, Shearer LS. Nonvisualization of the intravenous pyelogram—a poor prognostic sign in Wilms' tumor? *J Pediatr Surg* 1979;**14**:825–30.

49 Green DM, Fernbach DJ, Norkool P, Kollia G, D'Angio GJ. The treatment of Wilms' tumor patients with pulmonary metastases detected only with computed tomography: a report from the National Wilms' Tumor Study. *J Clin Oncol* 1991;**9**:1776–81.

50 Bennington JL, Beckwith JB. Tumors of the kidney, renal pelvis, and ureter. In: Firminger HL, ed. *Atlas of Tumor Pathology*, Second series, Part 12. Washington DC: Armed Forces Institute of Pathology, 1975.

51 O'Toole KM, Brown M, Hoffmann P. Pathology of benign and malignant kidney tumors. *Urol Clin North Am* 1993;**20**:193–205.

52 Corey SJ, Andersen JW, Vawter GF, Lack EE, Sallan SE. Improved survival for children with anaplastic Wilms' tumors. *Cancer* 1991;**68**:970–4.

53 Beckwith JB, Palmer NF. Histopathology and prognosis of Wilms tumor: results from the first National Wilms' Tumor Study. *Cancer* 1978;**41**:1937–48.

54 D'Angio GJ, Green DM. Primary renal tumors of childhood. In: Holland JF, Frei E III, Bast RC Jr *et al.* eds. *Cancer Medicine*, Vol. 2, 3rd edn. Philadelphia: Lea and Febiger, 1993:2207–18.

55 Sahjpaul RL, Ramsay DA, de Veber LL, del Maestro RF. Brain metastasis from clear cell sarcoma of the kidney—a case report and review of the literature. *J Neurooncol* 1993;**16**:221–6.

56 Exelby PR. Wilms' tumor 1991: clinical evaluation and treatment. *Urol Oncol* 1991;**18**:589–97.

57 Weeks DA, Beckwith JB, Luckey DW. Relapse-associated variables in stage I favorable histology Wilms' tumor: a report of the National Wilms' Tumor Study. *Cancer* 1987;**60**:1204–12.

58 Burnett AL, Epstein JI, Gearhart JP. Spectrum of differentiation in pediatric epithelial tumors of kidney: report of two cases. *Urology* 1993;**42**:93–8.

59 Looi LM, Cheah   PL. An immunohistochemical study comparing clear cell sarcoma of the kidney and Wilms' tumor. *Pathology* 1993;**25**:106–9.

60 Rainwater LM, Hosaka Y, Farrow GM *et al.* Wilms' tumors: relationship of nuclear deoxyribonucleic acid ploidy to patient survival. *J Urol* 1987;**138**:974–7.

61 O'Meara A, Gururangan S, Ball R, Kay E, Kelsey A. Ploidy changes between diagnosis and relapse in childhood renal tumours. *Urol Res* 1993;**21**:345–7.

62 Gearhart JP, Partin AW, Leventhal B, Beckwith JB, Epstein JI. The use of nuclear morphometry to predict response to therapy in Wilms' tumor. *Cancer* 1992;**69**:804–8.

63 Gururangan S, Dorman A, Ball R *et al.* DNA quantitation of Wilms' tumour (nephroblastoma) using flow cytometry and image analysis. *J Clin Pathol* 1992;**45**:498–501.

64 Douglass EC, Look AT, Webber B *et al.* Hyperdiploidy and chromosomal rearrangements define the anaplastic variant of Wilms' tumor. *J Clin Oncol* 1986;**4**:975–81.

65 Kramer SA. Surgical management of pediatric neoplasms. In: Marshall FF, ed. *Operative Urology.* Philadelphia: WB Saunders, 1991:547–54.

66 Leape LL, Breslow NE, Bishop HC. The surgical treatment of Wilms' tumor: results of the National Wilms' Tumor Study. *Ann Surg* 1978;**187**:351–6.

67 Richey ML, Kelalis PP. Surgical complications following nephrectomy for Wilms' tumor. *Dialog Pediatr Urol* 1991;**14**:5–7.

68 Kramer SA. Complications of Wilms' tumor and neuroblastoma. In: Marshall FF, ed. *Urologic Complications: Medical and Surgical, Adult and Pediatric*, 2nd edn. St Louis: Mosby Year Book, 1990:421–442.

69 Mesrobian H-GJ. Wilms' tumor: past, present, future. *J Urol* 1988;**140**:231–8.

70 Othersen HB Jr, DeLorimer A, Hrabovsky E *et al.* Surgical evaluation of lymph node metastases in Wilms' tumor. *J Pediatr Surg* 1990;**25**:330–1.

71 Dykes EH, Marwaha RK, Dicks-Mireaux C *et al.* Risks and benefits of percutaneous biopsy and primary chemotherapy in advanced Wilms' tumour. *J Pediatr Surg* 1991;**26**:610–12.

72 McLorie GA, McKenna PH, Greenberg M *et al.* Reduction in tumor burden allowing partial nephrectomy following preoperative chemotherapy in biopsy proved Wilms' tumor. *J Urol* 1991;**146**:509–13.

73 Greenberg M, Burnweit C, Filler R *et al.* Preoperative chemotherapy for children with Wilms' tumor. *J Pediatr Surg* 1991;**26**:949–53.

74 Saarinen UM, Wikström S, Koskimies O, Sariola H. Percutaneous needle biopsy preceding preoperative chemotherapy in the management of massive renal tumors in children. *J Clin Oncol* 1991;**9**:406–15.

75 Zuppan CW, Beckwith JB, Weeks DA, Luckey DW, Pringle KC. The effect of preoperative therapy on the histologic features of Wilms' tumor: an analysis of cases from the Third National Wilms' Tumor Study. *Cancer* 1991;**68**:385–94.

76 Zoeller G, Pekrun A, Lakomek M, Ringert R-H. Wilms' tumor: the problem of diagnostic accuracy in children undergoing preoperative chemotherapy without histological tumor verification. *J Urol* 1994;**151**:169–71.

77 Tournade MF, Com-Nougué C, Voûte PA *et al.* Results of the Sixth International Society of Pediatric Oncology Wilms' Tumor Trial and Study: a risk-adapted therapeutic approach in Wilms' tumor. *J Clin Oncol* 1993;**11**:1014–23.

78 Green DM, Breslow NE, Beckwith JB *et al*. Treatment outcomes in patients less than 2 years of age with small, stage I, favorable-histology Wilms' tumors: a report from the National Wilms' Tumor Study. *J Clin Oncol* 1993;**11**:91–5.

79 Green DM, Jaffe N. The role of chemotherapy in the treatment of Wilms' tumor. *Cancer* 1979;**44**:52–7.

80 Larsen E, Perez-Atayde A, Green DM *et al*. Surgery only for the treatment of patients with stage I (Cassady) Wilms' tumor. *Cancer* 1990;**66**:264–6.

81 Hanna MK, Samowitz HR. Rationale for partial nephrectomy in selected cases of Wilms' tumor. *Dialog Pediatr Urol* 1991;**14**:3–4.

82 Ritchey ML, Kelalis PP, Breslow N *et al*. Surgical complications after nephrectomy for Wilms' tumor. *Surg Gynecol Obstet* 1992;**175**:507–14.

83 Breslow N, Sharples K, Beckwith JB *et al*. Prognostic factors in nonmetastatic, favorable histology Wilms' tumor: results of the Third National Wilms' Tumor Study. *Cancer* 1991; **68**:2345–53.

84 Grundy P, Breslow N, Green DM *et al*. Prognostic factors for children with recurrent Wilms' tumor: results from the Second and Third National Wilms' Tumor Study. *J Clin Oncol* 1989;**7**:638–47.

85 Green DM, Breslow NE, Li Y *et al*. The role of surgical excision in the management of relapsed Wilms' tumor patients with pulmonary metastases: a report from the National Wilms' Tumor Study. *J Pediatr Surg* 1991;**26**: 728–33.

86 D'Angio GJ, Breslow N, Beckwith JB *et al*. Treatment of Wilms' tumor: results of the Third National Wilms' Tumor Study. *Cancer* 1989;**64**:349–60.

87 Clausen N. Late recurrence of Wilms' tumor. *Med Pediatr Oncol* 1982;**10**:557–61.

88 Finklestein JZ, Norkool P, Green DM, Breslow N, D'Angio GJ. Diastolic hypertension in Wilms' tumor survivors: a late effect of treatment? A report from the National Wilms' Tumor Study Group. *Am J Clin Oncol* 1993;**16**:201–5.

89 Argueso LR, Ritchey ML, Boyle ET Jr *et al*. Prognosis of children with solitary kidney after unilateral nephrectomy. *J Urol* 1992;**148**:747–51.

90 Evans AE, Norkool P, Evans I, Breslow N, D'Angio GJ. Late effects of treatment for Wilms' tumor: a report from the National Wilms' Tumor Study Group. *Cancer* 1991;**67**:331–6.

91 Breslow NE, Norkool PA, Olshan A, Evans A, D'Angio GJ. Second malignant neoplasms in survivors of Wilms' tumor: a report from the National Wilms' Tumor Study. *J Natl Cancer Inst* 1988;**80**:592–5.

92 Macklis RM, Oltikar A, Sallan SE. Wilms' tumor patients with pulmonary metastases. *Int J Radiat Oncol Biol Phys* 1991;**21**:1187–93.

93 Cosentino CM, Raffensperger JG, Luck SR *et al*. A 25-year experience with renal tumors of childhood. *J Pediatr Surg* 1993;**28**:1350–4.

94 Green DM. Effects of treatment for childhood cancer on vital organ systems. *Cancer* 1993;**71**:3299–305.

95 Green DM, Finklestein JZ, Tefft ME, Norkool P. Diffuse interstitial pneumonitis after pulmonary irradiation for metastatic Wilms' tumor: a report from the National Wilms' Tumor Study. *Cancer* 1989;**63**:450–3.

96 Montgomery BT, Kelalis PP, Blute ML *et al*. Extended followup of bilateral Wilms' tumor: results of the National Wilms' Tumor Study. *J Urol* 1991;**146**:514–18.

97 Blute ML, Kelalis PP, Offord KP *et al*. Bilateral Wilms' tumor. *J Urol* 1987;**138**:968–73.

98 Hamida MB, Bedrossian J, Pruna A *et al*. Wilms' tumor and renal transplantation: a case report and literature review. *Transplant Proc* 1993;**25**:2346–7.

99 Shaul DB, Srikanth MM, Ortega JA, Mahour GH. Treatment of bilateral Wilms' tumor: comparison of initial biopsy and chemotherapy to initial surgical resection in the preservation of renal mass and function. *J Pediatr Surg* 1992;**27**:1009–14.

100 Beckwith JB. Precursor lesions of Wilms' tumor: clinical and biological implications. *Med Pediatr Oncol* 1993;**21**:158–68.

101 White KS, Kirks DR, Bove KE. Imaging of nephroblastomatosis: an overview. *Radiology* 1992;**182**:1–5.

102 Fernbach SK, Feinstein KA, Donaldson JS, Baum ES. Nephroblastomatosis: comparison of CT with US and urography. *Radiology* 1988;**166**:153–6.

103 Cormier PJ, Donaldson JS, Gonzalez-Crussi F. Nephroblastomatosis: missed diagnosis. *Radiology* 1988;**169**:737–8.

104 Shapiro E, Strother D. Pediatric genitourinary rhabdomyosarcoma. *J Urol* 1992;**148**:1761–8.

105 Mandell LR. Ongoing progress in the treatment of childhood rhabdomyosarcoma. *Oncology* (Williston Park, NY) 1993;**7**: 71–83.

106 Mostofi FK, Morse WH. Polypoid rhabdomyosarcoma (sarcoma botryoides) of the bladder in children. *J Urol* 1952;**67**:681–7.

107 Kodet R, Newton WA Jr, Hamoudi AB *et al*. Childhood rhabdomyosarcoma with anaplastic (pleomorphic) features: a report of the Intergroup Rhabdomyosarcoma Study. *Am J Surg Pathol* 1993;**17**:443–53.

108 Boyle ET Jr, Reiman HM, Kramer SA *et al*. Embryonal rhabdomyosarcoma of bladder and prostate: nuclear DNA patterns studied by flow cytometry. *J Urol* 1988;**140**:1119–21.

109 Crist WM, Garnsey L, Beltangady MS *et al*. Prognosis in children with rhabdomyosarcoma: a report of the Intergroup Rhabdomyosarcoma Studies I and II. *J Clin Oncol* 1990;**8**: 443–52.

110 Shapiro DN, Parham DM, Douglass EC *et al*. Relationship of tumor-cell ploidy to histologic subtype and treatment outcome in children and adolescents with unresectable rhabdomyosarcoma. *J Clin Oncol* 1991;**9**:159–66.

111 Pappo AS, Etcubanas E, Santana VM *et al*. A phase II trial of ifosfamide in previously untreated children and adolescents with unresectable rhabdomyosarcoma. *Cancer* 1993;**71**: 2119–25.

112 Lee W, Han K, Harris CP, Meisner LF. Detection of aneuploidy and possible deletion in paraffin-embedded rhabdomyosarcoma cells with FISH. *Cancer Genet Cytogenet* 1993;**68**:99–103.

113 Pizzo PA, Horowitz ME, Poplack DG, Hays DM, Kun LE. Solid tumors of childhood. In: DeVita VT Jr, Hellman S, Rosenberg SA, eds. *Cancer: Principles and Practice of Oncology*, 3rd edn. Philadelphia: JB Lippincott, 1989: 1647–54.

114 Chan HSL, Thorner PS, Haddad G, Ling V. Immunohistochemical detection of P-glycoprotein: prognostic correlation of soft tissue sarcoma of childhood. *J Clin Oncol* 1990;**8**: 689–704.

115 Schwab M, Alitalo K, Klempnauer K-H *et al*. Amplified DNA with limited homology to *myc* cellular oncogene is shared by human neuroblastoma cell lines and a neuroblastoma tumour [Letter]. *Nature* 1983;**305**:245–8.

116 Mitani K, Kurosawa H, Suzuki A et al. Amplification of N-myc in a rhabdomyosarcoma. Jpn J Cancer Res 1986;77: 1062–5.

117 Garson JA, Clayton J, McIntyre P, Kemshead JT. N-myc oncogene amplification in rhabdomyosarcoma at release [Letter]. Lancet 1986;1:1496.

118 LaQuaglia M. Genitourinary rhabdomyosarcoma in children. Urol Clin North Am 1991;18:575–80.

119 Fletcher BD, Kaste SC. Magnetic resonance imaging for diagnosis and follow-up of genitourinary, pelvic, and perineal rhabdomyosarcoma. Urol Radiol 1992;14:263–72.

120 Hays DM, Shimada H, Raney RB Jr et al. Clinical staging and treatment results in rhabdomyosarcoma of the female genital tract among children and adolescents. Cancer 1988;61: 1893–903.

121 Leuschner I, Newton WA Jr, Schmidt D et al. Spindle cell variants of embryonal rhabdomyosarcoma in the paratesticular region: a report of the Intergroup Rhabdomyosarcoma Study. Am J Surg Pathol 1993;17:221–30.

122 Raney RB Jr, Gehan EA, Hays DM et al. Primary chemotherapy with or without radiation therapy and/or surgery for children with localized sarcoma of the bladder, prostate, vagina, uterus, and cervix: a comparison of the results in Intergroup Rhabdomyosarcoma Studies I and II. Cancer 1990;66:2072–81.

123 Maurer HM, Gehan EA, Beltangady M et al. The Intergroup Rhabdomyosarcoma Study-II. Cancer 1993;71:1904–22.

124 Hays DM. Bladder/prostate rhabdomyosarcoma: results of the Multi-Institutional Trials of the Intergroup Rhabdo-myosarcoma Study. Semin Surg Oncol 1993;9: 520–3.

125 LaQuaglia MP, Ghavimi F, Herr H et al. Prognostic factors in bladder and bladder–prostate rhabdomyosarcoma. J Pediatr Surg 1990;25:1066–72.

126 LaQuaglia MP, Ghavimi F, Heller G et al. Mortality in pediatric paratesticular rhabdomyosarcoma: a multivariate analysis. J Urol 1989;142:473–8.

127 Blyth B, Mandell J, Bauer SB et al. Paratesticular rhabdomyosarcoma: results of therapy in 18 cases. J Urol 1990;144:1450–3.

128 Raney RB Jr, Hays DM, Lawrence W Jr et al. (for the Intergroup Rhabdomyosarcoma Study Committee). Paratesticular rhabdomyosarcoma in childhood. Cancer 1978;42: 729–36.

129 Raney RB Jr, Tefft M, Lawrence W Jr et al. Paratesticular sarcoma in childhood and adolescence: a report from the Intergroup Rhabdomyosarcoma Studies I and II, 1973–1983. Cancer 1987;60:2337–43.

130 Rodary C, Gehan EA, Flamant F et al. Prognostic factors in 951 nonmetastatic rhabdomyosarcoma in children: a report from the International Rhabdomyosarcoma Workshop. Med Pediatr Oncol 1991;19:89–95.

131 Kay R. Prepubertal testicular tumor registry. Urol Clin North Am 1993;20:1–5.

132 Connolly JA, Gearhart JP. Management of yolk sac tumors in children. Urol Clin North Am 1993;20:7–14.

133 Brosman SA. Testicular tumors in prepubertal children. Urology 1979;13:581–8.

134 Kramer SA, Wold LE, Gilchrist GS, Svensson J, Kelalis PP. Yolk sac carcinoma: an immunohistochemical and clinico-pathologic review. J Urol 1984;131:315–18.

135 Rushton HG, Belman AB. Testis-sparing surgery for benign lesions of the prepubertal testis. Urol Clin North Am 1993;20:27–37.

136 Rushton HG, Belman AB, Sesterhenn I, Patterson K, Mostofi FK. Testicular sparing surgery for prepubertal teratoma of the testis: a clinical and pathological study. J Urol 1990;144: 726–30.

137 Tsuchida Y, Endo Y, Saito S et al. Evaluation of alpha-fetoprotein in early infancy. J Pediatr Surg 1978;13:155–6.

138 Klein EA. Tumor markers in testis cancer. Urol Clin North Am 1993;20:67–73.

139 Thava V, Cooper N, Egginton JA. Yolk sac tumour of the testis in childhood. Br J Radiol 1992;65:1142–4.

140 Wold LE, Kramer SA, Farrow GM. Testicular yolk sac and embryonal carcinomas in pediatric patients: comparative immunohistochemical and clinicopathologic study. Am J Clin Pathol 1984;81:427–35.

141 Gonzalez-Crussi F, Roth LM. The human yolk sac and yolk sac carcinoma: an ultrastructural study. Hum Pathol 1976;7:675–91.

142 Shirai T, Itoh T, Yoshiki T et al. Immunofluorescent demonstration of alpha-fetoprotein and other plasma proteins in yolk sac tumor. Cancer 1976;38:1661–7.

143 Kurman RJ, Scardino PT, McIntire KR, Waldmann TA, Javadpour N. Cellular localization of alpha-fetoprotein and human chorionic gonadotropin in germ cell tumors of the testis using an indirect immunoperoxidase technique: a new approach to classification utilizing tumor markers. Cancer 1977;40:2136–51.

144 Nogales-Fernandez F, Silverberg SG, Bloustein PA, Martinez-Hernandez A, Pierce GB. Yolk sac carcinoma (endodermal sinus tumor): ultrastructure and histogenesis of gonadal and extragonadal tumors in comparison with normal human yolk sac. Cancer 1977;39:1462–74.

145 Kaneko M, Takeuchi T, Tsuchida Y, Saito S, Endo Y. Alpha-fetoprotein and other serum proteins synthesized by endodermal sinus tumor transplanted into nude mice. Gann in Im 1980;71:14–17.

146 Kramer SA. Pediatric oncology update. Probl Urol 1990;4: 606–23.

147 Leonard MP, Jeffs RD, Leventhal B, Gearhart JP. Pediatric testicular tumors: the Johns Hopkins experience. Urology 1991;37:253–6.

148 Cortez JC, Kaplan GW. Gonadal stromal tumors, gonadoblastomas, epidermoid cysts, and secondary tumors of the testis in children. Urol Clin North Am 1993;20:15–26.

149 Dilworth JP, Farrow GM, Oesterling JE. Non-germ cell tumors of testis. Urology 1991;37:399–417.

150 Srikanth MS, West BR, Ishitani M et al. Benign testicular tumors in children with congenital adrenal hyperplasia. J Pediatr Surg 1992;27:639–41.

22   Office Practice of Paediatric Urology
J.L.Edens, K.M.Gil and L.R.King

Introduction

In paediatric urology, when dealing with congenital anomalies in neonates, infants and young children it is essential to gain rapport quickly with the parents and with the children themselves when they are old enough to respond. The surroundings should be as non-threatening as possible (Fig. 22.1): wood is better than chrome; pictures and cartoon figures should be used liberally for decoration. Whenever possible, medical paraphernalia such as otoscopes, blood pressure cuffs, syringes and needles should be kept out of sight. Many children have ear infections and one look at a wall-mounted otoscope may be enough to cause terror and crying which prevents all but the most cursory physical examination.

Try to gain the trust of children by talking to them directly. Ask what is the matter or how school is going. Most children do not respond very much at this point. Then ask if it is all right to ask their mother or father about them and get the history.

Since most diseases, even if not known to be inherited, have at least a slight familial tendency, get a good family history. Uncle Joe may have lost a kidney, and the family are terrified at what enuresis may portend. Primary reflux, infantile renal cystic disease and enuresis are clearly inherited and many other lesions, such as pelviureteric junction (PUJ) obstruction, crop up frequently in occasional families [1]. We have one family in whom urethral valves, primary reflux, obstructive megaureter and PUJ obstruction have been encountered over six generations.

The history of the present illness may amount to no more than the chief complaint in an infant (or fetus) or may be a seemingly endless litany in children with multiple urinary tract infections (UTIs), incontinence or hypospadias. Try to find out how urine specimens were collected and how much time went by before the specimen or culture was processed. Was the child symptomatic when the infection was detected? How has the incontinence been treated? What is the pattern of wetting? What is the dry interval? Is the child a girl, and always a little damp? This suggests an ectopic ureter or short urethra. Is the child dry when uninfected? Children with frequent infections occasionally present because of 'incontinence'.

In other words, take your time and follow-up as much as necessary. It may take a lot of effort to clarify the pattern of wetting or break down 'she is infected all the time' into the true pattern. I usually ask a child directly about pain during the physical examination, and ask them to point where it hurt, or hurts. Perineal or suprapubic pain during voiding tends to confirm a UTI. Periumbilical pain is very common in children, and often a cause cannot be found. On the other hand, such discomfort has urological origins, such as PUJ obstruction, in about 4% of such patients.

Look at the genitalia. Palpate the testes in boys and feel for cord thickening which suggests a hernia. If a hydrocele is present, try to squeeze the fluid into the peritoneum to demonstrate a communication, and to palpate the testis. If the hydrocele does not reduce, and the testis cannot be felt, get an ultrasound done. Infant hydroceles are almost always reabsorbed by the age of 2 years, but hydroceles in older children persist, and tend to enlarge gradually, so should usually be treated when they are relatively small.

If the testes are thought to be cryptorchid, examine the inguinal area by compressing the inguinal canal with one hand. With the other, palpate the testis and try to milk it into the scrotum. If the testis cannot be felt, it may still be within the canal and visible on ultrasound. If the testis is still not visualized, there is a 60% chance that it is present at or above the internal ring. Conversely, about 40% of 'impalpable' testes will have been lost to torsion, sometimes before descent has occurred. Pex the opposite testis if the impalpable testis is found to be absent.

If neither testis is palpable, a follicle-stimulating hormone (FSH) stimulation test is required to see if at least one testis is present. Measure the baseline testosterone level and then stimulate the testis with 500 IU/day for 3 days. The presence of a testis is signalled by a five to eightfold increase in serum testosterone. Alternately, one can give a therapeutic dose of FSH, usually 70 IU/kg twice a week for 3 weeks, remeasuring the testosterone during

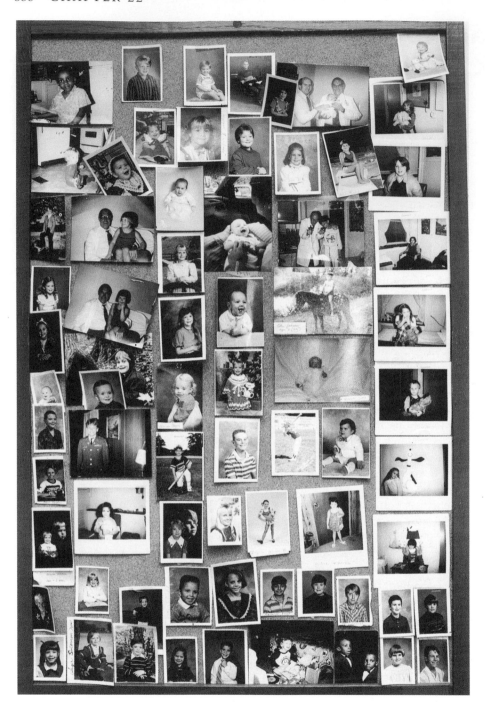

Fig. 22.1 We keep bulletin boards with photographs of patients. Children like to see themselves on return visits, and new patients are reassured when they realize they are not the only ones with a disease.

the second week. About 30% of bilaterally cryptorchid testes will descend. Hormonal stimulation works best in children with hypopituitarism or some syndrome affecting the hypothalamus, and can be used to differentiate retractile testes from those that are truly undescended.

Hypospadias is a common anomaly affecting two or three boys per 1000. The risk in first-degree relatives is about 14%. If the testes are descended and no hernia are present sex is not in question, though a rare true hermaphrodite may have normal male genitalia except for an undescended gonad. If hypospadias and cryptorchidism are associated it is safest to do a karyotype to make sure the boy is a genetic male.

In girls, look at the genitalia. An ectopic ureter can seldom be detected but coughing or straining may cause leakage from the urethra. Look at the spine. There is normally a dimple at the base of the coccyx, but other pits, bulges, hairs, café-au-lait spots and haemangioma may be clues to the presence of a closed meningocele, lipomeningocele or tethered cord (Fig. 22.2). Examine the

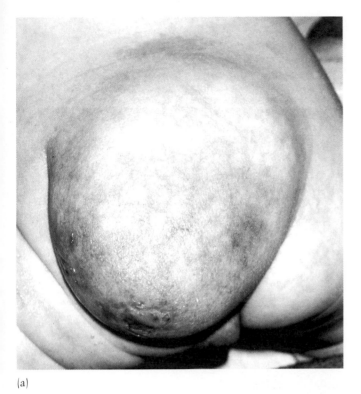

(a)

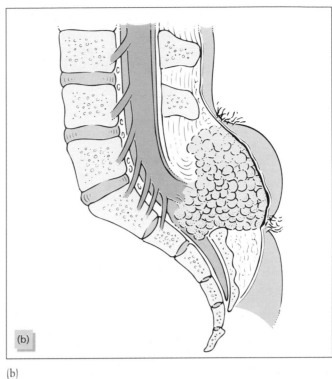

(b)

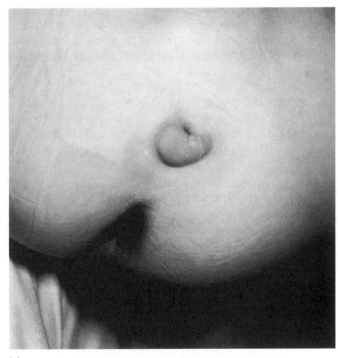

(c)

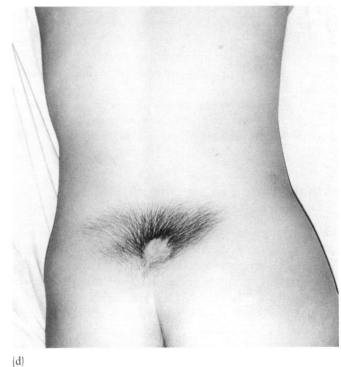

(d)

Fig. 22.2 Examination of the back is an important part of the physical examination (a, b). A lipomeningocele is usually obvious. Tethered spinal cords, which may result in incontinence, are often subtle but usually manifest by a dimple connecting the spinal cord to the skin (c) or a hairy nevus (d). Other clues include minor degrees of spinal deformity (e, f), hair, café-au-lait spots or a V-shaped gluteal cleft.

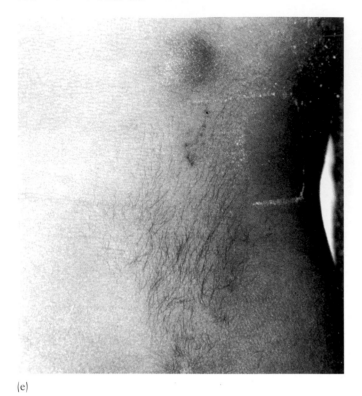

(e)

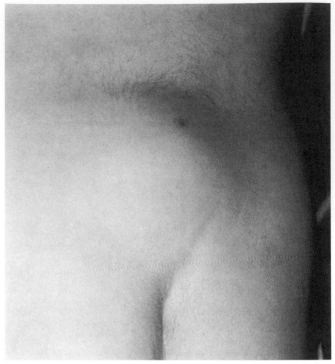

(f)

Fig. 22.2 *Continued.*

legs for symmetry and observe gait. Refer the child to a neurologist who will image the spinal cord to make sure it is normal.

Be sure to look at the growth chart. Check the blood pressure if this has not been done even if you have to send the baby to the nursery where a Doppler stethoscope is available.

Urinalysis and urine culture

Children often present with a vague history of UTI; there are few symptoms but positive cultures. The question of infection hangs on the method of urine collection and the handling of the specimen. Did a girl clean the genitalia before voiding, and sit with her legs apart to collect a mid-stream sample? Was the urine refrigerated before bringing it in? Was a culture done expeditiously, or did the urine incubate at room temperature before plating? Parents can answer some of these questions, but not all.

If you do not know the referring physician, and the child was not sick, it is usually best to assume that the urine grew contaminants. Explain this to the parents and ask them to do home cultures with uricults (Fig. 22.3), or to bring the child in whenever he or she is ill. Get fresh urine in the clinic and plate it immediately; as a cross-check, also get a urinalysis done. UTIs are possible with few white blood cells (WBCs), but this is unusual except in children

with a neurogenic bladder. Many, on intermittent catheterization, will have WBCs in the urine, but negative cultures. As the urologist, you are the last resort. If unexpected pyuria is present, get more fresh urine after routine cleansing. Recently we saw an asymptomatic girl with a history of UTI with 32 WBC/hpf. On a repeat urine there were 0–2 WBC/hpf! The technique of urine collection is very important in females, especially older girls, where WBCs are normally present in vaginal secretions.

Be alert to the possibility of misleading urinalyses and cultures. Know how the urine was collected and how it was processed. It is very hard to convince parents that a little girl has not had UTIs when they come in after five or six positive cultures, but this scenario is actually fairly frequent.

Many potential patients now present before birth. Sonograms are reviewed, the parents are counselled about the possible diagnosis and what to expect by way of evaluation after birth. We make every effort to get the neonate on antibacterial prophylaxis in case reflux is present, hoping to prevent a first infection and the generalized renal scarring that may result according to the 'big bang' theory. The ultrasound is repeated and a cystogram performed 2 or 3 days after birth. If reflux is absent, and the hydronephrosis persists, a renal scan with frusemide is usually the next step to try to distinguish non-obstructed dilatation from obstruction. We usually get this scan performed as quickly as possible, at a few days of age, to allay parental anxiety and to make an exact diagnosis if

Colony density chart

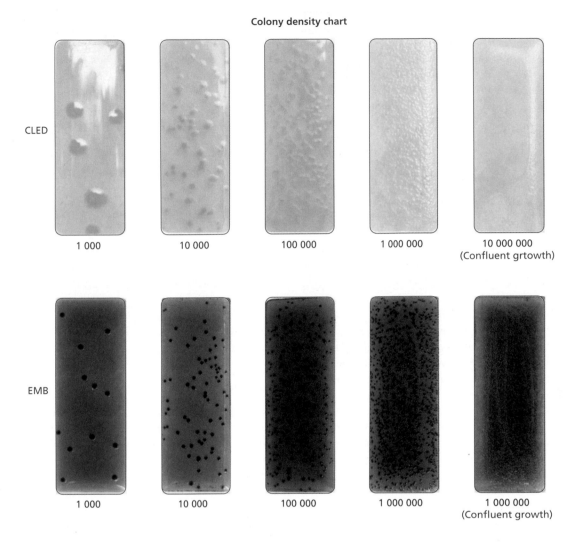

Fig. 22.3 Urocults are home culture kits used to detect bacteriuria in children with recurrent urinary infections without symptoms or with non-specific symptoms. Colony counts greater than 100 000 bacteria/cm³ usually indicate that a UTI is present.

possible. The kidney is immature, but the proportion of function in the dilated kidney and drainage characteristics persist with growth in our experience [2].

Hydronephrosis presenting in older children — as haematuria, pain, UTI or a mass — is managed in the same manner. We now see very few such cases between 1 and 6 years of age, suggesting that most are now being detected *in utero* and treated soon after birth.

UTI is a very common presenting complaint, especially in girls after toilet training. In male neonates, UTIs are usually associated with a normal urinary tract and seem to be mostly ascending infections secondary to non-circumcision. The converse is true of female infants. Many (45%) have reflux or upper tract obstruction, so girls are

evaluated by cystogram and upper tract imaging after a first infection until they are toilet trained.

Cystography is the most important imaging study. The catheter can be inserted almost painlessly, but the technician doing the study needs to be experienced — in catheterization and in putting patients and their parents at ease. A conventional radiographic study, using spot film technique with films during voiding, is preferred in males because the urethra must be seen to exclude obstruction. A better case can be made for isotope or nuclear cystography as the initial study in females, as the radioactivity images the urinary tract during the entire study and is therefore more accurate in detecting reflux, which is the most common anomaly found. Grade I reflux into the ureter only is not detected, and ureteroceles are usually not seen. However, hydronephrosis, and usually hydroureters and ureteroceles are well seen on real-time ultrasound, which is why the sonogram is now used for upper tract imaging in most patients. Sonography does not give any information about renal function, so a renal scan is usually performed if hydronephrosis is found. Multicystic kidneys often have a large medial cyst and smaller peripheral cysts on ultrasound, and mimic PUJ obstruction. The reverse is also occasionally seen, when apparent typical PUJ obstruction on ultrasound proves to be a functionless cystic dysplastic kidney on the scan. Frusemide urograms are recommended to assess function when either diagnosis seems most likely.

Incontinence

Toilet training is a rather mystifying event to parents and, we suspect, to most doctors. Every mother and grandmother seems sure she understands it, and tends to generalize her own experiences. Our own prejudice is that children simply more or less copy their parents or siblings when they are old enough to get the idea. In any case, girls train earlier than boys, perhaps because young children are with their mother more. Ninety per cent or more are dry in the daytime by the age of 3 years, and over 95% by 3.5 years. This is the earliest age that we like to treat diurnal wetting as the child must be old enough to realize that he or she is 'different' from his or her peers, and that there is a problem. Wetting and perineal dampness must predispose to UTI by allowing bacterial colonization, because about 50% of the girls we see with daytime wetting have a history of UTI. Those with a history of infections are screened by history to make sure they are wet when not infected, because, of course, infection is a common cause of urge incontinence and associated dysuria may make a child hold their urine and only void a small amount very frequently.

Children with a history of UTI, mostly girls, are screened with a voiding cystourethrogram (VCU) and ultrasound. When possible, sonography is used to estimate the thickness of the bladder wall. A thickened bladder wall suggests sphincter dyssynergia, especially if the parents volunteer that the child squats abruptly in an attempt to prevent urine leakage. However, bladder hyperactivity — spontaneous contractions — is another common explanation. Those with reflux and those with a history of many UTIs are placed on antibacterial prophylaxis. Oxybutynin is also used in small doses when reflux is present, as considerable evidence exists to show that lowering the intravesical pressure ameliorates or stops the reflux [3,4]. In the main, however, we treat daytime wetting with behaviour modification techniques. The children and their families are evaluated and treated by a psychologist, as described below.

Clinical evaluation

Following a thorough urological evaluation to rule out UTI, physiological anomalies or other medical complications, a child with daytime wetting is referred for behavioural management of his or her symptoms. While some parents merely want a 'magic bullet' for their child's symptoms, many are reluctant to administer medication to their child and are pleased to be offered a behavioural alternative. The first visit generally involves a comprehensive clinical interview where the focus is primarily upon behavioural patterns rather than potential psychopathology or emotional disturbance. Empirical research investigating the role of emotional disturbance in the development of non-organic enuresis has consistently failed to find a significant relationship between the two [5–10]. Thus, we feel a more problem-focused approach is warranted.

Begin the interview by briefly engaging the child in conversation to help allay his or her fears regarding the evaluation. It is useful to assure the child that, although the problem may seem embarrassing or difficult to talk about, it is actually quite common. Encourage the child to answer questions during the inteview and continue to actively engage the child in the interview process throughout the session. It is surprising how often even a young child can provide more accurate information about wetting patterns than can parents.

Presenting problem

Although the presenting problem may be well described in the referral, reassess this area through talking to both the child and the parents. Inconsistencies in symptom report may become evident and should be more thoroughly evaluated to gain an accurate symptom picture (i.e. wetting frequency or the quantity of voided urine may be over- or underreported). Also, parents who are unsure of actual wetting patterns may offer grossly inaccurate estimates of their child's behaviour in an attempt to respond to the clinician's questions. Beyond that, a great deal of non-verbal information can be gleaned from family members during problem description. For example, parents who are frustrated with their child or a child who is experiencing conflict with his or her parents may indicate these feelings through facial expressions, intonation and body posturing long before such problems will be verbally endorsed, and these types of unresolved conflicts can have a strong, negative impact upon treatment course and outcome. What are all of the symptoms (wetting, soiling, leaking, urgency) and temporal issues (diurnal, nocturnal or during school) related to the problem? How does the child feel about the problem?

Developmental history

It is important to assess whether the child has generally met developmental milestones. Enuresis in a 7-year-old with pervasive developmental delays may represent a maturational lag which will be overcome later, while the same symptoms in a healthy child points to a need for treatment. In particular, assess when and how toilet training was undertaken and the degree of success the child had with it. Does the child truly have secondary wetting? Although most children undergo fairly typical toilet training, assessment sometimes reveals a child who was never adequately trained and may, in fact, have had a lifelong problem despite parental report to the contrary. If the child is young, a simple refresher course of toilet training may be adequate to correct the symptoms.

Medical history

Briefly assess the child for both prior urological and general medical difficulties, as they may have been temporally related to the onset of wetting. Did symptom onset coincide with a UTI or major medical problem? It is often useful to question parents about latent UTI symptoms which may have heralded the onset of secondary wetting. Some children are relatively asymptomatic or simply do not complain of symptoms, but thorough probing may yield clues about symptom aetiology. This is also a good time to assess food allergies, eating and drinking habits, as well as a family history of incontinence.

Previous management

Although most childen we see have no prior history of formal medical treatment for the daytime wetting and/or enuresis, almost every parent has tried various strategies on their own. Praise, punishment, fluid restriction, nappies and regular voiding are commonly tried. Discussion of past strategies prevents duplication of unsuccessful treatments, and also gives the clinician an excellent opportunity to highlight two important issues to parents. First, parental feelings of failure can be assuaged by explaining why past attempts at treatment did not succeed. For example, parents may report having tried a urine alarm for 1 week without success. This probably 'failed' because the 1-week trial was far too brief a period for any child to achieve or maintain nighttime dryness. This discussion may also help give parents and the child a sense that they will be able to overcome this problem if given appropriate techniques. Second, this is a good opportunity to explain clearly what treatments should not be undertaken and why (e.g. fluid restriction for a child prone to UTIs). Parental attitudes toward the wetting can also be indirectly assessed at this time. As they discuss past methods of treatment, attitudes usually becomes clear. Parents run the gamut from being tolerant or almost indulgent of wetting to ridiculing and humiliating the child, and this has clear implications for treatment. Indulgent parents must be encouraged to request that the child take responsibility for the behaviour, while ridiculing parents must provide the child with a

supportive atmosphere in which to practice and learn appropriate toileting skills.

Psychosocial functioning

It is very important to gain some understanding of how the child is functioning in general, both prior to and after the onset of the wetting problem. How is the child doing academically and socially in school? Assess whether the child is suffering negative consequences of wetting at school, such as teasing by peers or restroom privilege refusal by teachers. Unfortunately, in our experience both are fairly common. This portion of the interview is also an excellent time to involve the child in the discussion. Parents are sometimes unaware of the full extent of difficulties the child may face outside the home secondary to enuresis. Also discuss the general pattern of family life. Do both parents live in the home? Do they both work, during what hours? How are other family members responding to the wetting problem? By evaluating the child's psychosocial functioning, a clinician is better able to determine whether the wetting is symptomatic of larger family or social problems. Finally, ascertain what types of things the child likes to do or play with. This can be useful later when trying to identify reinforcers for dryness.

Management

Despite the prevalence of daytime enuresis in children, there is a paucity of empirical literature evaluating different paradigms for treatment of the disorder. While early therapeutic interventions involved the use of traditional psychotherapy for enuretics, outcome studies comparing this mode of treatment to no-treatment control groups have not revealed significant differences in cure rates between the two groups [7,11,12]. Behavioural strategies for the management of day wetting, such as Kegel exercise training, timed voiding and contingency management, have enjoyed more success both clinically and empirically.

Kegel exercise training

Although originally developed to treat stress incontinence in adults via strengthening of the urinary sphincter [13], Kegel exercises have also been shown to be effective in treating children suffering from wetting and soiling via the same physiological mechanisms [10]. In a study of the ease of training and effectiveness of these exercises in treating diurnal enuresis, Schneider et al. [14] demonstrated a 60% cure rate using only 2 hours of professional time.

Although the concept of training a small child to voluntarily contract pelvic muscles may sound like an unwieldy task to many adults, most children are able to learn the exercises fairly rapidly. First, in order to assess whether the child can already strongly contract the pelvic muscles, ask the child and/or parent if they can stop a stream of urine. If they can, they are already effectively able to do the exercise, and all that remains is to have them consistently practice that skill while not urinating to improve sphincter tone.

For a child who cannot stop a stream of urine (and many cannot), several tactics can be used to teach this skill. For a school-age child, it is generally adequate to ask that she or he practice learning how to stop a stream of urine for a few days. Ask the child to pay attention to what he or she does to make the stream slow down or stop, and to think about what the body feels like as those muscles are contracted. This is generally sufficient to help the child understand how to contract the pelvic muscles. For a younger child, developmentally delayed child or a child who continues to have difficulty with the muscle contractions, palpation of the suprapubic muscles can reveal appropriate muscle contraction and help to indicate to the child which muscles should feel tense during the exercise. We instruct children to make their 'whole body relaxed and jiggly like a bowl of jelly', then to tighten up as if they were trying to hold their urine 'during a long car trip'. Several repetitions of this exercise are generally sufficient to help a child achieve appropriate muscle contraction.

For a child who is particularly difficult to train, electromyogram-assisted (EMG) biofeedback of the perineal area can be used to assess and assist in the training of Kegel exercises. Portable biofeedback equipment which can be programmed to play music or other interesting sounds usually helps to allay a child's fears of being monitored.

Once the child understands how to contract their pelvic muscles consistently, instruct the child to practice the exercises three times a day in sets of 10. The child should tighten the pelvic muscles for 5–10 s followed by a 5 s rest. It may be helpful to demonstrate this in session, instructing the child to complete a series of 10 Kegel exercises while the clinician counts aloud. Compliance with the exercises can be facilitated by having the child designate when he or she will exercise (i.e. before school, right after school and before bed), and having him or her keep a posted record of their practice.

Kegel exercise training is the treatment of choice in our clinic, but other methods of training are sometimes cited in the literature. Bladder retention training, developed by Kimmel and Kimmel [15], involves having the child consume increasing amounts of fluid while practicing retention of the fluid over increasing periods of time. However, while this treatment tends to increase functional bladder capacity, its impact upon wetting is equivocal [16–18]. In addition, there are several programmes throughout the USA that utilize extensive, multimethod approaches to the treatment of enuresis [19,20], although a complete discussion of their methods is beyond the scope of this chapter. While these programmes offer impressive success rates (76–91%) [19,20], their programme length and degree of labour intensiveness precludes their use for all but the most intractable cases.

Timed voiding

In conjunction with the use of Kegel exercises, regularly scheduled voiding at 60 or 90 min increments helps to train children to develop a normal voiding reflex [10]. We recommend purchasing the child an inexpensive wrist watch which can be programmed to chime at the appropriate interval, thus allowing the child to be responsible for maintaining their voiding schedule. School-age children may report that they are not permitted to leave the classroom at the scheduled intervals to void, but contact with the teacher to explain the medical treatment generally resolves this problem.

Urine alarms

It is not uncommon for a child with diurnal enuresis to wet at night also, but by first treating the day wetting the nocturnal enuresis may spontaneously remit. For a child who continues to wet at night, the urine alarm [21] is often the treatment of choice. The alarm consists of a moisture-sensitive probe which can be placed on the child's underwear or night clothes. The probe activates an alarm near the child's head when urine is voided. In use for over 40 years, this treatment has been shown to be initially effective in 75–90% of children who use it for more than 17 weeks [22–25]. There is evidence that approximately one-third of these children may relapse within the first year of treatment [26], but retreatment generally results in permanent symptom remission [27]. Ironically, the exact mechanisms by which the urine alarm successfully treats nocturnal enuresis remain unclear [28].

The urine alarm is, by far, the most well-researched method of non-pharmacological treatment for enuresis. The charges by psychoanalytic psychologists that treatment with a urine alarm will result in more serious symptom substitution have been clearly refuted [29], and it has been shown to be more effective than treatment with imipramine [8]. Adjunctive treatments, such as shaping the child toward appropriate behaviour via reinforcement of successive approximation, punishment, scheduled wakenings [30], overlearning [31] and cleanliness training [30], have been recommended for use with the urine alarm to facilitate treatment, yet research has shown that these adjuncts do not significantly improve the effectiveness of the urine alarm [28,32]. Moreover, most such adjuncts are much more inconvenient for both child and parents. However, cleanliness training is one exception [30]. For some night wetters, the experience of sleeping in wet bedding does not seem to be particularly distressing. Unfortunately, for parents, the excessive cleaning and washing becomes extremely burdensome. To help clarify to the child his or her responsibility for assisting in treatment, it is important to require that the child consistently complete cleanliness training whereby the bedroom is restored to its original condition by changing sheets and night clothes, and laundering the soiled ones. This practice need not be handled as a punishment, but merely as one of the child's responsibilities.

Compliance issues

Perhaps the biggest problem with any type of treatment is non-compliance with the treatment protocol by either parents or the child. Treatment non-compliance by the child tends to be rare, because children are generally embarrassed by their wetting and are eager to work toward a solution for the problem. However, young children often forget to do their exercises, void hourly or place the urine sensor in their night clothes. In addition, they may not fully understand the techniques. Thus, it is imperative that parents initially monitor some of their child's behaviour to ensure correct and consistent use of the strategies.

Unfortunately, in our clinical practice we have found parents tend to be the most frequent offenders, admitting that they had run out of time or patience with the child or the programme. To help circumvent such difficulties, it is paramount that the parents be clearly informed that these treatments initially require some monitoring, reminding and general attention on their part. They may be frustrated initially, particularly if immediate results are not seen. However, the key to each protocol is consistent and correct practice of the behaviours. If these two criteria are not met, the programme is doomed to failure. Troubleshooting for potential problems, such as family situations which will impede the completion of the programme, is useful. In fact, even simple strategies, like providing sheets for parents to record dry days or checklists of wet or dry hours, may help circumvent poor programme follow-through.

Persistent day wetting

Most patients do well with behaviour modification, but wetting persists in about 20%, often because of limited attention span or lack of familial support. These children then get a trial of oxybutynin, if that has not been used before, starting at 2.5 mg three times a day with the dosage increasing 1 mg every 10 days until the child becomes dry or tolerance is reached. If this is not successful, we often try Sudafed® or Marax®, α-adrenergics, to tighten the internal sphincter before we resort to urodynamics. Urodynamic testing puts the child in a very abnormal situation, and it is

hard for them to cooperate. For that reason, we often start with a relatively non-invasive flow rate and EMG, using paste-on electrodes. If sphincter dyssynergia is demonstrated, we then treat with diazepam, starting with 2 mg three times a day. Results are often prompt and dramatic.

In general, if medication helps and the child becomes dry, he or she needs to stay on whatever is working for about 4 months. After this period of time most get in the 'habit' of staying dry (voiding normally) and 80% can come off medication without recurrence of wetting. Twenty per cent need to be treated for a longer period.

Many patients with neurogenic bladder and a few with obstruction, such as those with the neurogenic–non-neurogenic bladder syndrome, need to empty completely by intermittent catheterization to stay dry and to prevent infection. A clean rather than sterile technique is employed. The meatus is washed and the lubricated catheter inserted after the hands are washed, without gloves. This may help in preventing latex sensitization. Children are taught to do this themselves whenever possible, and to jiggle the catheter around and push on the bladder to get out the last drops before the catheter is removed. We like to maintain these patients on antibacterial prophylaxis with sulfa, nitrofurantoin or nalidixic acid even when reflux is absent. However, it is getting the bladder completely empty at least once or twice a day that really prevents UTI.

A subset of these children, particularly boys with sensate genitalia, are afraid to catheterize and are afraid of the catheter. One of the authors (KMG) teaches such children to accept intermittent catheterization.

Intermittent self-catheterization

Accepting intermittent self-catheterization

From a psychological standpoint, there are multiple reasons why a child might have difficulty accepting intermittent catheterization. Some children develop fear, or a conditioned aversion, to catheterization. This response may be due to a previous unpleasant exposure to catheterization or other medical procedure (e.g. VCU). Some children may be conditioned by parents to view the genitalia as 'private' and 'not to be touched'. As a result of these prior negative experiences, the child may resist all efforts to teach self-catheterization by refusal and displays of anxiety. Most of these children have never acquired the skill of self-catheterization since their anxiety prohibited appropriate training in the techniques.

A second major reason why children may not self-catheterize is poor compliance. Several factors could contribute to this non-compliance. The child may be too young (less than 6 or 7 years old) or developmentally delayed, and thus is unable understand the importance of regular self-catheterization, to comprehend or implement the actual instructions, and to remember to do self-catheterization on their own. The child could have feelings that interfere with conducting regular self-catheterization such as embarrassment at school. Some children with chronic illnesses (e.g. renal disease) may avoid dealing with catheterization because of an underlying difficulty accepting the chronic nature of their health problems. Another possibility is that the parents themselves may not be providing consistent encouragement and support. The parents may have low educational levels or not be medically sophisticated. They could have multiple other demands on their time and emotional resources (e.g. other children). In our experience, it is also possible that the parents' attitudes and feelings about the need for their child to do intermittent self-catheterization are communicated to the child. Although many parents are able to adjust to the idea of the need for self-catheterization, other parents are anxious or uncomfortable with the idea, and can unintentionally convey these negative perceptions to the child. Children with compliance problems often have the ability to self-catheterize and exhibit no fear, but they do not do intermittent catheterization on a consistent basis.

A careful assessment of the factors leading to an inability to accept self-catheterization is necessary as behavioural treatment is markedly different depending upon the underlying problem. The assessment usually involves a careful history with the child and parents, consultation with professionals who have attempted to teach self-catheterization (e.g. a paediatric urology nurse clinician) and direct observation of the child attempting to self-catheterize.

In the history with the child, it is important to assess prior experiences with catheterization and other medical procedures. Is this a child who has intense fear of all medical procedures such as immunization, or are the fears specific to catheterization? Has the child been held down and catheterized forcibly by medical staff in the past? Does the child report fear, pain or other feelings of uncomfortableness when describing their experiences with catheterization? What seems to increase or decrease their fear (e.g. mother holding hand, father praising child)? What does the child remember from earlier experiences with catheterization? What is the child's attitude toward self-catheterization and what do they think their parents think about it? Does the child have many phobias and fears unrelated to medical procedures such as fear of storms, the dark or separation from parents? This information can help to tailor treatment to the needs of the child. For example, a child with many fears might need more intensive treatment than a child with a circumscribed fear of catheterization.

In the history with the parents or guardian, it is important to get their impression of what they think the problem is with their child accepting catheterization (e.g. 'He is just stubborn' or 'She says it hurts'). What happened during the first attempts to teach self-catheterization and what has happened since then? What efforts have the parents made to get the child to self-catheterize? Are the parents expecting a young child to be responsible for this new behaviour on their own without providing proper support? For an adolescent, is the parent overly involved or overprotective? Have the parents threatened or punished the child for not catheterizing? What are the parents' attitudes toward self-catheterization (e.g. 'Why is my child different from other children?' 'This is a terrible problem that must be kept secret from others')? Is the parent convinced of the need for their child to self-catheterize or are they feeling ambivalent about it? This information can help to involve the parent appropriately in treatment. Some parents might need to learn how to motivate their child effectively whereas others might need to learn how to foster independence.

In addition to this information, a general psychosocial and developmental history is important. What is the child's school class and intellectual level? Is the child in any special classes at school for learning or behavioural problems? Are there any behavioural problems at home with chores, homework, siblings or other self-care tasks such as bathing? What is the home environment? Is the family disorganized, chaotic and full of conflict, or cohesive and supportive? Has the child been physically or sexually abused? It is also helpful to try to understand the relationship of the child to each parent and other family members. Many behavioural interventions with children require involvement of one or more family members. Although we used to assume that boys might do best with their fathers helping them learn self-catheterization, and girls might do best with mothers, in our experience we have found it is best to remain open as some girls work best with their fathers and some boys with their mothers, and sometimes a grandparent is the best resource.

To determine the child's response to previous attempts to learn self-catheterization, it is useful to consult with staff who have attempted to train the child. In our clinic, this is usually one of the paediatric nurses. The nurse's observations can be very helpful in determining what is the best treatment course. For example, some children have difficulty learning the skill because of poor coordination.

Although much information can be gained by interviewing the child, parent and staff, we always also directly observe the child to see the child's response. This is especially helpful in determining the degree of anxiety. Some children display obvious signs of distress such as crying or statements of fear, pain or discomfort. Physical tension can sometimes be noticed in the muscles of the legs, arms, face or other areas of the body. Some children will refuse to do even simple things such as hold the catheter. Usually refusal is an indication of anxiety and should not be viewed as manipulative or 'bad' behaviour. Some children easily perform the catheterization while being observed and this suggests that if anxiety does plays a part, it is not with learning the skill but in maintenance of self-catheterization on a regular basis.

Systematic desensitization for anxiety and conditioned aversion

The programme for treating anxiety about self-catheterization usually incorporates several behaviour therapy techniques including systematic desensitization, practice assignments and gradual shaping (or teaching) of the new skill [33]. The basic rationale for these procedures is that a child's conditioned fear can be eliminated by gradually substituting a relaxation response for the fear reaction while the child is slowly and systematically exposed to the feared situation. In some cases, medical necessity may prohibit this slow and gradual approach and then other tactics may be needed.

First, a psychologist teaches the child general relaxation procedures including progressive muscle relaxation, imagery and other brief relaxation strategies. Biofeedback equipment is used to assist the child in learning to recognize muscle tension and relaxation. Sensors are typically placed on the quadriceps muscles and feedback in the form of tones or lights is provided. The child is taught to use the feedback as a signal to stop and go through a brief relaxation technique (i.e. stop, take a deep breath and whisper the word relax while exhaling). The feedback can be very useful in helping the child, staff and parent know when the child is tense and when the child has actually learned how to relax. Usually, two to three 1 h sessions in the biofeedback laboratory (or area outside the clinic) are devoted to teaching relaxation and biofeedback.

Next, the task of self-catheterization is broken down into several smaller steps. These typically include: washing hands, gathering materials (catheter, wipes, gel, cup, mirror for girls), getting into a comfortable position (sitting for boys, semireclining with legs apart for girls), cleansing the urethra, touching the catheter to the opening, inserting the catheter part way, inserting the catheter until urine flows, waiting until the bladder is empty and removing the catheter when the urine flow stops. Because the rationale of desensitization is to proceed slowly and until the child masters each step, the steps can be further enumerated, if necessary. During each session in this phase of treatment, a new step (or steps) is explained and, as the child completes the step, the child is couched by the psychologist in relaxation and provided with biofeedback. Usually, the first few steps can be combined into one session. However, several sessions may be needed for the successful completion of later steps. The training can continue in a com-

fortable setting with the psychologist until the child is ready to progress to working in a clinic room. Usually, when the child is ready to begin to insert the catheter, a paediatric nurse is present to help guide the child in the proper technique. In our experience, a total of six to eight weekly sessions may be needed until the child successfully inserts the catheter for the first time. A few additional sessions focusing on both anxiety reduction and long-term compliance may be necessary to get from this first success to daily intermittent self-catheterization (see below).

Throughout treatment the child is given things to practice at home in between each session. At first, the child is instructed to practice daily with a relaxation audiotape. As the child is working through the steps of the desensitization hierarchy, he or she is instructed to practice the steps at home. Records of practice are usually kept and these can be star or sticker charts for younger children.

Usually from the very beginning the parents are involved in treatment. Initially, their role is to encourage practice at home with the relaxation audiotape and to help the child keep records. During sessions with the psychologist and in the clinic, the parent often sits in and observes, but does not have an active role until about the fourth to sixth session when the parents begin to assume the role of relaxation coach during sessions. At this time, the biofeedback equipment can be very helpful in helping parents recognize tension in their child and use it as a cue to remind the child to stop and relax. At this phase of treatment the parent will also help the child complete steps of the catheterization programme at home.

Reinforcement can be used to supplement the programme and help maintain a focus on the positive aspects. It is best to use social praise or rewards (being able to play a favourite game with mummy or daddy), access to privileges (being able stay up later) or small token gifts for the child. Eventually, the natural reinforcers (staying dry, more peer approval) should take over to maintain the behaviour and these extra reinforcements can be stopped.

We have used these procedures successfully with children as young as 6 years old, and one of these case studies containing more details is published [34]. We have also had cases that were not responsive to this approach. Obstacles that we have encountered have included parents not being able to bring the child consistently for sessions or to follow the programme consistently at home and parents not being convinced of the need for self-catheterization despite physician advice. Adolescents can sometimes be treated effectively without consistent parental support; however, it is very difficult to treat younger children if the parents are not involved.

Compliance enhancement

For children who have poor compliance but no anxiety

related to self-catheterization, different training procedures are needed. For most of these children, the programme can use straightforward reinforcement procedures similar to those used for other compliance problems such as not doing homework or chores, or not following parental instructions [35].

It is a major step for a child (or anyone) to go from not catheterizing at all to self-catheterizing three to four times each day, every day for possibly their entire lives. To get to this goal successfully, it is helpful to have the child gradually build up to it, if this is medically possible. First, the rationale for the programme must be explained to the child and parents. The programme can be described as a means to give the child added motivation and support to accomplish an important goal. The programme starts with setting an easily attainable goal (e.g. self-catheterizing once each day in the morning on school days) that is gradually increased from week to week. A calendar, diary or sticker chart can be used to record successful completion of the goal. Potential rewards are identified to reinforce the child's compliance. Again, it is best for these to be social in nature, privileges or small token rewards. Both the child and the parents are involved in setting the initial goal and agreeing to the system of providing incentives. It is important for the family to meet weekly with a psychologist or other trained professional to monitor progress, increase the goals and to tackle obstacles that may interfere with accomplishing goals. Many parents may have the impression that they tried this type of approach on their own or with the advice of a health care provider. This programme might seem relatively simple; however, it often requires professional expertise to be done effectively.

We have used this type of programme successfully with children from 7 to 16 years old. Some children have not responded to this behavioural intervention alone and have required more intensive psychological therapy. One recent adolescent with kidney disease, for example, was not compliant with self-catheterization and taking his medications. We determined that the child was non-compliant secondary to depression and had difficulty accepting his chronic illness. In cases such as this, additional psychological treatment is necessary.

Intermittent catheterization can also be used in children, usually girls, who have normal anatomy and bladder function, yet frequently develop UTIs despite antibacterial prophylaxis. We tend to cystoscope such patients for a one-time calibration of the urethra, using dilatation, and to rule out cystitis cystica. If breakthrough infections persist we teach these children to catheterize and to instill 30 g of dilute acetic acid or dilute betadine once or twice a day.

Enuresis

About 10% of children still wet the bed at least occasionally at the age of 5 years. The problem is worldwide. Enuresis is more common in boys than girls, in depressed socioeconomic populations and in dysfunctional families. It is also more common in black children and in premature infants, even correcting for the age from conception. In short, there are probably many causes of bed wetting, and we are not very good at sorting them out. Enuresis is highly familial. If one parent wet the bed to an age where it is remembered as a problem the risk in a child is about 50%. If both parents were enuretic, the risk rises to about 80%.

In most of the world, lacking money for medication, enuresis is treated by fluid restriction before bedtime and often by giving the child something salty to eat just before they go to bed. In Korea, the child must go to a neighbour to beg the salt, adding an element of embarrassment. In Poland, salted herring is often chosen. In the USA, not many children will eat herring but salty potato chips may be tried if the child can eat them without drinking.

The reward system has many proponents. The child keeps a calendar and gets a star for each dry night. After so many dry nights a prize, usually previously agreed upon and something the child wants, is awarded. As the wetting occurs when the child is asleep it is hard to explain how this technique can work, but it has its proponents.

For treatment to be successful, the child must be old enough to realize that the bed wetting is a problem, and be motivated to try to stay dry. One can determine if an effort is being made by making sure that no fluids are imbibed for 1–1.5 h prior to bedtime.

Many medicines and treatment regimens can be successful, but none are more than 65–70% successful in individual patients. The best are imipramine, deamino-D-arginine vasopressin (DDAVP) and the alarm system. The alarm system needs to be used for an average of 17 weeks before a child will stay dry without it. Since children are sound sleepers, the alarm usually awakens a parent or a sibling who must then take the patient to the bathroom. At times, the alarm awakens everyone but the enuretic child. This factor obviously limits its usefulness, but it is a non-pharmacological method of treatment which has withstood the 'test of time' and is a reasonable mode of treatment if the family can endure it.

We tend to treat enuretics pharmacologically, with fluid restriction before bedtime and imipramine or DDAVP. Imipramine is both a mild anticholinergic and an α-adrenergic so it tightens the internal sphincter while relaxing the bladder; this is a useful combination. We start with 25 mg at bedtime, and occasionally give 75 mg in a sustained release formulation in older children. If the imipramine is effective, we continue it for 4 months before stopping therapy. If the imipramine is not effective or if the child is unable to tolerate the medication, we next recommend DDAVP, 10 µg in each nostril at bedtime.

DDAVP is a synthetic antidiuretic hormone and reduces urine output markedly for 5–6 h, thus promoting dryness. One month of therapy is clearly too little to get into the habit of staying dry, so we are currently using DDAVP until the child has been dry for 4 months prior to a trial off therapy. The dosage of DDAVP may also be increased, but the medication is relatively expensive.

Most children that become dry on medication stay dry when therapy is discontinued, but 20–25% need longer treatment periods. This is not much of a disadvantage once a medication that will prevent wetting has been identified.

Procedures in the clinic

As previously mentioned, one likes the clinic environment to be as non-threatening as possible. Painful procedures should usually be performed under general anaesthesia, although there are a few exceptions. Infant circumcisions can reasonably be performed under local anaesthesia when the parents decide they want their baby circumcised (Fig. 22.4). We have found that when we talk parents out of circumcision they will often return wanting the procedure when the boy has become too large to do in restraints and a general anaesthesia is then required. We now counsel the parents against routine circumcision but do not try to dissuade them when they are adamant. One to 3 ml of 1% xylocaine is used as a dorsal nerve block and infiltrated around the base of the penis with the boy on a circumcision restraint board. A Gomco clamp is then employed. No complications are likely when the bell selected is the proper size to cover the glans, which prevents the removal of too much skin. The clamp is tightened for 5 min or more to crush the skin edges to seal them together and prevent bleeding. Circumcisions are not performed in the clinic when other children are within hearing distance.

There are a few other procedures which can sometimes be performed in the clinic under local anaesthesia. A very small urethral fistula can be cauterized. The area is anaesthetized, a needle electrode placed in the fistula, and the skin lining destroyed by fulguration. Similarly, meatotomies may be done under local anaesthesia. Most meatal stenosis results from the effect of the very alkaline urine that is formed on the exposed meatus of circumcised infants, which may cause inflammation and subsequent scarring. The lack of a foreskin clearly predisposes to meatal stenosis, but the adhesions are usually filmy. The meatus is anaesthetized with xylocaine or ethylene chloride. A small haemostat is inserted into the meatus and the jaws spread. If this manoeuvre, which takes only an instant, does not resolve the problem a formal meatotomy is required.

Finally, older children with nerve deficits and little or no feeling in the genitalia and lower abdomen can be cystoscoped without anaesthesia. A parent usually stays with the child to help keep him or her calm.

More invasive or longer procedures are virtually always performed in the operating room under general anaesthesia. Most diagnostic procedures, orchidopexies and hypospadias repairs are now performed on an outpatient basis, as are most laparoscopic operations. These children have a full hospital history and physical, haematocrit, urinalysis and paediatric anaesthesia inspection on a day prior to surgery. Very few problems have been encountered, but we often prefer to keep the hypospadias patients overnight as a '23 h admission' so that the parents can familiarize themselves with the care of catheters or drip tubes.

Conclusion

Office paediatric urology has a lot in common with veterinary medicine. The patient must be put at ease if at all possible. Frightening equipment should be kept out of sight, and used only when the patient has been prepared. Physiologically, children are not 'little adults' or midgets, and they should not be treated that way. If you can get the child on your side, they will put up with a surprising amount of discomfort. On the other hand, procedures, especially invasive procedures, should only be performed on indication. There is no such thing as a 'routine' examination; every child does not need a cystogram, although this is the most frequent invasive radiological study needed. Ultrasound can replace intravenous

Fig. 22.4 Circumcision is not medically necessary, but does protect against neonatal UTI. All the other health benefits of circumcision are provided by teaching older boys to retract the foreskin to cleanse the glans when they are taking a bath. The foreskin is adherent to the glans at birth. Full retractability should not be expected until 5 or 6 years of age.

> Was any one at the time of his call already circumcized? Let him not seek to remove the marks of circumcision. Was any one at the time of his call uncircumcized? Let him not seek circumcision. For neither circumcision counts for anything nor uncircumcision, but keeping the commandments of God.
> **1 Corinthians**

urography in many, if not most, situations. Sonography has changed paediatric urology significantly in the past decade, as most babies with hydronephrosis now present before birth. The major challenge in paediatric urology today is to utilize presumptive antenatal diagnosis to prevent renal damage and to optimize eventual renal function.

The clinic setting is the environment in which the urologist meets the patient and the family, and interacts with them. If the child has a serious problem, this contact is of overwhelming importance. If the urologist is to embark on a series of complex procedures, of uncertain outcome, as in exstrophy or neurogenic bladder, clinic contacts are of vital importance because it is there that rapport is established. Most difficulties in treatment arise if the family has not been prepared for the occasional unfavourable result of therapy. The initial rapport, gained in the clinic, helps both doctor and patient to overcome such difficulties.

References

1 Noe HN, Wyatt RJ, Peeden JN Jr, Rivas ML. The transmission of vesicoureteral reflux from parent to child. *J Urol* 1992;**148**:1869–71.
2 Chung S, Majd M, Rushton HG, Belman AB. Diuretic renography in evaluation of neonatal hydronephrosis: is it reliable? *J Urol* 1993;**150**:765–8.
3 Homsy YL, Nsouli I, Hamburger B, LaBerge I, Schick E. Effects of oxybutynin on vesicoureteral reflux in children. *J Urol* 1985;**134**:1168–71.
4 Seruca H. Vesicouteral reflux and voiding dysfunction: a prospective study. *J Urol* 1989;**142**:494–8.
5 Tapia F, Jekel J, Domke H. Enuresis: an emotional symptom? *J Nerv Ment Dis* 1960;**130**:61–5.
6 Kolvin I, Taunch J, Currah J *et al.* Enuresis: a descriptive analysis and controlled trial. *Dev Med Child Neurol* 1972;**14**:715–26.
7 Sacks S, DeLeon G, Blackman S. Psychological changes associated with conditioning functional enuresis. *J Clin Psychol* 1974;**30**:271–6.
8 Wagner W, Johnson S, Walker D, Carter R, Wittmer, J. A controlled comparison of two treatments for nocturnal enuresis. *J Pediatr* 1982;**101**:302–7.
9 Werry (1967-look up in J counsel & develop '87 5, 265).
10 Rutter M. *Helping Troubled Children.* New York: Plenum Press, 1976.
11 Werry J, Cohrssen J. Enuresis: an etiologic and therapeutic study. *J Pediatr* 1965;**67**:312–31.
12 DeLeon G, Mandell W. A comparison of conditioning and psychotherapy in the treatment of functional enuresis. *J Clin Psychol* 1966;**22**:325–30.
13 Burgio KL, Whitehead WE, Engel BT. Urinary incontinence in the elderly. *Ann Int Med* 1985;**104**:507–15.
14 Schneider MS, King LR, Surwit RS. Kegel exercise and childhood incontinence: a new role for an old treatment. *J Pediatr* (in press).
15 Kimmel H, Kimmel E. An instrumental conditioning method for the treatment of enuresis. *J Behav Ther Exp Psychiatry* 1970;**1**:121–3.
16 Doleys C, Ciminero A, Tollison J, Williams C, Wells K. Dry-bed training and retention control training: a comparison. *Behav Ther* 1977;**8**:541–8.
17 Starfield B. Functional bladder capacity in enuretic and nonenuretic children. *J Pediatr* 1967;**70**:777–81.
18 Starfield B. Enuresis: its pathogenesis and management. *Clin Pediatr* 1972;**11**:343–50.
19 Whelen J, Houts A. Effects of a waking schedule on primary enuretic children treated with full-spectrum home training. *Health Psychol* 1990;**9**:164–76.
20 Scharf M. *Waking Up Dry: How to End Bedwetting Forever.* Cincinnati: Writer's Digest, 1986.
21 Mowrer O, Mowrer W. Enuresis: a method for its study and treatment. *Am J Orthopsychiatry* 1938;**8**:436-59.
22 Abramson H, Houts A, Berman J. The effectiveness of medical and psychological treatments for childhood enuresis. Presented to the Annual Meeting of the Society for Psychotherapy Research, Wintergreen, VA, June 1990.
23 Doleys D. Behavioral treatments for nocturnal enuresis in children: a review of the recent literature. *Psychol Bull* 1977;**84**:30–54.
24 Houts A, Leibert R. *Bedwetting: a Guide for Parents and Children.* Springfield: Charles C. Thomas, 1984.
25 Johnson S. Enuresis. In: Daitzman R, ed. *Clinical Behavior Therapy and Behavior Modification.* New York: Garland, 1980: 81–142.
26 Morgan R. Relapse and therapeutic response in the conditioning treatment of enuresis: a review of recent findings on intermittent reinforcement, overlearning, and stimulus intensity. *Behav Res Ther* 1978;**16**:273–9.
27 Forsythe W, Redmond A. Enuresis and the electric alarm: study of 200 cases. *Br Med J* 1970;**1**:211–13.
28 Houts A. Nocturnal enuresis as a biobehavioral problem. *Behav Ther* 1991;**22**:133–51.
29 Baker BL. Symptom treatment and symptom substitution in enuresis. *J Abnorm Psychol* 1969;**74**:42–9.
30 Azrin N, Sneed T, Foxx R. Dry-bed training: rapid elimination of childhood enuresis. *Behav Res Ther* 1974;**12**:147–56.
31 Young G, Morgan R. Conditioning treatment of enuresis: auditory intensity. *Behav Res Ther* 1972;**11**:411–16.
32 Fournier J, Garfinkle B, Bond A *et al.* Pharmacological and behavioral management of enuresis. *J Am Acad Child Adolesc Psychiatry* 1987;**26**:849–853.
33 Hersen M, Bellack AS. *Handbook of Clinical Behavior Therapy.* New York: Plenum Press, 1985.
34 Gil KM, Perry G, King L. The use of biofeedback in a behavioral program designed to teach an anxious child self-catheterization. *Biofeedback Self Regul* 1988;**13**:347–55.
35 Forehand RJ, McMahon RJ. *Helping the Noncompliant Child: a Clinician's Guide to Parent Training.* New York: Guilford Press, 1981.

Section 3
Urodynamic Disorders

Section 3a
Upper Urinary Tract

23 Anatomy of the Urinary Tract

J.A.Gosling and J.S.Dixon

The kidneys

Each kidney is of a characteristic shape possessing superior and inferior poles, a gently convex lateral border and an indented medial border. The anterior and posterior surfaces are usually smoothly convex, although marked lobulation, a normal feature before birth and during the first postnatal year, may occasionally persist into adult life. The kidney of an adult weighs 135–150 g and measures approximately 11 cm from pole to pole, 6 cm from lateral to medial border and 3 cm from anterior to posterior surface. Frequently, the left kidney is a little longer and more slender than the right. The medial border of each kidney presents an oval aperture, the hilum, which is traversed by the proximal parts of the urinary tract and by the renal vessels, lymphatics and nerves. The kidneys lie in the retroperitoneal tissues and their precise orientations are determined by the topography of the muscles of the posterior abdominal wall. As the kidneys are applied to the medial slopes of the paravertebral gutters, their anterior surfaces are directed laterally as well as forwards. The diverging lateral borders of the psoas major muscles cause relatively wide separation of the inferior poles of the kidneys. In addition, the anterior curve of the lumbar spine results in the inferior poles lying on a more anterior plane than the superior poles.

Perirenal tissues

Each kidney is closely invested by a continuous covering of fibrous tissue, the renal capsule. In the living, this capsule exerts tension upon the renal parenchyma, and causes kidney substance to bulge through an incision into the capsule. Each kidney within its capsule is embedded in a mass of adipose tissue lying between the peritoneum and the posterior abdominal wall (Fig. 23.1). The fat immediately adjacent to the renal capsule is named the 'perirenal fat'. This adipose tissue is enclosed by the renal fascia, which is itself covered both anteriorly and posteriorly by the pararenal fat. The renal fascia possesses anterior and posterior layers which subdivide the retro-

peritoneal tissues on each side of the midline into three potential spaces. The posterior space (posterior pararenal space) contains only fat and this can be traced laterally into the anterolateral abdominal wall where it is in continuity with a layer of adipose tissue lying between the transversalis fascia and the peritoneum. The intermediate space (perirenal space) contains the kidney and suprarenal gland together with the perirenal fat. The anterior space (anterior pararenal space) is a more extensive compartment and, unlike the posterior and intermediate spaces, extends across the midline from one side of the abdomen to the other. This anterior space is bounded by the anterior layer of the renal fascia of each kidney and by the parietal peritoneum. It contains the ascending and descending colon, the duodenal loop and the pancreas. A detailed description of the renal fascia will serve to clarify the foregoing account.

The anterior and posterior layers of the renal fascia merge superior to the suprarenal gland where they become continuous with the diaphragmatic fascia. Traced medially, the anterior layer blends with the connective tissue around the aorta and inferior vena cava while the posterior layer fuses with the psoas fascia. Inferior to the kidney, the two layers of renal fascia continue into the iliac fossa in the shape of a cone whose apex is directed inferiorly. In this region the two layers are relatively thin and ill defined. The ureter leaves the perirenal space obliquely by piercing the medial aspect of the fascial cone. On the lateral side of the cone the two layers of renal fascia combine to form a single layer, the lateroconal fascia, which can be traced posteriorly to the ascending or descending colon before fusing with the peritoneum of the paracolic gutter. The clinical significance of the renal fascia relates to the fact that, as it forms a closed compartment, it tends to limit the spread of effusions and exudates originating from the kidney. Such effusions are prevented from crossing the midline and tend to spread inferiorly towards the iliac fossa. The fat within the perirenal space is of relevance to radiological investigations since adipose tissue is radiolucent in comparison with renal tissue.

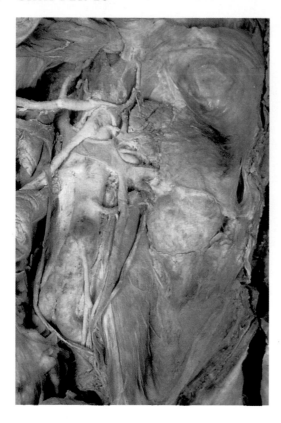

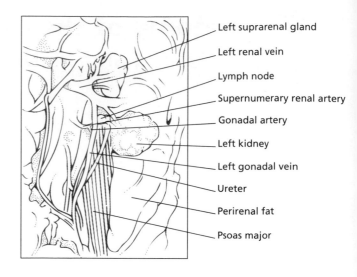

Left suprarenal gland

Left renal vein

Lymph node

Supernumerary renal artery

Gonadal artery

Left kidney

Left gonadal vein

Ureter

Perirenal fat

Psoas major

Fig. 23.1 Renal blood vessels and perirenal tissues. The left kidney illustrated in this dissection has a supernumerary artery. The digestive organs have been removed or displaced, but the left kidney and suprarenal gland remain *in situ*. Some of the perirenal fat has been removed to reveal the lower half of the kidney.

Anatomical relations of the kidneys

The posterior relations of the two kidneys are very similar and can be described collectively. However, because of the asymmetry of the digestive organs, the anterior relations of each kidney require separate descriptions.

Posterior relations of the kidneys

The 12th rib is a most useful landmark since this bone provides a guide to the location of most of the muscles, fasciae, nerves and vessels which comprise the kidneys' posterior relations. Anteroposterior radiographs usually depict the 12th rib dividing the renal outline into small superolateral and large inferomedial areas. (Because of its higher position, the left kidney is usually also related to the 11th rib.)

The medial borders of the kidneye lie anterior to the upper lumbar transverse processes. Textbook descriptions frequently state that the kidneys' inferior poles lie 2–3 cm superior to the supracristal plane (the plane passing through the uppermost parts of the iliac crests and transecting the body of the 4th lumbar vertebra). In some individuals, however, especially those of short broad stature, the interval between the costal margin and the bony pelvis may be relatively narrow. As a result, the kidneys are likely to

extend as far as or even below the supracristal plane. It must also be borne in mind that, in the living, the location of the kidneys fluctuates vertically in response to body position (such as erect or supine) and to movements of the diaphragm.

Attached to the ribs, to the vertebrae and to the ilia are muscles which, together with their associated fasciae and ligaments, form the principal posterior relations of each kidney (Fig. 23.2). The posterior aspect of a kidney can usefully be considered as four areas, each of which relates to one particular muscle. The uppermost area, superolateral to the 12th rib, is in contact with the diaphragm. The region inferomedial to the rib can be subdivided into three areas which from medial to lateral sides relate to the psoas major, the quadratus lumborum and the transversus abdominis muscle. However, since the inferior renal pole sometimes extends as far as the iliac fossa, the iliacus muscle and its fascial covering (the fascia iliaca) may also lie posterior to this part of the kidney.

The psoas major, clothed by the psoas fascia, occupies the furrow between the bodies and transverse processes of the lumbar vertebrae. The quadratus lumborum arises from the iliolumbar ligament and the adjacent part of the iliac crest and passes superiorly, tapering as it does so, to insert into the 12th rib (Fig. 23.2). The lumbar fascia (thoracolumbar or thoracodorsal fascia) attaches to the

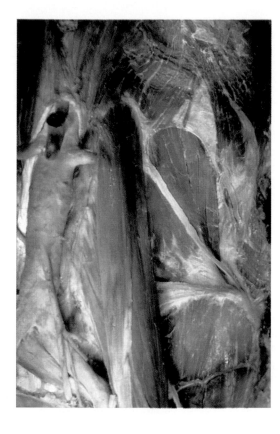

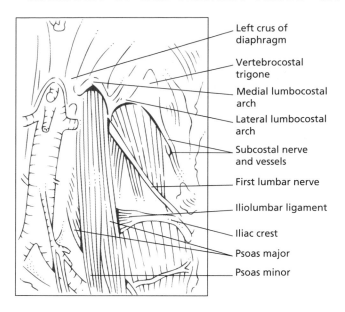

Left crus of diaphragm

Vertebrocostal trigone

Medial lumbocostal arch

Lateral lumbocostal arch

Subcostal nerve and vessels

First lumbar nerve

Iliolumbar ligament

Iliac crest

Psoas major

Psoas minor

Fig. 23.2 Muscles posterior to the left kidney: close up of the left paravertebral gutter showing the quadratus lumborum muscle, part of the diaphragm and psoas major, and the subcostal and 1st lumbar nerves.

lumbar vertebrae as three distinct layers, the anterior and middle of which enclose the quadratus lumborum muscle. The posterior layer is anchored to the spinous processes and all three layers fuse near the lateral border of quadratus lumborum to provide the aponeurotic origin for the transversus abdominis and internal oblique muscles.

As previously noted, the posterior aspect of each kidney superolateral to the 12th rib is related to the diaphragm. Not only does this part of the diaphragm take attachment from the vertebrae and ribs but it also arises from thickenings of the psoas fascia and the anterior layer of the lumbar fascia (specifically from the medial and lateral lumbocostal arches respectively; Fig. 23.2). Furthermore, there is often a triangular aperture of variable size, the vertebrocostal trigone (Fig. 23.2), situated between the vertebral and costal origins of the diaphragmatic musculature. Through this defect the perirenal tissues may be in direct contact with the pleura. It should also be noted that the inferior sulcus of the parietal pleura, the costodiaphragmatic recess, approaches the midline horizontally at the level of the disc between the last thoracic and the 1st lumbar vertebra. Therefore, the costodiaphragmatic recess of the pleura extends inferior to the medial part of the 12th rib and the pleural cavity may be opened in this situation during posterior surgical approaches to the kidney or suprarenal gland.

Other posterior relations of the kidney include the subcostal nerve and vessels and the 1st lumbar nerve (or its

iliohypogastric and ilioinguinal branches). These structures run parallel to the last rib and pass across the anterior surface of the quadratus lumborum and the aponeurosis of the transversus abdominis (see Fig. 23.2).

Anterior relations of the right kidney

The right suprarenal gland surmounts the upper pole of the right kidney and lies within the perirenal fat. The medial border of the kidney is associated, from above downwards, with the inferior vena cava, the renal vessels and the proximal part of the urinary tract.

The remaining structures relating to the right kidney all lie external to the renal fascia. Moving inferiorly from the superior pole, the organs include the liver, the duodenum, the colon (Fig. 23.3) and coils of jejunum or ileum. The peritoneum of the great sac is reflected from the anterior surface of the kidney on to the visceral surface of the liver to form the hepatorenal pouch (Morison's pouch). Superior to this peritoneal recess, the uppermost part of the kidney is related to the bare area of the liver. The second part of the duodenum (the descending duodenum) is closely apposed to the renal hilum and its retroperitoneal location places it in jeopardy when the anterior aspect of the renal pedicle is surgically exposed. The retroperitoneal ascending colon reaches the anterior aspect of the kidney (Fig. 23.3) and gains a mesentery (the transverse mesocolon) as it turns to the left to become the transverse colon. Inferior to the

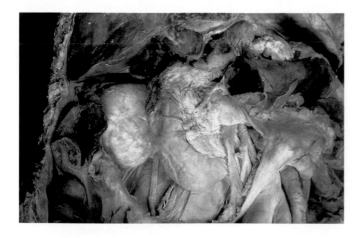

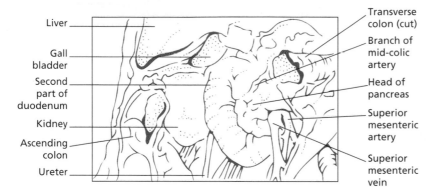

Fig. 23.3 Anterior relations of the right kidney. A portion of the transverse colon has been resected together with the perirenal tissue anterior to the kidney.

transverse colon and mesocolon, a small area of the right kidney adjacent to the lower pole is related to coils of jejunum or ileum lying within the infracolic compartment of the peritoneal cavity. This part of the kidney's anterior surface is occasionally crossed by the right colic artery and vein. It should not be forgotten that the caecum and vermiform appendix are notoriously variable in position and may be related to the anterior aspect of the right kidney.

Anterior relations of the left kidney

The left suprarenal gland is related to the superior pole and medial border of the kidney as far as the renal hilum (Fig. 23.4). Inferiorly, the medial border of this kidney is related to the renal and suprarenal vessels, the urinary tract and the left gonadal vein.

Beyond the confines of the renal fascia, the spleen is related to the superolateral aspect of the left kidney's anterior surface (Fig. 23.5). The tail of the pancreas, accompanied by the splenic vessels, lies horizontally across the hilum of the kidney. The splenic vein is usually situated posterior to the pancreas accompanied superiorly by the tortuous splenic artery. Above the superior border of the pancreas, the kidney presents an area lying between the suprarenal gland and the spleen which forms part of the

stomach bed in the floor of the lesser sac (omental bursa). Inferior to the pancreas, the anterior surface of the kidney is covered medially by coils of jejunum and more laterally by the transverse mesocolon and the commencement of the descending colon. Finally, the lower pole of the left kidney is often crossed by the superior left colic vessels.

Renal blood vessels

The most usual vascular arrangement of each kidney consists of a single renal artery, derived from the abdominal aorta, accompanied on its anterior aspect by a renal vein terminating in the inferior vena cava. As each artery approaches the kidney, it divides into approximately five branches which enter the renal hilum. In the renal sinus the arteries are usually arranged anterior and posterior to the urinary tract. These arteries pierce the walls of the sinus between the attachments of the minor calyces and are accompanied by renal veins similar in number and arrangement. The veins usually continue as far as the renal hilum before uniting anterior to the urinary tract to form a single renal vein. Variations from the above-described pattern are common and are of particular importance in the case of the arteries. Both supernumerary and polar arteries are frequently encountered. A supernumerary renal artery

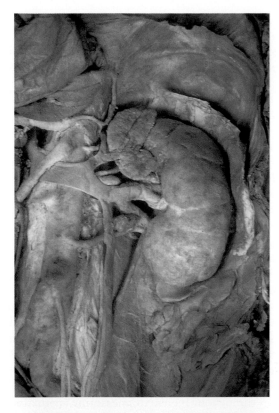

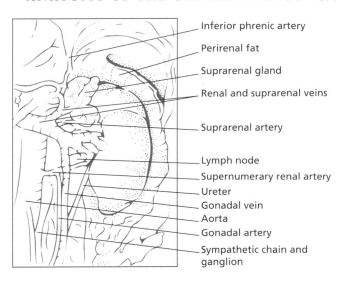

Inferior phrenic artery
Perirenal fat
Suprarenal gland
Renal and suprarenal veins
Suprarenal artery
Lymph node
Supernumerary renal artery
Ureter
Gonadal vein
Aorta
Gonadal artery
Sympathetic chain and ganglion

Fig. 23.4 Medial relations of the left kidney. This dissection illustrates the suprarenal gland, the renal and gonadal vessels and the ureter.

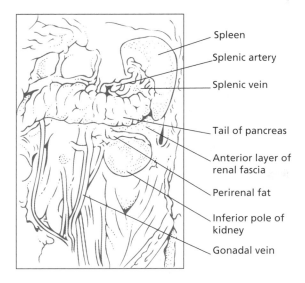

Spleen
Splenic artery
Splenic vein
Tail of pancreas
Anterior layer of renal fascia
Perirenal fat
Inferior pole of kidney
Gonadal vein

Fig. 23.5 Anterior relations of the left kidney. The pancreas, the splenic vessels and the spleen lie anterior to the left kidney.

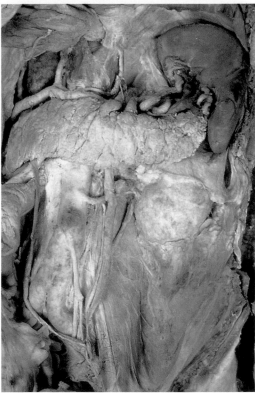

is one which has its origin in the aorta at a level above or below that usually occupied by the renal artery. Alternatively, such vessels may arise from other sites including the common or internal iliac arteries or, more rarely, from the lumbar, gonadal, phrenic, median sacral or external iliac vessels. Supernumerary renal arteries are present in approximately 20% of individuals. In some texts, such vessels are often described as 'anomalous', 'aberrant' or 'accessory' — terms which are inappropriate as these arteries are relatively common and form part of the essential blood supply to the kidney. Usually, supernumerary vessels traverse the renal hilum and pierce the renal substance from within the sinus, but they may occasionally enter the kidney directly by way of the medial border of the organ either above or below the hilum. The latter vessels are examples of polar arteries which provide the principal blood supply to the polar segments of renal parenchyma; ischaemia and necrosis may follow their ligation. The latter events are explained by drawing attention to an important feature of intrarenal vascular anatomy — a kidney normally consists of five segments, each supplied and drained by its own artery and vein. While effective anastomoses link adjacent segmental veins, the arteries are distributed exclusively to their own segments.

The calyces and renal pelvis

The proximal parts of the urinary tract consist of the minor and major calyces and the renal pelvis. The minor calyces attach to the renal parenchyma around the bases of a variable number (7–14) of conical renal papillae which form the tips of the renal pyramids. The renal capsule covers not only the external surface of the kidney but also continues through the hilum to line the sinus and fuse with the adventitial coverings of the minor calyces. Each minor calyx is a trumpet-shaped structure which surrounds either a single papilla or, more rarely, groups of two or three papillae.

The minor calyces unite with their neighbours to form two or possibly three larger chambers, the major calyces. The latter usually fuse with each other to form a single funnel-shaped renal pelvis, which tapers as it passes inferomedially, traversing the renal hilum to become continuous with the ureter.

The renal sinus contains, in addition to the proximal part of the urinary tract, several arteries and veins and a small quantity of adipose tissue which is continuous through the renal hilum with the perirenal fat. The renal blood vessels within the sinus are accompanied by lymphatic channels and a plexus of autonomic nerves.

The pelviureteric region and the ureter

Normally it is not possible to determine precisely the position where the renal pelvis ceases and the ureter begins. Consequently the precision implied by the phrase 'pelviureteric junction' to describe this area is anatomically invalid and the term 'pelviureteric region' is preferable. This region is usually extrahilar in location and normally lies adjacent to the lower part of the medial border of the kidney. In some individuals, however, the entire renal pelvis lies inside the sinus of the kidney and, as a consequence, the pelviureteric region is situated either in the vicinity of the renal hilum or completely within the renal sinus. Each ureter descends from the pelviureteric region to the ureterovesical opening and in adult males may be 30 cm in length. The length of the left ureter commonly exceeds that of the right by 2–3 cm to accommodate the higher position of the left kidney. In assessments of the diameter of the ureter, it has often been stated that the ureteric lumen is relatively narrow in three anatomical locations, namely, at the pelviureteric region, at the level of the pelvic brim and at the ureterovesical junction. While the lumen of the ureter at its vesical end is undoubtedly less distensible than that of the remainder, the evidence purporting to show normally occurring narrow segments in the proximal parts of the ureter is insubstantial. Such evidence is based on studies of fetal material and on the results of X-ray investigations. Regarding the latter, it must be borne in mind that techniques employed during radiographic examinations often impose upon the urinary tract artefactual conditions which may themselves produce misleading results. The external diameter of the ureter at postmortem is relatively uniform throughout its length, measuring approximately 5 mm in width. The living ureter is of similar uniform dimension except at those times when easily visible peristaltic contraction waves occur.

Approximately half of the length of each ureter lies on the posterior abdominal wall while the distal portion is situated within the confines of the true pelvis. The abdominal portion descends in the retroperitoneal tissues and pursues a relatively straight course inclining slightly forwards and towards the midline. After crossing the pelvic brim, the ureter continues extraperitoneally along the pelvic floor. The pelvic portions of the two ureters initially curve in a posterolateral direction and then pass forwards and medially (Fig. 23.6). The terminal portions of the ureters approach each other as they reach the posterior vesical wall; the degree of distension of the bladder determines their mutual separation which can range from 2.5 to 5.0 cm.

The abdominal ureter

Posterior relations of the ureters

The principal posterior relation of the ureter within the abdomen is the psoas major muscle. The anterior surface of this muscle is covered by the psoas fascia which also encloses the psoas minor muscle (if present) and the genitofemoral nerve. Occasionally, a supernumerary renal artery may cross posterior to the ureter to reach the inferior pole of the kidney. The skeletal structures lying posterior to the psoas major, which are of interest radiologically, are

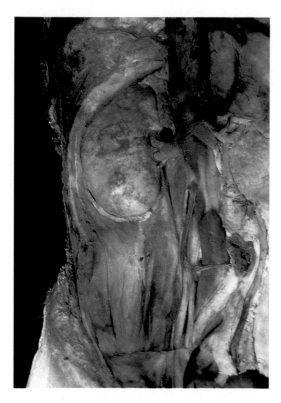

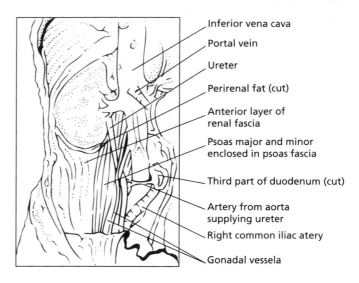

Inferior vena cava

Portal vein

Ureter

Perirenal fat (cut)

Anterior layer of renal fascia

Psoas major and minor enclosed in psoas fascia

Third part of duodenum (cut)

Artery from aorta supplying ureter

Right common iliac atery

Gonadal vessela

Fig. 23.6 This dissection illustrates the abdominal course of the right ureter, most of which lies on the psoas fascia. The ureter is crossed anteriorly by the gonadal vessels.

the lumbar transverse processes and the sacroiliac joint. It is often stated that the course of the ureter passes anterior to the tips of the transverse processes and to the sacroiliac joint space. However, considerable variations occur and urograms frequently depict the ureter either superimposed on the transverse processes some distance medial to their tips or lying beyond their lateral extremities. As a corollary, the ureter not infrequently runs either medial or lateral to the line of the sacroiliac joint.

Anterior relations of the right ureter

The proximal part of the right ureter and pelviureteric region are covered on their anterior aspects by the second (descending) part of the duodenum (Fig. 23.7). Inferior to the duodenum, the ureter lies posterior to the parietal peritoneum and is crossed by the root of the mesentery of the small intestine. Several retroperitoneal blood vessels cross its anterior aspect including the right colic, right gonadal and ileocolic arteries and veins, and occasionally a supernumerary renal artery. Anterior to the parietal peritoneum, within the infracolic compartment of the abdominal cavity lie coils of small intestine. The vermiform appendix may also be found adjacent to the ureter in this situation.

Anterior relations of the left ureter

On the left the proximal ureter (and pelviureteric region)

are covered anteriorly by the body of the pancreas. Below the inferior border of this organ, the ureter descends posterior to the parietal peritoneum as far as the root of the sigmoid mesocolon. On its anterior aspect, the ureter is often closely accompanied by the inferior mesenteric vein. The superior part of this vein often raises a ridge of peritoneum in the region between the fourth part of the duodenum (ascending duodenum) and the inferior pole of the left kidney. The ridge forms the lateral boundary of a peritoneal recess, the paraduodenal fossa, and in the course of its descent the ureter passes immediately lateral to this fossa. As on the right, the left ureter is crossed anteriorly by several retroperitoneal blood vessels which include the gonadal artery and vein, the superior and inferior left colic arteries and the sigmoid arteries. The peritoneal cavity overlying the left ureter is filled with coils of small intestine and usually part of the sigmoid colon.

The pelvic ureter

Within the true pelvis, each ureter follows a curved path along the lateral aspect of which it is related to the muscles, nerves and vessels of the pelvic wall and floor. Medially, the pelvic portion of the ureter is related to the peritoneum and to specific parts of the digestive and reproductive systems. In both sexes, the ureters enter the pelvis by passing anterior to either the common or external iliac artery. Thereafter, each ureter initially follows the internal iliac artery in a downwards and backwards

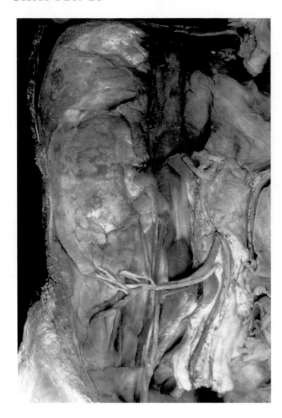

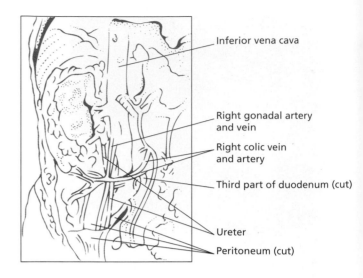

Fig. 23.7 Right ureter and right colic vessels. The latter cross anterior to both the ureter and the gonadal vessels. The colic vessels may supplement the blood supply to the ureter.

direction before the two structures gradually diverge as the ureter curves forwards. Although the ureter has no direct contact with the bony pelvis, its relationships to certain bony landmarks are relevant to radiographic studies. From the region of the sacroiliac joint, the ureter descends along the anterior border of the greater sciatic notch as far as the ischial spine. The ureter then turns forwards and overlies the medial aspect of the obturator foramen.

Ureteric relations in the male

In the male, the ureter crosses the medial aspect of the obturator nerve and artery and the superior vesical artery to reach the lateral part of the levator ani muscle (Fig. 23.8). On its medial aspect, the ureter is immediately adjacent to the peritoneum throughout all but the last 1–2 cm of its course within the male pelvis. On the left side it lies initially in the floor of the intersigmoid recess between the two limbs of the sigmoid mesocolon. Both ureters relate to those parts of the alimentary tract which occupy the peritoneal cavity of the true pelvis, namely, the sigmoid colon and rectum and possibly the ileum and vermiform appendix. On each side, the ureter and ductus deferens converge near the lateral angle of the bladder where the ductus crosses above the ureter and then turns downwards on its medial aspect. Thereafter, the ductus deferens descends posterior to the base of the bladder. Prior to its

passage through the bladder wall, the ureter has the tip of the seminal vesicle as a close medial relation. In this location, the ureter is surrounded by a plexus of veins and a network of autonomic nerves derived from the pelvic plexus.

Ureteric relations in the female

In the female pelvis, the lateral relations of the ureter are similar to those in the male. However, two additional features require description. The first of these is the uterine artery whose close proximity to the ureter is of well-recognized surgical importance. At its origin from the internal iliac artery, the uterine artery may lie close to the lateral aspect of the ureter. However, it is the distal part of the artery's course which is of particular clinical relevance. The ureter and the more laterally placed uterine artery run parallel courses for a short distance along the lateral pelvic wall. The artery then turns medially and crosses the anterosuperior aspect of the ureter, continuing medially towards the ureterine cervix. The uterine artery is accompanied by uterine veins which also cross the ureter in their course to the internal iliac vein.

The second feature is the relationship between the ureter and the ovary. Suspended from the posterior surface of the broad ligament by its own mesentery, the ovary of nulliparous women usually lies in the ovarian fossa in

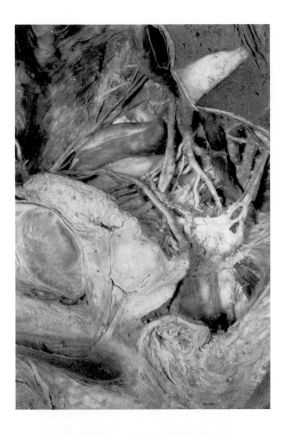

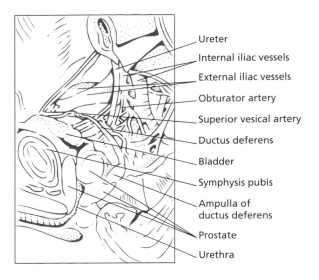

Fig. 23.8 Pelvic portion of the male ureter. The pelvis has been sectioned in the midline and the rectum and peritoneum have been removed to reveal the right ureter from its medial aspect.

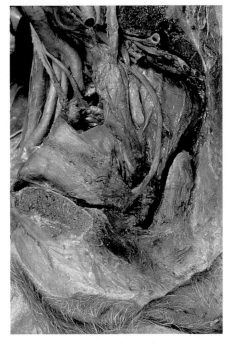

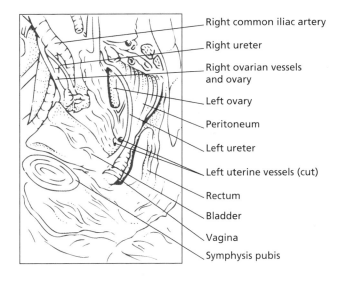

Fig. 23.9 The ureter, ovary, vagina and bladder. The viscera of the female pelvis are illustrated from the left side, including the entire pelvic portion of the left ureter. The relationship of the ureter to the vagina is clearly shown.

contact with the peritoneum of the lateral pelvic wall, in the angle between the external and internal iliac vessels (Fig. 23.9). The ureter descends in the posterior boundary of the ovarian fossa and is therefore closely related to the ovary and its vessels (Fig. 23.9). In parous women, however, the position of the ovary is inconsistent so the relationship between this organ and the ureter is correspondingly more variable.

The medial aspect of each ureter is in contact with the peritoneum as far as the root of the broad ligament.

Through the peritoneum it is related to the digestive organs previously named in the section on the male ureter. Below the root of the broad ligament, each ureter lies 1.5–2.0 cm lateral to the uterine cervix and a similar distance superior to the lateral fornix of the vagina. Anterior to the cervix, the ureters incline towards each other and may lie adjacent to the anterior vaginal wall. Because the uterus and vagina are commonly displaced to one or other side of the midline, one ureter may be more closely related to the cervix and vagina than the other. As the ureters pass between the vagina and the bladder they are surrounded by extensive networks of veins and by numerous autonomic nerves derived from the pelvic plexuses. As in the male, the terminal parts of the ureters approach each other before entering the posterior aspect of the wall of the urinary bladder.

Blood supply and lymphatic drainage

The calyces and the renal pelvis receive their blood supply via minute branches from the renal arteries within the renal sinus; the renal veins receive the venous drainage from these parts of the urinary tract. Each ureter obtains arterial branches — which are often quite long despite their small diameter — from several sources. Although the precise arrangement of vessels is very variable, the general pattern can be described by considering the ureter in three portions.

The uppermost third is supplied by branches that arise from the renal artery, supplemented by vessels from the gonadal and colic arteries. The vascularization of the intermediate portion of the ureter is subject to considerable variation. Usually this segment is supplied by one or more vessels which originate directly from the aorta, although the iliac and gonadal arteries are also potential sources of supply. In a small proportion of individuals, the blood supply may be provided solely by minute peritoneal vessels. The pelvic portion of the ureter receives arterial contributions from the vesical arteries, augmented by branches of the uterine or middle rectal arteries.

The small arteries supplying the ureter are adherent to the overlying peritoneum and, on reaching the viscus, subdivide into ascending and descending branches which form a plexus in the ureteric adventitial coat. The venous plexus of the ureteric adventitia drains both proximally to the renal and gonadal veins and distally to the uterine veins and the vesical venous plexus.

The lymphatic channels of the ureter follow the course of the arteries and carry the lymph predominantly in proximal or distal directions to the lumbar and pelvic lymph nodes.

Innervation

The upper urinary tract receives efferent and afferent innervation from both the sympathetic and parasympathetic parts of the autonomic nervous system. The sympathetic contribution is derived from the lower thoracic and upper lumbar segments (T11 to L2) of the spinal cord and passes to the kidney and upper ureter by way of the thoracic and lumbar splanchnic nerves and then via the coeliac, superior hypogastric and renal plexuses. The parasympathetic nerves originate in the sacral portion of the spinal cord, from the 2nd, 3rd and 4th segments. These fibres travel by way of the pelvic splanchnic nerves to the pelvic plexuses of nerves to reach the juxtavesical parts of the ureters. Parasympathetic nerves destined for the proximal parts of the ureters and calyces ascend in the hypogastric (presacral) nerves. There is considerable intermingling of the different types of autonomic nerves so that it is impossible to separate them by gross dissection.

The urinary bladder

Although the urinary bladder is highly variable in shape it is convenient to consider the viscus as a tetrahedron possessing an anterior, an inferior and two posterolateral angles. The anterior angle (the apex) is directed forwards and upwards and is attached to the urachus, a fibrous cord ascending in the extraperitoneal tissues of the abdominal wall as far as the umbilicus. The two posterolateral angles are those regions in which the ureters pierce the bladder wall; the inferior angle corresponds to the bladder neck and the associated internal urethral meatus.

As a tetrahedron the urinary bladder also possesses four surfaces which are readily discernible in the contracted organ. The two inferolateral surfaces conform to the pelvic walls and floor to which they become more closely related as bladder distension increases. The posterior surface, or base, of the bladder is small and varies in size to only a minor degree as the organ fills and empties. This surface extends between the entrances of the ureters into the bladder wall and the posterior aspect of the bladder neck. The superior surface (often called the fundus) varies the most in shape and area, expanding upwards and forwards as the organ fills. It is worth noting that in some texts the term 'fundus' is applied to the base of the bladder.

When viewed from within, the mucosa lining the lumen of the bladder presents three distinct apertures, namely the internal ureteric orifices and the internal urethral meatus. These lie relatively close to one another and delimit the trigonal region of the bladder. The two lateral orifices appear to be slit-like and are formed by the internal openings of the ureters. Frequently these two orifices are connected by a prominent ridge known as the interureteric bar. Extending inferomedially from the ureteric orifices are a pair of ridges corresponding to the lateral edges of the trigone which extend as far as the internal urethral meatus.

The latter lies in the midline and forms a circular aperture on the lumenal aspect of the bladder neck region.

With the exception of the trigone, the bladder mucosa is comparatively rugose in the undistended organ, but becomes smoother as filling proceeds. The trigone is characterized by a relatively flattened appearance with a smooth urothelial covering and retains its appearance and size irrespective of the degree of distension of the bladder.

Relations of the urinary bladder in the male

The inferolateral surfaces of the bladder are related to the fascia and to the walls and floor of the pelvis. The fascia consists of the connective tissue between and around the pelvic organs, inferior to the peritoneum. The lateral pelvic walls are formed by the obturator fasciae. The latter give attachment to the levator ani muscles which together form the pelvic floor. Both levator muscles are covered on their superior aspects by a further layer of fascia (the pelvic fascia). Several nerves and blood vessels course in the fascia adjacent to the inferolateral surfaces of the bladder. The nerves include the obturator nerves and part of the pelvic plexus of autonomic nerves. The arteries related to the surfaces of the bladder are the superior vesical arteries (which continue anteriorly as the obliterated umbilical

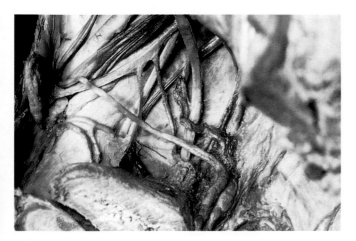

arteries) (Fig. 23.10). The obturator veins accompany the obturator arteries; the vesical veins form a network of venous channels, the vesical venous plexus, which lies adjacent to the bladder's inferolateral surface.

Applied to the lateral parts of the bladder base are the seminal vesicles and the ampullae of the ducti deferentes (Fig. 23.11). These structures are covered by peritoneum which continues for a short distance from the superior surface of the bladder on to its base. This peritoneum caps the seminal vesicles before being reflected at the rectovesical pouch on to the anterior surface of the rectum. When the rectum is distended its ampulla lies in close contact with the base of the bladder. However, when the rectum or bladder, or both, are relatively empty, coils of intestine frequently intervene and occupy the rectovesical pouch.

The whole of the superior surface of the bladder and the median portion of its base are covered by peritoneum and are related to intestines consisting of the ileum, sigmoid colon and rectum. Between the bladder and the pubic bones lies the retropubic space (Fig. 23.12) containing adipose tissue, and the puboprostatic and pubovesical ligaments. As bladder filling occurs the organ comes to occupy more of the retropubic space. Further filling results in the superior surface of the bladder extending above the pubis thereby displacing the peritoneum from the anterior abdominal wall. Thus the anterior aspect of the distended bladder is in direct relation with the abdominal wall without the intervention of peritoneum.

Relations of the urinary bladder in the female

The female bladder neck lies at a slightly lower level than in the male and therefore the inferolateral surfaces of the bladder are more closely applied to the pelvic walls and floor. The fascia, nerves and blood vessels related to the inferolateral surfaces are as described in the male. Inferiorly the bladder is in contact with the vesical venous plexus and the medial borders of the two levator ani muscles. The posterior relations of the female bladder are the cervix of

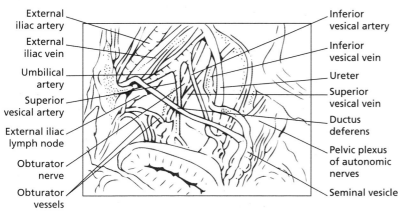

External iliac artery
External iliac vein
Umbilical artery
Superior vesical artery
External iliac lymph node
Obturator nerve
Obturator vessels

Inferior vesical artery
Inferior vesical vein
Ureter
Superior vesical vein
Ductus deferens
Pelvic plexus of autonomic nerves
Seminal vesicle

Fig. 23.10 Vesical vessels and nerves: the arterial supply, venous drainage and autonomic innervation of the male bladder.

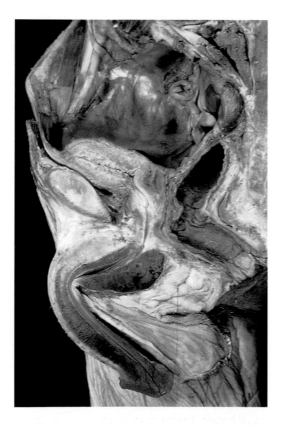

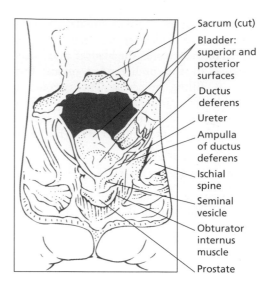

Sacrum (cut)

Bladder:
superior and
posterior
surfaces

Ductus
deferens

Ureter

Ampulla
of ductus
deferens

Ischial
spine

Seminal
vesicle

Obturator
internus
muscle

Prostate

Fig. 23.11 Posterior aspect of the male bladder. The sacrum and rectum have been removed to reveal the bladder and prostate. The peritoneum has been excised.

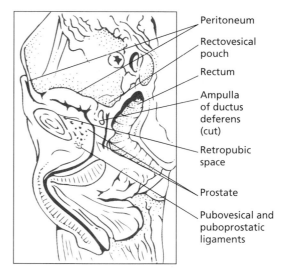

Peritoneum

Rectovesical
pouch

Rectum

Ampulla
of ductus
deferens
(cut)

Retropubic
space

Prostate

Pubovesical and
puboprostatic
ligaments

Fig. 23.12 A median sagittal section through the male pelvis to show the midline structures related to the bladder.

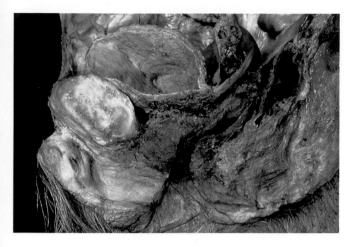

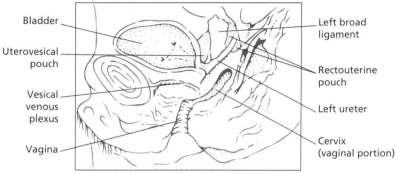

Bladder

Uterovesical
pouch

Vesical
venous
plexus

Vagina

Left broad
ligament

Rectouterine
pouch

Left ureter

Cervix
(vaginal portion)

Fig. 23.13 Relations of the female bladder. The pelvic wall and floor have been removed from the left side to reveal the anterior, inferior and posterior relations of the bladder. The bladder, vagina and rectum have been opened, but part of the left ureter remains *in situ*.

the uterus and the vagina (Fig. 23.13). The extravaginal portion of the cervix lies against the superior part of the base of the bladder while the anterior vaginal wall is in contact with most of the remaining area of the bladder base. The superior relations of the female bladder are somewhat variable because both the size and the position of the uterus are subject to alteration. The non-gravid uterus normally inclines forwards and upwards and lies on the posterior part of the superior surface of the bladder. The remainder of the superior surface of the bladder is related to coils of intestine. However, the body of the uterus may be retroverted and directed towards the rectum and sacrum thereby leaving the entire superior surface of the bladder in contact with the intestines.

Between the bladder and the pubic bones lies adipose tissue, the pubourethral and pubovesical ligaments and numerous veins. As in the male, vesical filling results in direct contact between the superior surface of the female bladder and the anterior abdominal wall above the pubic symphysis. The peritoneum from the anterior abdominal wall continues on to the superior surface of the bladder but extends posteriorly only as far as the isthmus of the uterus, on to which it is reflected to form the uterovesical pouch.

Blood supply of the urinary bladder

In both sexes the arterial supply to the bladder is provided by branches of the internal iliac arteries. The largest branches are usually the superior vesical arteries (Fig. 23.14) which run anteriorly along the lateral pelvic walls before dividing into two or more terminal vessels which extend medially to reach the bladder. Additional branches arise from the internal iliac arteries and all of these are involved in the supply of blood to the inferior aspects of the bladder wall. These vessels include the inferior vesical, obturator and inferior gluteal arteries. In the female, the uterine and vaginal arteries also contribute to the vascular supply of the bladder.

Venous blood from the bladder passes into the extensive plexuses of veins that lie within the pelvis in both sexes. The vesical venous plexus lies in the fascia close to the neck of the bladder and communicates with the prostatic or vaginal plexuses of veins. Blood from these plexuses drains directly into the internal iliac veins although anastomoses with the ovarian, superior rectal and sacral veins provide alternative routes to the inferior vena cava.

Lymphatic drainage

Most of the lymph originating in the wall of the urinary

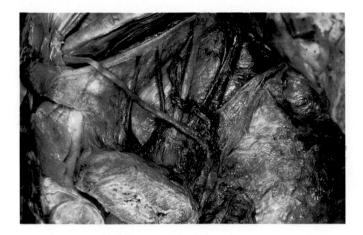

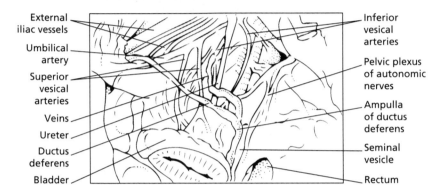

External iliac vessels

Umbilical artery

Superior vesical arteries

Veins

Ureter

Ductus deferens

Bladder

Inferior vesical arteries

Pelvic plexus of autonomic nerves

Ampulla of ductus deferens

Seminal vesicle

Rectum

Fig. 23.14 Blood vessels and nerves of the lateral pelvic wall. Structures related to the lateral aspect of the male blader are displayed by removal of the extraperitoneal adipose tissue.

bladder is conveyed to the external iliac group of lymph nodes. In addition lymph from the base and the infero-lateral surfaces of the bladder may pass directly to lymph nodes alongside the internal iliac or common iliac vessels; lymph from the bladder neck may pass into sacral nodes situated posterior to the rectum.

Peripheral innervation

The bladder receives an autonomic innervation derived from the left and right pelvic plexuses and these nerves usually accompany the principal vascular supply. That part of each pelvic plexus specifically related to the urinary bladder is sometimes designated the 'vesical plexus of autonomic nerves'. This plexus receives input from the pelvic splanchnic nerves which are derived from the 2nd, 3rd and 4th sacral segments of the spinal cord. In addition, the inferior hypogastric (presacral) nerves carry fibres from the 10th thoracic to the 2nd lumbar segments of the cord which also contribute to the formation of the vesical plexus.

The urethra

The male urethra

The male urethra is considered in four sections, namely the preprostatic, prostatic, membranous and penile (or spongy) parts (see Fig. 23.12). The preprostatic urethra possesses a stellate lumen and is approximately 1–1.5 cm in length, extending almost vertically from the bladder neck to the base of the prostate gland.

The prostatic urethra is approximately 3–4 cm in length and tunnels through the substance of the prostate gland. It is continuous above with the preprostatic urethra and emerges from the prostate slightly anterior to the apex of the gland. Throughout most of its length the posterior wall possesses a midline ridge, the urethral crest, which projects into the lumen causing it to appear crescentic in transverse section. The urethral crest is most prominent at about the midpoint of the prostatic urethra and here is named the verumontanum (or colliculus seminalis). The orifice of the prostatic utricle, flanked on either side by the openings of the two ejaculatory ducts (Fig. 23.15), is located on the summit of the verumontanum. The utricle is a blind-ending sac about 6 mm long extending upwards and backwards into the prostatic substance. The gutters on either side of the urethral crest are termed the 'urethral sinuses' and receive the openings of the pro-static ducts. In contrast, numerous mucous glands open around the entire circumference of the prostatic urethra.

The membranous part of the male urethra extends from

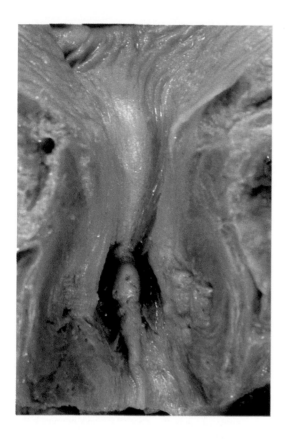

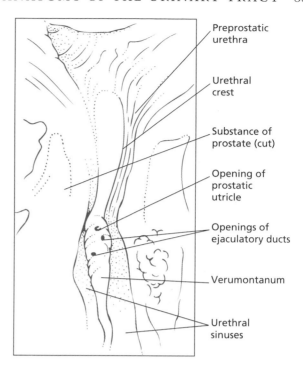

Preprostatic
urethra

Urethral
crest

Substance of
prostate (cut)

Opening of
prostatic
utricle

Openings of
ejaculatory ducts

Verumontanum

Urethral
sinuses

Fig. 23.15 Posterior wall of the preprostatic and prostatic urethra. The substance of the prostate has been incised in the midline anterior to the urethra and the two portions of the gland have been drawn apart to reveal the posterior wall of the urethra.

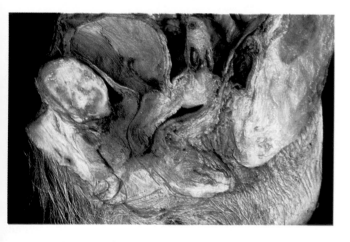

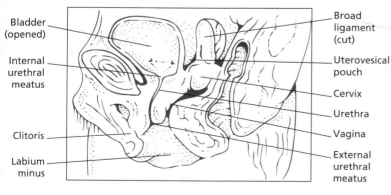

Bladder
(opened)

Internal
urethral
meatus

Clitoris

Labium
minus

Broad
ligament
(cut)

Uterovesical
pouch

Cervix

Urethra

Vagina

External
urethral
meatus

Fig. 23.16 Median section through the female pelvis. From the internal meatus the urethra extends downwards and forwards between the symphysis pubis and the vagina, and terminates at the external meatus.

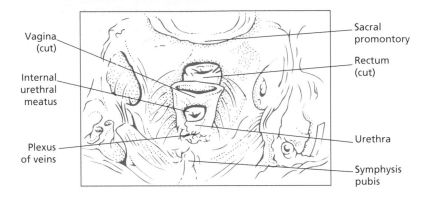

Vagina
(cut)

Internal
urethral
meatus

Plexus
of veins

Sacral
promontory

Rectum
(cut)

Urethra

Symphysis
pubis

Fig. 23.17 A dissection of the female pelvis to demonstrate the relationship of the urethra to the vagina. The entire length of the urethra has been preserved and is seen to be closely related to the anterior vaginal wall and to pass posterior to the symphysis pubis.

the prostate gland to the bulb of the penis, passing between the muscles of the pelvic floor. It is relatively indistensible and measures about 1 cm in length. Embedded in the adventitia of the membranous urethra on its posterior aspect are the two bulbourethral (Cowper) glands. The ducts of these glands accompany the urethra into the bulb of the penis to open through the floor of the penile urethra.

The penile or spongy part is the longest portion of the male urethra, extending for approximately 15 cm from the penile bulb to the external meatus. After piercing the roof of the bulb the urethra dilates to form the intrabulbar fossa and curves downwards and forwards to take up a central position within the corpus spongiosum. From the intra-bulbar fossa the penile urethra narrows to a transverse slit before dilating again within the glans penis to form the navicular fossa. Throughout most of its length the roof and floor of the penile urethra are in mutual contact. However, within the glans the lateral walls are in apposition and in this region (and at the external meatus) the urethra forms a vertical slit.

Along most of its length the penile urethra is surrounded by erectile tissue, but this arrangement is modified at both the proximal and distal ends. The initial 1 cm or so is devoid of erectile tissue on its dorsal aspect while in the

glans, erectile tissue is more abundant dorsally and laterally than ventrally.

The female urethra

The female urethra extends for a distance of 3-4 cm from the internal urethral orifice of the bladder to the external urethral meatus (Fig. 23.16). From the bladder neck the urethra inclines anteroinferiorly, lying behind the symphysis pubis before passing through the pelvic floor. The pubococcygeus parts of the levator ani muscles attach to the posterior aspect of the pubic bones. The most medial components of the two pubococcygeus muscles extend posteriorly towards the vagina leaving a midline hiatus through which the urethra passes (Fig. 23.17). These fibres have no attachment to the urethra, but insert into the lateral walls of the vagina and together form the so-called 'sphincter vaginae'. Throughout its length the urethra is embedded in the adventitial coat of the anterior vaginal wall. The mucosal surface of the urethra possesses a posterior midline ridge (the urethral crest) which projects anteriorly giving the lumen a crescentic slit-like appearance in transverse section. The external urethral meatus opens into the vestibule and is in the form of an anteroposterior slit with rather prominent margins.

24 Structure of the Upper Urinary Tract
J.A.Gosling and J.S.Dixon

Introduction

This chapter provides a brief review of the structure of the upper urinary tract, based on light and electron microscope observations of normal human postoperative material.

Histologically the wall of the upper urinary tract comprises three layers: (i) an inner mucosal layer (consisting of urothelium and its supporting lamina propria); (ii) a muscular layer; and (iii) an outer adventitial layer of connective tissue (Fig. 24.1). The most important component relating to urine transport is the muscle coat and so this will be described in detail. Significant differences occur in the architecture of the musculature within the wall of the calyces, pelvis and ureter. Two morphologically and histochemically distinct types of smooth muscle cell are present in certain regions of the upper urinary tract [1,2]. One type appears similar to smooth muscle found elsewhere, while the other possesses a number of unusual features and is referred to as atypical smooth muscle.

Distribution of smooth muscle cells in the renal calyces and pelvis

Atypical smooth muscle cells

In humans, atypical smooth muscle cells occur in the region of attachment of each minor calyx to the renal parenchyma. These morphologically distinctive cells are not arranged into compact bundles, but form a thin sheet of muscle which covers each minor calyceal fornix. These cells also extend across the renal parenchyma, which lies between the renal attachments of the minor calyces. Thus, each minor calyx is in effect connected to its neighbours by a thin layer of atypical smooth muscle. In the wall of each minor calyx, atypical smooth muscle cells are arranged longitudinally and form a discrete layer confined to the inner aspect of the muscle coat. This inner layer is closely applied to and interconnects with bundles of typical smooth muscle (see below). This arrangement continues

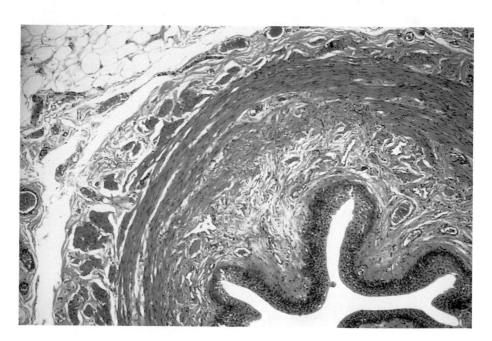

Fig. 24.1 In transverse section the wall of the ureter is seen to consist of three histological layers: a mucosa, a muscle coat and an adventitia. (H & E; ×50.)

throughout the walls of the major calyces and renal pelvis (Fig. 24.2). However, in the pelviureteric region this configuration ceases so that the proximal ureter is devoid of a morphologically distinct inner layer of smooth muscle. Individually, atypical cells are separated from one another for much of their length by quantities of connective tissue. In addition, histochemical studies have shown that these cells differ from typical upper urinary tract smooth muscle in that they are devoid of non-specific cholinesterase. Although the physiological significance of this intracellular enzyme is not known at present, it is a useful means by which to distinguish the two types of smooth muscle cell.

Typical smooth muscle cells

Typical spindle-shaped smooth muscle cells are grouped together into compact bundles which are first in evidence in the distal part of each minor calyx. These bundles lie external to the atypical muscle cell layer and extend throughout the major calyces and renal pelvis. In the pelviureteric region these bundles are directly continuous with those which form the muscle coat of the ureter. In the major calyces and renal pelvis these muscle bundles are closely related on their inner aspects to the layer of atypical smooth muscle.

Individual bundles lie in various directions although the majority tend to be circularly disposed. These compact bundles of smooth muscle frequently branch and connect with adjacent muscle fascicles, thus forming a plexiform arrangement of intercommunicating muscle bundles. In the pelviureteric region there is no localized thickening of

muscle, so that a pelviureteric sphincter does not exist anatomically [3]. Typical smooth muscle cells forming the outer layer of the muscle coat of the renal pelvis and major calyces are rich in non-specific cholinesterase and are thus easily distinguished from the atypical cell layer.

The ureteric muscle coat

The muscle coat of the ureter is composed entirely of typical smooth muscle cells and is fairly uniform in thickness throughout its length, with a width of about 800 µm. The muscle bundles which constitute this musculature are frequently separated from one another by relatively large amounts of connective tissue (Fig. 24.3). Branches which interconnect muscle bundles are common and result in frequent interchange of muscle fibres between adjacent bundles. Due to this extensive branching, individual muscle bundles do not spiral around the ureter as has often been described, but rather form a complex meshwork of interweaving and interconnecting smooth muscle bundles. In addition, unlike the gut, the muscle bundles are so arranged that morphologically distinct longitudinal and circular layers cannot be distinguished. However, in the upper part of the ureter, the inner muscle bundles tend to lie longitudinally while those on the outer aspect have a circular or oblique orientation. In the middle and lower parts of the ureter additional outer longitudinally orientated fibres are also present. As the ureterovesical junction is approached the ureteric muscle coat consists predominantly of longitudinally orientated muscle bundles [4].

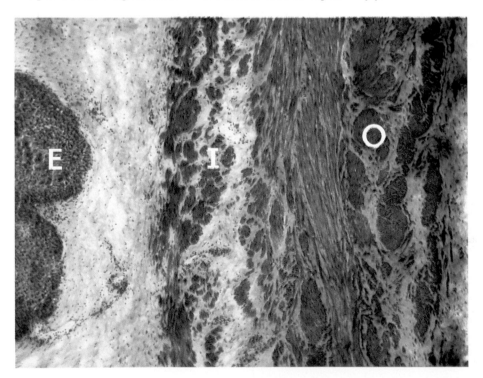

Fig. 24.2 The wall of the renal pelvis in transverse section. Compact bundles of smooth muscle form the outer layer of the muscle coat (O) while numerous atypical muscle cells lie on the inner aspect (I). E, urothelium. (Masson trichrome stain; ×100.)

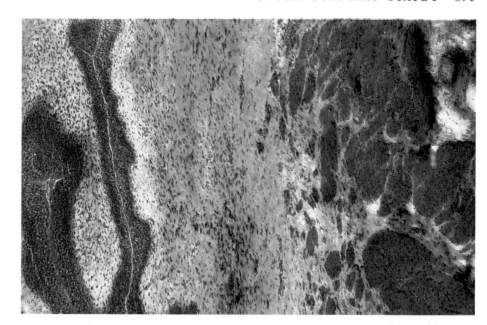

Fig. 24.3 The muscle coat of the ureter consists of a meshwork of smooth muscle bundles, widely separated by connective tissue. Note the absence of an inner layer of morphologically distinct (atypical) smooth muscle cells. (Masson trichrome stain; ×100.)

Fine structure of atypical smooth muscle cells

In the electron microscope the atypical smooth muscle cells are readily identified because of their wide separation from one another by collagen and elastic fibrils. Individual cells are extremely elongated and irregular in outline and often possess lateral protrusions or branches (Fig. 24.4). In addition many cells possess rounded or angular projections of sarcoplasm which enhance their irregular appearance. Each cell is surrounded by a basal lamina, which is often discontinuous over those regions of the sarcolemma where angular projections occur. Caveolae (flask-shaped micropinocytotic vesicles) do not occur in such projections, but are present at other regions of the cells' surfaces. The myofilaments of such cells are identical in type to those found in other upper urinary tract smooth muscle. However, within each cell the myofilaments are frequently arranged in elongated bundles separated by areas containing granular reticulum and small mitochondria. This contrasts with their arrangement in typical smooth muscle cells, in which the myofilaments generally occupy the major part of the sarcoplasm. Many of the atypical cells possess areas

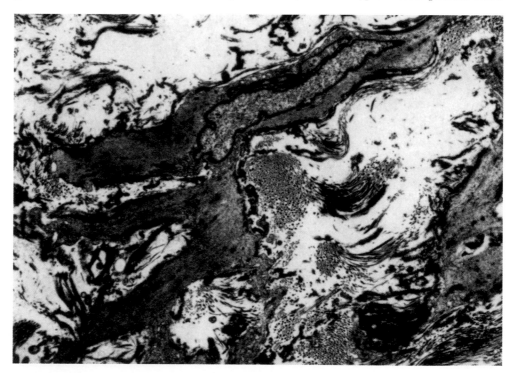

Fig. 24.4. Electron micrograph of an atypical smooth muscle cell from the renal calyx. The cell possesses several irregular branches and is surrounded by collagen and elastic fibres. (×6400.)

within their sarcoplasm which contain clusters of electron-dense glycogen granules.

Frequently, an elongated sarcoplasmic projection from one cell extends out to form an intercellular junction with a similar protuberance from an adjacent cell. At the junctional region the opposing cell membranes are separated by a gap of not more than 20 nm without any intervening basal lamina (Fig. 24.5). Junctions of this type are similar to the regions of close approach that occur between ureteric smooth muscle cells.

Fine structure of typical smooth muscle cells

As described above, the outer aspect of the muscle coat of the calyceal and pelvic wall and also the muscle coat of the ureter consists of typical smooth muscle cells arranged into compact bundles. Such bundles are composed of closely opposed smooth muscle cells separated from their neighbours by relatively little intervening connective tissue (Fig. 24.6). Each smooth muscle cell possesses sarcoplasm packed with longitudinally orientated myofilaments together with numerous electron-dense bodies. Mitochondria are scattered at random throughout the sarcoplasm while scant granular reticulum and Golgi membranes tend to cluster at either pole of the single elongated nucleus. Rows of caveolae interspersed with electron-dense regions are observed at the sarcolemma of each smooth muscle cell. Individual smooth muscle cells are surrounded by a basal lamina except at regions of close approach where a gap of 15–20 nm separates adjacent cell membranes in the absence of intervening basal lamina

material. Such regions are frequently observed between adjacent smooth muscle cells within a muscle bundle. Apart from such regions, the narrow intercellular spaces contain occasional collagen fibres while elastic fibres are very rarely observed.

Innervation of the upper urinary tract

The muscle coat of the calyceal wall, the renal pelvis and the ureter receives a dual autonomic innervation by both noradrenergic and cholinergic nerve fibres [5,6]. Some of these nerves directly innervate smooth muscle cells within the wall of the upper urinary tract while others form dense perivascular nerve plexuses. Nerve fibres containing vasoactive intestinal polypeptide (VIP), neuropeptide Y (NPY), substance P (SP), calcitonin gene-related peptide (CGRP) and tyrosine hydroxylase (TH) have recently been reported in the wall of the human ureter and it seems probable that some of these neuropeptides coexist with known neurotransmitters such as noradrenaline and acetylcholine [7,8]. Nerves containing SP and CGRP are mainly distributed to blood vessels and to the submucosal layer and are probably sensory in function. The density of innervation throughout the ureteric wall gradually increases in a proximodistal direction so that the juxtavesical segment of each ureter is relatively richly innervated [7]. Ganglion cells do not occur in the wall of the upper urinary tract.

Autonomic nerves in the wall of the upper urinary tract presumably have a modulatory function on the contractile activity of the muscle coat. However, it is generally

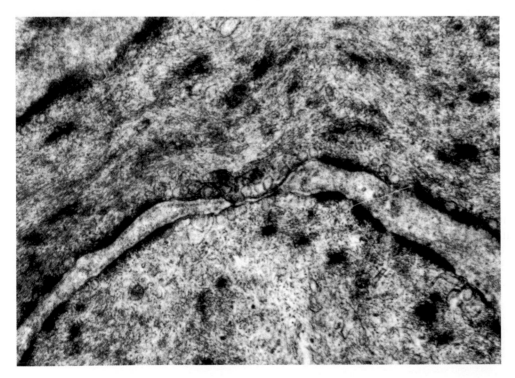

Fig. 24.5 A region of close approach between two ureteric smooth muscle cells where a gap of 15–20 nm separates the opposing cell membranes. At the periphery of the 'junction' the basal lamina of one cell is reflected back to become continuous with that of its neighbour. (×35 200.)

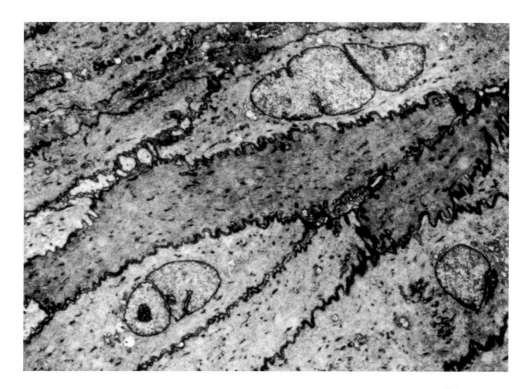

Fig. 24.6 In the ureteric muscle coat typical spindle-shaped smooth muscle cells are closely apposed with very little intervening connective tissue. Each cell is packed with longitudinally orientated myofiloments. (×4100.)

believed that they are not directly responsible for the propagation of contraction waves. Indeed, there is considerable experimental evidence to support this view. First, the electrical activity measured in the ureteric wall during peristalsis together with the rate of propagation of contraction waves are characteristic of smooth muscle and not nervous activity. Secondly, the ratio of axon terminals to smooth muscle cells is extremely low. Thirdly, it has been shown that ureteric peristalsis continues *in vivo* in the presence of nerve-blocking agents such as tetrodotoxin and *in vitro* in denervated ureteric segments.

Ureteric peristalsis

It is well known that under normal conditions contraction waves originate in the proximal part of the upper urinary tract and propagate in an anterograde direction towards the bladder. However, the mechanism involved in the initiation of these contractile events has been the subject of much controversy in the past. One theory proposes that smooth muscle contraction is initiated by the stretching forces exerted by the luminal contents on the muscle coat contained within the walls of the renal calyces and pelvis. However, there is now a considerable body of experimental evidence which demonstrates that the urinary tract possesses spontaneously active regions consisting of pacemaker muscle cells which initiate and exert a controlling influence on the peristalsis activity of the ureter [9,10].

From a morphological viewpoint, it seems likely that the smooth muscle cells which occur at the attachment of each minor calyx and which are structurally distinct from those elsewhere may act as pacemaker sites. Since each minor calyx possesses such cells (and is linked across the renal parenchyma to other calyces by similar cells), the number of pacemaker sites within a given system is related to the number of minor calyces. It seems probable that the normal sequence of events begins with the initiation of a contraction wave at one of the several minor calyceal pacemaker sites. Once initiated, the contraction is propagated through the wall of the adjacent major calyx and activates the smooth muscle of the renal pelvis. To what extent the inner layer of atypical cells acts as pacemaker (or as a preferential conduction pathway) remains to be determined. The proximal pacemaker site for successive contractions usually changes between the minor calyces, although sometimes the same minor calyx will initiate consecutive contractions before the site changes.

Functionally, the proximal location of these pacemaker sites ensures that, once initiated, contraction waves are propagated away from the kidney, thereby avoiding undesirable pressure rises directed against the renal parenchyma. In addition, since several potential pacemaker sites exist, the initiation of contraction waves is unimpaired by partial nephrectomy because the minor calyces spared by the resection remain *in situ* and continue their pacemaking function.

Each contraction wave extends across the renal pelvis as far as the pelviureteric region, and it seems likely that the onward transmission into the ureter is dependent upon the volume of fluid contained within the renal pelvis. At high urine flow rates, every contraction wave reaching the pelviureteric region is propagated as a ureteric contraction wave. At low flow rates not all renal pelvic contractions are transmitted to the ureter. Only when a sufficient quantity of urine has accumulated in the renal pelvis does a pelvic contraction wave propagate distally beyond the pelviureteric region. Thus, the pelviureteric region acts as a 'gate', allowing ureteric peristalsis to occur only when the volume of each bolus of urine propelled from the renal pelvis is above a critical amount.

In summary, ureteric peristalsis is apparently dependent upon two mechanisms within the proximal part of the urinary tract. First, contraction waves in the renal pelvis are initiated by spontaneously active pacemaker sites located within the wall of each minor calyx. Secondly, a regulating mechanism at the pelviureteric region determines whether each contraction of the renal pelvis is propagated into the ureter. The latter event is related to urine flow and probably depends upon the stretching forces or tension generated in the wall of the pelviureteric region. It is not yet known whether a malfunction of one or both of these mechanisms is involved in the aetiology of functional obstruction of the upper urinary tract.

Contraction waves are thought to be propagated across the renal pelvis and along the ureter by means of myogenic conduction, resulting from electrotonic coupling of one muscle cell to its immediate neighbours.

In several other organs in which myogenic conduction is known to occur, adjacent smooth muscle cells are normally linked by means of the nexus, or gap junction. This specialized region is thought to provide a low-resistance pathway allowing electrotonic spread of excitation from one cell to another. It is surprising, therefore, that upper urinary tract smooth muscle is typified by a relative paucity of this type of cell–cell contact. However, regions of close approach (with a cell–cell gap of about 20 nm) are extremely numerous between ureteric smooth muscle cells. Thus it seems probable that it is intercellular junctions of this type (rather than gap junctions) which are responsible for the conduction of contraction waves from one ureteric smooth muscle cell to the next.

The direction of propagation is normally from the renal pelvis towards the bladder, as dictated by the pacemaker mechanism in the minor calyces. Since muscle cells may conduct from one cell to the next in either direction, the direction of propagation may sometimes be reversed, resulting in retrograde contraction waves.

References

1 Dixon JS, Gosling JA. The musculature of the human renal calices, pelvis and upper ureter. *J Anat* 1982;**135**:129–37.
2 Rizzo M, Pellegrini MSF, Riccardi RA, Ponchietti R. Ultrastructure of the urinary tract muscle coat in man. *Eur Urol* 1981;**524**:171–7.
3 Notley RG. Electron microscopy of the upper ureter and the pelvi-ureteric junction. *Br J Urol* 1968;**40**:37–51.
4 Notley RG. Electron microscopy of the lower ureter in man. *Br J Urol* 1970;**42**:439–45.
5 Schulman CC. Electron microscopy of the human ureteric innervation. *Br J Urol* 1974;**4**:609–23.
6 Gosling JA, Dixon JS, Humpherson JR. *Functional Anatomy of the Urinary Tract*. London: Gower Medical, 1982.
7 Edyvane KA, Trussell DC, Jonavicius J, Henwood A, Marshall VR. Presence and regional variation in peptide-containing nerves in the human ureter. *J Auton Nerv Syst* 1992;**39**:127–38.
8 Allen JM, Williams G, Rodrigo J et al. Neuropeptide Y (NPY) containing nerves in mammalian ureter. *Urology* 1990;**35**:81–6.
9 Constantinou CE. Renal pelvic pacemaker control of ureteral peristaltic rate. *Am J Physiol* 1974;**226**:1413–16.
10 Constantinou CE, Djurhuus JC. Urodynamics of the multicalyceal upper urinary tract. In: O'Reilly PH, Gosling JA, eds. *Idiopathic hydronephrosis*. Berlin: Springer Verlag, 1981:16–43.

25 Physiological Response of the Upper Urinary Tract to Chronic Experimental Obstruction

C.E.Constantinou and J.C.Djurhuus

Introduction

Hippocrates writing about the upper urinary tract describes its structure and function as follows:

> ... the ureters penetrate the kidneys, which resemble the heart and are concave, but each kidney has its own cavity turned towards the great veins (renal pelvis), running to the bladder, in which the urine is collected after being conducted by the vessels to be filtered through the kidneys because of their sponge like composition ...

Hippocrates' concept of the ureters drawing up urine from the bladder to be filtered by the kidneys has been significantly modified by modern physiological science. In this chapter we will consider the function of the urinary tract with particular emphasis on an examination of the physiological characteristics that correspond to the anatomy. Because the main focus of this section of the book is on urodynamic disorders of the upper urinary tract we emphasize mainly those aspects that are of functional importance and relate to pathology produced by ureteric or urethral obstruction.

We will first briefly outline the basic physiological mechanisms involved with the generation of urine transport in the normal urinary system. Subsequently, we will consider the important influence of ureteric and bladder obstruction on the function of the ureter and pelvis with particular attention on the conditions under which the upper urinary tract is most at risk. Data from experimental approaches specifically designed to evaluate ureteric obstruction will be used to illustrate the physiological process. Similarly, data from experimental observations of urethral obstruction will be provided and upper urinary tract pressure–flow examinations presented.

It is now becoming routine clinical practice to evaluate bladder outlet obstruction by performing comprehensive diagnostic testing, the results of which are used to identify the important functional characteristics that define the lower urinary tract. Such an approach, made using a series of tests collectively termed urodynamics, produces a means of quantifying the function of the lower urinary tract, thus making it possible to compare the effects of surgical or pharmacological intervention. Upper urinary tract urodynamic testing has not developed to the same extent in practice or research. We present in this chapter some of the important new clinical and experimental studies on the function of the upper urinary system that have been undertaken in recent years and review the current state of the art in evaluating obstruction.

As the study of clinical urodynamics has progressed, urethral obstruction is now expressed in terms of pressure–flow measurements and it is appropriate to apply the lessons thus learned to the upper urinary tract. Such application is becoming necessary, as pharmacological treatment for the effects of detrusor instability and obstruction is becoming more widespread with the introduction of adrenergic antagonists, that ultimately have a systemic effect. Conversely, there are now emerging therapies for the pharmacological treatment of lower urinary tract symptoms such as enuresis that rely on modulation of urine production. For these reasons it is important to be aware of the relative and corresponding analogies in the physiological and pharmacological response of the upper and lower urinary systems and the factors that are common. Chapter 24 will deal specifically with the pharmacological action on the upper urinary system. We hope that after reading the physiological material given in this chapter the reader will be more aware of the many different physiological functions that the calyces, pelvis, ureter, vesico-ureteric junction and ultimately the bladder and urethra play in urine transport. Such a functional understanding of the role of these structures will be useful in the interpretation of the outcome of surgical and pharmacological intervention.

Basic physiological process

While urine production by the kidney is a relatively continuous process, its transport from the renal pelvis to the bladder is accomplished by discreet and irregular ureteric peristaltic contractions. Such peristaltic contractions by the ureter are responsible for the propulsion of a urine bolus to the bladder. The volume of a urine bolus varies enormously, from a few drops to several millilitres. The ureteric contractions are initiated by the triggering mechanism of the renal pelvis which forms the urine bolus. Once a bolus is formed and introduced through the pelviureteric junction (PUJ), it is propelled by the contracting ureteric walls behind the bolus and the relaxed ureteric walls at the leading edge of the bolus. The bolus propagates along the entire length of the ureter and is injected into the bladder through the specialized structural configuration of the vesico-ureteric junction (VUJ).

The triggering mechanism of ureteric peristalsis, the pacemaker system, is species dependent. The term pacemaker system is used in this chapter to describe the histologically organized region, or regions, of cells that are distributed in the calyces and pelvis. These regions, whose atypical histological characteristics have been described in Chapter 24, are not similar to the well-defined nodes controlling the heart, but are instead distributed in pelvic and ureteric smooth muscle endowing it with automaticity. The distribution of pacemaker cells is primarily at the most proximal regions of the calyx, thereby making it possible to initiate contractions at the origin of the upper urinary tract. The anatomical organization of the pacemaker system depends primarily on whether the kidney is unicalyceal or multicalyceal. Simply stated, mammals such as dogs, rabbits and rats have a unicalyceal kidney and thus a pacemaker system that surrounds the proximal regions of the calyx interconnected with the inner layer of the pelvis. Larger mammals such as the pig and human have a multicalyceal kidney and therefore possess a number of organized pacemaker regions around each calyx and also the pelvis. These individual regions collectively constitute the calyceal pacemaker system whose function is to coordinate drainage from each calyx to the renal pelvis. In the unicalyceal kidney the pelvis is comparatively small and resides mostly intarenally, resulting in a low-compliance pelvis. In the multicalyceal kidney the pelvis is mostly extrarenal, resulting in a higher capacity compliant pelvis. With this very simplified anatomical description of the configuration of the pacemaking system in mind we will consider below some relevant aspects of the mechanism for the initiation and control of upper urinary tract transport particularly as affected by obstruction.

Pacemaker control of ureteric peristalsis

The schematic diagram given in Fig. 25.1 illustrates our conceptual understanding of the physiological pacemaker mechanism responsible for the initiation of the upper urinary tract transport. In Fig. 25.1 we stress the importance of the frequency distribution in the different regions of the calyx and pelvis, particularly relating the organization of the process synchronization in the multicalyceal kidney.

Pacemaker control in the unicalyceal kidney

It will be helpful to consider first the physiological mechanisms of pacemaker control taking place in the unicalyceal kidney. This is because the unicalyceal kidney constitutes the principal unit and the multicalyceal system can be considered as a group of parallel kidneys. Extensive literature exists, which was obtained using electrical and hydrostatic methods, to show that in the unicalyceal kidney ureteric peristaltic contractions are triggered by the pacemaker system distributed throughout the renal calyx [1–6]. It has been shown that ureteric and renal pelvic peristalsis are directly controlled by the pacemaker system located at the pelvicalyceal border [7,8]. By measuring the time intervals between peristaltic contractions detected from electromyograms (EMGs) it was found that the duration of these intervals was an integral multiple of the time interval between renal pelvic contractions. The inherent time interval of the pacemaker region was demonstrated from data obtained from studies obtained under *in vivo* conditions [2,9].

Pacemaker control in the multicalyceal kidney

In the multicalyceal kidney the timing of these contractions is hierarchically organized with calyceal pacemaker(s) having the highest inherent frequency and the pelvic pacemaker regulating ureteric peristalsis [10,11]. Figure 25.1 illustrates the fundamental differences between the physiological features of the unicalyceal and multicalyceal collecting systems and highlights our current state of knowledge in the organization of the pacemaking system in each type of kidney. The mechanism of integration between calyces has been examined by Yamaguchi *et al.* [11] who demonstrated the presence of a narrow spectrum of spontaneous rhythmic activity and a heterogeneous means of phase locking between calyces. This study was done using a perfused kidney *ex vivo* and recording from individual calyces and the pelvis. The advantage of this approach is that the infundibula connecting the calyces with the pelvis are not disrupted by instrumentation. The calyces contract at considerably higher frequencies compared to the pelvis (approximately two times the frequency) and calyceal contractile frequency is independent of flow rate [11]. The heterogeneous calyceal synchronization observations reported by Yamaguchi *et al.* [11] have been disputed on the basis of a study of the multicalyceal porcine kidney using an *in vitro* preparation by Morita *et al.* [12] who found that the contraction rhythm of each calyx was different, suggesting the presence of

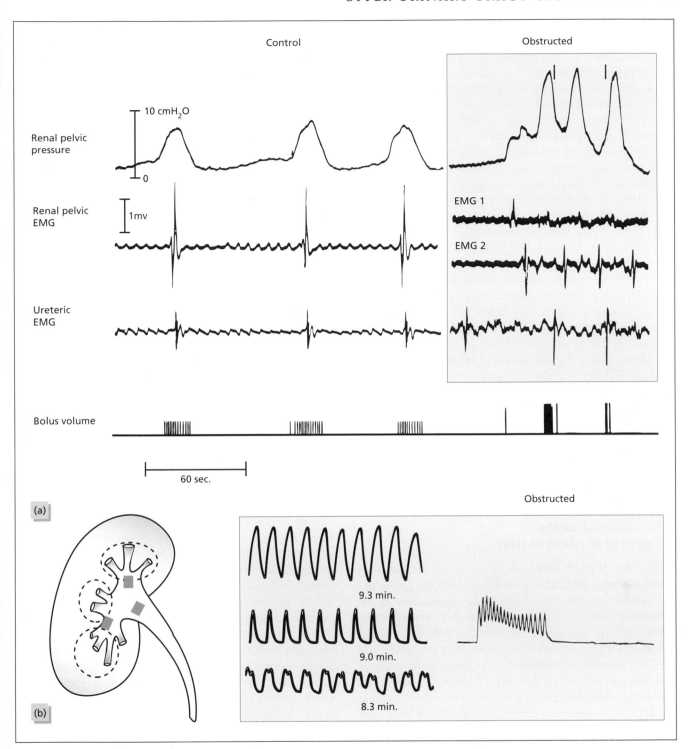

Fig. 25.1 Pacemaking process in the calyceal, pelvic and ureteric structures. This schematic diagram shows that all regions of the calyx and pelvis are capable of spontaneous rhythmic contractions. These contractions can be measured as (a) variations of pressure in the intact kidney under *in vivo* conditions, or (b) isometric contractions *in vitro* in small tissue strips. Unlike the calyx and pelvis, the ureter does not possess pacemaking cells allowing spontaneous contractions and therefore requires an external mechanical or electrical stimulus to generate a contraction.

independent multiple pacemaker systems. Furthermore, the peristaltic time intervals of the renal pelvis and ureter were irregular and it was not possible to determine with any accuracy which of the calyceal contractions were propagated across the pelvis to the ureter. Evidently the precise timing mechanism of integration of the calyceal and pelvic rhythm in triggering peristaltic contractions is not fully understood and requires further study.

A confounding factor in characterizing the mechanism of calyceal integration is urine flow rate and the behaviour of the kidneys under various conditions of urine production or diuresis. On one hand the mechanical behaviour of calyceal activity has been linked with modulation of the urine concentration function of the papillae, while on the other hand the presence of mechanoreceptors, reported by Kopp [13] as showing activation of renorenal reflexes, may be interpreted as contributing to higher level calyceal regulation. It is evident that the ramifications of changing urine flow rate spread over many aspects of the physiological status of the entire urinary tract.

Our focus here, however, will be centred on the influence of flow in producing changes in the urodynamic parameters. Indeed there is abundant evidence to suggest that the extent and duration of diuresis plays an important part in determining peristalsis in both the unicalyceal and multicalyceal kidney [14–17]. It is therefore possible that diuresis may act as an overall form of temporal synchronizer to coordinate the frequencies of calyceal contractility. It is suggested that the role of diuresis does not stop in the regulation of peristaltic rate but also plays an important part in determining the hydrostatic isolation of the upper urinary tract from the hydrostatic pressures of the bladder [18–20] and probably in facilitating the transport of bacteria to the renal pelvis [21]. In considering the role of diuresis on the mechanism of renal pelvic isolation from the bladder it is important to consider each circumstance separately.

Experimental ureteric and urethral obstruction

Because the kidney functions in part on the basis of hydrostatic pressure gradients to filter blood the prevailing renal pelvic pressure should ideally be maintained at the low level of a few centimetres of water. Our current understanding of the changes in hydrostatic pressures taking place in the upper urinary tract of patients are essentially based on invasive measurements performed in extreme cases where the need for intervention is clinically mandatory. For ethical reasons there are few reliable normal percutaneous nephrostomy measurements performed in practice and reported in the literature. As a consequence, reliable functional data are obtained using indirect methods such as radionucleotide renography, pyelography, echography and magnetic resonance imaging (MRI).

For these reasons animal models have become the principal method for obtaining information about dysfunction of the upper urinary system. Using animal models it is possible to establish a reliable starting point, time scale and sequence of pressure changes as a result of the obstruction. To a considerable extent this chapter focuses on experimental observations carried out using the pig as an experimental model because of its analogy with the human in terms of its gross anatomical urinary tract configuration, bladder innervation and function. Two distinctly separate experimental approaches were used to illustrate the effect of obstruction, first ureteric obstruction, producing unilateral hydronephrosis, and subsequently urethral constriction resulting in detrusor instability and associated bilateral damage to the kidneys.

Ureteric obstruction

To produce the kind of partial ureteric obstruction that can reasonably approximate clinical obstruction we used the method of ureteric external compression originally described by Ulm and Miller [22]. This was done by the implantation of a ureteric segment within the psoas muscle which induces a mild reproducible obstruction thereby allowing chronic studies to be performed. With such a model changes are uniform and reproducible, and results obtained have provided important new information about the impact of the development of obstruction on ureteric physiology [10,23]. EMG and hydrodynamic measurements were done by periodic monitoring of the renal pelvis using extracellularly implanted electrodes.

Analysis of pelvic pressures under such conditions shows that hydrostatic pressure alone cannot in absolute terms be used to differentiate the normal pelvis from the obstructed, although there is a trend towards elevation in the bascline of the obstructed pelvis. Analysis of the EMG record obtained from human studies during surgery reveals other useful information regarding the effects of obstruction; Figs 25.2 and 25.3 show the sequence of changes of peristaltic transport in terms of both pressure and conduction of ureteric contraction. Figure 25. 2 shows a record from a mildly hydronephrotic kidney demonstrating the transmission of pelvic contractions to the conus and in the ureter. In severe hydronephrosis or in cases of PUJ obstruction there are marked signs of a lack of coordination between peristaltic activity measured at each site in the pelvis. Indeed, in severe cases there is total lack of coordination reflecting disintegration of renal pelvic muscle. Figure 25.3 shows a sample of a recording illustrating the relative changes in the coordination of pelvic contractility. Further comparison between the pressure recordings of the mildly and severely obstructed kidney shows poorly differentiated pelvic pressures suggesting poor propagation of the pacemaker-initiated contractions.

There are many possible explanations that can be proposed to account for this outcome. Among these, it has been suggested that there is a variation in the transmission velocity of the actual peristaltic impulse, the *de novo*

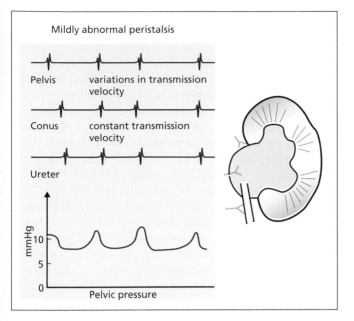

Fig. 25.2 EMG activity of the renal pelvis and ureter in human hydronephrosis. Recordings were made at the locations shown schematically in the inset. In the enlarged pelvis, in the absence of mild hydronephrosis, pelvic and ureteric contractions are coherent. In the early stages of hydronephrosis transmission is anterograde but pelvic/ureteric activity transmission times vary. Pelvic and ureteric activity may be virtually coincident or it may be incoherent , where pelvic contractions occur after the ureter has contracted.

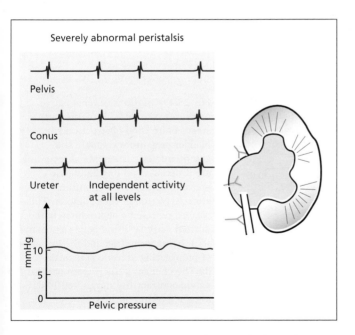

Fig. 25.3 EMG activity in a patient with severe hydronephrosis. Severe incoordination between peristaltic activity at different sites of the pelvis is demonstrated. This type of incoherent contraction accords poorly differentiated pressure waves that are not correlated with the EMG.

pacemaking activity due to changing excitability of the pelvis, and a changing hierarchy of the site of origin from one calyx to the other. Failure to coordinate contraction between different parts of the pelvis in severe hydronephrosis, observed in both experimental and clinical cases [24], is associated with split muscle bundles by proliferating fibrous connective tissues, suggesting the generation of isolated islands of the remaining smooth muscle. In making these considerations it is appropriate to bear in mind the similarity in the response of the bladder to obstruction, which has been more extensively studied than that of the pelvis and ureter (see below).

Urethral obstruction

Clinical and experimental evidence indicates that prolonged partial bladder outlet obstruction can become a risk factor in producing detrusor instability and upper urinary tract deterioration. Gradual partial obstruction can be found in patients with a diverse range of pathology ranging from benign prostatic hypertrophy (BPH) through prostate cancer to spinal cord injury. The sensory manifestations of partial obstruction, such as urgency and frequency, are considered to be associated with detrusor instability which invariably is the presenting symptom in many patients. There is an absence of the analogous sensory manifestation in slow upper urinary tract deterioration and with the exception of extreme pathology such deterioration is inevitably silent.

The diagnosis of bladder outlet obstruction has become straightforward using modern urodynamics criteria, primarily because of the accessibility of the bladder and urethra to catheterization and measurement. The upper urinary tract is not as readily accessible without highly invasive methods. As a result the consequences of bladder outlet obstruction in producing hydronephrosis are not as accurately chronicled in relation to the severity of detrusor instability and the development of pressures in the pelvis are not very well correlated with the onset, progression and severity of detrusor instability.

To chronicle the relative impact of urethral obstruction on the upper urinary tract, observations were made using adult female pigs instrumented with chronic implantable telemetry [25,26]. Renal pelvic pressure and bladder pressure were simultaneously monitored. Pelvic pressure was measured using a tube that was inserted as a nephrostomy through the parenchyma to the renal pelvis. Urethral compression was produced by the implantation of an artificial urethral sphincter whose cuff was placed around the proximal part of the urethra and the pump in a subcutaneous pocket in the perineum. The reservoir was filled to a pressure of $20\,cmH_2O$ and placed in the intraperitoneal cavity. Before closure of the animal the artificial sphincter was inactivated with the cuff empty, thus providing free and unimpaired voiding. After a period of 1 week the sphincter cuff was activated to allow voiding to occur naturally while telemetric monitoring of the bladder and pelvic pressures was made.

Consequences of detrusor instability on renal pelvic pressures

The gradual development of urethral obstruction is reflected as progressive alterations in the urodynamic function of both the bladder and pelvis. Such gradual changes in function are recognizable as deviations from the normal unobstructed wave forms in the shape of bladder and pelvic pressures. Using the telemetric method described above, we were able to chronicle such changing pressure patterns simultaneously in the bladder and pelvis with particular emphasis on their characteristics during detrusor instability and micturition.

Figures 25.4 and 25.5 demonstrate the urodynamic ramifications of the development of detrusor instability from the early stages of urethral obstruction and at approximately the same bladder volume. Figure 25.4a shows a regular pattern of renal pelvic contractions and a stable bladder pressure which was monitored 7 days after the activation of the artificial sphincter. Figure 25.4b, obtained 14 days after obstruction and under the same conditions, shows that the bladder pressures continue to be

stable while renal pelvic pressures become intermittent and characteristic of obstruction. These changes in pelvic pressure pattern are similar to those observed with partial ureteral obstruction [10,24].

An important observation made from such measurements is that the renal pelvis is adversely affected by the obstruction before the bladder shows evidence of detrusor instability. The onset of detrusor instability is characterized by rhythmic variations in bladder pressure.

During the early stages of urethral obstruction detrusor instability is present only when bladder filling is approaching capacity and is reduced when the bladder is emptied (Fig. 25.5). As the influence of urethral obstruction persists, detrusor instability is detected at lower and lower bladder volumes (Fig. 25.6). As Figs 25.5 and 25.6 show, obstruction produces frequent detrusor contractions during filling and an elevated micturition pressure. The corresponding renal pelvic pressures are marked by periods of low-pressure peristaltic phases followed by periods of consecutive peristaltic contractions. This is best illustrated by Fig. 25.7 where the time scale has been expanded.

The development of these renal pelvic pressure changes occurs prior to changes in the filling pressures of the bladder, and this raises a number of important questions as to the mechanism of upper urinary tract deterioration due to partial obstruction. We consider the nature of these renal pelvic patterns of contractility to be changes that are

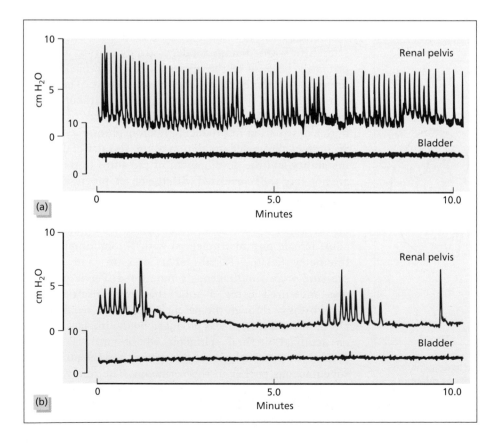

Fig. 25.4 Variations of renal pelvic pressures recorded during the early stages of urethral obstruction while bladder pressure was stable and compliant. Two segments of recording are illustrated. (a) Regular pelvic pressure contractions monitored 7 days after activation of the sphincter. This pattern represents approximately the normal activity of the pelvis associated with bolus formation and the initiation of propagating ureteric peristalsis. (b) The change in the pattern of renal pelvic contractility monitored 14 days after activation of the sphincter. The pattern illustrated here is intermittent and is associated with long periods of aperistalsis. Under such conditions bolus formation and peristalsis occur when larger amounts of urine fill the pelvis than is found in the unobstructed state.

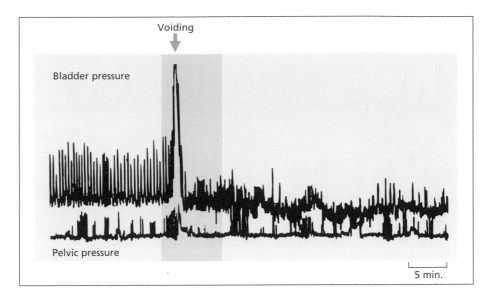

Fig. 25.5 Bladder and pelvic pressure monitored 2 weeks after partial ureteric obstruction. The arrow shows a micturition contraction associated with elevated detrusor pressures. Detrusor instability is shown prior to micturition which subsides after voiding. Note that the intermittent pattern of pelvic activity is maintained throughout the filling and voiding phase of the bladder.

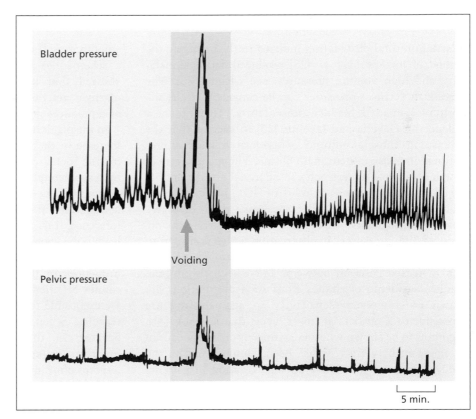

Fig. 25.6 Pattern of bladder and urethral pressures following prolonged (5 weeks) obstruction. The recording was obtained under similar conditions to those shown in Fig. 25.5. Note that the rhythmic pressure variations of the pelvis have been practically obliterated and micturition produced an elevation in pelvic pressure suggestive of disruption of ureteric emptying via the VUJ or transmission of detrusor pressures.

intrinsic to the smooth muscle of the pelvis and ureter and not the result of pacemaking system disruption. Our justification in coming to this conclusion is based on the fact that when studied *in vitro*, small tissue segments obtained from various regions of the obstructed renal pelvis and ureter exhibit this pattern of contractile activity [27]. In addition this pattern of activity has been demonstrated previously in observations made using EMG recordings made from hydronephrotic human kidneys as well as from

obstructed pigs [24]. The mechanisms involved in this type of asynchronous activity in the renal pelvis, sometimes termed incoherence or discordination of conduction, are not clearly understood and systematic studies are needed to identify whether the origin of these changes are direct or indirect outcomes of obstruction.

The response of the bladder to obstruction has been extensively investigated most recently by Jorgensen *et al.* [28] and Speakman *et al.* [29].

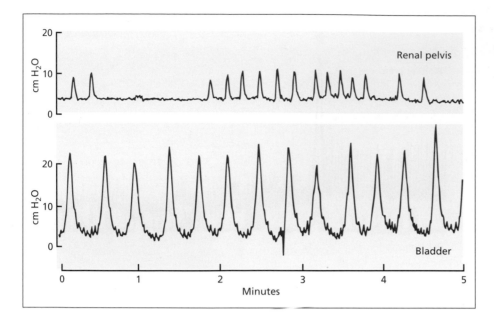

Fig. 25.7 Consequences of obstruction on the pattern of renal pelvic and bladder pressures. Bladder pressure is shown here to be constantly changing at a rate of approximately 3/min during filling. These detrusor contractions occur at a time when the bladder should be at a low pressure (as illustrated in Fig. 25.4). These contractions are interpreted to represent typical detrusor instability and are the result of the obstruction produced by the sphincter. The upper trace shows the corresponding renal pelvic pressures representative of early changes to urethral obstruction. Note that detrusor pressures due to instability are not transmitted to the pelvis and the bladder is hydrodynamically discontinuous and isolated from the pelvis.

Partial urethral obstruction induced in the pig using the method of Jorgensen *et al.* [28] produced detrusor instability and high voiding pressures (see Chapter 33). The increase in detrusor pressures can be considered to be the result of increased bladder musculature. There is now evidence by Gabella and Uvelius [30] to suggest that the increase in muscle volume is associated with a proportional increase in neuronal volume. The relative rate of growth of muscle hypertrophy to neuronal growth and its relevance to detrusor instability has not yet been established. Indeed, studies by Speakman *et al.* [29] have shown that progressive slow onset of obstruction in the pig produces high pressures, an observation which is similar to those demonstrated above. In the pig, hypertrophy is linked with increased collagen between and within the muscle bundles; segments of tissues from such preparations are known to show supersensitivity to agonists and are responsive to K-openers at lower levels than controls [31]. It remains to be shown whether analogous changes occur in the upper urinary tract as has been demonstrated in the bladder. Detrusor instability and denervation in patients with BPH has been shown to have a diminished response to electrical nerve stimulation and loss of intrinsic nerves on microscopy in a manner that is analogous to the pig model [32]. Based on these observations, Sethia *et al.* [33] suggested that unstable contractions result from changes in the detrusor rather than from increased reflex excitation. The observations of Speakman *et al.* [29] and Gosling *et al.* [34] in the pig and human are not consistent with those of Gabella and Uvelius [30] who did not observe a loss of nerve fibres in the hypertrophied bladder. It has been proposed that the chronology by which obstruction produces detrusor instability is based on the principle that progressive denervation causes physiological changes in the smooth muscle of the bladder. Supporting evidence for such a schema has been provided by Sethia *et al.* [33] who showed that bladder transection, which removed the extrinsic activation of the detrusor thereby denervating it, also produces detrusor instability and supersensitivity.

In the pig detrusor, Fujii [35] has shown that the apparent increase in the electrical coupling between cells accounts for the increased contractile activity seen in strips. Such increased coupling in the renal pelvis and ureter may be responsible for the discordination of propagating ureteric contractions and consequent loss of hierarchy [10,24]. By inference, it is suggested that such enhanced activity could lead to the spontaneous generation of ureteric peristalsis or unstable contractions of the whole bladder. Central influences in the development of neuronal hypertrophy cannot be ruled out particularly because Steers *et al.* [36] were not able to stop the development of a hypertrophied response when the ganglia were decentralized. This is because in the course of normal development the innervated tissue influences growth [37]. Thus, muscle hypertrophies due to stretch and the consequent increased work due to the obstruction stimulates nerve growth factors (NGFs) to be generated [38]. The neurotrophic factor characterized in the bladder wall is an NGF and its levels have been shown to increase during hypertrophy produced by obstruction [39].

There is now emerging evidence that growth factors may be identified that are specific to the response of the kidney to obstruction and perhaps to the pelvis and ureter. It may thus be possible in the future to study the functional response of the urinary tract to obstruction by examining the specific growth factors produced in response to the obstruction rather than the pressures associated with it [40].

Pressure–flow considerations

In analysing urodynamic studies dealing with lower urinary tract obstruction the relationship between voided flow rate and bladder pressure is considered to be the function characterizing the degree of obstruction. A similar but more complex relationship has also been derived for flow between the pelvis and bladder. Aspects of the pyelouretic pressure–flow interaction were reported by Mortensen and Djurhuus [41], demonstrating the presence of a relationship made up of four well-defined phases. Specific details of each phase define the physiological response of the system and are illustrated in Fig. 25.8. The first phase, representing a normal urine flow rate, takes place under low pressure with well-defined separated urine boluses. The second phase, associated with a high urine flow rate, is marked with increased pelvic pressure and there is ureteric filling so that individual boluses become connected to each other. Although transport still occurs in the isolated boluses, the net effect is an inhibition of passive filling and the ureter becomes dilated. In the third phase, when the flow is so high that the renal pelvis overdistends and thus inhibits bolus formation, peristaltic contractions become insufficient due to reduced contraction force leading to leakage between the boluses. In the fourth phase the ureter functions more like an open tube. A high baseline frequency causes an increased pressure response to elevations in urine production rate

(Fig. 25.9). A low peristaltic frequency causes a low-pressure response to increases in flow.

A theoretical analysis of several features of the pressure–flow relationship was conducted using the transected ureter, independently confirming the above results obtained from experimental preparations, by varying the urine flow rate [19,42]. It is interesting that also in the transected ureter flow begins when the renal pelvic pressure reaches the opening pressure. When flow rates increase, the boluses progress from an isolated state, through a leaky state, to a state of open-tube flow. Ureteric diameters, which at low levels of diuresis are small, become dilated at higher flow levels, producing the open-tube flow. Consequently, at high levels of diuresis the resistance to flow is theoretically determined by the resistance of the VUJ. According to work by Bisballe et al. [43], the transport of urine from the pelvis to the ureter is furnished by a pressure gradient and not by segmental active dilatation. His findings support the observations of Mortensen and Djurhuus [41] and the theoretical analysis of Griffiths [42], that the renal pelvic pressure drives ureteric flow. However, Bisballe et al. [43] do not discuss the contribution of active ureteric peristalsis to flow. Such an active contribution is expected to affect the value of the resistance to flow by the ureter. In accord with a recent analysis of data from Chen et al. [44], Mortensen et al. [45] indicate that transection of the ureter linearizes the relationship between renal pelvic pressure and ureteric flow. These findings further support the hypothesis that the ureter presents a varying resistance to ureteric flow because in its absence pressure and flow are related by a constant impedance [44].

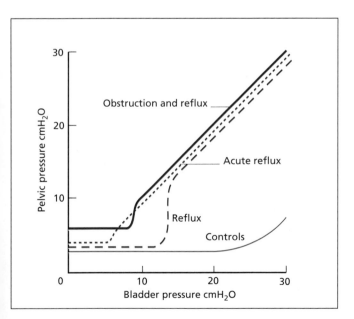

Fig. 25.8 Pressure–flow relationship in the upper urinary tract relative to obstruction and flow rate. Obstruction is shown to produce an elevated pelvic pressure baseline and an almost linear relationship between the bladder and pelvic pressures. (Redrawn from [41].)

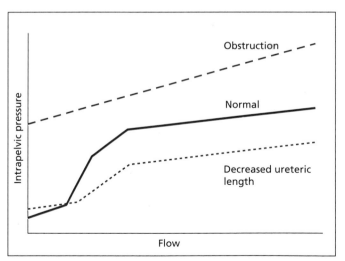

Fig. 25.9 Influence of peristaltic frequency on the pelvic pressure–flow relationship. A high peristaltic frequency causes an increased response to elevations in urine production rate and a low peristaltic frequency causes a proportionally low-pressure response to flow. (Redrawn from [41].)

Impact of reflux and obstruction on the pressure–flow relationship

In considering the pressure–flow relationship examined above, the occurrence of reflux was not taken into account. Although this subject is examined in detail in Chapter 30, it is appropriate to highlight some observations that are relevant to the material presented here. Because spontaneous reflux occurs in about one-third of some species of pigs, it has become a good experimental model for the study of the ramifications of obstruction on the dynamics of the pyeloureter. Using a sophisticated model, Jorgensen [46–48] studied the pressure–flow relationship in obstruction and reflux. Figure 25.10 schematically illustrates the cumulative findings, showing that acute and chronic reflux without obstruction causes an increase in the renal pelvic pressure which occurs at a lower bladder pressure in cases of acute reflux than is observed with chronic reflux.

Chronic reflux with obstruction causes a decrease in the magnitude of reflux-producing bladder pressure. The comparative outcome of Jorgensen's longitudinal study is schematically illustrated in Fig. 25.11; perhaps more significantly this study has shown that spontaneous reflux disappears with maturation as long as there is no obstruction. Evidently it is maintained in the presence of bladder outlet obstruction. Unroofing of the VUJ causes chronic reflux which in turn renders the upper and lower urinary tracts equibaric. However, this interesting experimental study has clearly shown that long-term persisting reflux is not important functionally to the kidney. On the other hand, the situation radically changes in the presence of simultaneous reflux and obstruction producing progressive deterioration of the upper urinary tract musculature and ultimately a compromise of renal function.

Pressure–flow relationship at early stages of chronic obstruction

It has been shown repeatedly that the pressure of the renal pelvis is not affected by micturition in the unobstructed bladder under normal levels of hydration. Examination of the results presented show that although the renal pelvis exhibits contractile characteristics consistent with obstruction, and the micturition pressures have consequently increased, there is no transmission of micturition pressures to the pelvis [26]. This has been shown in Figs 25.5–25.7 which illustrate sporadic renal pelvic pressure activity and a cystometrogram which is characteristic of a partially obstructed and unstable system. Regardless of the presence of spontaneous detrusor contractions, the sporadic contractile pattern of renal pelvic contractions in early hydronephrosis are not changed. Furthermore it is clear that during voiding, when detrusor pressure increases considerably, there is no evidence of associated transmission to the pelvis (see Fig. 25.5). It is thus clear that at early stages of partial urethral obstruction, the pattern of renal pelvic contractility and the pacemaker mechanism of initiating peristalsis change perceptibly before the detrusor pressures show evidence of instability. On the basis of these observations it appears that upper tract changes are not produced directly by transmitted high bladder pressures such as those that may be induced by transmission of detrusor instability or voiding contractions to the kidney. The only sign of increased pressures were observed during micturition which is not considered here to be of sufficient duration or frequency to produce significant distraction. Therefore, there appears to be no direct hydrodynamic explanation for the observed hydronephrotic changes in the upper urinary tract produced by partial urethral obstruction under normal hydration levels [49,50]. The importance of high hydration levels should not be underestimated. This is because, as with the controls where the urethra is undisturbed, the hydrodynamic isolation of the upper urinary tract from high detrusor instability and voiding pressures breaks down when hydration changes [15,18,20,21,51,52].

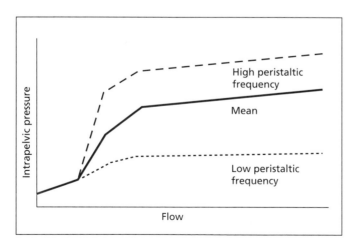

Fig. 25.10 Relationship between pelvic pressure and bladder pressure relative to reflux and obstruction. As shown in the controls, increased bladder pressures below 20 cmH$_2$O (1.96 kPa) do not affected pelvic pressure. In cases of reflux without obstruction, renal pelvic pressure is affected by bladder pressure at a lower threshold. Chronic reflux with obstruction further lowers the threshold at which bladder pressure affects renal pelvic pressure. (Redrawn from [47].)

Progressive alterations in pelvic and bladder pressure with sustained urethral obstruction

It has already been demonstrated that sustained urethral obstruction causes marked changes in the character of the pattern of the pressure wave forms of the renal pelvis as well as those of the bladder (see Fig. 25.11). Comparison of normal pelvic pressures (see Fig. 25.4) with those with a

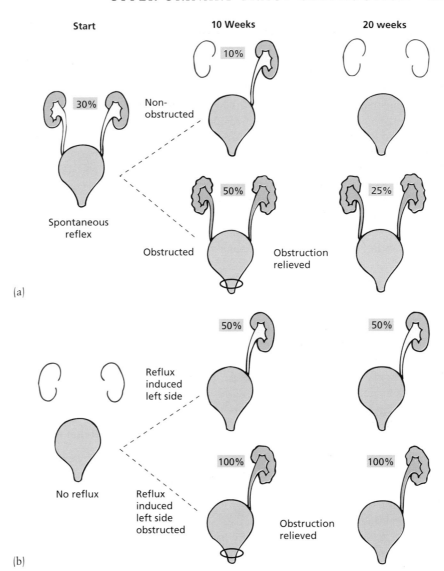

Start   10 Weeks   20 weeks

10%

30%   Non-obstructed

Spontaneous reflex

50%   25%

Obstructed   Obstruction relieved

(a)

50%   50%

Reflux induced left side

No reflux   Reflux induced left side obstructed

100%   100%

Obstruction relieved

(b)

Fig. 25.11 Schematic representation of a longitudinal study of the effects of spontaneous and induced reflux. (a) The occurrence of spontaneous reflux and its disappearance with maturation is illustrated relative to obstruction. (b) The cause of induced reflux (left), its maintenance in case of an unobstructed bladder (centre) and its impact on renal function in case of obstruction (right). (Data from [47].)

sustained obstruction (see Fig. 25.10) clearly shows that the renal pelvic contractile pattern undergoes an alteration in frequency and total duration of time over which the pelvis sustains high levels of pressure. The normal period of pressure prolongation can be from a few seconds to a few minutes. It can, therefore, be concluded that chronic urethral obstruction changes the character of the renal pelvis to such an extent that it approximates the functional characteristics of the bladder in terms of a prolonged filling phase followed by infrequent emptying. Indeed careful examination typically shows that prolonged obstruction also produces analogous changes in the contractile wave form of the bladder as well. The principal change in the obstructed bladder is the loss of lower amplitude detrusor instability contractions and the emergence of low-frequency sustained pressures. Under sustained and prolonged partial obstruction, the bladder and renal pelvic

pressures end up with contractile wave forms that possess similar characteristics, thereby suggesting that there may be a common process responsible for inducing thses events.

Clinical considerations

With ambulatory monitoring of the upper urinary system becoming available in a clinical setting it is appropriate to consider to what extent the observations made above can be used in practice. It is hoped that the experimental observations provided will point out a number of important issues that should be considered in the clinical interpretation of pelvic pressures, particularly those obtained by connecting pressure-monitoring devices on the access provided by the insertion of a nephrostomy tube. Thus, in observing renal pelvic pressures of the hydronephrotic kidney it is expected that the true baseline of the pelvis may be difficult to obtain given the slow nature of its contractility. On the other hand, a renal pelvic pressure that undergoes constant oscillation in pressure may represent a viable system. A drained pelvis may demonstrate little evidence of contractility in the short term and it may require some time to fill before any sign of activity can be detected, as the results of sustained obstruction have demonstrated. This is important, considering that when there is an acute obstruction the strategy of the urologist is to relieve it immediately after diagnosis. This is usually done by removal of the obstruction, and part of the patient preparation or the treatment *per se* may decompress the upper urinary tract above the obstruction in order to save kidney function, relieve symptoms or enhance the prospects of resolution.

It is now thought that the physiological impact of an obstruction and its potential to inflict damage depends on a variety of factors. Apart from the fundamental effect produced by the degree of obstruction, the site — whether it is a high or low obstruction — may influence the transport mechanism in terms of the mobilization of escape routes, the fluid load, and in that the pressure response in high obstructions makes the system more susceptible to flow changes than in low obstructions. A stone impacted in the ureter may or may not cause obstruction, for even when large stones are impacted total obstruction is extremely rare. Urine that may even exceed normal output can be transported across the site of obstruction. In general, impacted stones cause significant changes in the transport function of the ureter. Thus, above the site of the obstruction the frequency of peristalsis increases to the maximum frequency as dictated by the pacemaker activity of the calyces. In the beginning, pressure waves are easy to discern, often with increased amplitude, while later only small undulations may be present signifying pronounced peristaltic activity, although it is non-coaptive and without pressure relief. This hyperactive activity was shown by Bisballe *et al.* [43] to be transmitted at times around the obstruction and to some degree below it. Below the obstruction itself the peristaltic activity has a considerably lower frequency, suggesting that in this region the obstruction site has become a pacemaker for the remainder of the ureter.

Relief of acute obstruction by drainage

It is a well-known established clinical experience that decompression above the obstruction or creation of a new obstruction below the original one may enhance stone passage. Frequently the manipulation with a probe to catch stones suddenly causes spontaneous passage. The reason is that insertion of the probe distal to the obstruction creates a new obstruction distal to the existing obstruction, causing an equalization of peristaltic activity across the obstruction thus facilitating stone passage.

Decompression above the obstruction immediately relieves high-frequency peristalsis. This is a ureteric response to compression leading to total drainage of urine; then the peristaltic activity decreases proximally and the peristaltic activity ceases totally. Experimental studies by Tsuchita *et al.* [51] have shown that a ureter without a pacemaker and containing urine in the lumen, is devoid of peristaltic activity for at least 24 h after ablation of the pacemaker. Thereafter some spontaneous activity may emerge but essentially the normal ureter is driven from the pacing region.

Experimental studies where the ureter has been resected and inverted show that peristalsis is also inverted and becomes retrograde only if the pacemaker has been inverted. As the pressure–flow studies have shown above, the resistance of the ureter to the intrusion of urine is very low, and only few centimetres of water pressure are sufficient to unstick the ureter and allow flow to occur. As a consequence, the decompressed ureter may have little or no peristaltic activity and the site of the acute obstruction is then relaxed and scanty fillings may lead to peristalsis that can propagate and relieve the internal obstruction.

Relief of chronic obstruction

The experimental studies described earlier have shown that peristaltic activity increases provided there is some remaining function in the upper urinary tract. In more chronic stages where the hypertrophy and, to some extent, the hyperplastic state is reversed, then the musculature is split up into islands of more or less independent pacemakers producing spontaneous activity. It remains to be shown whether these events also produce changes in the innervation and receptor organization in the upper urinary tract as observed in the obstructed bladder [34,52–58].

Decompression of a chronically obstructed system may gradually show some restoration of peristalsis similar to the restoration seen after reconstruction of experimental hydronephrosis. In the acute phase of decompression of a chronic obstruction little or no peristaltic activity is present, suggesting that the process is not purely mechanical. Stenting of the ureter, as it is generally performed in relieving 'stein strasse', is a combination of chronic ubiquitous ureteric obstruction and decompression. The insertion of the catheter minimizes any local increase in obstruction induced by stone fragments enabling stone passage. Effectively, decompression above the stone fragments prevents hyperperistalsis and coordinated peristalsis is ensured in a ureter where the effect of local obstruction has been minimized and stone fragment passage is enhanced.

Conclusion

The above basic and experimental observations provide a framework to improve our understanding of the physiological processes involved in the transport of urine in the upper urinary system. It is evident that there are many unknown factors involved in the accommodation and compensation of the renal pelvis, ureter and bladder to even low levels of urethral compression. Atlhough the reported observations were made for far shorter time spans than, say, those of chronic obstructions seen in BPH, the data provided suggest that pressure alone is not sufficient in defining the physiological action of the upper urinary tract. As seen in the EMG measurements, the conduction in the pelvis becomes incoherent as a response to obstruction. Such incoherence can be the product of neuromuscular changes affecting the coordination and coupling of the urinary tract smooth muscle. Emerging evidence from studies of the bladder of obstructed experimental preparations suggests changes in the regulation and density of receptors (see Chapter 33). Unfortunately, analogous observations for the ureter and pelvis in an animal model that is comparable to the human are incomplete.

References

1 Gosling JG, Constantinou CE. The origin and propagation of upper urinary tract contraction waves; a new *in vitro* methodology. *Experientia* 1976;**32**:666–7.

2 Constantinou CE. Renal pelvic pacemaker control of ureteral peristaltic rate. *Am J Physiol* 1974;**226**:1413–19.

3 Zawlinski VC, Constantinou CE, Burnstock G. Ureteral pacemaker potentials recorded with the sucrose gap technique. *Experientia* 1975;**31**:931–3.

4 Constantinou CE, Yamaguchi O. Multiple coupled pacemaker system in the renal pelvis of the unicalyceal kidney. *Am J Physiol* 1981;**241**:412–18.

5 Constantinou CE. Velocity gradient and contraction frequency of the pyeloureteral system. *Experientia* 1979;**35**:444.

6 Golenhofen K, Hannappel J. Normal spontaneous activity of the pyeloureteral system in the guinea pig. *Pflugers Arch* 1973;**341**:256–70.

7 Tsuchida S, Morita M, Harada T, Kimura Y. Initiation and propagation of canine renal pelvic peristalsis. *Urol Int* 1981;**36**:307–14.

8 Saeki H, Morita M, Weiss R, Miyagawa I. The role of ureteral peristaltic rate and bolus volume on increasing urine flow. *Urol Int* 1986;**41**:174–9.

9 Constantinou CE, Hrynczuk JR. Urodynamics of the upper urinary tract. *Invest Urol* 1976;**14**:233–40.

10 Constantinou CE, Djurhuus JC. Pyeloureteral dynamics in the intact and chronically obstructed multicalyceal kidney. *Am J Physiol* 1981;**241**:398–411.

11 Yamaguchi O, Constantinou CE. Renal calyceal and pelvic contraction rhythms. *Am J Physiol* 1989;**257**:R788–95.

12 Morita M, Ishizuka G, Tsuchida S. Initiation and propagation of stimulus from the renal pelvic pacemaker in the pig kidney. *Invest Urol* 1981;**19**:157–60.

13 Kopp UC. Renorenal reflexes: role of substance P and prostaglandins. *NIBS* 1993;**8**:228–32.

14 Struthers RW. The role of manometry in the investigation of pelviureteral function. *Br J Urol* 1969;**4**:129.

15 Constantinou CE, Tsuchida S, Kavaney PB, Hayman WP, Govan DE. Simulated vesicoureteral reflux: comparison between the normal and hydrostatically bypassed ureterovesical junction as a function of urine flow rate and bladder pressure. *Urol Int* 1974;**29**:265–79.

16 Yamaguchi O. Transport efficiency of ureteral peristalsis correlated to pacemaker activity of renal pelvis. *Invest Urol* 1978;**16**:99–105

17 Djurhuus JC, Constantinou CE. Assessment of pyeloureteral function using a flow and cross-sectional diameter probe. *Invest Urol* 1979;**17**:103–7.

18 Harada T, Constantinou CE. Renal pelvic pressure isolation from passive and active bladder pressures in the rat. The facilitating effect of urine flow rate. *Urol Int* 1992;**48**:284–92.

19 Griffiths DJ, Constantinou CE, Mortensen J, Djurhuus JC. Dynamics of the upper urinary tract. II. The effect of variations of peristaltic frequency and bladder pressure on pyeloureteral pressure/flow relations. *Phys Med Biol* 1987;**32**:823–33.

20 Smyth TB, Shortliffe LM, Constantinou CE. The effect of urinary flow and bladder fullness on renal pelvic pressures in a rat model. *J Urol* 1991;**146**:592–6.

21 Issa MM, Shortliffe LM, Constantinou CE. The effect of bacteriuria on bladder and renal pelvic pressures in the rat. *J Urol* 1992;**148**:559–63.

22 Ulm AH, Miller F. An operation to produce experimental reversible hydronephrosis. *J Urol* 1962;**88**:337–41.

23 Djurhuus JC, Nerstrom B, Inversen-Hansen R, Gyrd-Hansen N, Rask-Andersen H. Dynamics of upper urinary tract. I. An electrophysiological *in vivo* study of renal pelvis in pigs: method and normal pattern. *Invest Urol* 1977;**14**;465.

24 Djurhuus JC. Aspects of renal pelvic function. PhD thesis, University of Copenhagen, Copenhagen, 1980.

25 Djurhuus JC, Frokjaer J, Munch Jorgensen T *et al*. Regulation of renal pelvic pressure by diuresis and micturition. *Am J Physiol* 1990;**259**:R637–44.

26 Constantinou CE, Djurhuus JC, Vercesi L, Ford AJ, Meindl JD. Model for chronic obstruction and hydronephrosis. In: Tumbleson ME, ed. *Swine in Biomedical Research*, Vol. 3. London: Plenum Press, 1986:1711–24.

27 Mensah-Dwumah M, Djurhuus JC, Constantinou CE. Hydronephrotic alterations in calyceal and renal pelvic pacemaker function of the *in vitro* pyeloureteral system. *Urol Int* 1980;**35**(3):161–6.

28 Jorgensen TM, Djurhuus JC, Jorgensen HS. Experimental bladder hyperreflexia in pigs. *Urol Res* 1983;**11**:239–40.

29 Speakman MJ, Brading AF, Gilpin CJ *et al*. Bladder outflow obstruction — a cause of denervation supersensitivity. *J Urol* 1987;**138**:1461–6.

30 Gabella G, Uvelius B. Urinary bladder of rat: fine structure of normal and hypertrophic musculature. *Cell Tissue Res* 1990;**262**:67–79.

31 Foster CD, Speakman MJ, Fujii K, Brading AF. The effects of cromakalim on the detrusor muscle of human and pig urinary bladder. *Br J Urol* 1989;**63**:284–49.

32 Harrison SCW. Bladder instability and denervation in patients with outflow obstruction. *Br J Urol* 1987;**60**:519–22.

33 Sethia KK, Brading AF, Smith JC. An animal model of non obstructive instability. *J Urol* 1990;**143**:1243–6.

34 Gosling JA, Gilpin SA, Dixon JS, Gilpin CJ. Decrease in the autonomic innervation of human detrusor muscle in outflow obstruction. *J Urol* 1986;**136**:50–4.

35 Fujii K. Evidence of ATP as an excitatory transmitter in guinea pig, rabbit and pig urinary bladder. *J Physiol* 1988;**404**:39–52.

36 Steers WD, Ciambotti J, Erdman S, deGroat WC. Morphological plasticity in efferent pathways to the urinary bladder of the rat following urethral obstruction. *J Neurosci* 1990;**10**:1943–51.

37 Steers WD, deGroat WC. Effect of bladder outlet obstruction on micturition reflex pathways in the rat. *J Urol* 1988;**140**:864–71.

38 Purves D, Snider WD, Voyvodic JT. Trophic regulation of nerve cell morphology and innervation in the autonomic nervous system. *Nature* 1988;**336**:123–8.

39 Steers WD, Tuttle JB, Creedon DJ. Neurotrophic influence of the bladder following outlet obstruction: implications for the unstable detrusor [Abstract]. *Neurourol Urodyn* 1989;**8**:395–6.

40 Sharmat K, Ziyadeh FN. The emerging role of transforming growth factor β in kidney diseases. *Am J Physiol* 1994;**35**:F829–42.

41 Mortenson J, Djurhuus JC. Aspects of pyeloureteral pressure flow relations. In: Tumbleson ME, ed. *Swine in Biomedical Research*, Vol. 3. London: Plenum Press, 1986:1745–51.

42 Griffiths DJ. Dynamics of the upper urinary tract. Peristaltic flow through a distensible tube of limited length. *Phys Med Biol* 1987;**32**:813–22.

43 Bisballe S, Djurhuus JC, Mortensen J, Jorgensen TM. Pyeloureteral hydrodynamics—the pelviureteral junction resistance in the pig. *Urol Int* 1983;**38**:55–7.

44 Chen J, Djurhuus JC, Constantinou CE. Urethral impedance in the pig. *Neurourol Urodyn* (in press).

45 Mortensen J, Frokiaer J, Tofft HP. Renal pelvis pressure flow relationship in pigs after transsections of the ureter. *Scand J Urol Nephrol* 1984;**18**:329–33.

46 Jorgensen TM. Dynamics of the urinary tract in long term vesico-ureteric reflux and infravesical obstraction in pigs, IV-VI. *Scand J Urol Nephrol* 1985;**19**:173–202.

47 Jorgensen TM, Djurhuus JC. Experimental vesicoureteric reflux in pigs. In: Tumbleson ME, ed. *Swine in Biomedical Research*, Vol. 3. London: Plenum Press, 1986:1737–44.

48 Jorgensen TM. Pathogenic factors in vesicoureteral reflux. *Neurourol Urodyn* 1986;**5**:153–83.

49 Ohlson L. Morphological dynamics of ureteral transport: I. Shape and volume of constituent urine fractions. *Am J Physiol* 1989;**256**:R14–23.

50 Ohlson L. Morphological dynamics of normal ureteral transport: II. Peristaltic patterns in relations to flow rate. *Am J Physiol* 1989;**256**:R24–34.

51 Tsuchita S, Harada T, Nishizawa O, Noto H. *The Function of the Renal Pelvis and Ureter*. Sasaki Co., 1994.

52 Kato K. The functional effects of long term outlet obstruction on the rabbit urinary bladder. *J Urol* 1987;**137**:1291–4.

53 Ekstrom J, Malmberg L, Oberg S. Unilateral denervation of the rat urinary bladder and reinnervation: a predominance for ipsilateral changes. *Acta Physiol Scand* 1986;**127**:223–31.

54 Gabella G. Hypertrophy of visceral smooth muscle. *Anat Embryol (Berl)* 1990;**182**:409–24.

55 Lindner P, Mattiasson A, Persson L, Uvelius B. Reversibility of detrusor hypertrophy and hyperplasia after removal of infravesical outflow obstruction in the rat. *J Urol* 1988;**140**:642–6.

56 Mattiasson A, Ekstrom J, Larsson B, Uvelius B. Changes in the nervous control of the rat urinary bladder induced by outflow obstruction. *Neurourol Urodyn* 1987;**6**:37–45.

57 Mattiasson A, Uvelius B. Changes in contractile properties in hypertrophic urinary bladder. *J Urol* 1982;**128**:1340–2.

58 Purves D. *Body and Brain: a Trophic Theory of Neural Connections*. Cambridge, MA: Harvard University Press, 1988.

26 Pathophysiology of Obstruction: Role of Novel Vasoactive Compounds

F. A. Gulmi, D. Felsen and E. D. Vaughan, Jr

Introduction

The study of ureteric obstruction can be divided into the effects of the occlusion of one or both ureters, referred to as unilateral ureteric occlusion (UUO) and bilateral ureteric occlusion (BUO), respectively. The model for UUO has stood the test of time, enduring for at least the last quarter of a century. Its reproducibility facilitates the comparison of data between investigators. In the first part of this chapter we will discuss several vasoactive mediators and how they may be involved in the classic triphasic changes of renal bloodflow and ureteric pressure that occur after UUO and BUO. Changes in tubule function will also be discussed. The second half of the chapter will explore the changes in extracellular matrix and cellular composition of the obstructed kidney and how such changes may be involved in the pathophysiology of obstruction.

Several systems of vasoactive compounds have been examined for their role in obstructive uropathy. Among those previously reviewed [1,2] are angiotensin II and bradykinin, eicosanoids (prostaglandins and thromboxanes) and platelet-activating factor (PAF). Newly described roles for nitric oxide (NO) (also known as EDRF or endothelium-derived relaxing factor) and atrial natriuretic peptide (ANP) will be discussed in more detail.

Vasoactive mediators

Angiotensin II and bradykinin

Angiotensin II is an octapeptide derived from a precursor peptide angiotensin I by the action of angiotensin-converting enzyme (ACE). The many biological effects of angiotensin II have been described in several reviews [3,4]. The active vasoconstrictor angiotensin II can be antagonized at its receptor by peptide and non-peptide analogues. ACE inhibitors, which prevent the formation of angiotensin II, include captopril and enalapril. In contrast, the action of bradykinin, a non-peptide vasodilator, is enhanced by ACE inhibitors because converting enzyme normally metabolizes bradykinin to less active metabolites. Administration of angiotensin II usually results in decreased renal bloodflow.

Eicosanoids (prostaglandins and thromboxanes)

The metabolites of arachidonic acid (5, 8, 11, 14, eicosatetraenoic acid) are numerous. Among these are: cyclooxygenase-derived prostaglandins (PG) — PGE_2, $PGF_{2\alpha}$, PGD_2, PGI_2 (prostacyclin) and thromboxanes (TxB_2); lipoxygenase-derived leucotrienes; and cytochrome P450-derived products. For a more complete discussion of arachidonic acid metabolism see reviews in Norris [5] and Baird and Morrison [6]. In the kidney, PGE_2 and PGI_2 are primarily vasodilators, whereas TxB_2 is a vasoconstrictor.

Platelet-activating factor

PAF is a vasoactive lipid [7] produced by both inflammatory cells and by glomeruli and mesangial cells. PAF has a variety of biological effects including platelet aggregation, bronchoconstriction and haemoconcentration. When given intrarenally, PAF decreases renal bloodflow, glomerular filtration rate (GFR) and urinary volume [7].

Nitric oxide (endothelium-derived relaxing factor)

In 1980, Furchgott and Zawadski [8] reported that the vasodilatory effects of acetylcholine were mediated by a smooth muscle relaxation factor contained within the endothelial cells called EDRF. Over the ensuing years EDRF was identified as NO. NO is synthesized in the endothelial cells from the amino acid L-arginine by the enzyme NO synthase [9]. NO has been shown to cause an increase in renal bloodflow independent of PGs [10]. Ercan et al. [11] have demonstrated that removal of the endothelium with Triton X-100 potentiated the vasoconstrictor effects of angiotensin II, noradrenaline and phenylephrine, suggesting an integral role for NO in balancing intrarenal vasoactive forces. Ito et al. [12] have described an antagonistic effect of NO on angiotensin II in the isolated microperfused rabbit afferent arteriole. L-NMMA (L-N^G-monomethyl-L-arginine) is an analogue of L-arginine that competitively inhibits the conversion of L-arginine to NO [13], an effect that can be exploited in experimental protocols studying the haemodynamic effects of NO.

Atrial natriureteric peptide

Jameison and Palade [14] first characterized the existence of granules within the cardiac atrial myocytes which were not found in the ventricular myocytes. In 1983 Debold and associates [15] demonstrated a prolonged diuresis and natriuresis in normal rats when given the extract of rat atria intravenously. This substance with time has come to be known as ANP. ANP is a 28 amino acid peptide and is released into the circulation in response to atrial stretch [16,17]. Therefore, ANP has been shown to be elevated in conditions associated with either acute or chronic extracellular volume overload, i.e. acute saline loading, congestive heart failure and renal failure prior to dialysis. ANP has also been shown to increase during paroxysmal atrial tachycardia [16]. The majority of receptors for ANP within the nephron are located within the glomerulus and the collecting duct [16,17].

ANP has several effects including vascular smooth muscle relaxation, vasodilatation, natriuresis and diuresis. The natriuretic action has been shown to be caused by an increase in GFR through afferent arteriole vasodilatation and efferent arteriole vasoconstriction, as well as increasing the glomerular capillary ultrafiltration coefficient (k_f), and finally through an inhibition of the glomerular tubular feedback mechanism [17].

Effects of ureteric obstruction on renal bloodflow, ureteric pressure and tubular function

The effect of ureteric obstruction on renal bloodflow and ureteric pressure differs in unilateral obstruction and bilateral obstruction.

The acute unilateral occlusion of a ureter will result in a characteristic triphasic relationship between renal bloodflow and ureteric pressure [18] (Fig. 26.1). Phase 1 is characterized by a rise in both ureteric pressure and renal bloodflow lasting approximately 1–1.5 h. This is followed in phase 2 by a decline in renal bloodflow and a continued increase in ureteric pressure lasting until the fifth hour of occlusion. Phase 3 ensues with a further decline in renal bloodflow accompanied by a progressive decrease in ureteric pressure. Haemodynamically, phase 1 is characterized by an initial afferent arteriole vasodilatation, followed by an efferent vasoconstriction in phase 2 and finally afferent arteriole vasoconstriction in phase 3 [18].

The patterns of changes of renal bloodflow and ureteric pressure are not the same following bilateral renal obstruction or unilateral obstruction of a solitary kidney. The renal bloodflow after BUO follows a pattern similar to that of UUO for the first 90 min. However, the renal bloodflow between 1.5 and 7 h of BUO is significantly lower than the renal bloodflow during UUO for the same hours post-obstruction [19]. This is also reflected by a greater renal vascular resistance in BUO than UUO during the same time period. At 24 h of obstruction renal bloodflow declines to the same level in both BUO and UUO [19].

The ureteric pressure follows a similar pattern during UUO and BUO for the first 4.5 h of ureteric obstruction, i.e. a steady progressive rise in pressure. However, after 4.5 h of BUO the ureteric pressure remains elevated, in contrast to the progressive decline below this level in the UUO model. In the BUO model the ureteric pressure remains significantly elevated above control values after 24–48 h of obstruction. Interestingly, this occurs despite both the UUO and BUO groups achieving similar renal vascular resistances at 24 h post-occlusion [19,20]. In contrast to UUO, the glomerulus in BUO passes through phases 1 and 2, and seems to remain in phase 2 (i.e. pre-glomerular vasodilatation and post-glomerular vasoconstriction), explaining the persistent rise in ureteric pressure at 24 h of BUO.

Acute UUO results in a decrease in sodium, potassium and solute excretion and an increase in urine osmolality [21]. Suki and associates, utilizing renal artery constriction during acute UUO along with either water or saline diuresis, demonstrated a decrease in urinary sodium excretion [22]. There is a more complete reabsorption of sodium in the proximal nephron secondary to a decrease in the flow rate. There is also an increase in the back-diffusion of free water in the collecting duct, thus ultimately increasing free water loss from the obstructed kidney. This would result in a diminished delivery of filtrate to the distal nephron [22]. For a further discussion of solute handling in both UUO and BUO, see p. 414.

Role of vasoactive substances in the pathophysiology of obstruction

Angiotensin II and bradykinin

The initial hyperaemia seen with acute UUO is not affected by ipsilateral renal denervation, α- and β-receptor blockage, contralateral nephrectomy or chronic renin suppression with sodium chloride loading and/or deoxycorticosterone administration prior to obstruction [23]. Gilmore [24] postulated an autoregulatory phenomenon resulting in an afferent vascular myogenic response to increases in interstitial and tubular pressure from acute

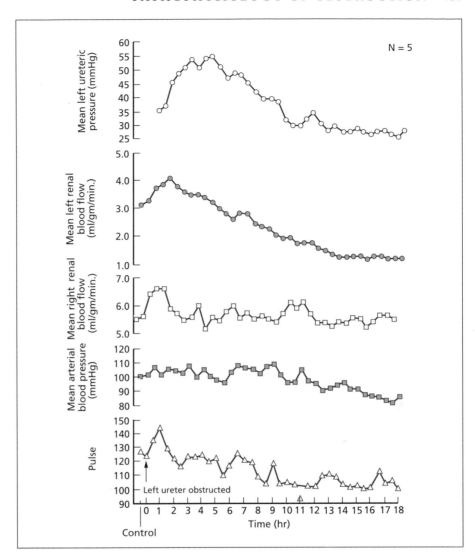

Fig. 26.1 The triphasic relationship between ipsilateral renal bloodflow and left ureteric pressure during 18 h of left ureter obstruction in the dog. In phase 1 (0–1.5 h), bloodflow and ureteric pressure rise together (hyperaemic phase). In phase 2 (1.5–5 h), bloodflow begins to decline while ureteric pressure continues to rise. In phase 3 (5–18 h), bloodflow and ureteric pressure decline in tandem. L-NMMA, L-*N*G-monomethyl-L-arginine, an arginine analogue. (Redrawn from [18].)

ureteric obstruction. Moody *et al.* [25] administered Sar[1]-Ala[8] angiotensin II (an angiotensin II inhibitor) and did not alter the initial hyperaemia after ureteric occlusion, suggesting that the autoregulatory mechanism is not mediated by angiotensin II. Several other studies utilizing either angiotensin II blockade, renin depletion or inhibition of ACE did not significantly alter the autoregulatory phenomenon [26–28].

Several investigators have demonstrated an increased release of renin by the ipsilateral kidney in acute UUO [23,29]. However, Vaughan *et al.* were unable to show any improvement in renal bloodflow with a 14-day regimen of desoxycorticosterone acetate (DOCA) and salt loading and showed a documented decrease in post-ureteric occlusion renal vein renin samples [23]. When saralasin is infused prior to ureteric occlusion there was a persistent decline in renal bloodflow 5 h post-obstruction, again arguing against angiotensin II as the humoral mediator of late phase post-UUO vasoconstriction [25,30]. However, saralasin itself has

been shown to have some vasoconstrictive effects and may mask the blockage of angiotensin II and the subsequent vasodilatation one might expect.

Utilizing agents without vasoconstrictive effects has provided support for angiotensin II as the humoral mediator of vasoconstriction in the late phase of UUO. Yarger *et al.* [30], utilizing captopril, were able to demonstrate an improvement in renal function post-UUO. This was irrespective of the administration of captopril either before or after the release of obstruction. Because captopril also increases serum levels of the vasodilator kinins, the experiments were performed using carboxypeptidase B and trasylol, inhibitors of kinin production. In the presence of kinin inhibitors and captopril, renal function still improved post-UUO. Franke and McDougal [31] administered enalapril, another ACE inhibitor, during UUO and were able to demonstrate an improvement in renal plasma flow and GFR during obstruction.

Yarger *et al.* [32] have also implicated the kinin–

kallikrein system in post-obstructive renal haemodynamics. Kinins are usually vasodilators; however, they are also known to stimulate the production of TxA_2. Aprotinin is a known inhibitor of the kinin system. Therefore, by administering aprotinin pre-obstruction, Yarger et al. were able to demonstrate a significant improvement in both GFR and renal bloodflow in the UUO kidney. When indomethacin was administered prior to aprotinin there was an improvement in post-obstructive renal function. However, when indomethacin and captopril were administered prior to aprotinin, there was no further improvement in renal function with the administration of aprotinin. This suggests that aprotinin may also affect the formation of angiotensin II and the kinin–kallikrein system may contribute to the post-obstructive renal vasoconstriction by generating both vasoconstrictor eicosanoids and angiotensin II.

Prostaglandins and thromboxanes

Several studies have demonstrated increased levels of PGE_2 and TxA_2 in UUO in rabbits [33,34]. Utilizing isolated perfused hydronephrotic rabbit kidneys after 72 h of ureteric obstruction, several investigators were able to demonstrate increased levels of PGE_2 and TxA_2 in response to an infusion of bradykinin, a known stimulator of the PG system [34]. Whinnery et al. [35] demonstrated increased levels of both TxB_2 (a chemically stable metabolite of TxA_2) and PGE_2 in the renal papilla, and increased levels of only TxB_2 in the cortex of UUO kidneys. After 2 h of UUO, both PGE_2 and TxB_2 were elevated; however, after 18 h of UUO, there was only an increased production of TxB_2. Yanagisawa et al. [36] demonstrated an increase in prostanoid production from glomeruli of kidneys following ureteric occlusion compared to production in the contralateral kidney.

In vivo, inhibitors of arachidonic acid metabolism have been used to probe the role of eicosanoids in the triphasic response of UUO. Allen et al. [37], using indomethacin (a cyclooxygenase inhibitor), were able to attenuate the initial rise in renal bloodflow after acute UUO. This was accompanied by a diminished initial rise in ureteric pressure after acute UUO, suggesting an unopposed vasoconstriction or the lack of an exaggerated vasodilatation of the afferent arteriole with indomethacin administration. In experiments testing the effectiveness of indomethacin or imidazole (a thromboxane synthetase inhibitor), Yarger et al. [30] demonstrated a decrease in the vasoconstriction post-UUO with the administration of imidazole. This vasodilatation was not observed when indomethacin was given post-UUO. The administration of imidazole selectively blocked TxB_2 production and permitted the continued synthesis of the vasodilator PGs, PGE_2 and PGI_2, and thus improvement in post-obstruction

renal function was observed. However, the administration of indomethacin blocked the production of all vasoactive arachidonic acid metabolites, and hence there was no beneficial effect on renal function in the obstructed kidney. Therefore, it may be that a balance between the vasodilator and vasoconstrictor eicosanoids during acute UUO is responsible for the overall renovascular tone. However, not all studies confirm those carried out in rats.

Loo et al. [38,39], utilizing a specific inhibitor of TxA_2 synthetase, OKY-046, selectively inhibited the production of TxA_2 during UUO in dogs and rabbits. This was documented by a 90% reduction in urinary TxB_2 production with no effect on urinary PGE_2 production. Despite this inhibition of TxA_2 synthesis, there was no improvement in ipsilateral renal bloodflow after 18 h of UUO. The use of a thromboxane synthetase inhibitor can lead to a short-lived build-up of the vasoconstrictor PGH_2, the precursor of TxA_2. Therefore, the failure of the TxA_2 synthetase inhibitor to change the haemodynamic response to obstruction could be due to the substitution of one vasoconstrictor (TxA_2) for another (PGH_2). To address this question experiments were also carried out with SQ-29548, a thromboxane and PGH_2 receptor blocker. In these experiments SQ-29548 was able to block the vasoconstrictor effect of an intravenously administered stable TxA_2 analogue; however, there was a persistent decrease in renal bloodflow following UUO [40]. Thus, species differences have been noted in studying the effects of eicosanoid synthesis inhibitors in the renal response to obstruction.

The previous studies have addressed the involvement of angiotensin II and eicosanoids in the response to UUO. Studies of BUO have also been carried out. Purkesón and Klahr [41] studied rats undergoing unilateral release of BUO. Those animals treated with either enalapril or OKY-046 after relief of obstruction demonstrated mild improvement in GFR and renal bloodflow. However, pretreatment of the animals for 48 h prior to obstruction markedly improved both the GFR and renal bloodflow post-obstruction. When the inhibitors were administered simultaneously there was an even greater increase in GFR then when either inhibitor was administered alone, suggesting a significant contribution by angiotensin and TxA_2 to the glomerular vascular tone during BUO. Harris and associates [42] studied C-inulin clearance in rats administered OKY-046 after the release of 24 h BUO and were able to demonstrate an improvement of post-obstructive GFR in previously irradiated animals. Imidazole also has been shown to improve GFR and effective renal plasma flow in the post-obstructed kidney [43].

Platelet-activating factor

The involvement of PAF in both UUO and BUO has been

studied. A PAF antagonist, SRI-63441, was administered intravenously and its efficacy against PAF administered intrarenally was confirmed. Administration of SRI-63441 prior to the onset of UUO in dogs had no effect on the renal haemodynamic response to UUO [40], suggesting that PAF is not involved in the haemodynamic response to UUO. Reyes and Klahr found that administration of a PAF antagonist enhanced the decreased GFR and renal bloodflow associated with BUO in rats, suggesting a vasodilatory role for PAF in BUO [44].

Nitric oxide

Lanzone et al. [45] demonstrated that the administration of L-NMMA prior to UUO significantly attenuates the initial rise in renal bloodflow. Upon discontinuation of L-NMMA, the initial rise in renal bloodflow was restored within 10 min. The addition of L-arginine to the L-NMMA infusion abrogated the fall in renal bloodflow caused by the administration of L-NMMA alone. These data provide strong evidence for the role of NO in reducing renal vascular resistance after ureteric occlusion. Previous micropuncture studies have shown an increase in glomerular capillary hydrostatic pressure after ureteric occlusion. It is conceivable that the physical stretch of the vascular endothelium as a result of the increase in hydrostatic pressure stimulates the release of NO.

Since both eicosanoids and NO have been shown to be involved in the initial hyperaemia of UUO, studies were undertaken to determine the interaction of these two systems in UUO. Schulsinger et al. [46] studied acute ureteric occlusion and L-arginine infusion in dogs that were pretreated with meclofenamate (a cyclooxygenase inhibitor), thus preventing PGs from contributing to the haemodynamic effects of UUO. After the administration of meclofenamate obstruction was induced and no rise in renal bloodflow and ureteric pressure was observed, confirming previously reported data [46]. However, the administration of L-arginine after 140 min of UUO restored renal bloodflow and ureteric pressure to control values. The administration of L-arginine in the absence of obstruction, with or without PG synthesis inhibition, did not alter renal haemodynamics. This emphasizes the importance of UUO in activating the NO system, possibly by up-regulating NO synthase activity. This study demonstrates that the NO system stimulated by UUO is capable of superseding the PG system and thus sustain increases in renal bloodflow and hence ureteric pressure after obstruction. At present, the exact interaction between the NO and PG systems is not well understood. Chou et al. [47] and De Nucci et al. [48] have shown that endothelin, a potent vasoconstrictor, stimulates the release of prostacyclin and NO, both vasodilators. Perhaps it is a balance between these vasoactive substances that explains the haemodynamic

continuum of early renal vasodilatation and late renal vasoconstriction seen in the acute UUO model.

Reyes et al. [49] have shown that the administration of L-arginine improves GFR and renal bloodflow in BUO, suggesting a decrease in the production of NO during BUO may be responsible for the observed decline in GFR and renal bloodflow during BUO. Von Lutterotti et al. [50] demonstrated elevated levels of prorenin in dogs after 48 h of BUO. Prorenin is believed to have vasodilator rather than vasoconstrictor effects within the kidney [51–53]. A positive relationship between plasma prorenin and post-obstruction effective renal plasma flow and GFR was established. Perhaps prorenin is another vasoactive hormone contributing to the overall hormonal environment and thus vascular tone during BUO.

Atrial natriuretic peptide

A major role for ANP is in the setting of bilateral obstruction [54]. Several investigators had postulated the build-up of a 'substance' during BUO that is excreted by the contralateral kidney in UUO. This substance would allow the glomerulus to remain in a state of afferent arteriolar vasodilatation and efferent arteriolar vasoconstriction, i.e. phase 2, and not permit the glomerulus to progress into phase 3 or afferent vasoconstriction in association with efferent vasoconstriction [19,55]. Wilson and Honrath [56] utilizing cross-circulation techniques were able to demonstrate the accumulation of a 'natriuretic substance' in BUO rats not found in UUO rats. The blood from BUO rats induced a natriuresis and diuresis when infused into the UUO rats [56]. Harris and Yarger, utilizing similar techniques, were also able to demonstrate the existence of a circulating natriuretic factor in BUO rats [57,58].

Fried et al. [59] demonstrated elevated levels of plasma ANP in rats after 24 h of BUO. However, ANP was not elevated in those rats with UUO [59]. Gulmi and associates demonstrated an augmented release of ANP in a prospective study of nine patients with BUO [20]. ANP causes afferent arteriolar vasodilatation and efferent arteriolar vasoconstriction, actions which could explain the persistent increase in ureteric pressure and decline in renal bloodflow observed after 7 h of BUO. Himmelstein and associates have demonstrated enhanced production of prostacyclin after 24 h of BUO [60]. With the administration of indomethacin, the increase in renal vascular resistance seen in BUO was blunted by 35–50% despite elevated ANP levels. Thus, the glomerular vascular tone during BUO may not be the direct effect of ANP, but rather an ANP-induced increase in eicosanoid production.

Classically, upon release of UUO there is no diuresis or natriuresis. Gulmi et al. [61] were unable to demonstrate an increase in urine output or sodium excretion after the release of 48 h of UUO from an ipsilateral kidney. The contralateral kidney, in fact, demonstrated an increase in sodium reabsorption during the post-release period. However, other investigators have demonstrated an increase in sodium excretion and fractional excretion of sodium from the ipsilateral kidney after UUO [62] but they were unable to show an increase in urine output post-release of obstruction. Harris and Yarger also failed to demonstrate a diuresis and natriuresis after the release of 24h of UUO. They attributed the failure of post-obstructive diuresis occurring in the ipsilateral kidney post-release of UUO to a greater percentage of non-functioning outer cortical nephrons compared to the situation in BUO (40% in BUO vs 84% in UUO) and to a decrease in the delivery of sodium and water to the distal nephron [63].

Gulmi *et al.* were unable to demonstrate an increase in plasma ANP during 48h of UUO in dogs [61]. Perhaps it is this lack of accumulation of ANP in the blood during UUO that is responsible for the absence of a post-obstructive diuresis and natriuresis in UUO. The fact that the contralateral kidney is excreting the fluid volume prevents atrial stretch and hence the stimulus for ANP secretion into the bloodstream. Wilson [64], utilizing the UUO model, was unable to obtain a post-obstructive diuresis upon release of UUO when there was an intact contra-lateral kidney. However, when the same animals were volume expanded with hypotonic saline after the relief of obstruction there was a marked diuresis and natriuresis from the ipsilateral kidney. This was not from a redistri-bution of filtration from deep to superficial nephrons during obstruction. Rather, it is believed that volume expansion may exaggerate an underlying defect in water reabsorption in the distal nephron induced by obstruction of the kidney. This reinforces the importance of volume expansion to the post-obstructive diuresis phenomenon.

Harris *et al.* [65] were able to improve post-obstruction GFR in the ipsilateral kidney after UUO with saline loading. This was associated with an increase in urinary cyclic guanosine monophosphate (cGMP) levels from the ipsilateral kidney. The administration of ANP to non-saline-loaded animals resulted in the same improvements in GFR and cGMP excretion as the saline-loaded animals. Saline loading has been shown to increase endogenous ANP levels and urinary cGMP excretion in both animals and humans [20,66]. It is, perhaps, the volume expansion that is stimulating endogenous ANP excretion and causing the post-obstructive diuresis and natriuresis in these animals. ANP may also help to preserve renal function in the post-obstructive ipsilateral kidney when volume expanded by helping to maintain GFR via afferent arteriolar vaso-dilatation.

Upon release of BUO there is a substantial and sustained decrease in both GFR and renal bloodflow. This decrease in GFR has been shown to last from 18h to 4 days after the release of the obstruction [67,68]. However, in both of these studies the animals were deprived of food and water once ureteral obstruction was induced. Gulmi *et al.* [61] were able to demonstrate a trend towards an improvement in GFR after the release of obstruction within 12h associated with a normalization in serum creatinine and blood urea nitrogen (BUN) which occurred in animals volume expanded with normal saline after the induction of BUO. This was accompanied by an elevation in serum ANP after 48h of obstruction. Again, because ANP causes afferent arteriole vasodilatation and efferent vasoconstriction, its presence may have a protective effect on glomerular functions by preventing vasoconstriction of the afferent arteriole that would further decrease GFR in the later phases of obstruction. Renal bloodflow, however, remained decreased 12–18h after release of BUO [61,68].

The release of BUO is characterized by a marked diuresis, natriuresis and kaliuresis [20,67]. This diuresis and natriuresis can last for several days in the patient, accompanied by a loss in body weight of up to 3.6kg [20,69]. This salt-wasting state requires close monitoring of the patient's fluid status, electrolytes and blood pressure. Initially, patients will have a low plasma renin activity secondary to the expanded extracellular fluid space [21]. Plasma renin activity will increase in all patients after the release of obstruction secondary to excretion of extracellular fluid volume. There seem to be several factors responsible for this phenomenon. Studies have shown an effect of obstruction itself on renal tubular function decreasing the kidney's ability to retain salt and water [70-72]. However, cross-circulation studies by Wilson and colleagues have suggested the existence of a natriuretic substance accumulated during BUO that may be responsible for post-obstruction diuresis and natriuresis [56]. Gulmi *et al.* [61] have described an increase in plasma ANP in dogs volume expanded during 48h of BUO. This was associated with an increase in body weight and pulmonary capillary wedge pressure, both indicators of an expanded extracellular fluid space, and hence indicated atrial stretch as the mechanism for the secretion of ANP. A second group in this study, not volume expanded, did not have elevated plasma ANP levels; however, the animals still underwent a modest post-obstructive diuresis and natriuresis. The salt and water loss was greater and more sustained in the volume-expanded group of animals than the non-volume-replete group. This lends support to a dual mechanism for the phenomenon of post-obstructive diuresis and natriuresis, i.e. a direct tubular effect of BUO on the kidney, enhanced by a hormonal environment that is the result of an expanded extracellular volume state.

Conclusion

The experiments described above demonstrate that both

established and newly described vasoactive compounds are involved in the response of the kidney to UUO and BUO. The renal response to UUO and BUO differs and this is reflected in the differential involvement of mediators in response to either UUO or BUO. It is important to note that although the initial increase in renal bloodflow associated with phase 1 of UUO can be eliminated, there has been no similar finding in phase 3 of UUO. No single mediator has been found which can account completely for the persistent decrease in renal bloodflow which follows UUO. The search for these elusive mediators continues.

Cellular infiltrates and extracellular matrix changes in UUO/BUO

The changes in renal bloodflow, GFR and tubular function appear to be mediated by vasoactive compounds in the kidney. Cellular elements in the kidney may play an important part in generating these vasoactive compounds. The first evidence for changes in the cellular composition of the obstructed kidney were those of Nagle et al. [73–75]. In these studies, it was demonstrated histologically that at 1 day following UUO in the rabbit the interstitial space contained fibroblasts and occasional mononuclear cells. By the fourth day following obstruction there were many more mononuclear cells in the interstitium. Between days 7 and 32 there was a progressive widening of the cortical interstitial space and fibroblast proliferation.

Nagle's findings were followed by the studies of Needleman and co-workers. Needleman's group showed that there were major changes in arachidonic acid metabolism in the obstructed kidney. Microsomal preparations of the obstructed kidney showed increased arachidonic acid metabolism to eicosanoids, in particular to the vasoconstrictor TxA_2, not found in the contralateral kidney [76]. Furthermore, ex vivo perfusion of obstructed kidneys demonstrated a time-dependent increase in eicosanoid synthesis, as well as the appearance of a time-dependent increase in release of TxA_2 [34]. Subsequent electron microscopic analysis of obstructed kidneys showed the presence of interstitial fibroblasts and macrophages [77]. Reversal of the obstruction decreased the numbers of macrophages but not the numbers of fibroblasts. Stimuli such as endotoxin, which are known to stimulate eicosanoid synthesis and release from macrophages, were effective stimulants of exaggerated eicosanoid and TxA_2 synthesis in the perfused kidney. The contralateral kidney and the cat kidney, both of which do not histologically demonstrate macrophage infiltration, do not respond to endotoxin and do not show the same exaggerated eicosanoid release. Further studies using nitrogen mustard to prevent infiltration of macrophages into the kidney decreased the exaggerated eicosanoid synthesis in the obstructed ex vivo perfused kidney [78].

Diamond et al. [79] have recently used immunohistochemical techniques to localize macrophages in the obstructed kidney. Using monoclonal antibodies to rat macrophages they demonstrated the presence of macrophages in the peritubular cortical interstitial space. By 96 h there was a 20-fold increase in the number of interstitial macrophages. These results complement those of Klahr and his associates who used sieving techniques to separate glomeruli from other renal compartments followed by incubation with monoclonal antibodies. Using this technique they demonstrated an increased number of macrophages and suppressor T-lymphocytes in the cortical and medullary interstitium and a decrease in the numbers of macrophages in glomeruli during a 72 h period of obstruction [80]. Irradiation of rats with BUO led to decrease in macrophage numbers and reversals of the decreased renal function [81].

Changes in vasoactive compounds and the cellular composition of the kidney may also have an impact on the fibrotic process which accompanies obstruction. Gonzalez-Avila et al. [82] have shown increases in collagen in the rat kidney following obstruction. Collagen was demonstrated both histologically and biochemically, and in biochemical studies was shown to be increased almost threefold. Collagenolytic activity of the obstructed kidney was decreased 10-fold. Immunohistochemical studies by Sharma et al. [83] in rabbit kidneys obstructed for 16 days, showed increases in interstitial collagens I and III. Collagen IV, laminin and fibronectin, normally found in association with the basement membrane, are also found in the interstitial space following obstruction. Increased mRNA for collagen monomers indicates increases in synthesis; collagen degradation was not studied.

Regulation of the synthesis of collagen and extracellular matrix (ECM) is complex. Both angiotensin II and TxA_2, which have been implicated in the haemodynamic response to UUO, may be involved in changes in the ECM. TxA_2 has been shown to affect ECM synthesis in vitro [84]. Angiotensin II-induced hypertension is associated with interstitial accumulation of collagens [85]. One cytokine which has been shown to be involved in several aspects of the regulation of ECM is transforming growth factor β (TGF-β) [86,87]. TGF-β is a multifunctional cytokine found as several different isoforms. TGF-β_1 has been the best studied; TGF-β_2 is similar to TGF-β_1 in many respects. The synthesis of active TGF-β is a multistep process and involves the intermediate formation of a latent TGF-β complex [88]. Activation of the latent complex determines the availability of active TGF-β and thus is a critical step in the control of TGF-β's bioactivity. Many TGF-β-binding proteins have been described, some of which may function as receptors for TGF-β. TGF-β is involved in cell proliferation, differentiation and the control of ECM [86,87,89]. It has been shown to stimulate the synthesis of

ECM components, as well as to inhibit ECM degradation. Inhibition of ECM degradation results from the direct action of TGF-β to inhibit synthesis of the proteolytic enzymes of ECM degradation, and also from effects of TGF-β on activating the synthesis of inhibitors of the proteases [89]. In glomerulonephritis and other fibrotic disease models, antibodies to, or antagonists of, TGF-β have been shown to ameliorate the fibrotic condition [90,91]. Two studies have demonstrated increased TGF-β mRNA expression in the acute response to UUO [92,93]; however, these studies did not measure active protein. Recent studies by Diamond *et al.* [79] have demonstrated immunohistochemical localization of TGF-β in acute UUO in association with interstitial macrophages. However, the involvement of both TGF-β and interstitial macrophages in the chronic response to UUO remains to be determined.

References

1 Loo MH, Felsen D, Weisman SM, Marion DN, Vaughan ED Jr. Pathophysiology of obstructive nephropathy. *World J Urol* 1988;**6**:53–60.

2 Klahr S, Purkerson ML. The pathophysiology of obstructive nephropathy: the role of vasoactive compounds in the hemodynamic and structural abnormalities of the obstructed kidney. *Am J Kidney Dis* 1994;**23**:219–23.

3 Goldfarb DA. The renin–angiotensin system. New concepts in regulation of blood pressure and renal function. *Urol Clin North Am* 1994;**21**:187–94.

4 Messerli FH, Weberm A, Brunner H. Angiotensin-II receptors: new targets for anti-hypertensive therapy. *Clin Cardiol* 1997;**20**:3–6.

5 Norris SH. Renal eicosanoids. *Semin Nephrol* 1990;**10**:64–88.

6 Baird NR, Morrison AR. Amplification of the arachidonic acid cascade: implications for pharmacological intervention. *Am J Kidney Dis* 1993;**21**:557–64.

7 Camussi G, Salvidio G, Tetta C. Platelet-activating factor in renal diseases. *Am J Nephrol* 1989;**9**(Suppl. 1):23–6.

8 Furchgott RF, Zawadski JV. The obligatory role of endothelial cells in the relaxation of arterial smooth muscle by acetylcholine. *Nature* 1980;**288**:373–6.

9 Gibaldi M. What is nitric oxide and why are so many people studying it? *J Clin Pharmacol* 1993;**33**:488–96.

10 Romero JC, Lahera V, Salom MG, Blondi ML. Role of the endothelium-dependent relaxing factor nitric oxide on renal function. *J Am Soc Nephrol* 1992;**2**:1371–87.

11 Ercan ZS, Soydan AS, Turker RK. Possible involvement of endothelium in the responses of various vasoactive agents in rabbit isolated perfused kidney. *Gen Pharmacol* 1990;**21**:205–9.

12 Ito S, Johnson CS, Carretero OA. Modulation of angiotensin II-induced vasoconstriction by endothelium-derived relaxing factor in the isolated microperfused rabbit afferent arteriole. *J Clin Invest* 1991;**87**:1656–63.

13 Lahera V, Salom MG, Miranda-Guardiola F, Moncada S, Romero JC. Effects of NG-nitro-L-arginine methyl ester on renal function and blood pressure. *Am J Physiol* 1991;**261**:F1033–7.

14 Jameison JD, Palade GE. Specific granules in atrial muscle cells. *J Cell Biol* 1964;**23**:151–72.

15 De Bold AJ, Salerno TA. Natriuretic activity of extracts obtained from hearts of different species and from various rat tissues. *Can J Physiol Pharmacol* 1983;**61**:127–130.

16 Cogan MG. Atrial natriuretic peptide. *Kidney Int* 1990;**37**:1148–60.

17 Maack T, Okolicany J, Koh GY, Price DA. Functional properties of atrial natriuretic factor receptors. *Semin Nephrol* 1993;**13**:50–60.

18 Moody TE, Vaughan ED Jr, Gillenwater JY. Relationship between renal blood flow and ureteral pressure during 18 hours of total unilateral ureteral occlusion. Implications for changing sites of increased renal resistance. *Invest Urol* 1975;**13**:246–51.

19 Moody TE, Vaughan ED Jr, Gillenwater JY. Comparison of the renal hemodynamic response to unilateral and bilateral ureteral occlusion. *Invest Urol* 1977;**14**:455–9.

20 Gulmi FA, Mooppan UMM, Chou S-Y, Kim H. Atrial natriuretic peptide in patients with obstructive uropathy. *J Urol* 1989;**142**:268–72.

21 Editorial review. Pathophysiology of obstructive nephropathy. *Kidney Int* 1980;**18**:281–92.

22 Suki WN, Guthrie AG, Martinez-Maldonado M, Eknoyan G. Effects of ureteral pressure elevation on renal hemodynamics and urine concentration. *Am J Physiol* 1971;**220**:38–43.

23 Vaughan ED Jr, Shenasky JH II, Gillenwater JY. Mechanism of acute hemodynamic response to ureteral occlusion. *Invest Urol* 1971;**9**:109–18.

24 Gilmore JP. Influence of tissue pressure on renal blood flow autoregulation. *Am J Physiol* 1964;**206**:707.

25 Moody TE, Vaughan ED Jr, Wyker AT, Gillenwater JY. The role of intrarenal angiotensin II in the hemodynamic response to unilateral obstructive uropathy. *Invest Urol* 1977;**14**:390–7.

26 Cadnapaphornchai P, Aisenbrey GA, McCool AL, McDonald KM, Schrier RW. Intrarenal humoral substances and hyperemic response to ureteral obstruction. *Kidney Int* 1974;**6**:29A.

27 Potkay S, Gilmore JP. Autoregulation of glomerular filtration in renin depleted dogs. *Proc Soc Exp B iol Med* 1973;**143**:508–13.

28 Gagnor JA, Rice MK, Flamenbaum W. Effect of angiotensin converting enzyme inhibition on renal autoregulation. *Proc Soc Exp Biol Med* 1974;**146**:414–18.

29 Vander AJ, Miller R. Control of renin secretion in the anesthetized dog. *Am J Physiol* 1964;**207**:537–46.

30 Yarger WE, Schocken DD, Harris RH. Obstructive nephropathy in the rat. Possible roles for the renin angiotensin system, prostaglandins and thromboxanes in postobstructive renal function. *J Clin Invest* 1980;**65**:400–12.

31 Franke JJ, McDougal WS. The mechanism of the preservation of renal function during obstruction by enalapril. *J Urol* 1991;**145**:329A.

32 Yarger WE, Newman WJ, Klotman PE. Renal effects of aprotinin after 24 hours of unilateral ureteral obstruction. *Am J Physiol* 1987;**253**:F1006–14.

33 Morrison AR, Nishikawa K, Needleman P. Unmasking of thromboxane A_2 synthesis by ureteral obstruction in the rabbit kidney. *Nature* 1977;**267**:259–60.

34 Reingold (Felsen) DF, Watters K, Holmberg SW, Needleman P. Differential biosynthesis of prostaglandins by hydronephrotic rabbit and cat kidneys. *J Pharmacol Exp Ther* 1981;**216**:510–15.

35 Whinnery MA, Shaw JO, Beck N. Thromboxane B_2 and prostaglandin E_2 in the rat kidney with unilateral ureteral obstruction. *Am J Physiol* 1982;**242**:F220–5.

36 Yanagisawa H, Morrissey J, Morrison AR, Klahr S. Eicosanoid

production by isolated glomeruli of rats with unilateral ureteral obstruction. *Kidney Int* 1990;**37**:1528–35.

37 Allen JT, Vaughan ED Jr, Gillenwater JY. The effect of indomethacin on renal blood flow and ureteral pressure in unilateral ureteral obstruction in awake dogs. *Invest Urol* 1978;**15**:324–7.

38 Loo MH, Marion DN, Vaughan ED Jr, Felsen D, Albanese CT. Effect of thromboxane inhibition on renal blood flow in dogs with complete unilateral ureteral obstruction. *J Urol* 1986;**136**:1343–7.

39 Loo MH, Egan D, Vaughan ED Jr *et al*. The effect of the thromboxane A_2 synthesis inhibitor OKY-046 on renal function in rabbits following release of unilateral ureteral obstruction. *J Urol* 1987;**137**:571–6.

40 Felsen D, Loo MH, Marion DN, Vaughan ED Jr. Involvement of platelet activating factor and thromboxane A_2 in the renal response to unilateral ureteral obstruction. *J Urol* 1990;**144**:141–5.

41 Purkerson ML, Klahr S. Prior inhibition of vasoconstrictors normalizes GFR in postobstructed kidneys. *Kidney Int* 1989;**35**:1306–14.

42 Harris KPG, Yanagisawa H, Schreiner GF, Klahr S. Evidence for 2 distinct and functionally important sites of enhanced thromboxane B_2 synthesis after bilateral ureteral obstruction in the rat. *Clin Sci* 1991;**81**:209–13.

43 Cadnapaphornchai P, Bondar NP, McDonald FD. Effect of imidazole on the recovery from bilateral ureteral obstruction in dogs. *Am J Physiol* 1982;**243**:F532–6.

44 Reyes AA, Klahr S. Role of PAF in renal function in normal rats and rats with bilateral ureteral obstruction. *Proc Soc Exp Biol* 1991;**198**:572–8.

45 Lanzone JA, Gulmi FA, Chou S-Y, Mooppan U, Kim H. Inhibition of endothelium derived relaxation factor (EDRF) attenuates early renal vasodilation in acute unilateral ureteral obstruction (UUO). *J Urol* 1993;**149**:500A.

46 Schulsinger D, Gulmi FA, Chou S-Y, Mooppan U, Kim H. Endothelium-derived nitric oxide (ED-NO) participates in the renal vasodilation induced by acute unilateral ureteral obstruction (UUO). *J Urol* 1993;**149**:500A.

47 Chou S-Y, Dahhan A, Porush JG. Renal actions of endothelin: interaction with prostacyclin. *Am J Physiol* 1990;**259**:F645–52.

48 De Nucci GR, D'Orleans-Juste P, Antunes E *et al*. Pressor effects of circulating endothelin are limited by its removal in the pulmonary circulation and by the release of prostacyclin and endothelium-derived relaxing factor. *Proc Natl Acad Sci USA* 1988;**85**:9797–800.

49 Reyes AA, Martin D, Settle S, Klahr S. EDRF role in renal function and blood pressure of normal rats and rats with obstructive uropathy. *Kidney Int* 1992;**41**:403–13.

50 von Lutterotti N, Gulmi F, Marion D *et al*. Increased plasma prorenin but not renin after bilateral ureteral ligation in dogs. *Kidney Int* 1991;**39**:901–8.

51 Lenz T, Sealey JE, Maack T *et al*. Half-life, hemodynamic, renal and hormonal effects of prorenin in cynomolgus monkeys. *Am J Physiol* 1991;**260**:R804–10.

52 Lenz T, Sealey JE, Lappe RW *et al*. Infusion of recombinant human prorenin into rhesus monkeys: effects on hemodynamics, renin–angiotensin–aldosterone axis and plasma testosterone. *Am J Hypertens* 1990;**3**:257–61.

53 Sealey JE, von Lutterotti N, Rubattu S *et al*. The greater renin system. Its prorenin-directed vasodilator limb. Relevance to diabetes mellitus, pregnancy and hypertension. *Am J Hypertens* 1991;**4**:972–7.

54 Gunning ME, Brenner BM. Natriuretic peptides and the kidney: current concepts. *Kidney Int Suppl* 1992;**38**:S127–33.

55 Bricker NS, Bourgoignie JJ, Klahr S. A humoral inhibitor of sodium transport in uremic serum. *Arch Intern Med* 1970;**126**:860–4.

56 Wilson DR, Honrath U. Cross-circulation study of natriuretic factors in postobstructive diuresis. *J Clin Invest* 1976;**57**:380–9.

57 Harris RH, Yarger WE. The pathogenesis of post-obstructive diuresis. *J Clin Invest* 1975;**56**:880–7.

58 Harris RH, Yarger WE. Urine-reinfusion natriuresis: evidence for potent natriuretic factors in rat urine. *Kidney Int* 1977;**11**:93–105.

59 Fried TA, Lau AT, Ayon MA, Stein JH. Elevation of atrial natriuretic peptide (ANP) levels in ureteral obstruction in the rat [Abstract]. *Clin Res* 1986;**34**:596A.

60 Himmelstein SI, Coffman TM, Yarger WE, Klotman PE. Atrial natriuretic peptide-induced changes in renal prostacyclin production in ureteral obstruction. *Am J Physiol* 1990;**258**:F281–6.

61 Gulmi FC, Marion DN, Matthews GJ, von Lutterotti N, Vaughan ED Jr. Atrial natriuretic peptide enhances the recovery of renal function and prolongs the diuresis after release of bilateral ureteral obstruction. *J Urol* 1990;**143**:239A.

62 Buerkert J, Martin D, Head M, Prasad J, Klahr S. Deep nephron function after release of acute unilateral ureteral obstruction in the young rat. *J Clin Invest* 1978;**62**:1228–39.

63 Harris RH, Yarger WE. Renal function after release of unilateral ureteral obstruction in rats. *Am J Physiol* 1974;**227**:806–15.

64 Wilson DR. The influence of volume expansion on renal function after relief of chronic unilateral ureteral obstruction. *Kidney Int* 1974;**5**:402–10.

65 Harris KPG, Purkerson ML, Klahr S. The recovery of renal function in rats after release of unilateral ureteral obstruction: the effects of moderate isotonic saline loading. *Eur J Clin Invest* 1991;**21**:339–43.

66 Hirth C, Stasch J-P, John A *et al*. The renal response to acute hypervolemia is caused by atrial natriuretic peptides. *J Cardiovasc Pharmacol* 1986;**8**:268–75.

67 McDougal WS, Wright FS. Defect in proximal and distal sodium transport in post-obstructive diuresis. *Kidney Int* 1972;**2**:304–17.

68 Buerkert J, Head M, Klahr S. Effects of acute bilateral ureteral obstruction on deep nephron and terminal collecting duct function in the young rat. *J Clin Invest* 1977;**59**;1055–65.

69 Robards VL Jr, Ross G Jr. The pathogenesis of postobstructive diuresis. *J Urol* 1967;**97**:105–9.

70 Massey SG, Schainuck LI, Goldsmith C, Schreiner GE. Studies on the mechanism of diuresis after relief of urinary-tract obstruction. *Ann Intern Med* 1967;**66**:149–58.

71 Maher JF, Schreiner GE, Waters TJ. Osmotic diuresis due to retained urea after release of obstructive uropathy. *N Engl J Med* 1963;**268**:1099–104.

72 Jaenike JR. The renal functional defect of postobstructive nephropathy: the effects of bilateral ureteral obstruction in the rat. *J Clin Invest* 1972;**51**:2999–3006.

73 Nagle RB, Bulger RE, Cutler RE, Jervis HR, Benditt EP. Unilateral obstructive nephropathy in the rabbit I. Early morphologic, physiologic and histochemical changes. *Lab Invest* 1973;**28**:456–67.

74 Nagle RB, Bulger RE. Unilateral obstructive nephropathy in the rabbit II. Late morphologic changes. *Lab Invest* 1978;**38**:270–7.

75 Nagle RB, Johnson ME, Jervis HR. Proliferation of renal

interstitial cells following injury induced by ureteral obstruction. *Lab Invest* 1976;**35**:18–22.

76 Needleman P, Wyche A, Bronson SD, Homberg S, Morrison AR. Specific regulation of peptide-induced renal prostaglandin synthesis. *J Biol Chem* 1979;**254**:9772–9.

77 Okegawa T, Jonas PE, DeSchryer K, Kawasaki A, Needleman P. Metabolic and cellular alterations underlying the exaggerated renal prostaglandin and thromboxane synthesis in ureter obstruction in rabbits. Inflammatory response involving fibroblasts and mononuclear cells. *J Clin Invest* 1983;**71**:81–90.

78 Lefkowith JB, Okegawa T, DeSchryver K, Needleman P. Macrophage-dependent arachidonate metabolism in hydronephrosis. *Kidney Int* 1984;**26**:10–17.

79 Diamond JR, Kees-Folts D, Ding G, Frye JE, Restrepo NC. Macrophages, monocyte chemoattractant peptide-1 and TGF-β_1 in experimental hydronephrosis. *Am J Physiol* 1994;**266**: F926–33.

80 Schreiner GF, Harris KPG, Purkerson ML, Klahr S. Immunological aspects of acute ureteral obstruction: immune cell infiltrate in the kidney. *Kidney Int* 1988;**34**:487–93.

81 Harris KPG, Schreiner GF, Klahr S. Effect of leukocyte depletion on the function of the postobstructed kidney in the rat. *Kidney Int* 1989;**36**:210–15.

82 Gonzalez-Avila G, Vadillo-Ortega F, Perez-Tamayo R. Experimental diffuse interstitial renal fibrosis. A biochemical approach. *Lab Invest* 1988;**59**:245–52.

83 Sharma AK, Mauer SM, Kim Y, Michael AF. Interstitial fibrosis in obstructive nephropathy. *Kidney Int* 1993;**44**:774–88.

84 Bruggeman LA, Horigan EA, Horikoshi S, Ray PE, Klotman PE.

85 Johnson RJ, Alpers CE, Yoshimura A *et al*. Renal injury from angiotensin II-mediated hypertension. *Hypertension* 1992;**19**: 464–74.

86 Border WA, Noble NA. Cytokines in kidney disease: the role of transforming growth factor-β. *Am J Kidney Dis* 1993;**22**: 105–13.

87 Border WA, Ruoslahti E. Transforming growth factor-β in disease: the dark side of tissue repair. *J Clin Invest* 1992;**90**:1–7.

88 Wakefield LM, Smith DM, Flanders KC, Sporn MB. Latent transforming growth factor-β from human platelets: a high molecular weight complex containing precursor sequences. *J Biol Chem* 1988;**263**:7646–54.

89 Bruijn JA, Roos A, de Geus B, De Herr E. Transforming growth factor-β and the glomerular extracellular matrix in renal pathology. *J Lab Clin Med* 1994;**123**:34–47.

90 Border WA, Okuda S, Languino LR, Sporn MB, Ruoslahti E. Suppression of experimental glomerulonephritis by antiserum against transforming growth factor β1. *Nature* 1990;**346**:371–4.

91 Giri S. Effect of antibody to transforming growth factor β on bleomycin induced accumulation of lung collagen in mice. *Thorax* 1993;**48**:959–66.

92 Kaneto H, Morrissey J, Klahr S. Increased expression of TGF-β mRNA in the obstructed kidney of rats with unilateral ureteral ligation. *Kidney Int* 1993;**44**:313–21.

93 Sawczuk IS, Hoke G, Olsson CA, Connor J, Buttyan R. Gene expression in response to acute unilateral ureteral obstruction. *Kidney Int* 1989;**35**:1315–19.

Thromboxane stimulates synthesis of extracellular matrix proteins *in vitro*. *Am J Physiol* 1991;**261**:F488–94.

27 Principles of Management of Dilatation
H.N.Whitfield

In the past decade methods of investigating the function of the upper urinary tract have become increasingly sophisticated. There is increasing recognition of the importance of differentiating measurements of function of the renal parenchyma from measurements of function of the pelvicalyceal system. Overall renal parenchymal function can be quantified biochemically in a number of ways: radioisotopic methods may be used to measure total renal function, effective renal plasma flow and to quantify individual renal function. The behaviour of the collecting system can be measured with precision urodynamically or with radioisotopes. This ability to distinguish between renal parenchymal function and the function of the collecting system has highlighted the importance of differentiating structure and function. No longer is it justifiable to make inferences about function from the study of the anatomy, whether that be radiological anatomy or the anatomy demonstrated at the time of surgery. When accurate methods of measuring overall and individual renal parenchymal function are available, clinical decisions as to whether to pursue medical management or to undertake conservative or ablative surgery should not be made on the basis of guessing parenchymal function from the thickness of parenchyma, either seen radiologically or inspected and palpated at the time of surgery.

The aim of the urologist must always be to conserve nephrons whenever possible, and the poor correlation between radiological anatomy and renal function should now be well recognized. Dilatation of the upper urinary tract demonstrated radiologically is not synonymous with obstruction. Any temptation to intervene surgically to produce more normal radiological appearances must be resisted in the absence of evidence of functional impairment and the prospect of conserving or restoring nephron function.

Much work has been concentrated on understanding the structure of the upper urinary tract in health and disease. Such studies have contributed to an appreciation of the many possible factors which influence the development of upper urinary tract disorders. The behaviour of the upper urinary tract may be influenced by infection, by drugs, by hormones and by the way in which the lower urinary tract functions, but it is difficult if not impossible to quantify these, although they undoubtedly have an important influence on the structure and function of the diseased upper urinary tract. Any or all of these factors can contribute to changes in the capacity of the collecting system and to changes in the compliance of the walls of the calyces, pelvis and ureter. The capacity of the system and the compliance of its walls are obviously both fundamentally important and may influence the physiology of both the renal parenchyma and of the collecting system, but neither capacity nor compliance can be measured *in vivo*. Thus, although methods of investigation and diagnosis have improved, there are still areas in which ignorance persists and the hope must be that further developments will occur which will enable a diagnosis to be reached on the basis of a broader appreciation of the pathophysiology.

However, it is not only new diagnostic methods that are needed: wider application of the methods of investigation which are already available can help to improve the management of the patient. Although controversy surrounds many aspects of the management of, for example, vesicoureteric reflux, this topic is a good example of the importance of studying urodynamic urological problems from every possible angle, epidemiological, experimental and clinical. It is not beyond the bounds of possibility that the epidemiologist will be able to identify the unborn child who is at risk and that this could be confirmed or refuted by studying the infant *in utero*, and where evidence of damaging reflux is found, surgery on the fetus before renal damage has occurred may become a real possibility.

Many urodynamic problems of the upper urinary tract remain unresolved and many questions unanswered. However, a critical approach to the management of patients with these disorders is essential if the benefits of improved diagnostic techniques are to be realized. In the absence of objective evidence to support them, observations based on intuition are unreliable and unnecessary, since although our state of knowledge is incomplete, there is no excuse for ignoring the advances which have been made and which enable clinical decisions to be based on a solid foundation of established fact.

28   Pelviureteric Junction Obstruction
P.H.O'Reilly

Introduction

Pelviureteric junction (PUJ) obstruction (or idiopathic hydronephrosis) is a congenital condition of unknown aetiology resulting in variable degrees of loin pain and obstructive uropathy. It may be acute (Dietl crisis), but is more often chronic or intermittent (Fig. 28.1). It can present at any age, afflict either sex and may be unilateral or bilateral. Accurate assessment of the condition is vital because many cases showing apparent obstruction are not obstructed and do not require intervention. Conversely, where genuine obstruction is proven, surgical correction will be required. This chapter describes the aetiology, pathogenesis, clinical features, diagnosis, management and outcome of idiopathic hydronephrosis.

Aetiology

Table 28.1 shows a historical list of suggested aetiologies for PUJ obstruction. Physiological constriction has been described in the 5–6 cm stage of the human fetus; adherence of the ureter to the renal pelvis [1] and delayed ureteric canalization [2] have both been reported as possible embryological causes. Various abnormalities found at operation or on intravenous urography (IVU) have also been implicated (Fig. 28.2). It is not at all uncommon to find kinks, angulations and adhesions in this area, although there is no evidence to suggest that these are anything other than secondary phenomena; their correction alone at surgery will not guarantee cure for what is in most cases an intrinsic urodynamic abnormality. High insertion into a square-shaped renal pelvis is frequently noted on urography, and it has been suggested that an overdistensible renal pelvis may be the precursor to peristaltic abnormalities [3]. One of the commonest findings at surgery is that of aberrant lower pole renal vessels, which cross the PUJ and, in some cases, appear to be the obstructing lesion. Usually these are the inferior branches of the bifurcating anterior division of the renal artery, with its accompanying veins, crossing anterior to the ureter. They

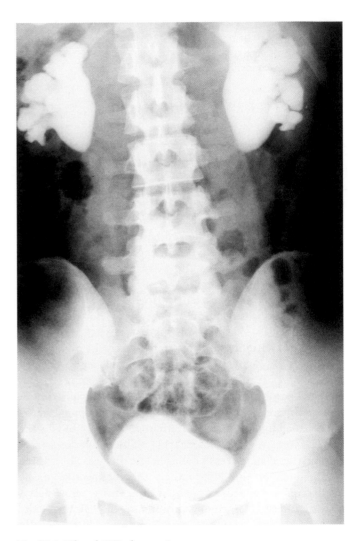

Fig. 28.1 Bilteral PUJ obstruction.

are found in 25–35% of cases. Smith *et al.* [4] reported an 80% cure rate in 19 patients with PUJ obstruction treated by ureterolysis and transposition of the vessels (the Chapman procedure). In contrast, Novak reported a 91% failure rate in patients treated by division of the vessels alone [5].

Table 28.1 Previously suggested aetiologies for PUJ obstruction.

Physiological constriction
Adherence of ureter to pelvis
Delayed canalization

Fetal folds
Ureteric papilloma
Vesicoureteric reflux

Kinks
Angulations
Adhesions

High ureteric insertion
Square-shaped renal pelvis

Aberrant vessels

Regional excess of longtitudinal muscle
Absence of muscle at the PUJ
Cuff of collagen at the PUJ
Generalized (secondary) pelvic collagen infiltration

Ureteric tumour
Ureteric stone
Postinflammatory scarring
Secondary (postoperative) stricture

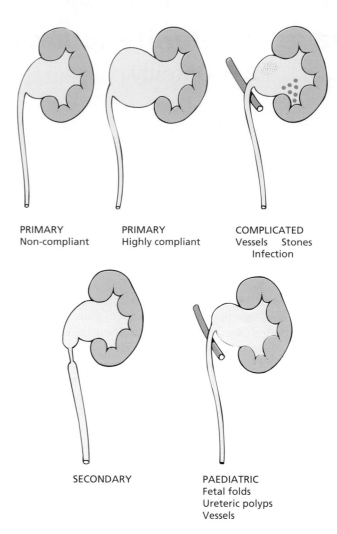

Fig. 28.2 Types of idiopathic hydronephrosis.

In a classic experiment to investigate this situation, Djurhuus placed electromyography (EMG) leads above and below aberrant vessels in a state of antidiuresis and demonstrated normal constant transmission of activity with none of the dysfunction to be expected if the vessels were the causative agent [6]. In contrast, during forced diuresis, compression by the vessel could aggravate an existing state of hydronephrosis.

Morphological studies have also been unsuccessful in demonstrating a convincing aetiology for idiopathic hydronephrosis. Murnaghan suggested that a regional excess of longitudinal muscle fibres might be a barrier to peristalsis [7], while Foote *et al.* reported an absence of muscle fibres at the PUJ [8]. Notley [9] and Hanna *et al.* [10] reported an obstructing cuff of collagen at the junction of the renal pelvis and ureter, but this was not supported by the detailed light and electron microscopy work of Gosling and Dixon in Manchester [11]. These workers also demonstrated an excess of collagen but this was not limited to the area of the PUJ; rather, this connective tissue infiltration extended throughout the entire renal pelvis proximal to the PUJ, ending abruptly at the PUJ, where the narrowed segment of ureter was found to be histologically entirely normal. It was suggested that Notley's and Hanna's findings might be explained by concentration on a limited area of pathological specimens without wider reference to the proximal tissues. Gosling and Dixon consider these changes to be a secondary consequence of an unknown functional disorder, and have provided supportive evidence for this theory from similar independent studies of the lower tract in infravesical obstruction [12].

The above aetiological considerations are applicable to all cases of PUJ obstruction. Some findings are exclusive to the disease in children. Johnston *et al.* [13] have reported cases of hydronephrosis secondary to the presence of fetal folds, ureteric polyps, ureteric papillomas and vesicoureteric reflux. He has also reviewed the existence of coexisting developmental abnormalities such as congenital heart disease, imperforate anus and myelodysplasia, and abnormalities of the contralateral kidney including congenital absence, cystic dysplasia and bilateral hydronephrosis. It seems from his studies that, in children, a variety of obstructive lesions can be associated with hydronephrosis and that 'the primary agent may be reinforced yet obscured by secondary developments so that it may or may not be possible to determine which precedes which' [14]—possibly the wisest words yet written on the aetiology of PUJ obstruction.

Acquired forms of obstruction at the PUJ include benign polyps, urothelial malignancy, stone disease and postinflammatory or postoperative scarring or ischaemia.

Pathogenesis

In addition to structural considerations, attention to the urodynamic features of the condition will help to guide the clinician towards accurate diagnosis and appropriate management (Fig. 28.3). In the normal kidney, pacemakers in the minor calyces initiate contraction waves which pass distally down the renal pelvis towards the ureter. Their transmission depends on urine flow rates. At low rates, proximal contractions may falter and fade away without reaching the distal pelvis. With increasing diuresis, contractions are transmitted to the distal renal pelvis and coupling, or direct transmission of contraction from the renal pelvis to the upper ureter, occurs. At moderate flow rates, 1 : 1 coupling is achieved, and the renal pelvis can be regarded as pacing ureteric peristalsis (Fig. 28.3a). At high flow rates, in the absence of any obstructive lesion, open tube flow will occur.

A crucial concept to the understanding of PUJ obstruction is the appreciation that, under normal circumstances, the renal pelvis delivers urine to a proximal ureter which is open and receptive, and able to accept delivery, so that it will be stretched as it accepts the urine, stimulating distal bolus transmission by peristalsis. In idiopathic hydronephrosis, the ureter is *not* open and receptive to the delivery of renal pelvic urine; the pressure required to open the PUJ for bolus delivery may be higher than normal, and passive ureteric filling is not seen on screening. The distal pelvis is dissociated from the proximal ureter and, with increasing dilatation, the proximal pelvis becomes dissociated from the distal pelvis, making transmission of pacemaker-induced contractions ineffective (Fig. 28.3b). Thus, peristaltic transmission and bolus volume are both reduced, grossly interfering with the efficiency of urine transport.

These abnormalities predispose to the further accumulation of urine in the renal pelvis and further dilatation of the pelvicalyceal system.

While such explanations are appropriate to the condition during obstructive episodes, it remains unclear what factors influence or determine the age of onset, severity, intermittency or self-limiting features of idiopathic hydronephrosis. Until the aetiology itself is determined, these aspects are likely to remain unclear.

Presentation and clinical features

PUJ obstruction is commoner in males than females, and the left side is more frequently affected than the right. Bilateral dilatation is found in 8–25% of reported series. The condition may present in the intrauterine fetus, the octogenarian geriatric or any intervening age group.

The current widespread use of prenatal ultrasound has resulted in a large number of cases of hydronephrosis being diagnosed before birth. The subject of neonatal hydronephrosis is a contentious one, opinions being divided between those who advocate a wait, watch and evaluate policy, to those who recommend early surgery in all cases. The majority verdict at present favours a conservative approach, with serial postnatal radionuclide and ultrasound evaluation to determine those cases who require surgery.

Occasionally a palpable flank mass may be found in the neonate or toddler. Small children may complain of non-specific abdominal pain—an important diagnostic point. It is rare for young children to localize the pain of PUJ obstruction to the flank or loin, rather it tends to be of a more anterior or general abdominal nature.

In older children and adults, loin or upper quadrant abdominal pain is the most common presentation. This

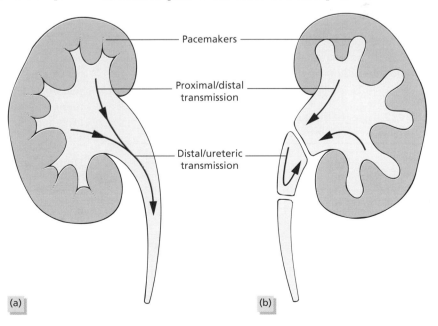

Fig. 28.3 Mechanism of urine transport in (a) the normal kidney and (b) in PUJ obstruction.

may occasionally follow minor blunt trauma which causes symptoms disproportionate to the degree of injury. Not uncommonly, young men present with loin pain after drinking large volumes of beer on a Friday or Saturday night, under which circumstances a profound diuresis may occur to stress the unsuspecting PUJ. Haematuria, or urinary tract infections, are other common clinical features. A relatively small proportion of patients will, during investigation of uraemia, be found to have bilateral hydronephrosis or hydronephrosis in solitary kidneys. In contrast to the above features, hydronephrosis is often detected as a chance finding during investigation of unrelated problems (e.g. ultrasound scanning for cholelithiasis).

In a prospective study of 50 consecutive cases of idiopathic hydronephrosis in Stepping Hill Hospital, Stockport [15], 28 were male and 22 female, with an age spread of 6–64 years (mean 43 years). Eight were children under 16 years old. The presenting features are shown in Table 28.2: 38% of cases were 'complex'—seven (14%) had coincidental renal calculi, seven (14%) had hydronephrosis in solitary kidneys and five (10%) had bilateral hydronephrosis.

Diagnosis

The diagnosis of idiopathic hydronephrosis depends initially on the radiographic detection of a dilated renal pelvis. If ultrasound is the first procedure to demonstrate dilatation it may be necessary to proceed to urography for further information; ultrasound will not demonstrate a normal ureter and, sometimes, not even a dilated one. Some information on the extent of dilatation, the site and nature of an obstructing lesion, and the presence of a functioning contralateral organ will be required to help management decisions. If urography is the first test to demonstrate dilatation, ultrasound scanning will add little, and progress towards other diagnostic procedures discussed below will be required. Once dilatation is detected, it becomes necessary to determine the significance of the

Table 28.2 Presenting complaints in 50 consecutive cases of idiopathic hydronephrosis.

Symptom	Number
Pain only	38
Pain and UTI	4
Pain on drinking	2
Haematuria only	2
Haematuria on exercise	1
Haematuria (traumatic)	1
Renal colic	1
Chance finding	1

UTI, urinary tract infection.

finding and whether it is evidence of a genuine obstruction, or a static non-obstructive dilatation reflecting some prior renal event which is no longer a threat to renal function. If there is one indisputable message from the work done in this sphere during the 1970s and 1980s, it is that *dilatation does not equal obstruction*. Where dilatation is found on urography or ultrasound without any organic explanation for it, further studies are indicated to distinguish non-obstructive harmless hydronephrosis from truly obstructive damaging hydronephrosis.

It is tempting to derive clues from IVU or ultrasound alone, at the stage when the dilatation is first discovered. Well-preserved parenchymal thickness and non-dilated calyces may be good, qualitative indicators of preserved renal intergrity, but they disclose nothing about urine flow or the effect of prevailing urodynamic conditions on the nephron. It was recognition of the need for dynamic rather than static data which stimulated the development of diuresis urography, diuresis renography, radionuclide parenchymal transit time studies (PTTS) and perfusion pressure–flow studies, (PPFS).

Diuresis urography

If the early films of an IVU series show evidence of renal pelvic dilatation, the supervising radiologist should be prepared to intervene by administering an intravenous injection of 40 mg of the diuretic frusemide at the 10 or 15 min stage. Rapid washout of contrast on fluoroscopy will exclude significant obstruction. Conversely, a considerable increase in the dimensions of the renal pelvis with no ureteric filling may indicate possible obstruction and the need for further investigation. Whitfield and colleagues described a computer-assisted assessment of the resultant images, dividing the responses into three groups according to the increase in pelvic size: (i) more than 22% increase indicated obstruction; (ii) 10–22% increase was equivocal; and (iii) less than 10% increase excluded obstruction [16]. Because of the logistics of running a busy radiology department, and possibly because of the development of more specialized methods of assessment, diuresis urography has not been widely adopted in clinical use.

Diuresis renography

This test is now widely accepted for the evaluation of upper tract dilatation [17–20] and is described in Chapter 6. Two techniques are currently recommended, the traditional F+20 procedure where the renogram is performed and frusemide given at 20 min after the radionuclide injection (Fig. 28.4), or the F–15 technique where the frusemide is given 15 min before the radionuclide to ensure maximal diuresis (Fig. 28.5). ^{123}I OIH and [^{99m}Tc] mercapto acetyl triglycine (MAG$_3$) are the radiopharmaceuticals of choice,

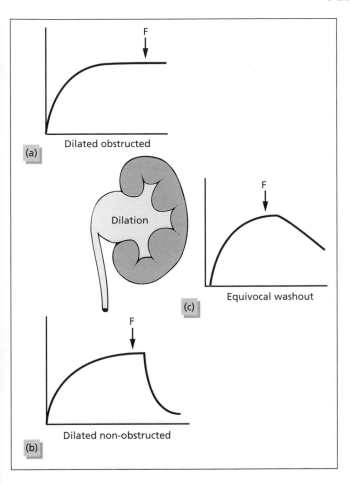

Fig. 28.4 Responses of diuresis renography showing: (a) F+20 dilated obstructed system; (b) F+20 dilated non-obstructed system; and (c) F+20 equivocal renography.

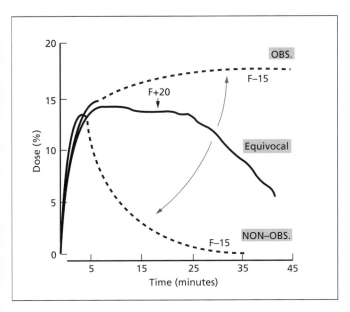

Fig. 28.5 Principle of the F–15 (maximal diuresis) renogram demonstrating its value in equivocal cases.

and give less technical problems and equivocal responses than [99mTc] diethylene triamine penta-acetic acid (DTPA). Attention to underlying renal function is necessary to ensure accurate interpretation of washout curves and to distinguish between a good diuresis with impaired washout through an obstructed ouflow tract, or poor diuresis and slow washout through a normal outflow tract. The work of Brown *et al.* investigating the correlation between renal function and diuretic responses demonstrated that for a flow rate of 10 ml/min to be achieved from frusemide, the single kidney glomerular filtration rate (GFR) must be greater than 16 ml/min [21]. Diuresis renography is widely used for the assessment of the dilated upper urinary tract, and attention to the choice of radiopharmaceutical, the use of the F–15 technique, and the roles of posture and bladder status have resulted in reliable results with very low equivocal responses.

Parenchymal transit time studies

This technique, using [99mTc] DTPA or 123I OIH relies on the ability to separate the renal parenchyma from the collecting system while replaying images from data acquired during gamma camera renography [22]. Subjective visual assessment or computer display of the renogram data as a functional image of the distribution of mean times can be used. Areas of interest are flagged over the whole kidney, the renal parenchyma and a vascular area. Activity–time curves are derived for each area. The process of deconvolution is then applied to the whole kidney and the parenchymal renograms, and retention functions are obtained. Thus, the transit times of radionuclide across both the whole kidney and the parenchyma alone can be calculated. In severe obstruction both are prolonged. In the dilated non-obstructed system whole kidney transit time will be prolonged, but parenchymal transit will not. Parenchymal transit times are specialized complex nuclear medicine procedures, and are usually reserved for major centres investigating equivocal cases, rather than as a first choice procedure.

Perfusion pressure–flow studies

Percutaneous puncture of a dilated urinary tract is now an everyday procedure in clinical uroradiological practice, so access for PPFS is much easier than it was when Whitaker popularized this test in the early 1970s [23]. The principle of the test is to perfuse contrast or saline through a nephrostomy tube, proximal to the suspected obstruction, at a fixed rate of 10 ml/min while measuring the pressure in the system. A bladder catheter should be *in situ* to avoid secondary effects of the bladder on the upper tract. If the pressure in the upper tract proximal to the obstruction stays below 15 cmH$_2$O (14.7 kPa) during perfusion, obstruction is excluded. If the pressure rises above 22 cmH$_2$O (21.6 kPa), obstruction is proven. The intervening range is equivocal. PPFS are invasive and complex, with their own technical problems and equivocal results. They are usually reserved for use in cases undiagnosed after using the other less invasive techniques available.

Correlation between available tests

Reported correlative studies have included comparisons between diuresis renography and gamma camera PTTS [24,25], PPFS (the Whitaker test) [26–30] and morphological features of operative specimens [31,32]. Correlation between diuresis renography and both PTTS and morphological changes have been good, while correlation with PPFS has been less rewarding, yielding variable and sometimes poor correlations. This should not be too surprising. The two tests investigate a renal capability by techniques which depend on dissimilar methods and are subject to differing clinical, experimental and statistical variations. In the 228 reported cases from such studies, the Whitaker test was equivocal or unsuccessful in 21, and diuresis renography unsatisfactory or equivocal in 31. In the remainder, there were two main types of discrepancies. Twenty one cases showed obstructed appearances on the diuretic renogram but not on PPFS. In two cases the hydronephrosis was intermittent and in the remainder it was specified in every case that the kidneys being examined were either grossly hydronephrotic or functioning very poorly, conditions under which diuresis renography is severely disadvantaged and unreliable. Some degree of function is necessary to get a significant amount of tracer into the collecting system and then to mount a sufficient diuretic response to influence the curve. If the system is vast, its volume will override the diuresis, and stasis will persist within the system, mimicking obstruction.

The other reported discrepancy concerned 46 cases in which the diuretic renogram did not show obstruction, but the Whitaker test did. Thirty two of these cases came from one study [26]. There are several possibilities for this discrepancy. One is the interpretation of the curves. One must be highly critical of the slope of the washout curve, so that one person's 'normal' is not, in fact, another person's 'equivocal'. For a curve to be non-obstructed, washout after frusemide must be as good as that in a normal study. Anything less should be regarded as equivocal or partially obstructed. A second possibility may be found in the fact that urinary outflow tracts undoubtedly have their own individual maximum flow-rate potentials. An individual PUJ might be able to transport urine efficiently at 5 or 7 ml/min, giving a non-obstructive diuresis renogram if the flow rate is less than 9 ml/min but an obstructed Whitaker test, if the PUJ decompensates at 9 or 12 ml/min.

The diuretic response might be variable and is directly proportional to the underlying renal function. As mentioned above, for 95% confidence limits single kidney GFR must be 16 ml/min or more to achieve a diuretic response of 10 ml/min. This must be remembered by workers assessing the washout responses to assist interpretation of results, especially if the Whitaker test is also used in the same patient and comparison of the two procedures is required.

All of the above procedures should be available to clinicians managing this condition.

Management

Patients with painful hydronephrosis and/or unequivocal obstruction on objective testing require surgical or endoscopic correction of the abnormality. The only exception to this statement is the rare case with asymptomatic, stable, 'compensated' hydronephrosis who has a dilated system and may demonstrate an obstructive diuresis renogram, but who has entirely stable function and refuses surgery. Such cases should be watched with care and followed with interval diuresis renograms and plain films to avoid silent atrophy, deteriorating function, development of renal calculi or the possibility of pyonephrosis.

Management of the emergency case

It is rarely necessary to perform emergency surgery in PUJ obstruction. Surgery for this condition requires precise technique, undamaged tissues, an uninfected field, a waterproof anastomosis and a minimal chance of postoperative infection if the desired objectives of surgery are to be achieved. If the patient presents with acute symptoms, these are most likely to be caused by secondary infection or sudden decompensation of the PUJ with acute hydronephrosis, and the conditions for optimum surgery do not pertain. The management of choice in new cases of acute hydronephrosis is decompression of the system by percutaneous nephrostomy or cystoscopic retrograde pyelo-ureteroscopy and insertion of a double-J stent, to allow the acute phase to settle pending later confirmation of the diagnosis and elective surgery (Fig. 28.6).

Ablation or conservation in PUJ obstruction

The prime objectives of surgery are to relieve symptoms and to preserve renal function. If obstruction has caused extensive stone disease or chronic infection, with severe renal damage, huge dilatation and a thin cortex, or the patient has had repeated unsuccessful operations, nephrectomy may be required. In the absence of stones and infection, however, severe dilatation and an apparently thin cortex should not be assumed to be a sign of irreversible

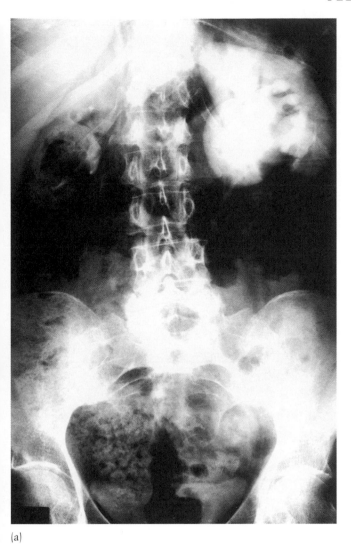

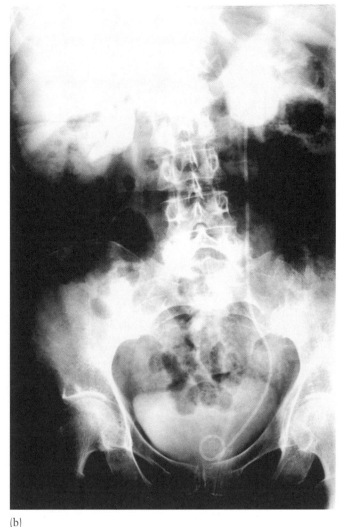

(a)

(b)

Fig. 28.6 (a) Acute PUJ obstruction. (b) Appearances 1 week after decompression with a double-J stent.

damage. Sometimes, dilatation is so gross that the cortex appears thin yet, after decompression of the system, the cortex–pelvis ratio changes dramatically and functional recovery is often surprisingly good (see below). The only certain way to assess potential or actual recovery of obstructive renal failure is to relieve it and repeat the measurements. It has been shown that such recovery occurs in two phases [33]. The initial or tubular phase consists of changes in fractional water and electrolyte excretion which occurs during the first few days following relief of obstruction and is completed in virtually all cases by 2 weeks (Fig. 28.7a,b). Plasma creatinine also improves during this early tubular phase (from tubular secretion of creatinine rather than an increase in GFR). The GFR, as measured by DTPA, iohexol and creatinine clearance, recovers more slowly between 2 weeks and 3 months, by which time recovery is complete (Fig. 28.7c). If doubt

exists, therefore, a period of decompression by nephrostomy or double-J stent is indicated, with repeated radionuclide studies after a minimum of 2 weeks and later (6 weeks, 3 months) if required.

Surgery

Presurgical considerations

If ureteric visualization has not been achieved by urography, preoperative retrograde ureteropyelography will be required before proceeding to definitive surgical correction, in order to exclude a more distal lesion such as a lucent stone or primary megaureter, which may mimic PUJ obstruction on urography, ultrasound and diuresis renography.

Traditionally, a reconstructive procedure has been performed by open surgery, using one of the various types of pyeloplasty. Minimally invasive alternatives in which the pelvi-ureteric junction is incised from an antegrade or

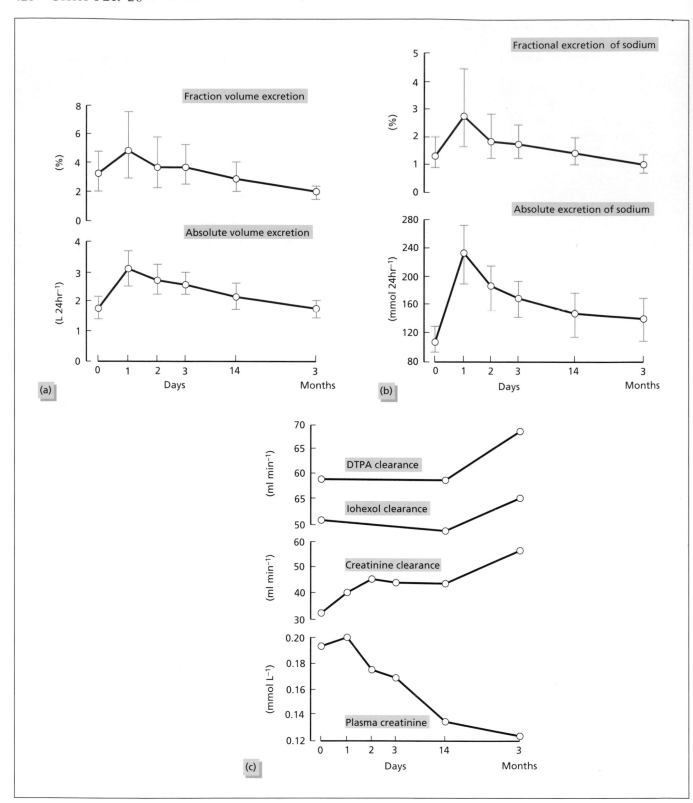

Fig. 28.7 Biphasic recovery after relief of chronic obstruction. (a) Absolute and fractional volume excretion. (b) Absolute and fractional sodium excretion. (c) GFR (measured by DTPA, iohexol and creatinine clearance) and plasma creatinine excretion. All show measurements taken during obstruction (day 0), 24 h after relief of obstruction (day 1) and on subsequent days (up to 3 months).

retrograde approach have been gaining popularity. Few reports of the long term success rates have been published and therefore the role of these procedures is not yet fully determined.

All the available corrective procedures are directed towards producing circumstances to effect the efficient delivery of a bolus of urine from the renal pelvis to the upper ureter, where stretch will initiate its onwards peristaltic transport.

Incision

The extraperitoneal flank incision is the approach of choice for pyeloplasty in adults. In children, an anterior extraperitoneal incision is sometimes preferred. A transperitoneal approach should be reserved for cases where there have been previous loin incisions, for bilateral cases or for PUJ obstruction in horseshoe kidneys where the PUJ is much lower and more medial than normal.

Nephrostomies, stents and drains

The use of stents, nephrostomies and drains are dictated by the individual surgeon's choice. Anderson and Hynes considered their operation to require neither splints nor drains. Many paediatric surgeons follow their lead, while most surgeons dealing with adults prefer a postoperative period of stent or nephrostomy drainage. The Cumming tube is a nephrostomy tube-cum-stent akin to a de Pezzer tube, with a thin tube 'tail' for splinting the anastomosis. It has the advantage that it diverts the urine, splints the suture line, allows a postoperative nephrostogram and can be removed on the ward without a further visit to the operating room. The current alternative is a double-J stent. The advantage of this is that it is internal and invisible and can reduce the hospital stay. Its disadvantages are: (i) that is may not be tolerated by the patient, causing intense trigonal irritation necessitating unscheduled and possibly undesirable removal after 1 or 2 days; (ii) the possibility of severe vesicoureteric reflux or infection which might compromise the anastomosis; and (iii) the need for a second procedure for its removal (although nowadays this can be done in a quick 5 min visit using local anaesthetic flexible cystoscopy).

It is generally considered that some form of stent or tailed nephrostomy is desirable after pyeloplasty, but the choice of which sort to use is for the supervising surgeon. What is not debateable is the need for some form of extrarenal drainage to prevent urinoma formation which, should it occur, is a disaster, leading to infection, anastomotic pressure or disruption and scarring. A large proportion of urinomas result in subsequent nephrectomy. The only debate here lies between sump and vacuum drains, again a matter of personal choice.

Choice of operation

The various operations which have been used for the correction of PUJ obstruction are listed in Table 28.3. The following are those which are in current use. The rest of the procedures listed are of historical value and do not feature in current practice.

Anderson–Hynes pyeloplasty

The most widely used of these is the dismembered pyeloplasty, usually the Anderson–Hynes technique. It involves excision of the site of obstruction and the PUJ, at the same time excising any redundant pelvis and reducing renal pelvic volume. The spatulated ureter is anstomosed to the inferior flap of the pelvis producing a wide open PUJ. The technique is appropriate to virtually all cases except those with a small tight intrarenal pelvis, or long segments of ureteric stricturing, and also allows transposition of the PUJ where there are associated aberrant vessels (Fig. 28.8).

Foley Y-V plasty

The Foley Y-V plasty is most useful in small renal pelvises and ureters with high insertions. It does not allow transposition of lower pole vessels (Fig. 28.9).

Culp–DeWeerd spiral flap

Several procedures have been developed to produce a flap of renal pelvis which can be turned down to anastomose to the adjacent ureter for bridging long segments of narrow or strictured ureter associated with PUJ obstruction. The Culp–DeWeerd spiral flap procedure is the one most commonly employed (Fig. 28.10).

Outcome of management of PUJ obstruction

Non-obstructive hydronephrosis

Where objective studies such as diuresis renography or

Table 28.3 Operations for the correction of PUJ obstruction.

Nephroplasty
Fixation of aberrant vessels
Transposition of aberrant vessels
Denervation
Intubated ureterostomy

Y-V plasty
Spiral flap plasty
Dismembered pyeloplasty

Endopyelotomy

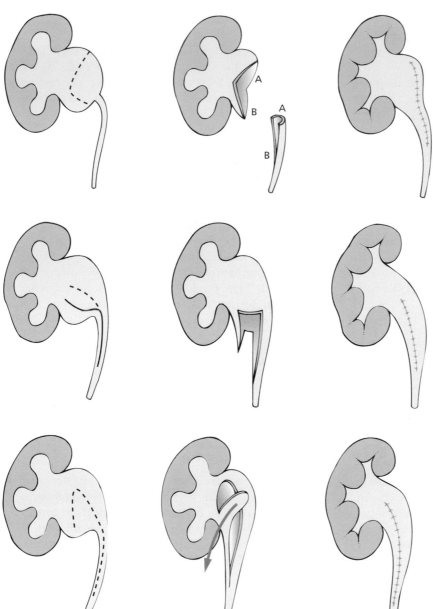

Fig. 28.8 Principle of the Anderson–Hynes (dismembered) pyeloplasty operation.

Fig. 28.9 Principle of the Foley Y-V pyeloplasty operation.

Fig. 28.10 Principle of the Culp–DeWeerd spiral flap operation.

PPFS indicate non-obstructive hydronephrosis, conservative management is indicated [34]. Of 50 consecutive cases followed by the author, 13 were non-obstructive. None of these, including four cases in solitary kidneys and six renal units with bilateral hydronephrosis, showed deterioration of function or progression to obstruction over a 5-year period, supporting reports from other centres. Of 250 children and adults in the literature, only one proceeded to pyeloplasty. However, vigilance is required to avoid missing the rare case of silent atrophy or intermittent hydronephrosis, and no patient with renal pelvic dilatation should be discharged until a suitable period of time with objective testing has taken place and the clinician is satisfied that he or she dealing with a stable condition.

Obstructive hydronephrosis

In most cases, pyeloplasty relieves symptoms and halts functional deterioration; in many cases, it leads to recovery of lost function. In the Stockport study [15], 30 obstructive cases were treated by dismembered pyeloplasty. One required secondary nephrectomy. Three others with normal function in solitary kidneys had unchanged postoperative function, leaving 26 cases. In eight cases improvement in split renal function measured by diuresis renography was less than 5%, which falls within the range of experimental error for this technique. There were 18 patients in whom preoperative function was significantly decreased. Postoperatively it improved significantly in 10

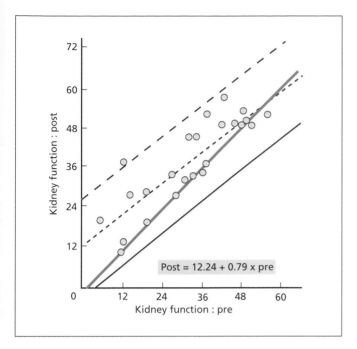

Fig. 28.11 Functional results of the Anderson–Hynes dismembered pyeloplasty procedure.

and remained the same in eight (Fig. 28.11) ($P < 0.0001$). Drainage improved in 22 of the 26 cases. It can be concluded that in addition to improving drainage in PUJ obstruction, pyeloplasty arrests functional deterioration in almost every case and improves function significantly in the majority.

Conclusion

PUJ obstruction is not a homogeneous disease entity. It may be primary or secondary, compliant or non-compliant, intrinsic or extrinsic, complicated (e.g. vessels, stones, bilateral or solitary kidney), secondary to scarring or fibrosis (e.g. after previous surgery) or, in children, associated with other problems (e.g. fetal folds, polyps, significant aberrant vessels, reflux). The techniques are now available to the urologist for accurate diagnosis and appropriate management. Identification of non-obstructed cases will avoid unnecessary surgery and allow conservative follow-up. Obstructed cases should proceed to interventional treatment, preferably using one of the available surgical procedures which will cope with all the aetiological factors, improve drainage, arrest deterioration and even restore renal function.

References

1 Ostling K. The genesis of hydronephrosis. Particularly with regard to the changes at the ureteropelvic junction. *Acta Chir Scand* 1942;**86**:72.

2 Ruano-Gil D, Coca-Payeras A, Tjedo-Mateau A. Obstruction and normal recanalisation of the ureter in the human embryo. Its relation to congenital ureteral obstruction. *Eur Urol* 1975;**1**:287.

3 Whitaker RH. Equivocal pelviureteric obstruction. *Br J Urol* 1975;**47**:771–9.

4 Smith JS, McGeorge A, Abel BJ, Hutchison AG. The results of lower polar renal vessel transposition (the Chapman procedure) in the management of hydronephrosis. *Br J Urol* 1982;**54**:95–7.

5 Novak R. Zur Bedeutung des abenierenden Gefasses bei der entstenung des Hydronephros. *Z Urol Nephrol* 1974;**67**:583–7.

6 Djurhuus JC. *Aspects of renal pelvic function*. PhD thesis, University of Copenhagen, Copenhagen, 1980.

7 Murnaghan GF. The mechanism of congenital hydronephrosis with reference to the factors influencing surgical treatment. *Ann R Coll Surg Engl* 1958;**23**:25.

8 Foote JW, Blennerhasset JB, Wigglesworth FW, MacKinnon KJ. Observations on the ureteropelvic junction. *J Urol* 1970;**104**:252–6.

9 Notley RG. Electron microscopy of the upper ureter and the pelviureteric junction. *Br J Urol* 1968;**40**:37–52.

10 Hanna MK, Jeffs RD, Sturgess JM, Barkin M. Ureteral structure and ultrastructure: the dilated ureter; clinicopathological correlation. *J Urol* 1977;**117**:28–35.

11 Gosling JA, Dixon JS. The structure of the normal and hydronephrotic upper urinary tract. In: O'Reilly PH, Gosling JA, eds. *Idiopathic Hydronephrosis*. Berlin: Springer Verlag, 1982:1–15.

12 Gosling JA, Dixon JS. Study of trabeculated detrusor smooth muscle in cases of prostatic hypertrophy. *Urol Int* 1980;**35**:351–5.

13 Johnston JH, Evans JP, Glassberg KI, Shapiro SR. Pelvic hydronephrosis in children: a review of 219 personal cases. *J Urol* 1977;**117**:97–102.

14 Johnston JH. Upper urinary tract obstruction. In: Innes Williams D, Johnston JH, eds. *Paediatric Urology*, 2nd edn. London: Butterworths, 1982:185–213.

15 O'Reilly PH. Idiopathic hydronephrosis: diagnosis, management and outcome. *Br J Urol* 1989;**63**: 569–74.

16 Whitfield HN, Britton KE, Henry WF, Wickham JEA. Frusemide intravenous urography in the diagnosis of pelviureteric junction obstruction. *Br J Urol* 1979;**51**:445–8.

17 O'Reilly PH, Testa HJ, Lawson RS, Farrar DJ, Charlton Edwards E. Diuresis renography in equivocal urinary tract obstruction. *Br J Urol* 1978;**50**:76–80.

18 O'Reilly PH, Lawson RS, Shields RA, Testa HJ. Idiopathic hydronephrosis. *J Urol* 1979;**121**:153–5.

19 O'Reilly PH. The diuresis renogram 8 years on: an update. *J Urol* 1986;**136**:993–9.

20 O'Reilly PH. Diuresis renography. Recent advances and recommended protocols. *Br J Urol* 1992;**69**:113–20.

21 Brown SCW, Upsdell SM, O'Reilly PH. The importance of renal function in the interpretation of diuresis renography. *Br J Urol* 1992;**69**:121–5.

22 Britton KE. Radionuclide studies. In: Whitfield HN, Hendry WF eds. *Testbook of Genitourinary Surgery*. Edinburgh: Churchill Livingstone 1985;67–103.

23 Whitaker RH. Pressure flow studies II In: O'Reilly PH, Gosling JA, eds. *Idiopathic Hydronephrosis*. Berlin: Springer Verlag, 1982:62–7.

24 Lupton EW, Lawson RS, Shields RA, Testa HJ. Diuresis

renography and parenchymal transit time studies in the assessment of renal pelvic dilation. *Nucl Med Commun* 1984;**5**: 451–9.

25 Cosgriff PS, Berry JM. A comparative assessment of deconvolution and diuresis renography in equivocal upper urinary tract obstruction. *Nucl Med Commun* 1982;**3**:377–84.

26 Hay AM, Norman WJ, Rice ML, Steventon RD. A comparison between diuresis renography and the Whitaker test in 64 kidneys. *Br J Urol* 1984;**56**:561–4.

27 Whitaker RH, Buxton Thomas MS. A comparison of pressure flow studies and renography in equivocal upper urinary tract obstruction. *J Urol* 1984;**131**:446–9.

28 Gonzales R, Chiou RK. Diagnosis of upper urinary tract obstruction in children. Comparison of diagnosis and perfusion pressure flow studies. *J Urol* 1985;**133**:646–9.

29 Senac MO, Miller JA, Stanley P. Evaluation of obstructive uropathy in children; radionuclide renography versus the Whitaker test. *Am J Roentgenol* 1985;**143**:11–15.

30 Kass ES, Majid M, Belman B. Comparison of diuretic renography and pressure flow studies in children. *J Urol* 1985;**134**:92–6.

31 Lupton EW, O'Reilly PH, Testa HJ *et al*. Diuresis renography and morphology in urinary tract obstruction. *Br J Urol* 1981;**51**:449–53.

32 English PJ, Testa HJ, Gosling JA, Cohen SJ. Idiopathic hydronephrosis in children. A comparison between diuresis renography and upper urinary tract morphology. *Br J Urol* 1982;**54**:603–8.

33 Jones DA, George NJR, Barnard PJ, O'Reilly PH. The biphasic nature of functional recovery following relief of chronic obstructive uropathy. *Br J Urol* 1988;**61**:192–7.

34 O'Reilly PH, Lupton EW, Shields RA *et al*. The dilated non-obstructive renal pelvis. *Br J Urol* 1981;**53**:205–10.

29 Extrinsic Ureteric Obstruction
H.N.Whitfield

Introduction

Radiological demonstration of dilatation of the upper urinary tract is not in itself sufficient evidence on which to base a diagnosis of obstruction. However, there are a number of occasions when extrinsic pressure upon the ureter from any one of a wide variety of causes results in dilatation and obstruction. With information from radioisotopic investigations and/or from urodynamic studies as well as radiological evidence, the decision can be made whether surgical intervention is necessary. This chapter deals with some of the less common causes of extrinsic ureteric obstruction, the management of which will largely depend on the underlying pathology in any individual case.

Retroperitoneal fibrosis

Retroperitoneal fibrosis (RPF) has intrigued urologists for several decades, ever since it was brought to their attention by Ormond in 1948 [1]. However, credit for the original description must go to Albarran who, nearly half a century earlier, had described the idiopathic variety of this condition [2]. Considerably later, Ormond provided a classification of the different types of RPF which can be encountered [3] (Table 29.1).

Idiopathic retroperitoneal fibrosis

Aetiology

In clinical practice the fibrosis which is encountered surgically can vary considerably. There may be just a thin sheet of fibrous tissue which scarcely seems to obstruct the ureter at all; on other occasions there are bulky masses. Such wide variations have encouraged speculation that different aetiologies may be responsible. A refuge for ignorance exists in the suggestion that there is an autoimmune mechanism. As methysergide can be shown experimentally to provoke fibrosis, this drug and other

Table 29.1 Classification of the different types of retroperitoneal fibrosis [3].

Benign	Malignant
Idiopathic	Retroperitoneal malignancy
Aortic aneurysm	Post-chemotherapy
Ureteric renal injury	
Post-irradiation	
Analgesic abuse	
Infection	

analgesics have been implicated. Resolving haematoma following trauma, urinary extravasation following renal or ureteric injury, periaortic fibrosis in association with aneurysmal dilatation and infection have all been suggested as possible causes [4–6].

Clinical features

Most patients present with a history of less than 12 months. The commonest symptom is pain, either in the flank, the back, the scrotum or the lower abdomen (Table 29.2). All series report a predominance in men in a ratio of

Table 29.2 Main presenting symptoms in 60 patients with idiopathic retroperitoneal fibrosis [8].

Presenting symptom	Percentage
Flank pain	42
Weight loss	38
Backache	32
Nausea and vomiting	32
Abdominal pain	28
Polyuria	18
Polydipsia	18
Malaise	18
Anorexia	15
Nocturia	13
Oliguria	10
Testicular pain	8
Frequency	8
Haematuria	2

3:1 [7,8]. Although isolated case reports have appeared of the condition occurring in children the majority are in adults between the ages of 40 and 70 years. Other presentations include fever, weight loss, malaise, renal failure and anuria. Hypertention is a common feature. The erythrocyte sedimentation rate (ESR) is invariably raised.

Investigations

An intravenous urogram is often the first investigation performed and, depending on the extent of the fibrosis, pelvicalyceal dilatation will be evident, together with some degree of ureteric dilatation above the upper limit of the fibrous plaque. Typically, the ureters are more medially placed than usual.

Retrograde ureterography is seldom necessary but was often performed before the advent of antegrade renal puncture techniques. Contrast is seen to flow smoothly and easily up the ureters and indeed there is no obstruction to the passage of a ureteric catheter or stent. The obstruction therefore seems to be functional, in preventing ureteric peristalsis.

A computed tomography (CT) scan (Fig. 29.1a–e) will demonstrate a retroperitoneal mass which may enhance a little after contrast. Coincidental pathology such as an aortic aneurysm would also be demonstrated but it is not possible to differentiate benign from malignant RPF. Increasing experience is being developed with the use of magnetic resonance imaging (MRI) which might enable differentiation to be made between benign and malignant disease. However, the relative merits of CT and MR scanning are not yet defined. In the early stages of the benign disease, gallium scintigraphy may demonstrate gallium uptake [9].

Pathology

The extent of the fibrous plaque in the retroperitoneum varies but most commonly extends most extensively over the lower lumbar vertebrae and upper sacrum. However, it is not uncommon for the fibrosis to extend right up into the renal hilum and down into the pelvis towards the vesico-ureteric junction (Fig. 29.2). Histologically, the material consists of dense collagenous tissue with perivascular inflammatory changes (Fig. 29.3). The ureteric wall itself may also be involved throughout its thickness with the same dense connective tissue. Because in malignant RPF mitotic cells appear infrequently it is easy to miss the diagnosis unless substantial biopsies are available for microscopy.

Management

Although aetiological factors are far from proven, any of the drugs that have been reported in relation to RPF should be discounted. If renal function is severely impaired an antegrade nephrostomy tube can quickly and easily be inserted under local anaesthesia. This technique has superseded prolonged retrograde ureteric catheterization.

Non-surgical treatment

Considerable reluctance has been expressed about treating patients with corticosteroids before a biopsy has been taken [8]. This stems from the fact that not only may a malignant process be missed in spite of a careful search but also that evidence suggests that steroids are less effective in reversing ureteric obstruction than surgery. Nevertheless, there is and always has been some support for using steroids as the primary treatment; if the obstruction resolves, the diagnosis of benign RPF is proven; if the obstruction remains, then little has been lost as the prognosis from a malignant retroperitoneal obstruction is usually very poor.

Initially, high doses of steroids should be prescribed, e.g. prednisolone 20 mg three times a day. The dose is reduced as rapidly as possible and titrated against renal function and the ESR. Even in those patients in whom surgery is performed, corticosteroid therapy is required on a long-term basis in order to prevent recurrent fibrosis. Patients will require life-long follow-up because flare-ups of the condition can occur.

Surgical treatment

There are two surgical approaches: intraperitoneal and extraperitoneal. The advantage of the extraperitoneal approach is that morbidity is less but ureterolysis can only be performed on one ureter. With an extraperitoneal approach it is possible to position the ureter more laterally and to suture the posterior parietal peritoneum over the psoas muscle and fibrous tissue in an attempt to ensure that the ureter remains free of the diseased area. However, evidence from one of the largest series suggests that an intraperitoneal approach, in which both ureters undergo lysis and are wrapped in omentum, provides a better solution [8].

Follow-up

Patients can be monitored and the steroid dose adjusted according to renal function and ESR. Serial CT scans are not necessary, though renal ultrasound may be a less invasive way of providing evidence of monitoring the ureteric obstruction.

Other forms of benign retroperitoneal fibrosis

Aortic aneurysms occur commonly but only in a minority

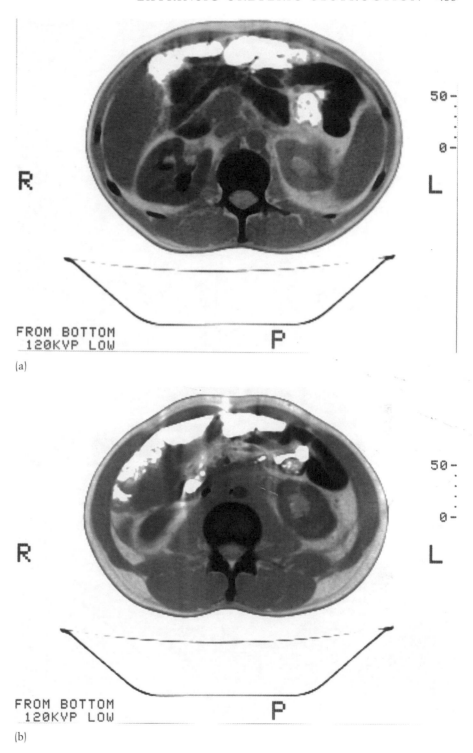

Fig. 29.1 (a) A contrast enhanced CT scan showing contrast within the right collecting system but no contrast within the collecting system of a dilated left renal collecting system, because of very poor renal function. (b) Contrast in the right ureter which lies alongside a peri-aortic mass.

(a)

(b)

is there significant ureteric obstruction. The reasons for this remain obscure [10,11]. It is usual that those patients in whom such a finding exists require surgery to the aneurysm, at which time the ureters will be released.

Retroperitoneal extravasation of urine may occur more often than is recognized. Patients with renal colic can, on intravenous urography, be seen to extravasate contrast when forniceal rupture occurs. It is at least theoretically possible that such urinary extravasation can track down and provoke fibrosis. This explanation for the more minor degrees of RPF that are sometimes encountered must remain speculative.

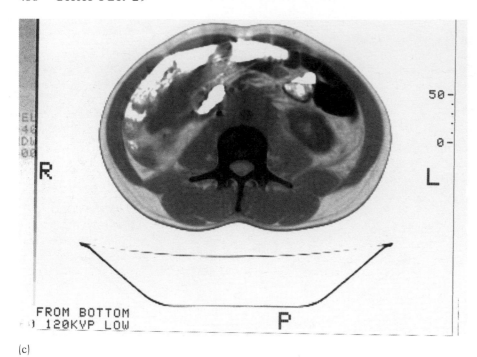

(c)

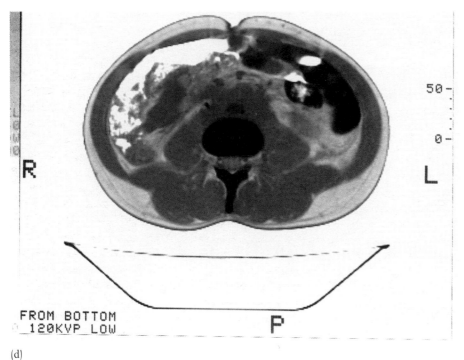

(d)

Fig. 29.1 *Continued.* (c,d) The right ureter becoming narrower and encased within the peri-aortic fibrotic tissue. Calcification is seen within the wall of the aorta which lies in the midline.

Less speculative is the ureteric obstruction which is occasionally seen in patients who have intraperitoneal infective processes such as ulcerative colitis, diverticular disease of the colon and Crohn's disease. It is arguable whether the desmoid tumour that occurs following surgery in patients with colonic carcinoma in familial polyposis coli and who subsequently develop a desmoid tumour (Gardener's syndrome) represent an example of benign or malignant RPF (Fig. 29.4). The argument is a semantic one. Such patients may require a ureterolysis which provides a difficult surgical challenge.

When irradiation has been given for a pelvic malignancy it is usual that the field included extends beyond the site of malignancy. On occasions ureteric devascularization occurs, leading to fibrosis, narrowing and obstruction, which must be resolved on an individual basis.

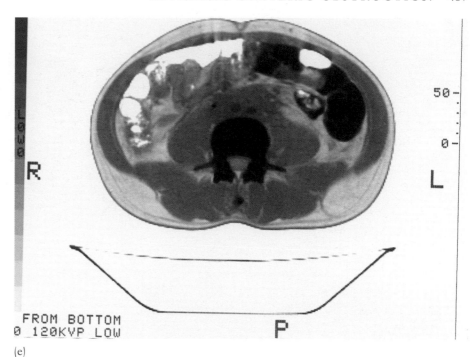

Fig. 29.1 *Continued.* (e) The right ureter encased within fibrous tissue, lying alongside the common iliac arteries. (Courtesy of Dr I Mootoosamy.)

(e)

Other causes of extrinsic obstruction of the ureter

Ovarian vein syndrome

The ureter may become obstructed at the site at which it is crossed by the ovarian vein. The obstruction may be intermittent and related to the onset of the menstrual cycle [12] and the large majority of patients are multiparous. Loin pain and evidence of upper urinary tract infection or obstruction may prove sufficient indications for surgery, which merely involves tying off one or both ovarian veins and, if necessary, lysing the ureter.

Aneurysmal obstruction

It is widely recognized that the perianeurysmal fibrosis associated with both abdominal aortic and iliac artery aneurysms may result in ureteric obstruction [13,14]. It is perhaps surprising that this problem is not encountered more frequently. The patient will usually complain of loin pain or backache, and although it is uncommon for renal function to be compromised, occasionally relief of the ureteric obstruction may be required prior to definitive treatment of the aneurysm.

Iatrogenic obstruction

The obstruction of a ureter at operation by the inadvertent positioning of a ligature may pass unnoticed. The complication may occur during a number of different operations but most commonly during a hysterectomy, although the same has happened during open prostatectomy, colposuspension, colonic resection and laparoscopic sterilization. Radiotherapy to the posterior abdominal wall may result in ureteric obstruction and has even been reported as being a common cause in some centres (S. Rocco Rosetti, personal communication).

Inflammatory diseases

Inflammatory diseases of the colon such as Crohn's disease, ulcerative colitis and diverticular disease may all cause ureteric obstruction, even in the absence of infection. In the presence of a retroperitoneal abscess from any one of these diseases or from other sources of intraperitoneal infection, periureteric fibrosis and obstruction may result.

Malignant diseases

A wide variety of malignant diseases extending from the pelvic organs or arising retroperitoneally higher up the posterior abdominal wall may cause ureteric obstruction, and the management of any individual case will depend on the nature of the malignant disease. Para-aortic node involvement and resultant ureteric obstruction may also occur with malignant disease arising from more distant sites, for example the breast. Retroperitoneal lymphomas are also a cause of ureteric obstruction.

It is important to establish a histological diagnosis as the nature of the treatment that is most appropriate and the potential for control or cure of the underlying malignant

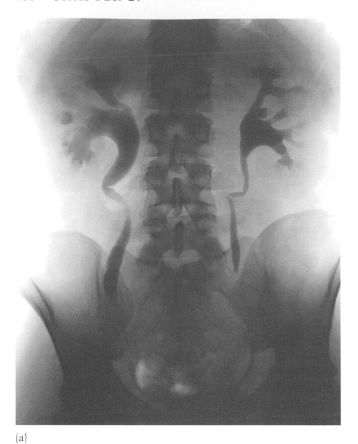

(a)

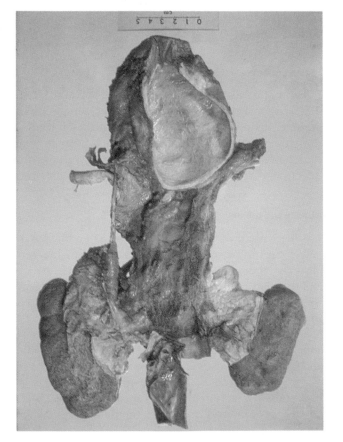

Fig. 29.2 (a) IVU showing bilateral ureteric obstruction at the level of the pelvic rim. (b) CT scan showing large intra-abdominal mass, the desmoid tumour.

(b)

disease will be entirely dependent on the pathology. Percutaneous needle biopsies, if necessary under CT control, or biopsies taken at the time of laparotomy and ureterolysis both provide adequate material for a histological diagnosis on which treatment can be based.

Female disorders

Dilatation of the right ureter during pregnancy is so common as to be normal. The weight of evidence suggests that this pregnancy-associated dilatation is more likely to be due to compression of the ureter by the gravid ureterus at the level of the pelvic brim than to hormonal changes. Endometriosis is an uncommon but not rare cause of ureteric obstruction and with medical treatment of the underlying condition the obstruction may resolve spontaneously. Ureteric prolapse and large ureterine fibroids have also been reported to cause ureteric obstruction.

Fig. 29.3 *Left*. Post-mortem *en bloc*. Illustration of extensive retroperitoneal fibrosis encasing both ureters. (Courtesy Dr M Pugh.)

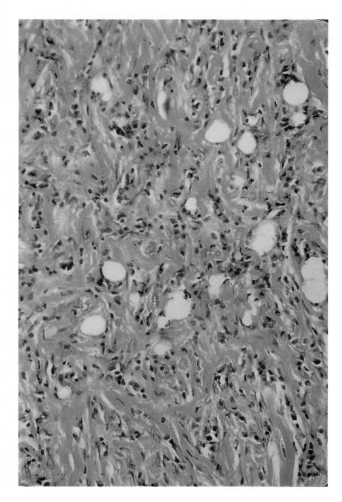

Fig. 29.4 Photomicrograph showing typical appearances of ideopathic retroperitoneal fibrosis. (Courtesy Dr MC Parkinson.)

References

1 Ormond JK. Bilateral ureteral obstruction due to envelopment and compression by an inflammatory retroperitoneal process. *J Urol* 1948;**59**:1072–9.

2 Albarran J. Rétention renal par peri-uréterite. Liberation externe de l'urétère. *Proces Verb Assoc Franc Urol* 1905;**9**:511–17.

3 Ormond JK. A classification of retroperitoneal fibrosis. *Urol Surv* 1975;**25**:53–7.

4 Stecker JF, Rawls HP, Devine CJ, Devine PC. Retroperitoneal fibrosis and ergot derivatives. *J Urol* 1974;**112**:30–2.

5 Harbrecht PJ. Variants of retroperitoneal fibrosis. *Ann Surg* 1967;**165**:388–401.

6 Kerr WS, Suby HI, Vickerty A, Fraley E. Idiopathic retroperitoneal fibrosis: clinical experiences with 15 cases 1956–1967. *J Urol* 1968;**99**:575–84.

7 Van Bommel EFH, van Spengler J, van der Hoven B, Kramer P. Retroperitoneal fibrosis: report of 12 cases and review of the literature. *Neth J Med* 1991;**39**:338–45.

8 Baker LRI, Mallinson WJW, Gregory MC *et al*. Idiopathic retroperitoneal fibrosis. A retrospective analysis of 60 cases. *Br J Urol* 1988;**60**:497–503.

9 Joekes AM, Hanley HG, Park JC. Retroperitoneal fibrosis. A follow-up assessment of surgical and medical treatment in 29 patients. In: Kuss R, Kegrain M, eds. *Siminaires d'Uro-Nephrologie*. Paris: Masson, 1975:171–82.

10 Boccon-Gibod L, Steg A. The value of corticotherapy for idiopathic retroperitoneal fibrosis. *Ann Urol* 1977;**11**:95–105.

11 Darke SG, Glass RE, Eadie DGA. Abdominal aortic aneurysm: perianeurysmal fibrosis and ureteric obstruction and deviation. *Br J Surg* 1977;**64**:649–52.

12 Polse S, Bobo E. Bilateral ureteral obstruction secondary to enlarged ovarian vein. *J Urol* 1969;**102**:305.

13 Abercrombie GF, Hendry WF. Ureteral obstruction secondary to aneurysm. *Br J Urol* 1971;**43**:170.

14 Abbott DL, Skinner DG, Yalowitz PA, Mulder D. Abdominal aortic aneurysms: an approach to management. *J Urol* 1973;**109**:987.

30 Vesicoureteric Reflux in Adults
A.R.Mundy

There has been relatively little interest in vesicoureteric reflux (VUR) in adults when compared with the flood of publications about VUR in children in recent years. This is presumably because most children with VUR grow out of it before their teenage years and therefore most urologists with a predominantly adult practice will only see five or six cases each year. However, the secondary effect of VUR, reflux nephropathy, previously called chronic pyelonephritis, is the second commonest cause of end-stage renal failure in adults in the UK, accounting for about 25% of patients who require dialysis or transplantation.

VUR occurs as a result of malfunction of the physiological valve at the vesicoureteric junction which normally prevents urine in the bladder from passing back into the ureter. This malfunction may be the result of a congenital malformation or it may be secondary to a disease process or therapeutic procedure which interferes with the function of a previously normal vesicoureteric junction (Table 30.1).

The presence of VUR *per se* is of no more than academic interest. The important factor is the effect that VUR has, or may have, on the function of the kidney that the affected ureter drains. The general view, as discussed in Chapter 17, is that VUR is potentially harmful to the kidney in the presence of urinary tract infection (UTI) or severe degrees of outflow obstruction. This view is supported by a substantial amount of excellent experimental work. It also seems likely, on the basis of the same experimental work, that VUR, in the absence of UTI or outflow obstruction is not harmful to the kidney in the short term (months). It remains to be seen whether the same is true in the long term (years). It is this area of ignorance of the long-term effects of sterile reflux that is responsible for the uncertainty surrounding the management of many adults with reflux.

Presentation

Primary VUR in adults, that is primary VUR that does not disappear during childhood, is about three times commoner in women than in men and usually presents during the

Table 30.1 The causes of vesicoureteric reflux (VUR) in adults.

Type of VUR	Cause
Primary	Congenital
Secondary	
Obstruction	Bladder neck/prostate
	Urethral stricture
Iatrogenic	Ureteric meatotomy for stone or ureterocele
	TUR—prostate
	TUR—bladder tumour
	Ureteroneocystotomy
	Radiotherapy
Neuropathic bladder	
Inflammatory	Urinary tract infection
	Tuberculosis
	Bladder stone
	Interstitial cystitis
	Bilharzia

TUR, transurethral resection.

third or fourth decade of life. Secondary VUR has a more even sex distribution and a wider age range of presentation with obstructive and iatrogenic causes predominating in men in middle and later life.

The most common presenting symptoms are those suggestive of recurrent UTI (80% of patients), which may or may not be bacteriologically proven, and loin pain (50%). These symptoms have often been present for several years before medical advice is sought and are not, of course, specific for VUR. In most instances, the diagnosis will only be made on the basis of the findings of an intravenous urogram (IVU) coupled with a high index of clinical suspicion.

Less commonly (15% of patients) the patient will present with hypertension, renal failure or proteinuria, having had an IVU which shows features suggestive of VUR as part of their preliminary investigation.

Diagnosis

On the basis of the presenting symptoms, most patients

will have an IVU and urine culture in the first instance. In the absence of reflux nephropathy, the IVU will almost certainly be normal (30% of patients) except perhaps for some ureteric dilatation (5%). At the other extreme, the kidney that has been destroyed by reflux neuphropathy will show non-function (30%). Between these two extremes, the damaged kidney will show varying degrees of cortical scarring and blunting of the calyces (25%) or, less commonly, global atrophy (10%).

Two other features may be present. First, a diverticulum may lie immediately lateral to the orifice of a refluxing ureter (15%). This is thought to arise as a consequence of the same malformation of the vesicoureteric junction that caused the VUR [1]. Secondly, complete duplication of the upper urinary tract may be associated with reflux into the ureter draining the lower renal moiety. A third, less frequent, association, rarely diagnosed on the basis of the IVU alone, is with ectopia of the ureteric orifice.

If these features are present, or if VUR is suspected despite a normal IVU, the diagnostic investigation is a micturating cystogram (MCG). If present, the VUR, which may be unilateral or bilateral in roughly equal proportions, is graded according to its severity (Table 30.2).

If reflux nephropathy is present, four additional investigations are important. The blood pressure should be measured; the urine should be examined for significant proteinuria; the serum creatinine should be measured; and a [^{99m}Tc] DMSA (dimercapto succinic acid) renal scan should be obtained to assess differential renal function. If the serum creatinine is elevated, the glomerular filtration rate should be estimated.

After these investigations, the patient's management is decided on the basis of the following.
1 The severity and frequency of the patient's symptoms.
2 Whether there is recurrent bacteriologically proven UTI.
3 Whether the VUR is unilateral or bilateral.
4 Whether there is radiological evidence of reflux nephropathy.

5 Whether there is significant hypertension.
6 The percentage contribution of the affected kidney to the total renal function if reflux nephropathy is present.
7 The total renal function if the VUR is bilateral and, if renal function is impaired, whether or not proteinuria is present. Proteinuria in a patient with VUR is an ominous prognostic feature indicating the rapid approach of end-stage renal failure [2].
8 The underlying pathology in a patient with secondary VUR.

Treatment

When treating primary VUR in children the urologist is mainly concerned with protecting the kidneys from the effects of urinary infection or, much less frequently, outflow obstruction, in the expectation that the child has an 80% chance that the VUR will disappear before puberty. The situation is different in adults as there is little or no chance that primary VUR will resolve. Thus in adults, the urologist is primarily concerned either with treating symptoms or with managing an already severely compromised urinary tract. Otherwise one is left to wonder what may happen to a less compromised urinary tract during the remaining 30–50 years of the patient's life.

In children there is no doubt that good medical treatment (with the emphasis on the word good), as described in Chapter 17, is satisfactory in the majority and that surgical correction of the VUR is unnecessary. The critical factor in good medical treatment is careful follow-up. This is difficult enough to achieve with concerned, intelligent parents of a paediatric patient over a period of 5–15 years. It is even more difficult to achieve in young adults who seem to think that they are immortal with a potential follow-up of 50–60 years. Thus the unanswered question as to whether or not long-term sterile reflux is harmful assumes great importance. It is tempting, when one is not sure which line of management to advise, to be rid of the problem by surgical correction of the VUR so that the risk of inadequate long-term follow-up is obviated.

Secondary VUR is usually less worrying as it is often transient, (as for example when it is a direct consequence of UTI), reversible (as for example when secondary to outflow obstruction or a bladder stone) or present in the middle-aged or elderly patient (e.g. outflow obstruction, post transurethral resection of the prostate or bladder tumour, post radiotherapy) when the life expectancy is considerably less than 50 years.

When considering the treatment of VUR, it is important to remember that many patients present with a history of recurrent UTI and that they may reasonably expect that their treatment will prevent them from suffering further episodes. This is not the case. Management of the patient with VUR is primarily concerned with reducing the

Table 30.2 One of the many schemes for grading the severity of VUR.*

Grade 1	Minor reflux into the lower ureter
Grade 2	Reflux up the full length of the ureter and into the renal pelvis but with only minor degrees of distension of the ureter
Grade 3	Gross reflux into a widely dilated ureter and renal pelvis

* More detailed schemes of grading VUR are probably unnecessary. It is currently felt that whenever the vesicoureteric junction is incompetent, bladder pressure is freely transmitted to the kidney and that the MCG appearances are therefore nothing more than a reflection of the ureter's response to that pressure.

morbidity of UTI, not the frequency, by confining any UTI that does subsequently occur to the lower urinary tract where it is less likely to do any harm.

As the question of the long-term effects of sterile reflux has yet to be answered, there are, at present, two groups of patients; a group whose treatment most urologists would probably agree about, irrespective of their views on sterile reflux, and a group whose treatment would be controversial.

Uncontroversial situations

Primary VUR (unilateral or bilateral), recurrent UTI, asymptomatic between attacks, no hypertension, good bilateral renal function. These patients are adequately treated by an appropriate course of antibiotics when infections occur, if they are infrequent (< 3/year), or by low-dose prophylactic antibiotics if infections occur more frequently. If, in the latter group, infections still occur or if, in either group, the infections regularly cause severe constitutional disturbances (due to acute pyelonephritis rather than acute cystitis) then ureteric reimplantation should be advised.

Primary or secondary VUR (unilateral or bilateral) with objective evidence of deterioration of the affected kidney(s). Reimplantation of the affected ureter(s) should be advised unless there is (in some patients with secondary VUR) a contraindication (see below).

Recurrent UTI associated with reflux into a ureteric stump following a previous simple nephretomy. Excision of the ureteric stump is recommended as this may be the focus of the infections.

Unilateral reflux (primary or secondary) into a non-functioning or poorly functioning kidney (contributing less than 15% of total renal function) with or without recurrent UTI, hypertension or severe symptoms and with a normal contralateral kidney. Nephroureterectomy is recommended. Associated hypertension may improve or resolve. Simple nephrectomy is not advised as pain or recurrent UTI may persist due to reflux into the ureteric stump. If there is reflux into the contralateral ureter then reimplantation of that ureter should be performed in conjunction with the nephroureterectomy.

Primary or secondary VUR, severe symptoms of loin pain on voiding, irrespective of recurrent UTI, hypertension or renal function. Reimplantation of the refluxing ureter(s) should be advised, bearing in mind that similar loin pain can occur, in the absence of VUR, in women with the urethral syndrome or detrusor instability.

Secondary reflux
1 *VUR into a transplanted kidney.* VUR does not seem to impair the function of a transplanted   kidney and an antireflux type of ureteroneocystotomy at the time of transplantation is not thought to be necessary. For the patient in whom VUR is noted after transplantation, the risks of ureteric ischaemia or vesicoureteric junction obstruction as a result of a second operation outweigh the advantage of correcting the VUR in most instances, even if the reflux is felt to be undesirable.

2 *VUR in a patient with a urothelial tumour.* This usually follows transurethral resection of a tumour close to or involving a ureteric orifice. In theory, VUR in this situation may lead to seeding of the tumour up the ureter. However, again in theory, surgical correction of the VUR may lead to seeding into the surgical field. The VUR is therefore best ignored. If the patient has a strong indication for operation and there is no contralateral reflux, transureteroureterosomy may (in theory) be preferable to reimplantation.

The presence of VUR may be a contraindication to the use of intravesical cytotoxic agents, depending on the agent to be used, and should therefore be excluded by an MCG before planning a course of this type of treatment.

3 *VUR in the neuropathic bladder.* The treatment of VUR in this situation is mainly the treatment of the associated vesicourethral dysfunction. In the absence of recurrent UTI or a high-pressure bladder (usually associated with obstruction due to detrusor–sphincter dyssynergia) (see Chapter 16) the VUR can usually be ignored.

4 *Other causes.* In other situations the cause should be treated, if possible, and the VUR itself, if it persists, should then be managed along the lines indicated above. If none of the above criteria apply, the VUR can probably be ignored.

VUR in patients with end-stage renal failure. On the one hand, bilateral nephroureterectomy might reduce the risk of recurrent UTI, improve voiding function and allow better control of hypertension. On the other hand, greater restriction of fluid intake would be necessary, anaemia may become more pronounced, there are the risks of the operation itself and none of the potential advantages may be realized. On balance, operation is probably best reserved for those patients with a definite indication and those who are about to be transplanted.

Controversial situations

As stated above, it is widely believed that VUR is not harmful to the kidney in the absence of urinary infection or outflow obstruction. Advocates of this view would therefore feel that the risks of operation do not justify surgical intervention unless there is a good indication.

The contrary view is that although it is proven that VUR only causes renal scarring in short-term experiments in pigs in the presence of urinary infection or extreme degrees of outflow obstruction, it is not proven that VUR does not cause less dramatic degrees of renal damage over a period of years in humans. Advocates of this view, and I am one, would feel that until it has been proved that long-term sterile reflux is indeed harmless, that the potential benefits of operative correction outweigh the minimal risks.

Thus, in addition to the situations discussed above, I would also advocate operative intervention in any patient with VUR who has impaired renal function (glomerular filtration rate < 80 ml/min when corrected to a body surface area of 1.73 m²) unless the degree of impairment is so severe that significant proteinuria has become established; and in any patient with normal renal function who has grade 2 or grade 3 reflux on the MCG and features of reflux nephropathy on the IVU.

On the other hand, if the patient presented with only one or two episodes of UTI and has a normal IVU then further follow-up is probably unnecessary. A female patient, and her general practitioner, should, however, be advised that her urine should be cultured regularly during any subsequent pregnancy.

Operative treatment

My preference is for the Cohen advancement type of operation [3]. If the patient has had a previous unsuccessful antireflux operation, this and other intravesical types of operation may not be possible because of scarring. In such cases a Leadbetter–Politano type of operation is to be preferred [4]. When there is a great deal of scarring around the terminal ureter, the Paquin technique of initially splitting the bladder down to the proposed site of reimplantation is useful [5].

Some urologists like to 'tailor' a widely dilated ureter before reimplanting it. Apart from hypothetical physiological reasons, the main practical indication for 'tailoring' is to make the reimplantation procedure easier in situations where there does not seem to be enough room in the bladder to reimplant two large ureters. In this situation I would prefer to reimplant one ureter and drain the other into the reimplanted ureter by transureteroureterostomy, as in my experience 'tailoring' is often not quite as neat and tidy an operation as line drawings by the advocates of this procedure would suggest.

In day-to-day practice urologists will always comfort their patients, will often palliate or relieve their symptoms but will only occasionally cure them. The surgical correction of VUR is one of those few situations when a cure can be offered. Nothing in life, let alone surgery, can be guaranteed and 3.5% of patients will have persistent reflux after their operation and 1.5% will develop obstruction at the site of reimplantation. However, a success rate of 95%, as any bookmaker will confirm, is good odds.

References

1 Hutch JA. Saccule formation of the ureterovesical junction in smooth walled bladders. *J. Urol* 1961;**86**:390–9.
2 Weston P, Stone AR, Bary PR, Leopold D, Stephenson TP. The results of reflux prevention on renal deterioration in adults with reflux nephropathy. *Br J Urol* 1982;**54**:677–81.
3 Cohen SJ. Ureterozystoneostomie. Eine neue Antireflux-technik. *Aktuelle Urol* 1975;**6**:1–6.
4 Politano VA, Leadbetter WF. An operative technique for the correction of vesico ureteric reflux. *J Urol* 1958;**79**:932–41.
5 Paquin JA. Ureterovesical anastomosis: the description and evaluation of a new technique. *J Urol* 1959;**82**:573–83.

Section 3b
Lower Urinary Tract

31 Structure of the Bladder and Urethra
J.A.Gosling and J.S.Dixon

Urinary bladder

The wall of the urinary bladder consists of three layers: (i) an outer adventitial layer of connective tissue which possesses in some regions a serosal covering of peritoneum; (ii) a smooth muscle layer (the detrusor muscle); and (iii) an inner layer of mucous membrane which lines the interior of the bladder.

Detrusor muscle

The muscle coat of the bladder is composed of relatively large diameter interlacing bundles of smooth muscle cells arranged as a complex meshwork (Fig. 31.1). Discrete layers of smooth muscle are not discernible although longitudinally oriented muscle bundles tend to predominate on the inner and outer aspects of the detrusor muscle coat. Posteriorly some of these outer longitudinal bundles extend over the bladder base and merge with the capsule of the prostate or with the anterior vaginal wall; other bundles extend on to the anterior aspect of the rectum to form the rectovesical muscle. Anteriorly some outer longitudinal bundles continue into the pubovesical ligaments and contribute to the muscular component of these structures. Exchange of fibres between adjacent muscle bundles within the bladder wall frequently occurs so that, from a functional viewpoint, the detrusor comprises a single unit of interlacing smooth muscle which, on contraction, will cause a reduction in all dimensions of the bladder lumen.

Ultrastructurally an electron-dense basal lamina surrounds each detrusor smooth muscle cell except at certain junctional regions. The most frequently observed type of junction between smooth muscle cells is the region of close approach at which an intercellular separation of 10–20 nm occurs over distances occasionally in excess of 1 µm. Junctions of the 'peg and socket' and 'intermediate' types are observed occasionally, but gap junctions (nexuses) are absent from the detrusor. Since electrotonic spread of

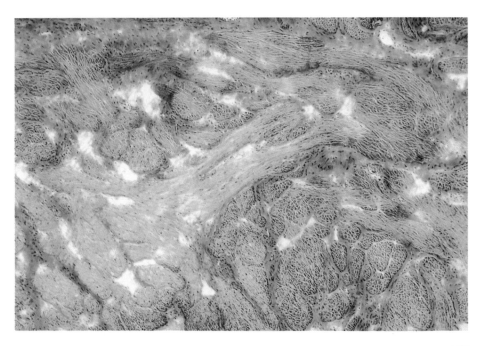

Fig. 31.1 An interlacing network of relatively large diameter smooth muscle bundles forms the human detrusor (Masson trichrome preparation; ×150).

447

excitation occurs in the smooth muscle of the bladder wall, the regions of close approach may represent the morphological feature which enables this physiological event to take place. Within each muscle bundle, the individual cells are closely packed together such that the basal lamina of one cell very often becomes confluent with that of its neighbours.

Ureterovesical junctions

The distal 1–2 cm of each ureter is surrounded by an incomplete collar of detrusor smooth muscle which forms a sheath (sheath of Waldeyer) separated from the ureteric muscle coat by a connective tissue sleeve. The ureters pierce the posterior aspect of the bladder and run obliquely through its wall for a distance of 1.5–2.0 cm before terminating at the ureteric orifices. This arrangement is believed to assist in the prevention of ureteric reflux since the intramural ureters are thought to be occluded during increases in bladder pressure. The longitudinally oriented muscle bundles of the terminal ureter continue into the bladder wall, and at the ureteric orifices become continuous with the superficial trigonal muscle [1].

A recent histological study of the ureterovesical junction in infants [2] has demonstrated an incomplete intermediate muscle layer (Fig. 31.2) lying between the intramural ureteric muscle coat and the surrounding detrusor muscle. It has been suggested that these clusters of tightly packed smooth muscle cells may represent a remnant of the mesonephric duct from which the ureter originates during fetal development.

Trigone

The smooth muscle of this region consists of two distinct layers, often termed the superficial and deep trigonal muscles. The latter is composed of muscle cells which are indistinguishable from those of the detrusor. Hence, this deep trigonal muscle is merely the posteroinferior portion of the detrusor muscle proper and confusion might be avoided if the term deep trigonal muscle was abandoned in favour of the more accurate definition of trigonal detrusor muscle.

The superficial trigonal muscle represents a morphologically distinct component of the trigone which, unlike the detrusor, is composed of relatively small diameter muscle bundles that are continuous proximally with those of the intramural ureters. The smooth muscle layer comprising the superficial trigone is relatively thin, but becomes thickened along its superior border to form the interureteric crest. Similar thickenings occur along the lateral edges of the superficial trigone. In both sexes the superficial trigone muscle becomes continuous with the smooth muscle of the proximal urethra, extending in the male along the urethral crest as far as the openings of the ejaculatory ducts.

Innervation of the detrusor muscle

The nerves supplying the bladder form the vesical plexus and consist of both sympathetic and parasympathetic components. The parasympathetic fibres arise from the 2nd to the 4th sacral segments of the spinal cord (nervi erigentes); the sympathetic fibres are derived from the lower two thoracic and upper two lumbar segments of the

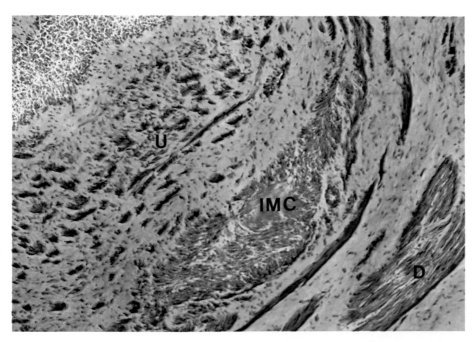

Fig. 31.2 In this section through the ureterovesical junction of a child an intermediate muscle component (IMC) is seen lying between the ureteric (U) and detrusor (D) muscle components (Masson trichrome preparation; ×200).

spinal cord. Small autonomic ganglia occur throughout all regions of the bladder wall (Fig. 31.3). These multipolar intramural neurones are rich in acetylcholinesterase and occur in ganglia composed of five to over 20 nerve cell bodies. Numerous preganglionic autonomic fibres form both axosomatic and axodendritic synapses with the ganglion cells. The majority of these preganglionic nerve terminals correspond morphologically to presumptive cholinergic fibres. Noradrenergic terminals also relay on cell bodies in the pelvic plexus and very occasionally on neurones within the intramural ganglia.

The urinary bladder (including the trigonal detrusor muscle) is profusely supplied with nerves which form a dense plexus among the detrusor smooth muscle cells. The majority of these nerves contain acetylcholinesterase (Fig. 31.4). Under the electron microscope, axonal varicosities adjacent to detrusor smooth muscle cells show features which are considered to typify cholinergic nerve terminals (Fig. 31.5), containing clusters of small (50 nm diameter) agranular vesicles together with occasional large (80–160 nm diameter) granulated vesicles and small mitochondria. Terminal regions approach to within 20 nm of the muscle

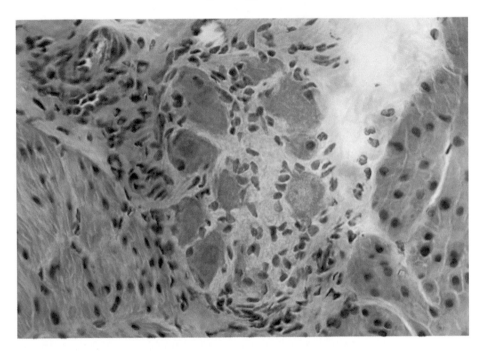

Fig. 31.3 A small autonomic ganglion is seen surrounded by detrusor muscle bundles (Masson trichrome preparation; ×600).

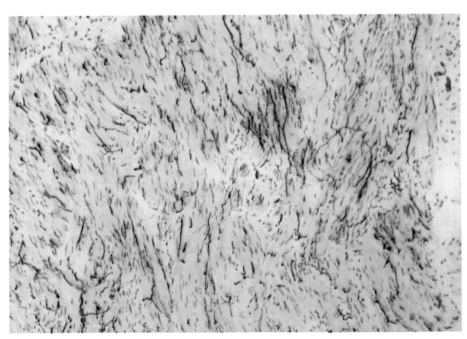

Fig. 31.4 A plexus of acetylcholinesterase-positive nerve fibres occurs among the detrusor muscle bundles (acetylcholinesterase preparation; ×150).

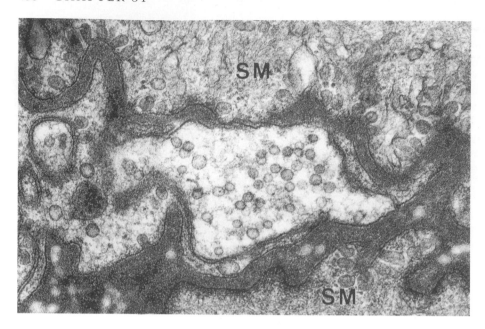

Fig. 31.5 An electron micrograph of a presumptive cholinergic nerve terminal lying adjacent to detrusor smooth muscle (SM) cells. The axonal varicosity contains numerous small electron-lucent vesicles. (×56 000).

cells' surfaces and are either partially surrounded by, or more often totally denuded of, neurilemmal cell cytoplasm. The human detrusor possesses a sparse supply of sympathetic noradrenergic nerves [3].

Nerves of this type generally accompany the vascular supply and only rarely extend among the smooth muscle cells of the urinary bladder. A further component plays a part in the autonomic innervation of the urinary bladder [4], which has been classified as a non-adrenergic, non-cholinergic nerve-mediated effect. It has been suggested that this 'peptidergic' response is due to the presence of a third type of effector nerve which provides an additional motor innervation to the bladder. Alternatively, it may be that cholinergic nerves supplying the detrusor release a second 'peptidergic' neurotransmitter or neuromodulator. While this third type of innervation has been established in some species, its presence in the human has yet to be confirmed.

Recent immunohistochemical studies have shown that vasoactive intestinal polypeptide (VIP) is present within nerves supplying the human detrusor muscle and also within many of the perivascular nerves of the bladder wall [5]. VIP is known to cause relaxation of smooth muscle and to act as an effective vasodilator. Of slightly greater frequency than VIP but otherwise alike in distribution is neuropeptide Y (NPY), distinct as a potent contractor of smooth muscle, and found to occur uniformly in the detrusor [5].

More recently it has been shown that some nerves supplying the human urinary bladder and ureters contain the inhibitory neurotransmitter nitric oxide [6], which is synthesized on demand within nerve terminals by the enzyme nitric oxide synthase. Nitrergic nerves are thought to be responsible for nerve-mediated smooth muscle relaxation in the lower urinary tract.

Innervation of the ureterovesical junctions

Numerous nerve fibres containing dopamine B-hydroxylase (DBH) have been demonstrated among the smooth muscle bundles of the intramural ureters [7] (Fig. 31.6), indicating that noradrenergic nerves play a major role in the control of the ureteric components of the ureterovesical junctions. Similar nerves are infrequent among the muscle bundles which form the detrusor component of the ureterovesical junction. The role played by the ureteric component of the ureterovesical junction in the prevention of ureteric reflux remains to be determined.

Innervation of the superficial trigone

Superficial trigonal muscle is associated with relatively few cholinergic (parasympathetic) nerves, while those of the noradrenergic (sympathetic) variety occur frequently. It should be emphasized that the superficial trigonal muscle forms a very minor part of the total muscle mass of the bladder neck and proximal urethra in either sex and is probably of little significance in the physiological mechanisms which control these regions.

Mucosa of the urinary bladder

The mucosa of the bladder is composed of an epithelium (the urothelium) supported by a layer of loose connective tissue, the lamina propria. The latter consists of loose fibroelastic connective tissue and forms a relatively thick

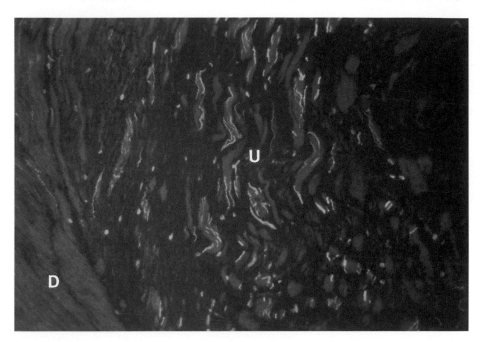

Fig. 31.6 Nerve fibres immunoreactive for DBH occur in profusion among the smooth muscle cells of the intramural ureter (U) while similar nerves are very infrequent among the adjacent detrusor muscle (D) (immunofluorescence preparation; ×200).

layer, varying in depth from 500 μm in the fundus and inferolateral walls to about 100 μm in the trigone. Small diameter bundles of smooth muscle cells also occur in the subepithelial connective tissue forming an incomplete and rudimentary muscularis mucosae. The connective tissue elements immediately beneath the urothelium, particularly in the region of the trigone, are densely packed. At deeper levels they are more loosely arranged, thus allowing the bladder mucosa to form numerous thick folds when the volume of fluid contained within the lumen is small. An extensive network of blood vessels is present throughout the lamina propria and supplies a plexus of thin-walled fenestrated capillaries lying in grooves at the base of the urothelium.

Non-trigonal urothelium is often up to six cells in thickness. These cells may be classified according to position and consist of highly differentiated superficial or luminal cells, one or more layers of smaller intermediate cells and a layer of undifferentiated basal cells [8]. The large superficial cells frequently bulge into the bladder lumen and are often binucleate. In contrast, the intermediate and basal cells are smaller and each contains a single darkly staining nucleus. The flattened urothelium of the trigone usually consists of only two or three layers of cells and a similar appearance prevails throughout the bladder when in the distended state.

In addition to the basal, intermediate and superficial cells described above, a fourth type of cell occurs in the urothelium of the human bladder neck and trigone. These flask-shaped cells extend throughout the depth of the urothelium and are characterized by the presence of numerous large membrane-bounded vesicles, each containing a central dense granule. Vesicles of this type are believed to be involved in the storage of amines and it seems likely that these cells belong to the so-called APUD (amine precursor uptake and decarboxylation) series which have a wide distribution throughout the body. The functional significance of cells of this type in the urothelium of the bladder is unknown at present.

Several morphological variations have been described in the mucosa of the bladder which, because of their occurrence in otherwise normal healthy adults, are not considered to represent pathological conditions. One of the most common epithelial variants are so-called Brunn' nests [9]. These consist of proliferations of morphologically normal basal urothelial cells which project into the underlying connective tissue of the lamina propria and are particularly frequent in the trigone. Mucus-secreting glands with single or branched ducts are another common feature of the bladder mucosa. When present, these structures are particularly numerous near the ureteric and internal urethral orifices. Non-keratinizing squamous metaplasia of the vaginal type also frequently occurs in the urinary bladder mucosa, especially over the trigone. This feature, while occasionally observed in males and in children, is more common in adult females.

Innervation of lamina propria

The bladder wall possesses a nerve plexus which extends throughout the lamina propria. The constituent nerves are cholinesterase positive (Fig. 31.7) and extend through the connective tissue unassociated with blood vessels. Some of the larger diameter axons are myelinated and others lie adjacent to the basal urothelial cells. This subepithelial nerve plexus of the bladder is assumed to subserve a

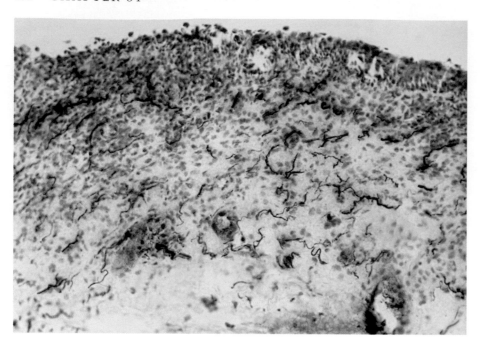

Fig. 31.7 Acetylcholinesterase-positive nerves occur in the lamina propria, forming a substantial subepithelial plexus (acetylcholinesterase preparation; ×400).

sensory function in the absence of any obvious effector target sites. The submucosal nerve fibres have been shown to contain VIP and also substance P, a well-recognized constituent of primary afferent sensory fibres [5].

Bladder neck

The smooth muscle of this region is histologically, histochemically and pharmacologically distinct from that which comprises the detrusor proper [10,11]. Hence, the bladder neck should be considered as a separate functional unit. The arrangement of smooth muscle in this region is quite different in males and females and consequently each sex will be described separately.

Male bladder neck

At the male bladder neck, the smooth muscle cells form a complete circular collar which extends distally to surround the preprostatic portion of the urethra. Because of the location and orientation of its constituent fibres, the terms internal, proximal or preprostatic urethral sphincter are suitable alternatives for this particular component of urinary tract smooth muscle. Distally, bladder neck muscle merges with, and becomes indistinguishable from, the musculature in the stroma and capsule of the prostate gland.

Innervation

In the male, bladder neck smooth muscle is supplied with cholinergic (parasympathetic) nerves and also possesses a rich noradrenergic (sympathetic) innervation [12]. A similar

distribution of autonomic nerves occurs in the smooth muscle of the prostate gland, seminal vesicles and ducti deferentes. On stimulation the sympathetic nerves cause contraction of smooth muscle in the wall of the genital tract resulting in seminal emission. Concomitant sympathetic stimulation of bladder neck muscle causes sphincteric closure of the region, thereby preventing reflux of ejaculate into the bladder. Although this genital function of the male bladder neck is well established it is not known whether the smooth muscle of this region plays an active role in maintaining urinary continence.

Female bladder neck

The female bladder neck also consists of morphologically distinct smooth muscle, since the large diameter muscle bundles characteristic of the detrusor are replaced in the region of the bladder neck by those of small diameter (Fig. 31.8). However, unlike the circularly oriented preprostatic smooth muscle of the male, the majority of muscle bundles in the female bladder neck extend obliquely or longitudinally into the urethral wall. The female does not, therefore, possess a smooth muscle sphincter at the bladder neck, and it is unlikely that active contraction of this region plays a significant part in the maintenance of female urinary continence.

Innervation

In contrast with the rich sympathetic innervation in the male, the smooth muscle of the female bladder neck possesses relatively few noradrenergic nerves, but is well supplied with presumptive cholinergic fibres. The sparse

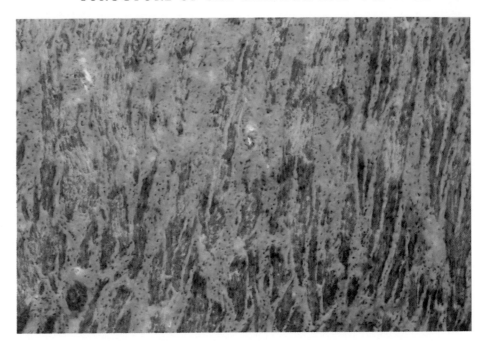

Fig. 31.8 The wall of the female bladder neck contains relatively small diameter muscle bundles, most of which are oriented longitudinally (compare with Fig. 31.1) (Masson trichrome preparation; ×150).

supply of sympathetic nerves presumably relates to the absence of a functional 'genital' portion incorporated within the wall of the female urethra. The role played by presumed cholinergic fibres in the bladder neck in either sex remains uncertain.

Male urethra

The male urethra may be considered in four regional parts: preprostatic, prostatic, membranous and penile. Except during the passage of fluid, the urethral canal is a mere slit; in the prostatic part the slit is transversely arched; in the membranous portion it is stellate; in the spongiose portion it is transverse; while at the external orifice it is sagittal.

Structure of the male urethra

Preprostatic urethra

The preprostatic urethra is approximately 1–1.5 cm in length, extending almost vertically from the bladder neck to the base of the prostate gland. The smooth muscle bundles of the preprostatic urethra are arranged circularly and are continuous proximally with bladder neck muscle and distally with the capsule of the prostate gland. The bundles which form this preprostatic or internal sphincter (sphincter vesicae) are separated by connective tissue containing many elastic fibres. Unlike the detrusor, the smooth muscle surrounding the proximal urethra possesses relatively few parasympathetic cholinergic nerves, but is richly supplied with sympathetic noradrenergic nerves (Fig. 31.9). Similar nerves also supply the smooth muscle of the prostate, ducti deferentes and seminal vesicles and are involved in causing smooth muscle contraction at the time

of ejaculation [13]. As previously mentioned, contraction of the preprostatic sphincter serves to prevent the retrograde flow of ejaculate through the proximal urethra into the bladder.

Prostatic urethra

The prostatic urethra is approximately 3–4 cm in length and extends through the substance of the prostate closer to the anterior than the posterior surface of the gland. It is continuous above with the preprostatic urethra and emerges from the prostate slightly anterior to its apex. Throughout most of its length the posterior wall possesses a midline ridge, the urethral crest, which projects into the lumen causing it to appear crescentic in transverse section. Distally the prostatic urethra possesses a layer of circularly disposed striated muscle cells which is continuous with a prominent collar of striated muscle (the rhabdosphincter) within the wall of the membranous urethra.

Membranous urethra

The membranous urethra is the shortest, least distensible and, with the exception of the external orifice, the narrowest section of the urethra. It descends with a slight ventral concavity from the prostate to the bulb of the penis, passing through the perineal membrane about 2.5 cm posteroinferior to the pubic symphysis. The wall of the membranous urethra contains a muscle coat which is separated from the urethral epithelium by a narrow layer of fibroelastic connective tissue. This muscle coat consists of a relatively thin layer of smooth muscle bundles which are continuous proximally with those of the prostatic urethra, together with a closely apposed outer layer of circularly

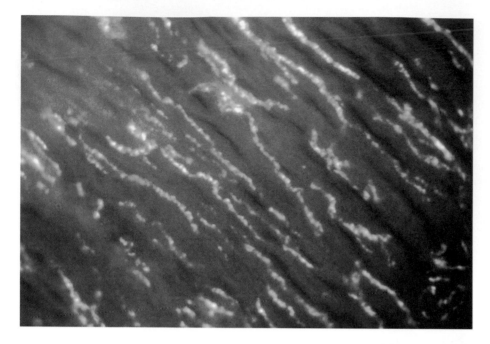

oriented striated muscle fibres which form the rhabdosphincter. The striated muscle fibres which comprise this rhabdosphincter (Fig. 31.10) are unusually small in cross-section with diameters of only 15–20 μm [14]. The fibres are physiologically of the slow twitch type [15], unlike the pelvic floor musculature which is a heterogeneous mixture of slow and fast twitch fibres of larger diameter [16]. Moreover, the rhabdosphincter is devoid of muscle spindles and is probably supplied by the pelvic splanchnic nerves, further distinguishing it from the periurethral levator ani muscle [17]. The slow twitch fibres of the external sphincter are capable of sustained contraction over relatively long periods of time and actively contribute to the tone which closes the urethra and maintains urinary continence.

Penile urethra

The penile or spongiose urethra is contained in the corpus spongiosum penis. It is about 15 cm long, and extends from the end of the membranous urethra to the external urethral orifice on the glans penis. The lumen is narrow, with a uniform diameter of about 6 mm for much of its length; it is dilated at its commencement (the intrabulbar fossa) and within the glans penis near its termination (the navicular fossa). The bulbourethral glands open into the spongiose section of the urethra about 2.5 cm below the perineal membrane.

Female urethra

The adult female urethra is approximately 4 cm long and 6 mm in diameter. It begins at the internal urethral orifice of the bladder and extends anteroinferiorly behind the

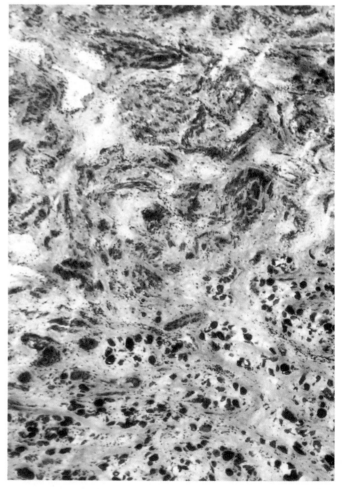

Fig. 31.10 The wall of the male membranous urethra contains an inner smooth muscle layer (on the right) and an outer layer of striated muscle, the rhabdosphincter (on the left) (Masson trichrome preparation; ×125).

symphysis pubis, embedded in the anterior wall of the vagina. It traverses the perineal membrane and terminates at the external urethral orifice. Except during the passage of urine the anterior and posterior walls of the urethra are in apposition, and the epithelium forms extensive longitudinal folds.

Structure of the female urethra

The wall of the female urethra comprises an outer muscle coat and an inner mucous membrane which lines the lumen and is continuous with that of the bladder. The muscle coat consists of an outer sleeve of striated muscle (the rhabdosphincter) together with an inner coat of smooth muscle fibres. The female rhabdosphincter is anatomically separate from the adjacent periurethral striated muscle of the anterior pelvic floor. The constituent fibres of this sphincter are circularly disposed and form a sleeve which is thickest in the middle third of the urethra. In this region striated muscle completely surrounds the urethra, although the posterior portion lying between the urethra and vagina is relatively thin (Fig. 31.11). The striated muscle extends into the anterior wall of both the proximal and distal thirds of the urethra but is deficient posteriorly in these regions. The muscle cells forming the rhabdosphincter are all of the slow twitch variety (Fig. 31.12). As in the male, cells of the rhabdosphincter are unusually small with diameters of about 15–20 µm. Although the thickness of the rhabdosphincter in the female is less than that of the male, its constituent fibres are able to exert tone upon the urethral lumen over prolonged periods, especially in relation to the middle third of its length. Periurethral striated muscle (pubococcygeus) aids urethral closure during events which

require rapid, albeit short lived, elevation of urethral resistance.

The smooth muscle coat extends throughout the length of the urethra and consists of slender muscle bundles, the majority of which are oriented obliquely or longitudinally. A few circularly arranged muscle fibres occur in the outer aspect of the smooth muscle layer and intermingle with the inner part of the rhabdosphincter. Proximally, the urethral smooth muscle is continuous with that of the bladder neck. This region in the female is devoid of a well-defined circular smooth muscle component comparable with the preprostatic sphincter of the male. When traced distally urethral smooth muscle bundles terminate in the subcutaneous adipose tissue surrounding the external urethral meatus. The smooth muscle of the female urethra is associated with relatively few noradrenergic nerves, but receives an extensive presumptive cholinergic parasympathetic nerve supply identical in appearance to that which supplies the detrusor [18]. From a functional viewpoint, in the absence of an anatomical sphincter, it seems unlikely that competence of the female bladder neck and proximal urethra is solely the result of smooth muscle activity. The innervation and longitudinal orientation of the majority of the muscle fibres suggest that urethral smooth muscle in the female may be active during micturition, serving to shorten and widen the urethral lumen.

Functional considerations

The urinary bladder performs a dual function—acting at times as a reservoir for fluid accumulating within its lumen, and at others as a contractile organ actively expelling its contents into the urethra. In the following

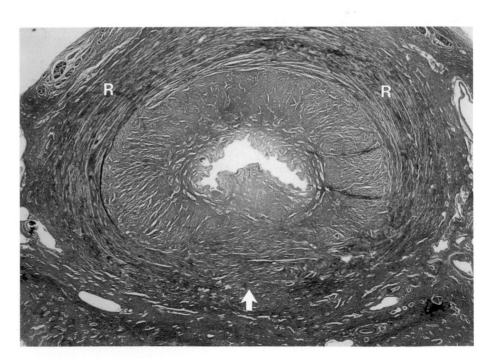

Fig. 31.11 A transverse section through the mid-portion of the female urethra. The circularly oriented rhabdosphincter (R) is incomplete posteriorly (arrow) and the urethral lumen appears as a transverse slit (Masson trichrome preparation; ×10).

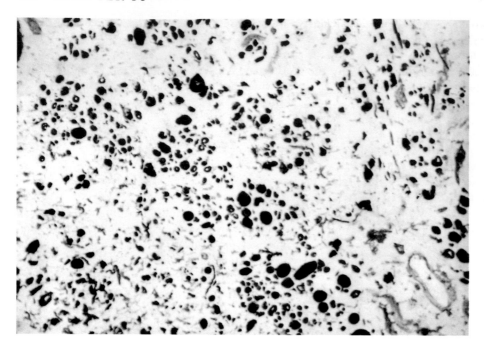

Fig. 31.12 A section through the female rhabdosphincter to show the rich acid-stable myosin adenosine triphosphate (ATP)-ase content of the constituent striated muscle fibres (myosin ATPase preparation; ×125).

account the tissue components and, where appropriate, their neurological control will be considered.

Continence of urine

To achieve urinary continence, the bladder acts as a passive reservoir retaining fluid because the forces acting on the urethra produce an intraurethral pressure greater than the bladder pressure. Several tissue components play a part in generating this urethral resistance, providing either an active or passive contribution. Since the smooth muscle of the bladder is replaced in the bladder neck region by a morphologically distinct type of smooth muscle, the detrusor muscle itself is not considered to play a part in closing the proximal urethra.

In the male, a distinct collar of circularly oriented smooth muscle occurs in the bladder neck and preprostatic urethra which is continuous distally with the muscular components of the genital tract. This smooth muscle sphincter is supplied by a rich plexus of sympathetic nerve fibres which, on stimulation, cause the sphincter to contract, thereby preventing retrograde flow of semen into the urinary bladder at ejaculation. Despite this well-defined genital role, it is not known whether the smooth muscle of the bladder neck region and preprostatic urethra play an active part in the maintenance of continence. Intramural collagen and elastic fibres within the wall of the bladder neck, proximal urethra and prostate generate passive forces which help to close the urethral lumen.

However, postoperative incontinence of urine does not usually follow radical surgical excision of the bladder neck, preprostatic urethra and the prostate gland, suggesting that these structures provide only a minor contribution to urinary continence.

In the female, a smooth muscle sphincter cannot be anatomically recognized in the wall of the bladder neck and proximal urethra. Consequently, it is even less likely that active smooth muscle contraction should be considered as an important factor in the continence of urine in women. However, the bladder neck and proximal urethra possess within their walls innumerable elastic fibres which are of particular importance in producing passive occlusion of the urethral lumen. Indeed, it has been suggested that the passive elastic resistance offered by the urethral wall is the most important single factor responsible for the closure of the bladder neck and proximal urethra in the continent woman.

In both sexes the urethra contains within its walls the rhabdosphincter, the location of which corresponds anatomically to the zone where maximal urethral closure pressure is normally recorded. This striated muscle sphincter is morphologically adapted to maintain tone over relatively long periods without fatigue and plays an important active role in producing urethral occlusion at rest. It remains to be determined, however, whether the force exerted by the sphincter is maximal at all times between two consecutive acts of micturition, or whether additional motor units are recruited during coughing, sneezing, etc., to enhance the occlusive force on the urethra during these events. The rhabdosphincter is innervated by nerve fibres which travel via the pelvic splanchnic nerves and not the pudendal nerves as often described. The clinical relevance of this arrangement is that pudendal blockade or neurectomy performed in order to reduce urethral resistance will not achieve the desired effect since the motor innervation of the striated sphincter remains unaffected by such procedures.

Concerning the role of periurethral muscle in the maintenance of continence, the medial parts of the levator ani muscles in both sexes are related to (but structurally separate from) the urethral wall. These periurethral fibres are innervated by the pudendal nerve and consist of an admixture of large diameter fast and slow twitch fibres. Therefore, unlike the rhabdosphincter, periurethral muscle possesses morphological features which are similar to other 'typical' voluntary muscles. This pelvic floor musculature plays an important part (especially in the female) by providing an additional occlusive force on the urethral wall, particularly during events which are associated with an increase in intra-abdominal pressure. In addition, the muscles provide support for the pelvic viscera.

Micturition

To enable fluid to flow along the urethra it is necessary for the pressure in the urinary bladder to exceed that within the urethral lumen. Under normal circumstances, in order to initiate micturition, a fall in urethral resistance immediately precedes a rise in pressure within the lumen of the bladder. This pressure rise is usually produced by active contraction of detrusor smooth muscle at the onset of micturition. The detrusor muscle coat consists of innumerable interlacing muscle bundles forming a complex meshwork of smooth muscle which, on contraction, reduces all dimensions of the bladder. The muscle coat is collectively involved and it is unnecessary to attach special significance to the precise orientation of individual bundles within the wall of the viscus.

The preganglionic nerve supply travels in the pelvic splanchnic nerves before synapsing on neurones located within the vesical part of the pelvic plexuses and also within the wall of the bladder. These peripheral neurones supply nerve fibres which ramify throughout the thickness of the detrusor smooth muscle coat. The profuse distribution of these motor nerves emphasizes the importance of the autonomic nervous system in initiating and sustaining bladder contraction during micturition. For micturition to occur the pressure differential between the bladder and urethra must overcome the elastic resistance of the bladder neck. Immediately prior to the onset of micturition, the tonus of the rhabdosphincter is reduced by central inhibition of its motor neurones located in the 2nd, 3rd and 4th sacral spinal segments. Such inhibition is mediated by descending spinal pathways originating in higher centres of the central nervous system. Concomitantly, other descending pathways activate (either directly or via sacral interneurones) the preganglionic parasympathetic motor outflow to the urinary bladder. This central integration of the nervous control of the bladder and urethra is essential for normal micturition.

References

1 Tanagho EA, Meyers FH, Smith RD. The trigone: anatomical and physiological considerations. 1. In relation to the uretero vesical junction. *J Urol* 1968;**100**:623–32.

2 Gearhart JP, Canning DA, Gilpin SA, Lam E, Gosling JA. A histologic and histochemical study of the ureterovesical junction in infancy and childhood. *Br J Urol* 1994;**72**:648–54.

3 Sundin T, Dahlstrom A, Norlen L, Svedmyr N. The sympathetic innervation and adrenoreceptor function of the human lower urinary tract in the normal state and after parasympathetic denervation. *Invest Urol* 1977;**14**:322–8.

4 Ambache N, Zar MA. Non-cholinergic transmission by post-ganglionic motor neurons in the mammalian bladder. *J Physiol (Lond)* 1970;**210**:762–83.

5 Scultety S. Neuropeptides in urology. *Urol Nephrol* 1989;**21**: 39–45.

6 Andersson K-E, Persson K. Nitric oxide synthase and nitric oxide-mediated effects in lower urinary tract smooth muscles. *World J Urol* 1994;**12**:274–80.

7 Dixon JS, Canning DA, Gearhart JP, Gosling JA. An immunohistochemical study of the innervation of the ureterovesical junction in infancy and childhood. *Br J Urol* 1994;**73**:292–7.

8 Jost SP, Gosling JA, Dixon JS. The morphology of normal human urothelium. *J Anat* 1989;**167**:103–15.

9 Jost SP, Gosling JA, Dixon JS. The fine structure of Brunn's nests in human bladder urothelium. *J Submicrosc Cytol Pathol* 1990;**22**:203–10.

10 Negardh A, Boreus LO. Autonomic receptor function in the lower urinary tract of man and cat. *Scand J Urol Nephrol* 1972;**6**:32–6.

11 Kluck P. The autonomic innervation of the human urinary bladder, bladder neck and urethra: a histochemical study. *Anat Rec* 1980;**198**:439–47.

12 Gosling JA, Dixon JS, Lendon RG. The autonomic innervation of the human male and female bladder neck and proximal urethra. *J Urol* 1977;**118**:302–5.

13 Learmonth JR. A contribution to the neurophysiology of the urinary bladder in man. *Brain* 1931;**54**:147–76.

14 Von Hayek H. Die muskulatur des beckenbodens. In: Alken CE, Dix VW, Goodwin WE, Wildbolz E, eds. *Handbuch der Urologie*, Vol I. Berlin: Springer Verlag, 1969:279–88.

15 Gosling JA, Dixon JS, Critchley HOD, Thompson SA. A comparative study of the human external sphincter and periurethral levator ani muscles. *Br J Urol* 1981;**53**:35–41.

16 Parks AG, Swash M, Urich H. Sphincter denervation in anorectal incontinence and rectal prolapse. *Gut* 1977;**18**: 656–65.

17 Donker PJ, Droes JThPM, van Ulden BM. Anatomy of the musculature and innervation of the bladder and the urethra. In: Williams DI, Chisholm GO, eds. *Scientific Foundations of Urology*, Vol II. London: Heinemann, 1976:32–9.

18 Ek A, Alm P, Andersson KE, Persson CGA. Adrenergic and cholinergic nerves of the human urethra and urinary bladder. A histochemical study. *Acta Physiol Scand* 1977;**99**:345–52.

32 Pharmacology of the Lower Urinary Tract
T.Hald and J.T.Andersen

Introduction

Pharmacological manipulation of bladder, urethral and prostate complaints has gained popularity over the last decades. The introduction of more specific drugs has contributed considerably to this trend. It is, however, important to establish a precise functional diagnosis prior to treatment. This implies that appropriate urodynamic methods are incorporated in the evaluation of potential candidates. It is equally important to realize that most of the drug regimens are aimed primarily at the relief of symptoms and do not change the underlying pathology, although they modify the pathophysiological manifestations.

Pharmacotherapy can be used as the only treatment modality, but will often attain its best results when combined with, for example, bladder and pelvic floor training, behavioural modifications, regulation of drinking habits or intermittent self-catheterization. All effective pharmacological treatment of voiding disorders are prone to cause side effects, and it is imperative that the patients are warned of this before beginning the treatment. It must be accepted that a number of patients drop out of the planned treatment either due to lack of effect or troublesome side effects.

Pharmacological treatment of bladder and urethral dysfunction

Pharmacological treatment can alter both the storage and the emptying function of the lower urinary tract. Storage function can be improved by: (i) inhibition of detrusor activity with increased bladder capacity; and/or (ii) stimulation of the urethral closure mechanism. Emptying function can be improved by: (i) stimulation of the detrusor contractility; and/or (ii) reduction of urethral outflow resistance. The drugs available may have peripheral action on the smooth musculature and/or the autonomic ganglia, or effects on the central nervous system.

Improvement of bladder storage

The main symptoms of disturbances in the bladder storage function are frequency, urgency and incontinence. The aetiology is most frequently an overactive detrusor function (frequently leading to urge incontinence) or an incompetent urethral closure mechanism (often leading to stress incontinence). The main principles of pharmacotherapy therefore aim at reducing detrusor contractility or stimulating the urethral closure mechanism.

Drugs inhibiting detrusor contractility

Detrusor contractility can be inhibited by several different drugs acting via different pharmacological mechanisms (Table 32.1).

Anticholinergics act by blocking the postganglionic

Table 32.1 Drugs inhibiting detrusor contractility — recommended daily dosages for adults.

Drugs	Effect	Dosage
Propantheline	Anticholinergic	15–30 mg t.i.d.
Methantheline	Anticholinergic	50–100 mg q.i.d.
Emepronium bromide	Anticholinergic	200–400 mg t.i.d./ q.i.d.
Dicyclomine	Anticholinergic + musculotrophic relaxant	20 mg b.i.d./t.i.d.
Oxybutynin	Anticholinergic + musculotrophic relaxant + local anaesthetic	5 mg b.i.d./t.i.d. (intravesically; diluted)
Flavoxate	Musculotrophic relaxant	200 mg q.i.d.
Imipramine	Anticholinergic + musculotrophic relaxant	25 mg t.i.d.
Doxepin	Anticholinergic + musculotrophic relaxant	25 mg t.i.d.
Prazosin	α-Blockade	0.5–2.0 mg t.i.d.

muscarine receptors, thereby reducing detrusor contractility. Some anticholinergics probably also exert a ganglion-blocking effect. Most anticholinergics can effectively block detrusor contractility after intravenous administration. The most widely used drugs are quaternary ammonium compounds, which have an uneven and generally poor absorption from the gastrointestinal tract. Therefore, the clinical effects are varying. Dose titration is necessary in the individual patient. In the elderly, significantly higher doses are often necessary with oral administration in order to obtain clinical effect. The therapeutic effect on detrusor contractility is frequently accompanied by moderate systemic anticholinergic side effects. None of the available drugs has been shown to have a selective effect on the urinary bladder [1]. In patients treated with clean intermittent catheterization/sterile intermittent catheterization for impaired bladder emptying and concomitant overactive detrusor function, anticholinergics may be administered intravesically in conjunction with the catheterizations. Clinically significant effects on the symptoms of overactive detrusor function have been reported with only a few systemic side effects [2,3]. In patients with idiopathic detrusor instability, placebo-controlled studies of the effect of anticholinergics have documented a considerable placebo effect [4]. This is probably due to the natural history of idiopatic detrusor instability.

Flavoxate has a papaverine-like 'direct' smooth muscle relaxant effect, but the mechanism of action is still not clear. The clinical effect of flavoxate in the treatment of overactive detrusor function is not well documented [5,6].

In vitro studies have demonstrated that certain calcium antagonists (e.g. nifedipine) can effectively block detrusor contractility [7,8]. Uncontrolled clinical trials have also shown an effect of nifedipine [9]. Treatment with calcium antagonists frequently give rise to side effects, mainly peripheral vasodilatation. Drugs with both anticholinergic and calcium antagonistic effect have been proven clinically effective in the treatment of overactive detrusor function [10]. Terodiline exerts both an anticholinergic and a calcium antagonistic effect [1]. A controlled double-blind trial has demonstrated a clinical effect of this drug and a low incidence of side effects [10]. However, reports on severe cardiac side effects have led to the withdrawal of these drugs from the market [11].

Tricyclic antidepressants exert both an anticholinergic and a direct muscle-relaxing effect. Furthermore, the urethral resistance is increased via α-receptor stimulation due to blocking of the re-uptake of noradrenaline in the adrenergic nerve terminals [12]. Therefore, tricyclic antidepressants are useful in the treatment of both motor urge incontinence and stress incontinence. Controlled trials have also documented a clinical effect of imipramine in the treatment of nocturnal enuresis [13]. In patients

suffering damage to the parasympathetic peripheral innervation of the bladder, uninhibited detrusor contractions can be caused by an increased activity in α-receptors. Treatment with α-receptor-blocking agents, therefore, may be effective in such patients [14].

Drugs stimulating the urethral closure mechanism

Stimulation of the α-receptors in the smooth musculature of the bladder neck and proximal urethra leads to an increase in urethral resistance and thereby a clinical effect on moderate stress incontinence caused by an incompetent urethral closure mechanism [15]. Ephedrine [16] and phenylpropanolamine [17] are the drugs most widely used (Table 32.2). These drugs do not specifically act on the urethra. Treatment is therefore frequently accompanied by slight side effects due to stimulation of the sympathetic nervous system (e.g. increase in blood pressure, exitation or insomnia [1]). Treatment with norfenefrine seems to carry few side effects [18].

Oestrogens are used in the treatment of stress incontinence in post-menopausal women. The mechanism of action is presumably a proliferation of the urethral epithelium, which thereby more effectively seals the urethra, and sprouting of new α-receptors [1].

Tricyclic antidepressants can also increase urethral pressure due to an α-receptor-stimulating effect [12]. Several uncontrolled trials have shown an effect of imipramine on stress urinary incontinence [19].

Improvement of bladder emptying

Disturbances of bladder emptying frequently lead to stranguria and urinary retention. Recurrent urinary tract infections, urge incontinence and/or overflow incontinence may also occur. Pharmacotherapy aims at increasing detrusor contractility and/or reducing urethral outflow resistance.

Table 32.2 Drugs stimulating the urethral closure mechanism— recommended daily dosages for adults.

Drugs	Effect	Dosage
Ephedrine	α- + β-Adrenergic stimulation	10–50 mg t.i.d.
Phenylpropanolamine	α-Adrenergic stimulation	50 mg b.i.d.
Norfenefrine	α-Adrenergic stimulation	15–30 mg t.i.d.
Imipramine	α-Adrenergic stimulation	25 mg t.i.d.
Oestradiol	Oestrogen + adrenergic stimulation	2 mg daily

Drugs stimulating detrusor contractility

The detrusor muscle is stimulated to contraction by parasympathomimetics, acetylcholinesterase inhibitors and prostaglandins. Available parasympathomimetics are carbachol and bethanechol. The effect of these drugs is short lasting due to a short half-life of the drugs in plasma. Theoretically parasympathomimetics may increase urethral resistance. This has been shown in animal experiments [12]. Treatment with carbacholine is now regarded as obsolete due to a pronounced nicotine effect via autonomic ganglia [20]. Patients suffering from peripheral denervation of the bladder often have an increased sensitivity to parasympathomimetics. Treatment with such drugs should therefore initially be given in relatively low doses [21].

Acetylcholinesterase inhibitors which reduce the degradation of acetylcholine are seldom used clinically for insufficient bladder emptying. A stimulating effect on the detrusor musculature of these drugs has been reported [22].

Prostaglandin (PG) $F_{2\alpha}$ and PGE_2 have been demonstrated to exert a stimulatory effect on the smooth musculature of the bladder in clinical uncontrolled trials [23,24]. Prostglandins are applied intravesically in dilution.

Drugs reducing the urethral outflow resistance

Functional infravesical obstruction may be caused by an increased activity in the smooth musculature around the bladder neck and the proximal urethra or increased activity in the urethral striated sphincter musculature. Drugs with a relaxing effect on these closure mechanisms are listed in Table 32.3. It is well documented that α-receptor-blocking agents reduce urethral resistance [1,14,15,25]. Prazosin has been the clinically most widely used α-blocking agent [1]. The classic side effects during treatment with α-receptor-blocking agents are orthostatic hypotension and tachycardia. New, more selectively acting α-blockers such as alfuzosin, terazosin and tamsulosin have fewer side effects. PGE_2 applied intraurethrally or intravesically has been shown clinically to relax the urethral closure mechanism [24].

Functional infravesical obstruction localized to the striated musculature (the external urethral sphincter and/or the periurethral musculature) can be treated with centrally acting muscle relaxants. Diazepam, Dantrium and baclofen have been used with a clinically good effect on this condition [1].

Dysfunction of the lower urinary tract due to side effects of pharmacological treatment

Several drugs commonly used for other disorders influence

Table 32.3 Drugs reducing urethral closure function—recommended daily dosages for adults.

Drug	Effect	Dosage
Prazosin†	α-Adrenergic blockade	0.5–2.0 mg t.i.d.
Alfuzosin	α-Adrenergic blockade	2.5 mg t.i.d.
Terazosin†	α-Adrenergic blockade	5–10 mg o.d.
Tamsulosin	α-Adrenergic blockade	0.4 mg o.d.
Prostaglandin E₂	Prostaglandin receptor stimulation	3–5 mg*
Baclofen	Polysynaptic inhibition	5–20 mg t.i.d.
Diazepam	Striated muscle relaxation	2–5 mg q.i.d.
Dantrolene	Striated muscle relaxation	50–40 mg o.d.

* Applied intraurethrally or intravesically in dilution.
† Dose titration required.

the function of the lower urinary tract. Treatment with such drugs thereby involves a potential risk of inadvertently inducing dysfunction of the bladder and urethra. The most commonly used drugs influencing lower urinary tract function are listed in Table 32.4. Drugs lowering the urethral pressure may produce or aggravate stress incontinence. Drugs increasing detrusor contractility may reduce the functional bladder capacity resulting in urinary frequency, urgency and urge incontinence. Drugs reducing detrusor contractility may provoke insufficient bladder emptying and urinary retention. Similar effects may be produced by drugs increasing the urethral resistance.

However, side effects in the lower urinary tract occur in relatively few patients. These side effects are most often seen in patients who a priori—due to local disorders—are predisposed to an unbalanced storage or emptying function of the bladder.

Guidelines and pitfalls

The innervation and the function of the lower urinary tract is extremely complex, and the spectrum of drugs influencing the bladder and urethral function is wide. A thorough diagnostic evaluation of dysfunctions of the lower urinary tract is thus mandatory for rational pharmacotherapy. In some cases, surgical treatment is clearly indicated. This applies to patients with infravesical

Table 32.4 Drugs with acknowledged and potential side effects on bladder and urethral functions.

Drug	Facilitate emptying		Facilitate storage	
	Detrusor contractility ↑	Outflow resistance ↓	Detrusor contractility ↓	Urethral closure mechanism ↑
α-Adrenergic blockers	0	+		
α-Adrenergic stimulators			0	+
Amphetamines				+
Anticholinergic antiparkinson drugs			+	
Antihistamines			+	
Atropine-like agents			+	
β-Adrenergic blockers	0			0
β-Adrenergic stimulators		0	0	
Bromocriptine			0	
Calcium antagonists			+	
Centrally acting muscle relaxants		0	0	
Cholinesterase inhibitors	0			
Digitalis	0			
Diphenylhydantoin		0	+	
Disopyramide			+	
Ganglionic-blocking agents			+	
Hydrallazine			0	
L-dihydroxyphenylalanine (L-DOPA)				+
Methyldopa		0		
Narcotics			0	
Oestrogens				+
Opiates			0	
Phenothiazines		0	+	
Progesterone		0		
Prostaglandin inhibitors			0	0
Prostaglandins	+	0		
Reserpine		0		
Testosterone	0			
Tricyclic antidepressants			+	+

+, acknowledged clinical effect; 0, effect *in vitro* or clinically uncertain effect.

obstruction due to benign prostatic hyperplasia (BPH), genital descensus and severe detrusor–external sphincter–dyssynergia. In patients with suspension defects of the bladder and stress incontinence, treatment is usually also surgical. In patients with defects not suitable for surgical treatment, in patients with slight or moderate stress incontinence and in idiopathic detrusor instability or functional infravesical obstruction, pharmacotherapy must be considered.

The extent of the evaluation before treatment is related to the clinical problems. Several studies have shown that a thorough history and a conventional urological/gynaecological study are an uncertain basis for evaluation of the pathophysiology. Thus, it has been shown that the symptom stress incontinence may be caused by both an incompetent urethral closure mechanism, detrusor instability and retention with overflow. In elderly persons suffering from urge incontinence, a thorough history, a micturition chart, a urinary culture, a pelvic examination and measurement of the residual urine volume will often give a safe knowledge of the underlying pathophysiology. In most cases detrusor instability will be the cause of the urge incontinence. However, the symptoms are frequently combined and therefore it is often necessary to undertake urodynamic investigations, cystoscopy and functional radiological studies of the lower urinary tract.

Much information regarding the influence of drugs on the lower urinary tract has come from *in vitro* studies using muscle strips or from *in vivo* studies using experimental animals. It is not possible, based on such investigations, to extrapolate to the possible clinical effects in humans. Nor is it possible, based on studies of healthy volunteers, to conclude safely on the effects of pharmacotherapy in patients with bladder or urethral dysfunction. The effect of several drugs is thus not documented in clinical controlled trials.

Pharmacotherapy frequently leads to satisfactory clinical effects, but it is extremely important to realize that no drugs presently available exert specific effects on bladder or urethral function. Therefore, treatment is frequently associated with systemic side effects, and these side effects can be unacceptable to the patients in relation to the intended effects. Therefore, pharmacotherapy demands frequent controls. Some patients will stop medication on their own initiative and accept the symptoms after a certain period of treatment [26]. This should also be seen in the light of the expenses of treatment. Treatment with the most frequently used anticholinergics involves a patient cost exceeding UK£20/month. Attention should further be drawn to the fact that pharmacotherapy is associated with a relatively high placebo effect and this effect should, of course, be taken advantage of.

In elderly patients, the usual drugs influencing the autonomic nervous system or the smooth musculature of the lower urinary tract may disrupt a normal voiding pattern, leading to difficult bladder emptying, urinary retention, frequency and/or urge incontinence. It is important to be aware of this risk, since discontinuation or change of pharmacotherapy may save the patient being referred for urological or gynaecological investigations.

It is not always possible, even by employing sophisticated investigative techniques, to clarify the underlying cause of bladder and urethral dysfunction, and sometimes the expected response of pharmacotherapy is not seen. This is probably due to the complex interaction between the sympathetic and parasympathetic innervation of the lower urinary tract. Furthermore, the status of the receptors in the target organ can be changed by other pathophysiological conditions (e.g. denervation, obstruction, etc.). Furthermore, the receptor status in the target organ can be changed during pharmacotherapy, and frequently it is necessary to use several drugs in the treatment of the same type of voiding dysfunction. Combinations of drugs may be beneficial. Without an adequate updated knowledge on the pathophysiology and clinical pharmacology of the lower urinary tract, rational pharmacotherapy is not possible.

Pharmacological treatment of benign prostatic hyperplasia

Pharmacological manipulation of prostatic complaints is not new. The use of anticholinergics for alleviating urgency at the risk of urinary retention and also of more or less specific α-blocking agents started decades ago. Plant extracts have been popular in many countries although the rationale has been unfirm and often absent.

Placebo effect

It is noteworthy that pharmacological treatment of BPH involves a considerable placebo effect. This is easy to understand realizing the unclear relationship between symptoms and pathophysiology. It is well documented that the symptomatology has a fluctuating course. The patient is prone to seek medical assistance at a time where he is most symptomatic and the natural course, along with the reassurance of a doctor's advice, will almost invariably cause the symptoms to subside in severity over the following months. Most publications dealing with spontaneous development as well as those involving controlled clinical trials with a placebo arm have substantiated this fact. The placebo effect may account for as much as 30–40% of improvement in symptom score. The more sophisticated pharmacological trials now allow for a period of placebo run-in in the patients who will receive active drugs in the study.

α-Blocking agents

The use of α-blockers started with the observations [27] that urinary retention could be relieved by phenoxybenzamine. The prostatic smooth muscle is richly innervated by α-sympathetic nerves [28]. This is also true for the bladder base and bladder neck. Phenoxybenzamine is not registered any longer in most countries due to observed carcinogenic effect in mice. Widespread use of prazosin [29] followed but a substantial number of patients did not tolerate the treatment due to orthostatic arterial hypotension.

Newer drugs have been developed with a more specific α-receptor-blocking effect, for example alfuzosin [30] and terazosin [31] and tamsulosin [32]. Systemic side effects (hypotension, nasal stuffiness, gastrointestinal motility) are less problematic with these drugs. Large series have shown a small flow rate increase, and a 10–15% better effect than placebo. The improvement seems to be durable at least over 1 year in those who respond from the outset. It would be logical to offer α-blockers to the troubled patient with uncomplicated BPH and a prostate with a high proportion of smooth muscle. A histological study of hyperplastic prostatic tissue found a correlation between smooth muscle content and response to α-blockers [33]. In a purely clinical setting this would indicate that the firm, small- to medium-sized gland would herald a good response but this remains to be proven. Recent studies indicate that the α-adrenoceptor which is most important in BPH stromal tissue is the α_{1c}-type [34]. Further development in manufacturing more selective drugs can be anticipated.

5α-Reductase inhibition

It is now recognized that the conversion of testosterone to dihydrotestosterone by the enzyme 5α-reductase is required to maintain maximum androgenic effect on the prostate. Lack of this enzyme leads to a characteristic inborn error with feminization of the external genitalia and a small underdeveloped prostate [35]. Large clinical trials have proven that the 5α-reductase inhibitor finasteride is able to shrink the prostate volume by 20–25%. The reduction is primarily in the epithelial element of the enlarged prostate.

The effect on symptomatology is markedly better than placebo and seems durable over at least 3 years in those patients who respond [36]. The flow rate improvement is in the order of 2–3 ml/s, but a substantial decrease in detrusor pressure has been observed [37]. Side effects involve gynaecomastia, erectile dysfunction and inspissation of semen, but are relatively rare and mostly of little consequence for this elderly population of males.

Studies are under way to develop drugs blocking both type I and II 5α-reductase enzyme.

Other hormonal manipulations

Reduction of testosterone effects on the prostate can be achieved by castration, gonadotrophin-releasing hormone agonists, gestogens and pure antiandrogens. The prostate response mimics that obtained with finasteride, but the side effects preclude a wider use of these drugs in a benign disease such as BPH [38].

It is known that oestrogens act together with androgens in the development of BPH. Therefore, some hope has been linked with the use of drugs that reduce oestrogen production. One such drug with an aromatase-inhibition effect has been tested [39]. Unfortunately, the reduction of serum oestrogens was overshadowed by the increase in serum androgens.

References

1 Andersson KE, Sjögren C. Aspects on the physiology and pharmacology of the bladder and urethra. *Prog Neurobiol* 1982;**19**:71–89.

2 Madersbacher H, Jilg G. Control of detrusor hyperreflexia by intravesical application of oxybutyin hydrochloride. *Paraplegia* 1991;**29**:84–90.

3 O'Flynn KJ, Thomas DG. Intravesical instillation of oxybutynin hydrochloride for detrusor hyperreflexia. *Br J Urol* 1993;**72**:566–70.

4 Meyhoff HH, Gerstenberg TC, Nordling J. Placebo—the drug of choice in female motor urge incontinence? *Br J Urol* 1983;**55**:34–7.

5 Dalaere KPJ, Michiels HGE, Debruyne FMJ, Moonen WA. Flavoxate hydrochloride in the treatment of detrusor instability. *Urol Int* 1977;**32**:377–81.

6 Stanton SL. A comparison of emepronium bromide and flavoxate hydrochloride in the treatment of urinary incontinence. *J Urol* 1973;**110**:529–32.

7 Husted SE. Activation mechanisms in the urinary bladder. Thesis, Arhüs University, 1984.

8 Formann A, Andersson KE, Henriksson L, Rud T, Ulmsten U. Effects of nifedipine on the smooth muscle of the human urinary tract *in vitro* and *in vivo*. *Acta Pharmacol Toxicol* 1978;**43**:111–18.

9 Rud T, Andersson KE, Ulmsten U. Effects of nifedipine in women with unstable bladders. *Urol Int* 1979;**34**:421–9.

10 Andersen JR, Lose G, Nørgård M, Stimpel H, Andersen JT. Terodiline, emepronium bromide or placebo for treatment of female detrusor overactivity? A randomised, double blind cross-over study. *Br J Urol* 1988;**61**:310–13.

11 Connolly MJ, Astridge PS, White EG, Morley CA, Cowan JC. Torsades de pointes, ventricular tachycardia and terodiline. *Lancet* 1991;**338**:344–5.

12 Wein AJ. Neuromuscular dysfunction of the lower urinary tract. In: Walsh PC, Retik AB, Stamey TA, Vaughan ED, eds. *Campbell's Urology*. Philadelphia: WB Saunders, 1992: 573–642.

13 Mahoney DT, Laferte RO, Mahoney JE. Observations on sphincter-augmenting effect of imipramine in children with urinary incontinence. *Urology* 1973;**1**:317–23.

14 Sundin T, Dahlstrøm A, Norlén L, Svedmyr N. The sympathetic innervation and adrenoceptor function of the human lower urinary tract in the normal state and after parasympathetic denervation. *Invest Urol* 1977;**14**:322–8.

15 Awad SA, Downie JW, Kiruluta HG. Alpha-adrenergic agents in urinary disorders of the proximal urethra. I. Sphincter incontinence. *Br J Urol* 1978;**50**:332–5.

16 Diokno AC, Taub M. Ephedrine in the treatment of urinary incontinence. *Urology* 1975;**5**:624–5.

17 Fossberg E, Beisland HO, Lundgren RA. Stress incontinence in females: treatment with phenylpropanolamine. *Urol Int* 1983;**38**:293-9.

18 Lose G, Lindholm P. Clinical and urodynamic effects of norfenefrine in women with stress incontinence. *Urol Int* 1984;**39**:298–302.

19 Gilja I, Rady M, Kovacic M, Parazadjer J. Conservative treatment of female stress incontinence with imipramine. *J Urol* 1984;**132**:909–10.

20 Taylor P. Cholinergic agonists. In: Gilman AG, Rall TW, Nies AS, Taylor P, eds. *The Pharmacological Basis of Therapeutics*. New York: Pergamon Press, 1990: 122–30.

21 Glahn BE. Neurogenic bladder diagnosed pharmacologically on the basis of denervation supersensitivity. *Scand J Urol Nephrol* 1970;**4**:13–24.

22 Philip NH, Thomas DG. The effect of distigmine bromide on voiding in male paraplegic patients with reflex micturition. *Br J Urol* 1980;**52**:492–6.

23 Bultitude MI, Hills NH, Shuttleworth KED. Clinical and experimental studies on the action of prostaglandins and their synthesis inhibitors on detrusor muscle *in vitro* and *in vivo*. *Br J Urol* 1976;**48**:631–7.

24 Andersson KE, Henriksson L, Ulmsten U. Effects of prostaglandin E_2 applied locally on intravesical and intraurethral pressures in women. *Eur Urol* 1978;**4**:366–9.

25 Whitfield HN, Doyle PT, Mayo ME, Poopalasingham N. The effect of adrenergic blocking drugs on outflow resistance. *Br J Urol* 1976;**47**:823–7.

26 Walter S, Meyhoff HH, Gerstenberg T, Nordling J, Hald T. Urinary incontinence in females. A long-term study on the effect of anticholinergics on overactive detrusor function. *Acta Obstet Gynecol Scand* 1984;**64**:159–61.

27 Caine M, Perlberg S, Meretyk S. A placebo-controlled double-blind study of the effect of phenoxybenzamine in benign prostatic obstruction. *Br J Urol* 1978;**50**:551–4.

28 Gosling JA. The distribution of noradrenergic nerves in the human lower urinary tract. *Clin Sci* 1986;**70**(Suppl. 14):36–65.

29 Kirby RS, Coppinger SWC, Corcoran MO, Chapple CR, Flannigan M, Milroy EJG. Prazosin in the treatment of prostatic obstruction. *Br J Urol* 1987;**60**:136–42.

30 Jardin A, Bensadoun H, Delauche-Cavalier MC, Attali P, BPH-ALF Group. Alfuzosin for treatment of benign prostatic hypertrophy. *Lancet* 1991;**337**:1457–61.

31 Lepor H, Henry D, Laddy AR. The efficacy and safety of terazosin for the treatment of symptomatic BPH. *Prostate* 1991;**18**:345–55.

32 Abrams P, Schulman CC, Vaage S and the European Tamsulosin Study Group. Tamsulosin, a selective α_{1c}-adrenoceptor antagonist: a randomized, controlled trial in patients with benign prostatic 'obstruction' (symptomatic BPH). *Br J Urol* 1995;**76**:325–36.

33 Shapiro E, Becich MJ, Hartanto V, Lepor H. The relative proportion of stromal and epithelial hyperplasia is related to the development of symptomatic benign prostatic hyperplasia. *J Urol* 1991;**147**:1293–7.

34 Lepor H *et al.* Alpha-1 adrenoceptor subtypes in the human prostate. *J Urol* 1993;**149**:640–2.

35 Imperato-McGinley J *et al.* Steroid 5-alpha-reductase deficiency in man. An inherited form of male pseudohermaphroditism. *Birth Defects* 1975;**11**:91–103.

36 Stoner E, Finasteride Study Group. The clinical effects of a 5-alpha reductase inhibitor, finasteride, on benign prostatic hyperplasia. *J Urol* 1992;**147**:1298–302.

37 Tammela TLJ, Kontturi MJ. Urodynamic effects of finasteride in the treatment of bladder outlet obstruction due to benign prostatic hyperplasia. *J Urol* 1993;**149**:342–4.

38 Hansen BJ, Hald T. Review of current medical treatment of benign prostatic hyperplasia. *Eur Urol* 1993;**24**(Suppl. 1):41–9.

39 Tunn UW, Schweikert HU. Aromatase inhibitors in the management of benign prostatic hyperplasia. In: Ackermann R, Schroeder FH, eds. *New Developments in Biosciences*, Vol. 5. *Prostatic Hyperplasia*. Berlin: De Gruyter, 1989:139–49.

33 Pathophysiology of Bladder Outflow Obstruction

A.F.Brading and M.J.Speakman

Introduction

The history of bladder outlet obstruction

Recognition of, and interest in, bladder outflow obstruction can be traced back to the earliest written records. The Ebers Papyrus dating from Egypt in 1550 BC contained the term 'retention of urine', which then included all urinary diseases. Obstruction to the outflow of urine in the male was recognized by the ancient Egyptians and Chinese and treated with catheters. Galen (AD 131–200) recorded various causes of lower urinary tract obstruction including 'morbid tumour, inflammation, fleshy callous, stone and clots'. Avicenna in Persia (AD 980–1037) noted that, especially in men, the bladder became 'corrugated' in obstruction—an early reference to trabeculation. The credit for understanding and demonstrating the significance of prostatic hyperplasia belongs to Morgagni (1682–1771), who at the age of 80, distinguished between prostatic abscess and prostatic hyperplasia which he believed to be a benign growth of the prostate. Excellent anatomical drawings of the bladder and urethral structure were produced by Leonardo da Vinci (1452–1519), but he failed to include the prostate. Vesalius (1514–1564), described longitudinal, transverse and oblique fibres in the bladder wall which he postulated made it capable of variation in its capacity. However, until Fallopius (1523–1562) identified its muscular nature, the bladder was regarded as a passive elastic structure, emptied by contraction of the abdominal wall musculature. Later, Spiegel gave the name detrusor urinae to the longitudinal fibres of the muscle coat (L. detrudere, to drive out). The association between bladder outflow obstruction and detrusor instability was recognized in 1786 by John Hunter when he commented 'The disease of the bladder arising from obstruction alone, is increased irritability, and its consequences, by which it admits of little distension, becomes quick in its action and thick and strong in its coats.' This shows clear reference to urgency, frequency and bladder hypertrophy. The difficulties in interpreting a patient's flow symptoms were understood by Guthrie (1843), when he stated 'On this point however, persons are always deceived. They never duly estimate the size of the stream they formerly made ... it is only when great change has occurred (after relief of obstruction) that the sufferer is aware of the fact.'

It was the abnormalities in bladder function that were studied first, the physiology of the normal bladder receiving little attention until the nineteenth century. In 1836, Guthrie's paper [1] showed that he appreciated that the bladder was a muscular organ, and that the function of the bladder was to expel urine. In the 1860s, Budge [2] stimulated the spinal cord in an experimental animal and observed that the bladder contracted. It was not until the end of the last century and the early part of this century, that Griffiths [3], Elliott [4] and Barrington [5,6], among others, performed carefully planned experiments studying the nerve supply to the bladder. Investigation of bladder function may have started in 1876 when Dubois [7] measured the static pressure in the bladder with an elastic catheter using the symphysis pubis as the baseline. The rate of flow was then recorded, first by Rehfisch [8] using a system in which urine displaced air from a closed vessel with the volume of air displaced being recorded. In 1933 true detrusor pressure was recorded by Denny-Brown and Robertson [9] when they also measured intra-abdominal pressure via a rectal line. This allowed detrusor function itself to be studied. In 1956, von Garrelts [10] pioneered simultaneous pressure–flow measurements and published a new method of recording the flow rate of urine using a pressure transducer.

Current understanding of the problem of micturition

In recent years, methods of measuring urethral pressures have evolved and X-ray video cystoscopy has been perfected to give us a fuller picture of the micturition process. We now realize that the urethra and its associated structures have to perform a very delicate balancing act, especially in upright animals such as ourselves. There must be sufficient resistance to urine flow to allow the bladder to fill without leaking, in spite of the effects of gravity and the frequent increases in intra-abdominal pressure, and at the same time the necessary mechanisms must be present to allow the urethra to change into a low-resistance pathway during voiding, so that the bladder can be emptied rapidly and at will, without an excessive rise in intravesical pressure.

The mechanisms that permit this are really quite complex, involving as they do autonomic reflexes which are activated voluntarily, and thus involve every possible level of the central and peripheral nervous systems as well as at least three types of effector systems—striated and smooth muscles, and the vascular filling of the urethral lamina propria. This degree of complexity inevitably means that many things can go wrong, leading to incontinence or outflow obstruction. In this chapter we will deal with the pathophysiology of outflow obstruction.

Pathophysiology of obstruction

It is clearly a bad thing for intravesical pressure to rise too high. Not only can this prevent filtration in the kidney, but it can lead to urinary reflux and kidney damage due to infection. However, if the urethral resistance does not drop at the right time to allow the contracting detrusor to expel its contents, the intravesical pressure cannot help but rise as a purely physical consequence [11]. Outflow obstruction can occur through external pressure acting on the urethra, through physical changes in the urethral wall and also through the failure of the control mechanisms to allow the normal drop in resistance.

When obstruction is progressive, little is known about the early stages. During these stages the increased voiding pressures may overcome the obstruction and allow apparently normal voiding without the development of symptoms, while resulting in progressive detrusor hypertrophy and smooth muscle disruption. The symptom presentation of bladder outflow obstruction depends on its cause, its severity, its speed of onset and on the presence of associated complications. Patients may present simply with obstructive symptoms or they may present with additional irritative symptoms, frequently associated with detrusor instability. Alternatively, patients may present suddenly with acute retention, often with little in the way of previous symptoms, or more slowly and less clearly with the complications of chronic retention.

In this chapter we will outline first the peripheral mechanisms involved in bladder filling and micturition to act as a point of reference. We will then discuss briefly the diagnosis of obstruction, and the factors responsible for it and, in more detail, the changes in the bladder structure and function that may result from obstruction.

Normal function

Bladder filling

The kidney produces urine by ultrafiltration of the blood, using a net filtration pressure of only some 20–30 mmHg (27–41 cmH$_2$O). This means that even small rises in pressure in the kidney tubule can readily block filtration. The pathway for urine flow from the kidney into the bladder is also a low-pressure pathway, and build-up of urine is prevented by waves of contraction that originate in the smooth muscle of the kidney pelvis and sweep down the ureters, propelling the urine into the bladder. The bladder thus has to fill at a low pressure. Failure to fill properly may be due to abnormalities in the bladder itself or its outlet.

The bladder wall smooth muscle

The wall of the bladder is composed largely of smooth muscle. When the bladder is empty, the bladder wall of humans can be more than 10 mm thick, but when full it can be as little as only 3–4 mm. This implies considerable reorganization of the smooth muscle during filling. An interesting study has been performed by Uvelius and Gabella [12] in which they examined this process in some detail in the guinea pig bladder. In humans and similar-sized animals such as pigs, the smooth muscles are arranged in large bundles, which may be as much as 1 mm or more in diameter, surrounded by connective tissue. Each bundle is subdivided into a number of smaller bundles, with a thinner layer of connective tissue surrounding them [13] (see Fig. 33.6a). It is possible in excised tissue to follow the large bundles by dissection for distances of 1 cm or more, and it is apparent that they form a 3D network in the bladder wall. During filling the individual cells within a bundle become longer and thinner. In the guinea pig they can change in length fourfold from an empty to a full bladder. The bundles themselves undergo rearrangement [12]. All this goes on without a significant increase in pressure, i.e. the bladder wall is very compliant. The organization of the connective tissue (collagen and elastin) has to allow this.

After micturition the normal bladder wall does not relax into a floppy structure, but adjusts itself to maintain the minimum surface area:volume ratio available to it during filling, a strategy which allows immediate build-up of pressure at whatever volume micturition is induced. The individual smooth muscle elements have spontaneous mechanical activity, which allows them to keep their appropriate length for whatever volume the bladder has. In spite of this continuous mechanical activity in the cells, which in smaller animals has been shown to be related to spontaneous action potential production [14,15], the intravesical pressure remains low, and this is almost certainly due to the fact that individual smooth muscle cells appear to be electrically coupled only to a few of their neighbours, which prevents synchronous activity and allows constant adjustment of the length of the smooth muscle cells without build-up of pressure. It has been suggested that a pressure rise in the bladder during filling is also prevented by continuous activation of an adrenergic inhibitory innervation [16]. Certainly sympathetic nerves do enter the bladder wall, and nerves can be demonstrated containing various peptides or amino acids such as vasoactive intestinal polypeptide (VIP) or γ-aminobutyric acid (GABA) that could be inhibitory [17], but there is at present no evidence of any inhibitory nerves acting on the detrusor smooth muscle. Inhibitory control of micturition is more likely to occur at the level of the intramural neurones in the parasympathetic pathway or at the spinal cord [18,19].

Bladder wall compliance

Since there is smooth muscle activity during filling, the question arises as to whether or not this can limit the compliance of the bladder. Compliance in humans is normally measured during bladder filling in urodynamic studies as the change in volume per unit change in pressure. Clinically a 'low-compliance' bladder is looked on as a bad sign. However, it has long been realized that compliance depends on the rate of bladder filling, and careful studies on animals have confirmed this [20,21]. This problem is particularly marked in neuropathic bladders [22,23], where faster filling rates during urodynamic measurements cause significant decreases in bladder compliance. Recently, compliance measured during natural bladder filling using ambulatory monitoring [22] showed that the low compliance measured during normal urodynamics disappeared during ambulatory monitoring, suggesting that it was an artefact of artificial filling, although in a similar study by Stott [23] significant decreased compliance was also seen in ambulatory monitoring on his patients. Such studies perhaps imply that there may be a significant contribution of the activity of bladder smooth muscle limiting compliance during rapid fill. It is interesting to note that in the organ bath, isolated strips of detrusor smooth muscle respond to sudden stretch by an increase in activity and tone, which, however, soon falls off towards the original basal level [24] (Fig. 33.1). Recent studies on isolated myocytes have revealed stretch-sensitive non-selective cation channels in the membrane, which allow the generation of an inward current that declines in time, and is thus just what is necessary to account for the strip behaviour [25].

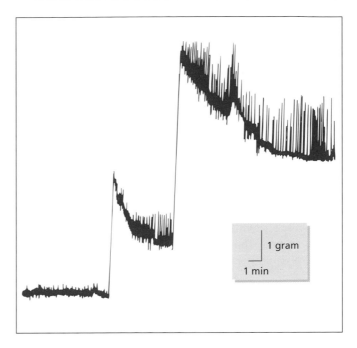

Fig. 33.1 Contractile activity recorded from a strip of pig detrusor in response to stretch. (Redrawn from [24].)

The urethra

During bladder filling, outflow resistance through the urethra remains high. Measurement of the urethral pressure profile shows that there is a high-pressure region beyond the bladder neck, and evidence suggests that this is generated in the urethral wall, and probably involves both smooth muscle tone and engorgement of the lamina propria with blood. Electromyography of the striated muscle in the urethral wall suggests that these muscles are continuously active during bladder filling [26], but increased activity in the striated sphincter and the pelvic floor is recruited as additional protection from increases in abdominal pressure during exercise or such things as coughing and sneezing [27]. The smooth muscle tone may be due largely to myogenic activity, although there may be involvement of some tonic excitatory sympathetic nerve activity [28,29].

Micturition

Sensory information

Although micturition is under voluntary control and can be initiated at will, normally a sensation of bladder fullness will trigger awareness of the need to micturate. Since there is little rise in intravesical pressure during filling in the normal bladder, the sensory information about bladder filling must be mediated by stretch receptors rather than pressure receptors in the bladder wall. If micturition is not initiated, the sensations change progressively from that of bladder fullness to urgency, and this information is used in the decision to induce micturition at an appropriate time and place.

Urethral relaxation

The first urodynamic manifestation of micturition is a fall in the urethral pressure. This is followed by a rise in intravesical pressure, which, when it is high enough to overcome the outflow resistance, results in urine flow. It is not yet entirely clear what causes the drop in urethral pressure. Reduction in activity of the striated urethral sphincter is seen [26], but the most important mechanisms seem likely to involve a fall in tone of the urethral smooth muscle brought about by a combination of a reduction in tonic excitatory nerve activity and activation of inhibitory nerves [29]. Nerve fibres containing many putative transmitters have been demonstrated in the human urethral wall [17], and in pigs, in which the urethral properties are similar, two functional excitatory neuronal inputs (one cholinergic and one adrenergic) and two inhibitory neuronal inputs (one nitrergic and one with an as yet unidentified transmitter) have been demonstrated [29].

Detrusor contraction

In the normal human, the excitatory input to the detrusor is through the parasympathetic system, and is mediated exclusively by activation of muscarinic receptors [30–32] (Fig. 33.2). This is in contrast to most other animals where there is a clear purinergic component of excitation which is dominant in the response to single shocks or low-frequency activation of the nerves (for reference see [13]). The muscarinic component becomes dominant at higher frequencies of nerve stimulation. In spite of the lack of purinergic innervation, the detrusor smooth muscle cells in humans possess the typical P2x purinoceptors that are activated in animal bladders [33] (Fig. 33.3).

Investigation of bladder outflow obstruction

Clinical evaluation

Bladder outflow obstruction results in major alterations in bladder structure and function, such as detrusor hypertrophy, elevated voiding pressures and detrusor instability. Investigation of obstruction, therefore, needs to elicit symptoms but must also attempt to reveal the underlying pathophysiological changes that can cause considerable damage before obvious symptoms are apparent. This requires a good clinical history with particular emphasis on the relative degree of obstructive and irritative symptoms. Obstructive symptoms are those which result directly from the blockage of the urethra or in later stages from failure of the detrusor to elevate pressure sufficiently. Irritative symptoms result from secondary changes occurring in the bladder in response to the obstruction. A symptom score can be valuable if future assessment of the patient is planned. Clinical examination of the abdomen and pelvis together with a digital rectal examination and neurological assessment should always be undertaken but sometimes

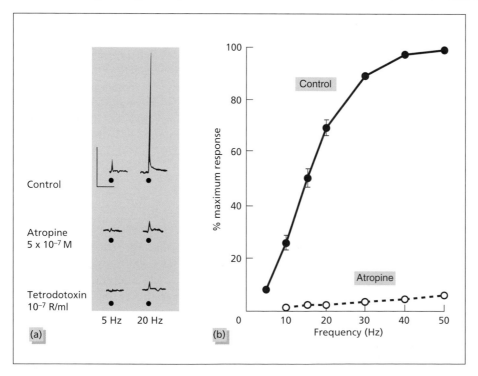

Fig. 33.2 Contractile response of strips of human detrusor in response to transmural stimulation of the intrinsic nerves (50 V, 0.05 ms pulses). (a) Individual responses to a 10 s train at 5 Hz and 20 Hz in control conditions, during an application of 5×10^{-7} mol/l atropine, and after perfusion with 10^{-7} g/ml tetrodotoxin to eliminate nerve-mediated responses. (b) Frequency response curve in control conditions and in the presence of 5×10^{-7} mol/l atropine. The curve obtained in the presence of tetrodotoxin is superimposed on that obtained in the presence of atropine. (Redrawn from [32].)

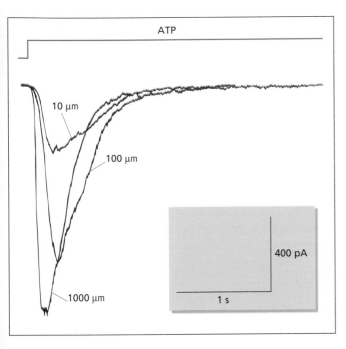

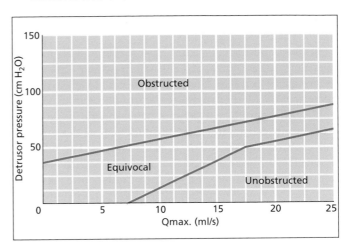

Fig. 33.4 The Abrams and Griffiths nomogram [35].

Fig. 33.3 Whole cell voltage clamp recording obtained from a single detrusor smooth muscle cell from human bladder. Responses to three different concentrations of adenosine triphosphate (ATP) are superimposed. ATP was applied by a concentration jump method. Note the large but transient inward current activated by the application of ATP. (Redrawn from [33].)

reveals little information about the cause or severity of obstruction. Urine analysis and appropriate laboratory investigations should be performed.

It is actually difficult to produce a reliable clinical diagnosis of outflow obstruction. A critical review of the problems has recently been published [34]. Although obstruction will be associated with a low flow rate during voiding, a low flow rate on its own cannot confirm obstruction since it could also be caused by poor detrusor contraction. Urodynamic evaluation can help to identify the presence or absence of obstruction by correlating the urinary flow rate with the voiding detrusor pressure. The nomogram of Abrams and Griffiths [35] can be useful (Fig. 33.4). Measurement of the maximum flow rate (Q_{max}) and detrusor pressure at Q_{max} allows a patient to be put into one of three categories: obstructed, unobstructed or equivocal. For the equivocal results, analysis of the whole pressure–flow relationship is necessary to reach a diagnosis. Urodynamic studies can also reveal abnormalities in filling such as detrusor instability or low compliance. It will identify increased or decreased bladder contractility (pressure) or reveal evidence of an atonic or areflexic detrusor.

However, the benefit of formal urodynamics in patient management, as opposed to clinical research, is still hotly debated. Some authors feel it offers much in the preoperative assessment [34,36,37] while others feel that it

helps little in individual patient evaluation [38]. Consequently, while in some units it is routine practice, in the majority it is rarely undertaken. Simple investigations, however, should be used in all patients. Two voiding flow rates on volumes greater than 200 ml allows the maximum flow and the flow pattern to be compared with other patients of a similar age, and an ultrasound post-micturition bladder residual volume estimation provides useful information about bladder emptying. Formal urodynamic evaluation should be reserved for patients with a high irritative symptom score in the presence of an unexpectedly high flow rate [39]. Assessment for renal tract stone disease or metastatic prostate carcinoma with a plain X-ray (kidneys, ureters and bladder), or for upper tract dilatation with renal ultrasound, is undertaken by most urologists. Cystoscopy will allow some assessment of the urethra and prostate and may show evidence of secondary changes in the bladder wall such as trabeculation or saccule formation, but usually adds little to the decision about the timing of surgical intervention.

Information about obstruction due to failure of the control mechanisms responsible for the drop in outlet resistance, such as external sphincter dyssynergia can be obtained using video cystourethrography. Measurements of urethral pressure profiles during voiding can also help to identify bladder outlet obstruction.

Diagnosis for clinical research

Advances in our knowledge of the aetiology and pathophysiology of bladder outflow obstruction clearly require more detailed investigations, and some attempt to classify patients into groups with similar pathophysiology. Without this, little advance will be possible in assessing the effectiveness of surgical or pharmacological treatment. Because of the different procedures used by individual urologists, it will be important to obtain cooperation between centres, and to establish some uniformity in the methods of assessing patients.

Elbadawi and his colleagues have recently published an important series of papers [40–43] in which they have attempted to correlate the results of careful urodynamic studies on 36 elderly patients (carefully selected to exclude those with neurological deficits or co-morbidity factors), with the ultrastructure of the bladder wall as determined from electron microscopy of cold cup biopsies. The subjects included symptom-free patients and those with various voiding dysfunctions. From the urodynamic studies (regardless of symptoms) they divided the patients into four major groups: detrusor overactivity, outlet obstruction, obstruction plus overactivity and neither overactivity nor obstruction. Each group had two subdivisions, one with normal contractility and the other with impaired contractility. The biopsies were studied separately (blindly) and catagorized into four patterns of ultrastructural features. Correlation of the two studies showed an absolute matching of the groups to the ultrastructural features. Those associated with the outflow obstruction will be described below, but the overall results demonstrate that, at least within the geriatric population, some grouping is possible.

However, the urodynamic tests were very extensive, taking from 1.5 to 3 h for each, the measurements were all performed by the same physician and measurements were repeated. The authors suggest that the ultrastructural patterns were straightforward and easy to recognize, and that detrusor biopsy is a potentially valuable tool for the clinical diagnosis and management of detrusor dysfunction. In this study outflow obstruction was defined arbitrarily as the presence during voiding of a pressure gradient of more than $10 \, cmH_2O$ in the supramembranous urethra of men or distal urethra of women, as determined by fluoroscopically guided micturitional urethral pressure profilometry. Detrusor contractility was defined as normal if there was a post-void residual volume of less than 50 ml, and impaired if it was more than 50 ml in the absence of straining and with no outlet obstruction or sphincter dyssynergia. With either of these, a post-void residual of more than 250 ml was used to define impaired contractility.

Changes that occur subsequent to obstruction

The best documented changes result from studies of obstruction due to prostatic hypertrophy, and from animal studies where obstruction is created artificially. In the animal work, acute obstruction produces massive changes but these will not be discussed since, although acute obstruction clearly occurs in man, the effects of untreated acute obstruction will not often be available for study. Progressive obstruction in animals is usually achieved by placing non-obstructing ligatures or rings around the urethras of young animals and allowing progressive obstruction during growth. Although these are good models, one should be aware that the progressive obstruction due to prostatic hypertrophy occurs in the older adult population in humans, and that age itself causes significant changes in the detrusor structure and function [44]. Nevertheless, in this section changes due to prostatic hypertrophy and experimental obstruction will be described almost exlusively. One should bear in mind, however, that many of the changes in bladder structure and function seen in various neuropathic bladders could result from a functional obstruction caused by impairment of the normal relaxation of the outflow resistance during micturition.

Clinical symptoms

The pathophysiological changes that occur subsequent to prostatic hypertrophy leading to outflow obstruction have been more carefully studied than other conditions. Clinically, apart from a poor stream, a common outcome for many patients is the development of urgency and frequency of micturition, and often detrusor instability [45,46]. Another, less common outcome is the development of a large residual urine and an 'atonic' bladder [47,48]. Experimental progressive outflow obstruction in the pig leads to conditions very similar to those seen in humans and with about the same incidence [49].

Instability

Urodynamic studies in patients with bladder outflow obstruction, secondary to prostatic hyperplasia, have revealed the presence of instability in more than 50% of patients [45,46,50–52]. This is characterized by inappropriate and involuntary rises in pressure during the filling phase of micturition and these contractions lead to the main symptomatic problems of urgency and urge incontinence.

Detrusor instability is also seen in outflow obstruction produced by causes other than prostatic hypertrophy, such as bladder neck stenosis and urethral stricture [46,53]. It has been suggested that the instability is not due to the obstruction *per se*, but rather to the older age of these patients [54]. Abrams [55], found instability in 35% of men aged between 40 and 50 years and in 65% of men over 70 years old. Andersen *et al.* [56] also showed a high incidence of detrusor instability (63%) in asymptomatic men aged between 60 and 70 years.

Further support for the link between instability and increasing age comes from studies in women, in whom outflow obstruction is rare, where the incidence of instability is 27% below 65 years and 38% over this age [57]. In addition, it has been reported that the inci-

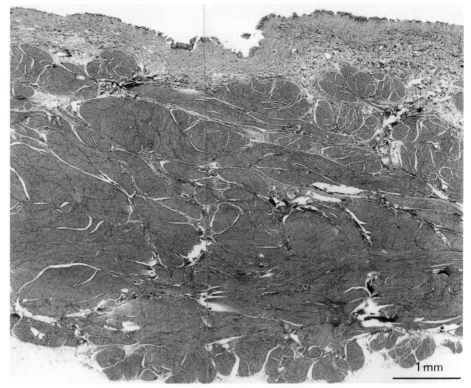

(a)

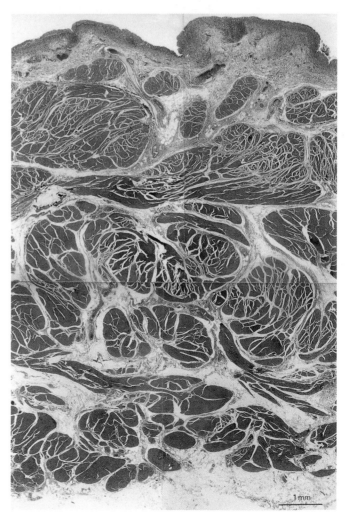

Fig. 33.5 Full-thickness sections of human bladder from (a) a normal, and (b) an obstructed unstable bladder at the same magnification. Note in (b) the large increase in wall thickness, the increased connective tissue between the smooth muscle bundles and the infiltration of connective tissue within the muscle bundles. Scale bar, 1 mm. (Reproduced from [32].)

(b)

dence of instability is similar in obstructed and unobstructed patients, who present with the complex of symptoms associated with prostatic enlargement [55]. Doubt remains, therefore, about the nature of the correlation between bladder outflow obstruction and detrusor instability. However, a gradual denervation may well explain the pathogenesis in both obstruction and increasing age.

Histological findings

Gross changes in bladder wall structure

In the unstable group, the bladder wall thickens and trabeculations are often seen [58,59]. Trabeculations are not, however, diagnostic of outflow obstruction. In Elbadawi's geriatric population, 50% of the unobstructed overactive bladders were trabeculated, and only five out of the seven obstructed bladders were trabeculated. Individual smooth muscle cells enlarge and there is an increase in connective tissue between the large and small muscle bundles, and eventually with time this penetrates between the smooth muscle cells [32] (Figs 33.5 and 33.6). Similar changes seem to occur not just in humans but also in all the experimental models of outflow obstruction in different species [32,60–62].

Cell structure

In the animal models, individual smooth muscle cells

increase in size after outflow obstruction. The diameter of the cells in cross-sections studied by electron microscopy are larger, but it is difficult without 3D reconstruction to be certain that this is not due to changes in cell shape during fixation. However, in our laboratory the dimensions of cells enzymatically isolated from normal and obstructed bladders confirm this hypertrophy, and measurements of cell capacitance suggest that the cell surface area is significantly increased. In Elbadawi's geriatric population, biopsies from the obstructed groups showed non-uniformity of smooth muscle size, with frequent hypertrophic muscle cells standing out by their distinctive profiles, which were often bizarre and branched [43]. The cells are separated by larger spaces and the intermediate junctions less well developed [43,58]. In the overactive obstructed group there were a large number of unusual junctions between the cells, including protrusion cell junctions and ultraclose abutments, both features characteristic of the overactive destrusor whether or not obstructed. We have also seen many such junctions in obstructed pig detrusors. These junctions might allow electrical interaction between the cells.

Extracellular matrix and compliance

There is increased collagen infiltration both around the muscle bundles and between the cells in the obstructed bladders, and increased elastin is often seen. Elbadawi found a particularly large increase in elastin in the bladder

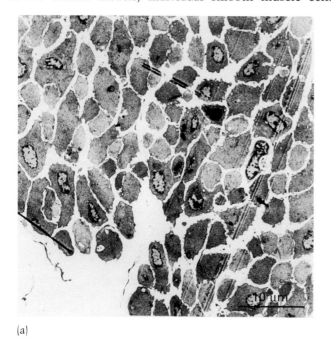

(a)

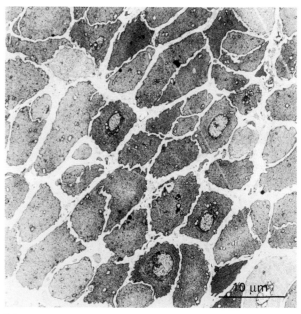

(b)

Fig. 33.6 Electron micrographs of smooth muscle cells from (a) control human detrusor, and (b) detrusor from an obstructed bladder at the same magnification. Note the increase in cross-sectional area of the smooth muscle cells in the obstructed bladder. (Reproduced from [32].)

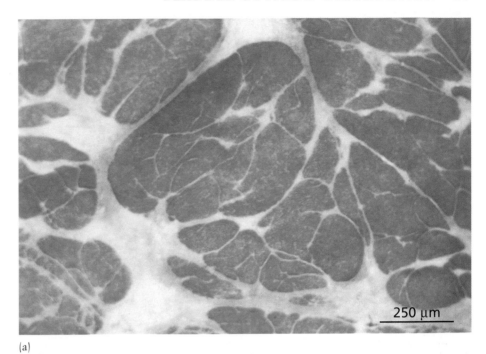

(a)

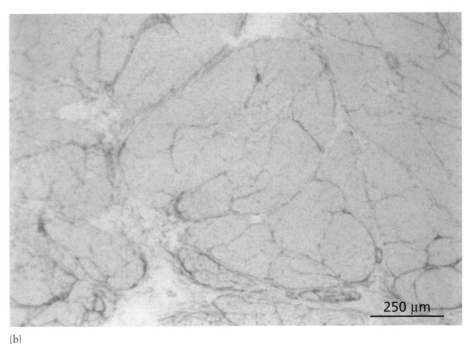

Fig. 33.7 Light micrographs of two adjacent sections of normal human detrusor: (a) stained with Masson trichrome (smooth muscle pink, collagen darker blue/grey), (b) stained for elastin. Note the thin covering of the smooth muscle bundles with elastic fibres. Scale bar, 250 μm. (Reproduced from [63].)

(b)

of one man with chronic retention. Figure 33.7 shows two adjacent sections of normal human bladder, one stained with Masson trichrome to show the collagen, and the other to show the elastin distribution at the edges of the bundles. Figure 33.8 is from a human bladder showing bundles with patches of extensive smooth muscle loss, with greatly increased collagen and elastin in these areas. Increase in these extracellular elements is likely to have effects on the compliance of the bladder wall. Collagen is extremely inextensible and the normal high compliance requires an arrangement of the fibres so that they become wound in helices around the smooth muscle cells when they shorten, and can thus allow lengthening without a drop in compliance. Extra deposition of collagen is likely to decrease compliance, whereas deposition of elastin could help to keep compliance low.

Two studies recently have tried to assess the contribution of the smooth muscle as opposed to the tissue matrix elements (elastin and collagen) to bladder wall compliance [63,64]. In these studies the effects of a slow stretch of

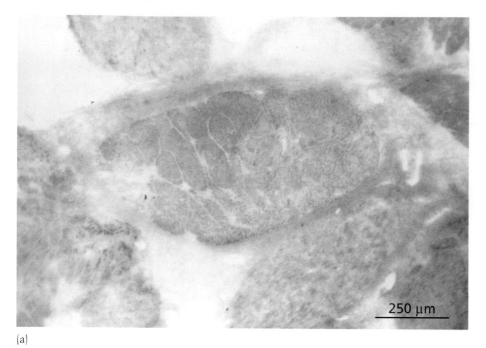

(a)

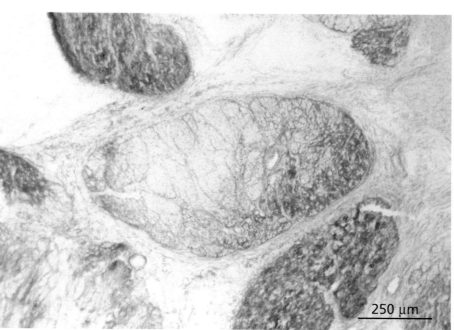

(b)

Fig. 33.8 Light micrographs of two adjacent sections of abnormal human detrusor (from a neuropathic bladder): (a) stained with Masson trichrome (smooth muscle pink, collagen green), (b) stained for elastin. Note the loss of smooth muscle and its replacement with collagen and elastic fibres. Scale bar, 250 μm. (Reproduced from [63].)

isolated strips of smooth muscle have been studied, at rates comparable to the stretching that would be obtained in medium fill cystometry. The studies have been carried out with the smooth muscle cells active (normal physiological saline) and in calcium-free, high-magnesium saline in which there is no contribution of smooth muscle tone. In one study strips from control guinea pig bladder were compared with strips taken from an animal with hypertrophied 'low-compliance' bladders subsequent to

bladder outflow obstruction [64]. In the other study, control strips from human bladder were compared with strips from non-compliant neurogenic bladders [63]. Although in both cases there was some evidence that activity in the smooth muscle cells could reduce the compliance of the strips, differences between the control and the low-compliance bladders appeared to be due to the 'passive' properties of the strips rather than to differences in the behaviour of the smooth muscle cells, suggesting that changes in the composition of the extracellular matrix are more important in reduced compliance than changes in the smooth muscle properties.

Innervation

Another notable histological finding in obstruction is a progressive decrease in the acetylcholinesterase-positive nerves [49,65]. In normal tissues there is a dense network of varicose nerve terminals that penetrates the smooth muscle bundles, and electron microscopy suggests that most cells receive a close innervation. Careful studies in animal and human tissues suggest that in bladders from animals with outflow obstruction, denervation may develop in a patchy manner. Occasionally, the same section will show muscle bundles with apparently normal innervation adjacent to others that are virtually totally denervated [66] (Fig. 33.9).

Physiological findings

Responses to nerve stimulation and agonist application

Studies on strips of smooth muscle demonstrate that transmural nerve stimulation is less effective at activating the smooth muscle from obstructed animals than from normal animals, although the smooth muscles from obstructed humans [31,32], pigs [49,67] and rabbits [68] show increased sensitivity to direct activation of the smooth muscle with excitatory agents such as high-potassium, muscarinic agonists and direct smooth muscle electrical stimulation [32] (Fig. 33.10).

Spontaneous activity

Studies on the spontaneous activity of smooth muscle strips from unstable bladders in both pigs and humans show significant changes from normal tissue [69].

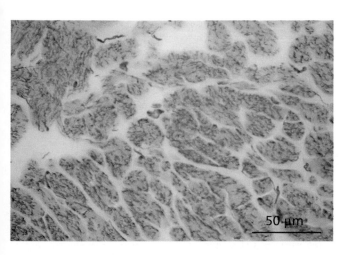

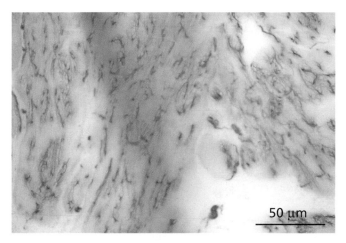

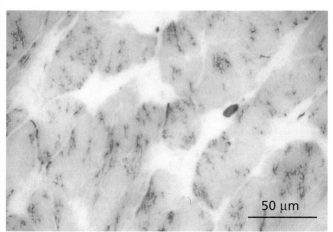

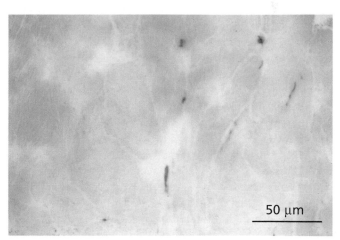

Fig. 33.9 Light micrographs from obstructed guinea pig detrusor stained for acetylcholinesterase, which is present on nerve fibres. Top right, from a normal guinea pig. The other three micrographs are from the bladder of the same guinea pig 10 weeks after a silver ring had been placed around the urethra to create a progressive obstruction. Note some degree of denervation in all the micrographs, but almost complete denervation of some muscle bundles. Scale bar, 150 μm. (Reproduced from [62].)

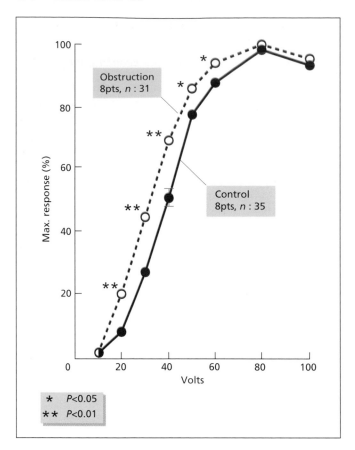

Fig. 33.10 Response of strips of human detrusor to direct activation of the smooth muscle cells with single shocks (100 ms) in the presence of tetrodotoxin to block nerve impulses. Note the increased sensitivity of muscle from obstructed bladders. (Reproduced from [32].)

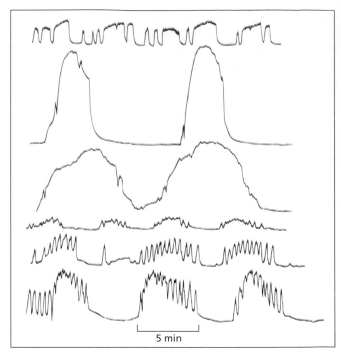

Fig. 33.11 Spontaneous activity recorded from strips of detrusor taken from pigs with outflow obstruction. Note the irregular and fused contractions. Scale bar, 5 min.

Normally, spontaneous contractions rise from the baseline and fall back to it. Only a minority of strips from normal human bladder show spontaneous activity. There is little evidence of fused tetanic contractions, and little basal tone. Strips from unstable bladder show a greater tendency for spontaneous mechanical activity and this is of a more irregular pattern, often with fused tetanic contractions, and elevated baseline tone (Fig. 33.11). It is probable that this is a manifestation of more synchronous behaviour of the smooth muscle cells. There is evidence in the pig [15] that electrical continuity between the cells is increased in the unstable bladder, which could account for the increased synchronous activity. Increased electrical connectivity has been seen in other smooth muscles, both associated with increased luminal distension (pregnant uterus [70], obstructed gut [71]) and denervation (vas deferens [72]). Denervation has also been shown to cause depolarization of smooth muscle, which might account for the increased sensitivity to depolarizing agents in muscle from unstable bladders [73].

Contractility

Although there is clear hypertrophy of the detrusor with prolonged outflow obstruction, the maximum contractile force produced by detrusor strips from experimentally obstructed bladders does not usually increase. The response varies depending on the duration and severity of the obstruction and the species. Most commonly the force per unit weight of tissue is less than in normal strips, which is consistent with the observation of increased connective tissue content.

Cause of bladder instability

The hypothesis has been put forward [74] that denervation is a necessary prerequisite for the development of bladder instability. It has been suggested that the smooth muscle response to denervation (i.e. increased excitability and electrical conductivity) is what allows small focuses of activity to spread into a synchronous contraction of the bladder wall, leading to a rise in intravesical pressure. Experimental functional denervation of the bladder in the pig by bladder transection also leads to bladder instability [75], and denervation has been seen in unstable bladders from neuropathic patients [76]. In these cases there is no physical outflow obstruction and the bladder is not hypertrophied. Hypertrophy seems to be a response to increased contractile demand on the bladder wall and can be induced by forced diuresis (sucrose feeding or untreated diabetes). It is therefore unlikely that hypertrophy and instability are directly related. On the other hand, there does seem to be a relationship between outflow obstruction and denervation, the obstruction being causative. It is possible that the important factor is the prolonged increased intravesical pressure during micturition. This could cause periodic ischaemic episodes in the detrusor, which might damage the intramural ganglion cells. It is interesting to note that the rat is the only animal in which obstruction is not associated with denervation, and it is also the only model in which there are no ganglion cells in the bladder wall [61].

Cause of frequency and urgency

Frequency and urgency are symptoms associated with outflow obstruction and it is interesting to speculate why this might be so. Frequency could be due to the drop in contractility of the bladder wall leading to incomplete emptying, or to the unstable contractions triggering a micturition reflex. With respect to urgency, it is known from urodynamic investigations that urgency is not necessarily associated with any increase in bladder pressure, nor does the pressure generated during micturition cause urgency, nor indeed do the spontaneous pressure rises that occur in the unstable bladder necessarily trigger urgency.

A recent hypothesis about urgency proposed by Coolsaet et al. [77] is that it may result from asynchronous activity in the bladder wall, where contraction of some parts will lead to stretching of adjacent areas. It has been shown that the bladder contains sensory nerves that respond to rapid stretching [78] as well as fibres that fire progressively during the filling of the bladder. During normal filling, the degree of excitation of the bladder muscle may increase [79], either through the direct effects of stretch, or through increasing activity of motor nerves. If this increased level of excitation does not result in asynchronous activation, then the sensory fibres activated by bladder filling may trigger the sensation of fullness, but if asynchronous contraction of parts of the wall occur, this may cause rapid stretch of adjacent areas and trigger urgency by activation of the sensory fibres responding to rapid stretch. Activity affecting the whole wall as triggered during the micturition reflex will result in synchronous activation and a rise in pressure, but will not trigger the rapid stretch receptors, and will relieve urgency. The increased electrical conductivity of the unstable bladder will clearly predispose it to significant contractions of parts of the bladder, and increase urgency. The clinical observation that anti-muscarinic drugs can decrease urgency and frequency suggests that the increased excitability of the bladder

during filling is caused to some extent by increasing activity in the motor nerves.

Conclusion

Although there may be many causes of bladder outflow obstruction, it seems clear that the rise in intravesical pressure that results leads in some way to changes in the bladder wall, regardless of the causes of the obstruction. These changes can add to the comparatively trivial symptom of a poor stream, the more distressing ones that develop with detrusor instability, urgency and urge incontinence. It is possible that some of the changes in the bladder muscle are irreversible and this may be of considerable clinical importance when considering benign prostatic hyperplasia, since there is no consensus of opinion on the correct timing for operation. Many patients may still have their operation deferred for long periods while on the waiting list for admission to hospital. It is important to know if such delays increase the likelihood of persistent instability after the relief of the obstruction. If particular changes could be identified on simple day-case biopsy then prioritization for transurethral resection of the prostate would be appropriate.

References

1 Guthrie GJ. *On the Anatomy and Diseases of the Urinary and Sexual Organs.* London: Churchill, 1836:181.
2 Budge. In: *Henle's Zeitschrift fur rat. Med.*, Vol. xxi. 1864:174.
3 Griffiths J. Observations on the urinary bladder and urethra. *J Anat Physiol* 1891;**25**:535–49.
4 Elliot TR. The innervation of the bladder and urethra. *J Physiol* 1907;**35**:367–45.
5 Barrington FJF. The relation of the hindbrain to micturition. *Brain* 1921;**44**:23–53.
6 Barrington FJF. The component reflexes of micturition in the cat. *Brain* 1931;**54**:177–88.
7 Dubois P. Uber den Druck in der Harnblase. *Dtsch Arch Klin Med* 1876;**17**:148–63.
8 Rehfisch M. Uber den mechanisms des Harnblasenveer-schlusses und der Harnentleerunh. *Virchows Arch [A]* 1987; **150**:111.
9 Denny-Brown D, Robertson EG. On the physiology of micturition. *Brain* 1933;**56**:149–90.
10 von Garrelts B. Analysis of micturition—a new method of recording the voiding of the bladder. *Acta Chir Scand* 1956;**112**:326–40.
11 Griffiths DJ. Effects of bladder outlet obstruction. *Prospectives* 1992;**2**:1–4.
12 Uvelius B, Gabella G. Relation between cell length and force production urinary bladder smooth muscle. *Acta Physiol Scand* 1980;**110**:357–65.
13 Brading AF. Physiology of bladder smooth muscle. In: Torrens MJ, Morrison JFB, eds. *The Physiology of the Lower Urinary Tract.* New York: Springer Verlag, 1987:161–91.
14 Callahan SM, Creed KE. Electrical and mechanical activity of

the isolated lower urinary tract of the guinea-pig. *Br J Pharmacol* 1981;**74**:353–8.

15 Fujii K. Electrophysiological evidence that adenosine triphosphate (ATP) is a co-transmitter with acetylcholine (ACh) in isolated guinea-pig rabbit and pig urinary bladder. *J Physiol* 1987;**394**:26.

16 Eaton AC, Bates CP. An *in-vitro* study of normal and unstable human detrusor muscle. *Br J Urol* 1982;**54**:653–7.

17 Crowe R, Burnstock G. A histochemical and immuno-histochemical study of the autonomic innervation of the lower urinary tract of the female pig. Is the pig a good model for the human bladder and urethra? *J Urol* 1989;**141**:414–22.

18 Morrison JFB. Reflex control of the lower urinary tract. In: Torrens M, Morrison JFB, eds. *The Physiology of the Lower Urinary Tract*. New York: Springer Verlag, 1987:193–236.

19 Morrison JFB. The functions of efferent nerves to the lower urinary tract. In: Torrens M, Morrison JFB, eds. *The Physiology of the Lower Urinary Tract*. New York: Springer Verlag, 1987:133–60.

20 Klevmark B. Motility of the urinary bladder in cats during filling at physiological rates. (ii) Effects of extrinsic bladder denervation on intramural tension and on intravesical pressure. *Acta Physiol Scand* 1977;**101**:176–84.

21 Coolsaet BLRA. Bladder compliance and detrusor activity during the collection phase. *Neurourol Urodyn* 1985;**4**:263–73.

22 Webb RJ, Griffiths CJ, Ramsden PD, Neal DE. Measurement of voiding pressures on ambulatory monitoring: comparison with conventional cystometry. *Br J Urol* 1989; **65**:152–4.

23 Stott MA. *Compliance in the neuropathic bladder*. MD thesis, University of Bristol, 1990.

24 Sethia KK. *The pathophysiology of detrusor instability*. DM thesis, University of Oxford, 1988.

25 Wellner MC, Isenberg G. Stretch-effects on whole-cell currents of guinea-pig urinary bladder myocytes. *J Physiol* 1994;**480**:439–48.

26 Fowler CJ, Fowler C. Clinical neurophysiology. In: Torrens M, Morrison JFB, eds. *The Physiology of the Lower Urinary Tract*. New York: Springer Verlag, 1987:309–32.

27 Bo K, Stien R. Needle EMG registration of striated urethral wall and pelvic floor muscle activity patterns during cough, Valsalva, abdominal, hip adductor, and gluteal muscle contractions in nulliparous healthy females. *Neurourol Urodyn* 1994;**13**:35–42.

28 Macneil HF, Turner WH, Brading AF. The physiology of the pig urinary sphincter. *Neurourol Urodyn* 1991;**10**:351–2.

29 Bridgewater M, Macneil HF, Brading AF. Regulation of tone in pig urethral smooth muscle. *J Urol* 1993;**150**:223–8.

30 Sibley GNA. A comparison of spontaneous and nerve-mediated activity in bladder muscle from man, pig and rabbit. *J Physiol* 1984;**354**:431–43.

31 Speakman MJ. *Studies on the physiology of the normal and obstructed bladder*. MS thesis, London University, 1988.

32. Sibley GNA. *The response of the bladder to lower urinary tract obstruction*. Thesis, University of Oxford, Oxford, 1984.

33 Inoue R, Brading AF. Human pig and guinea-pig bladder smooth muscle cells generate similar inward currents in response to purinoceptor activation. *Br J Pharmacol* 1991;**103**:1840–1.

34 Nielsen KK, Nordling J, Hald T. Critical review of the diagnosis of prostatic obstruction. *Neurourol Urodyn* 1994;**13**:201–17.

35 Abrams PH, Griffiths DJ. The assessment of prostatic obstruction from urodynamic measurements and from residual urine. *Br J Urol* 1979;**51**:129–34.

36 Abrams PH. The urodynamic changes following prostatectomy. *Urol Int* 1978;**33**:181–6.

37 Andersen JT. Prostatism III. Detrusor hyperreflexia and residual urine. Clinical and urodynamic aspects and the influence of surgery on the prostate. *Scand J Urol Nephrol* 1982;**16**: 25–30.

38 Frimodt Moller PC, Jensen KM-E, Iversen P, Madsen PO, Bruskewitz RC. Analysis of presenting symptoms in prostatism. *J Urol* 1984;**132**:272–6.

39 Speakman MJ, Sethia KK, Fellows GJ, Smith JC. A study of the pathogenesis urodynamic assessment and outcome of detrusor instability associated with bladder outflow obstruction. *Br J Urol* 1987;**59**:40–4.

40 Elbadawi A, Yalla SV, Resnick NM. Structural basis of geriatric voiding dysfunction. I. Methods of prospective ultrastructural/ urodynamic study and overview of findings. *J Urol* 1993;**150**: 1650–6.

41 Elbadawi A, Yalla SV, Resnick NM. Structural basis of geriatric voiding dysfunction. II. Aging detrusor: normal versus impaired contractility. *J Urol* 1993;**150**:1657–67.

42 Elbadawi A, Yalla SV, Resnick NM. Structural basis of geriatric voiding dysfunction. III. Detrusor overactivity. *J Urol* 1993;**150**:1668–80.

43 Elbadawi A, Yalla SV, Resnick NM. Structural basis of geriatric voiding dysfunction. IV. Bladder outlet obstruction. *J Urol* 1993;**150**:1681–95.

44 Gilpin SA, Gilpin CJ, Dixon JS, Gosling JA, Kirby RS. The effect of age on the autonomic innervation of the urinary bladder. *Br J Urol* 1986;**58**:378–81.

45 Abrams PH, Farrar DJ, Turner-Warwick R, Whiteside CG, Feneley RCL. The results of prostatectomy: a symptomatic and urodynamic analysis of 152 patients. *J Urol* 1979;**121**:640–2.

46 Andersen JT. Detrusor hyperreflexia in benign infravesical obstruction. A cystometric study. *J Urol* 1976;**115**:532–4.

47 Ball AJ, Feneley RCL, Abrams PH. The natural history of untreated prostatism. *Br J Urol* 1981;**53**:613–16.

48 Claridge M, Shuttleworth KED. The dynamics of obstructed micturition. *Invest Urol* 1964;**2**:188–99.

49 Speakman MJ, Brading AF, Gilpin CJ *et al.* Bladder outflow obstruction—a cause of denervation supersensitivity. *J Urol* 1987;**138**:1461–6.

50 Abrams PH, Feneley RCL. The significance of the symptoms associated with bladder outflow obstruction. *Urol Int* 1978;**33**: 171–4.

51 Bates CP. Continence and incontinence. A clinical study of the dynamics of voiding and of the sphincter mechanism. *Ann R Coll Surg* 1971;**49**:18–35.

52 Bates CP. *Continence and incontinence*. MD Thesis, University of Oxford, 1973.

53 Turner-Warwick R, Whiteside CG, Worth PHL, Milroy EJG, Bates CP. A urodynamic view of clinical problems associated with bladder neck dysfunction and its treatment by endoscopic incision and trans-trigonal posterior prostatectomy. *Br J Urol* 1973;**45**:44–59.

54 Abrams PH. The pathophysiology of male bladder outflow obstruction. In: Whitfield HN, Hendry WF, eds. *Textbook of Genito-urinary Surgery*. Edinburgh: Churchill Livingstone, 1985:370–84.

55 Abrams PH. *The investigation of bladder outflow obstruction in the male*. DM Thesis, University of Bristol, 1977.

56 Andersen JT, Jacobsen O, Warn-Petersen J, Hald T. Bladder

function in healthy elderly males. *Scand J Urol Nephrol* 1978;**12**:123–7.

57 Abrams PH. Detrusor instability and bladder outlet obstruction. *Neurourol Urodynam* 1985;**4**:317–28.

58 Gilpin SA, Gosling JA, Barnard RJ. Morphological and morphometric studies of the human obstructed, trabeculated urinary bladder. *Br J Urol* 1985;**57**:525–9.

59 Dixon JS, Gilpin CJ, Gilpin SA *et al*. Sequential morphological changes in the pig detrusor in response to chronic partial urethral obstruction. *Br J Urol* 1989;**64**:385–90.

60 Elbadawi A, Meyer S, Malkowicz SB *et al*. Effects of short-term partial bladder outlet obstruction on the rabbit detrusor: an ultrastructural study. *Neurourol Urodyn* 1989;**8**:89–116.

61 Gabella G, Uvelius B. Urinary bladder of rat: fine structure of normal and hypertonic musculature. *Cell Tissue Res* 1990;**262**: 67–9.

62 Williams JH, Turner WH, Sainsbury GM, Brading AF. Experimental model of bladder outflow obstruction in the guinea-pig. *Br J Urol* 1993;**71**:533–54.

63 German K. *Compliance studies in the human neuropathic bladder*. MS thesis, London University, 1994.

64 Macneil HF, Brading AF, Williams JH. Cause of low compliance in a guinea-pig model of instability and low compliance. *Neurourol Urodyn* 1992;**11**:47–52.

65 Gosling JA, Gilpin SA, Dixon JS, Gilpin CJ. Decrease in the autonomic innervation of human detrusor muscle in outflow obstruction. *J Urol* 1986;**136**:501–4.

66 Williams JH. *Physiological and pharmacological studies of bladder outflow obstructidon*. MS thesis, University of Wales, 1992.

67 Sibley GNA, Smith JC. Detrusor instability: an experimental model in the obstructed pig. *Proc Joint International Continence Society Urodynamics Society Meeting*, 1983;**2**: 219–20.

68 Harrison SCW, Ferguson DR, Doyle PT. Effect of bladder outflow obstruction on the innervation of the rabbit urinary bladder. *Br J Urol* 1990;**66**:372–9.

69 Foster CD, Speakman MJ, Fujii K, Brading AF. The effects of cromakalim on the detrusor muscle of human and pig urinary bladder. *Br J Urol* 1989;**63**:284–94.

70 Garfield RE, Merrett D, Grover AK. Gap junction formation and regulation in myometrium. *Am J Physiol* 1980;**239**: C217–28.

71 Bortoff A, Sillin LF. Changes in intracellular electrical coupling of smooth muscle accompanying atrophy and hypertrophy. *Am J Physiol* 1986;**250**:C292–8.

72 Westfall DP, Lee TJ-F, Stitzel RE. Morphological and biochemical changes in supersensitive smooth muscle. *Fed Proc* 1975;**34**:1985–9.

73 Westfall DP. Supersensitivity of smooth muscle. In: Bulbring E, Brading AF, Jones AW, Tomita T, eds. *Smooth Muscle: an Assessment of Current Knowledge*. London: Edward Arnold, 1983:285–309.

74 Brading AF, Turner WH. The unstable bladder: towards a common mechanism. *Br J Urol* 1994;**73**:3–8.

75 Sethia KK, Brading AF, Smith JC. An animal model of non-obstructive instability. *J Urol* 1990;**143**:1243–6.

76 German K, Bedwani J, Davies J, Brading A, Stephenson TP. What is the pathophysiology of detrusor hyperreflexia? *Neurourol Urodyn* 1993;**12**:335–6.

77 Coolsaet BLRA, Van Duyl WA, Van Os-Bossagh P, De Bakker HV. New concepts in relation to urge and detrusor activity. *Neurourol Urodyn* 1993;**12**:463–72.

78 Iggo A. Tension receptors in the stomach and the urinary bladder. *J Physiol* 1955;**128**:593–607.

79 Van Duyl WA. Spontaneous contractions in urinary bladder smooth muscle preliminary results. *Neurol Urodyn* 1985; **4**:301–7.

Clinical Evaluation of Bladder Outflow Obstruction

J. Reynard and P. Abrams

Introduction

Bladder outflow obstruction (BOO) is a frequently encountered problem in clinical urological practice. It is most commonly due to prostatic enlargement secondary to benign prostatic hyperplasia (BPH). Outflow obstruction is thought to be central to the pathophysiology of BPH. Indeed, Lepor has stated [1] that 'the clinical manifestations of BPH are related entirely to BOO'. The majority of treatments for BPH are designed to relieve BOO and included among the American Urological Association (AUA) list of indications for transurethral resection of the prostate (TURP) is 'intractable symptoms due to prostatic obstruction' [2]. Other causes of BOO include prostate cancer, urethral stricture and dyssynergic bladder neck obstruction. This chapter will concentrate on the evaluation of BOO secondary to BPH, but will also discuss the assessment of these other conditions. The clinical evaluation of BOO is based on an assessment of symptoms, physical examination and urodynamic investigation.

Symptom assessment

Symptoms play a major role in the clinical evaluation of BOO. Patients present with symptoms and are concerned with their resolution. For most urologists, an analysis of presenting symptoms is the mainstay by which a presumptive diagnosis of BOO is made. The nature and severity of symptoms remains the major criteria by which a decision is reached to recommend treatment designed specifically to relieve BOO. Furthermore, the relief of symptoms is the main way in which the efficacy of therapy for BPH and other causes of BOO is judged, irrespective of whether that therapy results in improvement in urinary flow rate or in pressure–flow relationships.

Traditionally, the symptoms of BPH are divided into obstructive and irritative types. The obstructive symptoms are thought to arise as a direct consequence of obstruction to the prostatic urethra and include reduced flow, hesitancy, intermittency, straining, terminal dribbling and feeling of incomplete bladder emptying. The irritative symptoms of frequency, nocturia, urgency and urge incontinence are believed to result from detrusor instability which is thought to arise secondary to BOO. In the case of urethral stricture, a marked reduction of flow is often the dominant symptom. Dyssynergic bladder neck obstruction characteristically occurs in a younger age group than that of BPH, and the patient often a gives a long history of symptoms [3].

In recent years a number of symptom scores have been designed to assist in the assessment of men with BPH. Boyarsky et al. [4] developed the first such score and this was followed by that of Madsen and Iversen [5], Fowler et al. [6], Hald et al. (the Danish score) [7] and the AUA symptom score [8]. The AUA and Danish scores [9] have been validated by formal psychometric testing. The contents of each of these scores is shown in Table 34.1. There is clearly considerable variability in the symptoms which have been selected for each system. More recently the International Continence Society (ICS) has carried out a study to assess the relationship between lower urinary tract symptoms and BOO and this has led to the development of the ICS male questionnaire which includes 20 questions covering a broad range of urinary symptoms [10]. Though a formal ICS symptom score has not as yet been developed, the questionnaire has also been validated by formal psychometric testing.

The AUA symptom score has been adopted by the World Health Organization as the international prostate symptom score or IPSS [11]. The AUA and Danish scores include a bother factor which allows a measure of the degree to which the symptoms influence quality of life. Symptom scores introduce the concept of quantification of symptoms and allow accurate documentation of the presenting complaints, both features being important as a means of expressing change after treatment for BPH. Of the AUA score it has been said that it 'powerfully discriminates between BPH and control subjects' [8] and the Danish score is said to 'assist in creating a solid base for the indication for ... treatment of BPH' [7]. At the International

Table 34.1 Symptoms included in current symptom scores for BPH.

	Boyarsky *et al.* score [4]	Madsen–Iversen score [5]	Fowler *et al.* [6]	Danish [7]	AUA [8]
Hesitancy	0–3	0 or 3		0–3	
Poor flow	0–3	0–4		0–3	0–5
Intermittency	0–3	0 or 3	1–5		0–5
Straining		0 or 2	1–5	0–3	0–5
Terminal dribble	0–3				
Incomplete emptying	0–3	0–4		0–3	0–5
Frequency	0–3	0–3	1–5	0–3	0–5
Nocturia	0–3	0–3		0–3	0–5
Urgency	0–3	0–3		0–3	0–5
Dysuria	0–3		1–5	0–3	
Incontinence		0 or 2			
Post-micturition dribble			1–5		0–5
Stress incontinence				0–3	
Incontinence not on activity or urge				0–3	

Consultation on BPH in Monaco in 1995 [11], it was recommended that the IPSS be used as part of the basic evaluation of all patients with prostatism.

The traditional concept of BPH leading to BOO and so causing the symptoms of prostatism has, however, been questioned in recent years. Hald [12] from Copenhagen has summarized the relationship between BPH, BOO and symptoms in his well-known 'rings', emphasizing that some patients have BPH and symptoms but no obstruction (Fig. 34.1). The evidence for the existence of such a population of patients comes from several studies. Castro *et al.* [13] found no correlation between symptom severity on total symptom score and urethral resistance, expressed as P_{ves}/Q_{max}^2 where P_{ves} is intravesical pressure and Q_{max} is maximum flow rate. Abrams and Feneley [14] found that 33% of men with prostatism did not have BOO on pressure–flow studies. Similarly, Andersen *et al.* [15] observed that symptoms were not significantly associated with increased bladder outflow resistance. These findings have been confirmed by several other studies, which have shown that approximately 25% of men with prostatism who are admitted for prostatectomy, do not have BOO [16–19]. There are several different methods by which BOO can be defined (see pressure–flow studies), and it could be argued that the lack of correlation between symptoms and BOO is simply due to a lack of consensus regarding which definition of BOO should be adopted. This would not, however, appear to be the case. Whatever technique is used for defining BOO, be this the Schafer nomogram [20,21], the group specific urethral resistance factor (URA) [22], micturition pressure profilometry [23] or the Abrams-Griffiths nomogram (J. Reynard and P. Abrams, personal communication), symptom scores are not correlated to the presence or severity of obstruction. Most studies that have considered the irritative symptoms of prostatism have reported a better correlation between these symptoms and the presence of detrusor instability [13–15]. Neal *et al.* [24] also found that irritative symptoms were associated with elevated detrusor pressure at maximum flow, as well as with detrusor instability.

The lack of specificity between symptoms and BOO is further emphasized by the presence of both irritative *and* so-called obstructive symptoms in women. A recent study

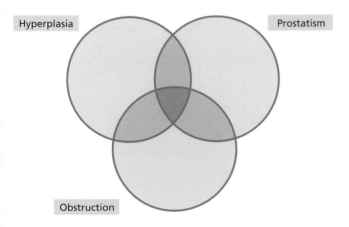

Fig. 34.1 Hald 'rings' showing the relationship between BPH, symptoms of prostatism and bladder outflow obstruction.

[25] has shown that women with no urodynamic evidence of BOO complained of similar symptoms to those reported by men, whose symptoms were supposedly due to BOO secondary to BPH. However, in an unselected group of elderly men and women, Chai *et al.* [26] did find a significantly higher mean obstructive score in men compared with women. This study also found weak stream and straining to be significantly more common complaints of men than women, but all other urinary symptoms occurred with similar frequency in the two sexes.

Studying the relationship between individual symptoms and BOO, Abrams and Feneley [14] found that hesitancy was significantly associated with the presence of BOO. In this study, 77% of men with high urethral resistance had hesitancy, whereas only 42% of men with low urethral resistance complained of hesitancy. Furthermore, this study found that a complaint of poor flow was also significantly associated with the presence of BOO, poor flow being reported by 80% of men with high urethral resistance, but by only 60% of men with low urethral resistance. Conversely, Andersen *et al.* [15] could find no correlation between a complaint of poor flow and increased urethral resistance.

Relatively little work has been carried out on the specificity or positive predictive value, with regard to BOO, of the other 'obstructive' symptoms of prostatism. Reynard *et al.* [27] and van Venrooij *et al.* [21] found that the symptom of intermittency, which is included in the Madsen–Iversen, Fowler and AUA symptom scores, was not specific for BOO defined both by the Abrams–Griffiths nomogram and URA. The inclusion of straining as a symptom of BPH seems to derive from the work of Susset *et al.* [28] who concluded that 'patients with obstructive disease ... usually required the added pressure provided by straining'. However, Reynard *et al.* [29] also found that there was no significant difference in the proportion of men complaining of straining among those with obstruction and those without obstruction. There was no significant difference in the frequency of straining (as measured by rectal catheter during free flow studies) in men with and

without BOO. Furthermore, there was poor agreement between the symptom of straining and objective evidence of its presence during voiding. From this study, it was concluded that straining was not a reliable symptom of BOO. Few attempts have been made to explore the relationship between the feeling of incomplete bladder emptying and BOO, despite its inclusion in all symptom scores for BPH apart from that of Fowler *et al.* [6]. Both Andersen *et al.* [15] and vanVenrooij *et al.* [21] were unable to demonstrate a relationship between a complaint of incomplete bladder emptying and BOO. With regard to terminal dribbling, Reynard *et al.* [30] found no correlation between this symptom and the presence of outflow obstruction.

As symptoms are of major importance in the evaluation of suspected BOO and they form the basis upon which a decision to offer treatment is made, it is important to know how effective treatment for BOO is in relieving these symptoms. If a symptom was 100% specific for BOO, then effective relief of obstruction would be expected to lead to resolution of the symptom in all cases. Conversely, one would be more cautious in diagnosing BOO on the basis of a symptom which failed to resolve in a high proportion of men after relief of obstruction by prostatectomy. Table 34.2 shows the effect of prostatectomy on a variety of symptoms commonly associated with BPH. The chance of improvement of hesitancy and poor flow is good, 80% of men reporting resolution of these symptoms after prostatectomy. As stated above, there is evidence of an association between these symptoms and BOO. However, prostatectomy has a less favourable effect on the symptoms of urgency, nocturia and frequency and this is consistent with the fact that there is no association between these symptoms and BOO. Clearly, no diagnostic tool is 100% specific or sensitive and one would not expect this to be the case with symptoms and symptom scores. The urologist should be aware of the poor specificity of symptoms as diagnostic tools. Nonetheless, since symptoms are an integral part of the assessment of BOO and are used as indications for obstruction-relieving surgery, only those

Table 34.2 Symptom relief after prostatectomy. Figures represent the percentage of patients complaining of a symptom before prostatectomy who had persistence of this symptom after surgery*.

	Persistence of symptom (%)		
	Abrams *et al.* [31]	Neal *et al.* [32]	Doll *et al.* [33]
Poor flow	9	22	15
Hesitancy	12	16	11
Dribbling	—	50	27
Frequency	31	—	24
Nocturia	44	33	20
Urgency	40	46	—
Urge incontinence	36	33	—

* Length of follow-up: Abrams *et al.* [31], 'at least 4 months'; Neal *et al* [32], mean 11 months; Doll *et al* [33], mean 12 months.

symptoms with a close correlation to BOO should be used to assist in the diagnosis of this condition because men without BOO are less likely to experience resolution of their symptoms after TURP [34].

Given the poor association between many symptoms of prostatism and BOO, and the fact that no symptom scores have been urodynamically validated, the value of currently available symptom scores for the diagnosis of BOO secondary to BPH must also be questioned. The symptoms included in these scores are not necessarily the most important in terms of BOO and the methods used in their construction is questionable. For example, the AUA score was based on data from men with 'clinically defined BPH' although 'no standard diagnostic evaluation was imposed' [8]. Similarly, the Danish score was constructed on the basis of the 'known symptoms of BPH' [7] and that of Madsen and Iversen from the symptoms 'widely accepted as frequent complaints in patients with BPH' [5]. Such selection criteria are somewhat arbitrary. Furthermore, in the symptom score of Madsen and Iversen, some symptoms are allotted greater importance than others. These so-called weighted symptoms include hesitancy, intermittency, straining and incontinence. Although the weighting of symptoms is likely to be a valid principle as not all symptoms are likely to be equally important, there is no evidence that those selected by Madsen and Iversen are more significant in terms of the pathophysiology of BPH than the non-weighted symptoms.

It is now generally accepted that there is no correlation between the presence or severity of outflow obstruction and symptoms [20,21,23], and that symptom scores have no diagnostic value with regard to specific pathophysiological conditions of the lower urinary tract. For this reason Abrams [35] has recently argued that we should move away from the use of such terms as 'prostatism', which imply a specific pathophysiological basis for particular groups of symptoms, towards the use of a less specific term such as 'lower urinary tract symptoms'. Having been somewhat negative about the diagnostic capabilities of symptoms and symptom scores it is none the less important to appreciate that they have an important role both in defining and quantifying symptom severity, and this has been particularly important in the assessment of the new treatment modalities for prostatic outflow obstruction.

In summary, the nature of presenting symptoms in BPH is of some prognostic value with regard to the outcome of prostatectomy. The variable outcome in relation to individual symptoms is probably at least partly explained by the variable relationship between symptoms and BOO. Some symptoms are only weakly associated with BOO and it is therefore hardly surprising that they fail to improve after surgery designed specifically to relieve obstruction. A clear distinction must be drawn between BPH as a histological process causing prostatic enlargement and the pathophysiological mechanism by which it causes symptoms. It is quite possible that this mechanism is not solely related to BOO, and it is likely that in a proportion of patients BPH is an associated rather than a causative factor with regard to their symptoms. Better understanding of the pathophysiology of lower urinary tract symptoms and in particular of their relationship to BOO, will hopefully improve our ability to diagnose BOO and allow a more selective approach to the treatment of BPH.

Physical examination

Physical examination yields relatively limited information in the evaluation of BOO, but nonetheless it is important since abnormalities either due to, or causing, outflow obstruction may be detected. Thus, the bladder is often easily palpated in high-pressure chronic retention [36] and although phimosis and meatal stenosis are rare causes of BOO in the adult male, the external genitalia should not be overlooked. On rectal examination, the finding of a hard, nodular prostate is suggestive of prostatic carcinoma which may well cause outflow obstruction.

The assessment of prostatic size by digital rectal examination is, in the outpatient setting, inaccurate [37] and, because prostatic size is traditionally thought not to be related to symptom severity or the degree of BOO, little attention has been paid to prostate volume estimation in the evaluation of BOO. However, prostatic size assessed by examination under anaesthesia and cystourethroscopy is correlated to urodynamic parameters of BOO [13,38]. Furthermore, a recent study [39] using transrectal ultrasound (TRUS) to measure prostatic volume, has found that total prostate volume and in particular the volume of the central part of the prostate (Fig. 34.2) are correlated to the presence of BOO. In this study, men with BOO defined on the basis of the Abrams–Griffiths nomogram [40] had significantly larger total gland volumes than those with equivocal or no obstruction (median 45 vs 34 ml). The difference between central zone volumes (the central zone representing the volume of hyperplastic tissue in BPH [41]) in men with BOO (median 32 ml) compared to those with equivocal or no obstruction (median 13 ml) was even more marked. Although Bosch et al. [42] found only weak correlations between total gland volume and various parameters of BOO, Kaplan et al. [43] have confirmed the association between transition zone volume and detrusor pressure at peak flow. These findings may have important implications. Outcome after prostatectomy is more likely to be favourable in men with urodynamically proven BOO [19,32,44]; because central zone volume and BOO are closely correlated, the volume of this part of the prostate volume may also be of prognostic value. At least one study has reported better outcome in men with larger total prostatic volumes [32] but the relationship between zonal

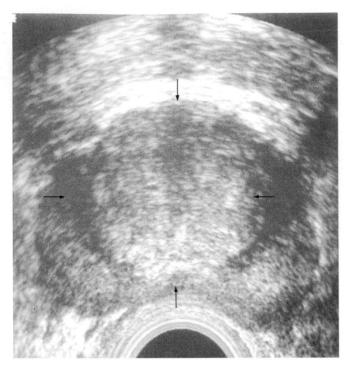

Fig. 34.2 Transrectal ultrasound of prostate showing clearly defined 'central zone' of prostate (arrows), representing the volume of hyperplastic tissue.

volumes and outcome of TURP has not as yet been explored. The advent of TRUS has improved both the accuracy and ease of measuring prostatic volume. As Kaplan *et al.* have stated [43], the estimation of prostatic size or zonal volume may serve as a useful proxy for evaluating worsening obstruction.

Urodynamic investigation

Urodynamic studies have come to occupy an increasingly important place in the assessment of suspected BOO. They are functional tests of the lower urinary tract and describe micturition in terms of several basic mechanical measurements, i.e. pressure, flow and voided volume.

Urodynamic studies may be classified into three groups of increasing complexity: uroflowmetry, pressure–flow studies and complex urodynamics.

Uroflowmetry

The recording of free flow rate was actually preceded by techniques that measured bladder pressure during voiding. In 1882 Mosso and Pellacani [46] described 'Le Pletismographe', a device which measured bladder pressure throughout the course of micturition. In 1897 Rehfisch [47] described a technique by which voided volume, measured by air displacement, could be plotted against time, although he did not measure flow rate. However, Drake [48] was responsible for the development of the first uroflowmeter, allowing urine flow rate to be simultaneously plotted against time. von Garrelts [49] introduced electronic recording of the flow rate, making such measurements easy, accurate and reproducible. von Garrelts proceeded to describe the pattern of urinary flow in normal people and in those with disorders of the prostate and with urethral strictures. Modern flowmeters are direct descendants of those developed by von Garrelts. They are now computerized so that a print-out of a variety of voiding parameters is given including maximum and average flow rate, voided volume and voiding times. None the less, computerized flowmeters are subject to artefacts (Fig. 34.3) which the computer may fail to recognize. In a review of over 20 000 flow traces comparing manual reading of flow variables with the computerized read-out from the flowmeter, Grino *et al.* [50] found a difference of more than 3 ml/s in 9% of traces. Thus, visual inspection of the flow curve trace to identify artefacts remains an important part of the interpretation of data from this test.

Voided volume is also thought to be important in the interpretation of the data from such studies. It is generally held that flow studies of voided volume below 150 ml are not interpretable although the basis for this is obscure. Reynard and Abrams [45] have analysed the predictive value of Q_{max} for BOO for both low and high volume voids. Their results suggest that low volume uroflowmetry (less

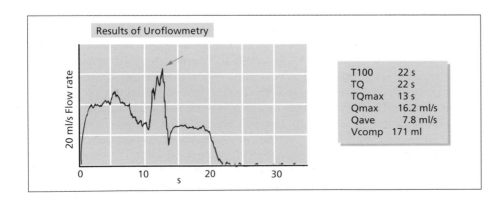

T100	22 s
TQ	22 s
TQmax	13 s
Qmax	16.2 ml/s
Qave	7.8 ml/s
Vcomp	171 ml

Fig. 34.3 Flow rate tracing with 'wag' artefact (arrow) due to patient voiding directly into centre of flowmeter during the course of flow.

than 150 ml) provides equivalent information, when compared with high volume flows, with regard to the diagnosis of BOO.

The most useful parameter of lower urinary tract function measured by uroflowmetry is Q_{max}. Q_{max} is dependent on the volume of voided urine. Since the relationship between Q_{max} and voided volume is non-linear, it is difficult to define a minimum 'normal' flow rate. Thus, a variety of nomograms plotting Q_{max} against voided volume have been developed. Different populations of men have been used for the development of these nomograms. The Siroky et al. nomogram [52] was constructed from flow measurements in normal (asymptomatic) men below the age of 50 years. Two Liverpool nomograms have been developed, one for normal men below the age of 50 and one for men aged 50 years and over [53]. By using the Liverpool nomograms it is thus possible to make some allowance for the deterioration of flow that is regarded as a normal phenomenon of ageing. The Bristol nomogram [54] (Fig. 34.4) and that of Jorgensen et al. [55] were based on flow recordings in asymptomatic men aged more than 50 years. With these nomograms a patient's flow rate can be related to a normal reference range.

A number of studies have assessed the ability of uroflowmetry to differentiate men with BOO from those with no outflow obstruction. Although there is evidence of a correlation between poor urinary flow rate and the presence of BOO [56], a low flow rate is not specific for outflow obstruction. In many series a large percentage of patients have low flows, but no obstruction. Schafer et al. [17] suggested that approximately 25% of men with a low flow rate are not obstructed. Chancellor et al. [57] found that uroflowmetry was unable to distinguish between BOO

and impaired detrusor contractility. Conversely, patients with normal flow rates can have outflow obstruction. Gerstenberg et al. [58] reported that 7% of men with maximum flow rates above 15 ml/s had BOO on pressure–flow studies and the majority benefited both symptomatically and in terms of flow rate improvement following TURP. Iversen et al. [59] also found so-called 'high flow–high pressure' BOO (with Q_{max} more than 15 ml/s) in approximately 25% of patients referred with symptoms of prostatism and similarly these patients benefited from prostatectomy.

There is evidence that multiple free flow studies may improve the ability of uroflowmetry to diagnose BOO [51]. Using a cut-off level for Q_{max} of 10 ml/s (a value below this level indicating the presence of BOO), specificity and positive predictive value of Q_{max} for outlet obstruction were 71 and 79% respectively on void 1, increasing to 96 and 93% respectively on void 4. This study suggests that considerable improvement in specificity and positive predictive value of Q_{max} for BOO can be achieved by performing multiple free flow studies and by carefully selecting an appropriate 'cut-off' level (though whether pressure–flow studies are not necessary will depend on what level of specificity and positive predictive value is deemed acceptable in clinical practice). This could be especially useful for urologists with limited facilities for complex urodynamic studies (i.e. pressure–flow studies).

The pattern of the urinary flow rate curve can in some cases be of diagnostic value. Although low flow is not specific for BOO, a prolonged 'plateau'-type of flow pattern is suggestive of a urethral stricture. Reynard et al. [30] have found that the presence of terminal dribbling on flow traces (Fig. 34.5) had an 88% positive predictive value for the presence of BOO. Intermittency during urinary flow

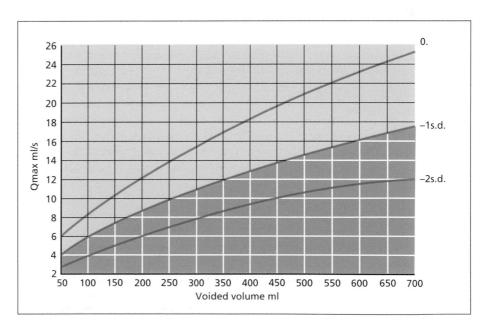

Fig. 34.4 The Bristol nomogram, plotting maximum flow rate against voided volume.

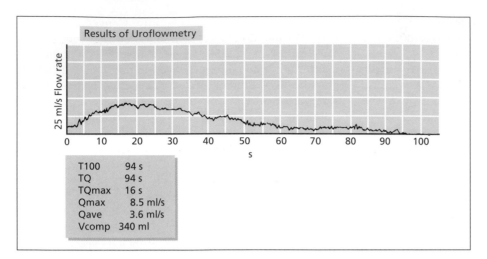

T100	94 s
TQ	94 s
TQmax	16 s
Qmax	8.5 ml/s
Qave	3.6 ml/s
Vcomp	340 ml

Fig. 34.5 Flow rate trace showing terminal dribbling.

(defined as stopping and starting of flow more than once) was also associated with the presence of BOO, having a positive predictive value of 92% for obstruction [27].

The ability of uroflowmetry to predict the outcome of prostatectomy has been the subject of much debate. Abrams [60] demonstrated an improved success rate of prostatectomy when uroflowmetry was used in the preoperative assessment, men with low flow having a greater likelihood of a good outcome. Jensen *et al.* [56] found that 91.5% of patients with a Q_{max} below 15 ml/s had a favourable symptomatic outcome after prostatectomy, compared to 70.5% of men whose preoperative flow rate was above 15 ml/s. Some studies, however, have been unable to demonstrate an association between preoperative flow rate and outcome [32,61,62].

Single flow uroflowmetry lacks sufficient sensitivity and specificity to allow a diagnosis of BOO to be made with confidence, and it is unable to predict with accuracy which patients will and will not benefit from surgery. None the less, uroflowmetry provides a visual record of the act of micturition and can provide evidence that an abnormality is present. Multiple free flow studies may improve specificity and predictive value for Q_{max} for BOO.

Pressure–flow studies

Mosso and Pellacani [46] were the first to measure bladder pressure during micturition and demonstrated that the rise in bladder pressure at the onset of micturition was not accompanied by a rise in intra-abdominal pressure. Rehfisch [47] carried out the first pressure–flow studies of voiding. von Garrelts [49] described the technique of pressure–flow studies as we know it today and the basic principles of performing this investigation remain essentially the same. P_{ves} is measured via a urethral or suprapubic catheter. There is no evidence that a fine catheter has a material effect on pressure–flow relationships of the urethra [63]. Indeed Reynard *et al.* [64] have shown that an 8 Ch urethral

catheter does not have an obstructive effect on the male urethra. Given the compressive nature of obstruction in BPH, this is not to be expected [65]. Abdominal pressure (P_{abd}) is usually measured intrarectally. The detrusor pressure (P_{det}) is calculated electronically by subtracting the abdominal pressure from the intravesical pressure (Fig. 34.6). The pressures can be recorded by fluid-filled catheters connected to external pressure transducers, placed at the level of the superior border of the symphysis pubis and zeroed to atmospheric pressure. Catheter-tip transducers can also be employed. They are simple to use, but correct levelling to eliminate gravitational artefacts can be difficult, and checking zero pressure once the catheter is in position is difficult or impossible. Automated, computerized data analysis is available with modern equipment, but it is still important to inspect the pressure–flow curves for the presence of artefacts.

Several studies have addressed the reproducibility of pressure–flow studies. In 12 healthy female volunteers, the coefficient of variation of studies repeated within a 2-month period was 18% for Q_{max} and 24–31% for P_{det} at maximum flow [66]. In patients with BPH there is a very close correlation between studies repeated during the same session [67]. Two studies suggest that though there is intraindividual variability in pressure–flow parameters on repeat studies, this seldom leads to a change in the clinical grade or diagnosis of BOO [64,68]. Thus it would seem that pressure–flow studies are reproducible.

The purpose of pressure–flow studies in men with symptoms of prostatism is to establish the presence or absence of obstruction, grade its severity and provide information about the cause of the obstruction. In order to establish if BOO is present and thus to grade its severity, obstruction must first be defined. Traditionally, outflow obstruction has been defined in terms of urethral resistance and a number of urethral resistance factors have been developed [63,69,70]. These factors were based on the theory that flow through the urethra is determined by the

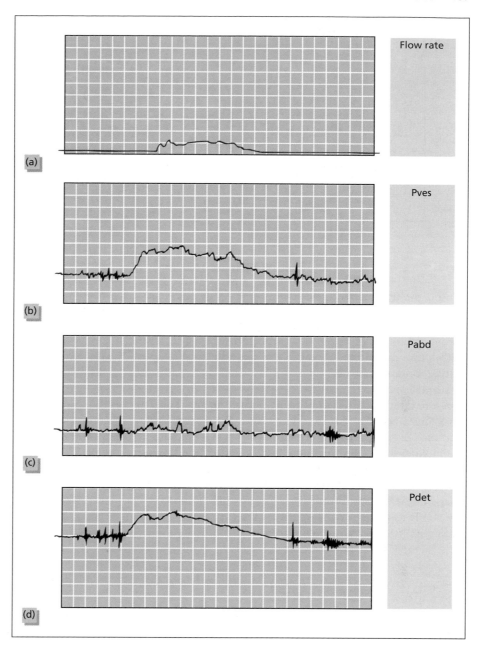

Fig. 34.6 Combined pressure–flow plot of voiding. (a) Q=flow rate; (b) Pves= intravesical pressure; (c) Pabd=abdominal pressure; (d) Pdet=detrusor pressure.

same principles governing flow through rigid tubes. However, current concepts suggest that the bladder outlet behaves as a distensible tube [71,72]. Furthermore, in recent years we have come to appreciate that the pressure source during voiding, the detrusor, is not a passive source of pressure, but rather that it behaves like other contractile tissue [72–74]. The force of contraction (equivalent to P_{det}) and the speed of contraction (equivalent to the flow rate) are inversely related (Fig. 34.7) as determined by the Hill equation [75]. In the case of the bladder, the relationship between these two parameters is known as the bladder output relation (BOR). The pressure developed by the bladder is dependent on both the power of the detrusor and the conditions of the bladder outlet. For given outflow

conditions, the pressure and flow rate increase with increasing detrusor contractile power. For a given detrusor power, a narrow bladder outflow leads to a high detrusor pressure at low flow, and for a wide outflow high flow occurs at low pressure [76]. At zero pressure the flow is limited by the maximum contraction speed of the detrusor. Similarly, when flow is shut off, P_{det} after an initial increase does not continue to rise, but reaches a maximum value determined by the strength of the detrusor.

All current methods of assessing BOO are centred around the relationship between P_{det} and flow during voiding, the so-called urethral resistance relation (URR) which essentially represents the resistance to flow due to the outlet of the bladder. The URR is derived from the simultaneous

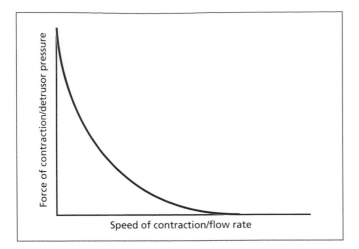

Fig. 34.7 The Hill relationship showing the inverse relationship between the force of contraction of muscle (equivalent to detrusor pressure) and the speed of contraction (equivalent to flow rate).

measurement of P_{det} and flow rate (Fig. 34.8). The URR shows the minimum P_{det} needed to keep the urethra open during voiding, and this pressure is called the minimum urethral opening pressure. However, the minimum pressure often occurs at the end of micturition and the term 'opening pressure' is therefore potentially confusing. Because of this, the International Continence Society standardization committee [77] has called the lowest pressure occurring during actual recorded flow the 'minimum voiding detrusor pressure'. As well as being characterized by a minimum pressure at which flow occurs, the URR can also be described in terms of its slope. Different types of obstruction have characteristic

minimum voiding P_{det} and slopes. In urethral stricture the minimum voiding P_{det} is low, but the slope of the URR is very steep [78] (see Fig. 34.8). This corresponds to a constrictive type of obstruction. In BPH, minimum voiding P_{det} is characteristically elevated and the slope of the URR tends to be less steep. This indicates a compressive type of obstruction [78]. Thus, generally speaking, the URR can be described by two parameters: a minimum voiding pressure and the slope of the curve. By simplifying the URR to a single parameter, the older urethral resistance factors fail to take into account the minimum voiding P_{det} and therefore they do not indicate the general pressure at which voiding takes place. Current methods of describing pressure–flow relationships of the urethra give a more complete picture of pressure and flow during voiding and all are based on the concept that, in terms of flow, the urethra behaves as a distensible tube. There are three such methods: the Abrams–Griffiths nomogram, the URA method and the linear passive URR method.

The Abrams–Griffiths nomogram [40] was the first method to be published. The pressure–flow plot is divided into three regions (Fig. 34.9) representing obstructed outflow conditions, no outflow obstruction and an area between the two in which the patient is said to be equivocally obstructed. Patients who fall within the equivocal area may be more precisely categorized from the minimum voiding P_{det} and the slope of the pressure–flow plot. The patient is said to be unobstructed if the mean slope of the curve is less than $2\,cmH_2O$ per ml/s and the minimum voiding detrusor pressure is less than $40\,cmH_2O$. If the slope of the pressure–flow curve is more than $2\,cmH_2O$ per ml/s or the minimum voiding P_{det} is greater than $40\,cmH_2O$, then the patient is said to be obstructed.

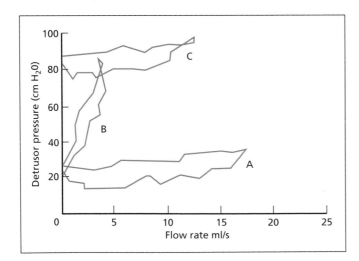

Fig. 34.8 Urethral resistance relation derived from plotting detrusor pressure against simultaneously measured flow rate in A, a normal case; B, a urethral stricture; and C, a man with obstructive BPH.

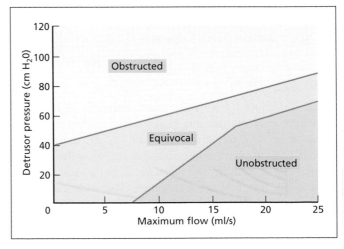

Fig. 34.9 The Abrams–Griffiths nomogram of detrusor pressure at maximum flow plotted against maximum flow. Patients who fall above the upper line are obstructed, those falling between the two lines are described as equivocally obstructed, and those who fall below the lower line are said to be unobstructed.

The two other well-established methods of defining BOO are those of URA [22] and linear passive URR [79]. Both methods also grade the severity of obstruction. In the first method URA, the urethral resistance factor is calculated from the point of intersection of the pressure–flow plot with the pressure axis (Fig. 34.10). URA thus represents the minimum voiding P_{det} and the units of URA are the same as those of pressure (i.e. centimetres of water). Simplification of the pressure–flow plot to a single parameter is justified in this situation because the method was designed specifically to define and grade BOO in a single type of obstruction (so-called 'group specific')—that due to BPH which is known characteristically to be associated with a high minimum voiding P_{det} [79]. By this method, outflow obstruction is defined as a value of URA of 30 cmH$_2$O or above.

Linear passive URR simplifies the pressure–flow plot to a straight line drawn between the two points representing P_{det} at maximum flow and the minimum voiding P_{det} [79]. The pressure–flow diagram is divided into seven bands from 0 to VI, representing increasing severity of obstruction (Fig. 34.11). The pressure–flow plot for an individual patient ideally falls within one of these seven bands, so allowing the severity of obstruction to be categorized. If the line crosses from one band to another, the band containing the maximum flow and pressure gives the best approximation of the degree of BOO. Patients whose pressure–flow plots fall into bands 0 and I are said to be unobstructed and in bands II–VI they are classified as obstructed.

Although each of the three methods divide the pressure–flow curve in similar ways, there are slight differences between the methods and as a consequence not all patients are classified identically. However, it has been shown that 74% of patients with BPH are similarly classified when all three methods are applied to their pressure–flow curves

[80]. Thus, whatever method is employed for defining the presence or absence of obstruction, consistent results can be expected in the majority of cases. This is hardly suprising given the similar theoretical basis of the various methods.

More recently, two other methods of grading the severity of BOO have been developed. An obstruction index (OBI) is a weighted sum of the average height and slope of the passive URR [81]. Detrusor-adjusted mean passive URR (DAMPF) is the pressure where the linear passive URR curve crosses a standardized BOR representing detrusor contractility [82]. It is specifically designed to give a measure of obstruction that is independent of detrusor contractile strength. Both methods can distinguish small differences in the severity of obstruction and thus offer a degree of refinement in the analysis of pressure–flow data. However, neither has as yet been widely used.

Several studies have addressed the ability of pressure–flow studies to predict outcome of TURP and they have reported that the symptomatic outcome of surgery is better in men with urodynamically proven BOO [19,32,44]. In a study of operative outcome in 139 men, Jensen [44] reported a satisfactory symptomatic outcome in 93% of the men with BOO, while only 78% of those in the unobstructed group had a satisfactory outcome. Rollema and van Mastrigt [19] studied outcome in relation to preoperative urodynamic findings in a small study of 29 men. They found that 70% of the unobstructed patients remained symptomatic after TURP, whereas only 20% of the obstructed patients failed to improve symptomatically.

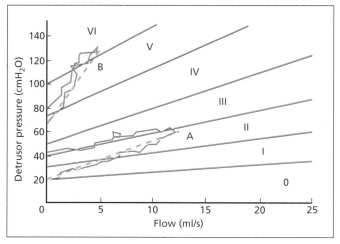

Fig. 34.11 Linearized passive urethral resistance relation, Linear PURR, with the pressure–flow plot divided into seven bands from 0–VI representing increasing severity of obstruction. A straight line is drawn between the two points corresponding to the detrusor pressure at maximum flow and the minimum voiding detrusor pressure. Patient A falls within band II and is thus mildly obstructed. Patient B falls in band VI and is severely obstructed.

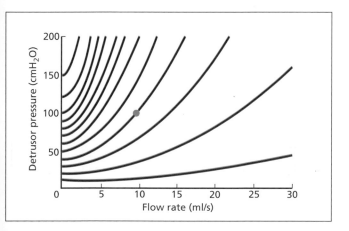

Fig. 34.10 The group specific resistance factor, URA. The red dot represents a point of voiding when the detrusor pressure is 100 cmH$_2$O and the flow rate is 10 ml/s. The value for URA at this point is 40 cmH$_2$O.

In a prospective study of 215 men selected for TURP on the basis of flow rates below 15 ml/s, Neal *et al.* [32] reported poor outcome in 21% of the group with high voiding pressures and in 36% of the group with low pressures. However, as Neal's group has pointed out, most of the patients with low voiding pressures also did well. It would therefore seem that pressure–flow studies are unable to predict outcome in individual cases. Nonetheless, they can provide some prognostic information with regard to outcome of TURP.

Cystometry

Cystometry is the technique by which the pressure–volume relationship of the bladder is measured. It allows the measurement of bladder capacity and bladder compliance. Detrusor overactivity, the presence of involuntary detrusor contractions, may also be seen. Detrusor overactivity is called detrusor instability when there is no apparent neurological cause. Detrusor instability has been reported in approximately 45–75% of men with symptomatic BPH [31,32,83] and there is a weak association between high voiding pressures (suggesting the presence of BOO) and the presence of detrusor instability [24]. However, detrusor instability is also found in healthy elderly males and one study has suggested a prevalence of detrusor instability of 53% in the absence of BOO [84].

There is evidence to suggest that urethral obstruction may be a causative factor in detrusor overactivity. Experimental urethral obstruction in animals has been shown to lead to detrusor overactivity [85]. It has been suggested that this may be due to denervation super-sensitivity secondary to the obstruction [86–88]. Relief of BOO in the pig leads to a reversal of this detrusor supersensitivity [89]. Furthermore, following TURP, detrusor instability is reversed in 54–69% of men with BPH [14,31,90–92] although the rate of reversal of detrusor

instability seems to be dependent on age. Andersen [83] found that the reversal of detrusor instability after TURP was lower in elderly patients compared with younger patients. In a more recent study the reversal rate of detrusor instability was only 9% in a small group of men whose mean age was 80 years [93]. Thus, the association between BOO and detrusor instability is complex and is not specific. There may well be different types of detrusor instability, some due to BOO and others occurring in its absence.

Cystometry forms an important part of the evaluation of suspected BOO since the presence of preoperative detrusor instability is associated with a poor symptomatic outcome after TURP, although for the individual patient the presence of detrusor instability cannot predict a poor outcome with accuracy [92,94,95].

Complex urodynamics

Urethral pressure profilometry

Measurement of urethral pressure was first described by Bonney in 1923 [96]. Brown and Wickham introduced perfusion profilometry in 1969 [97] and this is currently the most widely used technique for measurement of urethral pressure profile (UPPs). In this method fluid is perfused at a constant rate of 2 ml/s through an 8 Ch urethral catheter as it is slowly withdrawn along the course of the urethra. The fluid exits the catheter through eye holes located 2–3 cm proximal to the catheter tip. As the catheter meets the compressive zones of the urethra, the pressure required to maintain constant flow increases. This pressure is recorded as the UPP. More recently, microtip pressure transducers have been used for measuring UPPs [98]. In clinical practice three parameters are measured: the maximum urethral pressure (MUP), the maximum urethral closure pressure (MUCP) and the functional profile length (Fig. 34.12). According to the standardization committee of the

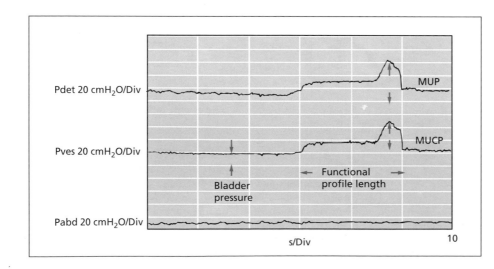

Fig. 34.12 Urethral pressure profile of a man with BPH. MUP; maximal urethral pressure, MUCP; maximal urethral closure pressure.

International Continence Society [77], the MUP is the maximum pressure of the measured profile, the MUCP is the difference between the MUP and P_{ves}, and the functional profile length is the length of the urethra along which the urethral pressure exceeds P_{ves}. The configuration of the profile varies between males and females. In the female, the bladder neck is often open at rest and so can be difficult to recognize on the UPP. The bladder neck is better defined in the male [65] and can often be identified as a small pressure peak immediately following the initial rise in pressure. Between the bladder neck and external sphincter lies the prostatic plateau, which in older men with prostatic enlargement may be several centimetres long. Static urethral pressure profilometry may be supplemented by pressure profilometry during voiding. Yalla et al. [99] have perfected this technique, known as micturitional pressure profilometry (MUPP) in which a triple lumen catheter is slowly withdrawn through the urethra while the bladder and urethral pressures are simultaneously measured.

The clinical value of urethral pressure measurements has been studied in some detail. Abrams and Torrens [100] observed a direct relationship between the prostatic area (the product of prostatic length and plateau) and the outflow resistance. Static urethral pressure profilometry is, however, regarded to be of limited value in investigating the presence and cause of BOO since it gives no information of the behaviour of the urethra during the course of micturition. MUPP has been used to establish the presence of obstruction and to localize its site. During micturition in the normal male there is an even fall in pressure along the urethra. In the presence of obstruction there is a marked pressure fall at the site of obstruction. Desmond and Ramayya [101] have found a good correlation between the results of MUPP and pressure–flow studies and the technique has been used in the assessment of BOO due to BPH, urethral strictures and bladder neck obstruction [99,102,103]. However, in the routine evaluation of a patient suspected of having BOO, UPPs have a limited role relative to simple pressure–flow studies.

Video urodynamics

Video urodynamics (VUDS) is the technique by which pressure–flow studies are combined with simultaneous fluoroscopic visualization of the lower urinary tract. A variety of commercial VUD equipment is available, some of which allows simultaneous display of pressure and flow traces with the radiographic image. This can then be recorded on videotape. The technique is essentially the same as that described for pressure–flow studies, but fluid containing a contrast medium is infused in place of normal saline.

VUDS gives added information to that obtained with routine pressure–flow studies. During the filling phase the contour of the bladder can be visualized, allowing assessment of the presence and degree of bladder trabeculation. Ureteric reflux may be seen. From the point of view of assessment of BOO, VUDS yields most information during the voiding phase. The measurement of pressure and flow allows the diagnosis of obstruction to be made and the voiding cystourethrogram can localize the site of obstruction. Failure of the bladder neck to open during voiding is suggestive of dyssynergic bladder neck obstruction. Reflux of contrast into the prostatic ducts and seminal vesicles suggests a membranous urethral obstruction such as a stricture or external sphincter–detrusor dyssynergia (although such reflux may also occur in chronic prostatitis).

The indications for VUDS in the case of suspected BOO have not been defined clearly. Although this technique provides the most precise means of investigation of lower urinary tract symptoms, the equipment is expensive and is not widely available. Furthermore, the information obtained is dependent on the skill of the urodynamic staff performing the study. Despite these limitations, VUDS is undoubtedly useful in the diagnosis of BOO secondary to dyssynergic bladder neck obstruction—indeed, definitive diagnosis of this condition is impossible without VUDS. Correct diagnosis of bladder neck obstruction is important because the appropriate treatment (by bladder neck incision) is less likely to lead to retrograde ejaculation than TURP [104]. This has obvious implications for the younger man. In the assessment of suspected BOO in the urodynamic unit at Southmead Hospital, Bristol, VUDS is used in all men below the age of 55 years, in those with a history suggestive of bladder neck obstruction, and in those patients presenting with symptoms of prostatism who have concomitant neurological disease.

Residual urine

Residual urine has been defined by the International Continence Society as the volume of fluid remaining in the bladder immediately following the completion of micturition [77]. The time interval between voiding and the estimation of residual urine volume should be as short as possible. Furthermore, one should be aware that the presence of ureteric reflux and bladder diverticula can influence the accuracy of measurement of residual urine.

There are a variety of techniques for measurement of residual urine volume. The most accurate and thus the 'gold standard' technique is by urethral catheterization, but as this method is invasive it is not used in routine clinical practice. When estimating residual urine volume by catheter, care must be taken to ensure that all of the residual urine is drained. Stoller and Millard [105] found that in practice the bladder was incompletely drained in

26% of cases with a mean of 76 ml remaining in the bladder.

In day-to-day practice, the most commonly used technique for estimating residual urine volume is transabdominal ultrasound. This has the advantage that it is simple to perform and is non-invasive. Several formulas can be used to calculate residual urine volume from the measurement of transverse, anteroposterior and sagittal dimensions. For clinical purposes the formula $0.52 \times$ height $\times$ width $\times$ anteroposterior diameter (the volume of an ellipsoid) is sufficiently accurate, with a correlation coefficient of 0.98 between the volume measured by ultrasound and that measured by catheter [106].

Assessment of post-void residual urine volume is important in the evaluation of suspected BOO, but care is required in the interpretation of its significance. There is some evidence to suggest that post-void residual urine volume is related to outflow obstruction. For example, there is a significant negative association between residual urine volume and Q_{max} [24] and relief of BOO by prostatectomy leads to a fall in residual urine [60,107]. However, several studies [58,108,109] have shown that there is wide variation in measured residual urine volume in an individual patient over a short period of time and in the very elderly the volume of residual urine has been shown to vary diurnally, being as much as 40% larger in the morning [110]. A single measurement of residual urine, therefore, is of limited value. Furthermore, although the presence of residual urine is generally taken to imply the presence of BOO, there is evidence to suggest that it may primarily be a reflection of abnormal detrusor function which may not necessarily be due to BOO. Thus, Abrams and Griffiths [40] found elevated residual urine in about 50% of men with prostatism who had no urodynamically demonstrable outflow obstruction and in another series 24% of patients with BOO had residual urine under 50 ml [111]. The finding of residual urine in both elderly men and women [110] adds weight to the suggestion that it may reflect an age-associated change in detrusor function.

Thus, although residual urine is associated with the presence of BOO, the association is not strong. For this reason and because of wide intraindividual variation, the presence and magnitude of residual urine cannot be used to diagnose or exclude the presence of BOO with any degree of certainty.

Cystourethroscopy

In the evaluation of BOO, cystourethroscopy can identify urethral and bladder pathology such as urethral strictures and bladder stones, but it is likely that evidence of these abnormalities would be identified by other investigations such as plain X-ray, ultrasound and urinary flow rate. Similarly, although prostatic size assessed by cystoscopy has been shown to correlate well with urodynamic parameters of BOO [38], the advent of TRUS has made estimation of prostatic volume much simpler and more accurate. Thus, in terms of diagnosis of BOO, cystoure-throscopy is of limited value in the routine case.

Radiology

Intravenous urography (IVU) is of limited value in the routine assessment of BOO [112–114]. It is inaccurate for the measurement of prostatic size [115] and although it can be used to estimate the volume of residual urine, ultrasound is easier, more accurate and safer [116]. The number of cases in which concomitant pathology is disclosed by the IVU is small, and its use for this purpose cannot be justified [117].

In the case of urethral stricture, urethrography is essential prior to urethroplasty [118]. Ascending urethro-graphy delineates the urethra distal to the stricture and the distal limits of the stricture. A micturating cystogram shows the bladder, bladder neck and urethra proximal to the stricture.

Conclusion

We have outlined the investigations that can be done in the evaluation of BOO. In clinical practice, however, there is wide variation in the tests which are employed in the assessment of patients presenting with 'prostatism'. Similarly, there is great variability in prostatectomy rates both nationally and internationally. Thus, in the USA age-adjusted prostatectomy rates vary threefold within small geographic areas and 1.7-fold between larger areas [119] and in England TURP rates vary from 2.8 to 29.2/10 000 males between health districts [120]. Although these differences are partly a reflection of variability in the resources available to the individual urologist, no doubt they also reflect differences of opinion regarding the extent to which patients presenting with 'prostatic' symptoms should be investigated together with differences of opinion regarding indications for prostatectomy.

Clearly, guidelines for investigation of men presenting with prostatism need to be developed. Symptoms have always been central to our management of BPH and until recently, since prostatectomy was the only effective treatment for BPH, symptom assessment was regarded as the only necessary preoperative evaluation. It was of little consequence if patients had BOO or not for the outcome of prostatectomy was favourable in the majority of cases. However, there has been recent concern regarding the morbidity and mortality of TURP and in particular the relatively high proportion of patients who undergo a repeat TURP several years after their first operation [34]. Furthermore, with the advent of new drugs and alternative surgical procedures for BPH, there are now more options for treating lower urinary tract symptoms. Given this, it would seem reasonable to make a more precise diagnosis before embarking on treatment. There is little sense in treating obstruction when the patient does not have obstruction. Prostatectomy may well be the most effective treatment for non-obstructive BPH, but until this is established (and as yet there is no evidence that this is the case) a more careful appraisal of symptoms is wise. As Blaivas has stated [121]:

> The concept remains that to develop rational therapies for the treatment of lower urinary tract disorders, such as BPH, we must understand the physiological mechanisms underlying symptoms. We must answer simple questions that are not so hard to answer with properly performed studies. Are symptoms in men with BPH due to prostatic obstruction? No one knows. Is it necessary to relieve obstruction for a successful outcome? No one knows. Is detrusor overactivity a result of obstruction, BPH or aging? No one knows.

We recommend that all patients presenting with symptoms of lower urinary tract should have an assessment of urinary flow rate and residual urine and that preferably at least two consecutive measurements should be made. An assessment of renal function should be made by measuring serum creatinine. For patients below the age of 50 years, those with a history of a neurological disorder, those with diabetes or previous pelvic surgery or trauma, a more extensive urodynamic investigation is recommended in the form of cystometry and pressure–flow studies, preferably with combined video cystourethrography. The use of pressure–flow studies in the 'routine' case of prostatism is open to debate. As stated above, several studies have suggested that patients with urodynamically proven BOO have a greater likelihood of a favourable outcome after TURP. Conversely, it has been argued that because pressure–flow studies cannot predict outcome in *individual* cases, they have no value in the evaluation of suspected BOO in routine clinical practice. This is, however, hardly suprising since in no other branch of medicine or surgery is a test able to predict the outcome of treatment with 100% accuracy. Ultimately the decision to perform pressure–flow studies rests with the individual urologist. It is difficult without larger studies of the prognostic role of pressure–flow studies to make definite recommendations about their routine use. It is, however, important to appreciate that without pressure–flow studies a diagnosis of BOO cannot be made with certainty. With the increase in the options available for treatment of BPH and BOO there is renewed interest in the pathophysiology of these conditions. Hopefully this will lead to future improvements in our clinical evaluation of BOO and so improve the results of treatment.

References

1 Lepor H. Non-operative management of benign prostatic hyperplasia. *J Urol* 1989;**141**:1283–9.

2 Mebust WK. Surgical management of benign prostatic obstruction. *Urology* 1988;**32**(Suppl.):12–15.

3 Turner-Warwick R, Whiteside CG, Worth PHL, Milroy EJG, Bates CP. A urodynamic view of the clinical problems associated with bladder neck dysfunction and its treatment by endoscopic incision and trans-trigonal posterior prostatectomy. *Br J Urol* 1973;**45**:44–59.

4 Boyarsky S, Jones G, Paulson DF, Prout GR. New look at bladder neck obstruction by the Food and Drug Administration regulators. Guidelines for the investigation of benign prostatic hypertrophy. *Trans Am Assoc Genitourin Surg* 1977;**68**:29–32.

5 Madsen PO, Iversen P. A points system for selecting operative candidates. In: Hinman HF, ed. *Benign Prostatic Hypertrophy*. New York: Springer Verlag, 1983:763–5.

6 Fowler FJ, Wennberg JE, Timothy RP et al. Symptom status and quality of life following prostatectomy. *J Am Assoc* 1988;**259**:3018–22.

7 Hald T, Nordling J, Andersen JT et al. A patient weighted symptom score in the evaluation of uncomplicated benign prostatic hyperplasia. *Scand J Urol Nephrol* 1991; **138**:59–62.

8 Barry MJ, Fowler FJ Jr, O'Leary MP et al. The American Urological Association symptom index for benign prostatic hyperplasia. *J Urol* 1992;**148**:1549–57.

9 Hansen BJ, Flyger H, Brasso K et al. Validation of the self-administered Danish Prostatic Symptom Score (DAN-PSS-1) system for use in benign prostatic hyperplasia. *Br J Urol* 1995;**76**:451–8.

10 Donovan JL, Abrams P, Peters TJ et al. The psychometric validity and reliability of the ICS male questionnaire. *Br J Urol* 1996;**77**:554–62.

11 Cockett ATK, Aso Y, Denis L et al. Recommendations of the international consensus committee concerning prostate symptom score (I-PSS) and quality of life assessment. In: Khoury S, Aso Y, Cockett ATK et al. eds. *Proceedings of the International Consultation on BPH, Monaco 1995*. Monaco. International Scientific Committee, 1991:626.

12 Hald T. Urodynamics in benign prostatic hyperplasia: a survey. *Prostate* 1989;**2**(Suppl.):69–77.

13 Castro JE, Griffiths HJL, Shackman R. Significance of signs and symptoms in benign prostatic hypertrophy. *Br Med J* 1969;**2**:598–601.

14 Abrams P, Feneley RCL. The significance of the symptoms associated with bladder outflow obstruction. *Urol Int* 1978;**33**:171–4.

15 Andersen JT, Nordling J, Walter S. Prostatism: the correlation between symptoms, cystometric and urodynamic findings. *Scand J Urol Nephrol* 1979;**13**:229–36.

16 Spangberg A, Terio H, Engberg A, Ask P. Quantification of urethral function based on Griffiths' model of flow through elastic tubes. *Neurourol Urodyn* 1989;**8**:29–52.

17 Schafer W, Rubben H, Noppeney R, Deutz FJ. Obstructed and unobstructed prostatic obstruction. A plea for urodynamic objectivation of bladder outflow obstruction in benign prostatic hyperplasia. *World J Urol* 1989;**6**:198–203.

18 McLoughlin J, Gill KP, Abel PB, Williams G. Symptoms versus flow rates versus urodynamics in the selection of patients for prostatectomy. *Br J Urol* 1990;**60**:303–5.

19 Rollema HJ, van Mastrigt R. Improved indication and follow-up in transurethral resection of the prostate using the computer program CLIM: a prospective study. *J Urol* 1992; **148**:111–16.

20 Ko DSC, Fenster HN, Chambers K *et al.* The correlation of multichannel urodynamic pressure–flow studies and American Urological Association Symptom index in the evaluation of benign prostatic hyperplasia. *J Urol* 1995;**154**: 396–8.

21 van Venrooij GEPM, Boon TA, Gier RPE. International prostate symptom score and quality of life assessment versus urodynamic parameters in men with benign prostatic hyperplasia symptoms. *J Urol* 1995;**153**:1516–19.

22 Griffiths DJ, van Mastrigt R, Bosch R. Quantification of urethral resistance and bladder function during voiding, with special reference to the effects of prostate size reduction on urethral obstruction due to benign prostatic hyperplasia. *Neurourol Urodyn* 1989;**8**:17–27.

23 Yalla SV, Sullivan MP, Lecamwasam HS *et al.* Correlation of American Urological Association symptom index with obstructive and nonobstructive prostatism. *J Urol* 1995;**153**: 674–80.

24 Neal DE, Styles RA, Ng T *et al.* The relationship between voiding pressures, symptoms and urodynamics in 253 men undergoing prostatectomy. *Br J Urol* 1987;**60**:554–9.

25 Chancellor MB, Rivas DA. American Urological Association symptom index for women with voiding symptoms: lack of specificity for benign prostatic hyperplasia. *J Urol* 1993; **150**:1706–9.

26 Chai TC, Belville WD, McGuire EJ, Nyquist L. Specificity of the American Urological Association symptom index: comparison of unselected and selected samples of both sexes. *J Urol* 1993;**150**:1710–13.

27 Reynard J, Lim C, Abrams P. The significance of intermittency in men with lower urinary tract symptoms. *Urology* 1996;**47**:491–496.

28 Susset JG, Rabinovitch H, MacKinnon KJ. Parameters of micturition: clinical study. *J Urol* 1965;**94**:113–21.

29 Reynard J, Peters T, Lamond E, Abrams P. The significance of straining in men with lower urinary tract symptoms *Br J Urol* 1995;**75**:148–53.

30 Reynard J, Lim C, Peters T, Abrams P. The significance of terminal dribbling in men with lower urinary tract symptoms. *Br J Urol* 1996;**77**:705–10.

31 Abrams PH, Farrar DJ, Turner-Warwick RT, Whiteside CG, Feneley RCL. The results of prostatectomy: a symptomatic and urodynamic analysis of 152 patients. *J Urol* 1979;**121**: 640–2.

32 Neal DE, Ramsden PD, Sharples L *et al.* Outcome of elective prostatectomy. *Br Med J* 1989;**299**:762–7.

33 Doll HA, Black NA, McPherson K *et al.* Mortality, morbidity and complications following transurethral resection of the prostate for benign prostatic hypertrophy. *J Urol* 1992;**147**: 1566–73.

34 Neal DE. Prostatectomy—an open or closed case. *Br J Urol* 1990;**66**:449–54.

35 Abrams P. New words for old—lower urinary tract symptoms for 'prostatism'. *Br Med J* 1994;**308**:929–30.

36 George NJR, O'Reilly PH, Barnard RJ, Blacklock NJ. High pressure chronic retention. *Br Med J* 1983;**286**:1780–3.

37 Meyhoff HH, Hald T. Are doctors able to assess prostatic size? *Scand J Urol Nephrol* 1978;**12**:219–21.

38 Andersen JT, Nordling J. Prostatism II. The correlation between cystourethroscopic, cystometric and urodynamic findings. *Scand J Urol Nephrol* 1980;**14**:23–7.

39 Reynard JM, Brewster SF, Peters TJ, Abrams P. The relationship between prostatic volume and bladder outflow obstruction in men with prostatism. *J Urol* 1994;**151**:314A.

40 Abrams P, Griffiths DJ. The assessment of prostatic obstruction from urodynamic measurements and from residual urine. *Br J Urol* 1979;**51**:129–34.

41 McNeal JE. The zonal anatomy of the prostate. *Prostate* 1981;**2**:35.

42 Bosch JLH, Kranse R, van Mastrigt R, Schroder FH. Reasons for weak correlation between prostate volume and urethral resistance parameters in patients with prostatism. *J Urol* 1995;**153**:689–93.

43 Kaplan SA, Te AE, Pressler LB, Olsson CA. Transition zone index as a method of assessing benign prostatic hyperplasia: correlation with symptoms, urine flow and detrusor pressure. *J Urol* 1995;**154**:1764–9.

44 Jensen KME. Clinical evaluation of routine urodynamic investigations in prostatism. *Neurourol Urodyn* 1989;**8**: 545–78.

45 Reynard J, Abrams P. Low volume uroflowmetry—useful or useless? *J Urol* 1996;**155**:394A.

46 Mosso A, Pellacani P. Sur les fonctions de la vesie. *Arch Ital Biol* 1882;**1**:97.

47 Rehfisch E. Uber den mechanismus des harnblasenver-schlusses und der harnentleerung. *Arch Pathol Anat Physiol* 1897;**150**:111–51.

48 Drake WM. The uroflowmeter: an aid to the study of the lower urinary tract. *J Urol* 1948;**59**:650–8.

49 von Garrelts. Analysis of micturition: a new method of recording the voiding of the bladder. *Acta Chir Scand* 1956; **112**:326–40.

50 Grino PB, Bruskewitz R, Blaivas JG *et al.* Maximum urinary flow rate by uroflowmetry: automatic or visual interpretation. *J Urol* 1993;**149**:339–41.

51 Reynard J, Lim C, Peters T, Abrams P. The value of multiple free-flow studies in men with BPH. *Br J Urol* 1996;**77**:813–18.

52 Siroky MB, Olsson CA, Krane RJ. The flow rate nomogram. I. Development. *J Urol* 1979;**122**:665–8.

53 Haylen BT, Ashby D, Sutherst JR, Frazer MI, West CR. Maximum and average urine flow rates in normal male and female populations—the Liverpool nomograms. *Br J Urol* 1989;**64**:30–8.

54 Kadow C, Howell S, Lewis, Abrams P. A flow rate nomogram for normal males over the age of 50. In: *Proceedings of the International Continence Society, 15th Annual Meeting, London,* 1985:138–9.

55 Jorgensen JB, Jensen KM-E, Bille-Brahe NE, Mogensen P. Uroflowmetry in asymptomatic elderly males. *Br J Urol* 1986; **58**:390–5.

56 Jensen KM-E, Bruskewitz RC, Iversen P, Madsen PO. Spontaneous uroflowmetry in prostatism. *Urology* 1984;**24**: 403–9.

57 Chancellor MB, Blaivas JG, Kaplan SA, Axelrod S. Bladder outlet obstruction versus impaired detrusor contractility: the role of uroflow. *J Urol* 1991;**145**:810–12.

58 Gerstenberg TC, Anderson JT, Klarskov P, Ramirez D, Hald T. High flow infravesical obstruction in the male. *J Urol* 1982; **127**:943–5.

59 Iversen P, Bruskewitz RC, Jensen KM-E, Madsen PO. Transurethral prostatic resection in the treatment of prostatism with high urinary flow. *J Urol* 1983;**129**:995–7.

60 Abrams PH. Prostatism and prostatectomy: the value of urine flow rate measurement in the preoperative assessment for operation. *J Urol* 1977;**117**:70–1.

61 Bruskewitz RC, Larsen EH, Madsen PO, Dorflinger T. 3-year follow-up of urinary symptoms after transurethral resection of the prostate. *J Urol* 1986;**136**:613–15.

62 Dorflinger T, Bruskewitz RC, Jensen KME, Iversen P, Madsen PO. Predictive value of low maximum flow rate in benign prostatic hyperplasia. *Urology* 1986;**27**:569–73.

63 Smith JC. Urethral resistance to micturition. *Br J Urol* 1968;**40**:125–56.

64 Reynard J, Lim C, Swami S, Abrams P. The obstructive effect of a urethral catheter. *J Urol* 1996;**155**:901–3.

65 Griffiths DJ. *Urodynamics. The Mechanics and Hydrodynamics of Lower Urinary Tract*, 1st edn. Bristol: Adam Hilger, 1980:107–8.

66 Sorensen S. Urodynamic investigations and their reproducibility in healthy postmenopausal females. *Scand J Urol Nephrol* 1988;**114**(Suppl.):42–7.

67 van de Beek, Rollema HJ, van Mastrigt R, Janknegt RA. Objective analysis of infravesical obstruction and detrusor contractility: appraisal of the computer program Dx/CLIM and Schafer nomogram. *Neurourol Urodyn* 1992;**11**:394–5.

68 Rosier PFWM, de la Rosette JJMCH, Koldewijn EL, Debruyne FMJ, Wijkstra H. Variability of pressure–flow analysis parameters in repeated cystometry in patients with benign prostatic hyperplasia. *J Urol* 1995;**153**:1520–5.

69 Bates P, Bradley WE, Glen E *et al*. Third report on the standardisation of terminology of lower urinary tract function. *Scand J Urol Nephrol* 1978;**12**:191–3.

70 Gleason DM, Bottaccini MR, Reilly RJ, Byrne JC. The residual stream energy is an index of male urinary outflow obstruction. *Invest Urol* 1972;**10**:72–7.

71 Griffiths DJ. Hydrodynamics of male micturition. I: theory of steady flow through elastic-walled tubes. *Med Biol Eng Comput* 1971;**9**:581–8.

72 Griffiths DJ. The mechanics of the urethra and of micturition. *Br J Urol* 1973;**45**:497–507.

73 Griffiths DJ. Urodynamic assessment of bladder function. *Br J Urol* 1977;**49**:29–36.

74 Schafer W. Detrusor as the energy source of micturition. In: Hinman F Jr, ed. *Benign Prostatic Hypertrophy*. New York: Springer Verlag, 1983:450–69.

75 Hill AV. The heat of shortening and dynamic constants of muscle. *Proc R Soc Lond [Biol]* 1938;**126**:136–95.

76 Schafer W. In: Krane RJ, Siroky MB, eds. *Clinical Neurourology*. Boston: Little Brown, 1991:111.

77 Abrams P, Blaivas JG, Stanton SL, Andersen JT. Standardisation of terminology of the lower urinary tract. *Neurourol Urodyn* 1988;**7**:403–27.

78 Schafer W. The contribution of the bladder outlet to the relation between pressure and flow rate during micturition. In: Hinman F Jr, ed. *Benign Prostatic Hypertrophy*. New York: Springer Verlag, 1983:470–96.

79 Schafer W. Basic principles and clinical application of advanced analysis of bladder voiding function. *Urol Clin North Am* 1990;**17**:553–66.

80 Abrams P. The objective evaluation of bladder outflow obstruction. In: Cockett ATK, Khoury S, Aso Y *et al*. eds. *Proceedings of the 2nd International Consultation on BPH, Paris 1993*. Paris: International Scientific Committee, 1993.

81 Kranse M, van Mastrigt R. The derivation of an obstruction index from a three parameter model fitted to the lower part of the pressure flow plot. *J Urol* 1991;**145**:261A.

82 Schafer W. A new concept for simple but specific grading of bladder outflow conditions independent from detrusor function. *J Urol* 1993;**149**:356A.

83 Andersen JT. Prostatism III. Detrusor hyperreflexia and residual urine. Clinical and urodynamic aspects and the influence of surgery of the prostate. *Scand J Urol Nephrol* 1982;**16**:25–30.

84 Andersen JT, Jacobsen O, Worm-Petersen J, Hald T. Bladder function in healthy elderly males. *Scand J Urol Nephrol* 1978;**12**:123–7.

85 Mostwin JL, Karim OM, van Koeveringe G, Brooks EL. The guinea pig as a model of gradual urethral obstruction. *J Urol* 1991;**145**:854–8.

86 Dixon JS, Gilpin CJ, Gilpin SA *et al*. Sequential morphological changes in the pig detrusor in response to chronic partial urethral obstruction. *Br J Urol* 1989;**64**:385–90.

87 Kato K, Monson FC, Longhurst PA *et al*. The functional effects of long-term outlet obstruction on the rabbit urinary bladder. *J Urol* 1990;**143**:600–6.

88 Speakman MJ, Brading AF, Gilpin CJ *et al*. Bladder outflow obstruction — a cause of denervation supersensitivity. *J Urol* 1987;**139**:1461–6.

89 Speakman MJ, Brading AF, Dixon JS, Gilpin CJ, Gosling JA. Cystometric, physiological and morphological studies after relief of bladder outflow obstruction in the pig. *Br J Urol* 1991;**68**:243–7.

90 Andersen JT. Detrusor hyperreflexia in benign infravesical obstruction. A cystometric study. *J Urol* 1976;**115**:532–4.

91 Rao MM, Ryall R, Evans C, Marshall VR. The effect of prostatectomy on urodynamic parameters. *Br J Urol* 1979;**51**:295–9.

92 Cote RJ, Burke H, Schoenberg HW. Prediction of unusual postoperative results by urodynamic testing in benign prostatic hyperplasia. *J Urol* 1981;**125**:69–2.

93 Gormley EA, Griffiths DJ, McCracken PN, Harrison GM, McPhee MS. Effect of transurethral resection of the prostate on detrusor instability and urge incontinence in elderly males. *Neurourol Urodyn* 1993;**12**:445–53.

94 Turner-Warwick RT, Whiteside CG, Arnold EP *et al*. A urodynamic view of prostatic obstruction and the results of prostatectomy. *Br J Urol* 1973;**45**:631–45.

95 Jensen KME, Jorgensen JB, Mogensen P. Urodynamics in prostatism III. Prognostic value of medium-fill water cystometry. *Scand J Urol Nephrol* 1988;**114**(Suppl.):78–83.

96 Bonney V. On diurnal incontinence of urine in women. *J Obstet Gynaecol* 1923;**30**:358.

97 Brown M, Wickham JEA. The urethral pressure profile. *Br J Urol* 1969;**41**:211–17.

98 Asmussen M, Ulmsten U. Simultaneous urethro-cystometry with a new technique. *Scand J Urol Nephrol* 1976;**10**:7–11.

99 Yalla SV, Sharma GVRK, Barsamian EM. Micturitional static urethral pressure profile: a method of recording urethral pressure profile during voiding and the implications. *J Urol* 1980;**124**:649–56.

100 Abrams P, Torrens MJ. Urethral closure pressure profile in the male. *Urol Int* 1977;**32**:137–45.
101 Desmond AD, Ramayya GR. Comparison of pressure/flow studies with micturitional urethral pressure profiles in the diagnosis of urinary outflow obstruction. *Br J Urol* 1988; **61**:224–9.
102 Yalla SV, Blute R, Bedford Waters W, Snyder H, Fraser L. Urodynamic evaluation of prostatic enlargement with micturitional vesicourethral static pressure profiles. *J Urol* 1981;**125**:685–9.
103 Yalla SV, Bedford Waters W, Snyder H, Varady S, Blute R. Urodynamic localisation of isolated bladder neck obstruction in men: studies with micturitional vesicourethral static pressure profile. *J Urol* 1981;**125**:677–84.
104 Reynard J, Abrams P. The role of bladder neck incision. *Eur Urol Update Ser* 1992;**1**:90–5.
105 Stoller ML, Millard RJ. The accuracy of a catheterised residual urine. *J Urol* 1989;**141**:15–16.
106 Roehrborn CG, Peters PC. Can transabdominal ultrasound estimation of postvoid residual (PVR) replace catheterisation? *Urology* 1988;**31**:445–9.
107 Schafer W. Urodynamics of micturition. *Curr Opin Urol* 1992;**2**:252–6.
108 Birch NC, Hurst C, Doyle PT. Serial residual urine volumes in men with prostatic hypertrophy. *Br J Urol* 1988;**62**:571–5.
109 Bruskewitz RC, Iversen P, Madsen PO. Value of post-void residual urine determination in evaluation of prostatism. *Urology* 1982;**20**:602–4.
110 Griffiths DJ, McCracken PN, Harrison GM, Gormley EA. Characteristics of urinary incontinence in elderly patients studies by 24-hour monitoring and urodynamic testing. *Age Ageing* 1992;**21**:195–201.
111 Griffiths HJ, Castro J. An evaluation of the importance of residual urine. *Br J Radiol* 1970;**43**:409–13.
112 Andersen JT, Jacobsen O, Strandgaard L. The diagnostic value of intravenous pyelography in infravesical obstruction in males. *Scand J Urol Nephrol* 1977;**11**:225–30.
113 Abrams P, Feneley RCL, Roylance JR. Excretion urography in the investigation of prostatism. *Br J Urol* 1976;**48**:681–4.
114 Abrams PH. Use of the intravenous urogram in diagnosis. In: Hinman F Jr, ed. *Benign Prostatic Hypertrophy.* New York: Springer Verlag, 1983:605–9.
115 Meyhoff HH. Transurethral versus transvesical prostatectomy. *Scand J Urol Nephrol* 1987;**102**(Suppl.):1–26.
116 Dadfar H, Zinsser HH. Bladder volumes from cystogram films. *Invest Urol* 1972;**9**:363–4.
117 Bauer DL, Garrison RW, McRoberts JW. The health and cost implications of routine excretory urography before transurethral prostatectomy. *J Urol* 1980;**123**:386–9.
118 Mundy AR. *Urodynamic and Reconstructive Surgery of the Lower Urinary Tract.* London: Churchill Livingstone, 1993.
119 Chassin MR, Brook RH, Park RE et al. Variations in the use of medical and surgical services by the medicare population. *N Engl J Med* 1986;**314**:285–90.
120 Donovan JD, Frankel S, Nanchahal K, Coast J, Williams M. *Epidemiologically Based Needs Assessment. Prostatectomy for Benign Prostatic Hyperplasia.* London: Department of Health, 1992.
121 Blaivas JG. Urinary symptoms and symptom scores. *J Urol* 1993;**150**:1714.

35   Urodynamic Disorders of the Urethra
J.G.Noble and T.J.Christmas

Introduction

Normal lower urinary tract function requires a competent urethral sphincter mechanism to provide urinary continence during bladder filling, and coordinated sphincter relaxation to allow unobstructed bladder emptying during voiding. The maintenance of this function depends upon a delicate interaction between the detrusor muscle, the bladder neck (and in the male the preprostatic sphincter) and the urethral sphincter mechanisms. Urethral dysfunction may therefore result in a failure of one or both of these roles leading to symptoms of urinary incontinence, obstructed voiding or a combination of the two.

The normal anatomy of the urethra differs considerably between the sexes and similarly the pathophysiological processes which may affect urethral function in each sex are different and should be considered separately. Urinary symptoms resulting from urethral dysfunction tend not to be specific and therefore require careful, planned investigation before treatment is initiated. This chapter reviews the investigation of urethral voiding dysfunction and the management of specific disorders in both sexes.

Investigation of urethral dysfunction

The degree of severity of a patient's urinary symptoms is a notoriously poor predictor of the extent of lower urinary tract dysfunction. While symptom scoring has attempted to quantify patients' responses to certain treatment regimens all patients should undergo careful evaluation of the lower urinary tract before treatment, especially where surgery is contemplated. Simple measures should include the analysis of a time–volume chart, the urinary flow rate (repeated on several occasions if possible) [1] and pad testing for a quantitative assessment of the degree of urinary incontinence. In many instances the correlation of an accurate clinical history and examination, simple urodynamic investigations and cystourethroscopy will provide an accurate diagnosis, For example urethral stricture. However, it is more usual to be uncertain of the diagnosis even after endoscopic assessment of the lower urinary tract and hence more complex investigations are indicated.

Urethrography

Voiding cystourethrography (VCU) is widely used as an anatomical investigation of the urethra in both children and adults. After filling the bladder with contrast, usually in retrograde fashion via a urethral catheter, voiding takes place in an upright position and spot films are taken of the urethra. Antegrade urethrography is often used to compliment VCU and allows better visualization of anterior urethral strictures. The contrast is injected slowly into the urethra, usually via a clamp or syringe device, and care must be taken not to use excessive force to overcome stricture obstruction; reflux of contrast into the periurethral vasculature [2], corpus cavernosum and spongiosum has been reported and may well complicate the images produced. Retrograde urethrography is difficult to perform in the female and is seldom indicated. The presence of urethral diverticula may accurately be defined with ultrasound obviating the need for contrast studies (see p. 499).

The primary indication for urethrography is in the assessment of urethral trauma or urethral stricture disease. While imaging of a stricture is usually clear, difficulties do occur occasionally due to misinterpretation of potential 'filling defects' within the urethra. These include the introduction of air bubbles into the urethra during instillation of contrast, the prostatic impression and, more importantly, that produced by the verumontanum and external sphincter spasm. However, narrowing of the anterior urethra with proximal dilatation is usually always pathological, making urethrography the investigation of choice in stricture disease. Extravasation of contrast following urethral trauma and the presence of false passages and false bladder necks are all clearly seen, especially on retrograde imaging.

Urodynamics

Our understanding of lower urinary tract dysfunction and the methods of investigation have evolved rapidly since the advent of urodynamic evaluation in the late 1960s [3]. While simple uroflowmetry may suggest that a bladder is either obstructed or decompensated, precise definition of the presence or absence of outflow obstruction using voiding cystometry is essential. Moreover, if voiding cystometry is combined with fluoroscopic assessment of the urethra, the so-called video cystometrogram (VCMG), then the precise definition of the site of obstruction may be visualized. In a similar way if a patient voids with low detrusor pressure in combination with low flow rates and an area of obstruction cannot be seen on fluoroscopy then poor detrusor function may be implicated as the cause of symptoms. This is especially useful in the diagnosis of male patients with bladder outflow obstruction in the absence of prostatic enlargement. VCMG will define clearly the characteristic video urodynamic appearances of bladder neck dyssynergia, and similarly in patients with neuropathic detrusor dysfunction the classic appearances of a 'fir tree' bladder combined with urinary outflow obstruction due to detrusor–sphincter dyssynergia can be demonstrated. The VCMG also provides an excellent method of assessing urinary incontinence. It accurately defines the presence or absence of abnormal detrusor activity during bladder filling and correlates the cysto-urethrographic appearances of the bladder outlet with detrusor pressure at the precise moment of urinary incontinence. The usual question as to whether leakage has occurred due to abnormal detrusor behaviour and/or inadequate sphincter activity can be answered and an assessment of bladder base descent during coughing can allow a reasoned selection of the correct surgical procedure.

Despite the fact that VCMG can reliably identify specific lower urinary tract disorders, problems of interpretation still commonly arise. Clearly, in a case where detrusor decompensation has occurred secondary to chronic bladder outflow obstruction, the degree of obstruction will be impossible to quantify accurately. To address this problem various mathematical derivations of the pressure–flow analysis have been devised in order to identify obstruction in the presence of poor detrusor function [4–7]. Similarly, our whole concept of understanding 'normal' detrusor function has been questioned with the advent of ambulatory urodynamics [8]. These complex urodynamic derivations are not utilized as yet in common urological investigation but obviously may become useful in the assessment of more complex urological cases. The details of these techniques are discussed in detail elsewhere.

Electromyography

While VCMG will allow accurate assessment of the majority of patients with uncomplicated urological disorders it is sometimes necessary to gain further information regarding the urethral sphincter mechanism, especially in cases where lower urinary tract symptoms are associated with neurological disease. Electromyography (EMG) studies the activity of the striated component of the urethral sphincter mechanism and when correlated with urodynamic data provides detailed assessment of urethral function and dysfunction. EMG may be performed using either surface or needle electrodes. Needle electrodes require more accurate placement than surface or patch electrodes but do provide a more detailed recording of sphincter activity. During bladder filling the activity of the urethral sphincter should gradually increase as pelvic floor muscles are recruited, the so-called guarding reflex, and then disappear just prior to and during voiding [9,10]. Absence of the guarding reflex and the loss of a sphincter 'flare' during a stop test suggest the presence of neurological dysfunction. EMG activity is increased in response to a number of stimuli including coughing, the Credé and Valsalva manoeuvres, the bulbocavernosus reflex and the stop test where the pelvic floor musculature is suddenly and voluntarily contracted during voiding.

Motor unit EMG studies the bioelectric potentials generated by skeletal muscle and may be studied with concentric needle electrodes placed into the urethral sphincter. The electrical discharge produced on the contraction of skeletal muscle fibres of a motor unit at depolarization is known as a motor unit action potential. The information may be recorded on an oscilloscope screen but is often converted into sound energy and can therefore be recorded as an audible sound. As the sphincter muscle contracts each individual motor unit fires at a more rapid rate and more motor units are recruited. The form of the EMG firings can be individually recorded and may be of significance in diagnosis. Although considerable expertise is required to interpret accurately the different forms of motor unit action potentials, EMG can be of use in detecting denervation or myopathy of the urethral sphincter. Interpretation of a motor unit EMG must be coupled with the known clinical and urodynamic data in reaching an accurate diagnosis [11].

Central, peripheral and spinal nervous pathways may be investigated with EMG utilizing sacral evoked responses. The efficiency of the sensory, spinal and motor nervous pathways is assessed using different sites of stimulation and recording. All of these investigations require specialized expertise and equipment and are therefore usually undertaken in specialist neurophysiology departments.

Urethral profilometry

During bladder filling the lumen of the urethra remains closed partly due to the elastic and muscular properties of the urethral wall and as a result of the effects of the sphincter active area. By measuring the resting urethral pressure an estimate of the ability of the urethra to prevent leakage of urine might be achieved. The term urethral profilometry is often used to refer to a variety of investigations which attempt to quantify urethral function and dysfunction based on this idealized concept.

The most commonly used investigation involves the measurement of the urethral closing pressure at various points along the urethra from the bladder neck to the meatus, thus generating a so-called static infusion urethral pressure profile (UPP). A fine diameter catheter containing side holes is passed into the bladder through which saline is infused at a predetermined rate. The catheter is withdrawn at a constant rate and the pressure required to force saline through the catheter is recorded as a UPP. This pressure is generated as a result of several factors including the compliance of the urethral wall, the resistance to the inflow of saline into the UPP catheter, the resistance of saline running into the bladder and out of the urethral meatus and artefacts generated by the UPP apparatus.

Despite the theoretical advantage of utilizing this test in the investigation of urethral dysfunction the exact diagnostic role of the static infusion UPP is poorly defined. Theoretically, areas of abnormally high urethral pressure at the level of the bladder neck, prostate and/or external urethral sphincter may indicate a site for urinary outflow obstruction and similarly low urethral pressures within the sphincter active area may reveal the cause of urinary incontinence. However, in clinical practice there is a considerable overlap between the results obtained from normal volunteers and patients with known urodynamic abnormalities and the reproducibility of results is very poor. Static infusion UPP does appear to be helpful in assessing the function of an artificial urinary sphincter and will reliably identify a non-functioning bladder neck where the urethral pressure within the proximal urethral segment is equal to that within the bladder and the pressure within the sphincter active area is generally lower than usual.

More complex urethral profilometry investigations have evolved from the static infusion UPP. Stress urethral profilometry is undertaken with dual pressure sensors — one within the bladder and one within the urethra — and is said to be useful in the diagnosis of genuine stress incontinence (GSI). During a cough test the urethral pressure should always exceed the intravesical pressure; this trend is reversed in patients with GSI. Dynamic or voiding profilometry is undertaken with dual sensors during both the filling and emptying phases of the micturition cycle, and micturition profilometry utilizes up to three sensors with the catheter slowly withdrawn during voiding. The maximal pressure drop should indicate the site of obstruction in this case.

While all of these tests are relatively simple to perform and have their protagonists they are generally not in widespread use as most of the information they provide may reliably be obtained with simple video urodynamics combined with endoscopic assessment of the urethra.

Ultrasound

While the mainstay of urethral imaging continues to involve antegrade and voiding urethrography for anatomical definition combined with urodynamic and elctrophysiological tests for functional assessment, in recent years the use of ultrasound has been employed increasingly and is proving to be of some clinical value, especially in the assessment of anterior urethral strictures [12–14].

The technique involves distention of the urethra with retrograde instillation of saline or by encouraging the patient to void against a penile clamp and imaging the periurethral tissue with 5 or 7 MHz linear array probes positioned over the penile and bulbar urethra. The potential advantage of sonography over conventional imaging techniques is based upon the fact that not only is the actual urethral stricture clearly visualized on ultrasound but the degree of periurethral scarring can also be assessed accurately. This has important diagnostic relevance in predicting the severity and prognosis of the stricture. In addition, the appearances of periurethral scarring seen in urethral stricture disease on ultrasound have been shown to correlate well with full-depth biopsy specimens taken at the time of subsequent urethroplasty [13].

Transrectal ultrasound (TRUS) has also proven beneficial in the investigation of urethral dysfunction in the male and, more recently, in the female patient [15–18]. TRUS provides detailed information regarding the bladder neck, preprostatic urethra and membranous urethra. Bladder neck and membranous strictures are easily identified using 7 MHz linear array probes and, similarly, the presence of an open bladder neck and/or good transurethral resection cavity after a bladder neck incision or transurethral resection of prostate (TURP) may suggest that recurrent symptoms following an operation may not be due to residual obstruction. Similarly, specific features of bladder neck dyssynergia have been described [19,20] and may provide a useful adjunct to urodynamic assessment in the investigation of voiding dysfunction in younger male patients.

Perineal ultrasound scanning has been used in the investigation of stress incontinence [21] with results comparable to those obtained with fluoroscopic techniques. The sonographic appearances of the normal female urethra were originally described by Hennigan and DeBose

[18] and previous to this ultrasound had been used effectively to image urethral diverticula [22,23]. More recently TRUS has been used to image the urethral sphincter in females with urodynamic evidence of obstructed voiding [24].

Ultrasound has also identified posterior urethral valves in neonates [25], urethral calculi [26], a urethral false passage [12], urethral foreign bodies [11] and urethral polyps [27].

There is undoubtedly scope for improving urethral anatomical and functional assessment by combining real-time ultrasound with voiding urodynamics, and several reports have alluded to this [28–30]. With the refinement of both urodynamic and sonographic apparatus the ability to investigate urethral function and dysfunction under more physiologically normal conditions will become possible.

Conclusion

Routine investigation of urethral dysfunction thus involves anatomical imaging of the urethral lumen with VCU and retrograde urethrography and of the periurethral structures with perineal ultrasound and/or TRUS. Functional assessment is best performed with VCMG, with EMG reserved for more complex and unusual cases where the diagnosis is uncertain using routine investigations. In the future magnetic resonance imaging (MRI) of the urethra may prove to be of benefit [31], but initial studies have failed to demonstrate any advantages over conventional techniques. Undoubtedly the refinement of imaging and urodynamic apparatus allowing the assessment of patients under more 'physiological' normal conditions will increase our understanding of urethral function both in normal and disease states.

Specific conditions associated with urethral dysfunction

The classification of lower urinary tract dysfunction has been the subject of considerable debate over many years. Classification of urodynamic disorders of the urethra can also prove to be difficult and often depends upon the emphasis of the investigator's own clinical area of interest and expertise. Urethral dysfunction may result in an inability to store urine during bladder filling resulting in urinary incontinence or alternatively in urinary outflow obstruction during voiding. Abnormalities causing urethral dysfunction may produce either of these phenomena at different anatomical levels within the urethra and thus classification of specific disorders can be confusing. In this section specific urodynamic disorders of the urethra are discussed on clinical, anatomical and urodynamic grounds and their clinical relevance in each sex is described (Table 35.1). The specific conditions of prostatic outflow obstruction in males and urinary incontinence in females are discussed in detail elsewhere.

Bladder neck dysfunction

Despite its importance in micturition the precise anatomical arrangement of the bladder neck is not known and is the subject of much debate [32,33]. In the male there is no doubt that a sphincteric type of mechanism exists proximal to the ejaculatory ducts to prevent the retrograde emission of semen into the bladder during ejaculation. The contraction of smooth muscle at ejaculation seems to be predominantly in response to sympathetic stimulation. Conversely, during voiding this area can be seen to funnel open on fluoroscopy allowing the bladder to empty in an

Table 35.1 Anatomical and urodynamic classification of urethral disorders.

Level of abnormality	Lesion causing urethral obstruction	Lesion causing urethral incompetence
Bladder neck	Bladder neck dyssynergia Bladder neck stenosis	Traumatic damage to bladder neck Bladder neck incompetence
Prostate	Benign prostatic hyperplasia Prostatic carcinoma Other prostatic tumours Prostatic cysts Prostatitis	
Urethral sphincter	Detrusor–sphincter dyssynergia Sphincter strictures Fowler syndrome	Sphincter incompetence
Urethra	Urethral strictures Posterior urethral valves Foreign bodies Urethral neoplasia	Urethral 'instability'

unobstructed fashion. The mechanism for relaxation of this so-called 'preprostatic sphincter' is unclear. It may open as a result of active smooth muscle relaxation or simply due to passive factors with simultaneous inhibition of sympathetic tone. The male bladder neck is known on clinical grounds to provide a cough-competent sphincter as demonstrated in men who have undergone pelvic fracture trauma to their external sphincter and yet remain continent. In the female, the bladder neck is poorly developed when compared to the male. Its relevance to continence is unclear but the fact that a proportion of asymptomatic young women have open bladder necks at rest suggests that it is not significant [34]. It can be seen, therefore, that any condition affecting the function of the bladder neck, particularly in male patients, may lead to significant urinary symptomology.

Bladder neck obstruction

The term 'bladder neck obstruction" is frequently used in clinical practice but is open to misinterpretation. It may be used specifically to indicate a functional abnormality of the bladder neck mechanism itself, which is better referred to as bladder neck dyssynergia. In the past it has been used very generally to denote bladder outflow obstruction with no distinction between proximal or distal urethral pathology. This is used rarely nowadays. More commonly, bladder neck obstruction may be used to refer to any obstructive lesion at the level of the blader outlet which of course includes all forms of prostatic disease. Many conditions can cause bladder neck obstruction and they can be classified as congenital, infective, neoplasic, iatrogenic, metabolic, neurogenic and psychogenic (Table 35.2). The specific disorders of bladder neck dyssynergia and prostatic outflow obstruction in males are discussed elsewhere.

Autonomic failure and bladder neck dysfunction

The precise role of the sympathetic nervous system in the control of continence and micturition in humans is controversial. However, there is some evidence in experimental animals to suggest that during bladder filling afferent information from detrusor muscle stretch receptors is conveyed to the central nervous system via the pelvic plexus. This activity may result in the inhibition of efferent transmission across the pelvic ganglia and may augment bladder filling by β-adrenergically mediated relaxation of the detrusor. In addition, continence may conceivably be enhanced by an α-adrenergic effect which increases tone in the proximal urethra. These concepts have, to a large extent, been supported by the study of patients with various forms of autonomic failure. The clinical disorders characterized by primary failure of the autonomic nervous system have been divided into

Table 35.2 The differential diagnosis of bladder neck obstruction.

Congenital
Congenital urethral valves
Congenital urethral hypoplasia
Obstructing embryological remnants

Infective
Prostatitis: acute/chronic bacterial
Non-bacterial
Prostatodynia
Infection at the level of the bladder neck, e.g. schistosomiasis
Postinfective urethral stricture
Urinary tract infection

Neoplasia
Bladder neck dyssynergia
Bladder neck hypertrophy
Extrinsic pelvic tumours, e.g. rectum
Pedunculated bladder tumours
Prostatic tumours: benign/malignant
Urethral carcinoma

Iatrogenic
Bladder neck fibrosis
Drug-induced bladder neck spasm, e.g. amphetamine abuse

Metabolic
Impacted urinary calculi

Neurogenic

Psychogenic

progressive autonomic failure (PAF) with multiple system atrophy (MSA), which mainly affects neurones in the central nervous system, and pan-dysautonomia and pure cholinergic dysautonomia in which the lesions seem to be mainly peripheral [35]. In patient with PAF and MSA the bladder neck has been shown to be completely incompetent; and in a patient with pan-dysautonomia the bladder neck has been found to be widely dilated during bladder filling. In contrast, a patient with a pure cholinergic deficit has been shown to have a bladder neck that remained tightly closed during filling [36].

Shy–Drager syndrome

The Shy–Drager syndrome is an uncommon neuromuscular disorder in which voiding dysfunction is associated with autonomic failure (orthostatic hypotension, anhydrosis, impotence) and cerebellar dysfunction. The neurological lesions are situated in the midbrain, caudate nucleus and intermediolateral columns of the thoracolumbar and sacral spinal cord [36,37]. Urinary symptoms usually include incontinence, frequency and an inability to void. Urodynamic assessment may reveal detrusor hyperreflexia in approximately one-third of patients and a similar proportion will exhibit poor compliance during bladder filling. On voiding, voluntary detrusor contraction is absent and bladder emptying is usually only achieved with significant abdominal straining. On fluoroscopy the bladder neck is usually seen to be open and EMG may reveal striated sphincter denervation in many cases. This observation provides a useful method of differentiating these patients from those with parkinsonian voiding dysfunction [38]. In Parkinson's disease, bladder neck function is not affected and striated sphincter denervation is unusual. Treatment of these patients centres around facilitating urine storage with clean intermittent self-catheterization (CISC), but this often becomes most difficult in advanced cases.

Autonomic hyperreflexia

Autonomic hyperreflexia may also be associated with bladder neck dyssynergia, although outflow obstruction is predominantly caused by detrusor (striated)–sphincter dyssynergia and is discussed later in this chapter (see 'Urethral Sphincter Dysfunction').

Traumatic bladder neck dysfunction

In the male, traumatic damage to the bladder neck either resulting from pelvic trauma or as part of endoscopic treatment for bladder outflow obstruction, usually results in ejaculatory failure but should not cause urinary incontinence providing there is adequate striated sphincter function. In the female, as already discussed, the precise role of the bladder neck in the maintenance of urinary continence is not known and therefore damage to the bladder neck should not necessarily result in urinary incontinence. Bladder neck stenosis resulting from previous damage to the bladder outlet (for example following endoscopic surgery) causes bladder outflow obstruction. The smooth muscle of the bladder neck is replaced by rigid, fibrotic scar tissue which prevents synergistic bladder neck relaxation during voiding. Treatment involves further endoscopic resection of the bladder neck, but subsequent restenosis is not unusual. This phenomenon is commonly seen following resection of small so-called 'fibrous' prostates and it may be that coexistent bladder neck dyssynergia and benign prostatic hyperplasia with inadequate attention to the bladder neck at the time of surgery may predispose to this complication.

Urethral sphincter dysfunction

Distal sphincter dysfunction usually occurs as a result of congenital or acquired neurological disease or trauma, so-called neuropathic vesicourethral dysfunction, or following direct trauma to the sphincter muscle.

Neuropathic urethral sphincter dysfunction

Neuropathic vesicourethral dysfunction may originate at a suprapontine, supraspinal, sacral or peripheral level. Although the effects on detrusor function vary considerably depending upon the level of the neurological lesion, sphincter dysfunction is usually associated with obstructed voiding caused by detrusor–sphincter dyssynergia. In general, suprapontine lesions are associated with contractile detrusor dysfunction, peripheral lesions with acontractile dysfunction and cord lesions with both. Other factors are also important in the genesis of urinary symptoms in association with neurological disease. These include vesicourethral sensation, the presence or absence of voluntary voiding control, the neurological status of the anorectum, lower limbs and abdomen, sexual function and general intelligence [39]. These factors may well influence the type of treatment offered to the patient for their urinary symptoms and should be assessed carefully before any treatment regimen is initiated.

Urethral sphincter function is usually spared in lesions above the level of the pons because detrusor–sphincter coordination is controlled at this level. Urodynamic assessment will demonstrate detrusor hyperreflexia in the absence of outflow obstruction and, therefore, patients are not at risk of upper tract damage. In patients with cord lesions, detrusor–sphincter coordination is often lost and outflow obstruction occurs secondary to detrusor–sphincter dyssynergia. These patients, therefore, often demonstrate both detrusor hyperreflexia and urinary outflow obstruction and are at considerable risk of upper tract damage. It is interesting to note that up to 50% of such patients have associated bladder neck incompetence although the mechanism for this is not clear.

In patients with so-called intermediate bladder dysfunction, associated urethral dysfunction is not uncommon. Vesicourethral dysfunction of this sort is only found in patients with cord lesions either due to spina bifida in the thoracolumbar region or extensive spinal injury. The detrusor is usually poorly compliant and contracts in an inefficient manner, often insufficient to promote voiding. The distal sphincter is usually of a fixed resistance, neither acting in a sysnergistic nor a dyssynergic manner. Thus, if sufficient detrusor contraction to overcome this resistance is present the patient becomes incontinent, if not urinary retention occurs. In these patients the bladder neck is incompetent and upper tract damage is unusual.

Static distal sphincter dysfunction is also seen in patients with acontractile bladders. Those with cord lesions usually have a low degree of urethral resistance and are usually incontinent, whereas those with peripheral lesions develop greater sphincter resistance. In this latter group large residual urine volumes are not uncommon.

In general, the urologist usually will treat patients with

either congenital cord lesions or those with spinal injuries, whereas patients with acquired neurological disorders rarely require surgical intervention. Urethral sphincter dysfunction may be improved by sphincterotomy or urethral stent insertion in patients with sphincter obstruction, or artificial sphincter insertion in those with incompetent sphincters. Palliative treatment with suprapubic catheterization, or continent or conduit urinary diversion may also be considered in neuropathic vesico-urethral dysfunction.

Spinal cord injury

Those patients with complete cord transection with urodynamic evidence of detrusor hyperreflexia and detrusor–sphincter dyssynergia with secondary upper tract damage should be considered for sphincterotomy, provided that permanent condom drainage is acceptable to the patient. If this option is unacceptable then intermittent catheterization should be employed. Associated detrusor dysfunction is usually managed with anticholinergic medication or a 'clam' cystoplasty. Those with urethral sphincter weakness or incompetence can be successfully treated with condom drainage, indwelling catheters or insertion of an artificial urinary sphincter (AUS). It is important to assess carefully the patient's suitability for an AUS on symptomatic, neurological, urodynamic and psychological grounds before such a procedure is undertaken.

Spina bifida

These patients usually follow the same urodynamic pattern as those with incomplete spinal cord injuries. The majority of those with cervical and upper thoracic lesions will usually respond to anticholinergic medication with or without CISC and rarely require sphincterotomy. Those with thoracolumbar or sacral spina bifida usually develop static urethral sphincter dysfunction and may require an AUS if urinary incontinence is the overriding symptomatic problem.

Parkinson's disease

This progressive degenerative neurological disorder has a reported incidence of 50 per 100 000 population. The onset usually occurs after 45 years of age with an equal sex distribution [40,41]. The pigmented neurones of the substantia nigra are predominantly affected leading to relative dopamine deficiency with respect to cholinergic activity within the corpus striatum. The reported prevalence of urinary symptoms in patients with Parkinson's disease varies between 25 and 75%. Murnaghan [42] reported a large series of patients with Parkinson's disease

and urinary symptoms and found that 'irritative' symptoms, i.e. daytime frequency, nocturia, urgency and urge incontinence, were more frequently encountered (30%) than symptoms of urinary outflow obstruction (10%). The most common urodynamic finding is that of detrusor hyperreflexia [42,43] with some studies reporting the incidence to be as high 75%. Detrusor–sphincter dyssynergia associated with detrusor hyperreflexia generally does not occur, although 'sphincter bradykinesia' in isolation has been reported in 11% of cases [44], Galloway [45] suggested that voiding dysfunction in Parkinson's disease was due largely to abnormally raised sphincter tone or 'sphincter tremor' and others have supported the view that symptoms are caused by detrusor–sphincter dyssynergia [46]. Other studies have refuted this concept arguing that, at least in male patients, symptoms are predominantly caused by detrusor hyperreflexia or bladder outlet obstruction due to prostatic hyperplasia [47]. It certainly is not clear whether patients retain voluntary sphincter control.

The overriding problem facing the clinician when investigating male patients is whether urinary symptoms are related to the effects of Parkinson's disease or whether they are caused by an existing pathological process (i.e. benign prostatic hypertrophy). Poorly sustained detrusor contraction with dyssynergic sphincter activity during voiding may be associated with Parkinson's disease but may reflect a decompensation of detrusor function as a result of long-term prostatic outflow obstruction. An incorrect interpretation of urodynamic data can therefore lead to a poor result from prostatectomy in patients with coexistent Parkinson's disease when compared to normal individuals.

One useful development in the investigation of male patients with coexistent Parkinson's disease and benign prostatic hyperplasia has been with the use of the short-acting dopamine agonist apomorphine. Subcutaneous administration of this drug allows urodynamic assessment of such patients in both 'on' and 'off' parkinsonian states, allowing the investigator to assess the underlying function of the lower urinary tract with minimal interference from the effects of Parkinson's disease [47]. Furthermore, detailed analysis of the data produced from such investigations has suggested that the predominant effect of Parkinson's disease may be on detrusor contractility rather than on urethral sphincter dysfunction [48]. Recently, it has even been suggested that associated urinary symptoms are no more prevalent than one might expect in patients of a similar age without Parkinson's disease [49]. Certainly the true effects of Parkinson's disease on lower urinary tract function are not known and the clinician and patient must be aware that surgical intervention may not improve, and indeed may worsen, urinary symptoms in this debilitating neurological disease.

Multiple sclerosis

Multiple sclerosis (MS) is associated with focal neuronal demyelination causing impairment of nerve conduction. It is predominantly a disease of the young and middle-aged and is more common in women. The symptoms caused by this process of demyelination are subject to exacerbation and remission. Because of the complex innervation of the lower urinary tract it is not surprising that urinary symptoms (frequency, urgency, urinary retention) are prevalent in MS and indeed may be the presenting features of the disease. It has been reported that 50–80% of patients with MS will complain of voiding symptoms at some time and in 10% urinary symptoms may be their sole complaint at the time of initial presentation. The urologist must therefore always harbour the possibility of MS as a cause of unexplained voiding symptoms in patients of this age group. The most common urodynamic abnormality identified in MS is that of detrusor hyperreflexia; it has been reported to occur in anything from 50 to 90% of cases [41,50,51]. Of these, up to 65% have associated detrusor–sphincter dyssynergia. Detrusor areflexia has also been reported in up to 40% of cases but these usually progress to detrusor hyperreflexia and bladder neck function in the male is generally not affected. Treatment consists of reducing filling bladder pressures with anticholinergic therapy and aiding bladder emptying with CISC.

Autonomic hyperreflexia

This condition only occurs in patients who have had complete cord transection above the 6th thoracic vertebra and results in exaggerated sympathetic activity (hypertension, bradycardia, etc.) in response to stimuli below the level of the lesion. It does not occur during the period of spinal shock following injury and the effects may be delayed for a period of up to 2 years. Detrusor–sphincter and bladder neck dyssynergia usually coexist and it must be remembered that any stimulus to the urinary tract during treatment may cause profound, life-threatening cardiovascular side effects. Any endoscopic surgery should therefore be undertaken under spinal anaesthesia with careful cardiovascular monitoring.

Cerebrovascular accidents

Detrusor–sphincter dyssynergia occasionally occurs following a cerebrovascular accident, but surgery is rarely indicated. Bladder emptying can usually be achieved with intermittent or permanent catheter drainage.

Transverse myelitis

The neurological and urinary symptoms may not stabilize in this condition for up to 2 years following the initial lesion, so that immediate intervention is contraindicated. Surgery is rarely indicated with most patients being successfully managed with CISC.

Female urethral dysfunction

The underlying pathophysiology of urinary outflow obstruction in female patients remains obscure but, at least in a proportion, there is an association with abnormal EMG activity within the urethral sphincter and lower urinary tract dysfunction [52]. This abnormal activity is typical of the type of repetitive, circuitous, self-excitatory activity that results from ephaptic excitation between muscle fibres. This activity may be responsible for inadequate relaxation of the urethral sphincter during voiding causing urinary outflow obstruction, detrusor decompensation and eventually detrusor failure and urinary retention [53]. Pseudomyotonia of the periurethral sphincter has been identified in patients with incontinence, in patients thought to have MS and in a series of children with urological symptoms and a variety of neurological conditions [54–56]. Further studies have indicated a possible association between polycystic ovarian disease and abnormal EMG activity within the urethral sphincter. An explanation for this highly localized abnormality could be that relative progesterone deficiency alters the stability of muscle cell membranes allowing circuitous excitatory pathways between muscle fibres to be established [57]. Treatment of female patients with this unusual condition usually involves empirical urethral dilatation or CISC, although further research into possible pharmacotherapy is clearly needed.

Traumatic urethral sphincter dysfunction

Direct damage to the muscle of the urethral sphincter is most commonly encountered following endoscopic resection procedures, although it may be associated with perineal trauma. The patient is usually left with a degree of cough incontinence but may be rendered totally incontinent if sphincter damage is complete. As with the case of neuropathic sphincter, urethral sphincter incompetence treatment should concentrate on the general health and suitability of each individual. AUS insertion may be indicated in some patients but simple condom drainage or catheter drainage may be more appropriate in others.

Urethral sphincter strictures are notoriously difficult to treat and are further discussed in the next section.

Urethral stricture disease

A review of the history of urological diseases and their treatment reveals that urethral strictures have been recognized as a cause of urinary symptoms since records began. The aetiology and treatment of urethral stricture disease has changed and evolved over many years. The crucial factor in deciding the most appropriate form of treatment for a stricture is based upon a knowledge of the aetiology and underlying pathology of the stricture and is discussed in detail elsewhere. In simple urodynamic terms, a urethral stricture presents an obstruction to the detrusor muscle during voiding resulting in compensatory hypertrophy of the bladder wall with trabeculation and sacculation and occasionally secondary changes in the upper tracts. The raised voiding pressures are simultaneously transmitted to the urethra proximal to the stricture causing dilatation of the urethra and blowing open of the mucous glands. In extreme cases this will accentuate any periurethral pathology and may lead to the formation of a urethral diverticulum or even a urethrocutaneous fistula [58]. The treatment of urethral strictures varies from simple urethral dilatation, optical urethrotomy, urethroplasty or, more recently, to the use of permanent metal stents [59]. These techniques are discussed in detail elsewhere.

Urethral strictures occurring within the sphincter-active area of the urethra are usually associated with previous urethral trauma, whether accidental or iatrogenic, and are notoriously difficult to treat. When such strictures result from previous bladder neck or prostatic surgery, problems of urinary incontinence are made worse because the patient cannot rely on a competent bladder neck mechanism to help urinary control. Dilatation of sphincter strictures often results in transient incontinence which resolves as the stricture narrows again. Endoscopic optical urethrotomy of the strictured sphincter must be undertaken with great care to avoid permanent sphincter damage and with each urethrotomy more scarring occurs, increasing incontinence for the patient and treatment difficulties for the urologist. Anastomotic or inlay one-stage urethroplasty is possible for treatment of sphincter strictures and more recently the use of permanent metal stents in conjunction with AUS insertion has been reported to be useful, especially in cases where the aetiology of the stricture is iatrogenic [60].

Urethral instability

The phenomenon of urethral instability is often referred to as a cause of urinary incontinence, especially in women, but is very poorly defined both on clinical and urodynamic grounds. During normal voiding the urethral sphincter relaxes several seconds prior to detrusor contraction and a similar pattern of events has been shown to occur in patients with detrusor instability [61,62].

The International Continence Society has defined urethral instability as an involuntary fall in urethral pressure resulting in urethral leakage in the absence of detrusor activity, and it has been implicated as the cause of urinary incontinence in approximately 2% of cases [63,64]. More commonly, the term is used to describe periodic falls in maximal urethral pressure which may not be related to clinically relevant incontinence. Up to 40% of urodynamically normal women demonstrate this phenomenon [65]. Urethral instability has also been shown to be associated with both sensory and urge incontinence [66]. The actual definition of this condition is therefore far from clear and its significance to normal or abnormal urinary tract function unknown.

References

1 Abrams P. The practice of urodynamics. In: Mundy AR, Stephenson TP, Wein AJ, eds. *Urodynamics: Principals, Practice and Application.* Edinburgh: Churchill Livingstone, 1984:127–41.

2 Mukerjee MG, Deshon GE Jr, Bruckman JA *et al.* Urethrovascular reflux and its significance in urology. *J Urol* 1974;**112**:608–9.

3 Bates CP. Continence and incontinence. *Ann R Coll Surg* 1971;**49**:18–35.

4 Griffiths D, von Mastrigt RV, Bosch R. Quantification of urethral resistance and bladder function during voiding, with special reference to the effects of prostatic size reduction on urethral obstruction due to benign prostatic hyperplasia. *Neurourol Urodyn* 1989;**8**:17–27.

5 Mundy AR, Stephenson TP, Wein AJ, eds. *Urodynamics: Principals, Practice and Application.* Edinburgh: Churchill Livingstone, 1984.

6 Schafer W. Urethral resistance? Urodynamic concepts of physiological and pathological bladder outlet function during voiding. *Neurourol Urodyn* 1985;**4**:161–201.

7 Yalla SV, McGuire EJ, Elbadawi A, Blavias JG. *Neurology and Urodynamics: Principals and Practice.* New York: Macmillan, 1988.

8 Webb R, Griffiths CJ, Ramsden PD, Neal DE. Measurement of voiding pressures on ambulatory monitoring: comparison with conventional cystometry. *Br J Urol* 1990;**65**:152–4.

9 Wein AJ, English WE, Whitmore KE. Office urodynamics. *Urol Clin North Am* 1988;**15**:609.

10 Wein AJ, Barrett DM. *Voiding Function and Dysfunction: a Logical and Practical Approach.* Chicago: Year Book, 1988.

11 O'Reilly PH, George NJR, Weiss RM. *Diagnostic Techniques in Urology.* Philadelphia: WB Saunders, 1990:335–51.

12 Gluck CD, Bundy AL, Fine C, Loughlin KR, Richie JP. Sonographic urethrogram: comparison to roentgenographic techniques in 22 patients. *J Urol* 1988;**140**:1404–8.

13 McAninch JW, Laing FC, Jeffrey RB Jr. Sonourethrography in the evaluation of urethral strictures: a preliminary study. *J Urol* 1988;**139**:294–7.

14 Merkle W, Wagner W. Sonography of the distal male urethra: a new diagnostic procedure for urethral strictures: results of a retrospective study. *J Urol* 1988;**140**:1409–11.

15 Fellows GJ, Cannell LB, Ravichandran G. Transrectal ultrasonography compared with voiding cystourethrography after spinal cord injury. *Br J Urol* 1987;**59**:218–21.

16 Shabsinge R, Fishman IJ, Krebs M. The use of transrectal

longitudinal real-time ultrasonography in urodynamics. *J Urol* 1987;**138**:1416–19.

17 Rifkin MD. Sonourethrography: technique for evaluation of the prostatic urethra. *Radiology* 1984;**153**:791–2.

18 Henigan HW, DuBose TJ. Sonography of the normal female urethra. *Am J Roentgenol* 1985;**145**:839–41.

19 Rickards D, Christmas TJ, Noble JG, Milroy EJG. Bladder neck dyssynergia in the male; a new finding on transrectal ultrasonography. *J Urol* 1991;**145**:369A.

20 Noble JG, Chapple CR, Rickards D *et al.* What is the pathophysiological basis of bladder neck dyssynergia? *Neurourol Urodyn* 1991;**10**:311–12.

21 Kohorn EI, Sciocia AL, Jeanty P, Hobbins JC. Ultrasound cystourethrography by perineal scanning for the assessment of female urinary incontinence. *Obstet Gynecol* 1986;**68**: 269–72..

22 Lee TG, Keller FS. Urethral diverticulum: diagnosis by ultrasound. *Am J Roentgenol* 1977;**128**:690–7.

23 Wexler JS, McGovern TP. Ultrasonography of female urethral diverticula. *Am J Roentgenol* 1980;**134**:737–41.

24 Rickards D, Noble JG, Milroy EJG, Fowler CJ. Ultrasound evaluation of the urethral sphincter in women with obstructed voiding dysfunction. *J Urol* 1992;**147**:221A.

25 Gilsanz V, Miller JH, Reid BS. Ultrasonic characteristics of posterior urethral valves. *Radiology* 1982;**145**:143–6.

26 Gaamelgaard J, Hastak SM. Ultrasonic detection of urethral calculus. *Br J Urol* 1983;**57**:589–91.

27 de Filippi G, Derchi LE, Coppi M, Biggi E. Sonographic diagnosis of urethral polyp in a child. *Paediatr Radiol* 1983;**13**:351–3.

28 Brown MC, Sutherst JR, Murray A, Richmond DH. Potential use of ultrasound in place of X-ray fluoroscopy in urodynamics. *Br J Urol* 1985;**57**:88–90.

29 Nishizawa O, Moriya I, Satoh S, Harada T, Tsushida S. A new video-urodynamics: combined ultrasonotomographic and urodynamic monitoring. *Neurourol Urodyn* 1982;**1**:295–301.

30 Perkash I, Friedland GW. Real-time gray-scale transrectal linear array ultrasonography in urodynamic evaluation. *Semin Urol* 1985;**3**:49–59.

31 Hricak H, Secaf E, Buckley DW *et al.* Female urethra: MR imaging. *Radiology* 1991;**178**:527–35.

32 El-Badawi A, Schenk EA. Dual innervation of the mammalian urinary bladder. *Am J Anat* 1966;**119**:405–28.

33 Gosling JA, Dixon JS, Lendon RG. The autonomic innervation of the human male and female bladder neck and proximal urethra. *J Urol* 1977;**118**:302–5.

34 Chapple CR, Helm CW, Blease S, Milroy EJG, Rickards D, Osbourne JL. Asymptomatic bladder neck incompetence in nulliparous females. *Br J Urol* 1989;**64**:357–9.

35 Bannister R. In: Bannister R, ed. *A Textbook of Clinical Disorders of the Autonomic Nervous System.* Oxford: Oxford University Press, 1983.

36 Kirby RS, Fowler CJ, Gosling JA, Bannister R. Vesico-urethral dysfunction in the Shy–Drager syndrome. *J Neurol Neurosurg Psychiatry* 1985;**48**:462–7.

37 Salinas JM, Berger Y, De La Roche R, Blavias JG. Urologic evaluation in the Shy–Drager syndrome. *J Urol* 1988;**135**: 741–6.

38 Berger Y, Salinas JM, Blavias JG. Urodynamic differentiation of Parkinson's disease and the Shy–Drager syndrome. *Neurourol Urodyn* 1990;**9**:117–18.

39 Mundy AR. Neuropathic vesicourethral dysfunction. In: Mundy AR, ed. *Urodynamic and Reconstructive Surgery of the Lower Urinary Tract.* Edinburgh: Churchill Livingstone, 1993:151–77.

40 Marsden C. Parkinson's disease. *Lancet* 1990;**335**:948–51.

41 Mundy AR, Blavias JG. Non-traumatic neurological disorders. In: Mundy AR, Stephenson TP, Wein AJ, eds. *Urodynamics: Principals, Practice and Applications.* New York: Churchill Livingstone, 1984:278–87.

42 Murnaghan GF. Neurogenic disorders of the bladder in Parkinsonism. *Br J Urol* 1961;**33**:403–7.

43 Andersen JT, Hebjorn S, Frimodt-Molter C *et al.* Disturbances of micturition in Parkinson's disease. *Acta Neurol Scand* 1976;**53**:161–4.

44 Pavlakis AJ, Siroky MB, Goldstein I *et al.* Neurological findings in Parkinson's disease. *J Urol* 1983;**129**:80–5.

45 Galloway NTM. Classification and diagnosis of neurogenic bladder dysfunction. *Probl Urol* 1989;**3**:1–24.

46 Fitzmaurice H, Fowler CJ, Rickards D. Micturition disturbance in Parkinson's disease. *Br J Urol* 1985;**57**:652–6.

47 Christmas TJ, Chapple CR, Lees AJ *et al.* Role of subcutaneous apomorphine in Parkinsonian voiding dysfunction. *Lancet* 1988;**2**:1451–3.

48 Noble JG, Christmas TJ, Malone-Lee J, Milroy EJG, Turner-Warwick RT. Change in detrusor contractility after apomorphine in parkinsonian voiding dysfunction. *J Urol* 1991;**145**: 361A.

49 Malone-Lee JG, Sa'adu A, Lieu PK. Evidence against the existence of a specific Parkinsonian bladder. *Neurourol Urodyn* 1993;**12**:341–2.

50 Blavias JG, Kaplan SA. Urologic dysfunction in patients with multiple sclerosis. *Semin Urol* 1988;**8**:159–66.

51 McGuire EJ, Savastano JA. Urodynamic findings and long term outcome management of patients with multiple sclerosis induced lower urinary tract dysfunction. *J Urol* 1984;**132**: 713–17.

52 Fowler CJ, Kirby RS, Harrison MJG. Decelerating burst and complex repetitive discharges in the urethral sphincter, associated with urinary retention in women. *J Neurol Neurosurg Psychiatry* 1985;**48**:1004–9.

53 Fowler CJ, Kirby RS. Electromyography of urethral sphincter in women with acute urinary retention. *Lancet* 1986;**1**:1455–7.

54 Butler WJ. Pseudomyotonia of the periurethral sphincter in women with urinary incontinence. *J Urol* 1979;**122**:838–40.

55 Potenzoni D, Juvarra G, Bettoni L, Stagha G. Pseudomyotonia of the striated urethral sphincter. *J Urol* 1983;**130**:512–13.

56 Dyro FM, Bauer SB, Hallett M, Khosholm S. Complex repetitive discharges in the external urethral sphincter in the paediatric population. *Neurourol Urodyn* 1983;**2**:39–44.

57 Fowler CJ, Christmas TJ, Chapple CR, Fitzmaurice Parkhouse H, Kirby RS, Jacobs HS. Abnormal electromyographic activity of the urethral sphincter, voiding dysfunction, and polycystic ovaries: a new syndrome? *Br Med J* 1988;**297**:1436–8.

58 Mundy AR. Urethral strictures. In: Mundy AR, ed. *Urodynamic and Reconstructive Surgery of the Lower Urinary Tract.* Edinburgh: Churchill Livingstone, 1993:183–251.

59 Milroy EJG, Chapple CR, Cooper JE *et al.* A new treatment of urethral strictures. *Lancet* 1988;**1**:1424–7.

60 Milroy EJG. Treatment of sphincter strictures using permanent urolume stent. *J Urol* 1993;**150**:1729–33.

61 Tanagho EA, Miller ER. Initiation of voiding. *Br J Urol* 1970;**42**:175–83.

62 Low JA. Urethral behavoir during the involuntary detrusor contraction. *Am J Obstet Gynecol* 1977;**128**:32–42.

63 International Continence Society. Fourth report on the standardisation of the terminology of lower urinary tract function. *Br J Urol* 1981;**53**:333–5.

64 Sand PK, Bowen LW, Ostergard DR. Uninhibited urethral relaxation: an unusual cause of incontinence. *Obstet Gynecol* 1986;**68**:645–8.

65 Tapp AJS, Cardozo LD, Versi E *et al*. The prevalence of variation in resting urethral pressure in women and its association with lower urinary tract function. *Br J Urol* 1988;**61**: 314–17.

66 Kulseng-Hanssen S. Prevelence and pattern of unstable urethral pressure in one hundred and seventy-four gynecologic patients referred for urodynamic investigation. *Am J Obstet Gynecol* 1983;**146**:895–900.

36 Benign Prostatic Hyperplasia
R.S.Kirby

Introduction

The prostate is unquestionably the organ of the body most frequently afflicted by disease in males beyond the age of 60 years, and the single most common pathological process involved is benign prostatic hyperplasia (BPH). This disorder is characterized by progressive increase in both glandular and fibromuscular tissue in the periurethral and transition zones of the prostate. Because the onset of this process is so gradual, many men fail to appreciate that anything is amiss with their lower urinary tract. Thus, they battle on stoically until obstruction is advanced or urinary retention supervenes, assuming that the associated quality of life impairment is an inevitable result of ageing.

Traditionally the remedy for BPH has been surgical, although perhaps less than 20% of symptomatic men ever actually undergo prostatectomy. In 1987 in the USA the number of transurethral resections of the prostate (TURP) performed per annum was almost 400 000, at an estimated healthcare cost of US$4.5 billion. Clearly, the economic implications of this disease are considerable and as the population in all industrialized countries continues to age, this burden seems bound to increase.

In the last few years there has been a flurry of activity directed to the development of a variety of new treatments other than surgery to relieve bladder outflow obstruction due to BPH. The driving forces behind this research include the altruistic wish to spare frail and elderly males the need for surgery, together with the perception that, with the demographic shift towards increasing longevity throughout the developed and developing world, a huge potential market exists for any product demonstrated to be both safe and effective.

A bewildering array of new pharmacological agents, implantable devices and energy-delivering machines have recently emerged, most of which have been greeted with considerable scepticism by the surgically oriented urological community. In this chapter the aim is to give an up-to-date background of the disease itself and review critically the latest developments in new treatment modalities.

Incidence

Autopsy studies have shown the first signs of histological BPH within the prostate in approximately 10% of males aged 40 years, with a steady increase in incidence of up to almost 90% in males over the age of 80 [1]. The proportion of men with palpable enlargement of the prostate is rather less and it is important to remember that histological evidence of BPH or palpable enlargement of the gland does not always correlate with clinically significant bladder outflow obstruction. In a recent study to evaluate the prevalence of the disease in Stirling, Scotland [2], using symptom evaluation, flowmetry and transrectal ultrasound (TRUS), a prevalence rate of 138 per 1000 men was found in men between 40 and 49 years, rising to 430 per 1000 men (i.e. 43%) in men beyond the age of 60 years. Of these around 50% were found to have quality of life impairment as a result of the effects of BPH on the activities of daily living [3].

Partly because BPH is so common it has been difficult to establish any definite risk factors for this disease. The primary risk factors are old age, circulating androgens, functional androgen receptors, Western diet, industrialized environment, hypertension and diabetus mellitus. BPH does seem most common in western industrial countries, especially among blacks, and the prevalence of symptomatic BPH is lowest in the Far East, particularly Japan and China. This has been assumed to be a racial phenomenon; however, it has been noted that South East Asians migrating to the USA acquire a higher rate of BPH than their counterparts remaining in South East Asia, which strongly suggests an environmental effect. A study from Japan has shown that the incidence of BPH is higher in men consuming large amounts of milk than in those with a low vegetable intake. Certain yellow vegetables and other elements of the Japanese diet, including soya beans, are known to contain phyto-oestrogens and it has been postulated that these may exert some protective effect [4]. It has also been suggested, but with little hard epidemiological evidence to corroborate it, that the incidence of BPH may be affected by other associated diseases. It has been proposed that BPH is more likely to develop in patients with insulin-dependent diabetes mellitus due to the effect of exogenous insulin-promoting androgen activity, which in turn stimulates prostatic growth [5]. Hypertension and cardiovascular disease have also been proposed as risk factors in BPH, although little firm evidence and no clear explanation has been offered for these associations.

Underlying molecular mechanisms

Despite the frequency of its occurrence, we still have surprisingly little knowledge of the fundamental causes of BPH at the cellular and molecular levels. Two factors, however, seem absolute prerequisites: (i) the presence of dihydrotestosterone (DHT), and (ii) an ageing factor.

The prostate requires the presence of adequate levels of circulating androgen in order to develop and grow [6]. The decapeptide luteinizing hormone-releasing hormone (LHRH) is released in a pulsatile fashion from the hypothalamus and stimulates the pituitary to secrete luteinizing hormone (LH). LH then acts directly on Leydig cells within the testes stimulating them in turn to secrete 95% of the 6–7 mg of testosterone produced in the body each day. The remaining 5% of daily testosterone production is either directly synthesized by the adrenal gland or produced by peripheral metabolism.

In the plasma, 98% of circulating testosterone is bound to a variety of proteins. The most important of these are human serum albumin and sex hormone-binding globulin (SHBG) [7]. As a consequence, only 2% or so of free testosterone is available to enter prostatic cells and it does so by a process of simple diffusion. Once within the cell, testosterone is rapidly metabolized by a series of prostatic enzymes. Over 90% is irreversibly converted to the major prostatic androgen, DHT, by a nicotinamide adenosine

dinucleotide phosphate (NADP)-dependent enzyme localized predominantly on the nuclear membrane and named 5α-reductase. The metabolite DHT is considerably more potent as an androgen within the prostate than testosterone itself, by virtue of its greater affinity for androgen receptors located within the nucleus. Binding of DHT to these androgen receptors produces a conformational change in the chromatin that facilitates transcription of specific sequences of DNA into mRNA. This sets off a complex but orderly series of events including signal-transducing protein synthesis, mRNA production and finally DNA synthesis and cell replication [8] (Fig. 36.1).

Ageing has a gradual but profound effect on both testicular function and androgen metabolism. Hypothalamic pituitary responsiveness is maintained — LH levels remain within normal limits and there is no loss of pulsatile diurnal variation in the ageing male — however, there is a decreased responsiveness of the testes to bioactive LH. In addition, there is an increased binding capacity of SHBG due to an increase in free plasma oestradiol levels, which stimulates synthesis of binding proteins by the liver. The consequence of these changes is an age-related decrease in free testosterone (Fig. 36.2), while free oestradiol levels are maintained, producing an increase of up to 40% in the ratio of free oestradiol to free testosterone.

Following the separate but simultaneous demonstrations by Bruchovsky and Wilson [9] and Anderson and Liao [10] that DHT is the major intracellular androgen in the prostate, several workers reported a three- or fourfold increase in DHT levels in BPH tissue compared with controls [11]. However, subsequent work by Walsh *et al.* [12] has cast doubt on these observations. Walsh's group in Baltimore demonstrated that differences between BPH and normal control tissue reflected the fact that the control

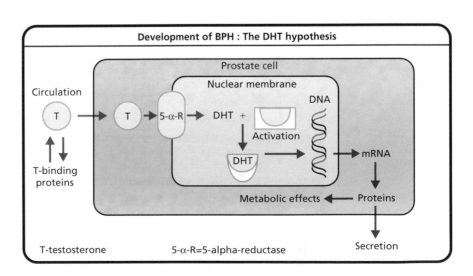

Fig. 36.1 Testosterone is metabolized to DHT within the cell and this more active androgen binds to androgen-receptor elements in the nucleus.

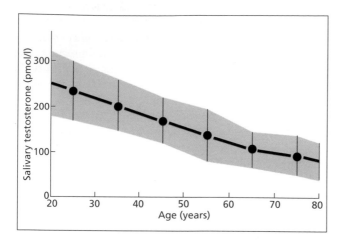

Fig. 36.2 Circulating testosterone levels decline with age.

material was obtained at autopsy, while BPH tissues were all freshly resected surgical specimens. Subsequently, it was shown that incubation of prostatic tissues at 37°C for several hours itself results in a marked decrease of intracellular DHT levels as a result of cell autolysis.

Although DHT levels may not be supranormal in BPH, 5α-reductase activity has been demonstrated to be greater in BPH tissue compared with controls. Moreover, there is evidence to suggest that androgen receptor levels are elevated in BPH [13], although the accurate measurement of these is still dogged by methodological problems. The sum of these changes may make the ageing prostate progressively suprasensitive to androgen stimulation.

In the dog, oestrogens have also been shown to be involved in induction of the androgen receptor, and the canine prostate contains abundant quantities of high-affinity oestrogen receptors [14]. Experimental hyperplasia of the prostate in young castrated dogs cannot be induced by androgens alone, but does occur following administration of oestradiol and DHT in combination [15]. In humans, however, although oestrogen receptors are present in BPH tissue and are most numerous in the nuclei of stromal cells, their levels are lower than those found in other peripheral tissues. As a consequence, although the alterations in the oestrogen:testosterone ratio associated with ageing remains an attractive hypothesis for the causation of BPH, additional factors almost certainly play a role.

BPH tissue contains a considerable amount of fibro-muscular stroma, and Franks and Barton [16] were the first to suggest that epithelial cells may be stimulated in some way by prostatic stroma to induce gowth. This has been termed 'epithelial reawakening'. Subsequently, Cunha [17,18], in an impressive series of experiments, recombined isolated mouse urogenital sinus mesenchyme (the embryonic prostatic stroma) with adult mouse bladder epithelium and transplanted these combined tissues

beneath the capsule of the kidney of the nude mouse. With the testes intact the epithelial cells differentiated and developed into mouse prostatic epithelium, an effect not seen when the nude mice were castrated. When similar recombinations were made using the same urogenital sinus mesenchyme, but epithelium from mice with testicular feminization syndrome (i.e. the tissue was deficient in androgen receptors), the epithelial tissue still differentiated and grew in intact nude mice. No development of prostatic epithelium occurred, however, if embryonic stroma from mice with testicular feminization syndrome was combined with normal bladder epithelium.

These experiments clearly demonstrated the differentiation and development of prostatic epithelium are indirectly controlled by androgens, through androgen-dependent mediators of stromal origin. Extensive research is currently directed towards the identification of these stimulatory mediators—paracrine growth factors produced by stromal cells which exert an influence on the physiological process within the epithelial cells—as they could clearly hold the key to the abnormal growth processes that characterize BPH.

The stromal mediators involved in the paracrine, and possibly autocrine, control of growth within the prostate are still to be identified conclusively. However, results from a number of institutions have confirmed that neither testosterone nor DHT has much effect on prostatic epithelial cell growth in culture. By contrast, epidermal growth factor (EGF) [19], insulin-like growth factor (IGF) and fibroblast growth factor (FGF) [20] have all been shown to have increased gene expression in BPH and exert a marked mitogenic effect on prostatic epithelial cells *in vitro*. By contrast, transforming growth factor β (TGF-β) may inhibit mitotic activity and thereby modulate the effects of other growth factors [21]. In addition, EGF receptors, which also have affinity for TGF-α, have been clearly demonstrated to be localized on the cell membrane of prostatic epithelial cells.

To summarize, the precise causes of BPH are still enigmatic and doubtless there is an interplay of a number of factors. Some of these have been identified: ageing is a prerequisite, as is the presence of the 5α-reduced form of testosterone, DHT. While DHT levels are probably not supranormal in BPH tissue, 5α-reductase activity and the density of androgen receptors may be significantly increased. Increasing oestrogens levels in later life may also play a role either by inducing androgen receptors or by decreasing the rate of epithelial or stromal cell death. Autocrine or paracrine growth factors may provide the mechanism for the stromal–epithelial interactions that may result in BPH nodule formation and slow, progressive bladder outlet obstruction. We can expect further elucidation of this complex but fascinating area over the next few years.

Histopathology

The microscopic features of BPH may be identified within the human prostate as early as the fourth to fifth decade of life. The characteristic changes in BPH are not simply an increase in cell population, but changes in the architecture of ducts and acini. Nodular hyperplasia is the characteristic histological feature in BPH and arises in two zones, the transition zone and the periurethral zone (Fig. 36.3). In most cases there are both diffuse and nodular components to transition zone enlargement. The diffuse enlargement appears to be an almost universal feature of the ageing process and increases gradually from 40 years onwards. The development of nodular hyperplasia is concentrated within the transition zone near the distal end of the bladder neck smooth muscle. Transition zone hyperplasia consists of large amounts of glandular tissue which arises by budding and branching from pre-existing prostatic ducts. These glands are surrounded by a variable amount of fibromuscular stroma. This type of hyperplastic proliferation is

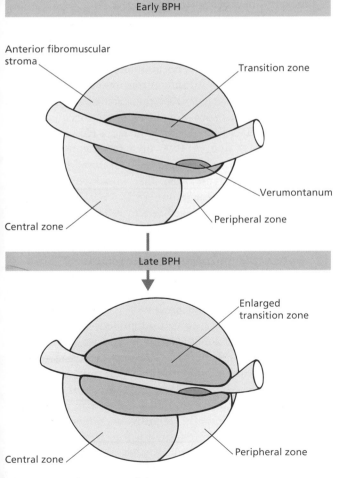

Transition zone hyperplasia in sagittal section

Early BPH

Anterior fibromuscular stroma

Transition zone

Verumontanum

Central zone

Peripheral zone

Late BPH

Enlarged transition zone

Central zone

Peripheral zone

Fig. 36.3 Zonal anatomy of the prostate.

a very unusual finding in either normal or diseased tissues in the adult human, and it has been suggested that such anomalous activity by stromal cells results from reversion to embryonic behaviour, perhaps through local stimulation by growth factors.

In addition, nodular hyperplasia arising within the periurethral zone may lead to a mass of tissue located dorsally at the bladder neck, so-called median lobe enlargement, but this is not usually the major component of bladder outflow obstruction in BPH. The majority of periurethral nodules consist mainly of stroma with an abundant pale ground substance interspersed with collagen fibres, but little or no glandular tissue.

Clinical features

One of the more puzzling featuers of BPH is the lack of a clear correlation between prostatic size and the presence or severity of outflow obstruction. There are probably several explanations for this: (i) bladder neck obstruction can occur in the absence of any prostatic enlargement whatsoever; and (ii) BPH is a non-uniform asymmetrical process and the enlargement of certain critical portions of the gland may be more important in producing outflow obstruction than others. Middle lobe enlargement, for example, may result in severe ball-valve type obstruction, while the rest of the gland remains relatively unenlarged. In addition, the degree of obstruction produced by transition zone hyperplasia may reflect the relative proportions of smooth muscle to glandular tissue within the gland. Prostatic smooth muscle is sympathetically innervated and its tone may therefore fluctuate with varying levels of neural activity. In general, however, for any given individual, progressive transition zone enlargement is associated with a gradual reduction in urine flow and the eventual development of symptoms and secondary effects of bladder outflow obstruction.

Symptoms

A patient's description of his symptoms are always important but caution should be exercised in their interpretation in relation to BPH. Diseases other than BPH may result in symptoms suggestive of bladder outflow obstruction. In addition, the onset of prostatic obstruction is so gradual that deterioration of urinary flow is often poorly appreciated by the patient. Objective confirmation of urine flow by means of uroflowmetry is therefore mandatory. Of late there has been an increasing vogue for the use of symptom scores [22,23], the latest of which, devised by a subcommittee of the American Urological Association (AUA) and now referred to as the international prostate symptom score (IPSS), also appraises the 'bothersomeness' of these symptoms (see Fig. 1.3, p.7). The symptoms associated with bladder outflow obstruction due to BPH are those of frequency, urgency and nocturia, associated with difficulty initiating micturition, a reduced urine flow and some post-micturition dribbling. Traditionally these symptoms have been subdivided into irritative and obstructive. It is easy to see that the obstructive symptoms are a reflection of the reduced distensibility of the prostatic urethra resulting in increasing impedance to urinary flow. The explanation for the irritative symptoms, however, seems more complex. Urodynamic evaluation in patients with BPH has consistently demonstrated a loss of bladder compliance and the presence of unstable detrusor contractions during filling in of up to 70% or so of patients [24]. Like other smooth muscle systems in the body, the detrusor responds to obstruction by smooth muscle hypertrophy and connective tissue infiltration [25]. In addition, there is a significantly reduced density of acetyl-cholinesterase-containing (presumptive parasympathetic) nerves; all of these developments may result in progressively decreased detrusor contractility.

Experimentally induced obstruction in the pig bladder has been shown to result in detrusor instability, and smooth muscle strips from these animals show an increased sensitivity to exogenously applied agonists, but a reduced sensitivity to intramural nerve stimulation [26]. These results suggest that secondary detrusor instability seen in bladder outflow obstruction may be partly the result of post-junctional supersensitivity secondary to partial denervation. Whether this supersensitivity occurs on the basis of an increased density of muscarinic receptors, or an alteration of the membrane potentials of smooth muscle cells themselves has yet to be established [27].

Physical examination

Although it has been accepted for some years that there is little correlation between prostatic size on digital rectal examination (DRE) and the degree of bladder outflow obstruction, it is interesting that the Baltimore Longitudinal Ageing Study [28] found a clear positive association between the presence of a palpably enlarged prostate on DRE and the risk of subsequently undergoing a prostatectomy. As already mentioned, however, not all men with a benignly enlarged prostate suffer outflow obstruction. It is clear, though, from TRUS examination that transition zone hyperplasia can occur without much overall enlargement of the prostate. In this context, it is of interest that Neal et al. [29] have found that patients with larger prostates fare better after TURPs than those with smaller glands. In addition, of course, diffuse induration within the gland or the discovery of a palpable prostatic nodule, either of which suggest the presence of a prostatic carcinoma, or a palpably distended bladder are important physical signs which need to be detected on physical examination, as they may influence critically an individual patient's management.

Investigations

Serology including prostate-specific antigen determination

Few would argue that urine microscopy, a full blood count, and urea, electrolyte and creatinine estimation is essential in the work-up of a patient with BPH, but the value of prostate-specific antigen (PSA) determination in this context, especially in older patients (>75 years), is more controversial. PSA values are, to some extent, a reflection of the volume of prostatic epithelium present and values above 4 ng/ml (Hybritech Tandem R assay) are common in BPH. Several investigators suggest that around 25–30% of patients with BPH have PSA values above the upper limit of normal, i.e. above 4 ng/ml [30]. Stamey et al. [31] have reported that serum PSA values rise in direct proportion to the volume of BPH tissue by 0.31 (±0.25) ng/ml per g of hyperplastic tissue. However, this does not take into account the marked variation in epithelial content between the prostates of different individuals.

A markedly raised PSA value, however, especially in a patient with a smaller prostate, should clearly alert the physician to the possibility of an occult A1 (T1A) or, more importantly, A2 (T1B) adenocarcinoma of the prostate. A careful TRUS with multiple ultrasound-guided biopsies, which include specimens from the transition zone, should be performed. The exact probability of a positive biopsy in this situation is still a matter of debate. However, recent studies of the value of PSA in screening for prostatic adenocarcinoma by Catalona et al. [32] found the positive biopsy rates in patients with PSA values between 4 and 10 ng/ml to be 22% (i.e. some 78% probably had a PSA which was moderately raised due to BPH). In the group of patients with PSA values greater than 10 ng/ml, 67% were found to have adenocarcinoma present on prostatic biopsy. The current recommendation is that younger patients (<75 years) with a PSA above 4 ng/ml, and especially those in whom there is a discrepancy between the PSA value and the volume of the gland on TRUS examination, should undergo systematic ultrasound-guided biopsy of the prostate to exclude adenocarcinoma. In cases of doubt, an alternative to an immediate biopsy is a period of 6–12 months' observation and repeat PSA determination. Carter et al. [33] have reported that a sequential rise of PSA of more than 20% or 0.75 ng/ml over 1 year may indicate the presence of a clinically significant adenocarcinoma; however, more data are required before recommendations can be made about the clinical value of the so-called PSA slope. The ratio of free to total PSA may also be helpful in distinguishing BPH from prostate cancer.

Uroflowmetry evaluation

Uroflowmetry is now so readily available that it is surprising that it has not become universal in the assessment of patients with prostatic obstruction. It is simple to perform, non-invasive and the apparatus is inexpensive when compared with, say, ultrasound equipment. Its disadvantages lie in a dependence on a voided volume of more than 150 ml, which is sometimes difficult for some patients with BPH to produce, and some variation between voids. In this context the use of the Siroky nomogram to correct for voided volume is sometimes helpful [34]. There is also a susceptibility to artefact from abdominal straining and movement. In spite of this, however, Abrams et al. [24] have shown that patients with a maximum flow rate below 10 ml/s are usually demonstrably obstructed if urodynamic evaluation is subsequently performed, while those with a maximum flow rate above 15 ml/s are generally unobstructed. Those patients in the 'grey zone' with maximum flows between 10 and 15 ml/s may be either obstructed or unobstructed and in cases of doubt there can be no substitute for pressure–flow urodynamics with or without radiology. Non-invasive uroflowmetry also provides the most effective way of either evaluating a patient during a period of watchful waiting or monitoring response to treatment. Increase in maximum or mean flows of more than 100% are common after prostatectomy and improvement in flow rates are usually mirrored by clinical and symptomatic response, unless detrusor instability persists.

Transabdominal ultrasound

Another important investigation available for the evaluation of BPH is the estimation of post-micturition residual volume, although it has been demonstrated by Bruskevitz et al. [35] that there is also a considerable coefficient of variation in this parameter. Protagonists of the intravenous urogram as a means of assessing residual urine have argued that it provided useful information on this count, but the forced diuresis resulting from the administration of intravenous contrast and the pressure to complete the study in order to vacate the radiograph room may often have produced erroneous results. In fact transabdominal ultrasound provides higher quality information about the residual urine volume and also assesses bladder wall hypertrophy and the presence of diverticula formation. In addition, intravesicular extension of the prostate (i.e. middle lobe enlargement) may be visualized, and with only moderate extra effort both kidneys may be scanned to include upper tract dilatation or other coincidental renal pathology. Although there is a statistically poor correlation between the value of residual urine volume and other urodynamic parameters of

obstruction or the outcome of surgery, a large residual urine volume (>300 ml) present on more than one evaluation suggests impending detrusor decompensation and is a risk factor for acute retention and should therefore prompt consideration of early surgical intervention.

Transrectal ultrasonography

A TRUS of the prostate using a 7 mHz biplanar probe is now increasingly being used by radiologists and urologists in the evaluation of patients with BPH. Apart from magnetic resonance imaging (MRI), it currently provides the most accurate means of measuring prostatic volume and can also demonstrate the true extent of transition zone and periurethral enlargement. Young men do not demonstrate sonographically well-defined central glandular anatomy until the end of the fourth decade, but after that transition zone adenomas develop in the majority of people with an estimated growth rate of 0.2 ml/year. The periurethral zone may also increase by an estimated 1.5% per year. Drach et al. [36] have reported an annual decrease in the mean flow rate of 0.2 ml/s per year which may be a reflection of this progressive transition zone hyperplasia. In addition, the peripheral zone of the prostate can also be scanned carefully for evidence of prostatic carcinomas, which, it should be remembered, in this location may not be sampled at TURP nor biopsies taken under ultrasound guidance.

Magnetic resonance imaging

MRI of the prostate, although often employed in the diagnosis and staging of prostate cancer, has until recently received scant attention as a means of evaluation of BPH. In fact the resolution achieved, especially with the new endorectal MRI coils, may be greater than TRUS and some of the images currently being produced of the prostate and seminal vesicles are spectacular. BPH increases the conspicuousness of the prostate on MRI; however, the MRI appearance depends on the ratio of glandular tissue to fibromuscular stroma. The peripheral zone therefore has a higher signal intensity than the central zone on T_2 imaging (Fig. 36.4). Precise information is available concerning prostate volumes and this has a lower coefficient of variability than measurement by TRUS. In addition, the degree of transition zone hyperplasia and the presence of coincidental peripheral zone adenocarcinomas may be assessed. It is doubtful, however, because of cost constraints, that this imaging modality will become widely used for the routine clinical assessment of patients with BPH; none the less, it is currently valuable as a research tool, especially for the evaluation of drug effects on the prostate.

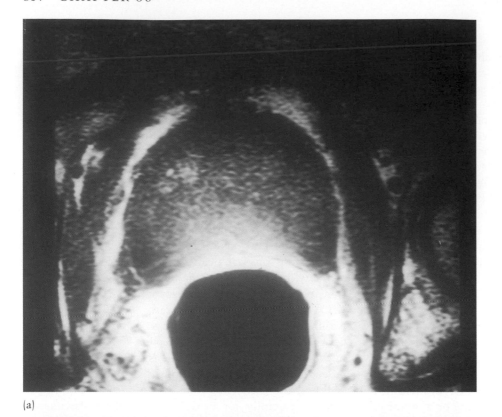

(a)

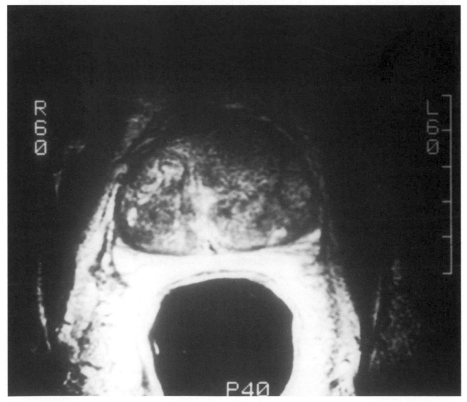

(b)

Fig. 36.4 MRI images of the prostate: (a) T_1- and (b) T_2-weighted images.

Urodynamics

Pressure–flow urodynamics with or without simultaneous vesicourethography during voiding still provides the gold standard in terms of determining the presence of bladder outlet obstruction due to BPH. While few would argue that it is essential in the assessment of complex cases (i.e. those with clinical BPH and urological disorders such as Parkinson's disease or multiple system atrophy), more controversy exists around the question of whether this investigation should be employed in routine patients with clinical BPH. Those advocating urodynamics to evaluate BPH on a routine basis point out that non-invasive uroflowmetry cannot distinguish high-pressure/low-flow obstruction from low-pressure/low-flow detrusor failure. In a recent study 24% of patients awaiting TURP were not judged to be truly obstructed when formal urodynamics was performed [37]. In addition, it has been estimated that up to 7% of patients presenting with symptomatic BPH have flow rates within the normal range. These patients have high-pressure/high-flow obstruction and often have a good outcome from surgery [38].

The critical question is whether or not the wider use of routine urodynamics will in fact improve the eventual outcomes of therapies for BPH such as transurethral surgery. Although it has been argued that a low voiding pressure may be a contraindication for prostatectomy, Neal et al. [29] were unable in a retrospective evaluation to clearly identify any urodynamic parameter that would predict a poor outcome from TURP. Jensen et al. [39] came to similar conclusions. In reality, patients with low-pressure/low-flow urodynamic findings, including many of those with chronic urinary retention, may respond well to reduction in outflow resistance by means of a TURP. At the moment, the case for more widespread use of invasive urodynamic testing must be regarded as unproven. The problem may lie in the fact that simultaneous voiding pressures and flow rates are not always a good measure of outflow obstruction, especially once detrusor decompensation has begun to develop. More sophisticated measurements of pressure–flow relationships, dynamic and mechanical resistance factors, detrusor work and contractility calculated from pressure–flow plots or derived from on-line computer analysis appear more valuable in this context and may merit wider use [40], perhaps with suprapubic placement of vesical pressure measuring lines, which allow repeated recordings of voiding in the same patient.

Differential diagnosis

A number of different conditions may mimic a diagnosis of BPH (Table 36.1). Irritative symptoms, such as frequency, nocturia and urgency of micturition, also occur in conditions other than BPH. Nocturia may be reported by patients with cardiac or renal conditions and these can be excluded at the outset by the measurement of nightly urine volumes by means of a voided volume diary chart. If irritative symptoms are present without an enlarged prostate or the presence of a residual volume, the

Table 36.1 The differential diagnoses of benign prostatic hyperplasia (BPH) and their related clinical features.

Conditions	Clinical features						
	Slow stream	Hesitancy	Nocturial frequency	Urgency	Haematuria	Urinary retention	Residual urine
BPH	+	+	+	(+)	(+)	(+)	+
Prostatitis, prostatodynia	(+)	–	(+)	(+)	–	(+)	–
Prostate cancer		(+)	(+)	(+)	(+)	–	+
Bladder neck constriction	+	+	+	+	–	(+)	+
Neuropathic or unstable bladder	(+)	–	+	+	–	–	(+)
Bladder ureteral stones	(+)	(+)	+	+	+	(+)	(+)
Bladder cancer	–	–	(+)	(+)	+	–	–
Cystitis	(+)	–	+	+	(+)	+	–
Urethral stricture	+	–	–	–	–	(+)	

+, usually present; (+), occasionally present; –, usually not present.

possibility of a neuropathic bladder, idiopathic detrusor instability, urinary tract infection or bladder stones must be considered, together with other conditions such as prostatitis and carcinoma *in situ* of the bladder.

Neuropathic involvement of the bladder is much more common in an age group likely to be affected by BPH than is currently recognized. Such conditions may be the result of subclinical cerebrovascular disease, central prolapse of an intervertebral disc, diabetes mellitus or neurological disorders such as multiple sclerosis, amyotrophic lateral sclerosis, Parkinson's disease or multiple system atrophy. Irritation caused by bladder stones or urinary tract infection must also be excluded.

Haematuria not uncommonly occurs in BPH as a result of bleeding from an enlarged and vascular prostate. If haematuria is present then transitional cell carcinoma or renal tumours must be carefully excluded by investigations including urinary cytology, intravenous urography and cystourethroscopy with biopsy. Urinary tract malignancy is less likely, however, if the bleeding occurs in the initial phase of micturition with a clear urine towards the end of voiding. Initial haematuria in combination with an enlarged prostate is usually the result of BPH.

The presence of residual urine after micturition may be the result of a number of conditions, including prostatic obstruction, but may also be due to weak or absent detrusor contractions. The differential diagnosis that often poses the most difficulty is urethral stricture; although this can be detected by means of retrograde urethrography or cystourethroscopy, such procedures will only have been performed if the condition is suspected. Hence, the diagnosis is sometimes made only once surgery is underway. Obviously, therefore, a urethral stricture is more likely to be misdiagnosed in the case of non-surgical management of BPH.

Management

History

The role of the prostate in causing infravesical obstruction and bladder dysfunction remained unappreciated for many centuries. Although Hippocrates is credited with the observation that 'bladder disorders are cured with difficulty in old men' there is little to suggest that he was in fact aware of the existence of the prostate itself. The term prostate is derived from the writings of Herophilus of Alexandria, from the word *prohistani* (to stand in front of), referring to its relation to the bladder.

The mainstay of treatment for advanced prostatic obstruction for more than 3000 years, right up to the final decades of the nineteenth century was intermittent catheterization. Alternative medical remedies also abounded including, among countless others, hemlock, ergot, strychnine, local heat, the application of perineal poultices and prostatic massage; but their main benefit must have been as a placebo. The dominant misconception through these early years was that chronic urinary retention was a condition in its own right due to an 'atony' of the bladder, rather than secondary to outlet obstruction. This theory could not be tested until the means became available for surgical removal of the obstructing tissue to determine whether or not the ability to void might be restored.

Selection for surgery

The indications for prostatectomy can be divided into absolute and relative. Absolute indications include repeated episodes of acute retention unresponsive to medical treatment and chronic retention due to prostatic obstruction with upper tract dilatation and renal impairment. Relative indications include severe symptoms, repeated haematuria due to BPH, recurrent urinary infections, large diverticula and bladder stone formation. Although the vast majority of patients will now be considered able to tolerate the regional or general anaesthesia necessary for prostatic surgery there are still some contraindications. The most common indication for surgery is moderate to severe symptoms, and ideally a symptom score should be obtained together with objective evaluation of uroflow and residual urine volume before a decision to operate is taken. Clearly, the greater the symptom score and associated bother factor, the lower the mean and maximum flow rate and the greater the post-void residual volume, the more likely the urologist will be to recommend surgical rather than medical relief of outflow obstruction.

Surgical procedures

Open prostatectomy

The surgical approach to the prostate was for many years adversely influenced by Hippocrates and Galen who declared that surgical opening of the bladder was invariably fatal and should always be avoided. Once this historical taboo was surmounted the numbers of patients treated by this means increased through the early years of the twentieth century and in modern practice there is an extremely low rate of morbidity and mortality. The first formal open prostatectomy was probably performed by WJ Bellfield in Chicago in 1886 via the transvesical route, although Magill in Leeds and Billroth in Austria also performed a similar procedure around this time. The operation was often complicated by haemorrhage and wound infection and resulted in considerable mortality in the early days. However, the technique was popularized in the UK by Sir Peter Freyer in 1901.

Open prostatectomy as a treatment for BPH is now mainly indicated for very large glands weighing in excess of 80–100 g. In fact only about 5% or less fall into this category, the remainder being effectively dealt with by TURP. Other relative indications for open prostatectomy include fixed adduction of the hips due to osteoarthritis or severe urethral stricture disease preventing urethral access for TURP. The best approach for this operation is via a transverse abdominal incision; the retropubic space being developed without opening the peritoneum.

Retropubic prostatectomy

Retropubic prostatectomy was developed by Terence Millin in 1945 [41]. The advantages of this procedure over the transvesical operation are: (i) that it gives a more direct approach to the prostate; (ii) by virtue of the fact that the bladder is not opened, vesicocutaneous urinary fistulas are less likely to occur; and (iii) suprapubic drainage can be avoided. In addition, the blood loss is less because better haemostatis can be achieved. The prostate is approached through a transverse incision in the anterior prostatic capsule after ligation of the overlying venous plexus. The adenoma is enucleated with a finger, and the prostatic urethra is divided under direct vision of the apex while care is taken to avoid injury to the distal and urethral sphincter. Any small tags of tissue are excised and a wedge of tissue is also removed from the posterior bladder neck, with care being taken not to injure the ureteric orifices. The trigonal mucosa is then mobilized distally to partially fill the defect and an irrigating urethral catheter is passed. The prostatic capsule is closed with a continuous absorbable suture and the catheter can usually be removed after 48–72 h, providing bleeding has stopped.

Transurethral prostatectomy

Technically the first transurethral resection of the prostate could be described as being performed by Ambrose Pare when he used an intraurethral sound to remove 'carnosities' from the prostatic urethra as early as the sixteenth century. However, it was not until the direct vision resectoscope was developed in the early twentieth century, initially by Reed and MacCarthy in the USA, that resutls improved; although problems with illumination and haemostasis made early procedures technically demanding. Perhaps the greatest step forward in the development of endoscopic urological surgery was the invention of Henry Hopkins of the rod lens for the endoscope [42].

The precise technique for TURP varies between surgeons. It is usual practice to resect the middle lobe initially, to facilitate irrigation flow. Care should be taken, however, not to undermine the bladder neck for fear of extravasation of irrigant. The lateral lobes are then resected sequentially, starting at the 10 o'clock position. This allows the lateral lobes to be dislocated dorsally from which they are easily resected piecemeal. Finally, the anterior prostate is resected and the remaining apical tissue cleared down to the level of the verumontanum. It is important to avoid lateral capsular and bladder neck perforation since this may lead to the TURP syndrome and also possibly result in damage to the neurovascular bundles posterolaterally. Scrupulous attention to haemostatis also reduces the morbidity of the procedure. At the end of the operation an irrigating catheter is passed and irrigation of the bladder is continued for 12–24 h postoperatively. The catheter is usually removed after 48 h.

Transurethral incision of the prostate

In patients with a small fibrous prostate in whom there is little or no projection of the middle lobe into the bladder or of the lateral lobes into the prostatic urethra, a full-thickness electrotome or laser incision may be made between the trigone and the verumontanum and the 7 o'clock position. If the incision is deep enough, the prostate will spring open and many cases will not require full prostatic resection. The procedure requires shorter hospitalization than TURP and is associated with a lower blood loss and a reduced incidence of bladder neck stenosis. Only about 20% or less of patients will suffer retrograde ejaculation after transurethral incision of the prostate compared with more than 50% after a resection, although patients should be counselled of this risk preoperatively. However, a significant number of patients undergoing bladder neck incision subsequently require a transurethral resection of the lateral lobes of the prostate, but this may be many years after the original operation.

Laser prostatectomy

Recently, a number of investigators [43–45] have developed a technique of transurethral laser ablation of the prostate. The use of lasers in the treatment of superficial bladder cancer and for the fragmentation of ureteric calculi has turned out to be more limited in application than originally anticipated. In the prostate, however, the protagonists of laser prostatectomy argue that the technique can obviate the troublesome bleeding that sometimes occur with TURP. The laser delivery systems involve deflecting the neodymium–yttrium aluminium garnet (YAG) laser beam through 90° to allow laser coagulation of laterally placed adenoma tissue. Three main categories of device have been developed.

1 The transurethral laser incision of the prostate (TULIP) probe which incorporates transurethral ultrasound imaging. This has now been abandoned.
2 The cystoscopically applied probes for visual laser

ablation of the prostate (VLAP) which are less complex and can be simply passed down the working channel of an ordinary cystoscope.

3 Interstitial laser devices.

Currently, the recommended dose of neodymium–YAG laser energy is 60 W for a total of 4 min in four separate locations and this is said to produce sufficient laser coagulation to result in a cavity which develops over the next 8–12 weeks. Early results suggest that the beneficial effects take a longer time to develop than after a TURP, dysuria may be troublesome for some months and the final flow rate is probably not quite equivalent to that achieved by TURP. However, clearly the technique is still being refined and the prospects for further improvement look promising.

Outcome following prostatectomy

Considering that the operation of prostatectomy is now over 100 years old it is surprising that we still have so little information about the outcomes that can be expected from these procedures. Flow rate improvement after either TURP or retropubic prostatectomy is generally dramatic, with enhancement of maximum and mean flow values of more than 100% being usual. Longer term follow-up, however, reveals some slight reduction in flow rate as the prostatic cavity shrinks, but the peak uroflow usually remains greater than 15 ml/s and this is associated with normalization of voiding pressures and reduction of the post-micturition residual volume. In spite of this not all patients benefit symptomatically from prostatectomy. Bruskevitz et al. [46] noted in a follow-up study of patients over 3 years after TURP, that at 1 year 84% of patients had symptomatic improvement; however, after 3 years only 75% remained improved. Nearly 10% of patients developed a bladder neck stenosis and this was more common in those with smaller prostates. In another study, Roos et al. [47] in a retrospective series of nearly 4500 patients followed up for at least 8 years, found a substantially higher incidence of reoperation (20%) in patients undergoing TURP, compared with those subjected to open prostatectomy (10%). Their data also suggested that there was an increased risk of later cardiovascular mortality in the TURP group compared with those undergoing open prostatectomy (relative risk 1.45). Although the reason for this is unclear, and differences in co-morbidity of patients selected for the two procedures in this restrospective study cannot be excluded, the AUA felt that the study raised sufficient question marks to embark upon a prospective study to assess the validity of these findings and compare TURP with other alternative therapies such as balloon dilatation and α-blockers.

Complications of prostatectomy

Although prostatectomy is a highly effective means of relieving infravesical obstruction and the morbidity is generally low, a number of complications may arise. Mebust et al. [48] have reviewed the immediate and postoperative complications of TURP in 3885 patients. The major complications encountered are discussed below.

Haemorrhage

One of the major causes of morbidity and mortality particularly associated with TURP as well as with retropubic prostatectomy is perioperative and postoperative haemorrhage. Preoperative assessment is important to prevent this complication. Although a preoperative clotting screen is not indicated in every patient undergoing TURP, any history of bleeding diathesis must be thoroughly investigated prior to surgery.

Anticoagulation therapy is only a relative contraindication to TURP. Providing that it is safe to temporarily discontinue therapy, warfarin can be stopped and more easily reversible systemic heparanization commenced. Aspirin is now widely used as a preventive measure for cardiovascular diseases and this should be discontinued at least 2 weeks prior to prostatectomy, since it may cause at least a twofold increase in perioperative and postoperative blood loss, and occasionally severe haemorrhage.

Transurethral resection syndrome

The transurethral resection (TUR) syndrome is characterized by neurological symptoms such as confusion and coma, bradycardia, shortness of breath, cyanosis, oliguria and acute hypertension. The aetiology of these disturbances is now thought to be due to the absorbtion of irrigating fluid through the veins within the prostatic capsule and from the extraperitoneal space. Absorption of the irrigation leads to hypervolaemia and dilutional hyponatraemia. In addition, absorbed glycine is metabolized to form free ammonia which is a potent neurotoxin. Glycine itself may cross the blood–brain barrier where it can act as an inhibitory neurotransmitter.

The TUR syndrome is fortunately uncommon with an incidence of less than 0.5%. It is more likely to occur after lengthy resections of large adenomas and for this reason it is generally recommended that resection should be discontinued after 60–90 min or earlier if extensive capsular penetration or open venous sinuses become apparent. The amount of fluid absorbed during TURP is related to the pressure of the irrigation solution and this should be kept to a minimum by lowering the height of the glycine bag throughout the procedure. If promptly recognized and treated TUR syndrome usually has no long-term sequelae.

Incontinence

Urinary incontinence may occur after TURP but the incidence is fortunately low. In the early postoperative period this may be due to overwhelming detrusor instability, which usually resolves spontaneously. If incontinence persists and occurs at moments when intra-abdominal pressure is raised (i.e. stress incontinence), this suggests that the distal sphincter mechanism has been damaged at the time of TURP. Endoscopy and video urodynamics at 6 months postoperatively may confirm the diagnosis and the best treatment in the longer term may involve insertion of an artificial urinary sphincter around the bulbar or membranous urethra (see Chapter 39). The results in these cases are usually satisfactory, but every effort should be made to avoid this complication by careful training of residents and scrupulous avoidance of resecting tissue distal to the verumontanum.

Sexual dysfunction

Retrograde ejaculation occurs in more than 50% of men after TURP and results from resection of the bladder neck. Some patients also experience an altered sensation of orgasm. All patients should be warned of these potential effects preoperatively and should provide a signed consent. In addition, a smaller number of patients complain of erectile impotence after TURP; however, it is often difficult to be certain that this is a direct consequence of surgery. In elderly males in whom age-related arteriogenic erectile dysfunction is a common problem, impotence may be incorrectly attributed to the TURP. It is conceivable, however, that in some patients the cavernous nerves and arteries that are periprostatic in location could be damaged by capsular perforation. Erectile impotence may be treated by intracavernosal pharmacotherapy with agents such as papaverine, phentolamine or prostaglandin E_1. If drug therapy is ineffective then implantation of inflatable penile prostheses may be an option in younger, fitter patients.

Urethral strictures

Urethral strictures may occur as a consequence of prostatic surgery. They have been reported in 1–12% of patients in large series of TURPs and may also occur after open prostatectomy. The incidence of these strictures can be reduced by careful attention to detail at the time of surgery. A urethrotomy should always be performed if the meatus or the urethra appear tight around the resectoscope sheath. The site of the stricture may be at any location between the bladder neck and urethral meatus, but meatal and bulbar strictures seem to be the most common. Their resolution may require optical urethrotomy or, if recurrent, reconstructive urethroplasty.

Reoperation and death

Death following prostatectomy should now be a rare event and most large series quote a postoperative mortality of TURP which is well below 1% [48]. Health insurance data, however, may provide a more representative picture and this has revealed a 'within 90-day mortality' of 1.5%, although some of these deaths must be due to unrelated co-morbidity in frail and elderly patients. The worrying excess mortality of TURP over open prostatectomy reported by Roos *et al.* [47] has already been mentioned, but this is retrospective data from the 1970s and may reflect a tendency for urologists to elect for transurethral rather than open surgery in those patients with significant co-morbidity.

Interventional treatment options

Partly because of the small but significant incidence of complications from prostatectomy, and because of concern, especially in younger patients, over retrograde ejaculation, a number of alternative interventional means of relieving infravesical obstruction have been, and are currently being, developed. Some, like cryotherapy, have largely been abandoned while other technologies such as balloon dilatation, hyperthermia and high-intensity focused ultrasound are so new that little objective data concerning their long-term efficacy, safety and outcome are yet available.

Balloon dilatation

Techniques for dilatation of the prostate have been in existence for many years. However, it was not until the nineteenth century that special instruments were developed for transurethral disruption of the prostatic urethra and bladder neck. Guthrie in 1830, Civiale in 1841 and Mercier in 1850 all designed metal dilators specifically to relieve prostatic outflow obstruction. In 1910 Hollingsworth described a procedure for the transvesical rupture of the anterior and posterior prostatic commissures without removal of the adenoma. However, the efficacy of all these techniques appeared to be short lived. Subsequently, in 1956 W Diesting developed a metal dilator, similar in concept to that of Mercier, invented more than a century before. This was designed to disrupt the anterior and posterior commissures as a treatment for bladder outflow obstruction due to BPH. He reported excellent results using this dilator, claiming 95% of patients to be cured with good long-term results [49]. Diesting's technique, however, never gained real popularity although there were sporadic reports of its use in the 1950s and 1960s.

In the 1980s, however, advances in balloon catheter technology and techniques of interventional radiology produced an alternative to surgery for the treatment of vascular obstruction and biliary strictures. Burhenne *et al.* [50] reported an assessment of balloon dilatation of the prostate in 10 male cadavers, and demonstrated an increase in the diameter of the prostatic urethra after a dilatation of 24 F (8 mm) for 30 s. The same author then dilated his own urethra to the same dimensions and reported an improvement of uroflow together with a reduction of nocturia!

Subsequently, Castenada *et al.* [51] performed balloon dilatation in an attempt to determine the optimal balloon dimensions and inflation time to produce long-term widening of the prostatic urethra. The first papers reporting clinical results in patients with symptomatic BPH began to appear in 1988 and 1990. Broadly, two types of prostatic balloon dilatation systems are currently available: one type utilizes a disposable endoscopic system to ensure correct positioning of the balloon so that the distal sphincter is not dilated; the other type of device employs a location balloon inflated in the bulbar urethra and a 'collar' on the prostatic balloon, which is palpable per rectum, to ensure that the device is corerctly located (Fig. 36.5).

There is now consensus that dilatation of the prostate to at least 75 F (28 mm) is necessary to produce any useful result and there is a trend towards even larger 90 F (30 mm) or even 105 F (33 mm) balloons. All the manufacturers recommend that the balloon inflation is maintained for at least 10 min.

The results achieved with these devices have been somewhat mixed. Early enthusiastic reports from the USA were countered by Gill *et al.* [52] who reported only modest improvement in their patients with this technique. A more recent report from the same group revealed virtually no urodynamic evidence of improvement in the majority of those obstructed patients who did not present with urinary retention, and virtually none in those who did [53]. What has emerged from a number of studies is the realization that balloon dilatation is only of any value in the smaller prostate and in those patients who do not have severe obstruction or prominent middle lobe enlargement. The technique is of no benefit in those patients with acute or chronic retention in whom a TURP will yield far better results.

Complications of balloon dilatation are usually relatively trivial, but bleeding may occur, necessitating bladder irrigation. Because post-dilatation prostatic oedema may occur it is best to insert a catheter for 24–48 h. However, there is no necessity for the patient to be hospitalized.

Although many patients will show a subjective symptomatic response not many show a parallel improvement in flow rates and residual urine parameters, and virtually none are unobstructed when studied later by urodynamic evaluation. It is doubtful that this technique will ever seriously challenge transurethral resection as a surgical option in the majority of patients with BPH, and in fact has now largely been abandoned.

Intraprostatic stents

M Fabian in 1980 was the first to suggest that bladder outflow obstruction due to BPH could be relieved by the insertion of a hollow metal spiral within the prostatic urethra without the need for resection of prostatic tissue. He reported the use of a stainless steel spiral which had an extension through the distal sphincter into the bulbar urethra to maintain its position. The device was inserted and could be exchanged or removed cystoscopically. Subsequently, in an attempt to resist encrustation with urinary precipitates, the spiral was modified by coating it with gold and it is now marketed under the trade name of Prostakath™ (Fig. 36.6).

A similar device (the Urospiral ™), which is slightly more flexible, retains the use of stainless steel and is also commercially available. Reports in the literature, however, suggest that the use of these devices is not always satisfactory as they may become displaced proximally into the bladder, or distally down the urethra. Moreover, uroflow values in patients with spirals *in situ* tend to diminish progressively with time. This suggests that encrustation may be occurring on many of these devices, and indeed we have recently observed the complete obstruction of a stainless steel spiral due to encrustation that required electrohydraulic lithotripsy to remove it [54] (Fig. 36.7).

In an attempt to overcome these twin problems of displacement and encrustation, two types of permanently

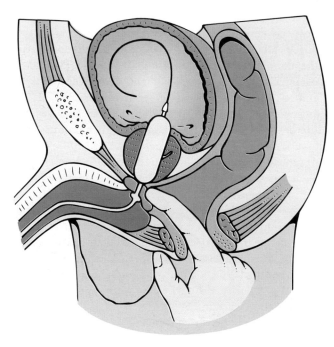

Fig. 36.5 Balloon dilatation of the prostate.

implanted metal stents have recently been developed. These are located within the prostatic urethra and then expanded to a diameter of more than 35 F (14 mm). After a period the stents become epithelialized, a feature which is suggested may protect them from encrustation. One variety of prostatic stent, the Urolume™ manufactured by Medinvent and marketed by American Medical Systems, is commercially available for the treatment of urethral strictures and is also being employed for the treatment of BPH.

The question of the long-term effects of metal implants in the wall of the urinary tract has yet to be fully addressed. In this respect, stainless steel may be a less than ideal material. The presence of chloride ions within the extracellular fluid renders any metal implant susceptible to corrosion; in animal experiments stainless steel implants have been demonstrated to exhibit corrosion in the majority of cases. Titanium may be more resistant to corrosion than stainless steel when implanted into the body and as a result has been developed for use of the Advanced Surgical Intervention balloon dilatation system. The length of the prostatic urethra is measured precisely and a stent of the correct dimensions selected. Under endoscopic control, the carrying balloon is inflated and the expanded stent is located just distal to the bladder neck [55] (Fig. 36.8). Longer term studies, however, have demonstrated a significant complication rate.

In conclusion, metal spirals and stents may constitute a useful alternative to the long-term catheterization in patients who are medically unfit for surgery. Their use, however, will inevitably be associated with the risks of

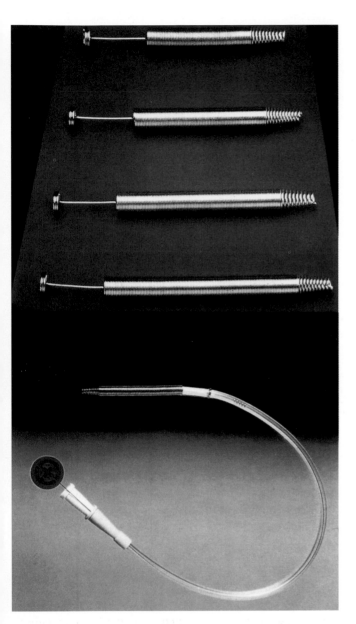

Fig. 36.6 Temporary intraprostatic stent.

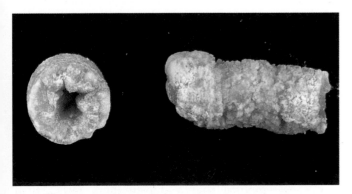

Fig. 36.7 Stones formed on an intraprostatic stent.

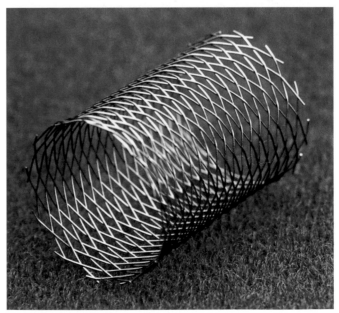

Fig. 36.8 Permanent intraprostatic stent.

encrustation where there is an interface between metal and urine for any duration. The metal spirals carry the advantage that they may easily be withdrawn and replaced, but with this comes the tendency towards spontaneous displacement. The advantage of the expandable stainless steel superalloy and titanium stents is their firm fixation and potential for complete epithelialization. However, they are not always easy to remove and careful long-term follow-up of their safety and efficacy in the prostatic urethra is necessary before their more widespread clinical use in less advanced cases of BPH can be advocated.

Hyperthermia

The concept that local heat may be beneficial in various pathological states dates back to Hippocrates who noted the therapeutic effect of hot steam baths. However, the possible tumouricidal effects of hyperthermia were not recognized until 1866 when the resolution of a sarcoma was reported after an attack of hyperpyrexia due to erysipelas. Histological changes after hyperthermia include swelling and fragmentation of the cytoplasm, rupture of the plasma membrane and ultimately complete cellular necrosis. Normal cells seem better able to repair themselves after heat damage than neoplastic cells. The degree of thermal damage to any tissue depends on the temperature and exposure time; temperatures below 39°C do not induce any injury and temperatures above 46°C irrevocably damage most cells. Temperatures between 40 and 45°C can perhaps be applied to selectively destroy neoplastic cells.

Transrectal microwave hyperthermia

The first scientific study of prostatic hyperthermia was in an animal model in which the prostate was treated by localized microwave hyperthermia administered transrectally with apparently safe and efficacious results. Subsequently studies of this treatment were commenced in patients which both prostatic carcinoma and BPH. Transrectal administration of microwaves was first directed at the human prostate as a treatment for carcinoma. The prostate was heated to 43°C using a transrectal microwave probe, while adjacent tissues were cooled to 32°C. Early results were encouraging with a reported reduction in both tumour mass and obstructive symptoms following this treatment [56].

The same apparatus was subsequently used to evaluate the effect of microwaves applied transrectally in BPH. A total of 29 patients with histologically proven BPH were studied, 11 of whom had an indwelling urethral catheter as a treatment for retention of urine. Each case was treated transrectally on an outpatient basis, without sedation, once every fortnight. The mean number of treatments required was 11.7 (range 4–18). There was symptomatic improve-

ment in voiding symptoms in all 18 cases without a catheter *in situ* and eight of the 11 catheterized patients were able to void after treatment. The therapy was reported to be well tolerated and was free of significant side effects [57].

The equipment used for transrectal microwave therapy was later modified by incorporating a cooling system to prevent thermal damage to the rectal wall. A 100 W 915 MHz microwave generator was employed. The temperature within the prostatic urethra was maintained at 42.5 ± 1°C for 60 min. TRUS showed no diminution in size of the prostate after treatment, however symptoms did seem to improve; although two patients developed a small prostatorectal fistula after treatment, both resolved with conservative management. Since then, a number of other devices have been developed and introduced into clinical use.

One of the more objective evaluations of transrectal microwave therapy reported to date has been undertaken using the Prostathermer™ (Model 99-D, Biodan Medical Systems); the study examined voiding parameters before and 4 weeks after treatment in 30 cases of BPH [58]. The changes in urinary symptoms did not reach statistical significance. The objective results were also poor with an improvement in the mean maximum flow rate of only 1.1 ml/s, which was not statistically significant. The increase in flow rate did, however, just reach statistical significance when corrected for the initial bladder volume according to the nomogram defined by Siroky and associates [34]. The post-micturition residual volume and the volume of the prostate itself assessed by TRUS were both unchanged following treatment with the Prostathermer™ and there was an overall improvement in only two of the 28 evaluable cases.

In spite of these disappointing results, transrectal hyperthermia does appear to be a safe procedure which is relatively free of side effects. A review of 435 cases of BPH treated by transrectal microwave using the Prostathermer™ resulted in the following complications: haematuria occurred in 1.4% of cases, urinary tract infection in 1.6% and epididymitis in 0.4%, together with rectal pain in 0.9% [59]. However, doubt has been cast upon the true efficacy of transrectal hyperthermia and an objective analysis of the longer term results of this treatment are still awaited. There is also a potential risk of the development of prostatorectal fistulas due to heat damage to the rectum and posterior prostate, and the technique has fallen from favour.

Transurethral microwave hyperthermia and thermotherapy

It has been argued that a transurethral, rather than transrectal, route for the administration of microwave hyperthermia might be more effective since the energy is being delivered more directly to the transurethral portion of the prostate, which is the area predominantly responsible for the obstruction in BPH. A number of transurethral applicators incorporating conventional microwave devices have recently been developed. The system developed by BSD Medical Corporation consists of a microprocessor-controlled microwave generator. During treatment the urethral temperature is monitored and the temperature within the substance of the prostate is regulated between 44 and 47.5°C.

In a series of 21 cases the treatment was well tolerated and not associated with significant long-term side effects. An average of 8.4 treatment sessions were utilized for each case with a mean treatment time per session of 56 min. There was a statistically significant decrease in the nocturnal frequency and in the post-micturition residual volume with some suggestion of a reduction in the volume of the prostate on TRUS, as well as an increase in the mean maximum flow rate from 11.0 to 15.9 ml/s. Pressure–flow cystometric studies were not performed and the median follow-up period was only 12.5 months. As in so many studies of the efficacy of microwave therapy, unfortunately, no control treated group was included in this study.

Another transurethral microwave applicator—the Prostatron™—has been developed by a group from Lyon, France. The antenna is mounted on a 20 F (6.7 mm) flexible catheter and a cooling device is included to reduce local thermal effects upon the urethral mucosa. This equipment has been shown to reliably heat the prostate above 46°C to a distance of 15 mm from the urethra, while the temperature of the rectal mucosa is monitored with three thermosensors and does not rise above 42.5°C during treatment. When transurethral microwave hyperthermia (or thermotherapy, as manufacturers term the treatment), using this apparatus, was applied prior to cystoprostatectomy, histological sections of the prostate showed evidence of thermal damage in the periurethral area with apparent preservation of the urethral mucosa itself.

An uncontrolled clinical trial, which evaluated 34 patients with outflow obstruction due to BPH before and 8 weeks after treatment with the Prostatron™, has shown a mean increase in the maximum flow of 5.1 ml/s. However, there was little change in the mean post-micturition residue or the mean prostatic length on TRUS. Of the 13 catheterized patients with acute retention of urine, six (46%) were voiding normally 3 months later. The main complication encountered was transient retention of urine [60]; this temporary but inconvenient complication occurs in up to 20–25% of patients and may last as long as 2 weeks after therapy. More recently a controlled study of Prostatron™ treatment versus 'sham' therapy has been reported by Ogden *et al.* [61] demonstrating objective improvement in the treated group compared with controls.

So far there is no conclusive evidence to suggest that any form of either hyperthermia or thermotherapy is capable of completely and permanently relieving prostatic outflow obstruction in the majority of patients, although some individuals do unquestionably respond to this therapy (Fig. 36.9). Symptomatic improvement, however, does seem to be produced in 60% or so of cases, and prostatic hyperthermia, particularly administered transurethrally, is an apparently safe and relatively inexpensive treatment that does not require inpatient stay. The therapy may in time prove more effective as technology advances. At present, further controlled studies using objective parameters are indicated to evaluate the long-term efficacy and

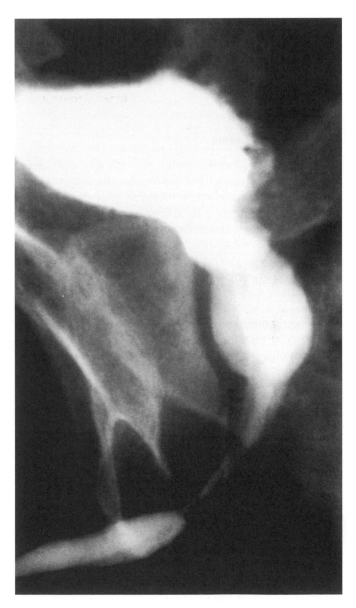

Fig. 36.9 Voiding cystourethrogram 6 months after treatment with the Prostatron™ thermotherapy device.

outcome of prostatic hyperthermia, perhaps utilizing higher temperatures, to elucidate its mechanism of action. In the meantime, it seems likely that this treatment will have some future role particularly in younger men and in those with small prostates and mild to moderate obstruction who wish to avoid the development of retrograde ejaculation induced by TURP. The technology has recently been approved in the USA.

Other forms of heat therapy including transurethral needle ablation (TUNA), high-intensity focused ultrasound (HIFU) and extracorporeal pyrotherapy are currently under evaluation. The last, however, has recently been abandoned.

Medical treatment options

The idea of 'a pill for the prostate' has long been an alluring one for patients, but has been regarded with scepticism by urologists for many years. There are, however, data accumulating now to suggest that a number of pharmacological agents may provide both a safe and effective treatment of BPH.

α-Adrenoceptor blockers

The search for non-hormonal pharmacological agents capable of reducing outflow obstruction by BPH began in the 1970s when α-adrenergic receptors were demonstrated within prostatic adenomas, the prostatic capsule and the bladder neck. Since the prostate in BPH contains a greater percentage of smooth muscle within its stroma (approximately 60%) than the normal prostate (45%) it has been suggested that the tone in this smooth muscle may be an important factor in the development of obstruction in BPH.

The autonomic innervation of the prostate has been evaluated by histological studies, radioligand binding and organ bath experiments. Both adrenergic and cholinergic nerves have been demonstrated within the prostate. Adrenergic fibres release noradrenaline which stimulates receptors of two types: α_1- and α_2-adrenoceptors. Both types of adrenoceptor are present within the prostate. Stimulation of adrenergic receptors within the smooth muscle element of the prostate has been shown to lead to an increase in the muscle tone in *in vitro* prostate strip experiments [62].

The contraction of smooth muscle within the prostate is inhibited by the addition of the α_1-specific antagonist prazosin but only mildly suppressed by the α_2-specific antagonist rauwolscine. These findings suggest that the α-adrenoceptors on prostatic smooth muscle cells which mediate contraction are predominantly α_1-adrenoceptors. Recently, evidence has emerged that the α_1-receptor itself has three subtypes: α_{1A}, α_{1B} and α_{1D}. The first of these seems to be the variety mainly involved in prostatic

smooth muscle tone, raising the possibility of prostate selective compounds [63].

Compounds in clinical use

Phenoxybenzamine

The first α-adrenergic blocker to be intensively investigated for efficacy in BPH was phenoxybenzamine at a dose of 10 mg twice daily. An uncontrolled, open label study reported symptomatic improvement in many cases, although there was no objective urodynamic evidence of improved outflow. A later placebo-controlled double-blind study of phenoxybenzamine taken for 14 days showed a significant improvement in urinary frequency, the maximum and mean flow rates and the urethral closure pressure but no reduction in post-micturition residual volume [64]. A similar placebo-controlled study also showed significant improvements in these parameters but highlighted the problems with side effects, including dizziness in 28.6% of the active treatment group as well as lethargy, palpitations, nasal congestion, visual disturbances and retrograde ejaculation [65].

Unfortunately, phenoxybenzamine, which is chemically related to nitrogen mustard, has been shown to induce gastric carcinoma in rats and is also mutagenic in mouse tissue culture. For this reason it is no longer generally available.

Prazosin

The first α_1-specific adrenoceptor to be studied was prazosin. This drug was initially introduced as an antihypertensive agent but it was soon noted to have some effect in BPH. Hedlund *et al.* [66] demonstrated a significant increase in mean and maximum flow rate and a reduction in post-micturition residual volume in a double-blind crossover study of 20 men. A larger study by Kirby *et al.* [67], involving 80 men for a 4-week treatment period, confirmed the improvement of symptoms and flow rate but reported no improvement in residual volume. A longer term double-blind study investigating 58 men with urodynamics before and after 12 weeks of treatment with prazosin or placebo revealed similar results and, in addition, a statistically significant reduction in maximum voiding pressure [68].

Alfuzosin

A double-blind placebo-controlled trial of the α-adrenoceptor alfuzosin administered twice a day in 31 cases of bladder outflow obstruction due to BPH has shown a statistically significant improvement in irritative symptoms but no alteration in urodynamic parameters [69].

However, a 6-month multicentre placebo-controlled trial without urodynamics other than flow rate showed significant improvement in voiding symptoms, mean flow rate and post-micturition residual volume [70], although there was a relatively high drop-out rate as a result of side effects. More recent studies have confirmed the longer term efficacy and tolerability of this agent, as well as its positive effects on the quality of life of patients with lower urinary tract symptoms due to BPH [71].

Indoramin

The first placebo-controlled clinical trial of the α-adrenoceptor blocker indoramin, at a dose of 50 mg twice daily, showed a remarkable improvement in the mean maximum flow rate from 8.5 to 18.5 ml/s [72]. However, a more recent multicentre controlled trial has reported a rather less dramatic improvement in the flow rate with indoramin, more in line with the 30% or so improvement reported for other α-adrenoceptor blockers [73].

Terazosin

The α_1-specific adrenoceptor blocker terazosin was initially developed as an antihypertensive therapy. A dose-ranging but uncontrolled study of this agent originally showed a significant improvement in symptoms as well as an increase in the maximum and mean flow rates [74]. A further trial evaluating the action of terazosin in 45 men with symptomatic BPH using a dose-titrating regimen confirmed a statistically significant and dose-related improvement in symptom scores and urinary flow rates. Side effects such as erectile dysfunction, tiredness, headache, palpitations and nasal congestion were encountered in some of the patients, leading to withdrawal from the trial in five cases. Continued therapy, however, over a period of up to 6 months showed a well-sustained therapeutic response to terazosin [75]. The results of a double-blind study show a good safety/efficacy profile [76]. The once a day dosing regimen with this compound is of some advantage.

Doxazosin

The new α_1-specific blocker, doxazosin, is structurally similar to prazosin, has a smoother onset of action and a longer half-life and is therefore also particularly suitable for a once a day dosage regimen. Dosage, as with all α-blockers, should be titrated up cautiously starting at 1 mg/day for 1 week, 2 mg/day for 4 weeks and finally to 4 mg/day. A multicentre placebo-controlled 12-week study of the effects of doxazosin (4 mg given once a day) has recently been reported [77] and has shown a significant improvement in symptoms together with an increase in the mean flow rate

and a reduction in maximum voiding pressure. Side effects, although present in a number of patients were usually tolerable and could usually be resolved by reducing the dosage. Interestingly, although doxazosin effectively lowers blood pressure in normotensive individuals it has only minimal, clinically insignificant effects in normotensive men with BPH [78].

Tamsulosin

The most recent addition to the urologist's armamentarium against BPH is a new α-blocker named tamsulosin. This agent, which can be administered once per day at a dose of 0.4 mg, exhibits about 30-fold selectivity for the α 1A subtype of adrenoceptor. A multicentre study of 313 patients with symptomatic BPH reported reasonable efficacy and no significant cardiovascular effects [79]. A close ranging study has confirmed the optimal dose to be 0.4 mg/day [80] and two recent studies have suggested that tamsulosin is better tolerated than other α-blockers [81,82]. These data suggest that the development of even more selective agents in the future may permit even more effective therapy of symptomatic BPH without the drawbacks of tiredness, dizziness and postural hypotension.

Endocrine therapy for BPH

John Hunter, one of the fathers of modern scientific surgery, observed as early as the eighteenth century that the prostate undergoes atrophy after castration. Almost certainly stimulated by this observation, Cabot [83] reported on the effects of bilateral orchidectomy for the treatment of bladder outflow obstruction due to BPH and described some symptomatic improvement. The assessment of this improvement, however, was totally subjective and it is not entirely clear whether or not some patients in these studies were in fact suffering from malignant rather than benign prostatic enlargement.

In more recent times, Peirson [84] reported shrinkage of the prostate with stilboestrol therapy in 10 out of 13 patients suffering from BPH, and noted symptomatic improvement in 70% of individuals. Geller et al. [85] used the progestational agent 17α-hydroxyprogesterone caproate—which also exerts potent antiandrogenic effects as a result of inhibition of pituitary gonadotrophin release—in six patients with BPH in an open study and claimed encouraging effects.

Another potent antiandrogen, flutamide, has been used in a similar context by Caine et al. [62], who provided evidence of an improvement of uroflow with this agent. In addition, some prostatic shrinkage was reported. More recently, Stone et al. [86,87] reported the preliminary results of a multicentre study of the use of flutamide in BPH. After 3 months' treatment a 23% reduction in prostatic volume was observed compared with no detectable alteration in the control group.

The effects of reversible androgen deprivation using LHRH analogues on patients with bladder outflow obstruction have been reported. Peters and Walsh [88], using nafarelin acetate, observed a mean reduction of prostatic volume of 25%, reaching a plateau at 4 months, with clinical improvement in three of nine patients. Bosch *et al.* [89] used either the LHRH agonist buserelin or cyproterone acetate in 12 patients with BPH and noticed a 29% reduction in gland volume by 12 weeks, but only a minimal improvement in urodynamic parameters.

Although many of the above studies can be criticized for the small numbers studied, their methodology and lack of controlled data, there seems little doubt that androgen deprivation will produce some reduction in prostate volume and a modest improvement in symptoms of outflow obstruction in at least a proportion of patients with BPH. The drawback, however, with all the therapeutic agents mentioned above, except possibly flutamide, is their detrimental effect on potency as a result of the induction of hypogonadism. For this reason these agents have almost exclusively been used for the treatment of malignant rather than benign prostatic disease.

5α-Reductase inhibitors

The discovery that testosterone is metabolized in the prostate to DHT by the enzyme 5α-reductase was originally made by Farnsworth and Brown in 1963 [90]. Subsequently, Bruchovsky and Wilson [9] suggested that DHT rather than testosterone is the main intracellular androgen that modulates prostatic growth. The studies of Imperato-McGinley *et al.* [91] involving patients with congenital deficiency of 5α-reductase confirmed that the females with this condition were unaffected, but males, who were born with ambiguous genitalia, subsequently masculinized and acquired normal libido and spermatogenesis but never developed prostatic enlargement. These observations raised the possibility that a compound similar in structure to testosterone could be synthesized which would competitively inhibit the conversion of testosterone to DHT. A drug which could produce effective inhibition of 5α-reductase would reduce intraprostatic DHT levels and might not only prevent the development of BPH but also induce remission in established disease, without interfering with potency, libido and other testosterone-dependent functions.

Finasteride

After extensive research, the compound finasteride was identified. This is a neutral 4-azasteroid, which appears to act as a pure 5α-reductase inhibitor without detectable

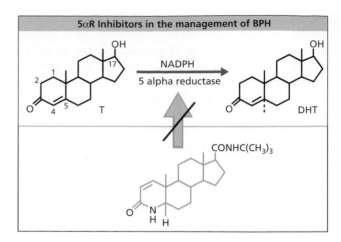

Fig. 36.10 Mechanism of action of finasteride.

androgen receptor-blocking properties (Fig. 36.10). In the rat, growth of the ventral prostate has been shown to be inhibited by 17β-NN-diethylcarbamoyl-4-aza-4-methyl-5α-androstan-3-one (4MA), a compound related to finasteride, and prostatic volume was reduced by 64% in a series of mature male beagles treated with this compound [92]. In the latter group of animals, histological study of the prostate after treatment showed flattening of epithelial cells with vacuolization of the cytoplasm and pycnosis of the nuclei.

In humans, finasteride has been shown to be a potent reversible inhibitor of 5α-reductase even at doses as low as 1.5 mg/day. A multidose safety and tolerability study, using 12.5 mg of the drug twice daily, demonstrated an 80% decrease of serum DHT from a baseline of 64 ± 16 ng/dl to 18 ± 17 ng/dl. Moreover, finasteride decreased intraprostatic DHT by nearly 90% [93]. Serum testosterone levels did not change significantly and there were no clinically important adverse effects. Importantly, there was no evidence of antiandrogenic action such as nipple tenderness or gynaecomastia, and no changes in libido or spermatogenesis or other toxicity was seen.

Phase 2 studies with finasteride have demonstrated shrinkage of the prostate volume of about 18% within 3 months using treatment at dosages of 5 mg/day, as well as improvements in uroflow and symptom scores. In a 6-month study the prostatic shrinkage detected was 28% [94].

In our own placebo-controlled urodynamic studies of finasteride in 69 patients with BPH, the drug produced a profound reduction in DHT levels in all patients treated [95]. There was also a statistically significant improvement in symptom score and urinary flow, together with a reduction of prostate volume of 14% after treatment for 1 year; PSA values also declined by a mean of 28%. The drug was well tolerated in almost all patients and side effects were trivial. Two patients complained of erectile impotence, but potency returned after stopping the medication. After 3 years' therapy in a subset of patients voiding pressures fell and uroflow improved to the unobstructed range for that age group [96].

Significant prostatic shrinkage occurred in just over 60% of patients treated, which suggests that not all forms of BPH are susceptible to treatment by 5α-reductase inhibition. Obviously it would be of value to be able to predict those patients likely to respond to this medication. However, it is still too early to evaluate which features, if any, can distinguish responders from non-responders. Clearly, the composition of the gland, that varies markedly in different individuals, may influence this. Those patients with prostatic enlargement that is predominantly glandular rather than stromal (fibromu-scular) might, on theoretical grounds, be expected to respond better to this modality of therapy, and currently it is believed that those patients with larger prostates are most likely to respond to treatment.

Phase 3 studies in the USA [97] on over 895 men with BPH have revealed similar improvements in uroflow and symptoms, and a mean reduction of prostatic volume of 19% in treated individuals. In these studies, the only important side effect was an incidence of loss of libido, ejaculatory disturbance and impotence in less than 5% of patients, which was reversible on stopping the medication. Open label continuation data is now available on these patients for up to 4 years showing well-maintained efficacy [98]. A recent 2-year placebo controlled trial of finasteride has been reported from Scandinavia [99], again confirming the efficacy and safety of this compound. In this study a rather higher percentage of men (19%) complained of sexual dysfunction on the active drug compared with placebo (10%), but fewer men suffered acute retention of urine requiring TURP. A subsequent metanalysis of several placebo-controlled studies has revealed that finasteride reduces the incidence of acute retention by 54%, and the need for surgery by 34%.

Several other 5α-reductase inhibitors are currently under development including a new compound from Glaxo. Some of these show activity against the two types of 5α-reductase enzyme (5α-reductase I and II) which may result in different biological effects. At the time of writing no placebo-controlled data of the efficacy of this compound in BPH is yet available.

Aromatase inhibition and antioestrogens

Aromatase is an enzyme complex responsible for the conversion of androgens to oestrogens. Aromatase is widely distributed in the reproductive tissues of both sexes in many species. In the human male oestrogen production occurs mainly by extratesticular aromatization of andro-stenedione to oestrone and of testosterone to oestradiol.

Immunocytochemical studies [100] have identified a predominant localization of oestrogen receptors in the stroma and ductal epithelium of the periurethral zone of the normal canine prostate. Moreover, recently it has been reported that aromatase activity in the human prostate is also highest in the periurethral zone [101] where the stromal form of BPH especially appears to develop. Experimental studies in dogs and monkeys have also indicated that prostatic stromal proliferation, induced by the adminis-tration of androstenedione, can be antagonized by the administration of an aromatase inhibitor.

The best known and most widely used aromatase inhibitors are aminoglutethimide and ketoconazole. However, neither of these agents was originally developed as an aromatase inhibitor. Ketoconazole is much more widely used as an antifungal agent and in most countries has been withdrawn as therapy for endocrine disorders. Aminoglutethimide is also used as a treatment for carcinoma of the prostate, with some clinical success, but there is disagreement over the precise mechanism of action of the drug. Lassitude, depression and gynaecomastia have all been associated with the use of aminoglutethimide and it has been argued that the adverse effects are too unpleasant to justify use of the drug. Ketoconazole has also been used in the treatment of carcinoma of the prostate, but again side effects have been troublesome; the most serious toxicity is hepatitis, which is usually reversible on discontinuation of the therapy, but occasionally may be fatal.

Neither aminoglutethimide nor ketoconazole is a selective inhibitor of aromatase. A range of more selective agents, however, is now under investigation but experience in BPH is still limited. Tunn and Schweikurt [102] reported some prostatic shrinkage in an uncontrolled study of 13 patients treated with testolactone at a dose of 200 mg/day. They also reported that preliminary results with a new aromatase inhibitor 1-methyl-androsta-1,4-diene-3,7-dione (1-methyl-ADD) were more encouraging, the compound producing significant reductions in plasma concentrations of both oestrone and oestradiol. However, Oesterling et al. [103] reported that aromatase inhibition was not an effective treatment for BPH in the dog, the only species other than humans in which BPH occurs spontaneously.

Perhaps a more logical approach would be to block the effects of oestrogens at target cells by means of anti-oestrogen therapy (i.e. an oestrogen-receptor antagonist). One report of the use of tamoxifen at a dose of 80 mg/day for 4 weeks demonstrated no useful effect; however, tamoxifen itself has activity as a weak oestrogen, and moreover 4 weeks' treatment is probably too short a period in which to detect an effect on the prostate. However, ICI have a new compound, ICI 183720, which is considerably more potent as an oestrogen-receptor blocker than tamoxifen and has no agonist oestrogenic properties. No reports of its use in BPH are available yet but it does seem possible that it may have some useful activity, perhaps if used in combination with a 5α-reductase inhibitor such as finasteride.

Conclusion

Because BPH is so prevalent there has been a tendency to ascribe virtually any urinary symptoms in elderly men to this disease. Careful evaluation is necessary in every case, however, to ensure that bladder outflow obstruction is in fact present and is the cause of the symptoms with which the patient presents.

The decision-making process involved in selecting a given treatment for an individual patient, whatever the pathology, always involves balancing the probabilities of producing a beneficial outcome against the risk of adverse effects. In addition, consideration also has to be made of the possible harmful consequences of electing not to treat, but simply employing a policy of watchful waiting. In the case of BPH our knowledge of the natural history of the condition is currently incomplete. Although most cases of BPH are assumed to be gradually progressive as a result of increasing transition zone hyperplasia, several studies [104,105] have suggested that this is not always the case. It would be particularly helpful in planning a rational treatment regimen to know which patients are at risk of developing complications such as acute retention, chronic retention, urinary tract infection and upper tract dilatation. Unfortunately, these data are almost completely lacking.

Until recently, decisions about the management of bladder outflow obstruction due to BPH involved a relatively simple choice between watchful waiting or prostatectomy, usually by the transurethral route. With the advent of an ever-increasing range of alternative therapies discussed in this chapter, life for the urologist is no longer so straightforward. Figure 36.11 is a graphical demonstration of the risk–benefit analysis of various treatment options for BPH, although sufficient information on outcome is not available for all modalities. As was said many years ago 'new treatments always work wonders for a while', and before embracing these new modalities too enthusiastically it must be remembered that there are a number of fundamental problems inherent in all non-surgical alternatives to prostatectomy.

1 Lack of tissue for pathological evaluation to rule out coexistent prostatic carcinoma.

2 Delay of definitive treatment and increased cost if prostatectomy is eventually required.

3 Increased capital cost and personnel requirement for multiple treatments (especially for hyperthermia and laser therapy).

4 Compliance for long-term pharmacological therapy.

5 Risk of retreatment as well as silently developing

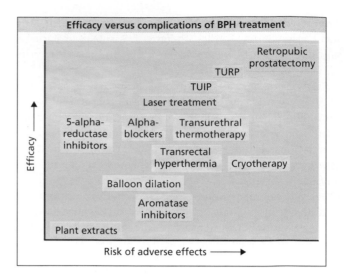

Fig. 36.11 Efficacy versus complications of various BPH treatments.

complications including renal impairment and bladder decompensation.

Only by properly conducted, placebo-controlled, long-term studies which also assess retreatment rates in sufficient numbers of patients will the true values and disadvantages of these competing therapies be revealed. Whether the next millenium will see the same inexorable increase in the number of TURPs performed annually across the world seen in the 1980s, or whether the role of the prostatectomy as the gold standard therapy for BPH will be supplanted by these alternatives, as lithotripsy has replaced open surgical renal stone extraction, only time will tell.

References

1 Berry SJ, Coffey DS, Walsh PC, Ewing LL. The development of human benign prostatic hyperplasia with age. *J Urol* 1984; **132**:474–9.

2 Garraway WM, Collins GN, Lee RJ. High prevalence of benign prostatic hypertrophy in the community. *Lancet* 1991;**338**: 469–71.

3 Tsang KT, Garraway WM. Impact of benign prostatic hyperplasia on general well-being of men. *Prostate* 1983;**23**:1–7.

4 Araki H, Watanabe H, Mishina T, Nakao M. High-risk group for benign prostatic hypertrophy. *Prostate* 1983;**4**:253–64.

5 Bourke JB, Griffin JP. Diabetes mellitus in patients with prostatic hyperplasia. *Br Med J* 1968;**4**:492–3.

6 Isaacs JT, Coffey DS. Changes in DHT metabolism associated with the development of canine benign prostatic hyperplasia. *Endocrinology* 1981;**108**:445–53.

7 Vermeulen A. *The Endocrine Function of the Human Testis.* New York: Academic Press, 1973.

8 Coffey DS. The endocrine control of normal and abnormal

growth of the prostate. In: Raifer J, ed. *Urologic Endocrinology*. Philadelphia: WB Saunders, 1986:170–93.

9 Bruchovsky N, Wilson JD. The conversion of testosterone to 5-alpha-androstan-17-beta-ol-3-one by rat prostate *in vivo* and *in vitro*. *J Biol Chem* 1968;**243**:2012–21.

10 Anderson KM, Liao S. Selective retention of dihydrotestosterone by prostatic nuclei. *Nature* 1968;**219**:277–9.

11 Siiteri PK, Wilson JD. Dihydrotestosterone metabolism in prostate hypertrophy. I. The formation of content of dihydrotestosterone in the hypertrophic prostate of man. *J Clin Invest* 1970;**49**:1737–45.

12 Walsh PC, Hutchins GM, Ewing LL. Tissue content of dihydrotestosterone in human prostatic hyperplasia is not supranormal. *J Clin Invest* 1983;**72**:1772–7.

13 Barrack ER, Bujnovsky P, Walsh PC. Subcellular distribution of androgen receptors in human normal, benign hyperplastic and malignant prostatic tissue: characterization of nuclear salt-resistant receptors. *Cancer Res* 1983;**43**:1107–16.

14 Trachenberg J, Hicks LL, Walsh PC. Androgen and estrogen receptor content in spontaneous and experimentally induced canine prostatic hyperplasia. *J Clin Invest* 1980;**65**:1051–9.

15 Walsh PC, Wilson JD. The induction of prostatic hypertrophy in the dog with androstanediol. *J Clin Invest* 1976;**57**:1093–7.

16 Franks LM, Barton AA. The effects of testosterone on the ultrastructure of the mouse prostate *in vivo* and in organ culture. *Exp Cell Res* 1960;**19**:35–50.

17 Cunha GR. Tissue interactions between epithelium and mesenchyme of urogenital and integumental origina. *Anat Rec* 1972;**172**:529–42.

18 Cunha GR. The role of androgens in the epithelio-mesenchymal interactions involved in prostatic morphogenesis in embryonic mice. *Anat Rec* 1973;**175**:87–96.

19 Davis P, Eaton CL. Binding of epidermal growth factor by normal, hypertrophic and carcinomatous prostate. *Prostate* 1989;**14**:123–32.

20 Mori H, Maki M, Oishi K, Jays M, Igaroshi K, Yoshida O. Increased expression of genes for basic fibroblast growth factor and transforming growth factor in human benign prostatic hypertension. *Prostate* 1990;**16**:71–80.

21 Martikainen P, Kyprianou N, Isaacs JN. Effect of transforming growth factor-beta on proliferation and cell deaths of rat prostatic cells. *Endocrinology* 1990;**127**:2963–8.

22 Madson PO, Iversen PA. A point system for selecting operative candidates. In: Hinman F Jr, Boyarsky S, eds. *Benign Prostatic Hypertrophy*. New York: Springer Verlag, 1983:763–9.

23 Boyarsky S, Jones G, Paulson DF, Front CR. A new look at bladder neck obstruction by the Food and Drug Administration regulators: guidelines for investigation of benign prostatic hypertrophy. *Trans Am Assoc Genito-urina Surg* 1977;**68**: 29–32.

24 Abrams PH, Griffiths DJ. The assessment of prostatic obstruction from urodynamic measurements and from residual urine. *Br J Urol* 1979;**51**:129–34.

25 Gilpin SA, Gosling JA, Barnard RJ. Morphological and morphometric studies of the human obstructed, trabeculated urinary bladder. *Br J Urol* 1985;**57**:525–9.

26 Speakman MJ, Brading AF, Gilpin CJ, Dixon JS, Gilpin SA, Goslins JA. Bladder outflow obstruction cause of denervation supersensitivity. *J Urol* 1987;**138**:1461–7.

27 Brading AF, Turner WH. The unstable bladder: towards a common mechanism. *Br J Urol* 1994;**73**:3–8.

28 Arrighi HM, Guess HA, Metter EJ, Fozard JL. Symptoms and signs of prostatism as risk factors for prostatectomy. *Prostate* 1990;**16**:253–61.

29 Neal DE, Ramsden PD, Sharples L *et al.* Outcome of elective prostatectomy. *Br Med J* 1989;**299**:762–7.

30 Oesterling JE. Prostate specific antigen: a critical assessment of the most useful tumour marker for adenocarcinoma of the prostate. *J Urol* 1991;**145**:907–23.

31 Stamey TA, Yang N, Hay AR *et al.* Prostate specific antigen as a serum marker for adenocarcinoma of the prostate. *N Engl J Med* 1987;**317**:909–16.

32 Catalona WJ, Smith DS, Ratliff TL *et al.* Measurement of prostate specific antigen in serum as a screening test for prostate cancer. *N Engl J Med* 1991;**324**(17):1156–61.

33 Carter BH, Pearson JD, Metter J *et al.* Longitudinal evaluation of prostate specific antigen levels in men with and without prostate cancer. *J Am Med Assoc* 1993;**267**:2215–20.

34 Siroky MB, Olsson CA, Krane RJ. The flow rate nomogram I: development. *J Urol* 1980;**123**:208–10.

35 Bruskevitz RC, Iversen P, Madsen PO. Value of postvoid residual urine determination in evaluation of prostatis. *Urology* 1982;**20**:602–4.

36 Drach GW, Layton TN, Binard WJ. Male peak urinary flow rate: relationship of volume voided and age. *J Urol* 1979;**122**:210–14.

37 Schou J, Poulson AL, Nordling J. The anatomy of a prostate waiting list: a prospective study of 132 consecutive patients. *Br J Urol* 1994;**74**:57–60.

38 Gerstenberg TC, Andersen JT, Klarskov P, Ramirez D, Halt T. High flow intra-vesical obstruction in men: symptomatology, urodynamics and the results of surgery. *J Urol* 1982;**127**:943–5.

39 Jensen KE, Bruskevitz RC, Iversen P, Madsen PO. Predictive value of voiding pressures in benign prostatic hyperplasia. *Neurol Urodyn* 1983;**2**:117–25.

40 Van Mastrigt R, Rollema HJ. The prognostic value of bladder contractility in transurethral resection of the prostate. *J Urol* 1992;**148**:1856–60.

41 Millin T. Retropubic prostatectomy: new extravesical technique. Report on 20 cases. *Lancet* 1945;**2**:693.

42 Hopkins HH. Optical principles of the endoscope. In: Berci G, ed. *Endoscopy*. New York: Appleton, Century Crofts, 1976:3–26.

43 Costello AJ, Bowsher WG, Bolton DM, Broslis KG, Burt J. Laser ablation of the prostate in patients with benign prostatic hyperplasia. *Br J Urol* 1992;**69**:603.

44 Norris JP, Norris DM, Lee RD, Rubenstein MA. Visual laser ablation of prostate: clinical experience in 108 patients. *J Urol* 1993;**150**:1612–14.

45 McCullough DL, Roth RA, Babayan RK *et al.* Transurethral ultrasound-guided laser-induced prostatectomy. *J Urol* 1993;**150**:1607.

46 Bruskevitz RC, Larsen EH, Madson PO. Three year follow-up of urinary symptoms after trans-urethra resection of the prostate. *J Urol* 1986;**136**:613–15.

47 Roos NP, Wennberg JE, Malenka DJ *et al.* Mortality and re-operation after open and trans-urethral resection of the prostate for benign prostatic hyperplasia. *N Engl J Med* 1989;**320**: 1120–4.

48 Mebust WK, Holtgrewe HL, Cockett ATK. Transurethral prostatectomy; immediate and postoperative complications: a cooperative study of 13 participating institutions evaluating 3885 patients. *J Urol* 1989;**141**:243–7.

49 Diesting W. Transurethral dilatation of the prostate: a new method in the treatment of prostatic hypertrophy. *Urol Int* 1956;**2**:158–71.

50 Burhenne HJ, Chisholm RJ, Quenville NF. Prostatic hyperplasia; radiological intervention. *Radiology* 1987;**152**: 655–7.

51 Castenada F, Reddy P, Wassermann N *et al.* Benign prostatic hyperplasia: retrogade dilatation of the prostatic urethra in humans. *Radiology* 1987;**163**:644–53.

52 Gill KP, Machan LS, Allison DJ, Williams G. Bladder outflow obstruction and urinary retention from prostatic hypertrophy treated by balloon dilatation. *Br J Urol* 1989;**64**:618–22.

53 McLoughlin J, Keane DF, Jager R *et al.* Dilatation of the prostate with a 35 mm balloon. *Br J Urol* 1991;**67**:177–81.

54 Holmes S, Kirby RS. Encrustation occuring on an intraprostatic spiral—a case report. *Br J Urol* 1992;**69**:322–3.

55 Kirby RS, Heard SR, Miller PD *et al.* Use of the ASI titanium stent in the management of bladder outflow obstruction due to benign prostatic hyperplasia. *J Urol* 1992;**148**:1195–7.

56 Yerushalmi A, Servadio C, Lieb Z , Fishslous Y, Rakowsky A, Stain JA. Local hyperthermia for the treatment of carcinoma of the prostate; a preliminary report. *Prostate* 1982;**6**:623–30.

57 Yerushalmi A, Fishelowitz Y, Singer D *et al.* Localized deep microwave hyperthermia in the treatment of poor operative risk patients with benign prostatic hyperplasia. *J Urol* 1985;**133**:873–6.

58 Strohmaier WL, Bichler KH, Fluchter SH, Wilbert DM. Local microwave hyperthermia of benign prostatic hyperplasia. *J Urol* 1990;**144**:913–17.

59 Lindner A, Golomb J, Siegel Y, Lev A. Local hyperthermia of the prostate gland for the treatment of benign prostatic hypertrophy and urinary retention. *Br J Urol* 1987;**60**:567–71.

60 Devonec MA, Berge N, Perrin O. Transurethral microwave heating of the prostate—or from hyperthermia to thermotherapy. *J Endocrinol* 1991;**5**:129–35.

61 Ogden CW, Reddy P, Johnson H, Ramsay JWA, Carter SStC. Sham versus transurethral microwave thermotherapy in patients with symptoms of benign prostatic bladder outflow obstruction. *Lancet* 1993;**341**:14–17.

62 Caine M, Perlberg S, Gordon R. The treatment of benign prostatic hypertrophy with flutamide (SCH 13521): a placebo controlled study. *J Urol* 1975;**114**:564–8.

63 Kirby RS, Pool JL. Alpha adrenoceptor blockade in the treatment of benign prostatic hyperplasia. *Br J Urol* 1997;**80**: 521–32.

64 Caine M, Perlnerg S, Meretyk S. A placebo-controlled double-blind study of the effect of phenoxybenzamine in benign prostatic obstruction. *Br J Urol* 1978;**50**:551–4.

65 Abrams PH, Shah PJR, Stone AR, Choa RG. Bladder outflow obstruction treated with phenoxybenzamine. *Br J Urol* 1982;**54**:527–30.

66 Hedlund H, Andersson KE, Ek A. Effects of prazosin in patients with benign prostatic obstruction. *J Urol* 1983;**130**:275–8.

67 Kirby RS, Coppinger SWC, Corcoran MO, Chapple CR, Flannagan M, Milroy EJG. Prazosin in the treatment of prostatic obstruction: a placebo-controlled study. *Br J Urol* 1987;**60**: 136–42.

68 Chapple CR, Scott M, Abrams P, Christmas TJ, Milroy EJG. A 12 week placebo-controlled double-blind study of prazosin in the treatment of prostatic obstruction due to benign prostatic hyperplasia. *Br J Urol* 1992;**70**:285–94.

69 Ramsey JWA, Scott GI, Whitfield HN. A double-blind controlled trial of a new alpha blocking drug in the treatment of bladder outlfow obstruction. *Br J Urol* 1985;**57**:657–9.

70 Jardin A, Bensadoun H, Delauche-Cavalier MC, Attali P. Alfusozin for treatment of benign prostatic hypertrophy. *Lancet* 1991;**337**:1457–61.

71 Italian Alfuzosin Study Group. Multicentre observational trial on symptomatic treatment of BPH with alfuzosin: clinical evaluation of impact on patient's quality of life. *Eur Urol* 1995;**27**:128–34.

72 Iacovou JW, Dunn M. Indoramin—an effective new drug in the management of bladder outflow obstruction. *Br J Urol* 1987;**60**:526–8.

73 Chow W, Hahn D, Sandhu D *et al.* Multicentre controlled trial of indoramin in the symptomatic relief of benign prostatic hypertrophy. *Br J Urol* 1990;**65**:36–8.

74 Fabricius PG, Weizert P, Dunzendorfer U, MacHannaford J, Maurath C. Efficacy of once-a-day terazosin in benign prostatic hyperplasia. a randomized placebo controlled clinical trial. *Prostate* 1990;**3**(Suppl.):85–93.

75 Lepor H, Knapp-Maloney G, Sunshine H. A dose titration study evaluating terazosin, a selective, once-a-day alpha-1 blocker for the treatment of symptomatic benign prostatic hyperplasia. *J Urol* 1990;**144**:1393–8.

76 Lepor H, Auerbach S, Puras-Baez A *et al.* A randomised, placebo-controlled multicentre study of the efficacy and safety of terazosin in the treatment of benign prostatic hyperplasia. *J Urol* 1992;**148**:1467–74.

77 Chapple CR, Carter P, Christmas TJ *et al.* A three month double-blind study of doxazosin as treatment for benign prostatic bladder outflow obstruction. *Br J Urol* 1994;**74**:50–6.

78 Kirby RS. Doxazosin in benign prostatic hyperplasia: effects on blood pressure and urinary flow in normotensive and hypertensive men. *Urology* 1995;**46**:182–6.

79 Abrams PH, Schulman CC, Vaage S and the European Study Group. Tamsulosin, a selective alpha$_{IC}$-adrenoceptor antagonist: a randomized, controlled trial in patients with benign prostatic 'obstruction' (symptomatic BPH). *Br J Urol* 1995;**76**:325–36.

80 Abrams P, Speakman M, Stott M, Arkell D, Pocock R. A close-ranging study of the efficacy and safety of tamsulosin, the first prostate-selective α_{1A}-adrenoceptor antagonist, in patients with benign prostatic obstruction. *Br J Urol* 1997;**80**: 587–96.

81 Buzelin JM, Fonteyne E, Kontturi M, Witjes WPJ, Khan A. Comparison of tamsulosin with alfuzosin in the treatment of patients with lower urinary tract symptoms suggestive of bladder outlet obstruction. *Br J Urol* 1997;**80**:597–605.

82 Lee E, Lee C. Clinical comparison of selective and non-selective α_{1A} adrenoceptor antagonists in benign prostate hyperplasia: studies on tamsulosin in a fixed dose and terazosin in increasing doses. *Br J Urol* 1997;**80**:606–11.

83 Cabot AT. The question of castration for enlarged prostate. *Ann Surg* 1896;**24**:265–309.

84 Peirson EL. A study of the effect of stilboestrol therapy on the size of the benignly enlarged prostate gland. *J Urol* 1946;**55**: 73–8.

85 Geller J, Bora R, Roberts T, Newman H, Lin A, Silva R. The treatment of benign prostatic hypertrophy with hydroxyprogesterone caproate. Effect on clinical symptoms, morphology and endocrine function. *J Am Med Assoc* 1965;**193**:121–8.

86 Stone N, Clejan S, Ray PS. A double-blind randomized controlled study of the effect of flutamide on benign prostatic hypertrophy: side effects and hormonal changes. *J Urol* 1989;**141**:307A.

87 Stone N, Ray PS, Smith JA. A double-blind radiological controlled study of the effect of flutamide on benign prostatic hypertrophy—clinical efficacy. *J Urol* 1989;**141**:240A.

88 Peters CA, Walsh PC. The effect of nafarelin acetate, a luteinizing hormone releasing hormone agonist, on benign prostatic hyperplasia. *N Engl J Med* 1987;**317**:599–604.

89 Bosch RJ, Griffiths DJ, Blom J, Schroeder FH. Treatment of benign prostatic hyperplasia by androgen deprivation: effects on prostate size and urodynamic parameters. *J Urol* 1989;**141**:68–72.

90 Farnsworth WE, Brown JR. Testosterone metabolism in the prostate. *Nat Cancer Inst Monogr* 1963;**12**:323–5.

91 Imperato-McGinley J, Guevro L, Gauteri T, Petersen RE. Steroid 5-alpha-reductase deficiency in a man: an inherited form of pseudohermaphroditism. *Science* 1974;**186**:1213–15.

92 Rasmusson GH, Reynolds GF, Utre T *et al*. Azasteroids as inhibitors of rat prostatic 5-alpha-reductase. *J Med Chem* 1984;**27**:1690–1701.

93 Geller J. Effect of finasteride, a 5-alpha reductase inhibitor on prostate tissue androgens and prostate specific antigen. *J Clin Endocrinol Metab* 1990;**71**:1552–5.

94 Stoner E. The clinical effects of a 5-alpha reductase inhibitor finasteride, on benign prostatic hyperplasia. *J Urol* 1992;**147**:1298–302.

95 Kirby RS, Bryan J, Christmas TJ *et al*. Finasteride in the management of benign prostatic hyperplasia—a urodynamic study. *Br J Urol* 1992;**70**:65–72.

96 Kirby RS, Vale J, Bryan J, Holmes K, Webb JAW. Long-term urodynamic effects of finasteride in benign prostatic hyperplasia: a pilot study. *Eur Urol* 1993;**24**:20–6.

97 Gormley GJ, Stoner E, Bruskevitz RC *et al*. The effect of finasteride in men with benign prostatic hyperplasia. *N Engl J Med* 1992;**327**:1185–91.

98 Stoner E, Members of the Finasteride Study Group. Three-year safety and efficacy data on the use of finasteride in the treatment of benign prostatic hyperplasia. *Urology* 1994;**43**(3):284–94.

99 Andersen JT, Ekman P, Wolf H *et al*. Can finasteride reverse the progress of benign prostatic hyperplasia? A two-year placebo-controlled study. *Urology* 1995;**46**:631–7.

100 Schulse H, Barrack ER. Immunocytochemical localization of oestrogen receptors in spontaneous and experimentally induced canine BPH. *Prostate* 1987;**11**:145–62.

101 Stone NN, Fair WR, Fishman J. Oestrogen formation in human prostate tissue from patients with and without BPH. *Prostate* 1986;**9**:311–18.

102 Tunn UW, Schweikurt HU. Aromatase inhibitors in the management of benign prostatic hyperplasia. In: Actermann R, Schröder FM, eds. *New Developments in Biosciences 5*. Berlin: de Gruyter, 1989:139–49.

103 Oesterling JE, Juniewicz PE, Walters JR. Aromatase inhibition in the dog. Effect on growth, function and pathology of the prostate. *J Urol* 1988;**139**:832–9.

104 Ball AJ, Feneley RCL, Abrams PH. The natural history of untreated 'prostatism'. *Br J Urol* 1981;**533**:613–16.

105 Craigen AA, Hickling JB, Saunders CRG, Carpenter RG. Natural history of prostatic obstruction. A prospective survey. *J R Coll Gen Pract* 1969;**18**:226–32.

37   Bladder Neck Obstruction
J.F.Jiménez-Cruz and E.Broseta

Introduction

The bladder neck, internal sphincter and external urinary sphincter play an important role in the mechanisms of urinary continence and micturition. The internal sphincter extends from the bladder neck into the proximal urethra in the adult female and to the membranous urethra in the male. It is composed of smooth muscle fibres. The origin and disposition of these fibres in the bladder neck have been much debated causing sharp disagreement among investigators.

Many different and, sometimes, opposite theories are still being discussed. Some authors claim that detrusor fibres are continuous with those of the bladder neck and proximal urethra. The bladder neck and urethral closure is secondary to the inherent tension of the urethral wall and the urethral length. When the detrusor contracts the bladder neck opens up [1–3]. Accordingly, these authors do not consider the bladder neck to be a sphincter or an anatomical and functional specific area. Other investigators consider the urethral musculature, the detrusor muscle and the trigonal muscle as different smooth muscle systems. Circular fibres from the trigonal muscle form the bladder neck, whereas other layers of this trigonal muscle extend into the urethra [4–7]. Finally, a mixed theory accepts the bladder neck as a special arrangement of fibres from the detrusor and trigonal musculature [8–10].

Therefore, the anatomical structure of the vesicourethral area, including the bladder neck, is still controversial. However, it is an increasingly accepted fact that the bladder neck works as a sphincter with an important contribution to the mechanisms of continence and bladder emptying. During bladder filling, the detrusor fibres are relaxed and the superficial trigonal muscle contracts to keep the trigonal base and the bladder neck fixed and closed. When the bladder detrusor contracts to empty, both the internal and external sphincters must open to allow the flow of urine. Contractions of the trigonal detrusor will produce a conical shape in the trigonal base opening the bladder neck [7,9]. Therefore, the normal opening mechanism of the bladder neck is related to detrusor and trigonal function.

All this muscular activity is under a direct neurological influence. In humans and animals, the hypogastric nerves produce the bladder neck closure. The electrical stimulation in a hypogastric nerve generates a rhythmic contraction of the bladder neck [11].

The isolated human bladder neck mainly contains α-adrenoceptors, basically from the α_1-type [12,13]. The bladder neck is then under a constant sympathetic stimulation that is inhibited by parasympathetic discharge during micturition, producing the opening of the bladder neck simultaneously with detrusor contraction [14].

Some in vitro studies have demonstrated an active nerve-mediated relaxation of smooth muscle around the bladder neck [15]. The neurotransmitter substance is non-cholinergic and non-adrenergic. Vasoactive intestinal polypeptide has been investigated to evaluate its influence on the relaxation of the bladder neck smooth muscle, but, to date, its role in the bladder neck functional activity has not been determined [16].

In 1834, Guthrie [17] described for the first time the outlet bladder obstruction due to organic narrowing of the bladder neck. A few years later, in 1913, Young [18] reported more than 50 cases of this pathology, the majority of them related to chronic infection and fibrosis. He also described the punch operation for bladder neck contraction. This disease was forgotten until 1933 when Marion [19] reviewed and characterized it as 'dysuric disturbances similar to those giving rise to hypertrophy of the prostate, disturbances caused by alterations of the bladder neck and which can not be attributed to nerve injuries'. Marion considered two different types of this disease affecting the bladder neck: an acquired type and a congenital form in infants and children. Since then, the aetiology and frequency of this disease have been controversial. It has been considered as a very common condition, mainly in children and women, who, in the 1950s and 1960s, frequently underwent surgical treatment.

A further re-evaluation of this entity and its treatment demonstrated a significant degree of overdiagnosis and failure of therapy. This led to it being accepted as an uncommon entity, using strict diagnostic criteria, or to doubt about its existence.

A large number of terminologies have been used to label this entity: Marion's disease, bladder neck stenosis, bladder neck obstruction, median bar and fibrous bladder neck contracture. While all these terms are used to suggest organic obstruction, other expressions describe non-organic dysfunction of the bladder neck: detrusor–bladder neck dyssynergia, bladder neck dyskinesia, dysfunctional bladder neck obstruction and internal sphincter dyssynergia.

We prefer to denominate this entity bladder neck obstruction instead of dyssynergia, because dyssynergia can be active (increased contraction from the bladder neck accompanying detrusor contraction) or passive (absence of relaxation of the bladder neck during detrusor contraction). In the majority of these patients it is very difficult to establish if the obstruction is due to active or passive dyssynergia.

A second denomination must be used to identify the aetiological factor responsible: primary when no apparent cause is demonstrated and secondary if the aetiological factor causing the dysfunction of the bladder neck is evident.

Aetiology

An obstruction in the bladder neck or in the vesicourethral junction without any other obstruction in the remaining urethra or prostatic enlargement may be considered as a bladder neck obstruction. Many factors have been implicated in the aetiology and pathogenesis of this entity, which is most often seen in young and middle-aged men but may also be present in older men [20–22].

Clasically, the obstruction has been attributed to a muscular hypertrophy or fibrous scarring of the bladder neck, but a dysfunction of the bladder neck mechanism has also been implicated. In some patients, the origin of bladder neck obstruction may not be established. In women, bladder neck obstruction is considered, to date, to be an uncommon process [23,24].

Fibrosis and scarring at the bladder neck level is usually secondary to surgery (prostatectomy) and chronic inflammatory changes. It would normally be an acquired type of bladder neck obstruction and must be separated from the primary type.

The aetiology of primary isolated bladder neck obstruction is controversial. Leadbetter and Leadbetter [25] consider that a fault in dissolution of mesenchyme of the bladder neck or the inclusion of abnormal amounts of non-muscular connective tissue could be the aetiological factors. They observed, with histological studies, hypertrophic smooth muscle affecting a part, or the entire circumference, of the bladder neck. Increased amounts of fibrous tissue and chronic inflammatory changes were also reported. Other investigators did not observe any increase in collagen fibres or fibrosis in patients with primary bladder neck obstruction [26,27]. Holm [28] in 1964 suggested this condition to be caused either by a defective opening of the vesical neck or by some inadequate correlation between the detrusor and the opening mechanism of the primary vesical neck trigonal muscle. Turner-Warwick et al. [9] consider that bladder neck obstruction in males is an intrinsic dyssynergia as a result of a dysfunctional arrangement of the bladder neck musculature inherent to its development. Apparently, there is no coordination between the activity of the detrusor and that of the bladder neck. Several aetiological mechanisms may be involved in this lack of coordination [29]. For Bates et al. [30], the obstruction is functional and due to the tightening of the bladder neck during micturition as the detrusor contracts. They found that in obstructed patients, the pressure in the bladder during micturition was always higher than at the outlet at rest. This fact means that, instead of the bladder neck being actively opened, it not only fails to open but appears to be actively tightened.

A sympathetic nervous system dysfunction has also been suggested by several investigators [31–33]. Micturition is a complex neurological mechanism. Integration of the outflow from spinal cord autonomic nuclei, spinal cord reflexes, ganglionic transmission and postganglionic neurotransmitter and receptor function are necessary for a coordinated micturition. A dysfunction of any component alone or in combination could produce bladder neck obstruction [34]. However, Parys et al. [35] evaluated sacral reflex latency in 25 patients with bladder neck obstruction. Their results did not indicate any underlying neuropathy.

Bladder neck obstruction as a consequence of inadequate detrusor contractility is not uncommon. Premature closure of the bladder neck due to failure in maintaining an adequate detrusor contraction has been observed in women with voiding dysfunction [20]. A reduced detrusor contraction to open the bladder neck could also produce a functional obstruction. A continual high tonus in the smooth muscle of the urethra causes a rigidity of the bladder neck in women [27].

In summary, primary bladder neck obstruction can be produced by a bladder neck dysfunction with either a failure to relax or an increased activity with voiding (dyssynergia). The exact aetiological factors that produce such dysfunction remain unclear (Table 37.1). In these patients fibrosis at the bladder neck level has not been histologically demonstrated.

Diagnosis

When Marion [19] described bladder neck obstruction the diagnosis was reached by a process of elimination.

Table 37.1 Aetiology of primary and secondary bladder neck obstruction.

Primary	Secondary
Congenital increase in connective tissue	Prostatectomy
Muscular lack of coordination	Benign prostatic hyperplasia
Neurological dysfunction hyperplasia	Prostatitis
Inadequate detrusor contractility	Neurogenic processes
Urethral high tonus	

Subsequently, it was based mainly on clinical manifestations, use of calibrating instruments and endoscopic visualization of the bladder neck and urethra. In spite of the use of sophisticated diagnostic methods like urodynamic tests and radiology aided synchronous pressure–flow studies, the diagnosis of primary bladder neck obstruction is still a hard task. The diagnosis is only confirmed by the improvement or relief of symptoms after bladder neck surgery. In secondary bladder neck obstruction, the diagnosis is less complex because the origin of such obstruction is more evident.

Symptomatology

No differencies can be found in the clinical manifestations of primary and secondary bladder neck obstruction. In the latter, symptoms have a shorter evolution and can be related to the aetiological factor(s).

In primary bladder neck obstruction, symptoms are vague, confusing and have a long duration. In some patients these symptoms date back to late childhood. A previous history of recurrent urinary infections is frequent, especially in females. Most patients complain of frequency, hesitation, weak or poor stream, post-micturition dribbling, urgency, nocturia, a feeling of incomplete bladder emptying, suprapubic or pelvic pain and discomfort. Chronic urinary retention is as uncommon as a dilated upper urinary tract and renal failure. Several patients may be practically asymptomatic with only minor changes in their voiding pattern. In women, symptoms are almost similar to those found in males.

Physical exploration is usually normal. The prostate in the young and middle-aged male must always be examined to detect prostatitis and prostate hypertrophy. In primary bladder neck obstruction, the size of the prostate should be related to the patient's age, with no significant enlargement. In women, cystoceles and/or urethroceles must be excluded from the diagnosis of primary bladder neck obstruction.

Urethral calibration with a catheter or bougie has not proved to be useful. From a theoretical standpoint, a rigid urethra must have an inner diameter lesser than 10 F to produce a significant degree of obstruction [36]. Calibration only indicates the limit of passive urethral wall stretching.

Therefore, since symptoms and physical exploration are rather nonspecific it is necessary to employ the aid of invasive techniques to obtain a diagnosis.

Radiological examination

To exclude organic and inflammatory conditions that could be considered the cause of the symptoms, an intravenous urography must be performed. This procedure may provide indirect evidence of bladder neck obstruction (changes in bladder morphology or post-voiding residual urine), but a normal exploration cannot exclude it.

Retrograde and voiding cystourethrography are informative about the morphology of the urethra and can rule out an anatomical obstruction. In the same way, narrowing of the bladder neck and lack or minimal funnelling of the trigone during micturition can be observed (Fig. 37.1), but this radiological pattern is not specific to primary bladder obstruction. It can be seen, for instance, with an isolated enlargement of the median lobe. In such cases, a careful examination in the lateral and anteroposterior positions will increase the diagnostic possibilities.

The diameter of the bladder neck can also be measured. In a primary obstruction the diameter during micturition is usually less than 6 mm [37]. To obtain the best information a synchronous pressure–flow study is also advisable. A similar anatomical evaluation is achieved with transrectal ultrasonography.

Endoscopic evaluation

Urethrocystoscopy alone is an urealiable tool in the diagnosis of primary bladder neck obstruction, since the bladder neck endoscopic appearance is usually normal in spite of the lack of proper opening during voiding. Only in secondary obstruction, when the outlet is fibrous and pinpoint, can endoscopic evaluation yield the diagnosis as in the case of urethral stenosis. Endoscopic bladder examination confirms the radiographic findings of trabeculation and/or diverticula, either due to bladder neck obstruction or another cause of urinary tract obstruction.

Urodynamic evaluation

Uroflowmetry is an important screening test for the detection of bladder outflow obstruction. A peak flow rate less than 15 ml/s suggests detrusor–urethral imbalance but it cannot differentiate bladder outlet obstruction from poor detrusor function. Thus, further urodynamic studies are necessary in these patients. In bladder neck obstruction cystometry will show a normal or increased detrusor pressure. If the detrusor is severely hypotonic as a conse-

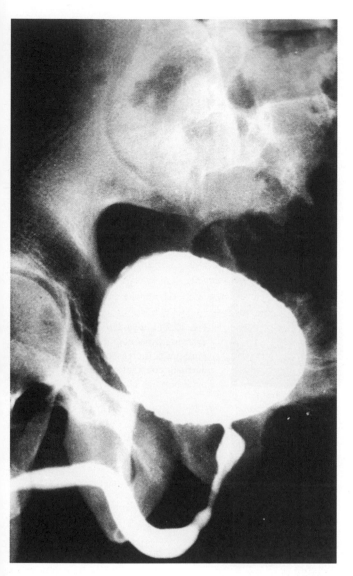

Fig. 37.1 Voiding cystourethrography showing an irregular bladder shape with a limited opening of the vesical neck and widening of prostatic urethra.

quence of obstruction, detrusor pressure will be low or absent and bladder neck obstruction cannot be diagnosed in these cases. Sphincter electromyography is a useful tool to rule out detrusor–striated sphincter dyssynergia. Urethral pressure profilometry is a static study used to determine the closing pressure in the passive urethra so it has no diagnostic value because the resting bladder neck and proximal urethral pressures are normal in patients with bladder neck obstruction [31].

Simultaneous pressure–flow video cystourethrography or video cystourethrosonography are the keys to confirm the diagnosis of primary bladder neck obstruction. Normal or high detrusor pressure and a low peak flow rate confirm outlet bladder obstruction. The site of the obstruction is determined by the appearance of a narrowed vesical neck

on voiding cystourethrography or video cystourethrography. The authors prefer the use of simultaneous pressure–flow video cystourethrosonography to evaluate patients with suspected obstruction of the lower urinary tract. The use of a transrectal linear array transducer obtains a saggital view of the bladder base plate, prostatic urethra and membranous urethra, which enables the bladder changes and voiding phase to be studied. Simultaneously, pressures are determined (Figs 37.2 and 37.3).

Taking into account the sympathetic influence in the activity of the bladder neck, once the basal measurements are made, an α-adrenergic blocking agent (intravenous phentolamine, 0.10–0.15 mg/kg body weight) can be administered to determine changes in the cystometry parameters, uroflowmetry and morphology of the bladder neck during voiding. As detrusor pressure remains unchanged and the bladder neck is wide open, an increase in the peak flow rate would suggest a primary bladder neck obstruction [32,38]. Poulsen et al. [38] consider that the phentolamine effect is proportional to the degree of bladder neck obstruction, with practically no change being observed in patients with normal bladder neck function.

A modification of the urethral pressure profilometry, the micturitional static urethral pressure profile, has been proposed [34,39] to establish directly the site and degree of bladder outlet obstruction. In primary bladder neck obstruction the static pressure profile during voiding shows a precipitous decrease in pressure at the bladder neck [39]. In animals, Cass and Hinman [40] suggest that constriction of the vesical neck of more than 50% of its cross-sectional area could produce a decrease in static pressure across the constricted bladder neck even at low flow rates. Such a decrease was not observed when the bladder neck was constricted to only one-third of its cross-sectional area. Thus, in patients with a mild degree of bladder neck obstruction a decrease in the static pressure could be not observed if they void with low urinary flow rates. In this situation additional increases in intravesical pressures by means of the Valsalva manoeuvre, augmenting the detrusor contractions, could accentuate the pressure decrease across the bladder neck [39]. Using the same technique, Woodside [34] describes two different patterns of bladder neck obstruction. If the bladder neck pressure increases during voiding, it indicates an obstruction by active dyssynergia. Conversely, if the bladder neck pressure remains unchanged during detrusor contraction associated with markedly elevated intravesical pressure, a passive failure of bladder neck relaxation is responsible for the obstruction. In both situations the basic functional abnormality remains unknown.

It is necessary to perform more studies in order to confirm these findings. Andersen et al. [37] introduced the maximum opening time as the most representative

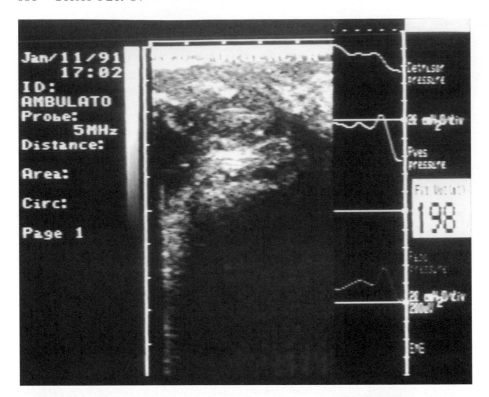

Fig. 37.2 Flow video cystourethrosonography. Bladder pressure is increased due to uninhibited detrusor contractions and the bladder neck remains closed.

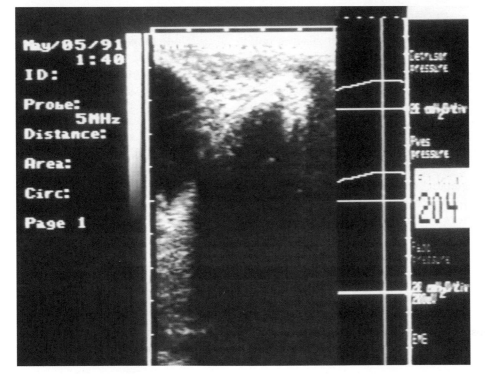

Fig. 37.3 Flow video cystourethrosonography. This female patient has closed bladder neck in spite of the increase in vesical pressure (30 cmH$_2$O).

pressure parameter in the diagnosis of bladder neck obstruction. It represents the interval between the previoiding rise in intravesical pressure and the time of peak flow rate. In patients with bladder neck obstruction it tends to be higher than in normal men or in those with benign prostatic hypertrophy. Gilja *et al.* [41] also observed a high detrusor pressure at the moment of bladder neck opening and a prolonged opening time in patients with primary bladder neck obstruction. All these findings need to be confirmed.

For primary bladder obstruction to be diagnosed, the following findings have to all be present.

1 A normal or high sustained detrusor contraction.
2 A reduced peak flow rate of 15 ml/s or less.
3 Complete relaxation of the external urethral sphincter during voiding.
4 Radiographic or sonographic evidence of obstruction at the bladder neck.
5 A lack of prostatic enlargement and urethral stricture.

In secondary bladder neck obstruction, the first four findings are always present, but their severity depends on the main cause of the obstruction.

Differential diagnosis

To establish the diagnosis of primary bladder neck obstruction it is necessary to rule out all of the causes that could produce an obstruction of the lower urinary tract, such as urethral valves or strictures, prostatic enlargement, neurogenic lesions, cysts and tumours. Radiological and urodynamic studies together with endoscopic examination are enough in the majority of patients to reach a proper diagnosis.

In other cases the achievement of a differential diagnosis is a more difficult matter because symptoms and investigations are confusing. In males with a prostatic median lobe and non-apparent prostatic enlargement, symptoms and urodynamic findings can be similar to those derived from primary bladder neck obstruction. However, urethrocystoscopy, voiding cystourethrography (both in the lateral and anteroposterior positions), sonography of the bladder and prostate and, in particular, video cystourethrosonography are useful in differential diagnosis (Figs 37.4 and 37.5).

In young males with suprapubic pain, frequency, urgency and an aching sensation in the testicles, chronic prostatitis must be suspected. Prostatic location cultures and cytology of the expressed prostatic secretions must be performed to exclude that diagnosis. Urethral hypertonia can be responsible for the symptoms and urodynamic and radiological changes observed in males with a first diagnosis of chronic non-bacterial prostatitis or prostatodynia. In such cases, this form of prostatitis produces a secondary bladder neck obstruction where no differential signs from a primary bladder neck obstruction are found [42,43].

George and Slade [44] reported young males with symptoms of prostatism and multiple somatic symptoms that they considered to be produced by psychological causes. Urodynamic evaluation demonstrated in these cases a reduced flow with poorly sustained detrusor contractions. Because of this low detrusor pressure, diagnosis of primary bladder neck obstruction cannot be established. A sympathetically mediated systemic anxiety state might conceivably produce the changes observed.

In female patients, a chronic urinary retention associated with frequency, overflow incontinence and recurrent urinary tract infection have also been associated with detrusor failure due to a psychological aetiology [45,46].

Management

Many different procedures have been used in the treatment of primary bladder neck obstruction: pharmacological agents, transurethral bladder neck incision, transurethral resection of the bladder neck and retropubic Y-V bladder neck plasty.

Pharmacological treatment

Pharmacological treatment is the main alternative to surgery. α-Receptor blocking agents have been used to modulate the overactivity of the α-receptors that are densely located at the bladder neck. The phentolamine test can be useful in screening out functionally obstructed patients of both sexes [31] and in the selection of those cases that would be successfully treated with α-blockers. Phenoxybenzamine and prazosin have been used in primary bladder neck obstruction; 50% of males treated improved with minimal or no side effects [22,26,32,47]. In female patients the results were similar [48].

In the latter study, six patients were treated with some degree of subjective and objective improvement but only three definitely benefited from the treatment.

We consider that α-blockers should be the first therapeutical option in patients with primary bladder neck obstruction. Surgery would then be reserved for those cases with poor results, side effects or who demand a definitive solution.

Surgery

The definitive treatment of primary bladder neck obstruction is surgery and transurethral bladder neck incision seems to be the best option. Transurethral resection of the bladder neck has no advantages and increases the risk of secondary fibrosis at the bladder neck level, retrograde ejaculation in males and incontinence in females. To date there does not appear to be any place for retropubic Y-V bladder neck plasty in the treatment of these patients.

Transurethral bladder neck incision

This technique was described in 1834 by Guthrie [17] and later reviewed by Beer in 1933 [49] with the introduction of transurethral diathermy. In the 1970s Turner-Warwick et al. [9] induced a widespread popularity for this technique.

The incision is performed from the 5 o'clock and/or 7

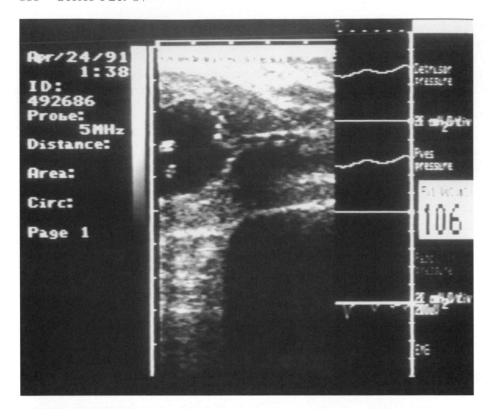

Fig 37.4 Flow video cystourethrosonography showing the thick wall of the detrusor. There is a limited opening of the bladder neck in spite of the detrusor contraction (60 cmH$_2$O).

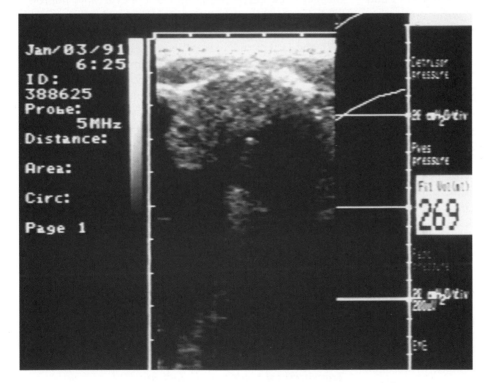

Fig. 37.5 Flow video cystourethrosonography. There is a high detrusor pressure (>150 cmH$_2$O) with a minimal opening of the vesical neck due to a prostatic median lobe.

o'clock position and from the trigone to the verumontanum extending through the bladder neck and prostatic tissue. The incision is gradually deepened as the capsule is reached. This incision tends to spring apart as the extravesical plane is approached, making it difficult to perform a complete second incision. Once the longitudinal incisions (one or two) have been performed, the endoscopic image from the verumontanum shows a completely open bladder neck.

An indwelling catheter drains the bladder for 24–48 h.

This procedure carries very few complications: peroperative and postoperative bleeding is scarce, epididymitis and urinary infection are uncommon and the two most significant complications are retrograde ejaculation and incontinence. The postoperative stay is usually short (2–14 days).

Results with a single or double incision are excellent. In a review from the literature with 275 males treated, good results were obtained in 84.3% of them ($P = 0.015$). A single incision was used in 68 out of 73 patients (93.1%) and a double incision in 164 out of 202 (81.8%). Retrograde ejaculation was observed in 23 out of 141 patients evaluated (16.3%) and was less frequent with a single incision procedure than with a double incision: 12.5 and 33.3%, respectively ($P = 0.3$) [50–53] (Table 37.2). These results are sufficient to indicate that a single incision, when correctly performed, is a better procedure than a bilateral incision. All patients must be informed about the risk of postoperative retrograde ejaculation linked to the procedure, although the reasons for this are still unknown.

In female patients with primary bladder neck obstruction, bladder neck incision has also been used with a high rate of success: 39 of 52 women were cured or improved their symptoms [27,48,54]. Incision at the 12 o'clock position avoids the risk of a vesicovaginal fistula which may follow a posterior or posterolateral incision. Moreover, it offers the best chance of subsequent retropubic repair in cases of incontinence.

The incision is made from the inner portion of the bladder neck, distally for 1–2 cm, to avoid possible damage in the intrinsic urethral sphincter. Incontinence is the most disturbing complication in female patients; levels of up to 15.2% postoperative incontinence following transurethral resection of the bladder neck have been reported [55], but 70% of these patients soon became continent without

further treatment, with a definitive incidence of 4.7%. With bladder neck incision the rate of incontinence is lower: 0–6.2% [27,48,54,56]. In some cases incontinence is only produced when a second incision is necessary due to a poor result of a previous procedure [26,53].

Argon lasers have been used to perform a precise incision in cases of a bladder neck obstruction. The argon probe provides a bloodless incision reducing the need for fulguration and, as a result, a lesser risk of scar. Treatment can be carried out on an outpatient basis without the aid of general or spinal anaesthesia. No postoperative urethral catheter is required [57]. Further results are necessary to evaluate this technique in the management of bladder neck obstruction.

Secondary bladder neck obstruction

Post-prostatectomy

Post-surgery bladder neck obstruction is an uncommon but disappointing complication of prostatic surgery. It is more frequently described after transurethral resection but is also found after open surgery. Millin [58] reported five cases of bladder neck obstruction in his first 75 consecutive patients. However, he eliminated this complication in subsequent patients by fixing the vesical mucosa across the bladder neck. Most bladder neck obstruction appears after surgery of prostates weighing less than 20 g [59,60].

The precise mechanisms of bladder neck obstruction are not clearly established yet. Experimental trauma limited to the bladder neck in dogs produces obstruction [60]. An extensive resection of the bladder neck or excessive fulguration or heat released from the loop can provoke serious injuries in a large enough portion of the bladder neck to produce a hypertrophic scar. Such a possibility is

Table 37.2 Results of transurethral bladder neck incision studies.

	Number	Incision	Good result	Retrograde ejaculation	Reference
	6	Double	6	6	Norlen & Blaivas [26]
	2	Single	2	0	Norlen & Blaivas [26]
	128	Double	96	6 of 27	Christensen et al. [50]
	38	Single	33	4 of 26	Moisey et al. [51]
	32	Double	32 }	3*	Hedlund & Ek [52]
	29	Single	29 }		Hedlund & Ek [52]
	4	Double	4	0	Yalla et al. [22]
	4	Single	4	0	Yalla et al. [22]
	32	Double	26	4 of 11	Delaere et al. [53]
Subtotal	202	Double	164 (81.1%)†	16/48 (33.31%)‡	
	73	Single	68 (93.1%)†	4/32 (12.5%)‡	
Total	275		232 (84.3%)†	23/141 (16.3%)‡	

*Three cases of retrograde ejaculation in 61 patients under double or single incision (not specified).
† $P = 0.015$.
‡ $P = 0.03$.

more common in small prostates because the bladder neck is neither dilated nor pushed aside as occurs when the prostate is large or intravesical. The degree of obstruction depends on the tissue injured: elevation of the posterior lip of the bladder neck or circumferential narrowing and rigidity. In its severest type, a diaphragm occludes the whole bladder neck down to a pinhole opening placed centrally [61].

The onset of symptoms due to bladder neck obstruction varies from a few weeks after prostatectomy to 10 years later [59,60]. The diagnosis is easily made either by urethroscopy or retrograde urethrography where the characteristic 'jet' or 'toothpaste' sign can be observed.

Transurethral incision of the prostate and bladder neck in small glands (less than 20–30 g) has been suggested as a primary treatment to avoid bladder neck obstruction [62]. If a transurethral resection is made in small glands, obstruction can be prevented by avoiding extensive resection or fulguration at the bladder neck plus a bladder neck longitudinal incision with a cold or electric knife. The bladder neck diameter is thus increased while reducing the risks of contractural healing [63].

We have observed in prostates less than 30 g, worse results with transurethral resection than those obtained with transurethral deep incision (going as far as the perivesical and pericapsule fat) from the trigone to the verumontanum, either at the 5 o'clock or 7 o'clock position. A few pieces of prostatic tissue must be resected to obtain a histological diagnosis.

Once the bladder neck obstruction has occurred the best treatment is a bladder neck incision with electric or cold knife (Sachse urethrotome). The recurrence rates, about 10%, are lower than those produced with a new transurethral resection [59].

Bladder neck dilatation obtains the worse results.

Benign prostatic hyperplasia

The prostate usually begins to be hyperplasic in the fourth decade of life, giving rise to hypertonia of the prostatic urethra associated with an increase in urethral resistance. The first effect could be a hyperstimulation of the urethral mucosa and the bladder neck with an increased activity at the α-receptors of this area. The excessive sympathetic activity and the push-back of the basal plate of the trigone from the fibroadenosis reduce the possibilities of the basal plate being turned into a cone, formed by the anterior and posterior lips of the bladder neck coming together as a result of the pull of trigonal fibres during detrusor contraction. So, simple elevation of the posterior lip of the bladder neck by a small enlargement of the median lobe can impair normal micturition more than a huge adenoma which lifts the trigone uniformly. The prostatic hypertrophy also leads to a narrowing of the prostatic

urethra. This hyperplasia does not occur uniformly in the different lobes and, therefore, the lumen of the prostatic urethra becomes distorted. These changes can be observed during urethroscopy, urethrography and urethroprostatic sonography.

Accordingly, the evidence of prostatic enlargement, including the median lobe, eliminates the diagnosis of primary bladder neck obstruction unless the symptoms date back several years. However, many patients older than 50 years with no evidence of significant prostatic enlargement had obstructive symptoms similar to those produced by primary bladder neck obstruction. Turner-Warwick et al. [9] used the term 'trapped prostate' for these patients. This entity is a combination of pre-existing bladder neck obstruction and a mild degree of prostatic enlargement. Each component by itself would not lead to clinical outlet obstruction.

In spite of the use of different studies including video urodynamic studies, the diagnosis of mixed obstruction is difficult.

Transurethral deep incision from the trigone to the verumontanum is an effective treatment for both primary and secondary obstruction. In selected cases with minimal symptoms α-blocker drugs can also be effective.

Prostatitis

Prostatitis is the most common urinary inflammatory syndrome in men under 40 years old. Four main forms have been described: bacterial (acute and chronic), non-bacterial and prostatodynia [64]. Both bacterial and non-bacterial chronic prostatitis have been associated with bladder neck obstruction but the precise relationship is not established yet [65,66].

Histological studies have revealed that inflammatory changes occur in bacterial and non-bacterial prostatitis. However, as these conditions affect only the prostate gland, it is difficult to accept that such inflammation could spread to produce an active obstruction at the bladder neck. Nonetheless, secondary fibrosis at the bladder neck has been reported following the development of a prostatic abscess [65].

When men diagnosed as having chronic non-bacterial prostatitis or prostatodynia were subjected to pressure–flow urodynamic assessment, patients were found to fall into two distinct clinical groups [42]. All patients showed an increase in the urethral pressure at rest and a narrowing of the prostatic urethra during voiding, both at the level of the prostate and the external urethral sphincter [42]. The majority of these patients also had a reduced urinary flow rate. However, in some patients, obstruction resulting from incomplete funnelling of the bladder neck was also observed. In such patients, urinary flow rate was always reduced. Thus, urethral hypertonia, as a result of overactivity of the sympathetic nervous system innervating the functional autonomic sphincter area, was the main cause of the symptoms and signs reported. It was suggested that the reported incomplete funnelling of the bladder neck during voiding implies a lack of coordination of, or the incomplete relaxation of, the sympathetically dependent urethral musculature [42,43]. In this case it would be a secondary bladder neck obstruction.

Another group of patients, mainly young men previously diagnosed as having prostatitis, have also been shown to have an isolated bladder neck obstruction. Such patients frequently experience prostatitis-like symptoms: irritative voiding symptoms (such as frequency or urgency accompanied by perineal, suprapubic and testicular discomfort) and obstructive symptoms.

Because it is not usual to find bladder neck obstruction in young men, such patients can easily be misdiagnosed as having prostatitis. However, urodynamic studies and video cystourethrography or video cystourethrosonography can reveal the typical signs of primary bladder neck obstruction. In such patients, bladder neck obstruction is an isolated pathology and it is not associated with prostatitis. Irritative symptoms are usually the result of detrusor instability secondary to the obstruction. Recurrent urinary infections are also a frequent consequence of incomplete bladder emptying. Misdiagnosis is therefore possible, but lower tract localization and colour Doppler transrectal ultrasound reveal normal findings.

In summary, bladder neck obstruction is an unusual complication of prostatitis. However, in patients with bladder neck obstruction and symptoms of prostatitis two possibilities can be considered.

1 In patients with prostatitis or prostatodynia, sympathetic dysfunction produces an increase in the intraurethral pressure and gives rise to obstructive and irritative symptoms.
2 Isolated bladder neck obstruction can be demonstrated in young men with symptoms similar to those of prostatitis, but the prostate is unaffected. Urologists should be careful in considering this possibility during diagnosis, so as to avoid inappropriate treatment and its inherent consequences.

Neurogenic processes

The bladder neck smooth muscle is under neurological influences from the sympathetic and parasympathetic systems, especially the former. The activity of both systems after spinal cord injury or in different diseases affecting the central nervous system is dependent on the lesion level, and in particular its relationship with the thoracolumbar sympathetic nuclei.

In acute spinal cord lesions detrusor areflexia and urethral sphincter hypoactivity are observed together with an increased urethral resistance probably due to smooth

muscle-enhanced activity. Patients with chronic spinal cord lesions above the thoracolumbar spinal nuclei with an intact cord below the level of lesion are prone to autonomic dysreflexia, a common syndrome associated with inappropriate activity of the bladder neck. Sympathetic reflex activity occurs as a result of the lack of cerebral regulatory influences that come from the injured area, resulting in an overridden parasympathetic-mediated bladder neck relaxation during detrusor contraction [34,67].

In patients with spinal cord lesions at the level of the thoracolumbar nuclei, the bladder neck and urethral smooth muscle are excluded from the sympathetic influence and remain a reflex activity that produces a dysfunction in the bladder neck.

When the spinal cord lesion is located between the thoracolumbar sympathetic nuclei and the parasympathetic sacral nuclei it results in an uninhibited excessive sympathetic discharge at the internal sphincter area. Consequently, a bladder neck obstruction would occur.

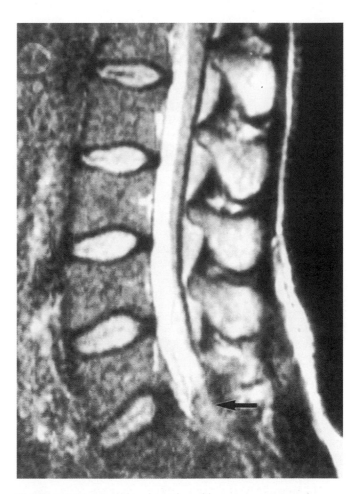

Fig. 37.6 A 35-year-old male with problems in erection and ejaculation. The urodynamic evaluation showed detrusor hyperreflexia and a residual urine volume greater than 300 ml. The MRI shows a spinal cord lipoma (the arrow marks the location of the tumour).

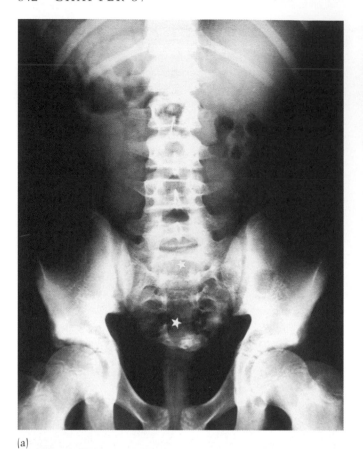

(a)

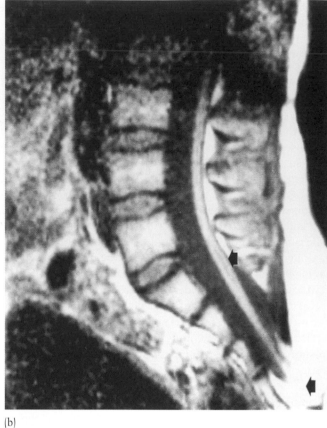

(b)

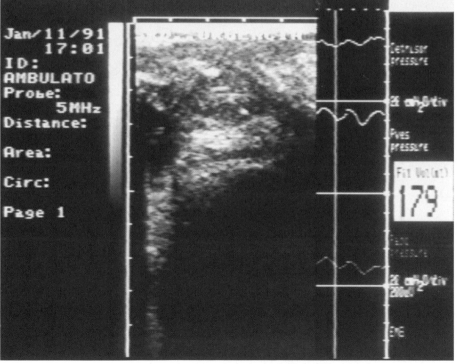

(c)

Fig. 37.7 A 12-year-old male with micturition problems and overflow incontinence. (a) A plain film of the urinary tract showing myelodysplasia (spina bifida) and coccyx agenesis. (b) MRI showing syringomyelia (upper arrow), sacral lipoma, tethered cord syndrome and epidermoid cyst (lower arrows). (c) Flow video cystourethrosonography showing uninhibited detrusor contractions (> 100 cmH$_2$O) without opening of the bladder neck.

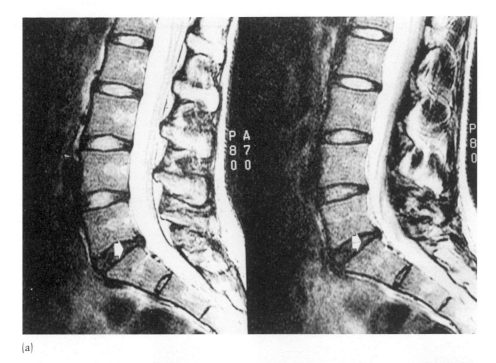

(a)

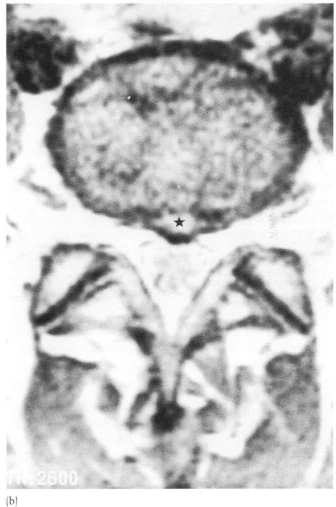

(b)

Fig. 37.8 A 16-year-old female referred because of recurrent urinary tract infections. (a) MRI showing spinal cord compression (white arrow). (b) MRI showing an intervertebral disc in the spinal canal (star).

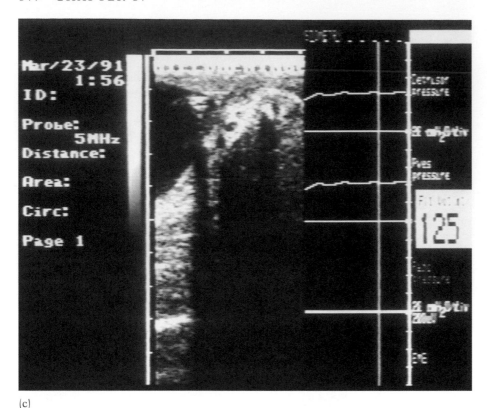

(c)

Fig. 37.8 *Continued.* (c) Flow video cystourethrosonography showing a hyperactive detrusor without opening of the bladder neck.

Patients with cauda equina lesions have detrusor areflexia and an increased urethral resistance. The damage to the parasympathetic system could result in unimpeded thoracolumbar sympathetic outflow, producing bladder neck obstruction. A similar situation is observed in patients with non-traumatic diseases affecting this spinal cord area. Pressure–flow studies have shown a low peak flow rate with reduced or absent detrusor pressure. The bladder capacity is increased and a high post-voiding residual urine and normal striated sphincter activity is the rule.

Therefore, a neurogenic process can be associated with functional bladder neck obstruction owing to a lack of appropriate inhibition of sympathetic innervation of the bladder neck observed in lesions above the thoracolumbar nuclei, where the obstruction is usually seen (detrusor hyperactivity with bladder neck dyssynergia). In these patients the urodynamic pattern is the same as that found in primary bladder neck obstruction. However, in spinal cord-injured patients a uroflowmetry is difficult to obtain.

On the other hand, in those injuries affecting the lower segments of the spinal cord, detrusor areflexia and bladder neck obstruction (closed bladder neck) are uncommon associations. Nevertheless, the introduction of new diagnostic methods such as the computed tomography scan and magnetic resonance imaging (MRI) has shown neurological disorders located in the lower spinal cord

segment that were responsible for bladder neck dysfunction in young and middle-aged patients with only urinary symptoms and, apparently, a primary bladder neck obstruction. Protrusion of intervertebral discs, tethered spinal cord syndrome and tumours such as lipomas (Figs 37.6–37.8) have been diagnosed. In all these patients no neurological symptoms were present and only urinary symptoms led them to seek medical advice. Therefore, we consider that newer methods (particularly MRI) must be included in the evaluation of patients who have been diagnosed with an apparent primary bladder neck obstruction.

Finally, in neurological patients with striated muscle overactivity, the bladder neck obstruction may occur secondary to spasticity of the striated muscle component existing in the vicinity of the bladder neck [10]. Hypertrophy of the detrusor resulting from prolonged distal obstruction has also been considered to produce obstruction at the bladder neck [68].

These types of bladder neck obstruction are usually mixed forms whose most important factor is the obstruction of the striated muscle [69].

In the treatment of neurological bladder neck obstruction, α-blocking agents can be used as the first alternative. Surgical incision of the bladder neck must be considered as a more definitive therapy when pressure in this area remains high or side effects are significant.

References

1 Lapides J. Structure and function of the internal vesical sphincter. *J Urol* 1958;**80**:341–53.

2 Woodburne RT. Structure and function of the urinary bladder. *J Urol* 1960;**84**:79–85.

3 Tanagho JA, Smith DR. Mechanism of urinary incontinence. I Embryologic, anatomic and pathologic considerations. *J Urol* 1968;**150**:640–6.

4 McNeal JE. The prostate and prostatic urethra: a morphologic synthesis. *J Urol* 1972;**107**:1008–16.

5 Droes JThPM. Observations on the musculature of the urinary bladder and the urethra in the human fetus. *Br J Urol* 1974;**46**:179–85.

6 Donker PJ, Droes JThPM, Van Ulden BM. Anatomy of the musculature and innervation of the bladder and the urethra. In: Williams DI, Chisholm GD, eds. *Scientific Foundations of Urology*, Vol. 1. Chicago: Year Book, 1976:32–9.

7 Khanna OMP, Barbieri EJ, Altamura M, McMichael R. Vesicourethral smooth muscle: function and relation to structure. *Urology* 1981;**18**:211–17.

8 Hutch JA. The internal urinary sphincter: a double loop system. *J Urol* 1971;**105**:375–83.

9 Turner-Warwick R, Whiteside CG, Worth PHL, Milroy EJG, Bates CP. A urodynamic view of the clinical problems associated with bladder neck dysfunction and its treatment by endoscopic incision and trans-trigonal posterior prostatectomy. *Br J Urol* 1973;**45**:44–59.

10 Gil Vernet D. *Morphology and Functions of Vesico-prostato-urethral Musculature.* Treviso: Ed Canova, 1968:245–69.

11 Ando M, Kihara K, Dato K, Sato T, Oshima H. Regulation of the bladder neck closure by lumbar splanchnic nerves at ejaculation in the dog. *Neurol Urodyn* 1993;**12**:91–2.

12 Owad SA, Bruce AW, Carro-Ciampi G, Downie JW, Lin M, Mark GS. Distribution of α-and β-adrenoceptors in human urinary bladder. *Br J Phamacol* 1974;**50**:525–9.

13 Kunisawa Y, Kawabe K, Niijima T, Honda K, Takenaka T. A pharmacological study of alpha-adrenergic receptor subtypes in smooth muscle of human urinary bladder base and prostatic urethra. *J Urol* 1985;**134**:396–8.

14 Krane RJ, Olsson CA. Phenoxybenzamine in neurogenic bladder dysfunction I. A theory of micturition. *J Urol* 1973;**110**:650–2.

15 Klarskow P, Gerstenberg TC, Ramirez D, Hald T. Non-cholinergic, non-adrenergic nerve mediated relaxation of trigone bladder neck and urethral smooth muscle *in vitro. J Urol* 1983;**129**:848–50.

16 Klarskov P, Holm-Bentzen M, Norgaard T, Ottesen B, Walter S, Hald T. Vasoactive intestinal polypeptide concentration in human bladder neck smooth muscle and its influence on urodynamic parameters. *Br J Urol* 1987;**60**:113–18.

17 Guthrie GJ. *Anatomy and Disorders of the Neck of the Bladder and of the Urethra.* London: Burgess and Hall, 1834.

18 Young HH. A new procedure (punch operation) for small prostatic bars and contracture of the prostatic orifice. *J Am Med Assoc* 1913;**60**:253–65.

19 Marion G. Surgery of the neck of the bladder. *Br J Urol* 1933;**5**:351–6.

20 Webster GD, Lockhart JL, Older RA. The evaluation of bladder neck dysfunction. *J Urol* 1980;**123**:196–8.

21 Mishra VK, Kumar A, Kapoor R, Srivastava A, Bhandari M. Functional bladder neck obstruction in males: a progressive disorder? *Eur Urol* 1992;**22**:123–9.

22 Yalla SV, Blute RD, Snyder H *et al.* Isolated bladder neck obstruction of undetermined etiology (primary) in the adult male. *Urology* 1981;**17**:99–108.

23 Farrar DJ, Whiteside CG, Osborne JL, Turner-Warwick RT. A urodynamic analysis of micturition symptoms in the female. *Surg Gynec Obst* 1975;**141**:875–81.

24 Axelrod SL, Blaivas JG. Bladder neck obstruction in women. *J Urol* 1987;**137**:497–9.

25 Leadbetter GW, Leadbetter WF. Diagnosis and treatment of congenital bladder neck obstruction in children. *N Engl J Med* 1959;**260**:633–41.

26 Norlen LJ, Blaivas JG. Unsuspected proximal urethral obstruction in young and middle-aged men. *J Urol* 1986;**135**:972–6.

27 Gronbaek K, Struckmann JR, Frimodt-Moller C. The treatment of female bladder neck dysfunction. *Scand J Urol Nephrol* 1992;**26**:113–18.

28 Holm HH. *The hydrodynamics of micturition.* PhD thesis, Copenhagen, 1964.

29 Gierup J, Ericsson NO, von Hedenberg Ch. Urodynamic studies in boys with disorders of the lower urinary tract. IV Congenital bladder neck obstruction. A pre and postoperative study. *Scand J Urol Nephrol* 1978;**12**:195–203.

30 Bates CP, Arnold EP, Griffiths DJ. The nature of the abnormality in bladder neck obstruction. *Br J Urol* 1975;**47**:651–6.

31 Awad SA, Downie JW, Lywood DW, Young RA, Jarzylo SV. Sympathetic activity in the proximal urethra in patients with urinary obstruction. *J Urol* 1976;**115**:545–7.

32 Kaneko S, Minami K, Yachiku S, Kurita T. Bladder neck dysfunction. The effect of the adrenergic blocking agent phentolamine on bladder neck dysfunction and a fluorescent histochemical study of bladder neck smooth muscle. *Invest Urol* 1980;**18**:212–18.

33 Booth CM, Shah PJR, Milroy EJG, Thompson SA, Gosling JA. The structure of the bladder neck in male bladder neck obstruction. *Br J Urol* 1983;**55**:279–82.

34 Woodside JR. Urodynamic evaluation of dysfunctional bladder neck obstruction in men. *J Urol* 1980;**124**:673–7.

35 Parys BT, Woolfenden KA, Parsons KF. The use of sacral reflex latencies in detrusor bladder neck dyssynergia. *Br J Urol* 1988;**61**:32–5.

36 Tanagho EA, McCurry E. Pressure and flow rate as related to lumen caliber and entrance configuration. *J Urol* 1971;**105**:583–5.

37 Andersen JT, Jacobsen O, Gammelgaard PA, Hald T. Dysfunction of the bladder neck: a urodynamic study. *Urol Int* 1976;**31**:78–86.

38 Poulsen EU, Kirkeby HJ, Djurhuus JCh. Urodynamic effect of acute alpha-receptor blockade in patients with bladder neck dysfunction. *Scand J Urol Nephrol* 1989;**23**:15–20.

39 Yalla SV, Sharma GVRK, Barsamian EM. Micturitional static urethral pressure profile: a method of recording urethral pressure profile during voiding and the implications. *J Urol* 1980;**124**:649–56.

40 Cass AS, Hinman F Jr. Constant urethral flow in female dog model. In: Hinman F Jr, ed. *Hydrodynamics of Micturition.* Springfield: Charles C Thomas, 1971:136–51.

41 Gilja I, Kovacic M, Radej M, Parazajder J. Functional

obstruction of bladder neck in men. *Neurol Urodyn* 1989;**8**:433–8.

42 Barbalias GA. Prostatodynia or painful male urethral syndrome? *Urology* 1990;**36**:146–53.

43 Hellstro, WJG, Schmidt RA, Lue TF, Tanagho EA. Neuromuscular dysfunction in nonbacterial prostatitis. *Urology* 1987;**30**:183–7.

44 George NJR, Slade N. Hesitancy and poor stream in younger men without outflow tract obstruction—the anxious bladder. *Br J Urol* 1979;**51**:506–9.

45 Fox M, Jarvis GJ, Henry L. Idiopathic chronic urinary retention in the female. *Br J Urol* 1976;**47**:797–803.

46 Deane AM, Worth PHL. Female chronic urinary retention. *Br J Urol* 1985;**57**:24–6.

47 Hedlund H, Andersson KE. Effects of prazosin in men with symptoms of bladder neck obstruction and a non-hyperplastic prostate. *Scand J Urol Nephrol* 1989;**23**:251–4.

48 Kumar A, Mishra VK, Kapoor R, Dalela D, Bhandari M. Functional bladder neck obstruction in females, a revisit. *Arch Esp Urol* 1991;**44**:1209–15.

49 Beer E. Discussion on surgery of the neck of the bladder. *Br J Urol* 1933;**5**:362–3.

50 Christensen MG, Nordling J, Andersen JT, Hald T. Functional bladder neck obstruction. Results of endoscopic bladder neck incision in 131 consecutive patients. *Br J Urol* 1985;**57**:60–2.

51 Moisey CU, Stephenson TP, Evans C. A subjective and urodynamic assessment of unilateral bladder neck incision for bladder neck obstruction. *Br J Urol* 1982;**54**:114–17.

52 Hedlund H, Ek A. Ejaculation and sexual function after endoscopic bladder neck incision. *Br J Urol* 1985;**57**:164–7.

53 Delaere KPJ, Debruyne FMJ, Moonen WA. Extended bladder neck incision for outflow obstruction in male patients. *Br J Urol* 1983;**55**:225–8.

54 Delaere KPJ, Debruyne FMJ, Moonen WA. Bladder neck incision in the female: a hazardous procedure? *Br J Urol* 1983;**55**:283–6.

55 Bhatnagar BNS, Barnes RW. Incontinence following transurethral resection of the bladder neck in the female. *Br J Urol* 1981;**53**:29–34.

56 Ray EH. Transurethral incision of the vesical neck. *J Kentucky State Med Assoc* 1967;**65**:41–2.

57 Adkins WC. Argon laser treatment of urethral stricture and vesical neck contracture. *Laser Surg Med* 1988;**6**:600–3.

58 Millin T. *Retropubic Urinary Surgery*. Edinburgh: Churchill Livingstone, 1947.

59 Sikafi Z, Butler MR, Lane V, O'Flynn JD, Fitzpatrick JM. Bladder neck contracture following prostatectomy. *Br J Urol* 1985;**57**:308–10.

60 Robinson HP, Greene LF. Postoperative contracture of the vesical neck. II Experimental production of contracture in dog: transurethral series. *J Urol* 1962;**87**:610–16.

61 Greene LF, Robinson HP. Postoperative contracture of the vesical neck. VI Prophylaxis and treatment. *J Urol* 1966;**95**:520–5.

62 Orandi A. Transurethral incision of the prostate. *J Urol* 1973;**110**:229–31.

63 Kulb TB, Kamer M, Lingeman JE, Foster RS. Prevention of postprostatectomy vesical neck contracture by prophylactic vesical neck incision. *J Urol* 1987;**137**:230–1.

64 Drach GW, Meares EM, Fair WR, Stamey TA. Classification of benign diseases associated with prostatic pain: prostatitis or prostatodynia [Letter]. *J Urol* 1978;**120**:266.

65 Duvie SOA. Bacterial prostatitis: an unusual cause of total urinary incontinence and its surgical management. *J Urol* 1988;**139**:139–41.

66 Arnold EP. Urodynamic significance of minor urological problems in the male. *Urol Clin North Am* 1979;**6**:193–7.

67 McGuire EJ, Wagner FM, Weiss RM. Treatment of autonomic dysreflexia with phenoxybenzamine. *J Urol* 1976;**115**:53–5.

68 Gibbon NOK. Later management of the paraplegic bladder. *Paraplegia* 1974;**12**:87–91.

69 Yalla SV, Blunt KJ, Fam BA, Constantinople NL, Gittes RF. Detrusor-urethral sphincter dyssynergia. *J Urol* 1977;**118**:1026–9.

38   Bladder Diverticula
A. Tajima and Y. Aso

Introduction

Vesical diverticulum is a condition in which the wall of the urinary bladder has an outward, cystic projecting area. It can be divided into two types: acquired and congenital. Acquired vesical diverticula are much more frequent than congenital vesical diverticula. Most cases of acquired vesical diverticula are accompanied by obstructive lesions of the lower urinary tract (Fig. 38.1). Congenital vesical diverticula, on the other hand, are mainly accompanied by vesicoureteric reflux or renal hypoplasia. These two types of bladder diverticula will be discussed separately because they can be understood more easily when treated as two different disease entities.

Acquired bladder diverticula

Pathogenesis

Acquired bladder diverticula occur more often in males than in females [1,2]. In most cases, the formation of this type of bladder diverticulum can be attributed to obstruction of the lower urinary tract, which is most often caused by benign prostatic hypertrophy [1]. Acquired bladder diverticula are seen in all age groups, but are most frequently seen in individuals between 60 and 65 years of age [1,2]. Patients with bladder diverticula often complain of symptoms caused by obstruction of the lower urinary tract, such as difficult urination, frequency and urinary retention. This condition is often accompanied by asymptomatic urinary tract infection.

Although bladder diverticula themselves do not manifest many symptoms [1], several characteristic symptoms are recognized. For example, the patients show urinary frequency only during the daytime, because the diverticulum serves as a reservoir when the patient takes a lying position at night. In addition, two-stage urination and discomfort or pain of the lower abdomen on the ipsilateral side of the diverticulum are characteristic symptoms of the bladder diverticula. In general, however, bladder diverticula show

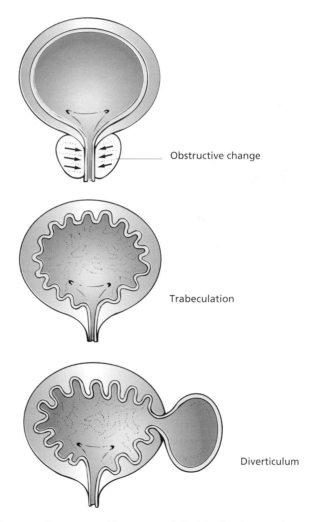

Obstructive change

Trabeculation

Diverticulum

Fig. 38.1 The process of formation of the bladder diverticulum. The diverticulum formation can be attributed to obstruction of the lower urinary tract, which is most often caused by benign prostatic hypertrophy.

few symptoms. For this reason, a high percentage of patients with this condition are incidentally detected during urography, ultrasonography or cystoscopy (Fig. 38.2).

In 85% of all cases, acquired bladder diverticula are

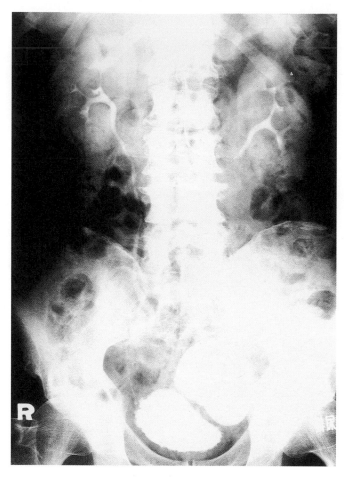

Fig. 38.2 An intravenous pyelogram of a man complaining of difficult urination and frequency which incidentally showed a large bladder diverticulum.

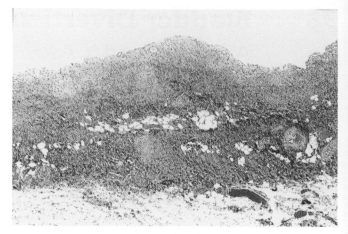

Fig. 38.3 The diverticulum wall contains little or no muscle layer.

located above or lateral to the ureteric orifice [1]. They are rarely located medial to the ureteric orifice or in the vesical trigone. It is also rare that this type of diverticulum is seen in the base of the bladder. The size of the diverticulum varies among individual cases and the diameter is over 5 cm in a relatively large number of cases [1]. It is not uncommon for the diverticulum to attain a larger size than the urinary bladder itself. The diverticulum tends to be multiple when it is accompanied by obstructive lesions of the lower urinary tract.

When observed by light microscopy, the wall of the diverticulum appears to be composed of the vesical mucosa which has protruded outwards through spaces in the muscle layer. The wall is very thin and contains little or no muscle layer (Fig. 38.3). The mucosal and submucosal layers of the diverticular wall often show signs of chronic inflammation and atrophy, which seem to be attributable to the reduced contractility of the wall and to decreased bloodflow [3]. It is not uncommon for bladder peridiverticulitis to develop, and the resultant adhesion of the diverticular wall to the surrounding tissue and organs makes complete surgical resection of the diverticulum difficult. In cases complicated by diverticular stones, the mucosa of the diverticular wall often shows hyperplasia, dysplasia or squamous metaplasia.

Complications

Major complications observed in patients with acquired bladder diverticula are hydronephrosis, stones and malignant tumours. Because of a high prevalence of obstructive lesions of the lower urinary tract in patients with acquired bladder diverticula, the incidence of hydronephrosis is relatively high in this group of patients. The diverticula themselves sometimes disturb urination. Since urine tends to stagnate within the diverticular cavity, diverticular stones are sometimes formed [1]. In cases complicated by diverticular stones, peridiverticulitis is most likely to occur, and squamous metaplasia of the diverticular mucosa is often noted.

The incidence of malignant neoplasms is reported to be high for bladder diverticula [1,3,4]. Although the exact cause for this tendency is unknown, chronic bloodflow disturbances and inflammation of the diverticular wall are thought to initiate the onset of malignant tumours. Care is needed when macroscopic or microscopic haematuria persists in patients with bladder diverticula.

Transitional cell carcinoma is the predominant histological type of the malignant tumours associated with bladder diverticulum. Squamous cell carcinoma is the second highest in incidence. Mixed-type carcinoma and adenocarcinoma are also seen, although their percentages are very low. The malignant potential appears to be high for the bladder diverticulum tumours [1]. Because the diverticular wall is thin, tumour often invades the surrounding organs when it is detected [5]. Thus, the prognosis of this cancer is usually poor [6]. It is therefore recommended that malignant tumours of the bladder diverticulum are treated by complete cystectomy after irradiation therapy [7].

Surgical management

Small bladder diverticula, which are not accompanied by infection, can be left untreated. In cases where the diverticulum is accompanied by infection, antibiotics are needed. The diverticulum needs to be resected if it is large enough to disturb normal urination or to cause massive residual urine or if the symptoms caused by the diverticulum (even when its size is small) cannot be controlled by conservative treatment. At the operation, the surgeon should not forget to treat obstructive lesions of the lower urinary tract as well. To facilitate the selection of an optimal operative procedure, it is essential to assess accurately the location and number of diverticula, the presence or absence of malignant tumour or stones (their location and number, if any) and the state of the lower urinary tract (in particular the prostatic urethra if the patient is male). To this end, cystoscopy is indispensable. It is also necessary to assess the anatomical relationship between the diverticulum and the ureter, and to evaluate the size of the diverticula and the presence or absence of residual urine. Excretory urography is also recommended.

Surgical treatment of bladder diverticula (i.e. bladder diverticulectomy) can be divided into three types depending on the route of approach to the diverticulum: (i) the intra- and extravesical (combined) approach; (ii) the intravesical approach; and (iii) the extravesical approach. For all three of these approaches the patient is in a supine position and epidural anaesthesia suffices. The lower abdominal midline incision is usually carried out from the umbilicus to immediately above the pubic symphysis, to expose the anterior wall of the urinary bladder.

The intra- and extravesical (combined) approach is suitable for larger diverticula (Fig. 38.4). In such cases the diverticular orifice must be first identified after opening the bladder. Subsequently, the diverticulum is filled with gauze or a balloon catheter, or the surgeon's finger is inserted into the diverticulum to serve as a landmark. The diverticulum is then freed from the surrounding tissue via the extravesical approach, to expose the diverticular neck adequately. The diverticulum is then resected at its neck, followed by two-layer suturing of the bladder wall using absorbable 2/0 sutures. In cases where the diverticular orifice is near the ureteric orifice, it is recommended that a 5 or 6 F ureteric catheter is indwelt into the ureter. The most troublesome complication during diverticulectomy is ureteric injury. This injury can be avoided by keeping a ureteric catheter in place. The urethral catheter needs to be kept in place for about 1 week after surgery.

The intravesical approach is suitable for smaller diverticula (Fig. 38.5). In such cases the diverticular orifice

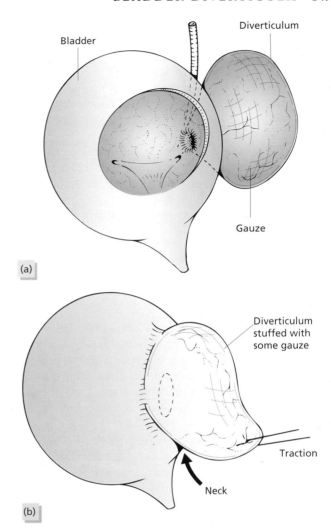

(a)

(b)

Fig. 38.4 The intra- and extravesical (combined) approach. (a) The diverticulum cavity is filled with gauze via the intravesical approach. (b) The diverticulum is freed via the extravesical approach, to expose the diverticular neck adequately.

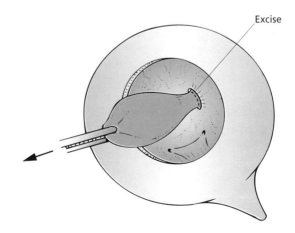

Fig. 38.5 The intravesical approach. The mucosa of the diverticular sac is pulled and everted using Allis forceps.

must be first located by opening the urinary bladder. Subsequently, the mucosal surface of the diverticular sac is pulled and everted using Allis forceps. The everted diverticulum is then resected at its neck, followed by bladder wall suturing using absorbable threads as mentioned above. If the diverticulum is small, the outer fibrous capsule can be left unresected, and only the mucosal layers of the diverticulum need to be freed and resected.

With the extravesical approach, diverticulum freeing is performed from the outside of the urinary bladder, which is not opened, and the diverticulum is resected at its neck (Fig. 38.6).

Operative results have not differed greatly among these three approaches.

Congenital bladder diverticula

Pathogenesis

As with acquired bladder diverticula, congenital bladder diverticula are formed more often in males than in females. However, congenital bladder diverticula are usually not accompanied by obstruction of the lower urinary tract. This type of bladder diverticulum is often located around the ureteric orifice and is often accompanied by vesicoureteric reflux.

There seems to be some causal relationship between this type of bladder diverticulum and vesicoureteric reflux. It is even more important to take precautions against infection in the case of congenital bladder diverticula than in acquired bladder diverticula. Giant diverticula are rarely formed below or behind the urinary bladder, sometimes disturbing urination [8,9].

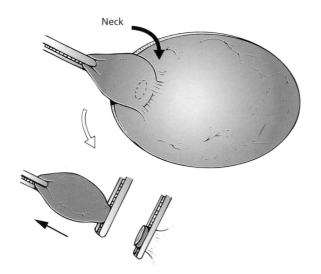

Neck

Fig. 38.6 The extravesical approach. The separation of the diverticulum is performed from the outside of the urinary bladder, which is not opened, and the diverticulum is resected at its neck.

The level of severity of congenital bladder diverticula varies among individual cases. Congenital bladder diverticula detected in the infantile period or childhood are often severe and accompanied by vesicoureteric reflux or renal hypoplasia [10–12]. Congenital bladder diverticula detected in adulthood during examination of mild vesicoureteric reflux or urinary tract infection are often less severe [13].

The muscle layer of the urinary bladder is thin in its region around the ureteric orifice. This is thought to serve as a precipitating factor for diverticulum formation [10]. The muscle layer above and lateral to the ureteric orifice is particularly weak and is likely to permit the vesical mucosa to prolapse and protrude. In early phases, the prolapsed mucosa protrudes when the intravesical pressure rises and it falls back (retreats) when the pressure decreases. Repetitions of the protruding and retreating cycles result in a gradual growth of the diverticulum, probably resulting in collapse of the reflux-preventing mechanism of the ureteric orifice, leading to vesicoureteric reflux. In some cases, the ureteric orifice is pulled into the diverticulum as it increases in size. Since bladder diverticulum is often accompanied by vesicoureteric reflux, most patients have acute or chronic urinary infection. If such cases are left untreated their renal function on the affected side will decrease and is eventually lost completely.

Some investigators attribute the fragility of the muscle layer around the ureteric orifice to abnormal development of ureteric buds [12,13]. It has also been reported that patients with a double renal pelvis often have bladder diverticula in the vicinity of the ureteric orifice [12,14]. Thus, there seems to be a close relationship among congenital bladder diverticula, vesicoureteric reflux and double renal pelvis [11]. Although genetic inheritance of congenital bladder diverticula has been suggested, the exact mechanism of this type of bladder diverticula is unknown.

When observed by light microscopy, the diverticular wall has little or no muscle layer. In addition, the wall has little or no capsule [12,15]. At the lower end of the ureter, facing the diverticulum, myofibrils show an approximately ring-shaped arrangement. At some points these fibres are interrupted by collagen fibres, resulting in marked narrowing of the ureteric lumen. The upper segment of the ureter is histologically intact, but the formation of hydroureter is found relatively frequently.

Complications

As mentioned above, congenital bladder diverticula are often accompanied by acute or chronic pyelonephritis. It is not uncommon that renal hypoplasia accompanies bladder diverticula in young patients or severe cases. Hydroureter, due to narrowing of the lower end of the ureter, is a relatively frequent complication [11,12]. It is not uncommon that the collapse of the reflux-preventing mechanism at the lower end of the ureter leads to the onset of both vesicoureteric reflux and hydroureter.

Surgical management

Operative procedures are selected depending on the severity of vesicoureteric reflux and the state of the ipsilateral kidney at the time of detection (in particular depending on the residual renal function). Some cases only require treatment of the accompanying infection [13], while others require diverticulectomy and ureteroneocystostomy. Cases where the renal dysfunction on the affected side seems to be irreversible are indicated for unilateral nephrectomy.

References

1 Fox M, Power RF, Bruce AW. Diverticulum of the bladder — presentation and evaluation of treatment of 115 cases. *Br J Urol* 1962;**34**:286–98.

2 Peterson LJ, Paulson DF, Glenn JF. The histopathology of vesical diverticula. *J Urol* 1973;**110**:62–4.

3 Target JH. Diverticula of the bladder, associated with vesical growths. *Trans Pathol Soc Lond* 1896;**47**:155–68.

4 Williams WR. Sarcoma of a diverticulum of the bladder. *Trans Pathol Soc Lond* 1883;**34**:152–6.

5 Ostroff EB, Alperstein JB, Young JD Jr. Neoplasm in vesical diverticula: report of 4 patients, including a 21-year-old. *J Urol* 1973;**110**:65–9.

6 Aubert J, Dombriz M, Dore B. Tumeur vesicale intradiverticulaire. *J Urol (Paris)* 1982;**88**:537–40.

7 Faysal MH, Freiha FS. Primary neoplasm in vesical diverticula: a report of 12 cases. *Br J Urol* 1981;**53**:141–3.

8 Taylor WN, Alton D, Toguri A, Churchill BM, Schillinger JF. Bladder diverticula causing posterior urethral obstruction in children. *J Urol* 1979;**122**:415.

9 Verghese M, Belman AB. Urinary retention secondary to congenital bladder diverticula in infants. *J Urol* 1984;**132**: 1186–8.

10 Allen NH, Atwell JD. The paraureteric diverticulum in childhood. *Br J Urol* 1980;**52**:264–8.

11 Atwell JD, Allen NH. The interrelationship between paraureteric diverticula, vesicoureteric reflux and duplication of the pelvicaliceal collecting system: a family study. *Br J Urol* 1980;**52**:269–73.

12 Tokunaka S, Koyanagi T, Matsuno T, Gotoh T, Tsuji I. Paraureteral diverticula: clinical experience with 17 cases with associated renal dysmorphism. *J Urol* 1980;**124**: 791–6.

13 Amar AD, Das S. Vesicoureteral reflux in women with primary bladder diverticulum. *J Urol* 1985;**134**:33–5.

14 Mackie GG, Stephens FD. Duplex kidneys: a correlation of renal dysplasia with position of the ureteral orifice. *J Urol* 1975;**114**:274–80.

15 Stephens FD. The vesicoureteral hiatus and paraureteral diverticula. *J Urol* 1979;**121**:786–91.

39 Management of Urinary Incontinence in the Male

R.S.Kirby

Introduction

Although urinary incontinence is far less common in men than in women, it is none the less quite commonly encountered. When present in severe form, although never life threatening, incontinence of urine can have a devastating effect on an individual's self image and quality of life. For example, a recent audit by the Royal College of Surgeons of England of the outcome of transurethral resection of the prostate (TURP) found that leaking incontinence, which occurred in as many as 6% of patients 3 months after TURP, was associated with considerable patient dissatisfaction about the outcome of surgery and had a strongly negative impact on the quality of life [1].

As described in Chapters 71–73 on neurogenic bladder dysfunction, the neurophysiological mechanisms controlling continence and micturition are not only complex, but also susceptible to disruption by a large number of disease processes. Detailed discussion of all these disorders is beyond the scope of this chapter; however, the diseases that need to be especially borne in mind can be divided into congenital causes, such as spina bifida and bladder exstrophy, as well as acquired causes, the most common of which are neuropathic in nature and include cerebrovascular accidents, multiple sclerosis and other spinal cord disorders such as paraplegia. A further important acquired cause of urinary incontinence in the male is iatrogenic injury to the urethral sphincter following procedures such as radical prostatectomy, TURP or abdominoperineal resection (APR) of the rectum. In addition, it must be remembered that ageing and associated senility alone will often result in urinary incontinence that may tip the balance between self-sufficiency and the requirement for permanent nursing care.

Assessment of the incontinent male

The assessment of men suffering from incontinence is of importance because accurate diagnosis and correct institution of therapy can be curative and thereby markedly improve the afflicted individual's quality of life. Moreover, urinary incontinence can be secondary to bladder outflow obstruction resulting in chronic urinary retention, and this form of incontinence can result in potentially reversible renal failure. A detailed history is crucial. For example, the onset of urinary leakage will often provide an important clue as to its causation. Gradual onset of predominantly nocturnal leaking is often the result of overflow incontinence due to chronic retention. Urge incontinence associated with severe frequency and a normal urinary stream and a past history of enuresis may be due to detrusor instability. Enquiries about other neurological symptoms including lower limb weakness and erectile dysfunction may provide the clue as to a neurogenic aetiology of the urinary leakage. Obviously the reported association with an operative procedure such as prostatectomy, either radical or transurethral, is strongly suggestive of an iatrogenic aetiology.

Physical examination should include a focused neurological examination, including some assessment of anal sphincter tone; although, admittedly, lower motor neurone lesions resulting in urinary incontinence are much less common than spinal or supraspinal neurological disorders, which are more likely to be associated with neurological signs in the lower limbs. Abdominal examination should be performed to detect a palpable bladder as well as a digital rectal examination (DRE), to assess prostatic size, shape and consistency. However, it should be remembered that chronic urinary retention due to bladder prostatic outflow obstruction can occur in the absence of any palpable enlargement of the prostate, particularly when middle lobe hyperplasia is the cause of obstruction.

Special investigations in affected patients should include a full blood count together with an assessment of the levels of urea, electrolytes and creatinine, to exclude anaemia or renal impairment, and a prostate-specific antigen (PSA) test to detect the presence of prostate cancer. Bladder ultrasound and uroflow rate determination is an important non-invasive way of evaluating lower urinary tract function in the male, although perhaps more applicable to patients presenting with simple bladder outflow obstruction, rather than urinary incontinence. Certainly an overdistended bladder coexistent with enlargement of the prostate would confirm a diagnosis of chronic urinary retention with overflow incontinence, and this would be in marked contrast to the findings expected in a neurogenic bladder due to an upper motor neurone lesion, which is usually associated with a thickened hypertrophic bladder of small capacity, albeit with a significant post-void residual urine volume. Urinary flow rate determination may also cast some light on the aetiology of incontinence; for example, in idiopathic detrusor instability the flow rate will usually be normal. In neuropathic bladder dysfunction flow rates are variable, but often there is a reduced and intermittent pattern produced by voiding achieved mainly by abdominal straining. In the severely incontinent patient with urethral sphincter weakness it may not be possible for the patient to store enough urine in the bladder to get any useful information from bladder ultrasound or flow rate determination.

Video urodynamics constitutes the gold standard means of evaluating men with incontinence and is capable of making the important distinction between detrusor over-activity and sphincter weakness. It can also identify those patients in whom a combination of both these abnormalities co-exist. The important components of urodynamic evaluation include the detrusor pressure rise seen during slow fill cystometry (Fig. 39.1), the ability of the sphincter to resist stress urinary incontinence with the patient standing. A not uncommon abnormality is an open bladder neck at rest (Fig. 39.2) in combination with an obvious loss of contrast during coughing. The patient is

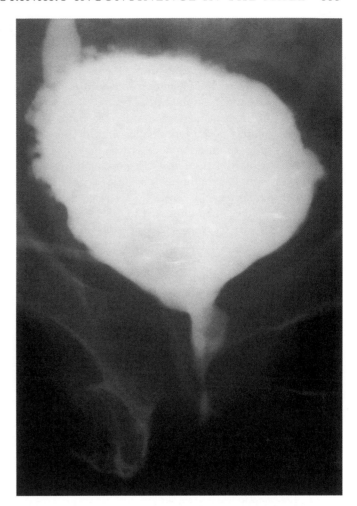

Fig. 39.2 A cystogram demonstrating an open bladder neck at rest in a male patient.

then asked to void, the maximum detrusor pressure during urinary flow as well as the maximum and mean urinary flow rate may then be evaluated. At the end of the study the presence of a residual urinary volume is assessed.

More detailed neurophysiological evaluation by sphincter electromyography (EMG) as well as the measurement of evoked response latencies may also be of value but should be performed by, or in conjunction with, an experienced neurophysiologist.

Management

Management of urinary incontinence in the male will depend on its underlying cause, as well as the nature of leakage, i.e. whether the incontinence is of the urge, stress or overflow variety.

Urge incontinence resulting from either neuropathic or non-neuropathic detrusor instability will often respond to a combination of bladder training and judicious use of anticholinergic therapy. Often the two treatment

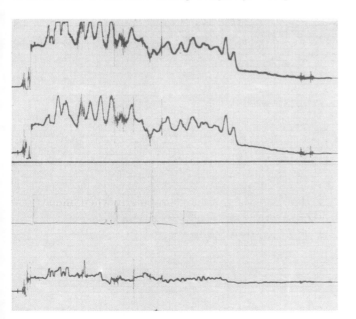

Fig. 39.1 A cystometrogram demonstrating unstable detrusor contractions in response to slow bladder filling.

modalities can be usefully employed together. Bladder training is best accomplished with the use of a voided volume chart combined with the help of a nurse counsellor. Anticholinergic agents in the form of propantheline, or more usually oxybutynin, have been shown in a number of randomized controlled studies to be more effective than placebo in the management of motor urge incontinence [2,3]. Unfortunately both these medications are limited by side effects due to interference with other cholinergic systems in the body, particularly dry mouth, blurred vision and constipation. On the horizon are new antimuscarinic drugs such as darifenacid, which is selective for the M3 muscarinic receptor. The improved tolerability may allow higher doses to be used to achieve better efficacy in the bladder while reducing the incidence of side effects. Detrusor instability in its severest form with associated urge incontinence is less common in men than in women, presumably as a result of the ability of the more powerful external urethral sphincter and pelvic floor to resist the unstable detrusor contractions.

When more conservative measures fail, a further option may be to raise the passive urethral resistance to deal with intractable stress incontinence. In females this can effectively be done by means of a sling-type procedure, but this is less effective in the male and usually the best solution is implantation of an artificial urinary sphincter. Control of sphincteric urinary incontinence with implantable prosthetic devices has evolved rapidly during the past few decades. The most significant contribution in this respect was the introduction in 1973 of an implantable sphincter mechanism that could be used not only in adults but also in children [4]. This hydraulic device, composed of silicone rubber, allowed for the placement of an inflatable cuff around the bladder neck or bulbar urethra. The original device was controlled by small pumps that were placed in the subcutaneous tissue within the scrotum. Unidirectional valves within the system directed fluid from a reservoir to and from the inflatable cuff.

Earlier attempts to control urinary incontinence with, for example the Rosen device, had unfortunately been far less successful [5]. Recently some have advocated the injection of Teflon paste or gax collagen periurethrally, but this has had only a very limited efficacy in resolving incontinence in the male [6].

The American Medical Systems (AMS) artificial urinary sphincter was developed as the AMS721 sphincter. This device produced mixed results in patients with various types of sphincteric incontinence. Although many patients did benefit from this implant the mechanical reliability and the erosion rate were unfortunately unexpectedly high. From 1977, therefore, a number of new devices were developed, culminating in the production in late 1982 of the device that has lasted the test of time for over a decade known as the AMS800 artificial urinary sphincter. The AMS800 control assembly contains the unidirectional valves, flow reservoir, on-and-off button and a deflate pump; it also allows for non-surgical delayed activation and complete control by the patient during cuff compression. The currently used device has a much improved cuff that has been constructed of a silicone-based material that is extremely resilient (Fig. 39.3).

Preoperative considerations

Patients with chronic urinary tract infections must be adequately managed before their operation and all should be given broad spectrum parenchymal antibiotics at the time of surgery as prophylaxis. The organism most often implicated with device infection is *Staphylococcus epidermidis* and prophylaxis should, therefore, be designed with this in mind. A combination of a cephalosporin and an aminoglycoside are the antimicrobials most often employed. Administration of oral antibiotics is continued up to a week after implantation, usually with a quinolone derivative.

Many patients with chronic urinary incontinence have varying degrees of pre-existing ammoniacal dermatitis around the perineum and it is often advisable to insert a catheter several days in advance of implantation and use hydrophilic creams to reduce bacterial counts on the perineal skin and to promote healing. Patients scheduled for uncomplicated bulbar urethral cuff implantation may be admitted to hospital on the morning of the surgical procedure, while those having a bladder neck operation are

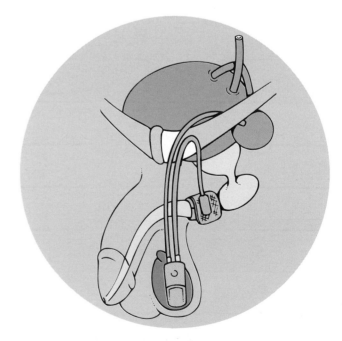

Fig. 39.3 The AMS800 artificial urinary sphincter located around the bulbar urethra.

usually admitted the evening before for a limited lower bowel preparation. Shaving the perineum is best left until just before surgery to avoid bacterial colonization of the small scratches and skin nicks that may occur during the shaving. On the operating table, patients receiving a bulbar urethral cuff implantation are placed in the lithotomy position, while those undergoing bladder neck cuff procedure are placed supine with the legs slightly apart.

The skin preparation is very important; an iodine-based product is preferred and a 5–10 min scrubbing time is advisable. Draping is performed in such a way to allow access to the lower abdominal wall and the perineum, and urethral catheters are inserted after skin preparation and draping. An antibiotic solution should be used frequently for irrigation during the procedure because of the considerable risks of infection in patients undergoing prostatic implantation; strict aseptic technique is essential. Ideally the number of people in the operating theatre at the time of implantation should be kept to an absolute minimum.

Operative technique

Bulbar urethral cuff implantation

A 12 or 14 F Foley catheter is inserted and the bladder emptied. Two incisions are made, one in the perineum in the midline over the bulbar urethra and another transversally on the lower abdominal wall, either to the right or to the left of the midline, depending on the site of the pump placement. Through the perineum incision the bulbocavernosus muscle is identified. Dissection should be carried out around the bulbocavernosus muscle and a plane established between it and the tunica albuginea of the corporeal bodies (Fig. 39.4). This plane of dissection is around 2 cm wide and as close as possible to the underlying tunica albuginea of the corporeal bodies. This plane allows

the placement of the cuff around the bulbocavernosus muscle and not directly onto the bulbar urethra, thereby reducing the risk of erosion. Particular care must be taken to avoid damaging the urethra, especially at the 12 o'clock position where the point of dissection is most difficult and the majority of urethral injuries occur.

If the urethra is inadvertently injured it may be possible to close the defect primarily with a fine absorbable suture; an alternative site along the urethra can then be selected for cuff placement. Unfortunately, some urethral injuries remain unrecognized at the time of surgery and these are probably a leading cause of early cuff erosion. Such an injury may be thermal as a result of diathermy coagulation leading to delayed tissue necrosis.

Once the urethral plane has been established the circumferential measurement is determined using the calibrated measuring strap (Fig. 39.5). A properly sized cuff which, for the bulbar urethra, is usually 2.5 or 5.0 cm in length, is passed, tab first, under the urethra (Fig. 39.6). The tab should be passed beneath the urethra towards the side

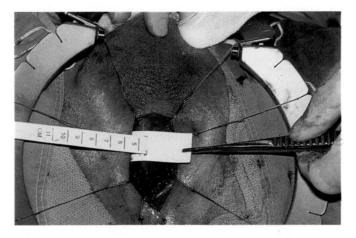

Fig. 39.5 A measuring strap is passed around the bulbar urethra.

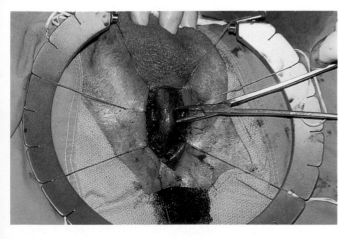

Fig. 39.4 The bulbar urethra is exposed through a perineal incision.

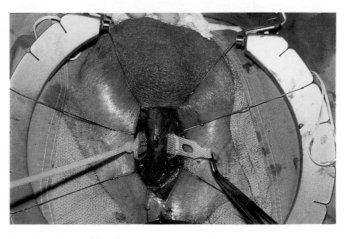

Fig. 39.6 The cuff is then passed around the urethra.

where the pump is to be placed, the tubing is then fed through the opening in the tab and the cuff snapped into place while gentle opposing traction is applied (Fig. 39.7). In some patients, particularly those who are wheelchair bound, or those who are enthusiastic cyclists, placement of the cuff around the bulbar urethra may result in episodes of incontinence when sudden pressure is exerted on the cuff which results in deflation. In such cases, when placement of the cuff around the urethra is still preferred, the attachment of the central tendon of the bulbar urethra may be incised. This allows a more proximal dissection of the urethra, up to the level of the urogenital diaphragm. Placement of the cuff around the urethra in this location will prevent direct pressure upon the cuff when the patient is seated, thus reducing the risk of these troublesome episodes of incontinence.

The cuff tubing is then drawn into the upper incision through the subcutaneous tissues and a balloon reservoir selected. In general the 61–70 cm H_2O reservoir is applicable to most patients, although if it is thought that there is a high risk of erosion a 51–60 cm H_2O reservoir may be a better choice. A 2 cm incision is then made into the rectus fascia and the unfilled reservoir located in the perivesical space extraperitoneally. The reservoir tubing is passed through a separate opening in the fascia and the balloon filled with 22 ml of saline or isosmotic contrast medium and the cuff pressurized. Once the cuff has been pressurized, the balloon is emptied and then refilled with exactly 20 ml of the same fluid.

The AMS800 pump mechanism is located in the subcutaneous tunnel on one or other side of the scrotum (Fig. 39.8). The pump is attached to the reservoir and cuff by means of so-called 'quick connect' connectors (Fig. 39.9) and the device then cycled to ensure that it is functioning satisfactorily. The wound is then closed in layers without the use of drains and a 12 or 14 F urethral catheter remains *in situ* postoperatively for 24–48 h. Before the patient leaves

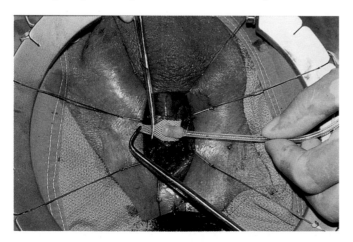

Fig. 39.7 The bulbar cuff is retained by snapping the tab into place.

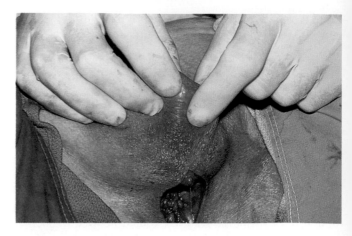

Fig. 39.8 The pump is located superficially in the scrotum.

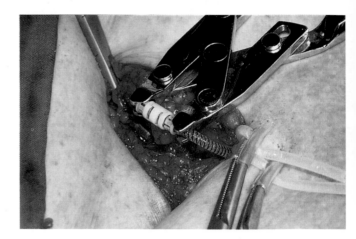

Fig. 39.9 'Quick connect' connectors are used to join the tubing.

the operating room, the cuff is emptied and the system deactivated by pressure on the deactivation button.

Bladder neck placement

In order to achieve bladder neck placement (Fig. 39.10), a Foley catheter is inserted and a lower abdominal transverse incision used. An extraperitoneal approach is utilized and the superficial vessels overlying the prostate are controlled either with sutures or diathermy. The endopelvic fascia is then incised on either side of the midline and care taken not to injure the deep dorsal vein. The plane between the posterior aspect of the prostate and membranous urethra and the rectum is then carefully developed, with particular care being taken not to injure the rectum in this location. This posterior dissection can be very difficult in reoperated cases, and in this situation it is sometimes helpful to open the bladder and, with the aid of a finger inside the bladder neck and prostatic urethra, to undertake the posterior dissection carefully. Once the area has been completely

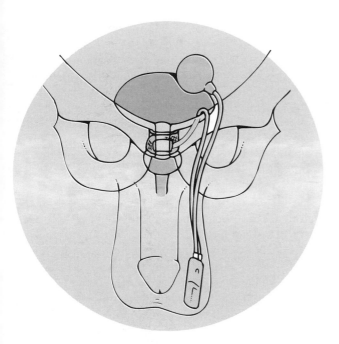

Fig. 39.10 Bladder neck placement of the AMS800 artificial urinary sphincter.

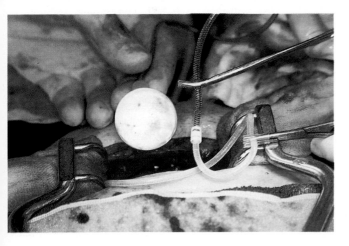

Fig. 39.11 The pressure reservoir is located in the prevesical space.

opened the width of the plane should be in the order of 2 cm, so the cuff will fit snugly without crimping. A tape is then passed around the bladder neck and the bladder filled with an antibiotic solution to identify any openings that may have been created during the dissection. If such an opening is detected it should be closed with several interrupted 000 or 0000 absorbable sutures.

As with the bulbar urethra, the bladder neck is circumferentially measured with a calibrated measuring strap. The catheter remains indwelling during this process, unless it is a large one, in which case it should be removed before the measurement of the bladder neck area. Once the

properly sized cuff has been passed beneath the bladder neck and snapped in place, the tubing from this sphincter component is then passed through one of the rectus muscles to the abdominal wall fascia on the side where the pump will be placed.

The pressure of the balloon reservoir is chosen on the basis of the quality of the tissue and the size of the cuff used. In most patients with bladder neck cuffs a 71–80 cm H_2O pressure balloon reservoir is chosen; however, with those patients who have tissues of substandard quality a 61–70 cm H_2O pressure reservoir may be employed. In general, the larger the cuff, the higher the pressure balloon reservoir selected. Cuff sizes range up to as high as 11 cm for placement around the bladder neck, although in most men an 8–9 cm H_2O cuff is adequate. The pressure balloon reservoir is placed in the prevesical space and its tubing penetrates the rectum muscle next to the tubing of the cuff (Fig. 39.11). Before the balloon is filled, the prevesical space is drained and the anterior abdominal wall is closed with an absorbable suture. Once the closure is complete the balloon is filled with either 22 ml of saline or isosmotic contrast medium and the cuff pressurized. Once the cuff has been pressurized, the balloon is then emptied and refilled with exactly 20 ml of fluid.

The cuff accommodates between 0.5 and 1.5 ml of fluid, depending on the length of the cuff. The artificial sphincter control assembly is placed in the deep subcutaneous pocket in the scrotum and connections between the control assembly and the balloon are established with a straight connector using a 'quick connect' system. As in the bulbar urethra, the cuff is left deactivated for at least 6–8 weeks. The patient's indwelling Foley catheter is removed 24–48 h after surgery and, if necessary, bladder emptying is augmented by intermittent catheterization.

Postoperative complications

Haematoma

One of the more common, but less significant, complications of sphincter surgery is the formation of a subcutaneous haematoma. However, scrotal haematomas cause the most concern because they may not only displace the pump into an unfavourable location, but also become secondarily infected. Most haematomas will resolve spontaneously but occasionally a large haematoma may be better drained to prevent discomfort and enhance the rapidity of healing. If at all possible haematomas should be avoided by careful dissection and scrupulous haemostasis.

Urinary retention

Another problem that is occasionally seen is incomplete voiding after implantation. In such circumstances it is important to check that the sphincter mechanism has been completely deactivated. Most patients, regardless of cuff location, will begin to void after a few 'in and out' catheterizations, but those with a bladder neck placement may require self-catheterization on an indefinite basis. Patients with a bulbar urethral cuff implantation are at more risk of urethral injury from repeated or prolonged urethral catheterization.

Cuff erosion

The most troublesome complication of sphincter surgery is cuff erosion and device infection. Although cuff erosion is far less common since the introduction of delayed activation devices, this problem still occurs from time to time. Erosion can occur at any time after implantation but is most common around 3–4 months after surgery. Cuff erosions occurring before activation usually are the result of unrecognized surgical injury to the urethral bladder neck.

Clinically, patients with cuff erosion may present with pain and swelling in the cuff or pump area, recurrent incontinence or urinary tract infection. Urethrography or urethroscopy will confirm erosion and surgical removal of the cuff is mandatory, especially if there is evidence of active infection. The cuff, pump and pressure reservoir should all be removed and an 18 or 20 F silicone Foley catheter inserted and retained for at least 10 days, until there is radiographic evidence of complete healing. Surprisingly, urethral strictures seldom seem to follow cuff erosion.

If the erosion is uncomplicated and there is no obvious evidence of infection, simply removing the cuff and using a stainless steel tubing plug to occlude the tube leading to the pump and reservoir temporarily can occasionally be successful. Generous irrigation of the surrounding area with antibiotic solutions and drainage may prevent subsequent infection around the device components and 3–6 months later a new cuff may be inserted. In the case of a urethral cuff, another location around the bulbar urethra should be selected; for bladder neck placement the same site can be used, but this can often be associated with technical difficulties.

Mechanical device malfunction

The mechanical reliability of the AMS800 artificial urinary sphincter is now remarkably good; however, recurrent or persistent incontinence may occur as a result of failure of cuff compression, cuff erosion, device malfunction due to fluid loss, tubing kink or pump malfunction. Other problems such as the wrong choice of pressure within the reservoir as well as previously undiagnosed detrusor instability will reduce bladder compliance and may contribute to failure. In general, however, over 80% of male patients with sphincter weakness can be expected to be completely continent following implantation of these devices, and probably 90% or more can expect to be sufficiently dry to be satisfied with the results obtained.

Conclusion

Incontinence of urine can be a socially and psychologically devastating disorder that can potentially wreck an individual's life. With iatrogenic incontinence, prevention is always better than cure and this will depend upon adequate urological training, satisfactory supervision and scrupulous technique. In incontinence due to neurological conditions of chronic retention, careful assessment and early institution of therapy is invaluable. For patients with sphincter weakness, implantation of an artificial sphincter is often the best option and the outcome is now usually acceptable. For end-stage incontinence unresponsive to medication and unsuitable for artificial sphincter implantation the only solution may be a permanent indwelling urinary catheter or one of the surgical options described in Chapter 73.

References

1 Emberton M, Neal DE, Black N et al. The effect of prostatectomy on symptom severity and quality of life. Br J Urol 1996;77:233–47.
2 Moisey C, Stephenson T, Brendler C. The urodynamic and subjective results of treatment of detrusor instability with oxybutinin chloride. Br J Urol 1980;52:472–6.
3 Gajewski JB, Awad JA. Oxybutinin versus propantheline in patients with multiple sclerosis and detrusor hyperreflexia. J Urol 1986;135:966–1000.
4 Scott FB, Bradley WE, Timm GW. Treatment of urinary incontinence by an implantable prosthetic sphincter. Urology 1973;1:252–9.
5 Rosen M. A simple implantable artificial sphincter. Br J Urol 1976;48:675–80.
6 Politano VA. Periurethral polytetrafluoroethylene injection for urinary incontinence. J Urol 1982;127:439–42.
7 Furlow WL, Barrett DM. Recurrent or persistent urinary incontinence in patients with the artificial urinary sphincter: diagnostic considerations and management. J Urol 1985;133:792–5.
8 Goldwasser B, Furlow WC, Barrett DM. The model AS800 artificial urinary sphincter: Mayo Clinic experience. J Urol 1987;137:668–71.

40 Disorders of Continence and Voiding in Females

G.R.Wahle and S.Raz

Introduction

Otherwise healthy women presenting to their healthcare provider with primary voiding complaints typically do so as a result of changes in the support of their pelvic floor. Although mechanisms of urinary continence remain incompletely understood, several factors can be identified which act in concert to maintain normal urinary control in women. These include measures which allow for compliant filling and low-pressure storage of urine in the bladder, and outlet resistance sufficient to prevent unintended leakage of urine. Causes of urinary incontinence related to the bladder, including processes that result in uninhibited detrusor activity or loss of normal compliance, are discussed in detail in other chapters of this book. Urinary incontinence related to the bladder outlet is by far more prevalent in women than in men [1], in whom it is most commonly related to surgical damage or neurogenic alterations. The most common source of clinically significant incontinence in women is outlet related, and results from compromised anatomical support of the bladder neck and proximal urethra, which leads to stress urinary leakage [2–4]. In addition, the forces involved in the pathophysiology of stress urinary incontinence in women are generally not isolated in their effects to the bladder outlet alone, but result in other associated manifestations of deficiencies of pelvic support, including cystocele, uterine prolapse, enterocele and rectocele [5].

Clinicians involved in the care of women should possess a clear, conceptual understanding of the anatomy and pathophysiology of pelvic support in order to evaluate effectively and treat the most common disorders of micturition, which result from pelvic floor relaxation. This chapter will therefore provide a basic overview of the anatomy and musculofascial support of the pelvic structures involved in voiding, discuss their importance in clinically significant disorders of urination resulting from pelvic prolapse and review general principles of surgical repair of outlet-related incontinence.

Anatomy of pelvic support

Bladder

The bladder is a hollow muscular pelvic organ, usually divided into three anatomical layers: the inner mucosa, middle smooth muscle detrusor and outer adventitia consisting of fat and connecting tissue. The mucosa consists of transitional cell epithelium and is continuous with the epithelium of the proximal urethra and both ureters. The muscular middle layer of the bladder is comprised of a smooth muscle mesh, occasionally described as being organized into three layers of orientation at the outlet or bladder neck: inner and outer longitudinal, and middle circular [6] (Fig. 40.1). The function and innervation of the bladder is understood better if it is thought of as having two divisions: the body and trigone. The body of the bladder is primarily involved in compliant distension during gradual ureteral filling resulting in low-pressure filling and storage of urine, and in the generation of efficient detrusor muscle contraction during voiding. The trigone is a triangular region at the floor and apex of the bladder formed by both ureteral orifices and the bladder outlet. It has a different embryological origin from the body of the bladder, and is described as having two muscular layers, superficial and deep, which are separate from the detrusor. The deep layer is a continuation of the fibromuscular outer layer, sometimes called the Waldeyer sheath, of the distal ureters, and the superficial layer is an extension of the inner ureteral musculature. The muscular layers of the trigone also continue distally into the posterior aspect of the proximal urethra [7]. The bladder is richly innervated by the autonomic nervous system. Cholinergic receptors from postganglionic parasympathetic fibres and β-adrenergic receptors from postganglionic sympathetic fibres predominate in the body of the bladder, while α-adrenergic receptors from the sympathetic system predominate in the trigone and proximal urethra [8] (Fig. 40.2).

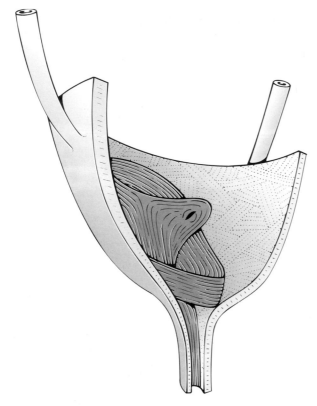

Fig. 40.1 Schematic coronal section of the bladder showing the circular orientation of the detrusor muscle fibres at the bladder neck and the continuation of the apical trigonal musculature into the anterior urethra.

Urethra

In the female, the urethra consists of a 4 cm tube of inner epithelium (transitional cells at the bladder neck and squamous cells at the meatus) and outer muscularis, including both smooth muscle in continuity with the trigonal musculature and striated muscle oriented in a circular layer particularly in the middle third [9]. The infolded epithelium is enclosed by a rich vascular sponge, which is in turn surrounded by a coat of smooth muscle and fibroelastic tissue (Fig. 40.3). The submucosa, consisting of loosely woven connective tissue scattered throughout with smooth muscle bundles and an elaborate vascular plexus, creates a 'washer effect' vital to the mechanism of continence [10]. Functionally, the integrity of the surrounding smooth muscle coat maintains this mechanism by directing submucosal expansile pressures inward towards the mucosa. Healthy, normal smooth muscle and vascular spongy tissue of the urethra together provide a major contribution to the closure mechanism of the urethra and are therefore of great importance in normal passive urinary continence. Striated muscle fibres extrinsic to the urethra at the level of the urogenital diaphragm provide reflex and voluntary sphincteric activity and primarily contribute to active continence.

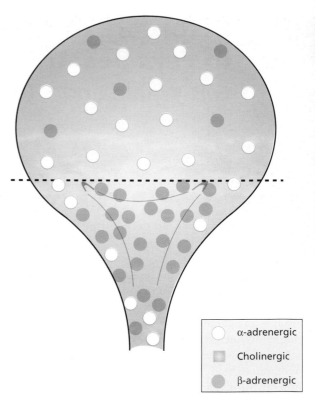

α-adrenergic

Cholinergic

β-adrenergic

Fig. 40.2 Distribution of autonomic receptors in the bladder and proximal urethra.

Sphincter structures

Bladder outlet resistance is a complex mechanism with contributions from the bladder neck and proximal urethral smooth musculature, anatomical support of the bladder base and urethra, and the striated muscle of the mid-urethral area in the female. A proximal or internal sphincter is often described as being formed by circular fibres of smooth muscle at the bladder neck and, in the male, proximal prostatic urethra. It is sometimes also referred to as the smooth muscle sphincter [9]. The distal or external sphincter is comprised of smooth muscle fibres, elastic tissue, intrinsic striated slow-twitch muscle fibres providing baseline tonic activity, and extrinsic striated fast-twitch fibres responsible for reflex and voluntary sphincteric activity [11]. It is sometimes referred to as the striated sphincter and is under partial voluntary control separate from anal sphincter function.

Musculofascial support of the bladder and urethra

The fascia associated with the levator ani muscle group plays a crucial role in maintaining pelvic support. The fascia of the pelvic floor is often described as having different layers, and the abdominal portion is usually referred to as the endopelvic fascia. In order to eliminate confusion, the authors prefer to avoid distinguishing

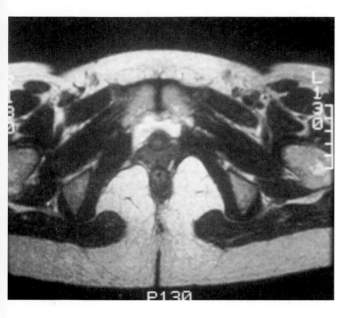

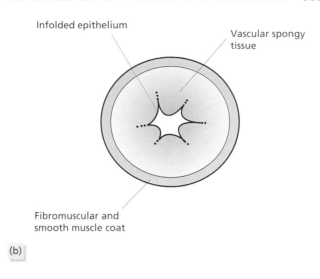

Fig. 40.3 The female urethra. (a) Magnetic resonance image of the female pelvis, showing the cross-sectional urethral anatomy. (b) Schematic cross-section of the urethra, showing the epithelium, spongy tissue and fibromuscular coat.

between the endopelvic and other layers of fascia of the levator musculature and will refer to them collectively as the levator fascia. Although the levator fascia (like the musculature) works in an integrated fashion to provide pelvic support, certain areas of the levator/endopelvic fascia have been described separately on the basis of their importance in the support of individual pelvic structures, and in the surgical correction of pelvic support defects. Four of these condensations, the pubourethral ligaments, the urethropelvic ligaments, the pubocervical fascia and the cardinal–sacrouterine ligament complex will be discussed in detail.

Pubourethral ligaments

The pubourethral ligaments are a condensation of the levator fascia which connect the inner surface of the inferior pubis to the mid-portion of the urethra [12] (Fig. 40.4). They support and stabilize the urethra and associated anterior vaginal wall, and divide the urethra into two halves: the proximal half, which is intra-abdominal and responsible for passive/involuntary continence, and the distal half, which is outside the abdomen. The striated muscle fibres of the external urethral sphincter are located just distal to these ligaments, resulting in this mid-urethral area being responsible for active/voluntary continence. The distal urethra functions mainly as a conduit, and damage to or resection of the distal-most third of the urethra usually results in no significant change in continence. In addition to the previously mentioned pubourethral ligaments,

fascial support of the urethra in its mid-portion is provided laterally on each side by segments of the levator fascia just below their attachments to the pubis (Fig. 40.4). These areas of levator fascia are continuous with the adjacent, more proximal urethropelvic ligaments (described below). The pubourethral ligaments and the lateral levator fascial support of the mid-urethra may be referred to collectively as the mid-urethral complex.

Urethropelvic ligaments

The most important source of anatomical support of the bladder neck and proximal urethra is from a two-layered condensation of the levator fascia which the authors refer to as the urethropelvic ligaments [13]. One layer, the peri-urethral fascia, is encountered just beneath the epithelium during vaginal surgery as a glistening white layer which covers the vaginal side of the urethra. It is continuous with the pubocervical fascia (discussed below) proximally under the vaginal side of the bladder (Fig. 40.5). The second layer of the urethropelvic ligament consists of the levator fascia covering the abdominal side of the urethra, which fuses laterally with the periurethral fascia and attaches as a unit to the tendinous arc of the obturator fascia along the pelvic side wall on each side (Fig. 40.6). These lateral fusions (one on each side) of the periurethral and levator fascia in the region of the bladder neck and proximal urethra provide critical elastic musculofascial support to the bladder outlet. These structures are therefore essential in providing passive continence in women, particularly during periods of increased intra-abdominal pressure. In addition, voluntary or reflex contractions of the levator or obturator musculature increase the tensile forces of these ligamentous areas improving outlet resistance and continence. The urethropelvic ligaments are considered by the authors

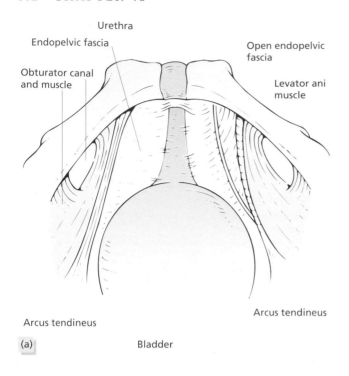

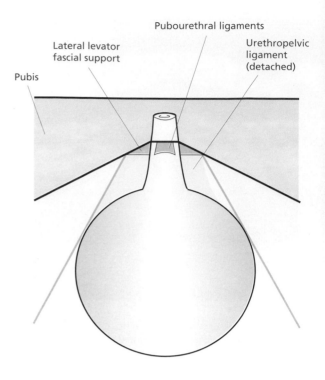

Fig. 40.4 (a) View of the pelvis from above, and (b) corresponding schematic diagram showing the musculofascial support of the bladder neck and proximal urethra, including the mid-urethral complex (pubourethral ligaments and lateral levator attachments of the mid-portion of the urethra) and the urethropelvic ligaments. The urethropelvic ligament is detached from the tendinous arc (arcus tendinus) on the right side.

to be of great importance in the surgical therapy of anatomical stress incontinence.

Pubocervical fascia

Just deep to the anterior vaginal wall in the region of the bladder base lies the pubocervical fascia, a layer of fascia formed from the fusion of the fasciae of the bladder wall and anterior vagina. It is continuous with the periurethral fascia distally, and fuses with the uterine cervix and cardinal ligament complex (discussed below) proximally (see Fig. 40.5). The pubocervical fascia fuses laterally with the levator/endopelvic fascia covering the abdominal side of the bladder in a manner similar to the ligamentous support of the bladder neck and proximal urethra. These lateral fusions, analogous to the urethropelvic ligaments and occasionally referred to as the vesicopelvic ligaments [14] (Fig. 40.7), attach laterally on each side of the pelvic wall at the tendinous arc to provide support at the base

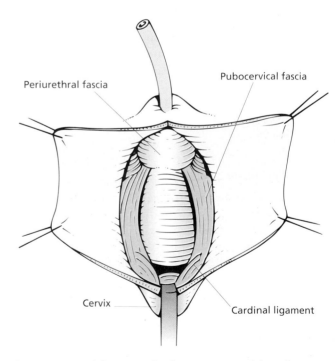

Fig. 40.5 View of the rectangle of anterior vaginal fascial support, found beneath the vaginal wall (shown retracted). The periurethral fascia, which forms the vaginal layer of the urethropelvic ligaments, is continuous with the pubocervical fascia proximally.

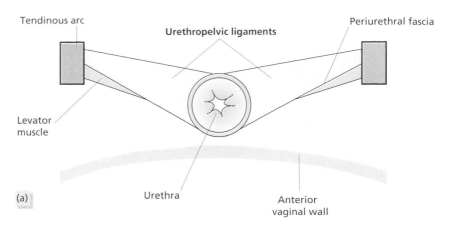

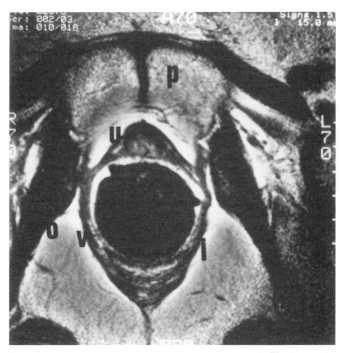

Fig. 40.6 The urethropelvic ligaments. (a) Schematic coronal section at the level of the proximal urethra, showing the two layers of the urethropelvic ligaments which enclose the urethra and fuse laterally to attach to the tendinous arc of the obturator fascia. (b) Magnetic resonance image of the urethropelvic ligaments, which stretch from the urethra to the tendinous arc of the obturator on each side. The vaginal lumen is round and distended by an intravaginal coil. l, levator musculature; 0, obturator muscle, p, pubic bone; u, urethra; v, vaginal wall (distended by coil).

of the bladder and the anterior vaginal wall. Attenuation of support of the bladder at the attachment of the pubocervical fascia to the pelvic wall results in a lateral (or paravaginal) cystocele defect (Fig. 40.8)

Cardinal–sacrouterine ligament complex

The anterior-most aspect of the cardinal–sacrouterine ligament complex fuses with the medial portion of the pubocervical fascia, which is continuous distally with the periurethral fascia. Thus, when viewed from a vaginal perspective with the epithelium removed, these structures together form a rectangle of anterior vaginal fascial support beneath the base of the bladder [5] (Fig. 40.9). Herniation of the bladder through a midline defect in this fascial rectangle results in a central cystocele defect (Fig. 40.8).

Pathophysiology of deficient pelvic support

Alterations in the normal support of pelvic structures may occur as the result of several processes. Congenital defects of pelvic support are uncommon and usually present in childhood. Traumatic or surgical injury may also cause various degrees of pelvic prolapse, as can heavy physical labour. Nulliparous women may experience genitourinary symptoms related to pelvic floor relaxation due to post-menopausal tissue atrophy [15]. Some authors have stressed the importance of denervation of the pelvic floor musculature in the genesis of pelvic relaxation [16].

The most common source of significant pelvic support deficiency appears to be related to trauma from childbirth and/or hysterectomy. The fact that stress urinary

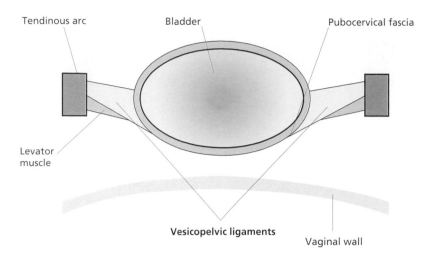

Fig. 40.7 The vesicopelvic ligaments. Analogous to the urethropelvic ligaments, these two-layered fusions of the levator fascia attach laterally to the tendinous arc to provide lateral support to the bladder base.

incontinence and other manifestations of pelvic support compromise more often occur during or shortly after menopause rather than at the time of obstetric or gynaecological trauma further implicates trophic changes from hormonal alterations in the loss of pelvic support [5].

Stress urinary incontinence is often the first symptom experienced during a gradual loss of pelvic support in women, and frequently leads them to seek medical attention. It occurs when intravesical pressure exceeds that of outlet resistance during periods of increased intra-abdominal pressure, such as during coughing, sneezing or straining. Prior to a detailed consideration of the patho-physiology of pelvic support defects, the forces responsible for maintaining outlet resistance in women will be reviewed.

Mechanisms of outlet resistance in women

Normal outlet resistance in the female is achieved by several factors working in concert which provide conti-nence both at rest and during stress. These factors can be organized into the following four categories.

Anatomical and functional urethral length

Anatomical urethral length is defined as the distance between the internal and external urethral meatus. Congenital anomalies and traumatic injuries resulting in the loss of a portion of urethra may result in incontinence. Functional urethral length refers to the total length of the urethra measured during urethral pressure profilometry in which urethral pressure exceeds bladder pressure [17] and therefore correlates better with the physiology of outlet continence. Certain observations argue against the clinical usefulness of the concept of urethral lengths. Twenty per cent of asymptomatic nulliparous women have open bladder necks at rest during transvaginal ultrasonography

[18], and up to 50% of normal continent women will demonstrate funnelling of the bladder neck and proximal urethra on straining cystograms [19]. Y-V plasty or incision of the bladder neck will not produce incontinence in women with otherwise healthy and well-supported outlets. As previously discussed, resection of the distal third of the female urethra does not typically influence continence. In addition, surgical elongation of a poorly coapted urethra will not restore continence. Despite these observations, certain critical lengths of healthy, functional urethra are required to provide the coaptation necessary to achieve passive continence and continence during abdominal stress. Although bladder neck suspension procedures do not change anatomical urethral length, their success in im-proving continence may be thought of as resulting from an increase in, or more accurately a restoration of, functional urethral length.

Closing forces of the urethra

As discussed previously, the healthy infolded urethral mucosa and spongy vascular tissue of the normal female urethra (both under trophic hormonal influence), surround-ed by a thin musculofascial envelope creates an effective coaptive seal, like the washer of a faucet [10]. The tensile forces of the urethropelvic ligaments (which enclose the urethra) and, indirectly, the levator musculature also result in compression of the proximal and mid-urethra. In addition, the resting tone of the striated musculature in the mid-urethral area provides further closing pressure to the urethra.

Pelvic floor muscular activity during stress

A sudden change in abdominal pressures will produce reflex contraction of the muscles of both the levator group and the urogenital diaphragm in neurologically intact

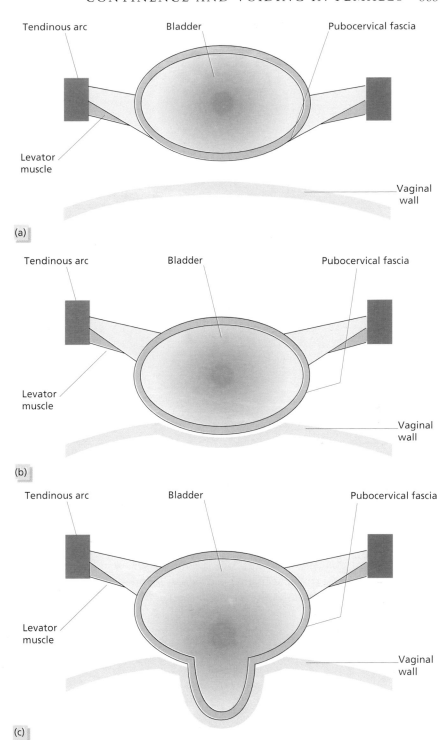

Fig. 40.8 Schematic diagram of anterior vaginal support defects. (a) Normal anterior vaginal support. (b) Compromise of support of the bladder at the attachment of the pubocervical fascia to the pelvis, resulting in a lateral cystocele defect. (c) Herniation of the base of the bladder through a separated, attenuated pubocervical fascia and the adjacent cardinal–sacrouterine ligament support, resulting in a central cystocele defect.

women, producing an increase in mid-urethral pressures. Voluntary or reflex contraction of the levator and obturator muscles will also increase tension on the urethropelvic ligaments, thereby elevating and compressing the proximal urethra [5] (Fig. 40.10).

Position and anatomical support of the outlet

A true valvular effect is created by the high retropubic fixation of the bladder neck and urethra in relation to the more dependent position of the bladder base. Limited posterior rotation of the bladder base against a well-supported urethra during stress will increase this valvular

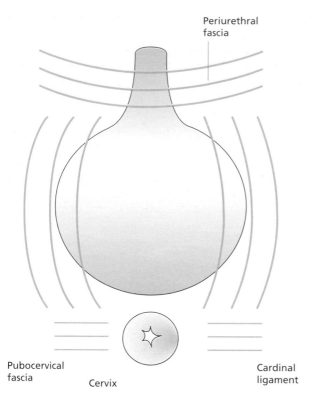

Periurethral fascia

Pubocervical fascia

Cervix

Cardinal ligament

Fig. 40.9 Schematic diagram of the rectangle of fascial support of the anterior vagina beneath the bladder.

during periods of abdominal stress, including coughing, sneezing, walking or straining. Processes that result in deterioration of these mechanisms can result in variable degrees of incontinence. Urethral function may be compromised due to atrophy of urethral spongy tissue secondary to menopausal hormonal changes, compromised neuromuscular function or damage from surgery, trauma or radiation therapy. Weakened levator musculature will not increase as efficiently mid-urethral pressures during stress. While loss of intrinsic urethral resistance and/or pelvic floor muscular activity can adversely influence continence, the most common process resulting in impairment of the mechanisms of outlet resistance in women is loss of anatomical support of the bladder neck and urethra. Pelvic floor relaxation and weakening of the urethropelvic ligaments and mid-urethral complex produces significant posterior and downward rotation of the urethra and bladder neck. This laxity will transfer the bladder neck and urethra to a dependent position in the pelvis, eliminating the previously described valvular function. Sudden increases in intra-abdominal pressures will facilitate funnelling and opening of a poorly supported outlet. In addition, intra-abdominal forces are not transmitted efficiently to the poorly supported proximal urethra due to its extra-abdominal location and to the loss of the backboard effect of the strong normal support of the urethropelvic ligaments.

The forces responsible for pelvic relaxation rarely affect only isolated anatomical zones, and stress urinary incontinence resulting from hypermobility of the bladder neck and urethra is therefore often accompanied by associated defects of pelvic support, including uterine prolapse, cystocele, enterocele and rectocele. In order to provide optimal treatment, the pelvic surgeon considering repair of the anatomy responsible for the incontinence must fully delineate the defects present and treat them in an integrated fashion.

effect of the bladder neck [5]. In addition, direct through transmission of intra-abdominal forces to the area of the proximal urethra in a well-supported woman will increase its resistance during periods of abdominal stress as well [20].

In a normal healthy woman, this complex set of interrelated compensatory mechanisms exists to maintain sufficient outlet resistance to prevent urine leakage, even

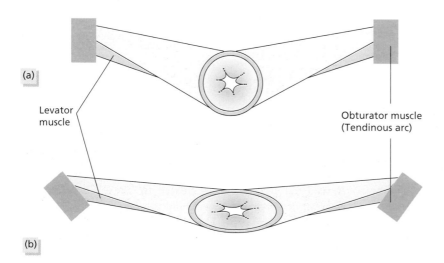

(a)

Levator muscle

Obturator muscle (Tendinous arc)

(b)

Fig. 40.10 Schematic diagram of the urethra and its supporting fascia (a) at rest and (b) during voluntary or reflex contraction of the obturator and levator musculature. The subsequent increase in tension on the urethropelvic ligaments and the mid-urethral levator support results in elevation and compression of the bladder neck and urethra.

Anterior vaginal wall relaxation

Bladder neck and urethral prolapse

As discussed previously, normal support of the bladder outlet in women is provided by the levator fascia in the region of the bladder neck and urethra which the authors refer to as the urethropelvic ligaments and mid-urethral complex. Bladder neck hypermobility resulting in stress urinary incontinence is most commonly related to attenuation of the urethropelvic ligaments and/or their attachment to the pelvic side wall at the tendinous arc of the obturator fascia. In general, little attention has been given to the support of the mid-portion of the urethra in the genesis of stress urinary incontinence. Video urodynamic evaluation reveals that in most patients with stress incontinence resulting from loss of pelvic support there is separation of the mid-portion of the urethra from its normal attachment to the underside of the symphysis pubis as well as hypermobility of the bladder neck and proximal urethra (Fig. 40.11). Although based on preliminary clinical work, the authors believe that further improvements in treatment may be achieved by incorporating concepts of mid-urethral support and use of the mid-urethral complex in designing and modifying surgical approaches for use in outlet-related incontinence.

Surgical procedures designed to restore an intrinsically normal but poorly supported outlet to a well-supported intrapelvic position can be expected to have an 80–90% rate of success in eliminating stress incontinence in women [21]. Although the importance of restoring anatomical position and support of the bladder neck and urethra in the treatment of stress incontinence is undeniable, one must keep in mind that the majority of women with bladder neck hypermobility do not experience significant incontinence. Intrinsic urethral function is critical to continence as well, and may make up for the loss of support of the bladder neck and proximal urethra. In fact, it is reasonable to argue that all woman with outlet hypermobility and stress incontinence have a component of intrinsic urethral dysfunction [22]. Conversely, anatomical support is not sufficient to achieve continence, and inadequate urethral resistance not uncommonly leads to nearly complete incontinence despite perfect support of the bladder neck and urethra.

Intrinsic urethral dysfunction

While an understanding of the anatomical support of the bladder neck and urethra is essential in considering female urinary continence, knowledge of the anatomy and intrinsic function of the urethra is also required. The plasticity of the highly efficient mucosal seal mechanism (see Fig. 40.3) normally allows perfect continence even when a grooved sound is inserted into the urethra. The intrinsic urethral tissues are affected by trophic hormonal influences, and lack of oestrogen at menopause may lead to thinning and flattening of the urethral epithelium, and atrophy of the vascular sponge with substitution by fibrous tissue. Multiple surgical procedures, pelvic trauma, radiation therapy and neurogenic disease may also impair the ability of the urethra to achieve or maintain a perfect

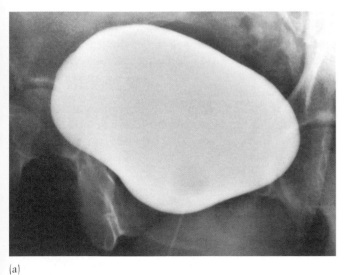

(a)

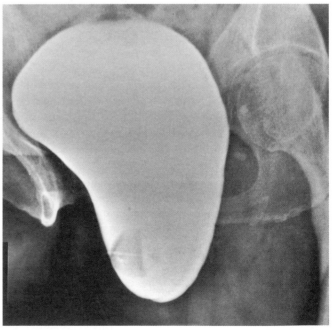

(b)

Fig. 40.11 Lateral upright cystogram (a) at rest and (b) during straining, showing hypermobility of the bladder neck and proximal urethra, as well as separation of the mid-urethra from the underside of the pubis.

seal. Outlet-related incontinence is frequently divided into anatomical incontinence (felt to be more common, present in up to 90% of cases of stress leakage at presentation), due to inadequate support of the bladder neck and urethra, and intrinsic sphincteric dysfunction, due to inadequacy of the urethra's contribution to resistance [5]. As previously discussed, when the continence mechanisms of intrinsic urethral function are compromised, stress incontinence may result despite adequate pelvic support. Simple bladder neck and proximal urethral suspension in this case is insufficient to achieve continence, and treatment must be aimed at providing urethral coaptation and compression (such as via sling procedures, injection of bulking agents into the envelope of the urethra or implantation of hydraulic sphincter devices) in addition to restoring anatomical support.

Cystocele

Hypermobility of the bladder neck and urethra is only one manifestation of anterior vaginal wall prolapse. Most women with stress urinary incontinence on the basis of bladder neck hypermobility have an associated cystocele which must also be addressed at the time of evaluation and treatment.

Many classification systems have been used to grade cystocele defects [23,24]. The authors prefer to describe four degrees of anterior vaginal wall prolapse. In grade I and II cystourethrocele, there is a mild to moderate degree of hypermobility of the anterior vaginal wall during straining. In grade III, the anterior vaginal wall reaches through the introitus on straining, and in grade IV the bladder base protrudes through the introitus.

Two different types of anterior vaginal wall support defects in the region of the base of the bladder can be identified: (i) lateral defects, due to loss or attenuation of the lateral (or paravaginal) attachment of the pubocervical fascia/vesicopelvic ligament at the tendinous arc of the obturator; and (ii) central defects, resulting from separation of the pubocervical fascia and cardinal ligaments in the midline, allowing herniation of the bladder base into the vagina (see Fig. 40.8). These two types of support compromise may occur in conjunction, as is seen in women with grade IV cystoceles who have, in general, combined lateral and central support defects, both of which must be corrected at the time of surgical repair (Fig. 40.12).

Surgical principles of the correction of stress incontinence

Urologists as a group have failed to recognize that stress incontinence is only one manifestation of pelvic prolapse, and that no single surgical procedure can be used to treat outlet incontinence effectively. Instead, patients presenting

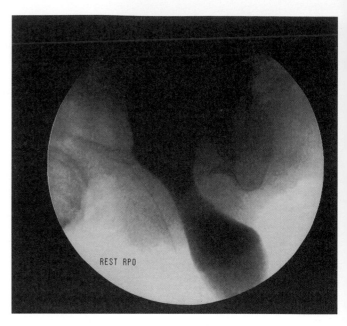

Fig. 40.12 Upright cystogram, showing grade IV cystocele with both lateral and central defects.

for surgical correction of their symptoms should be managed according to the degree of anterior vaginal wall prolapse and associated defects of pelvic support.

There have been many surgical techniques and modifications thereof described to treat stress urinary incontinence. Although success rates of abdominal and vaginal suspension procedures are similar [25,26], the morbidity of vaginal surgery is significantly less than procedures which involve an abdominal incision. When dealing with a patient with stress urinary incontinence who requires an abdominal incision for hysterectomy or other abdominal or pelvic disorder, the authors use a Burch suspension technique [27]. In all other cases the use of a vaginal approach to correct stress urinary incontinence is preferred.

Based on anatomical and pathophysiological principles, an algorithm using a group of previously described surgical procedures may be defined to approach the treatment of stress urinary incontinence and associated pelvic support defects [28].

Stress incontinence without significant cystocele

Several options for bladder neck suspension exist. As mentioned above, the authors prefer the use of a simple transvaginal procedure. Several principles of transvaginal suspension technique can be identified which must be strictly adhered to in order to ensure a successful outcome [21,22].

1 *Mobilization of the urethra and bladder neck from fixation and tethering.* This is important to ensure that the suspension can be performed without tension, and is particularly important when approaching patients with a history of previous anti-incontinence procedures.

2 *Placement of the suspension sutures in hardy tissues.* The authors feel that the most successful and durable suspensions will be achieved through placement of permanent suture material to include the portion of levator fascia which anchors the urethra and bladder neck to the tendinous arc of the obturator fascia and lateral pelvic wall (the urethropelvic ligament), as well as vaginal wall without epithelium, and pubocervical fascia [28,29].

3 *Precise placement of the bladder neck suspension sutures in the proper location.* Distal placement can result in urethral kinking; proximal placement can result in ineffective suspension; medial placement may lead to urethral obstruction; and lateral placement can result in ineffective suspension and may cause pain from the inclusion of the levator complex in the suspending suture [30].

4 *Satisfactory securing of the anchoring tissue.* The authors prefer the placement of helical sutures in the anchoring tissues, which results in more reliable anchoring than does incorporating only a loop of tissue, or the use of barrel knots or buttresses.

5 *Appropriate selection of the suprapubic punch puncture site.* The suspension sutures should be transferred and tied over an area of rectus fascia that is immobile to prevent positional changes in continence and avoid postoperative pain in the suprapubic area with activity [28]. This is accomplished easily by identifying the area of midline rectus fascia just above its insertion onto the pubis where the abdominal wall is thickest. Attachment of the suspension sutures to the pubic bone or its periosteum should be avoided in order to eliminate the potential risks of osteitis pubica or frank osteomyelitis [30].

6 *Fingertip guidance of the passage of the ligature carrier through the retropubic space.* This allows the surgeon to pass the carrier by scratching the superior margin of the pubis, prevents inadvertent perforation of the bladder or urethra and ensures correct position of the suspending sutures.

7 *Use of a double-pronged ligature carrier.* This reduces the number of passes through the retropubic space by half and provides a 1 cm fascial bridge over which the suspension sutures are tied [21].

8 *Injection of indigo carmine and cystourethroscopy after transferring the suspension sutures.* This will document bilateral ureteral efflux of urine, demonstrate the lack of damage to the bladder and urethra and confirm proper elevation of the bladder neck and proximal urethra when gentle traction is applied to the suspension sutures. Endoscopic examination of the bladder following placement and/or transfer of suspension sutures is mandatory when permanent suture material is used.

9 *Tying the suspension sutures over the fascia without tension.* A suspension procedure is designed to provide support and eliminate movement of the bladder neck and proximal urethra during abdominal straining. Undue tension is unnecessary and may cause chronic postoperative pain [30].

Stress incontinence with moderate cystocele

Traditional methods of cystocele repair, such as anterior colporrhaphy, correct central fascial defects, but do not address the underlying problem resulting in stress incontinence (lack of support of the bladder neck and proximal urethra) or lack of lateral support of the bladder base. Suspension of the bladder neck alone in the presence of a significant cystocele may lead to further voiding dysfunction, including obstruction from kinking between a mobile bladder and a supported outlet.

In patients with moderate cystocele due to a lateral defect, bladder neck suspension may be performed in conjunction with placement of suspending sutures in the lateral pubocervical fascia and cardinal ligaments in the region of the bladder base to restore lateral pelvic support and thereby repair the cystocele. This procedure, a 'four-corner' bladder and bladder neck suspension, involves transfer of the four supporting sutures to the suprapubic area where the sutures are tied independently over the midline suprapubic rectus fascia [31].

Stress incontinence with severe cystocele

In severe cystocele defects, there is in general a combination of bladder neck and proximal urethral hypermobility, detachment of the lateral bladder support from the pelvic wall and herniation of the bladder through a central defect in the pubocervical fascia and cardinal ligaments (see Fig. 40.11c). The urethral hypermobility is repaired with bladder neck suspension (or a sling procedure in intrinsic sphincter dysfunction), the lateral defect is addressed by applying permanent suspending sutures to the cardinal ligaments, pubocervical fascia and urethropelvic ligaments, and the central defect by reapproximation of strong pubocervical fasciae and the cardinal ligaments to the midline [28].

Bladder prolapse is commonly associated with other pelvic support defects, including enterocele, rectocele and uterine prolapse, which must be addressed at the time of surgical repair as well.

Intrinsic sphincter dysfunction

Options for treatment of intrinsic sphincter dysfunction include sling procedures, artificial sphincter devices [32] and injection of bulking agents into periurethral tissues.

Sling procedures have been described using synthetic material, autologous fascia and vaginal wall flaps to restore compression and coaptation of incompetent urethral tissues as well as support of the bladder neck and proximal urethra [33–35]. Periurethral injections do not address anatomical causes of incontinence, but may be appropriate for patients with good pelvic support and relatively 'pure' sphincteric incontinence; in particular, those who have failed previous attempts at surgical repair [28].

If intrinsic sphincter dysfunction is felt to be present, the authors generally address it through the use of a sling procedure, and prefer to use a vaginal wall sling rather than a pubovaginal fascial sling to avoid the morbidity of an abdominal fascial incision. Currently, we are using a modification of a previously reported vaginal wall sling procedure which does not involve the use of a formal buried flap of vaginal wall and epithelium. The preliminary rate of resolution of stress-related incontinence is more than 90%, and the incidence of unpredicted permanent retention is rare, occurring in only 1–2% of cases thus far [36]. In general, the authors do not recommend the placement of artificial sphincter devices in female patients, in whom sling procedures are highly effective and carry little risk.

Conclusion

Although stress urinary incontinence is frequently the incentive leading to a woman's initial visit to a physician, pelvic surgeons in general, and urologists in particular, have failed to recognize that stress urinary incontinence is only one manifestation of pelvic relaxation and have been remiss in addressing it without concomitant attention to the associated pelvic defects that often accompany it. By arming themselves with a fundamental grasp of the anatomy and pathophysiology of pelvic support, concerned clinicians will be able to address effectively their female patients who present with complaints related to deficiencies in pelvic support, and appropriately apply the current methods of evaluation and treatment of voiding dysfunction discussed in this and other chapters of this book.

References

1 Diokno AC, Brock BM, Brown MB, Herzog AR. Prevalence of urinary incontinence and other urological symptoms in the non-institutionalized elderly. *J Urol* 1986;**136**:1022.

2 Marshall VF, Marchetti AA, Krantz KE. The correction of stress incontinence by simple vesicourethral suspension. *Surg Gynecol Obstet* 1949;**88**:509.

3 Hodgkinson CP. Stress urinary incontinence. *Am J Obstet Gynecol* 1970;**108**:1141.

4 McGuire EJ, Lyton B, Pepe V, Kohorn EI. Stress urinary incontinence. *Obstet Gynecol* 1976;**47**:255.

5 Raz S, Little NA, Juma S. Female urology. In: Walsh PC, Retik AB, Stamey TA, Vaughan ED, eds. *Campbell's Urology*, 6th edn. Philadelphia: WB Saunders, 1992:2782–829.

6 Hutch JA. A new theory of the anatomoy of the internal sphincter and the physiology of micturition. *Invest Urol* 1965; **3**:36.

7 Tanagho EA, Pugh RCB. The anatomy and function of the ureterovesical junction. *Br J Urol* 1963;**35**:151.

8 Gosling JA. The structure of the bladder and urethra in relation to function. *Urol Clin North Am* 1979;**6**(1):31.

9 Redman JF. Anatomy of the genitourinary system. In: Gillenwater JY, Grayhack JT, Howards SS, Duckett JW, eds. *Adult and Pediatric Urology*, 2nd edn. St Louis: Mosby Year Book, 1991:3–62.

10 Staskin DR, Zimmern PE, Hadley HR, Raz S. The pathophysiology of stress incontinence. *Urol Clin North Am* 1985; **12**:271.

11 Elbadawi A. Neuromuscular mechanisms of micturition. In: Subbarao UY, ed. *Neurourology and Urodynamics*. New York: Macmillan, 1988:3–35.

12 Zacharin RF. The anatomic supports of the female urethra. *Obstet Gynecol* 1968;**21**:754.

13 Klutke C, Golomb J, Barbaric Z, Raz S. The anatomy of stress incontinence: magnetic resonance imaging of the female bladder neck and urethra. *J Urol* 1989;**143**:563.

14 Raz S. The anatomy of pelvic support and stress incontinence. In: Raz S, ed. *Atlas of Transvaginal Surgery*. Philadelphia: WB Saunders, 1992:1–22.

15 Stanton SL. Vaginal prolapse. In: Ras S, ed. *Female Urology*. Philadelphia: WB Saunders, 1983:229–40.

16 Snooks SJ, Swash M, Henry MM, Setchell ME. Injury to innervation of the pelvic floor sphincter musculature in childbirth. *Lancet* 1984;**2**:546.

17 Bruskewitz R. Urethral pressure profile in female lower urinary tract dysfunction. In: *Female Urology*. Philadelphia: WB Saunders, 1983:113–22.

18 Chapple CR, Helm CW, Blease S, Milroy EJG, Rickards D, Osborne JL. Asymptomatic bladder neck incompetence in nulliparous females. *Br J Urol* 1989;**64**:357.

19 Versi E, Cardozo LD, Studd JWW, Brincat M, O'Dowd TM, Cooper DJ. Internal urinary sphincter in maintenance of female continence. *Br Med J* 1986;**292**:166.

20 Enhörning G. Simultaneous recording of intravesical and intraurethral pressure. *Acta Chir Scand* 1961;**276**:3.

21 Siegel AL, Raz S. Surgical treatment of stress urinary incontinence. *Neurourol Urodyn* 1988;**7**:569.

22 Wahle GR, Young GPH, Raz S. Vaginal surgery for stress urinary incontinence. *Urology* 1994;**43**(4):416.

23 Hughes EC, Hughes EC, ed. *American College of Obstetricians and Gynecologists Book on Obstetric–Gynecologic Terminology*. Philadelphia: FA Davis, 1972.

24 Beecham, CT. Classification of vaginal relaxation. *Am J Obstet Gynecol* 1980;**136**:957.

25 Green DF, McGuire EJ, Lyton B. A comparison of endoscopic suspension of the vesical neck versus anterior urethropexy for the treatment of stress urinary incontinence. *J Urol* 1986; **136**:1205.

26 Spencer JR, O'Connor VJ, Schaeffer AJ. A comparison of endoscopic suspension of the vesical neck with suprapubic vesicourethropexy for treatment of stress urinary incontinence. *J Urol* 1987;**137**:411.

27 Burch JC. Urethrovaginal fixation to Cooper's ligament for

correction of stress incontinence, cystocele, and prolapse. *Am J Obstet Gynecol* 1961;**81**:281.

28 Raz S. Surgical therapy for urinary incontinence. In: Raz S, ed. *Atlas of Transvaginal Surgery*. Philadelphia: WB Saunders, 1992: 49–101.

29 Raz S, Sussman EM, Erickson DB, Bregg KJ, Nitti VW. The Raz bladder neck suspension: results in 206 patients. *J Urol* 1992;**148**:845.

30 Wahle GR, Young GPH, Raz S. Complications of vaginal surgery. In: Raz S, ed. *Female Urology*, 2nd edn. Philadelphia: WB Saunders, in press.

31 Raz S, Klutke CG, Golomb J. Four-corner bladder and urethral suspension for moderate cystocele. *J Urol* 1989;**142**:712.

32 Scott FB. The use of the artificial sphincter in the treatment of urinary incontinence in the female patient. *Urol Clin North Am* 1985;**12**(2):305.

33 Aldridge AH. Transplantation of fascia for relief of urinary stress incontinence. *Am J Obstet Gynecol* 1942;**44**: 398.

34 McGuire EJ, Lytton B. The pubovaginal sling in stress urinary incontinence. *J Urol* 1978;**119**:82.

35 Raz S, Siegel AL, Short JL, Snyder JA. Vaginal wall sling. *J Urol* 1989;**141**:43.

36 Young GPH, Wahle GR, Raz S. Modified vaginal wall sling. Presented to the American Urologic Association Eighty-Ninth Annual Meeting, 18 May, 1994.

Section 4
Infections and Inflammatory Diseases

41 Bacteriology of Urinary Tract Infection
R. Maskell

Introduction

At the present moment it is accepted that the normal urinary tract is sterile above the distal one-third of the urethra, which is colonized by a commensal flora of several bacterial species. These organisms fulfil a protective function, inhibiting by various mechanisms the access of other bacteria, principally the Gram-negative bowel organisms, to the bladder. The composition of this commensal flora varies between the sexes and at different stages of life. It is important to the treatment of urinary tract infection that the dynamic nature of the process is understood, both in the initial access of organisms to the proximal urethra and in the insubsequent movement to the bladder and paraurethral tissues (the prostate in men and the paraurethral glands in women) and sometimes to the kidneys. Without a clear understanding of this process, laboratory diagnosis is open to misinterpretation and antibiotics can be used incorrectly.

Pathogenesis and infecting organisms

While a few organisms that cause infection in the urinary tract (e.g. *Neisseria gonorrhoeae* or *Mycobacterium tuberculosis*) are obligatory pathogens, the great majority are constituents of the commensal flora of neighbouring structures, the bowel, perineum and distal urethra. Rarely, infection occurs by the haematogenous route, but the usual pathway is ascending.

Haematogenous infection

Table 41.1 lists those organisms that gain access to the urinary tract by the haematogenous route. In the neonatal period, bowel or vaginal organisms such as *Escherichia coli* or *Streptococcus agalactiae* (Lancefield group B) may invade the bloodstream of the infant during birth. Bacteraemia precedes the finding of a positive urine culture. Infection may occur, usually in severely ill or immunocompromised patients or those on broad-spectrum

Table 41.1 Organisms involved in haematogenous infection.

Bacteria	*Escherichia coli, Streptococcus agalactiae* (neonatal period)
	Staphylococcus aureus
	Salmonella spp.
	Mycobacterium spp.
	Brucella spp.
Parasites	*Schistosoma haematobium*
Fungi	*Candida* spp.
	Histoplasma duboisii
Viruses	Cytomegalovirus
	Adenovirus type 2
	Polyomavirus

antibiotics, secondary to bacteraemia with *Staphylococcus aureus* or *Candida* spp. This may result in the formation of multiple renal abscesses. In tuberculosis, salmonellosis, brucellosis and some virus infections the organisms are excreted in the urine in the course of a generalized infection. This does not imply that they necessarily give rise to symptoms or urinary tract inflammation. For example, urinary excretion of *Salmonella* spp. is usually asymptomatic but can cause clinical signs of urinary infection. Urinary tuberculosis is secondary to infection elsewhere in the body. Granulomatous lesions in the renal cortex may rupture into the tubular lumen, spreading infection to the pelvis, ureters and bladder.

Although viruria occurs during the course of many viral illnesses little is known about the frequency with which it causes symptoms. It seems likely, especially in children, that it may sometimes account for urinary symptoms for which no bacterial cause can be found [1].

Ascending infection

The commensal organisms which invade the urinary tract from below exist in equilibrium with others in their natural sites, fulfilling a beneficial function. The defensive properties of the commensal flora of the distal urethra against invasion by bowel organisms include production of inhibitors against potential pathogens, coaggregation of commensal species with each other or with potential pathogens [2], colonization of epithelial surfaces and competition for sites of adhesion [3]. The trigger for successful invasion of the urinary tract may be local trauma, such as occurs during sexual intercourse, failure of the washout mechanism resulting, for example, from impairment of bladder emptying, or direct introduction of organisms by catheters or instruments.

Antibiotics may also determine the ability of potential pathogens to gain access to the urinary tract and its adjacent structures. They have an effect on the commensal flora throughout the body. The nature of this effect depends upon the antibacterial spectrum and pharmacokinetic properties of the agent used and the duration of treatment. Important factors in the balance between benefit and harm in the use of antibacterial agents for treatment of urinary tract infection are the composition of the commensal flora of bowel and urethra, the site of infection (whether in the urine only or involving tissue), the presence of any predisposing mechanical factor such as impaired bladder emptying or an indwelling catheter and the duration of treatment.

Table 41.2 lists the principal factors that predispose to infection of the urinary tract by the ascending route. These factors are relevant to different extents in different age and sex groups. It follows that the bacteria likely to be responsible for urinary tract infection differ in a similar

Table 41.2 Factors that predispose to urinary tract infection by the ascending route.

Inefficient washout mechanism
  Low fluid intake
  Low urinary output (hot climate, renal failure)
  Infrequent or incomplete micturition

Poor bladder emptying
  Neuropathic bladder
  Bladder diverticulum
  Post-micturition residue (vesicoureteric reflux, chronic cystitis)

Obstruction of the bladder outlet
  Congenital urethral valves
  Urethral stricture
  Constipation
  Prostatic hypertrophy
  Bladder stone
  Periurethral inflammation

Mechanical introduction of organisms
  Catheterization or instrumentation
  Sexual intercourse

Direct spread of organisms from the bowel
  Diverticular disease
  Appendix abscess

way. In addition, as well as those organisms which commonly cause infection in the normal intact urinary tract, there are others of lower pathogenicity, for example *Staphylococcus epidermidis* and *Pseudomonas* spp., which can assume a pathogenic role in damaged urinary tracts or in severely ill or immunocompromised patients. Bacterial properties relevant to the ability of an organism to establish itself and multiply in the urinary tract or its adjacent structures include adhesiveness to uroepithelium, slime production, possession of somatic (O) and capsular (K) antigens, motility, growth rate, gaseous requirements, tolerance of an acid pH, toxin production, resistance to the antibacterial effect of some chemical constituents of urine or tissue and the balance of organisms within the commensal flora.

There is a body of *in vitro* and some *in vivo* evidence of the relevance of each of these factors but, at the time of writing, their importance relative to the clinical and mechanical factors listed in Table 41.2 is undetermined. Adhesiveness to uroepithelium occurs via attachment of bacterial fimbriae to glycolipid or glycoprotein receptors on the epithelial cell membrane. In the case of the most common urinary pathogen, *E. coli*, it is known that the fimbriae are of two types, mannose sensitive and mannose resistant, and that the latter can adhere to a disaccharide receptor on uroepithelial cells [4]. This receptor is related to the antigens of the P blood group system, and mannose-resistant fimbriae have therefore been called P fimbriae. It has been suggested that possession of P fimbriae is relevant to the ability of an organism to cause infection in the upper or lower urinary tract, and that this property might be useful in distinguishing renal from bladder infection [5]. However, the evidence is conflicting [6,7], and no useful clinical test has yet emerged. The difficulty of validating any test of bacterial virulence as evidence of renal involvement is that imaging techniques provide evidence only of postinfective damage. Definitive proof of the presence of bacteria in the kidney—to be of maximum clinical use this should be before structural damage has occurred—can only be obtained from culture of urine collected by a ureteric catheter.

Conflicting evidence in the field of adhesiveness studies may be due to differences in methodology or to extrapolation of findings in animal studies to humans. It is likely that bacterial adhesion is species and tissue specific. An example of the latter within the urinary tract is the ability of *Chlamydia trachomatis* to invade the squamous epithelium of the urethra but not the transitional epithelium of the bladder. When epithelium type changes, for example squamous metaplasia occurring in the trigone and proximal urethra as a result of inflammation, an organism such as *Gardnerella vaginalis*, which adheres to squamous epithelium in the vagina, could assume a pathogenic role there. This hypothesis is consistent with the finding that patients found to have *G. vaginalis* infection of the bladder always have a history of previous urinary tract infection with other urinary pathogens [8]. Change of epithelial type might also be partly responsible for the pathogenicity of lactobacilli in the proximal urethra and trigone, where the epithelium is transitional, whereas that of the distal urethra where they are commensals is squamous.

The ability of *S. epidermidis* to produce an outer glycocalyx matrix (slime) may be a factor in the pathogenicity of this organism in patients with urethral catheters or plastic implants such as J stents, or in tissue previously damaged by infection with more virulent organisms.

Growth rate is relevant to the ability of organisms such as *E. coli* to reproduce themselves sufficiently fast to counteract the mechanical washout effect of urine production and bladder emptying. Gaseous requirements account for the fact that anaerobes, which far outnumber aerobes in the bowel, only rarely cause urinary infection because they are unable to survive in the oxygen tension of urine. They, and more frequently capnophiles (carbon dioxide-requiring organisms), are known to cause infection in damaged and fibrotic tissue or in situations such as the heavily infected urine of patients with long-term indwelling catheters, where multiplying aerobes have the effect of reducing the oxygen tension.

Neisseria gonorrhoeae provides an example of the relevance of pH and resistance to inhibitory substances to pathogenicity. It is rapidly killed in acid urine, which is an important factor in preventing the extension of infection from the urethra to the bladder; it survives, however, in the relatively alkaline pH of prostatic secretions. It is also resistant to the inhibitory effect of spermine and zinc in these secretions.

The biochemical properties of an organism may determine the way in which the pathological process develops once it has gained access to the tissues of the urinary tract. For example, the ability of some organisms, in particular *Proteus* spp. and some staphylococci, to metabolize urea in the urine can result in deposition of struvite and carbonate-apatite as a friable matrix, in which living bacteria survive, in the renal substance [9]. This calcifies, often rapidly, forming an infection stone which may eventually fill the renal pelvis, the so-called staghorn calculus. The pathogenesis of prostatic calculi is probably similar.

Anything that affects the balance of organisms in commensal flora may determine that a harmless or beneficial organism assumes a pathogenic role. By selectively destroying some bacterial constituents of the bowel or urethral flora antibacterial agents may predispose to urinary tract infection. For example, broad-spectrum penicillins, by eradicating sensitive Gram-negative organisms in the bowel, enable resistant ones such as *Klebsiella* spp. or *Pseudomonas* spp. to invade the urinary tract. Furthermore, they destroy most of the commensal bacterial species in the urethra, thus removing their protective effect against invasion by bowel organisms. Other agents, in particular co-trimoxazole and the fluoroquinolones, although being less likely to select resistant Gram-negative bowel organisms, have a selective effect on the urethral flora. They kill most of the commensal bacteria with the important exception of the lactobacilli, which are intrinsically resistant to these agents [10]. They may multiply disproportionately and extend into the proximal urethra and paraurethral glands, causing inflammation and symptoms — the so-called urethral syndrome [11]. If trimethoprim is given without the sulphonamide component of co-trimoxazole, lactobacilli persist but so do many strains of *S. epidermidis*. This is relevant to infection with the latter organism which can occur in patients with indwelling catheters. The longer the course of antibiotic treatment the more likely it is that the balance of commensal flora will be affected. It follows, therefore, that treatment courses should be as short as is consistent with efficacy, that antibiotics should not be given to patients with inevitable bacteriuria (e.g. those with neuropathic bladders or long-term indwelling catheters) at times when they are well, and that when long-term low-dose prophylaxis is indicated an appropriate agent with a minimal effect on commensal flora should be used.

Figure. 41.1 summarizes the role of particular organisms as pathogens at different sites in and adjacent to the urinary tract.

E. coli

Overall this organism is the most frequent isolate from the urine of patients with urinary tract infection. It has its origin in the bowel, and the O serotypes isolated from the urine are those found to be present at the time in the bowel [12]. It is by far the most common pathogen found in patients outside hospital and those with a mechanically normal urinary tract. It also accounts for the majority, but a smaller percentage, of infections in hospitalized patients. The reasons for this, both mechanical and resulting from the use of antibiotics, have already been explained.

Proteus mirabilis

This is the most common species of *Proteus* isolated from urine. It accounts for fewer than 10% of infections in the general population, but the percentage rises in hospitalized or instrumented patients and in patients on antibiotics. The most important clinical connotation of infection with this organism is the formation of infection stones, and this possibility should always be considered in patients with persistent or recurrent *Proteus* infection.

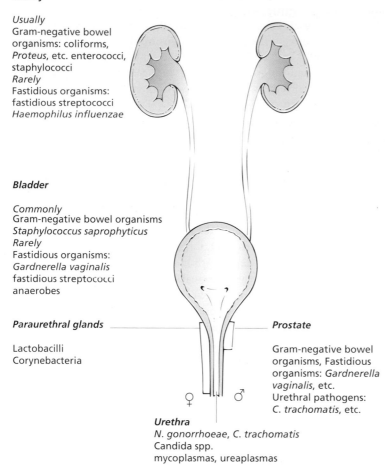

Kidney

Usually
Gram-negative bowel
organisms: coliforms,
Proteus, etc. enterococci,
staphylococci
Rarely
Fastidious organisms:
fastidious streptococci
Haemophilus influenzae

Bladder

Commonly
Gram-negative bowel organisms
Staphylococcus saprophyticus
Rarely
Fastidious organisms:
Gardnerella vaginalis
fastidious streptococci
anaerobes

Paraurethral glands

Lactobacilli
Corynebacteria

Prostate

Gram-negative bowel
organisms, Fastidious
organisms: *Gardnerella
vaginalis*, etc.
Urethral pathogens:
C. trachomatis, etc.

♀   ♂

Urethra
N. gonorrhoeae, C. trachomatis
Candida spp.
mycoplasmas, ureaplasmas

Fig. 41.1 Pathogens in the urinary tract
and its adjacent structures.

Other Gram-negative bowel organisms

These include *Klebsiella* spp., *Citrobacter* spp., *Pseudomonas* spp., species of *Proteus* other than *P. mirabilis*, *Morganella* spp. and *Providencia* spp. Together these organisms account for fewer than 5% of infections in the general population but the incidence rises in hospitalized patients, for the reasons already given. An additional problem can be contamination of urological instruments or infusion apparatus. Many of these bacterial species can survive for long periods on instruments or on the hands of attendants. Modern control of infection procedures should prevent such mishaps. Isolation of an unusual species such as *Pseudomonas cepacia* from urine or blood culture should always alert the microbiologist and clinician to the possibility of such nosocomial infection.

Staphylococci

Staphylococcus saprophyticus is the second most common urinary pathogen in young women. Infection with this organism is almost always confined to young, sexually active women; it occurs occasionally in older women and in children of both sexes [13]. It has been suggested that infection with this organism in a child may indicate sexual abuse [14]. The reservoir of this organism is unknown; there is some evidence that it colonizes the bowel and that such colonization may be related to the striking seasonal incidence of infection [13,15]. It causes acute infection with severe symptoms and the infection may involve the kidneys [16]. However, it is rarely associated with renal damage, possibly because it so seldom causes infection in childhood, when the likelihood of renal damage due to infection is greatest.

Staphylococcus epidermidis is a distal urethral commensal which causes infection in catheterized or instrumented patients or in those on broad-spectrum antibiotics. It can also be a secondary pathogen in patients with damaged urinary tracts. An explanation for infection with this organism should always be sought.

Staphylococcus aureus may infect the kidneys by the haematogenous route, causing multiple renal abscesses. It is also a very rare pathogen in damaged urinary tracts; an explanation for such infection should always be sought.

Many strains of staphylococci metabolize urea in urine and may, therefore, be associated with infection stone formation.

Enterococci

Both *Enterococcus faecalis* and *E. faecium* are bowel organisms which can be ascending urinary pathogens. They are seldom primary pathogens, occurring in hospitalized patients or those on antibiotics. *E. faecalis* has always accounted for a small proportion of urinary infections. The recent emergence of *E. faecium* is undoubtedly related to the use of broad-spectrum antibiotics. Unlike *E. faecalis*, it is intrinsically resistant to ampicillin, and the widespread use of vancomycin in hospital has led to development of resistance to that agent also [17]. This organism presents a new and serious problem. Patients may be severely ill and cross-infection is liable to occur.

Streptococci

Streptococcus agalactiae (Lancefield group B) is a well-recognized urinary pathogen. The reservoir is in the vagina, but the organism features in most studies of suprapubic aspiration of urine and it is clear that it can gain access to the bladder. When urine cultures are incubated in an atmosphere containing carbon dioxide (an atmosphere closer to that *in vivo* than air, which is customarily used) not only are more strains of *S. agalactiae* detected but other fastidious streptococci, such as *S. milleri* and *S. morbillorum*, can also be isolated [18]. The role of these organisms awaits further evaluation but there is anecdotal evidence that they have been isolated from the urine of some patients with damaged urinary tracts.

Corynebacteria

Non-diphtheria corynebacteria are now recognized as rare, but important, pathogens in the urinary tract. *Corynebacterium* group D2 is recognized as a secondary pathogen in the urine of patients with damaged urinary tracts and in those on broad-spectrum antibacterial therapy [19]. It is resistant to many of the commonly used agents. When appropriate culture techniques are applied to urine other, more sensitive, species of corynebacteria can be isolated. Such isolations include those from catheter specimens, those from patients with pyuria and some from patients with pathological conditions of the bladder or kidneys [20].

Fastidious organisms

This term is used to include those organisms that require culture or incubation techniques other than overnight incubation in air. Some are detected by 48 h incubation in an atmosphere containing carbon dioxide; some require special culture media.

Haemophilus spp.

Both *H. influenzae* and *H. parainfluenzae* are rare urinary pathogens in adults and children. They have been isolated from men with urinary symptoms [21] (possibly indicating an ability to invade the prostate) and from children with urinary tract abnormalities [22].

Gardnerella vaginalis

There is evidence that this vaginal organism can invade the urinary tract of both men and women. It has been isolated from ureteric urine [23] and from catheter urine and bladder biopsy specimens taken from patients with the chronic inflammatory changes of so-called interstitial cystitis [8].

Streptococcus pneumoniae, Aerococcus spp. and *Gemella haemolysans*

These organisms have occasionally been isolated from patients with suspected urinary tract infection.

Obligate anaerobes

Although anaerobic culture of urine is seldom undertaken nowadays, it is unlikely that such organisms could survive and multiply in the normal oxygen tension of urine. Anaerobic infection might occur in anoxic scar tissue or in the presence of large numbers of multiplying aerobes. The literature of the pre-antibiotic era, when severe urinary sepsis was common and anaerobic culture was undertaken, reported many such isolations [24].

Urethral pathogens

The pathogenicity of both *N. gonorrhoeae* and *Chlamydia trachomatis* in the urethra and its communicating tissues has already been discussed. Non-gonococcal urethritis is caused by *C. trachomatis* in about 30–50% of cases and by *Ureaplasma urealyticum* in a smaller percentage [25]. Because both these organisms can be isolated from symptom-free sexually active men and women, discussion as to their role continues. The search for other causative agents for urethritis and prostatitis has provided recent evidence that *Mycoplasma genitalium* may be one such pathogen. Studies have been hampered by the fact that some of these organisms are difficult to culture; the advent of the more sensitive method of polymerase chain reaction (PCR) has certainly provided evidence of the pathogenicity of *M. genitalium* [26]. The role of all these organisms in prostatic infection is still disputed. While Gram-negative bowel organisms (almost invariably *E. coli*) can be isolated from the urine of about one-third of men with the symptoms of prostatitis, organisms can only be isolated from the others if techniques capable of detecting the more fastidious species are employed. Determining the site of infection is bedevilled by the fact that prostatic infection arises by extension of pathogens from the urethra; the technique of transperineal biopsy [27] provides definite advantages over the three-glass technique (see below).

Lactobacillus spp.

There is evidence that these organisms can cause symptoms of urethral and paraurethral infection in a large number of women, in particular those who have been repeatedly treated with antibiotics [11]. The mechanism has already been explained. Evidence to the contrary can be explained either by the use of inappropriate controls [28] or of culture methods which do not detect the organism reliably [29]. The natural history of the association of urinary symptoms with this organism will not be elucidated until other careful long-term studies are undertaken. The fact that this has not been done is probably attributable to the reluctance of laboratories to accept that more complex procedures than those usually employed for urine culture are necessary. When conventional procedures are used, the symptoms of over 50% of the women who present to their doctors remain unexplained. Antibiotic treatment is usually prescribed and, far from improving, the situation often deteriorates.

Viruses and fungi

Viruria as a possible cause of urinary symptoms has already been discussed. There are few published data on the subject.

Candida spp., most often *C. albicans*, account for about 1% of urinary isolates in hospital practice. Fungal infection is always consequent upon treatment with broad-spectrum antibiotics and is most likely to occur in seriously ill or immunocompromised patients, those with damaged urinary tracts or indwelling urinary catheters. Colonization of the bladder urine occurs, and this may be followed by ascent of infection to the kidneys and invasion of the bloodstream.

Laboratory diagnosis of urinary tract infection

Because of the nature of the pathogenesis—the fact that most urinary pathogens are normal inhabitants of the commensal flora of adjacent areas—accurate laboratory diagnosis presents many problems. Methods of specimen collection and transport are of great importance. It is vital that the clinician should present the laboratory with adequate and relevant information and that the laboratory should apply the best possible techniques to the examination of the specimen. The laboratory findings should be interpreted in the light of the clinical information and presented to the clinician in a way that makes their meaning clear. At the present time many laboratories and clinicians fail on several of these counts. Urine specimens comprise at least 50% of the specimens submitted to laboratories and financial pressures on the latter are increasing. Requesting is often delegated to non-medical personnel, who may not provide the relevant information, and laboratory work and interpretation may be undertaken by junior staff who lack the necessary clinical knowledge. To state these problems is not to solve them.

Specimen collection and transport

Table 41.3 lists the various methods of collection of urine specimens from non-catheterized patients for the diagnosis of urinary tract infection. Different methods are appropriate for particular circumstances.

Suprapubic aspiration of urine from the bladder is the definitive method of diagnosis of bladder infection and is used, although not sufficiently widely, for collection of specimens from babies.

Ureteric catheterization is, at present, the only definitive method of confirming renal infection. It requires instrumentation under anaesthesia and is only appropriate, therefore, when there is a clear clinical need to confirm or exclude renal infection. One such situation might be the determination of a management protocol for a patient with renal calculi.

Careful aseptic bladder catheterization is the method of choice in patients with poor bladder control which makes midstream collection impossible or when contamination is very likely to occur. For these reasons it is often appropriate

Table 41.3 Methods of urine specimen collection.

Babies
 Suprapubic aspiration
 Clean catch specimen of urine
 Bag

Children
 Clean catch specimen of urine
 Midstream specimen of urine

Adults
 Midstream specimen of urine
 Three-glass test (before and after prostatic massage)

Elderly women
 Midstream specimen of urine
 Diagnostic catheter specimen of urine

for elderly women in hospital. The risk of introduction of organisms on the catheter is outweighed by the disadvantages of making a wrong diagnosis of infection. Any investigation necessitating bladder catheterization, such as cystoscopy or micturating cystourethrography, provides an opportunity for collection of a catheter specimen for culture. This can be particularly useful in young children.

Bags attached to the perineum are widely used for specimen collection from babies. Provided that the baby is kept in the upright position after application of the bag and that urine is drained immediately into a sterile container and refrigerated the findings may exclude infection. However, false-positive results are so common that this method should be discarded in favour of the clean catch specimen. The baby is held, by the mother or nurse, until it passes urine into a sterile dish, which is then decanted immediately into a laboratory container and refrigerated. This method can be used for children until they achieve the bladder control necessary for the use of the midstream method. There is evidence that after normal washing of the perineum there is little risk of contamination of the specimen in either sex [30,31].

The midstream specimen is used for the great majority of patients. The two important considerations for the correct use of this technique are that there should be sufficient urine in the bladder and that the patient should have good control of micturition. The problem of perineal contamination has often been overemphasized and it may be that it is only of real importance in patients with poor hygiene such as some elderly women. Urethral organisms may, in fact, be indicative of urethral infection; in the past they have often been dismissed as contaminants.

Catheter specimens can be collected from patients with indwelling catheters when there is a clinical indication for treatment.

Three consecutive early morning specimens of urine are required for the diagnosis of tuberculosis. Urine collected at the end of micturition is required for detection of the ova of *Schistosoma haematobium*.

Urine collected after prostatic massage—the three-glass test of Stamey [32]—has been used as a means of detecting prostatic infection. The results are not definitive and the test is not widely used in the UK. Transperineal biopsy [27] has advantages for this purpose but it remains a research tool at present.

All urine specimens should be refrigerated at 4°C immediately and transported to the laboratory as soon as possible. Refrigeration overnight, or even over a weekend, is still consistent with a meaningful culture result.

The addition of 1.8% boric acid to urine containers in order to prevent the multiplication of organisms between the collection and examination of specimens [33] has disadvantages. The concentration of boric acid may be excessive if the volume of urine passed is small, there is evidence that boric acid decreases the count of some bacterial species, and there is no evidence about its effect on fastidious organisms which are increasingly recognized as of importance.

Laboratory examination of urine

Detailed discussion of laboratory techniques would be out of place, but a summary of principles and current practice will enable clinicians to evaluate the service offered to them by the laboratory. Testing for protein has no place in the diagnosis of urinary tract infection. Many patients with bacteriuria do not have proteinuria.

Microscopy of urine for the presence of white blood cells should be undertaken using a method which gives a quantitative assessment of the white cell content of urine. For this reason examination of the centrifuged deposit is not appropriate. Cell counting in a haematological counting chamber is accurate, but time consuming. In recent years it has been superseded in many laboratories by the inverted microscope method [34].

Important considerations in urine culture are the medium or media used, the duration and atmosphere of incubation, the interpretation of the findings and the criteria for testing and reporting antibacterial sensitivities. While most of the aerobic bowel organisms are detected by commonly used primary isolation media incubated overnight in air, other more fastidious bacteria may require additional culture media, prolonged incubation or incubation in an atmosphere containing carbon dioxide. Such requirements have been outlined in the discussion of particular organisms above.

Counting of bacteria in urine has been firmly established in laboratories as a determinant of the presence or absence of urinary tract infection since Kass developed his criterion of significance [35]. The convenience of this practice— enabling inexperienced staff to report on and interpret urine cultures, often with no reference to the clinical circumstances — probably accounts for the fact that little attention has been paid to the large body of evidence supporting the significance of bacterial counts of fewer than 10^5/ml. This evidence has been reviewed [36] and has recently been revalidated in a large study of young women with acute urinary symptoms [37]. Also recently, bacteria have been demonstrated in low counts in bladder urine collected from babies by suprapubic aspiration, some of whom had urinary tract abnormalities [38]. High bacterial counts are the result of incubation of bacteria in bladder urine. They are not to be expected in other circumstances, for example in patients with intense frequency, patients excreting small numbers of bacteria from infection stones or patients with infection below the bladder (e.g. in the prostate, urethra or paraurethral glands). All these situations are clinically significant. It follows, therefore, that laboratories should use culture methods that detect low bacterial counts and should interpret their findings in the light of the clinical situation.

Dip-inoculation culture—the inoculation of a plastic spoon or slide coated with culture medium into a fresh midstream specimen before dispatch to the laboratory for incubation and interpretation—can be useful if there is unavoidable delay in specimens reaching the laboratory.

Antibacterial sensitivity testing

This should be undertaken on isolates deemed, in the light of the considerations outlined above, to be indicative of infection. The exceptions to this rule are isolates from patients with inevitable bacteriuria (e.g. those with indwelling catheters, neuropathic bladders or urinary diversions) at times when they are well and treatment is therefore contraindicated. The agents tested should be those appropriate for the treatment of urinary infection. In general, these should be cheap, orally administered agents, chosen in the light of the known sensitivities of urinary pathogens in the area. Other agents, including those given parenterally, should be tested and reported only for resistant organisms or for appropriate clinical situations. An important example of the latter is the testing of isolates from men against agents that penetrate prostatic tissue (co-trimoxazole, a tetracycline and, for resistant organisms, a quinolone). If the usefulness of antibiotics is to be maintained, clinicians should restrict the agents they prescribe to those reported by the laboratory.

Screening methods for detecting pyuria and bacteriuria

The increasing pressures on laboratories have already been referred to. While accurate microscopy and appropriate culture methods correctly interpreted remain the methods likely to yield the most information, they are time consuming and labour intensive. Laboratories are increasingly turning to the many automated methods and screening devices that are available [39].

Most widely used are the leucocyte esterase test for detecting the presence of white cells and the nitrite test for the detection of bacteriuria. Both these tests have been incorporated into dipsticks, which may also carry other tests, for example for the detection of proteinuria. Published reports of the sensitivity and specificity of these tests vary widely. Any test which depends upon bacterial metabolism such as nitrite production will, of course, only detect bacteria with this property. It is a major criticism of all such tests, and of a number of automated or semi-automated rapid screening tests for the detection of bacteriuria, that they have only been validated against conventional overnight aerobic culture, using the Kass criterion of significance. Many do not detect low-count bacteriuria and it has not been determined whether so-called false-positive tests are, in fact, indicative of this or of infection with fastidious organisms. The latter criticism also applies to detection of pyuria with apparently negative culture.

Nonetheless, such tests will continue to be widely used, at least to attempt to screen out negative specimens which do not require microscopy and culture. It is desirable, therefore, that improved tests should be developed and that they should be validated more thoroughly.

Antibody tests

These have been used to detect a serological response, with the object of distinguishing between upper and lower tract infection [40]. Attempts to detect a local immune response to infection in urine have given variable results [39].

Immunofluorescence test for *Chlamydia trachomatis*

Enzyme immunoassay of urine deposit has been shown to be almost as effective as a similar examination of a urethral swab for the detection of *C. trachomatis* [41,42]. It is used in some laboratories for the elucidation of apparently sterile pyuria.

References

1 Crowther P, Pead PJ, Pead L, Maskell R. Daytime urinary frequency in children. *Br Med J* 1988;**297**:855.
2 Reid G, McGroarty JA, Angotti R, Cook RL. Lactobacillus inhibitor production against *Escherichia coli* and coaggregation ability with uropathogens. *Can J Microbiol* 1988;**34**:344–51.
3 Chan RCY, Reid G, Irvin RT *et al.* Competitive exclusion of uropathogens from human uroepithelial cells by lactobacillus whole cells and cell wall fragments. *Infect Immun* 1985;**47**:84–9.
4 Kallenius G, Mollby R, Svenson SB, Winberg J, Hultberg H. Identification of a carbohydrate receptor recognised by uropathogenic *Escherichia coli*. *Infection* 1980;**8**(Suppl. 3):288–93.
5 Svanborg-Eden C, Eriksson B, Hanson LA *et al.* Adhesion to normal human uroepithelial cells of *Escherichia coli* from children with various forms of urinary tract infection. *J Pediatr* 1978;**93**:398–403.
6 Latham RH, Stamm WE. Role of fimbriated *Escherichia coli* in urinary tract infections in adult women: correlation with localisation studies. *J Infect Dis* 1984;**149**:835–40.
7 Majd M, Rushton G, Jantausch B, Wiedermann BL. Relationship among vesicoureteral reflux, P-fimbriated *Escherichia coli*, and acute pyelonephritis in children with febrile urinary tract infection. *J Pediatr* 1991;**119**:578–85.
8 Wilkins EGL, Payne SR, Pead PJ, Moss ST, Maskell R. Interstitial cystitis and urethral syndrome: a possible answer. *Br J Urol* 1989;**64**:39–44.
9 Nemoy NJ, Stamey TA. Surgical, bacteriological and bio-

chemical management of 'infection stones'. *Am J Med* 1971; **215**:1470–6.

10 Maskell R, Pead L. 4-fluoroquinolones and *Lactobacillus* spp. as emerging pathogens. *Lancet* 1992;**339**:929.

11 Maskell R, Pead L, Sanderson RA. Fastidious bacteria and the urethral syndrome: a 2-year clinical and bacteriological study of 51 women. *Lancet* 1983;**2**:1277–80.

12 Kennedy RP, Plorde JJ, Petersdorf RG. Studies on the epidemiology of *E. coli* infections. IV. Evidence for a nosocomial flora. *J Clin Invest* 1965;**44**:193–201.

13 Pead L, Maskell R, Morris J. *Staphylococcus saprophyticus* as a urinary pathogen. *Br Med J* 1985;**291**:1157–9.

14 Goldenring JM, Fried DC, Tames SM. *Staphylococcus saprophyticus* urinary tract infection in a sexually abused child. *Pediatr Infect Dis* 1988;**7**:73–4.

15 Hedman P, Ringertz O, Olsson K, Wollin R. Plasmid-identified *Staphylococcus saprophyticus* isolated from the rectum of patients with urinary tract infections. *Scand J Infect Dis* 1991;**23**:569–72.

16 Hedman P, Ringertz O. Urinary tract infections caused by *Staphylococcus saprophyticus*. A matched case control study. *J Infect* 1991;**23**:145–53.

17 Uttley AHC, George RC, Naidoo J *et al.* High level vancomycin resistant enterococci causing hospital infections. *Epidemiol Infect* 1989;**103**:173–81.

18 Collins LE, Clarke RW, Maskell R. Streptococci as urinary pathogens. *Lancet* 1986;**2**:479–81.

19 Soriano F, Fernandez-Roblas R. Infections caused by antibiotic-resistant *Corynebacterium* Group D2. *Eur J Clin Microbiol Infect Dis* 1988;**7**:337–41.

20 Maskell R, Pead L. Corynebacteria as urinary pathogens. *J Infect Dis* 1990;**162**:781–2.

21 Gabre-Kidan T, Lipsky BA, Plorde JJ. *Hemophilus influenzae* as a cause of urinary tract infections in men. *Arch Intern Med* 1984;**144**:1623–7.

22 Granoff DM Roskes S. Urinary tract infection due to *Hemophilus influenzae*. *J Pediatr* 1974;**84**:414–16.

23 Abercrombie GF, Allen J, Maskell R. *Corynebacterium vaginale* urinary tract infection in a young man. *Lancet* 1978; **1**:766.

24 Finegold SM, Miller LG, Merrill SL, Posnick DJ. Significance of anaerobic and capnophilic bacteria isolated from the urinary tract. In: Kass EH, ed. *Progress in Pyelonephritis*. Philadelphia: FA Davis, 1965:159–78.

25 Bowie WR. Urethritis in males. In: Holmes KK, Mardh P-A, Sparling PF, Wiesner PJ, eds. *Sexually Transmitted Diseases*, 2nd edn. New York: McGraw-Hill, 1989:627–39.

26 Horner PJ, Gilroy CB, Thomas BJ, Naidoo ROM, Taylor-Robinson D. Association of *Mycoplasma genitalium* with acute non-gonococcal urethritis. *Lancet* 1993;**342**:582–5.

27 Doble A, Furr PM, Walker MM, Harris JRW, Witherow RO'N, Taylor-Robinson D. A search for infectious agents in chronic abacterial prostatitis using ultrasound guided biopsy. *Br J Urol* 1989;**64**:297–301.

28 Brumfitt W, Hamilton-Miller JMT, Ludlam H, Gooding A. Lactobacilli do not cause frequency and dysuria syndrome. *Lancet* 1981;**2**:393–6.

29 O'Dowd TC, Ribeiro CD, Munro J, West RR, Howells CHL, Harvard Davis R. Urethral syndrome: a self limiting illness. *Br Med J* 1984;**1**:1349–52.

30 Saez-Llorens X, Umana MA, Odio CM, Lohr JA. Bacterial contamination rates for non-clean-catch and clean-catch midstream urine collections in uncircumcised boys. *J Pediatr* 1989;**114**:93–5.

31 Lohr JA, Donowitz LG, Dudley SM. Bacterial contamination rates in voided urine collections in girls. *J Pediatr* 1989; **114**:91–3.

32 Meares EM, Stamey TA. Bacteriological localization patterns in bacterial prostatitis and urethritis. *Invest Urol* 1968;**5**:492–518.

33 Porter IA, Brodie J. Boric acid preservation of urine samples. *Br Med J* 1969;**2**:353–5.

34 Maskell R. In: *Urinary Tract Infection*. London: Edward Arnold, 1982:24.

35 Kass EH. Bacteriuria and the diagnosis of infections of the urinary tract. *Arch Intern Med* 1957;**100**:709–13.

36 Maskell R. A new look at the diagnosis of infection of the urinary tract and its adjacent structures. *J Infect* 1989;**19**: 207–17.

37 Kunin CM, VanArsdale White L, Hua Hua T. A reassessment of the importance of 'low-count' bacteriuria in young women with acute urinary symptoms. *Ann Intern Med* 1993;**119**: 454–60.

38 Buys H, Pead L, Hallett R, Maskell R. Suprapubic aspiration of urine in children: a one year study. *Br Med J* 1994;**308**:690–2.

39 Morgan MG, McKenzie H. Controversies in the laboratory diagnosis of community-acquired urinary tract infection. *Eur J Microbiol Infect Dis* 1993;**12**:491–504.

40 Hajlem E, Schwan A, Lundell-Etherden I, Sandberg T. Antibody responses to *Staphylococcus saprophyticus* in urinary tract infection. *Scand J Infect Dis* 1990;**22**:557–60.

41 Caul EO, Paul ID, Milne JD, Crowley T. Non-invasive method for detecting *Chlamydia trachomatis*. *Lancet* 1988;**2**:1246–7.

42 Hay PE, Thomas BJ, Gilchrist C, Palmer HM, Gilroy CB, Taylor Robinson D. The value of urine samples from men with non-gonococcal urethritis for the detection of *Chlamydia trachomatis*. *Genitourin Med* 1991;**67**:124–8.

42   Pathology of Urinary Tract Infections
A. Mansoor and D. A. Levison

Kidney

Pyelonephritis

Pyelonephritis is a bacterial-induced inflammation of the renal pelvis, the calyces and renal parenchyma. It occurs in acute and chronic forms and affects one or both kidneys, usually in an irregular patchy fashion.

Acute pyelonephritis

In this condition there is acute suppurative inflammation of the pelvis, calyces and parts of the kidneys. Characteristically, the suppuration takes the form of pale linear streaks bordered by a red rim of congestion, extending radially from the tips of the papillae to the surface of the cortex (Fig. 42.1). In more advanced cases, adjacent lesions fuse to produce extensive abscesses. Even in the absence of obvious extensive suppuration, the renal parenchyma usually feels softer than normal. Obstruction to outflow can result in pyonephrosis where suppurative exudate fills the renal pelvis and calyces. Uncommonly, a perinephric abscess is formed between the renal capsule and Gerota fascia by extension of the suppurative inflammation. Microscopically the appearances are those of a typical acute inflammation involving the pelvis, the calyces and the kidney. Within the kidney there is extensive but focal tubular destruction with the tubules being replaced by areas of suppuration (Fig. 42.2). In the cortex there is striking sparing of glomeruli and large blood vessels despite the fact that these may be seen to be surrounded by intense acute interstitial inflammation. These microscopic changes tend to be more florid and more extensive, particularly if there is obstruction in the lower urinary tract. In cases with lower urinary tract obstruction and in cases of very severe inflammation in the absence of urinary obstruction, particularly if the patient is diabetic, renal papillary necrosis may occur (Fig. 42.3). In this condition the renal papillae appear macroscopically dull yellow in

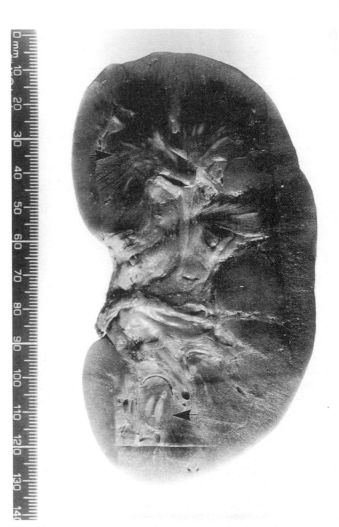

Fig. 42.1 Acute suppurative pyelonephritis. The upper and lower poles show linear streaks of suppuration in the medulla (arrow).

colour and are sharply demarcated from the viable parenchyma by a zone of congestion. Microscopically the necrotic papillae show the appearances of coagulative necrosis/bland infarction.

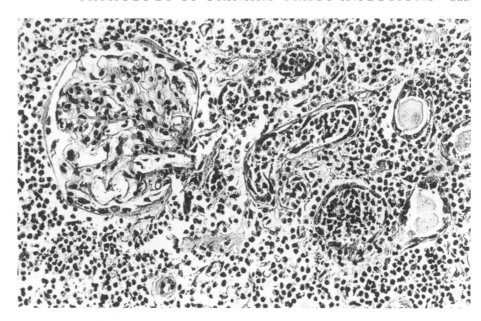

Fig 42.2 Acute suppurative pyelonephritis. Acute inflammatory infiltrate is present in the interstitium and disintegrating tubules with remarkable sparing of the glomerulus.

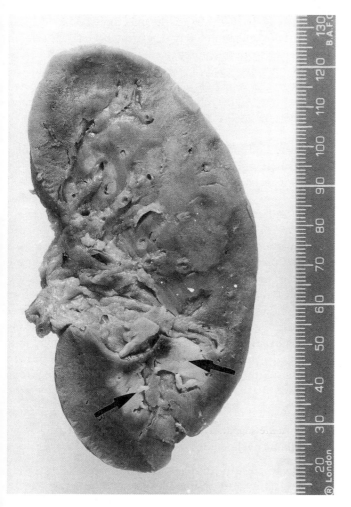

Fig. 42.3 Renal papillary necrosis. The necrotic papillae are more obvious in the lower pole (arrows).

Chronic pyelonephritis

Chronic pyelonephritis can be divided into two broad groups according to the underlying aetiology. In obstructive chronic pyelonephritis there is some form of urinary tract obstruction giving rise to recurrent infection and renal scarring. Reflux nephropathy or non-obstructive chronic pyelonephritis, on the other hand, is a relatively uncommon condition and is associated with underlying vesicoureteric and intrarenal reflux [1].

Renal scarring due to chronic pyelonephritis shows a number of distinctive macroscopic features. In contrast to the scarring of chronic glomerulonephritis or essential hypertension, the scars of chronic pyelonephritis are patchy and more irregular in size and the kidneys are unequally affected, one kidney often being very much more shrunken than the other. Diagnostically the most useful macroscopic feature of a chronic pyelonephritic scar is its close relationship to a deformed calyx (Fig. 42.4). Scarring of the pyramids always results in calyceal distortion and dilatation. Pyelonephritic scars are common in the upper and lower poles of the kidney, which are the usual sites of intrarenal reflux. The walls of the pelvis and calyces are usually thickened and granular. In the parenchyma, between the scarred areas, surviving kidney may appear normal or show changes of hypertension. The scarred areas themselves can be recognized as areas of thinning (involving cortex and medulla), with overlying surface depressions which are said to be shallower than those produced by ischaemia, but may actually be very similar. Chronic pyelonephritic kidneys are reduced in size.

Microscopically, provided the inflammation is not burnt out, the mucosa of the pelvis and calyces is thickened by granulation tissue and infiltrated by lymphocytes, plasma

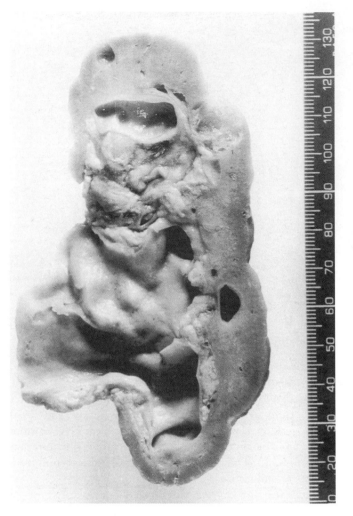

Fig. 42.4 Chronic pyelonephritis showing irregularly dilated and clubbed calyces with thinning of the overlying renal parenchyma. The renal pelvis is thickened and dilated.

cells and neutrophil polymorphs. In some cases, lymphoid follicles are prominent and contribute to the granularity of the surface (Fig. 42.5). In cases with florid inflammation, the surface epithelium may be lost and the pelvis and calyces lined by granulation tissue. In burnt out cases, one sees only scattered chronic inflammatory cells in the mucosa with fibrous thickening of the lamina propria. Sections of the scarred areas show very striking loss of tubules with corresponding interstitial fibrosis and variable patchy chronic interstitial inflammation (Fig. 42.6). Atrophic tubules often show marked thickening of their basement membranes. Sequestered portions of renal tubules often become dilated by inspissated colloid-like material, presenting an appearance resembling superficially that of thyroid tissue. Glomeruli are often remarkably well preserved. A proportion of the glomeruli, however, show ischaemic changes—initially partial collapse with wrink-

ling of the basement membranes and eventually complete collapse and hyalinization with obliteration of the enlarged Bowman's space by collagen. Periglomerular fibrosis (i.e. fibrosis developing outside the Bowman's membrane) is another feature most commonly seen in chronic pyelonephritis. Some patients, especially those with reflux nephropathy, develop a progressive renal disease with proteinuria, even in the nephrotic range. This is associated with a glomerular lesion, focal segmental glomerulosclerosis, which carries a poor prognosis [2,3]. The arteries show variable degrees of medial and intimal fibrous thickening—arteriosclerosis. Arterioles show variable hyaline thickening of their walls and luminal narrowing—arteriolosclerosis.

Xanthogranulomatous pyelonephritis

This is a well recognized but relatively uncommon variant of chronic pyelonephritis [4]. It is usually associated with *Escherichia coli* or *Proteus* infection and is thought to result from an inability of the macrophages to dispose efficiently of and completely digest the bacteria. It seldom occurs apart from the presence of stones in the renal pelvis. Macroscopically focal, often extensive, areas of the parenchyma are converted into fairly well-demarcated zones with a bright yellow colour (Fig. 42.7). Microscopically these areas are found to be populated by masses of distended macrophages, some of which have a clear cytoplasm and others of which have a more granular cytoplasm (Fig. 42.8). The granules, composed of indigestible bacterial debris, are periodic acid Schiff (PAS) positive, and diastase resistant. There are usually other chronic inflammatory cells, i.e. plasma cells and lymphocytes, mingled with these macrophages. This lesion can be mistaken by the inexperienced histopathologist as a clear cell carcinoma but the absence of glycogen in these clear cells, the lack of vascularity of the lesion, the lack of cytological atypia and the presence of abundant other chronic inflammatory cells should guide one to the correct histopathological diagnosis of xanthogranulomatous pyelonephritis. The kidney in this condition is not infrequently enlarged rather than shrunken. In contrast to standard chronic pyelonephritis, xanthogranulomatous inflammation can sometimes extend to involve the perinephric fat.

Tuberculous pyelonephritis

This always results from blood-borne spread of tubercle bacilli, usually from pulmonary lesions. Miliary tuberculosis can affect the kidneys and, as with other organs, these are studded with minute tubercles. In our experience, miliary tuberculosis tends to relatively spare the kidneys. Diffuse interstitial renal tuberculosis is a more recently

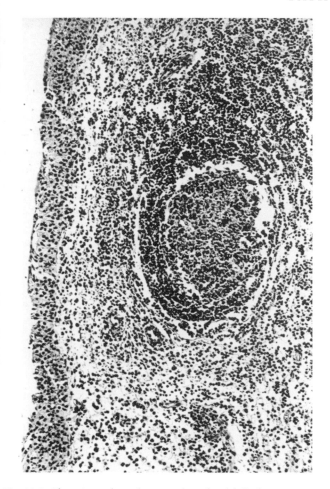

Fig. 42.5 Chronic pyelonephritis. A lymphoid follicle is present in the heavily inflamed lamina propria of the renal pelvis.

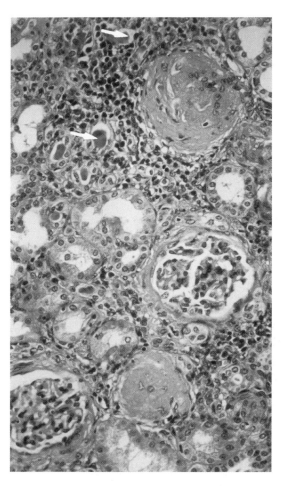

Fig. 42.6 Chronic pyelonephritis. There are atrophic tubules some with homogeneous casts (arrows) and interstitial inflammatory cell infiltration. The glomeruli show fibrous obliteration and periglomerular fibrosis.

described unusual cause of renal failure [5]. Of more importance numerically are the localized renal lesions of tuberculous pyelonephritis which may slowly extend to destroy the kidney (Fig. 42.9). This form of tuberculosis is thought to originate from small tubercles in the cortex which enlarge, caseate and coalesce and thus form an enlarging patch of caseation. These lesions often reach several centimetres in diameter, reach the renal pelvis and may discharge their contents, leaving a ragged cavity. Spread from tubercles which subsequently form in the wall of the renal pelvis occurs into the rest of the kidney and so the whole kidney can become involved. The ureter or renal pelvis may become obstructed by tuberculous lesions in their walls or by plugging with caseous material (Fig. 42.9). In this circumstance all the urine comes from the other kidney and it may well show no evidence of tuberculous infection. Tuberculous involvement of the renal pelvis often results in haematuria. The renal lesions also tend to suppurate giving rise to pyuria.

Microscopically a typical tuberculous lesion, in the kidney as elsewhere, has a caseous centre, surrounded by a mantle of epithelioid cells mixed with variable numbers of giant cells of the Langhans type (Fig. 42.10). Outside this there is a variable population of lymphocytes and fibrosis. In miliary tuberculosis some, at least, of the small granulomas may not show caseation. In the rare diffuse interstitial tuberculosis, the microscopic appearances are similar to those of miliary tuberculosis, but the lesions are widespread in the kidneys, the patient does not have other stigmas of miliary tuberculosis and presents with renal impairment.

Cytomegalovirus disease

This disease is best known in newborn infants and occurs either as a localized or generalized condition. It also occurs as an opportunistic infection at all ages in patients with various forms of congenital or acquired immunodeficiency.

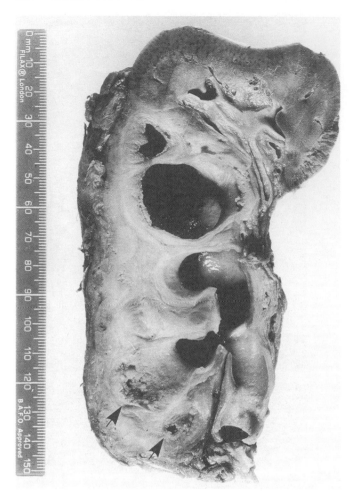

Fig. 42.7 Xanthogranulomatous pyelonephritis. Most of the renal parenchyma, except the upper pole, show fibrosis, loss of papillae and expanded calyces, some of which are lined by granular pale material (arrows).

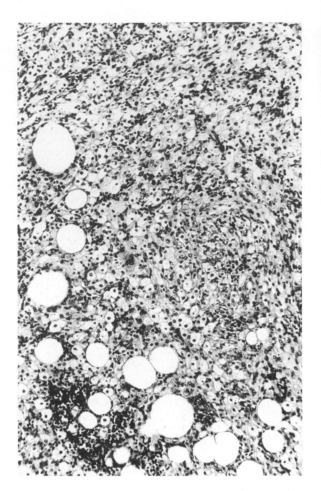

Fig. 42.8 Xanthogranulomatous pyelonephritis. There are sheets of foamy histiocytes with occasional multinucleated giant cells and other chronic inflammatory cells in the interstitium.

It is most commonly seen nowadays in patients on immunosuppressive drugs. Serological evidence of infection has been reported in over 50% of renal transplant patients. Colonized cells become greatly enlarged and show nuclear or sometimes cytoplasmic inclusions. Infection of the renal tubular cells does not appear to have much effect on renal tubular function.

Lower urinary tract

Cystitis

The term cystitis means simply inflammation of the urinary bladder. A variety of descriptive terms are applied to the macroscopic appearances, i.e. catarrhal, purulent and pseudomembranous. The latter is usually seen in association with chronic obstruction and hypertrophy of

the bladder. The pseudomembrane is composed of an admixture of fibrinous exudate and necrotic mucosa. The depth of necrosis is variable, usually being most pronounced over muscular ridges. Shreds of necrotic mucosa may be shed and passed in the urine. Such changes are usually observed when there is alkaline decomposition in the urine. In association with these changes there are often haemorrhages into the mucosa and these may become greenish or blackish. Microscopically the appearances are those of either acute or chronic inflammation confined usually to the mucosa. The proportions of various inflammatory cells vary from case to case but there is almost always an admixture of plasma cells and lymphocytes.

Mild catarrhal inflammation of the bladder can result from infection by typhoid bacilli. The bacilli may persist indefinitely in the urinary tract, the patient becoming a urinary carrier. Almost any anatomical abnormality in the urinary tract can predispose to the establishment of the carrier state. In some cases of coliform infection there is

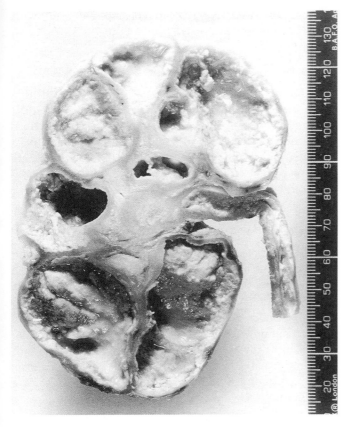

Fig. 42.9 Renal tuberculosis. Most of this kidney is replaced by large areas of caseation. The ureter is also lined by caseous material.

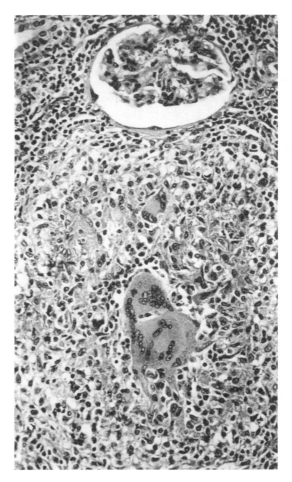

Fig. 42.10 Tuberculosis. There is an epithelioid cell granulomatous lesion with Langhans type giant cells. Caseous necrosis is not obvious in this histological section.

only a very mild inflammatory catarrhal reaction. Cystitis is occasionally a feature of gonorrhoea and here the inflammation is purulent in character.

Malacoplakia

This is a relatively rare variant of chronic cystitis and is characterized by the formation of numerous soft rounded plaques in the bladder wall [4]. These vary in size from 1 to 2 cm and have a pale, sometimes yellowish, appearance surrounded by a zone of congestion. The surface of these plaques often becomes ulcerated and invaded by bacteria. Microscopically the plaques are seen to be composed of cellular granulation tissue in which there are numerous large cells containing granules of various kinds and characteristic hyaline spheres with concentric markings known as Michaelis–Gutmann bodies. These inclusions usually stain positively for iron, positive with PAS, and also contain calcium salts. They are thought to be derived from breaking down bacteria. Lymphocytes and plasma cells are also always present in the lesion. Although its exact pathogenesis is not known, it is thought that the condition develops as the result of an inability of macrophages to dispose of the bacteria completely—as in xanthogranu-

lomatous pyelonephritis (see above). Malacoplakia less often involves other genitourinary sites such as the renal pelvis and parenchyma, ureter, prostate, testis and epididymis, broad ligament and endometrium. Even rarer is involvement of the colon, stomach, appendix, lymph nodes, brain, lungs, bones, skin and adrenals.

Tuberculosis

Tuberculosis in the bladder is relatively rare and is usually the result of spread of infection via the ureters from renal tuberculosis. Bacilli invade the mucosa and produce tubercles which coalesce and ulcerate. The base of the bladder, in particular, and sometimes the orifices of the ureters are involved. Sometimes the ulcers become large and the lining of the bladder considerably thickened.

Schistosomiasis

It is the Egyptian form of the disease due to *Schistosoma*

haematobium that involves the bladder. The adult parasites lie in the veins of the bladder and the eggs laid by the female pass into the surrounding tissues. Their presence stimulates the development of vascular granulation tissue which causes great thickening of the mucosa and submucosa. In some cases there are large numbers of eosinophil polymorphs in the inflammatory infiltrate. Multiple small nodules can often be seen on the mucosal surface and ulcers form fairly frequently. Pyogenic infections may be superadded and squamous carcinoma develops in a proportion of cases in Egyptians but has rarely been reported in infected Europeans. Schistosomal lesions also sometimes occur in the ureters and renal pelvis.

Unusual variants or sequelae of cystitis

Cystitis cystica and cystitis glandularis

A peculiar sequel of a few cases of chronic cystitis is the development of multiple small cysts containing clear fluid projecting from the mucosa into the lumen of the bladder. In cystitis cystica, foci of transitional epithelium become sequestrated deep to the surface and develop central cystic areas as a result of accumulation of mucin. Intestinal metaplasia can be seen in the epithelial cells lining these cysts, producing cystitis glandularis [6]. Identical changes are seen occasionally in the ureters and renal pelvis, where the terms ureteritis cystica and pyelitis cystica, respectively, are employed.

Interstitial (Hunner) cystitis

Classically the patient is female, the history of severe suprapubic pain, urinary frequency and haematuria, all unresponsive to medical therapy [7]. Ulcerated lesions develop anywhere in the bladder. Microscopically there are no pathognomonic features [8]. The ulcers are lined by fibrin and necrotic mucosa. The underlying tissue, including the muscle coat, shows oedema and non-specific chronic inflammation with numerous mast cells and fibrosis. The cause is not known but there is some evidence that suggests an autoimmune aetiology [9,10].

Eosinophilic cystitis

This is sometimes seen in women and children in association with allergic disorders and eosinophilia. Alternatively, it is seen in older men and is usually associated with bladder injury related to other conditions of the bladder or prostate [11].

Clinically it presents with severe and recurrent episodes of dysuria and haematuria. Cystoscopically the mucosa is diffusely oedematous and erythematous with broad-based polypoid swellings. Microscopically there is a dense inflammatory infiltrate rich in eosinophils, often with fibrosis and muscle necrosis.

Nephrogenic adenoma

This bladder lesion used to be regarded as a benign neoplasm. It is now thought most likely to represent a localized or diffuse metaplastic response of the urothelium to chronic inflammation. It is sometimes seen in combination with cystitis cystica. Histologically this lesion is composed of tubular structures lined by cuboidal cells, rather reminiscent of renal tubules.

Inverted papilloma

This lesion is a benign epithelial neoplasm. It shows no relationship to bladder carcinoma, but occasionally these two lesions may coexist. It is most commonly seen in adult and elderly males and is almost always located in the trigone, bladder neck or prostatic urethra. It is usually solitary and presents with haematuria and/or obstruction. Cystoscopy shows a polypoid lesion, with smooth contours, usually pedunculated. Microscopically there is invagination of epithelium beneath the normal surface urothelium, giving rise to trabeculae and anastomosing cords of bland transitional cells. However, sometimes they show multiple glandular formations resembling cystitis cystica and cystitis glandularis. This type probably arises on the basis of chronic proliferative cystitis [12]. Simple excision is adequate treatment.

Non-neoplastic polyps

Simple fibroepithelial polyps occur in relation to chronic inflammation in the bladder and ureter. In the bladder they can grow to a large size and are said to be particularly associated with schistosomiasis. In the ureter they are seen most often in the upper third, in the second and third decades of life, and are sometimes multiple. They have fibrovascular cores and are lined by normally looking transitional cell epithelium. Sometimes the core contains chronic inflammatory cells and some smooth muscle fibres continuous with the muscle fibres in the wall. In the ureter they may become ulcerated due to ischaemia, may cause obstruction or rarely intussusception of the ureter.

Polypoid cystitis is the name given to a lesion which sometimes complicates the presence of a catheter. It takes the form of polypoid swelling, oedema and redness of the posterior wall. Microscopically stromal oedema and congestion are the main features. Inflammation is minimal, and epithelial atypia is absent.

Urethritis

Bacteriological and other aspects of this condition are dealt with elsewhere. Pathologically, acute, subacute and chronic forms occur. Microscopically one sees correspondingly an acute or a chronic inflammatory infiltrate or an admixture of acute and chronic inflammation.

Prostatitis

Acute inflammation of the prostate usually results from spread of organisms from the urethra either in gonorrhoea or septic cystitis. Gonococcal prostatitis may pass into a chronic state in which the organisms persist for a long time in the tubules, the secretion of which remains infective. In prostatitis complicating septic cystitis, the inflammation of the prostate often proceeds to multiple foci of suppuration or the development of a large abscess, in which case the prostate may be extensively destroyed. Chronic persistent infection may also result. E. coli is the usual causative organism but other bacteria which commonly infect the urinary tract may be responsible.

In chronic prostatitis the prostate becomes diffusely scarred and shrunken. This may result in urethral obstruction and acute or chronic urinary retention. A variety of granulomatous lesions have been described in the prostate [13]. The most common diagnosis is non-specific granulomatous prostatitis where large aggregates of histiocytes, lymphocytes and plasma cells are seen around damaged and distorted prostatic ducts. Occasionally, a prominent eosinophilic infiltrate can also be present. Post-transurethral resection granulomatous prostatitis represents a reaction to altered epithelium and collagen due to surgical trauma. Histologically, there is a central area of fibrinoid necrosis surrounded by palisading epithelioid histiocytes. These lesions have to be distinguished from tuberculous prostatitis which results from spread of tubercle bacilli from the urinary bladder or epididymis and is characterized by caseous necrosis and the presence of acid alcohol-fast bacilli. Very rarely, patients with some systemic allergic disorder and eosinophilia can develop eosinophilic or allergic granulomatous prostatitis.

Acknowledgements

We wish to thank the Gordon Museum, Guy's Hospital, London, for the macroscopic pictures, the Department of Medical Illustration and Mr Asit Das, St Thomas' Hospital, London, for printing the microscopic pictures and Miss Marilyn Murphy who typed the manuscript.

References

1 Symmers WStC. In: KA Porter, RCB Pugh, ID Ansell, series eds *Systemic Pathology*, Vol. 8, 3rd edn. *The Kidney/The Urinary Tract*. London: Churchill Livingstone, 1992.

2 Cotran RS. Glomerulosclerosis in reflux nephropathy. *Kidney Int* 1982;**21**:528–34.

3 Torres VE, Velosa JA, Holley KE, Kelalis PP, Stickler GB, Kurtz SB. The progression of vesicoureteral reflux nephropathy. *Ann Intern Med* 1980;**92**: 776–84.

4 Heptinstall RH. *Pathology of the Kidney*, Vol. 3, 4th edn. Boston: Little, Brown, 1992.

5 Mallinson WJM, Fuller RW, Levison DA, Baker LRI, Cattell WR. Diffuse interstitial renal tuberculosis—an unusual cause of renal failure. *Q J Med* 1981;**50**:137–48.

6 Rosai J. *Ackerman's Surgical Pathology*, Vol. 1, 7th edn. St Louis: CV Mosby, 1989.

7 Pool TL. Interstitial cystitis. Clinical aspects and treatment. *Med Clin North Am* 1944;**28**:1008–15.

8 Lynes WL, Flynn SD, Shortliffe LD, Stamey TA. The histology of interstitial cystitis. *Am J Surg Pathol* 1990;**14**(10):969–76.

9 Holm-Bentzen M, Lose G. Pathology and pathogenesis of interstitial cystitis. *Urology* 1987;**29**(Suppl.):8–13.

10 Rosin RD, Griffiths T, Sofras F, James DCO, Edwards L. Interstitial cystitis. *Br J Urol* 1979;**51**:524–7.

11 Hellstrom HR, David BK, Shonnard JW. Eosinophilic cystitis. A study of 16 cases. *Am J Clin Pathol* 1979;**72**:777–84.

12 Kunze E, Schauer A, Schmitt M. Histology and histogenesis of two different types of inverted urothelial papillomas. *Cancer* 1983;**51**:348–58.

13 Epstein JI, Hutchins GM. Granulomatous prostatitis: distinction among allergic, non-specific, and posttransurethral resection lesions. *Human Pathol* 1984;**15**:818–25.

43 Principles of Management of Urinary Tract Infections

W.R.Cattell

Introduction

Urinary tract infection (UTI) is a common, distressing and sometimes life-threatening condition. Fortunately, the 30 years up to 1984 saw major advances in our understanding of the pathogenesis and natural history of the condition and this, plus the advent of many effective antibacterial agents, made it possible to define successful management policies in the majority of patients. In the 10 years since this text was last written significant new information has been added in terms of pathogenesis, natural history, diagnostic criteria and treatment schedules. As previously, therapeutic success requires accurate diagnosis and a clear understanding of the nature of the problem, its significance and factors governing the successful and safe use of antibacterial drugs.

Mode of presentation

Patients with UTI may present with symptoms, or be asymptomatic and diagnosed on the culture of a routine midstream specimen of urine (MSU). Symptomatic patients may have 'typical' or 'atypical' symptoms (Table 43.1). Patients should not be labelled asymptomatic without close questioning for symptoms resulting from infection such as nocturia, vague malaise or intermittent fever. These may be dismissed by the patient, yet effective treatment in such patients regularly improves their quality of life.

Table 43.1 Clinical (symptomatic) presentation of urinary tract infections.

Typical symptoms	Atypical symptoms
Frequency and/or dysuria	Abdominal or loin pain
±	Fever or rigors
Suprapubic or loin pain	Retention or incontinence
Fever or rigors	Haematuria
'Smelly' urine	*without*
Haematuria	Frequency and/or dysuria

The most common symptoms are dysuria and/or frequency. These symptoms must not, however, be considered synonymous with UTI, since several studies throughout the world have clearly shown that among women presenting with these symptoms, a significant number do not have bacteriuria as previously defined [1,2]. A confident diagnosis can only be made on the result of urine culture. In patients with a single isolated episode of uncomplicated frequency/dysuria, the question as to whether or not there is bacteriuria is of little long-term significance. In patients with recurrent or persisting symptoms, whether typical or atypical, establishing the diagnosis by urine culture is essential for successful management.

Longitudinal studies of patients with recurrent or persisting frequency/dysuria have shown that they fall into three major groups: (1) those who, whenever symptomatic, are bacteriuric; (2) those who, despite repeated, correctly timed urine cultures, are always abacteriuric; and (3) those who, when symptomatic are sometimes bacteriuric and sometimes not [3] (Fig. 43.1). Groups 1 and 3 may be considered as one population who get recurrent infection and respond to measures to control this. Group 2 belong to that group of patients who have abacteriuric frequency/dysuria. It cannot be overemphasized that this group can only be identified with careful longitudinal study with frequent urine cultures, whether of MSU or suprapubic aspiration (SPA) samples, at the onset of symptoms. Regrettably, few published studies of recurrent frequency/dysuria have recognized this requirement.

Cystitis and pyelonephritis

It is not possible on the basis of symptoms to distinguish confidently those patients who have infection confined to the bladder (cystitis) as opposed to those with extension of infection to the upper urinary tract (pyelonephritis). Thus, while in general high fever, loin pain and tenderness are associated with upper tract involvement, localization studies have shown a poor correlation between symptoms

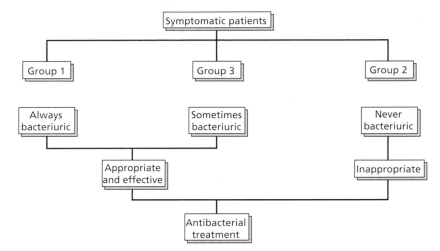

Fig. 43.1 Recurrent frequency/dysuria.

and the site of infection [4]. Nevertheless, bacteriuric patients with fever, loin pain and tenderness should be deemed to have pyelonephritis. In the previous edition of this textbook it was suggested that a distinction between patients with infection confined to the bladder as opposed to those with pyelonephritis had little merit. This view must be revised both in terms of management and long-term sequelae. Thus, there is now a consensus that patients presenting with acute clinical pyelonephritis should have renal imaging performed 6–8 weeks after successful treatment to exclude upper tract abnormalities predisposing to or complicating upper tract infection. Potentially more important is the recognition in recent years that acute pyelonephritis may be followed by the development of renal scars, even in patients with functionally and anatomically normal urinary tracts (see below) [5].

Diagnosis

By definition, UTI means the establishment and multiplication of organisms within the urinary tract. For practical purposes this means the presence of bacteria within bladder urine. Conversely, the continuing failure to demonstrate bladder bacteriuria excludes a diagnosis of UTI with a few exceptions. These include obstructed pyonephrosis when there is no communication between the obstructed segment and the remainder of the urinary tract, chronic bacterial prostatitis and abscess of the kidney. The belief that bacteria can 'hide' within the urinary tract for prolonged periods without bacteriuria is no longer acceptable, urine having a strong tendency to sustain bacterial growth.

Bladder bacteriuria

In the past 10 years the criteria upon which 'significant bacteriuria' is diagnosed have changed. Since the pioneering work of Kass [6] evidence for significant bacteriuria has been based on the demonstration of 100 000 or more ($\geqslant 10^5$) of the same organism per millilitre of urine. This blanket criterion is now recognized to be unacceptable especially in symptomatic young women and in men. A bacterial count of more than 10^5 of the same organism per millilitre of urine remains the benchmark for the diagnosis of bladder bacteriuria in *asymptomatic* patients. This level of bacteriuria has an accuracy of 80% on a single sample, increasing to more than 95% when demonstrated on two consecutive urine samples. Many women with symptomatic infection will also have bacterial counts of this order, but for many years there have been doubts regarding young women presenting with frequency dysuria. Several studies [1,2] indicated that less than 50% of these women have bacterial counts of 10^5 or more bacteria in their urine. It is now accepted that lower counts of coliform bacteria (100–1000/ml) associated with pyuria indicate bladder bacteriuria [7]. Even lower counts may be significant but require the demonstration of bladder bacteriuria in a sample obtained by SPA for confirmation. In males, bacterial counts of 10^3 or more of the same organism are now accepted as evidence of significant bacteriuria [8]. These modified criteria for the diagnosis of bladder bacteriuria are set out in Table 43.2.

'Low-count' bladder bacteriuria

A factor leading to 'low-count' bacteriuria may be the rate of urine flow and the frequency and completeness of bladder emptying [9]. A high rate of urine flow and frequent, complete bladder voiding may dramatically reduce bacterial counts [10] (Fig. 43.2). It follows that patients with symptoms of UTI who spontaneously embark on a high fluid intake may achieve a degree of bladder bacterial 'washout' such that MSUs on culture may yield bacterial counts less than 10^5/ml. It is essential that clinicians be aware of this. In symptomatic or high-risk

Table 43.2 Significant bacteriuria criteria in different groups.

Symptomatic women	10^2 or more *Escherichia coli*/ml of urine plus ≥ 8 pus cells/mm^3
	or
	$\geq 10^5$ of the same pathogenic organism/ml urine
	or
	Any organisms in SPA urine
Symptomatic men	$\geq 10^3$ pathogenic organism/ml urine
Asymptomatic patients	$\geq 10^5$ of the same organism in two consecutive MSUs

MSU, midstream specimen of urine; SPA, suprapubic aspiration.

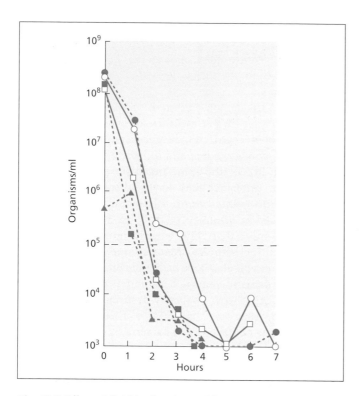

Fig. 43.2 Effect of fluid loading (300 ml/h) and hourly micturition on bacterial counts in urine. (Reproduced with permission from [10].)

asymptomatic patients with low bacterial counts it is essential to obtain MSUs when the patient first wakes in the morning when the washout effect is minimal, or to obtain urine by SPA before confidently excluding bladder bacteriuria.

Suprapubic aspiration

SPA of urine [11] is the acid test as to whether there is bladder bacteriuria or not. Normal bladder urine is sterile. Any growth of bacteria (save skin commensals) from urine obtained by SPA indicates bladder bacteriuria. Quantitative culture to establish significance is unnecessary. Whenever there is doubt, it is worth culturing urine obtained by SPA.

Mixed growth bacteria

A common point of confusion arises when the laboratory reports a mixed growth of bacteria with low counts of separate organisms. Most often this represents contamination of the sample during collection—a conclusion supported by the finding of large numbers of squamous epithelial cells on microscopy of the urine. However, in certain circumstances genuine bladder bacteriuria may be associated with low counts in the bladder urine and it is then no longer possible to distinguish between simple contamination versus contamination of a sample in which there is true 'low-count' bladder bacteriuria. Occasionally, urine samples are shown to contain mixed organisms in high counts. This may result from careless handling of urine samples after collection with post-voiding multiplication of organisms entering the sample via contamination. On occasion, there may truly be infection of the bladder with multiple organisms as, for example, with vesicocolic fistulas or neurogenic bladders. It cannot be overemphasized that careful attention to the collection of clean catch MSUs with careful instruction of the patient is essential if a clear diagnosis is to be obtained and waste of laboratory time and money is to be avoided.

Transient bacteriuria

The normal bladder has a considerable potential for spontaneous bacterial clearance, especially with high urine flow rates. It is probable that many women who develop typical symptoms and embark on a high fluid intake can effect fairly rapid bacterial clearance [12]. If the collection of an MSU in these women is delayed, significant bacteriuria may be missed. To diagnose the cause of recurrent frequency/dysuria it is thus critical to obtain urine for bacterial examination as early as is possible in the illness. Failure to do so may lead to patients being labelled as having the abacteriuric frequency/dysuria syndrome with consequential inappropriate investigation and management.

Pyuria

As criteria for the diagnosis of 'significant bacteriuria' have changed in the past 10 years, so have concepts regarding the definition and significance of pyuria. Traditional methods of recording pyuria on the basis of the number of white blood cells per high-powered field is now recognized to be inaccurate [13]. White blood counts must be expressed quantitatively per cubic millimetre of urine. This is facilitated by the development of automated laboratory techniques. A cut-off point of more than eight white blood cells per cubic millimetre of urine is defined as abnormal, indicating pyuria [14].

Pyuria *per se* is not diagnostic of urinary infection nor does its absence exclude UTI, particularly in asymptomatic patients. Alternative causes include renal stone disease and drug-induced kidney damage. It is now clear that the combination of pyuria and 'low-count' bacteriuria is highly suggestive of UTI in symptomatic young women and its association with bacterial counts of 10^2 or more of the same organism per cubic millimetre of urine is diagnostic in respect of coliform infections. 'Sterile' pyuria in symptomatic patients should raise the possibility of infection by fastidious organisms (see below). Persistence of pyuria in patients previously shown to be bacteriuric should alert the clinician to the possibility of some complicating factor such as the presence of stones or papillary necrosis. Tuberculosis of the urinary tract, although now uncommon in the UK, must still be considered in patients with sterile pyuria. Finally, sterile pyuria in symptomatic patients may result from interstitial cystitis (Hunner's ulcer).

Special staining of urine deposits for white cells and quantitation of white cell excretion rates enjoyed brief vogue in the past but have little place in clinical practice.

Special microbiological studies

The diagnosis of UTI on the basis of quantitative urine culture presupposes that appropriate microbiological methods are used. In recent years considerable attention has been focused on the possibility that symptomatic UTI may be due to fastidious organisms not normally isolated by conventional laboratory techniques. Maskell *et al.* [15] reported the isolation of *Lactobacillus, Corynebacterium* and *Streptococcus milleri* in patients with supposedly 'abacteriuric' frequency/dysuria, and claimed cure following treatment with appropriate antibiotics. This initial report generated considerable controversy and has led to many conflicting reports [16]. Attention has also been focused on *Chlamydia trachomatis* as a cause of 'abacteriuric' frequency/dysuria and impressive evidence in favour of this has been presented by Stamm *et al.* [17,18]. *Ureaplasma urealyticum* has also been recovered from the urinary tract in symptomatic patients and has been postulated as a possible cause of progressive kidney damage [19]. The precise role of these various organisms in producing symptomatic urinary tract infection or kidney

damage has yet to be firmly established. At this time it would seem prudent to undertake appropriate culture of urine obtained by SPA in persistently or repeatedly 'abacteriuric' symptomatic patients, and especially those with persistent pyuria, to exclude bladder bacteriuria due to fastidious organisms.

Significance of urinary tract infections

UTI may be an isolated event or a recurrent problem. It may be merely an unpleasant and distressing complaint or may result in serious kidney damage and even life-threatening septicaemia. The level of investigation and the principles of management in each individual must take account of this spectrum of significance.

Complicated versus uncomplicated infection

For the patient with symptomatic or asymptomatic infection the most burning question is, 'will this damage the kidneys?'. Thirty years ago it was widely believed that recurrent UTI could lead to progressive kidney damage in many adults. This view then give way to the believe that in adult life, if the urinary tract is anatomically and functionally normal, renal damage rarely if ever occurred as a result of UTI. This view has in turn been challenged in recent years. Thus, sequential computed tomography (CT) studies [5] have demonstrated the development of scars in kidneys previously shown to have evidence of bacterial interstitial nephritis. It may be relevant that a number of these patients had diabetes. The long-term functional significance of these scars both in terms of renal function and the possible development of hypertension is unclear. Suffice it to say that renal scars may develop occasionally in patients with acute pyelonephritis even in the presence of a normal intravenous urogram (IVU). Nevertheless, in the vast majority of patients with acute pyelonephritis and a normal IVU, serious kidney damage is unusual and rarely if ever leads to progressive kidney damage.

An exception to this are those patients who, while possibly having a normal IVU, have some associated condition such as sickle cell disease/trait or diabetes mellitus. Such conditions themselves may lead to renal damage, but there is in addition the suspicion that recurrent UTI may increase the potential for such damage. The same is possibly true of patients who abuse analgesics. Certainly such patients should be considered at greater risk and the control and prevention of recurrent infection must be seen as desirable in terms of protecting kidney function.

Quite a different situation exists in those patients who have an abnormality of the urinary tract such as renal stones, obstruction, polycystic kidneys or vesicoureteric reflux. Stones may result from urinary infection—the familiar mixed triple phosphate stone. Alternatively, patients with metabolic stone disease may develop UTI which may in turn graft triple phosphate on top of a metabolic core. In either instance, the stone may damage the kidney by its size or, more commonly, cause damage due to obstruction to all or part of the collecting system. Of much greater importance is the potential for the development of an obstructed pyonephrosis due to the combination of obstruction and infection. In this situation there may be rapid destruction of kidney tissue and the possibility of perirenal abscess and life-threatening septicaemia. All patients with renal stones, and particularly stones causing or likely to cause obstruction, who have been shown to have UTI must be considered high-risk subjects in respect of developing serious renal sepsis.

Subacute obstruction whether due to stones, pelvi-ureteric obstruction, ureteric stenosis, etc., predisposes both to extension of bladder bacteriuria to the upper urinary tract and, especially in the presence of a high-pressure system, to renal damage and septicaemia. Again, subjects with this combination must be considered high-risk patients. It is possible, but unproven, that patients with totally obstructed systems are prone to blood-borne infection. The evidence for this largely stems from animal experimentation. It is unclear as to how frequently this occurs in humans. Given this observation, the justification for prophylactic removal of a totally obstructed kidney in an otherwise healthy and asymptomatic patient with no history of UTI rests on slim evidence.

In children (see Chapters 17 and 44) the combination of vesicoureteric reflux and UTI has been clearly shown to predispose to renal scars and impaired kidney growth. The importance of reflux and infection in adults is unclear. Vesicoureteric reflux facilitates the ascent of bladder infection to the upper tracts, but whether or how often this results in further kidney damage is unclear. There are scattered references in the literature to the development of calyceal abnormalities and reduction of renal function in adults with acquired reflux [20] and infection, but conversely there are an equal number of studies reporting the follow-up of adults with recurrent infection and reflux

in whom no deterioration of function has been observed [21]. A recent study reporting vesicoureteric reflux in 76% of adults with a current UTI [22] has reawakened interest in this complicating factor. However, in the absence of any well-controlled prospective study of renal function in such patients with or without surgical correction of the reflux it is impossible to make a scientific judgement as to its contribution to progressive renal impairment.

This doubt regarding the effect of infection and reflux on function is a quite separate issue to the need to undertake surgery in patients with recurrent distressing *symptoms* in whom infection or symptoms cannot be controlled by medical management (see p. 603).

UTI assumes more than mere symptomatic significance in pregnant women (see Chapter 44) and in immuno-suppressed subjects. In the latter, whether receiving treatment as part of cancer chemotherapy, for the control of immunologically mediated disease or for the control of transplant rejection, infection may be more severe and more difficult to eradicate as a result of the partial paralysis of the host defence mechanisms. Patients also run the risk of developing life-threatening septicaemia.

Given these observations on the significance of UTI it is convenient to subdivide patients into those with complicated or uncomplicated UTI (Fig. 43.3). In uncomplicated cases the problem clearly relates to whether the patients have symptoms or not and to whether symptomatic attacks are isolated and rare or frequent and distressing. In the case of complicated UTI, whether symptomatic or asymptomatic, a new factor—renal damage and septicaemia—is introduced. This may alter life expectancy. This subdivision of patients with UTI defines for the clinician *and* the patient the nature of the problem and the need for and importance of aggressive treatment and long-term follow-up.

Natural history

Management policies for patients with UTI must take account not only of the significance of infection but also its natural history.

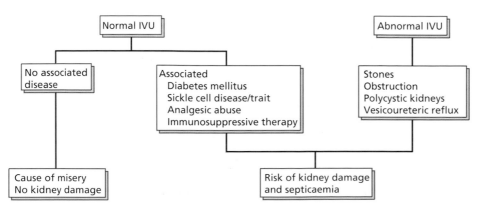

Fig. 43.3 Significance of recurrent UTI.

Single episodes

Single, isolated, never-repeated episodes of symptomatic or asymptomatic bacteriuria occur in a very large proportion of women at some time in their lives. If treated and the patient has no further symptoms, bacteriuria or other evidence of renal disease, it is of little importance and does not require further investigation.

Recurrent infection

Recurrent infection, whether symptomatic or asymptomatic, is of much greater importance both as a cause of misery and as a possible cause of kidney damage or septicaemia. Recurrent infection may be due to reinfection or to relapsing infection.

Recurrent reinfection

This is much the most common cause of recurrent UTI. Reinfection signifies that situation in which a patient with bacteriuria becomes abacteriuric, whether spontaneously or as a result of treatment, remains abacteriuric for weeks or months only to have a further episode of bacteriuria due to the same or a different organism (Fig. 43.4). The problem is not failure to eliminate organisms from the urinary tract but rather a failure in the patient's defence systems which allows repeated reinvasion of the tract. Reinfection may occur at frequent or infrequent intervals. It can only be diagnosed by careful serial urine culture, obtaining urine samples at the onset of symptoms and at 7–10 days after completing treatment. The organism most commonly responsible is *Escherichia coli*, and the identification of differences in *E. coli* strains may be based on patterns of antibiotic sensitivities or, more accurately, by serotyping.

In busy clinical practice this is made much easier by the use of flow charts in the case records (Fig. 43.5). The use of dip inoculum cultures which the patient can carry out at home as required at the onset of symptoms makes serial urine culture a practical proposition.

Relapsing infection

This is much less common than reinfection. It is defined as that situation in which bacteriuria is controlled during the administration of antibacterial therapy but there is recurrence *with the same organism* within 5–10 days of cessation of treatment (see Fig. 43.4). This implies a failure to eradicate the infection and is most often associated with stones, scarred kidneys, diverticula of the urinary tract, cystic disease, bacterial prostatitis or impaired host defence mechanisms as in the immunosuppressed subject. Again, diagnosis demands serial urine culture and attention to the bacterial species and antibiotic sensitivities. A diagnosis of relapsing bacteriuria demands careful review of the IVU to identify possible factors which make eradication of infection difficult.

Treatment failure

This is most correctly defined as that situation in which bacteriuria is not controlled during the administration of an antibacterial drug to which the organism has been shown to be sensitive on laboratory testing (see Fig. 43.4). It can only be diagnosed if urine cultures are performed during treatment. The causes of this are few—failure to take the drug, incorrect sensitivity testing in the laboratory or renal functional impairment of such a degree that adequate levels of the drug cannot be achieved in the urine.

Treatment failure should not be confused with the rare

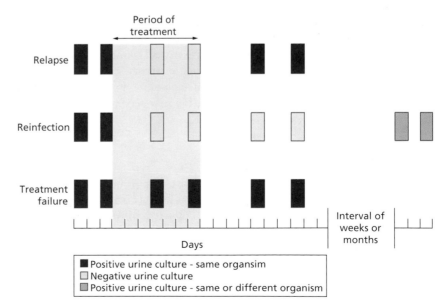

Fig. 43.4 Distinction between relapse, reinfection and treatment failure. (Reproduced with permission from [47].)

Date	4./3.81	13/8/81	10/9/81	22/x1/81	23/x1/81	26/x1/81	3/12/81		
Frequency	++	O	O	+/–	+/–	O	O		
Dysuria	++	O	O	+/–	+/–	O	O		
Suprapubic pain	O	O	O	O	O	O	O		
Loin	O	O	O	O	O	O	O		
Fever	O	O	O	O	O	O	O		
Vaginal discharge	O	O	O	O	O	O	O		
Other	O	O							
Urine									
MSSU	×	×	×	×			×		
Dip side						×			
SPA					×				
WBC	>100	<5	O	10	10		O		
Organism	>10^5 E.C.	O	O	>10^3 E.Coli	>10^3 E.Coli	O	O		
Sensitivties									
Cotrimoxazole	✓				✓				
Ampicillin	O				✓				
Nitro.	✓				✓				
Nalid	✓				✓				
Treatment	R$_x$ CoT. 5 days				R$_x$ Nitro 5 days				

Fig. 43.5 Flow sheet for documentation of symptoms, bacteriology and treatment.

situation in which, during treatment, bacteriuria with a different 'resistant' organism becomes apparent. Given that the initial bacterial species was correctly identified, this indicates an initial double infection, one of the bacterial species having been masked by the dominance of the other. During treatment, this second, and of necessity resistant, organism is unmasked. It is rare for drug resistance to develop during treatment. It is also of course possible, but rare, that there has been superinfection with a new second organism during treatment.

Special investigations

It cannot be overemphasized that the most important investigation in patients suspected of having UTI is quantitative urine culture of a carefully collected MSU. Unfortunately, patients are often inadequately instructed in the correct procedure for collecting an MSU (Table 43.3). Given the demonstration of bacteriuria, the need for further investigation must then take account of the particular circumstances of the individual patient.

Localization of infection

Following Kass' pioneer work on quantitative urine culture [6] there was a period of intensive research throughout the world on the natural history and management of UTI. During this period methods were developed to localize the site of infection (i.e. lower tract versus upper tract infection). Direct and indirect techniques were used [23]. The most direct technique was to undertake ureteric catheterization following bladder washout as described by Stamey et al. [24]. A simpler version, not allowing lateralization of upper tract infection and fraught with some inaccuracies, was developed by Fairley et al. [25], involving forced diuresis following bladder wash-out. A more indirect approach developed by Winiberg et al. [26] and later by Percival et al. [27] was to study serum antibacterial antibody. More recently, study of the bacterial antibody coating has been proposed as a method for localization of the site of infection [28]. Apart from the direct localization test of Stamey et al. these methods are not reliable.

Table 43.3 The correct procedure to collect an MSU.

In the female
- The bladder should be full ('desperate to go')
- Remove underpants and stand over the toilet pan
- Separate the labia using the left hand
- Clean the vulva front to back with a sterile swab
- Void downward into the toilet and continue until 'half done'
- Without stopping the urine flow the sterile container is plunged into the stream of urine with the right hand; only a small volume is required
- Complete voiding into the toilet

In the male
- The bladder should be full
- Retract the foreskin if present
- Clean the glans penis with a sterile swab
- Void into the toilet until 'half done'
- Without stopping the urine flow, the sterile container is plunged into the stream of urine
- Complete voiding into the toilet

The underlying theory behind such studies was that upper tract infection, as opposed to lower tract infection, was both potentially more damaging to the kidney and more difficult to treat. Time and experience have shown these concepts to be only half true. Thus, in terms of kidney damage it is now generally accepted that in general it is not whether the infection is upper or lower tract that determines kidney damage but rather whether it is complicated or uncomplicated. Similarly, save possibly with ultrashort treatment, it is now clear that the ease of treatment in uncomplicated cases differs little whether there is upper tract or lower tract infection. In terms of practical management it is more important to undertake serial urine culture before and after treatment to identify relapsing bacteriuria versus reinfection, since this distinction materially affects management.

Rarely, localization studies may be justified when a decision is being made as to the need for nephrectomy of a diseased kidney to control relapsing infection, or when relapsing infection occurs in males and doubt exists as to whether the site of infection requiring eradication is in the upper tract or in the prostate. In other instances localization studies are primarily research tools [29].

Intravenous urography

The casual and repeated use of IVUs in patients with recurrent UTI is to be deplored. IVU should only be undertaken if the clinician is quite clear as to what information is being sought and how this information may affect management. There is no need for IVU in women with a single episode of frequency dysuria. In males, in whom UTI is uncommon, it should be undertaken after the first episode of documented bacteriuria to define or exclude

some potentially treatable predisposing abnormality. In women who have two or more episodes of documented bacteriuria, IVU should be carried out for two main reasons: (i) to identify whether such patients have complicated or uncomplicated UTI and so define the possible natural history of the disease (see p. 595); and (ii) to identify possible factors predisposing to either relapse or reinfection, such as scarred kidneys, impaired bladder emptying, etc. The question being asked, therefore, is 'is the urinary tract normal or are there stones, obstruction, scarred kidneys, polycystic kidneys, impaired bladder emptying or evidence suggestive of vesicoureteric reflux?' It has been suggested [30] that because of the low yield of abnormal IVUs such a policy is mistaken. The author would disagree as, without this information, neither the clinician nor the patient is fully aware of the significance or likely natural history of the UTI. The hazard, unpleasantness and waste attached to undertaking IVUs does not relate to this first investigation but to the needless repetition of the IVU.

If the initial IVU is normal there is no point in repeating renal imaging unless there is some new unexpected clinical feature, for example acute loin pain, fever and oliguria in a patient with diabetes or sickle cell trait who may be suspected of having dropped off a papilla which is causing obstruction. In such situations renal ultrasound to define or exclude obstruction is the investigation of first choice. If there is suspicion of infected stone formation, and especially in patients with relapsing *Proteus* bacteriuria, plain renal tomography is the investigation of first choice.

If the IVU is abnormal (e.g. in patients with bladder outflow problems, ileal conduits or stones) it may be repeated if there is fear of the development of an obstructing lesion but again renal or pre- and post-micturition bladder ultrasound will usually suffice.

Ultrasound versus intravenous urography

In recent years it has been proposed that ultrasound of the kidneys and the bladder is sufficient for renal imaging of patients with recurrent urinary infection [31]. The author also believes this to be unacceptable. The purpose of the renal imaging is to identify abnormalities which may predispose to UTI, complicate the course of the infection or make treatment difficult. While ultrasound can, in the hands of the skilled operator, define renal size, the presence or absence of upper tract obstruction and impaired bladder emptying, it cannot clearly define renal anatomy and can miss renal stones. Most importantly, no clinician can confidently reassure a patient that their renal tract is normal on the basis of renal ultrasonography.

The special value of renal ultrasound is in the emergency imaging of patients who have severe loin pain to exclude upper tract obstruction. It is also of value in the follow-up of patients known to have stones or bladder outflow obstruction to define the development of or change in obstruction.

Cystoscopy

This investigation is widely abused. There is no place for cystoscopy in women with a single episode of uncomplicated frequency/dysuria. In both sexes it may be indicated where there is evidence on the IVU or ultrasound of bladder outflow obstruction, to define, in conjunction with urodynamic studies, the nature of the problem. It is indicated in patients over the age of 40 years who have overt haematuria with negative urine cytology, and is also indicated if the bladder or vesicoureteric junction looks abnormal on IVU.

Micturating cystourethrography

This should only be undertaken to assist in the evaluation of bladder outflow problems or possible urethral stenosis. In adults, the presence or absence of all but grade III vesicoureteric reflux is academic save where there is difficulty in controlling infection by medical means or where there is disabling loin pain during micturition. Undertaking micturating cystourethrography, except in these circumstances, does not alter management.

Urodynamic studies

Urodynamic studies are indicated to investigate impaired bladder emptying as in the non-infected patient, with the proviso that recurrent UTI may itself result in mild impairment of bladder emptying. Studies should not therefore be undertaken until an attempt has been made to control the infection for a period of some months.

Management

Single isolated episode of frequency/dysuria

In patients with an acute 'one-off' episode of cystisis it is desirable but in no way obligatory to obtain an MSU for culture prior to commencing antibacterial treatment. Many patients will already have tried self-treatment before seeking medical advice. Deferring antibacterial therapy is pointless. Treatment with a 'best bet' antibacterial drug should be given, preferably based on advice from the local laboratory as to the current pattern of drug sensitivities of urinary pathogens in the community. Drugs of first choice are a sulphonamide (e.g. sulphfurazole), nitrofurantoin, amoxycillin or trimethoprim in conventional dosage.

Duration of treatment

The duration of antibacterial therapy required to treat UTI has been the subject of considerable interest in recent years. It is abundantly clear that in the single acute episode in otherwise healthy women there is no advantage in treatment lasting for more than 7 days [32]. Controversy does exist, however, as to whether and how often this can be reduced to 3 days or even restricted to a single large dose of antibiotic. The use of a single dose [33] or a 3-day course [34] of treatment has many advantages — cost, convenience and a reduction in side effects due to disturbance of gut and vaginal flora. Single dose or short-course therapy requires explanation to the patient that while infection can be eliminated very quickly, symptoms due to inflammation may persist for 24–48 h after completing their treatment. Post-treatment urine culture at 7–10 days is essential. There is good evidence to suggest that in women with few, if any, previous attacks, who present within 2 days of developing symptoms, a single large dose of an antibiotic (amoxycillin, co-trimoxazole, kanamycin) or a 3-day course of regular drug dosage will suffice as significant tissue invasion and thus difficulty in eradication of infection is unlikely. An advantage claimed for single dose or 3-day therapy is that failure to eradicate infection identifies patients with some underlying renal abnormality requiring further investigation [35].

Asymptomatic bacteriuria

In men, the diagnosis of asymptomatic bacteriuria is uncommon in the absence of some abnormality of the urinary tract. It thus merits both treatment and further investigation. Women with asymptomatic bacteriuria must be subdivided into pregnant and non-pregnant groups.

Bacteriuria in pregnancy must always be treated and be shown to be eradicated by follow-up urine culture (see Chapter 45).

The question as to whether asymptomatic bacteriuria in non-pregnant women should be treated is controversial. If patients are known to have no anatomical or functional abnormality of the urinary tract and are truly asymptomatic, treatment is unnecessary. However, on first presentation it is impossible to distinguish between complicated and uncomplicated infection. A pragmatic approach is to treat the bacteriuria and to do a post-treatment urine culture. If bacteriuria is permanently eradicated and there is no persisting abnormality on routine chemical testing or microscopy of the urine, no further investigation is required. If bacteriuria recurs, an IVU should be carried out to establish whether there is complicated or uncomplicated infection. If there is evidence of anatomical or functional abnormality of the urinary tract, asymptomatic bacteriuria should be treated as for recurrent infection.

Recurrent infection

Recurrent or persisting infection is a much more serious problem both in terms of morbidity and the potential for kidney damage. Appropriate and effective management demands a clear definition of the problem. This requires careful history taking, serial urine culture and IVU. The management of recurrent UTI is primarily a medical problem, surgical intervention being rarely required. The first requirement is to distinguish between relapsing UTI and recurrent reinfection.

Relapsing bacteria

This implies failure to eradicate some nidus of infection within the urinary tract. It may simply reflect too short a treatment of an otherwise uncomplicated, usually upper tract, infection. It may, however, be associated with some situation in which it is difficult for antibacterial agents to reach and eradicate infection as, for example, in scarred or polycystic kidneys, renal stones or bacterial prostatitis. In patients presenting with UTI who subsequently relapse, the practical approach is to treat with a more prolonged (10–14 day) course of an antibacterial drug to which the organism is sensitive. An MSU must be obtained during treatment to ensure compliance and effectiveness of treatment and a further MSU 7–10 days' post-treatment. If there is further relapse the patient will require an IVU or a review of any previous IVU to seek a cause for relapse. If there are stones, the potential for their removal must be considered since it is virtually impossible to eradicate relapsing bacteriuria if there are infected stones. If there is no surgically treatable condition, the patient should be given intensive high-dose treatment with an aminoglycoside, a 5-quinolone such as ciprofloxacin or orfloxacin or one of the more recent penicillins in an attempt to get sufficient tissue/stone penetration to eradicate infection. If this fails, long-term suppressive therapy must be considered [36]. The treatment schedule is as with prophylactic therapy (see below) but the objectives are different. The purposes of suppressive treatment are to prevent frequently recurring episodes of distressing symptomatic infection, to prevent new or further stone formation and to prevent kidney damage in patients with papillary necrosis or potentially obstructive uropathy. If none of these apply, then the justification for treatment must be reconsidered. Patients with relapsing uncomplicated UTI do not require suppressive treatment. Such cases are rare. Suppressive treatment may be required indefinitely but it is worth stopping at yearly or 2-yearly intervals to check whether infection has been eradicted. If complicated by recurrent superinfection, suppressive therapy may have to be abandoned and symptomatic infections treated as they arise (see p. 602).

Recurrent reinfection

This poses a different problem—prevention of reinfection of a susceptible urinary tract. A rational approach to this requires consideration of the pathogenesis of UTI in general and the identification of predisposing factors in the individual.

Gut flora are the source of infecting organisms in the vast majority of cases, but little can be done at present to modify these. Whether, in the future, it will be possible to vaccinate against pilated bacteria—commonly believed to be especially uropathogenic—remains to be seen [37].

Periurethral colonization or 'build-up' with bacteria is believed to be a preliminary step in ascending infection [38]. It is doubtful whether special attention to perineal toilet, the wearing of tight jeans or underpants makes much difference to colonization, and obsessional attention to these is unnecessary. The use of bubble baths or disinfectants in bath water does seem to predispose to persistent or recurring infection and these are best avoided. Coexistent chronic vaginitis should be treated. In older women, hormone-deficient atrophic vulvitis may facilitate periurethral colonization and should be treated.

The factors determining the transuretheral passage of bacteria to the bladder (with the exception of catheterization) are poorly understood. It is probable that it is facilitated by coitus when periurethral bacteria may be massaged up the urethra, especially in the absence of vaginal lubrication. Patients should be advised to practice post-coital voiding in an attempt to evacuate any bacteria which may have been introduced to the bladder during intercourse. They should also ensure adequate vaginal lubrication using K-Y jelly if necessary. There is evidence that the use of a diaphragm with a spermicidal jelly predisposes to recurrent infection [39]. In such cases the use of alternative contraceptive measures should be considered. It is extremely doubtful whether functional urethral stenosis plays much part in the pathogenesis of UTI in most women. Certainly, there is little evidence that urethral dilatation or surgery is of any but very temporary symptomatic value.

Most probably the main factor predisposing to recurrent UTI is impairment of the normal bladder defence mechanisms. These are still poorly understood (see Chapter 54). In terms of practical management, the only manner in which bladder defences can be enhanced is to ensure optimum hydrokinetic clearance, i.e. a high rate of urine flow with frequent and complete bladder emptying [10]. In patients with impaired bladder emptying, the cause of this must be identified and, when appropriate and effective, surgical treatment carried out. If there is a large post-micturition bladder residual volume, there is little hope of preventing recurrent infection unless voiding can be improved. Patients should be taught double or triple micturition especially where there is vesicoureteric reflux. Patients with neurogenic bladders should be taught manually assisted voiding. Drug treatment to facilitate complete voiding is at present unsatisfactory. Constipation should be avoided as a loaded rectum may interfere with bladder emptying.

A practical regimen

All patients with recurrent reinfection must have the nature of the problem explained to them and their active participation in prophylaxis must be recruited. Without active 'self-help', management is likely to fail. Correctable pathogenic factors as mentioned above must be sought and eliminated. All patients must embark on a regimen of high fluids with frequent complete voiding and persist with this for at least 6–12 months after their last attack (Table 43.4).

Low-dose prophylactic antibacterial drug treatment

Such has been the success of low-dose treatment [40,41] that there has been a tendency to embark on drug treatment when the patient is first seen without attention to the conservative measures listed above. The author believes this is wrong. It is desirable to attempt to resolve the problem first without drug treatment. At any rate, fully successful drug treatment can only be achieved if these other measures are also taken during treatment. We believe, therefore, that low-dose prophylaxis should not be given until there has been an initial period of conservative management. Thus, we only introduce low-dose drug treatment if the patient has had two episodes of infection within 6 months despite attending to the high fluid regimen.

Low-dose prophylactic antibacterial drug treatment requires an initial 3–5-day course of conventional drug dosage to control the current infection. Dosage is then reduced to one dose last thing at night before retiring. Low-dose treatment was first introduced with a combination of trimethoprim and sulfamethoxazole [40], but since then co-trimoxazole itself, nitrofurantoin and trimethoprim alone have all been shown to be effective [41]. Treatment should be continued for 6–12 months. On cessation of treatment many patients will have no further trouble, but some do. The latter should be returned to low-dose treatment for a more prolonged period. Some may need prophylactic treatment indefinitely.

The emphasis is on low-dose treatment. Prolonged courses of full dosage of antibacterial drugs are wasteful and more likely to be complicated by fungal infections and the emergence of drug-resistant bacteria in the gut flora. Using low-dose treatment, the emergence of resistant strains in the gut flora with subsequent superinfection of the urinary tract and break-through infections are remarkably uncommon [41,42]. When they occur they should be treated with a conventional dose of another antibacterial drug to which the organism is sensitive and low-dose treatment should be reinstituted at the end of this treatment. The effectiveness of treatment is enhanced by continuing with a high fluid regimen.

It must be re-emphasized that there is no place for low-dose prophylactic treatment in patients with persistent or recurrent symptoms who are never shown to be bacteriuric.

In patients in whom recurrence of infection is clearly shown to be related to coitus, the overall load of prophylactic drug treatment can be reduced by taking a single dose of antibiotic only after intercourse.

When not to treat

While it may be felt desirable that the urinary tract be kept free of bacteria, this is not always possible and indeed measures to eradicate infection may be potentially more harmful than the presence of bacteriuria. The potential for eradicating infection and maintaining the urinary tract sterile in patients with dilated and poorly emptying systems (e.g. patients with ileal conduits or neurogenic bladders) is often small. The same applies to patients with multiple calculi which cannot be removed. If an initial attempt fails, the need for further treatment must be balanced against the hazards of multiple, possibly potentially nephrotoxic, drug treatments with the associated risk of the emergence of polyresistant organisms. In general, if there is a low pressure within the urinary tract, the potential for serious kidney damage is small. In these patients it is our practice not to continue attempts at treatment if there is rapid recurrence of infection or infection with a drug-resistant organism. Rather, we warn the patients to report immediately should they develop symptoms, especially loin pain or fever. Patients are then treated for this symptomatic attack. Patients with calculi should have regular yearly or 2-yearly plain X-rays to observe any change in the size or position of the stones which may predispose to obstructive nephropathy.

Table 43.4 Recurrent reinfection—management regimen.

High fluid intake	>2 litres per day
Bladder voiding	3 hourly by day
	Before going to bed
	After coitus
	Practise double micturition
Avoid vaginal sprays, chemicals in bath water, etc.	
Low-dose prophylaxis if further bacteriuria	

Role of surgery

Although it is traditional to refer patients with urinary infection, and especially recurrent infection, to urologists, the management of such patients rarely requires surgical skill.

Relapsing bacteriuria

There is undoubtedly a role for surgery in this condition when there are infected stones, infected malfunctioning kidneys, blind-ended ureters or large diverticula, all of which may harbour bacteria which cannot be eradicated by medical means. The decision to remove part or all of a kidney must, however, take account of residual renal function. It may be better to accept relapsing bacteriuria rather than seriously prejudice renal function.

Recurrent reinfection

Tempting as it may be, there is a very limited role for surgery in these patients which relates primarily to measures to improve bladder emptying. Save when there is manifest bladder outflow obstruction, there is no good evidence that urethral dilatation in women is of any value save as a means of giving temporary symptomatic relief. When there is organic bladder outflow obstruction, this requires conventional treatment. Reconstructive surgery to improve bladder emptying is dealt with elsewhere in this book (see Chapter 35).

Vesicoureteric reflux

In adults there is little indication for ureteric reimplant- ation except where there is gross reflux and an uncontrollable post-micturition bladder residue which prevents control of recurrent infection by medical means. High-pressure reflux likely to cause kidney damage in association with infection is more likely to be due to bladder overflow obstruction than to simple vesicoureteric reflux. Vesicoureteric reflux, while facilitating the spread of bladder bacteriuria to the upper tract, does not itself facilitate recurrent reinfection of the bladder except where there is a large post-micturition residue.

Bladder catheterization

The only sure way to avoid catheter-induced urinary infection is to avoid catheterization! Even with careful attention to technique, there is always a potential for the establishment of bacteriuria. The risk increases with indwelling catheters and every catheterization must be justified and the hazards recognized. A principle indication for isolated catheterization is to relieve a temporary obstruction or inability to void. Rarely, it is required to obtain a urine sample for culture in the elderly or infirm. It is required for micturating cystourography and urodynamic studies and these investigations must be clearly justified. A strictly aseptic technique must be employed and catheters must be passed gently. There is little evidence that lubricants containing antibacterial agents are of much value. In high-risk patients, for example those suspected of having acute oliguric renal failure, diagnostic bladder catherization should include the installation of 50 ml of a 1% solution of noxythiolin or polymyxin B (200 mg/l) or neomycin (40 mg/l) prior to removal of the catheter [43]. In males with a history of previous infection, and particularly where it is suspected that there may be chronic bacterial prostatitis, instrumentation of the urethra whether for catheterization or cystoscopy should be covered by antibiotic pretreatment continued for 72 h after the instrumentation.

Intermittent catheterization

Intermittent catheterization in the spinal cord injury patient and in patients with neurogenic bladders due to other causes has been shown to be safe and effective both in the UK and USA [44,45], but again requires careful training and supervision by a dedicated team.

Suprapubic drainage

This is gaining in popularity. Although not widely practised in the UK, it is likely to become more widespread with the development of new and better catheters.

Indwelling urethral catheters

These remain the safest technique for general use in patients who cannot void, are grossly incontinent or require contin- uous drainage for surgical reasons. It must be used conservatively and be practised carefully. It is mandatory that a closed catheter drainage system be employed. The perineum must be cleansed twice daily and kept dry. There is little evidence that prophylactic, intermittent or continuous irrigation with antibacterial agents has any advantage save possibly the use, in women, of a plastic sponge around the catheter abutting against the external urethral orifice which is kept impregnated with antiseptic solution [46].

Prophylactic oral antibiotics should not be given to patients on continuous drainage. If bacteriuria develops, provided there is free drainage, it need not be treated unless there is clinical evidence of tissue invasion—fever, suprapubic or loin pain. The need for the catheter should be reviewed and treatment given after it is removed. Should removal be impractical, the patient should be treated with a short course of antibacterial agents shown to be appropriate on laboratory sensitivity testing.

References

1 Mond NC, Percival A, Williams JD, Brumfitt W. Presentation, diagnosis and treatment of urinary tract infection in general practice. *Lancet* 1965;**1**:514–16.

2 Gallagher DJA, Montgomerie JZ, North DK. Acute infection of the urinary tract and the urethral syndrome in general practice. *Br Med J* 1965;**1**:622–6.

3 O'Grady FW, Charlton GAC, Kelsey Fry I, McSherry A, Cattell WR. Natural history of intractable 'cystitis' in women referred to a special clinic. In: W Brumfit, AW Asscher, eds. *Urinary Tract Infection*. London: Oxford University Press, 1973:81–91.

4 Fairley KF, Carson NE, Gutch RC *et al.* Site of infection in acute urinary tract infection in general practice. *Lancet* 1971;**2**:615–18.

5 Meyrier A, Condamin MC, Fernet M *et al.* Frequency of development of early cortical scarring in acute primary pyelonephritis. *Kidney Int* 1989;**35**:696–703.

6 Kass EH. Bacteriuria and the diagnosis of infection of the urinary tract. *Arch Intern Med* 1957;**100**:709–14.

7 Stamm WE, Counts GW, Running K *et al.* Diagnosis of coliform infections in acutely dysuric women. *N Engl J Med* 1982;**307**:436–58.

8 Lipsky BA. Urinary tract infections in men. *Ann Int Med* 1989;**110**:138–50.

9 O'Grady F, Cattell WR. Kinetics of urinary tract infection. II The bladder. *Br J Urol* 1966;**38**:156–62.

10 Cattell WR, Kelsey Fry I, Spiro FI *et al.* Effect of diuresis and frequent micturition on the bacterial content of infected urine. *Br J Urol* 1970;**42**:290–5.

11 Eykyn S, Newman CGH. Suprapubic puncture. *Br J Hosp Med* 1969;**2**:863–5.

12 Cattell WR, Brooks HL, McSherry MA, Northeast A, O'Grady F. Approach to the frequency and dysuria syndrome. *Kidney Int* 1975;**8**:138–43.

13 Stamm WE. Measurement of pyuria and its relation to bacteriuria. *Am J Med* 1983;**75**:53–8.

14 Stamm WE, Wagner KF, Amsal R *et al.* Causes of the acute urethral syndrome in women. *N Engl J Med* 1980;**303**:409–15.

15 Maskell R, Pead L, Allen J. The puzzle of 'urethral syndrome'; a possible answer? *Lancet* 1979;**1**:1058–9.

16 Brumfitt W, Hamilton Miller JMT, Ludlam H, Gooding A. Lactobacilli do not cause frequency and dysuria syndrome. *Lancet* 1981;**2**:393–5.

17 Stamm WE, Wagner KF, Amsal R *et al.* Cause of the acute urethral syndrome in women. *N Engl J Med* 1980;**303**:409–15.

18 Stamm WE, Running K, McKevitt M, Counts GW, Turck M, Holmes KK. Treatment of the acute urethral syndrome. *N Engl J Med* 1981;**19**:58–64.

19 Birch DR, Fairley KF, Pavillard RE. Unconventional bacteria in urinary tract disease. *Kidney Int* 1981;**19**:58–64.

20 Williams G, Wallace DM, Bloom HJG, Stevenson JJ. Vesico-ureteric reflux following interstitial irradiation of the urinary bladder. *Proc R Soc Med* 1971;**64**:64–6.

21 Gower PE. A longterm study of renal function in patients with radiological pyelonephritis and other allied radiological lesions. In: W Brumfitt, AW Asscher, eds. *Urinary Tract Infection*. London: Oxford University Press, 1973:74–9.

22 Wankowicz Z, Sulkin J, Przedlacki J. Retrospective analysis of own diagnostic and therapeutic protocol used in urinary tract infection (UTI) in years 1965–92 [Abstract XII]. International Congress of Nephrology, 1993:612.

23 Cattell WR, Charlton CAC, McSherry A, Kelsey Fry I, O'Grady FW. The localisation of urinary tract infection and its relationship to relapse, reinfection and treatment. In: W Brumfitt, AW Asscher, eds. *Urinary Tract Infection*. London: Oxford University Press, 1973;206–14.

24 Stamey TA, Govan DE, Palmer JM. The localisation and treatment of urinary tract infections. *Medicine (Baltimore)* 1965;**44**:1–36.

25 Fairley KF, Bond AG, Brown RB, Habersberger P. Simple test to determine the site of urinary tract infection. *Lancet* 1967;**2**:427–8.

26 Winiberg J, Anderson HJ, Hanson LA, Lincoln MD. Studies of urinary tract infection in infancy and childhood. *Br Med J* 1963;**2**:524–7.

27 Percival A, Brumfitt W, de Louvois J. Serum antibody levels as an indication of clinically inapparent pyelonephritis. *Lancet* 1964;**2**:1027–33.

28 Thomas VT, Shelokov A, Forland M. Antibody-coated bacteria in the urine and the site of urinary tract infection. *N Engl J Med* 1974;**290**:488–590.

29 Turck M. Importance of localisation of urinary tract infection in women. In: EH Kass, W Brumfitt, eds. *Infections of the Urinary Tract*. London: University of Chicago Press, 1978: 114–21.

30 Fowler JF, Pulaski ET. Excretory urography, cystography and cytoscopy in the evaluation of women with urinary tract infection. *N Engl J Med* 1981;**304**:462–5.

31 Spencer J, Lindsell D, Mastaorakou I. Ultrasonography compared with intravenous urography in investigation of urinary tract infection in adults. *Br Med J* 1990;**301**:221–3.

32 Kincaid-Smith P, Freedman A, Namura RS. Controlled trials of treatment in urinary tract infection. In: P Kincaid-Smith, KF Fairley, eds. *Renal Infection and Renal Scarring*. Melbourne: Mercedes Publishing Services, 1970:165–74.

33 Bailey RR, Abbott GD. Treatment of urinary tract infection with single doses of amoxycillin. *Nephron* 1977;**18**:316–20.

34 Charlton CAC, Crowther A, Davies JG *et al.* Three day and ten day chemotherapy for urinary tract infections in general practice. *Br Med J* 1976;**1**:124–6.

35 Lubis HR. Relationship of response to single dose therapy to the presence of abnormality of the urinary tract. In: RR Bailey, ed. *Single Dose Therapy of Urinary Tract Infection*. Sydney: Adis Health Science Press, 1983:40–1.

36 Cattell WR, Chamberlain DA, Fry IK, McSherry MA, Broughton C, O'Grady F. Long-term control of bacteriuria with trimethoprim-sulphonamide. *Br Med J* 1971;**1**: 377–3.

37 Jones GW, Rutter JM. Role of the K88 antigen in the pathogenesis of neonatal diarrhoea caused by *E. coli* in piglets. *Infect Immun* 1972;**6**:918–27.

38 Stamey TA. *Urinary Infections*. Baltimore: Williams & Wilkins, 1972;80–119.

39 Stamm WE, Hooton TM, Johnson JR *et al.* Urinary tract infections; from pathogenesis to treatment. *J Infect Dis* 1989; **159**:400–8.

40 O'Grady F, Chamberlain DA, Stark JE *et al.* Longterm low dosage trimethoprim-sulphonamide in the control of chronic bacteriuria. *Postgrad Med J* 1969;**45**(Suppl.):61–4.

41 Stamm WE, Counts GW, Wagner KF *et al.* Antimicrobial prophylaxis of recurrent urinary tract infection. *Ann Intern Med* 1980;**92**:770–5.

42 Pearson NJ, Towner KJ, McSherry MA, Cattell WR, O'Grady F. Emergence of trimethoprim resistant enterobacteria in patients

receiving longterm cotrimoxazole for the control of intractable urinary tract infection. *Lancet* 1979;**2**:1205–28.

43 Harper WES. An appraisal of 12 solutions used for bladder irrigation or instillation. *Br J Urol* 1981;**53**:433–8.

44 Guttman L, Frankel H. The value of intermittent catherisation in the early management of traumatic paraplegia and tetraplegia. *Paraplegia* 1966;**4**:63–83.

45 Lapides K, Diokno AC, Gould FR. Further observations on self-catherisation. *Am Assoc Genito-urin Surg* 1975;**67**: 15–17.

46 Gillespie WA, Lennon GG, Linton KB. Prevention of urinary infection in gynaecology. *Br Med J* 1964;**2**:423.

47 Cattell WR. In: GD Chisholm, ed. *Tutorials in Postgraduate Medicine — Urology.* London: Heinemann, 1980.

44 Urinary Tract Infection in Special Situations

P. Kincaid-Smith

Introduction

This chapter discusses urinary tract infections in a number of special situations; they are dealt with in the order of frequency with which they are usually encountered in clinical practice.

Recurrent urinary tract infection in adult women

Recurrent symptomatic urinary tract infection in women used to be the most frequent form of presentation seen in urinary tract infection. A major question which arose in these women was how far to proceed with investigations, because in the large majority no underlying cause for the urinary tract infection was uncovered. Partly for this reason, there was a tendency for doctors to regard these infections as being of no great significance although for the patient they often caused extremely painful and unpleasant symptoms and much marital discord as they were frequently precipitated by intercourse. The elucidation by Stamey [1] and others of the importance of vaginal and introital carriage of urinary tract pathogens preceding these infections has revolutionized the management of this type of infection, and in many cases the lives of the women concerned.

Presentation

The clinical presentation in women with recurrent urinary tract infection is almost always with symptoms of cystitis (namely dysuria and frequency), but the dysuria may be accompanied by severe strangury and tenesmus. Symptoms of pyelonephritis are infrequent. Symptoms typically occur in clusters of infections in close proximity to one another and are then followed by much longer intervals of remission of up to 6 months or more.

Investigations

While there is a tendency to investigate because of the recurrent nature of the symptoms, the likelihood of finding a significant underlying abnormality is small and is independent of any findings on intravenous urography [2]. Intravenous urography is the most commonly performed investigation and is clearly indicated if the patient has documented bacterial persistence (see p. 607) but has generally been regarded as unrewarding in recurrent urinary tract infection [3]. Likewise cystoscopy is not indicated because it is unlikely to reveal an abnormality unless there is persistent non-glomerular haematuria or some other independent indication for cytoscopy.

Course and management

In spite of the unpleasant symptoms associated with this type of infection, spontaneous improvement of the symptoms is often achieved by simple remedies such as increased fluid intake, alkali or even the time-honoured remedy of barley water. In a remarkable study of 219 women presenting with symptoms of urinary tract infection, Mabeck [4] demonstrated that 60% on placebo achieve a sterile urine within 4 weeks and 80% have a sterile urine in 5 months. Only 16% of women in Mabeck's study developed frequent recurrences (four or more over 30 months' follow-up). Stamey and colleagues demonstrated that trimethoprim-sulphamethoxazole in one-eighth of the regular therapeutic dose eradicated the bowel and vaginal carriage of urinary tract pathogens, and in a continued dosage of one-half of a tablet containing 40 mg of trimethoprim and 200 mg of sulphamethoxazole prevented recurrent infection [5].

The two treatments included in Stamey's study, namely trimethoprim-sulphamethoxazole and nitrofurantoin, have become the standard methods of prophylaxis of recurrent urinary tract infection in women. Nitrofurantoin works by eradicating infection from the bladder after this has occurred and not by altering the bowel flora by the eradication of urinary tract pathogens, which is the mechanism of action of the trimethoprim-sulphamethoxazole combination. Trimethoprim is thought by some to be as effective as the combination with sulphamethoxazole, but there is disagreement about this. Stamey demonstrated that trimethoprim was not nearly as effective in the eradication of *Escherichia coli* or *Klebsiella* from the bowel flora as the combination treatment [6].

Other antibacterial agents are less effective in the long term because of the emergence of bacteria in the bowel flora which are resistant to the drug in question. While some women need to take prophylaxis for many years to prevent recurrent infection, the majority achieve a long remission as a result of a course of 6 months' duration. They are then likely at some future time to have to use prophylaxis again for 6 months. Some women find prophylaxis effective if they take a dose only at the time of intercourse; however, intercourse is by no means invariably responsible for recurrence.

Urinary tract infection in pregnancy

Three types of infection may develop in pregnancy: asymptomatic bacteriuria, cystitis and acute pyelonephritis.

Bacteriuria in pregnancy, observed in many women who appeared otherwise healthy, was not generally treated unless symptomatic until the studies of Kass [7] showed that episodes of acute pyelonephritis could be prevented by the early detection and treatment of pregnancy bacteriuria. Kass also suggested that the incidence of prematurity and perinatal deaths could be reduced by treatment in early gestation [8]. This work led to numerous studies almost all of which confirmed the observation that acute pyelonephritis of pregnancy could be prevented in bacteriuric women by eradication of bacteriuria. Although several studies confirmed Kass' observation that certain complications of pregnancy such as prematurity and fetal loss were more frequent in the bacteriuric group [9,10], none was able to reduce their frequency. Two studies demonstrated a very high incidence of underlying urinary tract abnormalities on intravenous urograms in women with bacteriuria in pregnancy [9,11]. In one of these there were also significant differences in renal function between women with pregnancy bacteriuria and controls [9]. The increased incidence of prematurity, fetal loss and pre-eclampsia in bacteriuric women were attributed to these underlying renal abnormalities [9].

Presentation

Women with urinary tract infection in pregnancy may be asymptomatic and have the infection discovered as a result of a screening test or they may present with symptoms of cystitis or acute pyelonephritis.

Of women who are screened in early pregnancy and are found to have asymptomatic bacteriuria, about 40% develop symptoms of urinary tact infection later in that pregnancy. Although 50% of women with bacteriuria have a bladder localization on formal testing [12], if symptoms develop they are always those of acute pyelonephritis [9]. It is possible to document the ascent of infection from the bladder to the kidney during pregnancy [13]. Presumably there are factors in women with pregnancy bacteriuria which facilitate ascent of infection to the kidney because if bacteriuric women who are not pregnant develop symptoms of urinary tact infection they usually only have dysuria and frequency [14].

Women with acute pyelonephritis of pregnancy, while they develop similar symptoms to those of other women with acute pyelonephritis, generally seem to develop more severe symptoms, particularly if there is accompanying obstruction. Obstruction is most commonly due to so-called physiological dilatation of the ureter which becomes kinked at the pelvic brim, but can also be due to calculi.

Investigations

Investigations in pregnant women are obviously limited because of risks to the fetus from such procedures as radiographs.

Careful urine examination is of critical importance for the diagnosis of bacteriuria. Most studies have followed the recommendations of Kass that the bacterial count in two voided urine specimens should be above 100 000 for a diagnosis of bacteriuria. In using this definition some cases with true bacteriuria in the bladder urine will be missed. Eykyn did a study of 1000 consecutive pregnancies using needle aspiration of urine from the bladder [15]. She demonstrated lower bacterial counts and a higher prevalence (5.9%) of bacteriuria using this method than in other studies in London at the same time which were based on Kass' methodology and showed bacteriuria in only about 4% of pregnant women.

Demonstration of pyuria is obviously also important. The presence of heavy pyuria was one method used by obstetricians in the past to distinguish between bacteriuria and impending acute pyelonephritis. In a careful study of sequential urine specimens each month in a large series of bacteriuric women the author documented that a rising urinary leucocyte count is indeed found in women before they present with symptoms of acute pyelonephritis. We often observed extremely high leucocyte counts before symptoms appeared. In contrast, the 60% of women with bacteriuria who did not develop acute pyelonephritis did not show a progressive elevation of the urinary leucocyte count [16] (Fig. 44.1).

One of the most frequent abnormalities which we demonstrated on radiographs taken after the pregnancy was

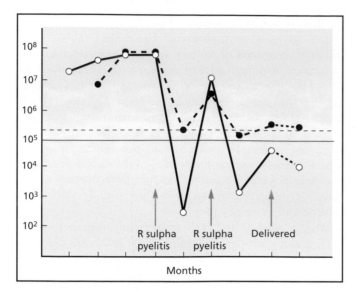

Months

Fig. 44.1 Graph of the changes in the bacterial count (o—o) and leucocyte excretion rate (●--●) in a patient receiving placebo tables. The horizontal lines indicate the levels which are usually accepted as the upper limit of normal for bacterial counts (100 000 organisms/ml) and leucocyte excretion rates (400 000 cells/h). Two clinical attacks of pyelonephritis occurred and the patient was treated with 2-week course of sulphamethoxydiazine (0.5 g daily), at the points indicated by arrows. The leucocyte excretion rate and bacterial count ran a closely parallel course, rising to high levels before the onset of symptoms on each occasion and falling steeply when treatment was given. An intravenous pyelogram showed the features of chronic pyelonephritis.

the presence of renal calculi (Table 44.1). A third of the calculi which were demonstrated were causing ureteric obstruction and subsequent renal parenchymal loss [17]. Such calculi can now be successfully removed during pregnancy using percutaneous techniques. In order to avoid severe symptoms during pregnancy due to an infected obstructed kidney and subsequent renal parenchymal loss it is desirable to detect and where possible treat these calculi during pregnancy. Imaging techniques such as ultrasound can be used without fear of harmful effects on the fetus, but there is a need to determine which women with pregnancy bacteriuria are likely to have renal calculi. There is a simple technique which makes this possible. Pyuria almost always accompanies bacteriuria associated with renal calculi. Patients who have renal calculi have an

Table 44.1 Radiographic lesions in 134 patients with pregnancy bacteriura.

Lesion	Number
Reflux nephropathy	27
Renal calculi	10
Duplex system	3
Miscellaneous	16

infection which is not easily eradicated and even when the bacteriuria responds temporarily to treatment the pyuria persists (see Fig. 44.1) and the infection relapses. Such patients should be carefully examined by ultrasound for renal or ureteric calculi.

Because underlying lesions are so frequently encountered in patients with pregnancy bacteriuria we believe that they should all have some form of renal imaging after the pregnancy. We prefer intravenous urography to ultrasonography because of better definition of the lesions. The most frequent lesion seen is reflux nephropathy (see Table 44.1).

Course and management

Clearly in pregnant women with bacteriuria in early pregnancy it should be possible to prevent the development of acute pyelonephritis and this alone is a strong argument for screening for pregnancy bacteriuria. When bacteriuria has been found, a variety of different treatments have been used. In early studies ampicillin, nitrofurantoin and sulphonamides were usually used, and more recently trimethoprim-sulphomethoxazole and amoxycillin are used. The choice of antibiotic is not as important as the disappearance of the bacteriuria. The bacteriuria usually disappears after a short course of treatment [18]. In up to a third of cases the bacteriuria recurs and some of these patients will require continuation of treatment for the remainder of the pregnancy. The relapse of infection during pregnancy provides a marker for those women who have an underlying lesion.

Acute pyelonephritis and renal abscess formation

Although acute pyelonephritis is relatively common and renal abscess formation is now rare, there is recent evidence based on new imaging techniques which suggests that these conditions may represent different stages in the same infective process involving 'lobes' of the renal parenchyma. A discussion of acute pyelonephritis as a 'special' form of urinary tract infection is warranted for two reasons. Acute pyelonephritis is the form of urinary tract infection which occurs in most cases of urinary tract infection in special situations with the exception of recurrent urinary tract infection in adult women. A discussion of acute pyelonephritis is also necessary as an introduction to renal abscess formation.

Acute pyelonephritis

Presentation

The presentation in acute pyelonephritis is with an acute febrile illness in which loin pain may be severe and is usually accompanied by tenderness. The urine shows pyuria and bacteriuria, but there may or may not be symptoms which suggest bladder involvement such as dysuria and frequency. Rigors are common and probably reflect bacteraemia. Other generalized features are common including nausea, vomiting and headache.

Acute pyelonephritis is most frequently seen in young women. In a consecutive series of 164 patients presenting to the emergency department of a major hospital, 142 were women with a mean age of 33 years [19]. A third of these young women showed an abnormality on intravenous urography. Only 22 patients were men and the mean age in the men was 46 years. Two-thirds of the males either had prostatitis or a radiographic abnormality. Reflux nephropathy was the most frequent predisposing abnormality in women and prostatitis the most frequent in men.

Investigations

The most important investigation is examination of the urine. The presence of leucocyte and/or bacterial casts in the urine is virtually diagnostic of parenchymal lesions of acute pyelonephritis. Urine culture most commonly reveals a pure culture of *E. coli*, which is found in 60–80% of cases. Insufficient attention has been paid to unusual and fastidious organisms as a cause of acute febrile pyelonephritis. Fraser *et al.* [19] reported *Ureaplasma urealyticum* as the second most frequent organism present in 5% of cases.

There has recently been increased interest in the use of new imaging techniques to document the extent of renal parenchymal involvement in acute pyelonephritis. Hodson, who made immense contributions to our understanding of renal parenchymal scarring in reflux nephropathy, described computed tomography (CT) appearances of areas of renal parenchymal involvement in acute pyelonephritis which resembled areas which he had previously documented in reflux nephropathy and which he named acute lobar nephronia [20,21].

In two recent studies of adults presenting with acute pyelonephritis, these cortical lesions of acute lobar nephronia have been documented in a high percentage of cases. In Fraser's study, renal parenchymal lesions of acute lobar nephronia were found in 55% of consecutive patients presenting to the emergency department of a major hospital [19]. In a study of patients referred to a nephrology service, which included nine diabetics and four malnourished/alcoholics, Meyrier *et al.* [22] reported similar lesions in 80% of cases. In both series late studies showed some persistent scarring. Only a small number were found in Meyrier's study, but a surprising 77% showed scars 6–12 months after the acute presentation in Fraser's study. There was a strong correlation between the presence of late scars and a particular cultural characteristic, namely suscep-

tibility to the presence of ethylenediamine tetra-acetic acid (EDTA) in the culture medium.

The high incidence of parenchymal lesions in patients with acute pyelonephritis and their persistence as scars in some patients probably indicates that some form of renal imaging should be carried out in acute pyelonephritis to document the extent of renal parenchymal involvement, both in the acute stage and as residual scars. Dimercapto succinic acid (DMSA) nuclear scanning and CT scanning demonstrate the lesions very clearly but they are less well seen on ultrasound scans.

Course and management

Acute pyelonephritis usually warrants admission to hospital and the administration of parenteral antibacterial agents. There is probably little advantage of the newer agents over the standard treatment which has been available for almost 30 years — gentamicin and ampicillin. Some of the newer agents which may be used are listed in Table 44.2; they may have some benefit in terms of side effects. Occasional patients suffer neurotoxicity affecting the 8th cranial nerve from gentamicin therapy. The duration of parenteral treatment of 5–7 days is usually adequate to eradicate infection. The cost of treatment can be considerably reduced by oral medication administered as an outpatient [23]. Stamm demonstrated that this is effective in a selected group of patients and that 2 weeks' oral medication is as effective as 6 weeks' treatment. He also showed that trimethoprim-sulphamethoxazole was significantly more effective than ampicillin. With treatment, the clinical symptoms of acute pyelonephritis resolve within a matter of 3–5 days.

The scars which may develop in the renal parenchyma as a result of acute pyelonephritis are small and probably have little significance in a patient who has one episode of acute pyelonephritis. They will almost certainly prove to have greater significance in recurrent acute pyelonephritis which occurs in the context of an underlying lesion, such as those discussed below. This has not yet been studied, but the reduction in renal size which accompanies acute pyelonephritis when the kidney is obstructed [17] probably represents the effect of extensive parenchymal scarring resulting from multiple areas of acute lobar nephronia.

Renal abscess formation

It is likely that a renal abscess forms in an area of acute lobar nephronia because of late or ineffective treatment or because of an underlying lesion which delays or prevents healing or because the patient is too debilitated to show an adequate response to treatment. Thus instead of healing the lesion progresses and liquefaction occurs.

Table 44.2 Antibiotics of use in acute pyelonephritis.

Pregnant patient	Parenteral therapy with:
	Gentamicin-ampicillin
	Cephtriaxone
	Trimethoprim-sulphamethoxazole
	Aztreonam
Non-pregnant patient (Severe symptoms)	Parenteral therapy with:
	Gentamicin-ampicillin
	Cephtriaxone
	Trimethoprim-sulphamethoxazole
	Aztreonam
	Imipenem-cilastin
	Ciprofloxacin
(Mild symptoms)	Consider oral therapy with:
	Trimethoprim-sulphamethoxazole
	Fluoroquinones

Presentation

The clinical presentation in a patient with a renal abscess is similar to that of acute pyelonephritis except that the symptoms are more severe and last longer. Instead of resolving in a matter of 3–5 days, resolution is slower and takes over a week on adequate management. A renal mass is present in a third of cases and about half the patients have septicaemia.

Investigations

Almost all cases of renal abscess are associated with Gram-negative pathogens, and the haematogenous Gram-positive infections which were more prevalent before adequate antibacterial therapy was available are now rare [24,25].

Although there has been a great interest in the appearance of abscesses with one or other of the new imaging modalities, the appearances which clearly distinguish an abscess from a well-defined area of acute lobar nephronia have not really been spelled out [24,25].

Many patients who develop renal abscesses have an underlying cause, the most frequent being diabetes and renal calculi. They are also more likely to develop in debilitated patients; thus in Meyrier's series of referred cases of acute pyelonephritis (which included diabetics and alcoholics) abscesses were documented, including two in diabetics whose clinical condition was so serious that it demanded nephrectomy. When the kidney was removed it contained abscesses, one being perinephric [22].

It seems likely that the renal abscess results from failure of resolution of an area of acute lobar nephronia which is particularly likely to occur in debilitated subjects or in the presence of obstruction. A perinephric abscess probably represents extension of pus into the perinephric fat in susceptible individuals, particularly those with diabetes or renal calculi.

Treatment

The treatment of renal abscess formation often warrants surgical intervention in addition to the same parenteral antibiotics which are used in acute pyelonephritis (see Table 44.2).

Urinary tract infection in patients with vesicoureteric reflux

There is a wealth of literature documenting the development of renal parenchymal scars in children with vesicoureteric reflux but it is not possible to review much of this extensive data here. There is little doubt that the gross cortical scarring previously called chronic atrophic pyelonephritis occurs as a result of a combination of vesicoureteric reflux in association with infection during early childhood [26]. Progressive scar formation is only occasionally recorded in older children and has not been clearly documented in adults, although it is possible that some of the focal scars discussed above which develop in acute pyelonephritis are associated with vesicoureteric reflux.

The benefit derived from surgical correction of vesicoureteric reflux to prevent further parenchymal scarring in childhood has recently been examined in two large prospective randomized controlled trials [27,28]. In neither study was there evidence that surgical correction of vesicoureteric reflux reduced subsequent scar formation. There was also no benefit in terms of better renal function or renal growth which could be attributed to surgical correction of vesicoureteric reflux.

Presentation

Children or adults with persistent vesicoureteric reflux who develop urinary tract infection are likely to present with symptoms and signs of acute pyelonephritis.

Investigations

The investigations are as for other patients with acute pyelonephritis. In view of the frequency of scar formation in children with vesicoureteric reflux, particular attention should be paid to the appearances of the renal parenchyma using newer imaging techniques. DMSA nuclear scanning has been widely used and is more appropriate in children than techniques such as CT scanning which involves exposure to irradiation.

Course and management

One very positive result of the large randomized controlled trials [27,28] was the demonstration that it is possible to virtually eradicate the risk of progressive scar formation in children using a small prophylactic dose of trimethoprim-sulphamethoxazole to prevent urinary tract infection. This is the recommended management at this time. Episodes of acute pyelonephritis should be treated as outlined above.

Urinary tract infection associated with ureteric calculi and other forms of obstruction

Ureteric calculi are the most frequent lesions encountered as a cause of ureteric obstruction and an infected obstructed kidney.

Presentation

The clinical features are those of a severe acute pyelonephritis which does not resolve when treated with antibacterial drugs alone. Although renal colic may be part of the presenting symptomatology it is often not present.

Investigations

When acute pyelonephritis does not respond promptly to appropriate antibacterial treatment, obstruction should be suspected and it should be the aim of investigations to detect the site and nature of the obstruction. Ultrasound is a quick non-invasive method which will usually, but not always, demonstrate dilatation of the ureter and pelvis above the obstruction. It may give a complete diagnosis or may need to be used in conjunction with other imaging techniques such as CT scanning.

Course and management

Once the cause of the ureteric obstruction is removed the infection will respond to appropriate treatment. The method used will vary with the nature of the obstruction, but most ureteric calculi can now be removed without open surgery and a number of other obstructive lesions can also be treated by percutaneous techniques. The management of infection stones is discussed below.

Persistent urinary tract infection associated with urological abnormalities

Stamey has drawn attention to a group of urological abnormalities which are associated with persistence of the same organism after appropriate treatment with antibacterial drugs [29]. He points out that this group of conditions includes all those in which a cure of infection can be achieved by surgical correction. Table 44.3 sets out the list of these conditions. The most frequent and most important is the so-called infection stone. It is not within the scope of this chapter to discuss the surgical management of many of

Table 44.3 Urological abnormalities associated with urinary tract infection, in which infection can be treated by surgical correction. Modified from [29].

Infected renal calculi
Chronic bacterial prostatitis
Unilateral infected reflux nephropathy
Infected pericalyceal diverticuli
Infected non-refluxing ureteric stump
Medullary sponge kidneys
Infected necrotic papillae
Infected urachal cysts
Vesicovaginal fistulas
Vesicointestinal fistulas
Ectopic ureter draining dysplastic renal segment
Foreign bodies

the conditions listed in Table 44.3, but infection stones and renal papillary necrosis will be discussed below.

Infection stones

Infection stones are struvite calculi which develop in the urinary tract in the presence of urea-splitting organisms, most frequently *Proteus mirabilis*. They can grow very rapidly and tend to fill the pelvis—the staghorn calculus—or the bladder.

Presentation

Patients with renal infection stones present with recurrent episodes of acute pyelonephritis. They show only a temporary response to appropriate antibacterial treatment because the infection is present within the stone and recurs as soon as treatment is stopped.

Course and management

This is one of the most important forms of urinary tract infection to be treated effectively by eradicating the infection and the calculus. The infection cannot be cured unless the calculus is removed or dissolved. Neglect of such patients leads to end-stage renal failure due to a combination of the effects of relative obstruction by the growth of the calculus around the calyces, which it eventually compresses, and by lesions of acute pyelonephritis on the renal parenchyma.

There are now many techniques for eradicating infection stones without open surgery which, in the case of a large staghorn calculus, was previously a serious operation which sometimes resulted in nephrectomy. Infection and recurrent stone formation recurs rapidly after removal or lithotripsy unless all the fragments are dealt with and as the fragments may be very small and adherent to the pelvic mucosa it may be impossible to remove them without using a method for dissolving the fragments. Renacidin, a compound introduced in 1959 [30] for the dissolution of struvite calculi, fell into disrepute because it was used under pressure and in the presence of infection. Stamey [31] reintroduced the technique of infusion of renacidin into the renal pelvis under strictly controlled pressure and with a urine maintained sterile by the use of antibacterial treatment. He reported excellent results [31] in terms of eradicating infection and small fragments of stone and preventing recurrence of the calculus; we can confirm similar results. Without renacidin infusion it is difficult to eradicate infection and the calculus thus recurs rapidly unless continuous full or 'suppressive' doses of antibacterial agents are used. The author was recently shown a patient who was about to be treated for the fourth time for a recurrent staghorn calculus after lithotripsy. These recurrent calculi could clearly have been prevented by using renacidin and eradicating infection.

Renal papillary necrosis

Renal papillary necrosis occurs in association with urinary tract infection mainly in two clinical contexts: analgesic nephropathy and diabetes.

Analgesic nephropathy

Analgesic nephropathy is a chronic form of renal papillary necrosis associated with abuse of 'over the counter' mixed analgesic compounds. It has almost disappeared from countries where sale of these compounds has been restricted, such as Scandinavia and Australia, but is still common in some countries where no such restrictions apply. A very similar lesion is seen in association with prolonged use of non-steroidal anti-inflammatory drugs.

Presentation

The patient is typically a middle-aged or elderly woman, with only one in five patients being male. There may be associated clinical features of the so-called analgesic syndrome, including psychiatric disorders, and peptic ulceration. In addition to renal papillary necrosis such patients may, after 20–30 years of heavy analgesic intake develop urothelial malignancies. The patient may present with macroscopic haematuria arising from the necrotic papillae (or an associated malignancy) but most commonly presents with recurrent intractable acute pyelonephritis which recurs rapidly after appropriate treatment. Infection is present within the necrotic debris in the pelvis and cannot be cured until the process of active papillary necrosis ceases. Gradual recovery occurs after cessation of analgesic (or non-steroidal anti-inflammatory drug) intake.

Investigations

The urine shows heavy pyuria which may at times appear to be sterile, but it is usual for relapse to occur with the same organism which is voided in the urine, which can also be cultured from papillary tissue . Sections of this papillary material provides the most secure diagnosis. However, the radiological appearances are characteristic [32]. In cases with urothelial malignancies, these are usually seen on the intravenous urogram but may require CT scanning. In cases associated with non-steroidal anti-inflammatory drugs the diagnosis may be more difficult because the radiographic features are not present because the papillae do not become detached. CT scans may, however, be helpful in confirming the diagnosis. Renal function is usually impaired and hypertension is usually present and may be severe. Intermittent obstruction may occur by papillae passing down the ureter. Such patients may die of septicaemia secondary to the infected obstructed kidney.

Course and management

If the analgesic or other drug intake ceases the papillary necrosis usually resolves and the pyuria and infection can be eradicated by antibacterial drugs. If drug intake continues renal function deteriorates to end-stage renal failure.

Diabetic renal papillary necrosis

Although occasionally nectrotic papillae may separate and pass down the ureter in diabetics with renal papillary necrosis, more commonly renal papillary necrosis in diabetes is an acute terminal event often associated with severe urinary tract infection and with acute renal failure.

Urinary tract infection in cystic disorders of the kidney

Autosomal dominant polycystic disease of the kidney

Urinary tract infection is a major clinical feature in this disorder. Infection is common and may be complicated and difficult to eradicate.

Presentation

Women with autosomal dominant polycystic disease of the kidney (ADPK) are much more likely than men to have urinary tract infection. Women with ADPK may have asymptomatic urinary tract infection or symptomatic cystitis, as may other women in the community. However, they often present with symptoms and signs of acute pyelonephritis which may be severe and difficult to eradicate once it is present within a cyst.

Renal calculi are a common complication of ADPK and these are often infection stones.

Investigations

Examination of the urine often reveals a sterile pyuria composed of mainly polymorphonuclear leucocytes in asymptomatic patients, but in those with symptoms of acute pyelonephritis the organism can usually be cultured from the urine and sometimes also from the blood. Renal function may deteriorate abruptly when a cyst enlarges and causes ureteric deviation or obstruction, as may occur with infection.

Management

The two drugs which are commonly used to treat acute pyelonephritis (gentamicin and ampicillin) penetrate cysts poorly. Lipid soluble drugs are more effective at penetrating cyst fluid. Drugs which are effective against most urinary tract pathogens and which penetrate cysts well are ciprofoxacin, norfloxacin, trimethoprim-sulphamethoxazole and chloram-phenicol. Treatment should be continued for 2 weeks [33].

Medullary sponge kidney

Urinary tract infection is a common manifestation in patients with medullary sponge kidney. Other clinical features include haematuria and renal calculi. Stamey [29] lists this as a cause of persistent bacterial infection and showed that the persistent infection was in a unilateral medullary sponge kidney and was cured by nephrectomy. We have not found medullary sponge kidney to be associated with persistent bacterial infection but have observed evidence of parenchymal involvement and destruction by lesions of acute pyelonephritis. Ekstrom [34] reviewed the clinical feature in patients with medullary sponge kidneys and stated that only 11% developed chronic pyelonephritis. All five cases which the author has personally seen at autopsy, including one young woman, showed scars radiating out from the area of the medullary 'cysts'. These scars resembled the parenchymal lesions which develop in scars following acute pyelonephritis.

Urinary tract infection in neurogenic disorders

Very high pressures may be generated within the bladder in a variety of neurogenic disorders, probably through the mechanism of detrusor hyperreflexia and contraction against a closed sphincter [35]. In the presence of infection and indeed perhaps due to high pressure without infection,

scars develop which are identical to those seen in reflux nephropathy.

Presentation

Symptoms are usually those of acute pyelonephritis in patients with neurogenic bladder disorders.

Investigations

Vesicoureteric reflux has been demonstrated in a high percentage of patients with neurogenic disorders [36]. Investigations should probably include a micturating cystourethrogram and cystometric studies to determine the voiding pressure. These patients are at a high risk of developing progressive renal parenchymal scars and infection stones; in 12% of cases infection stones are formed within 3 years of developing the neurogenic disorder [37].

Course and management

Patients with neurogenic disorders are very likely to develop urinary tract infection because of bladder catheterization and instrumentation. In patients with acute spinal injuries the closed drainage bag is the usual source of infections. Maizels and Schaeffer [38] were able to prevent the occurrence of this infection by intermittent instillation of hydrogen peroxide into the drainage bag. Pearman and England [39] achieved a very low rate of infection in paraplegic patients by instillation of kanamycin 150 mg and colistin 30 mg through the bladder catheter.

Episodes of acute pyelonephritis in adults with neurogenic disorders may be followed by large coarse focal scar formation similar in appearance to that seen in children with vesicoureteric reflux.

The combination of urinary tract infection, renal parenchymal scars and infection stones in these patients place them at high risk of deterioration to end-stage renal failure. Many are now entering dialysis programmes in spite of the fact that it should be possible to prevent deterioration if infection is controlled.

Urinary tract diversion procedures

Urinary tract diversion procedures such as an ileal loop or other form of pouch are commonly carried out in patients with high bladder pressures, including children with myelodysplasia. Urinary tract infection remains a very frequent occurrence in these patients even when the pressure has been reduced in this way.

Presentation

Continuing infection with high bacterial counts and

leucocyte counts in the urine are very frequent in patients with diversion of the urinary tract. Intermittent episodes of acute pyelonephritis occur and can be severely debilitating and eventually constitute a threat to renal function. Infection stones also commonly develop and grow and cause obstruction further threatening renal function.

Investigations

It is relatively easy to image the urinary tract by passing a catheter into the ileum and performing a retrograde study with contrast medium. If the urine constantly shows infection resistant to treatment, stones should be sought; CT scans may be necessary because of the anatomical distortion which exists in the skeletal system in some patients.

Course and management

Recurrent episodes of acute pyelonephritis in some of these patients can be very debilitating. It may be possible to prevent these with low-dose prophylactic treatment with trimethroprim-sulphamethoxazole but even in the absence of documented infection stones or other sources of recurrent or persistent infection it may be necessary to use long-term full-dose suppressive treatment. On the positive side this may transform the lives of these individuals and prevent the deterioration of renal function which otherwise seems inevitable.

Urinary tract infection in renal transplant recipients

Urinary tract infection may be introduced at the time of the transplant operation by infection of the donor kidney or by catheterization [40]. Screening for urinary tract infection in transplant recipients has revealed infection in about half of the patients [41]. Catheter infections can be reduced by closed drainage and by the use of agents such as chlorhexidine in the bag [42].

Presentation

Urinary tract infection after renal transplantation is often asymptomatic; however, it should be sought on a routine basis and treated because it may cause severe acute pyelonephritis which may occasionally be life-threatening. We have encountered particular problems in patients with polycystic disease where recurrent episodes have been sufficiently bad to warrant removal of the polycystic kidneys.

Course and management

In general, urinary tract infections do not constitute a serious problem after transplantation if the patients are monitored and infection is eradicated when it is detected.

There has been considerable interest in cytomegalovirus (CMV) infection which commonly occurs after renal transplantation. Richardson *et al.* [43] described a glomerulopathy associated with CMV infection and it has been suggested that this is associated with declining renal function [44]. CMV infection can now be prevented with a solution of anti-CMV immunoglobulin which has been used with success in heart, bone marrow and renal transplants [45].

Xanthogranulomatous pyelonephritis and malacoplakia

These two conditions may be different manifestations of the same process. The lesions are in some respects similar. Both lesions are most commonly seen in middle-aged women and there is an association with urinary tract infection in both. Xanthogranulomatous pyelonephritis is being reported with increasing frequency, perhaps as a result of the more widespread use of newer imaging techniques. It is usually associated with infection stones and with a urea-splitting organism.

Presentation

Both conditions present with loin pain, malaise and a renal mass with or without fever.

Investigations

These are mainly aimed at defining the extent of the lesions because surgical removal has been the treatment most frequently used. Lesions may be bilateral. The final diagnosis depends on typical pathological findings and again there are similarities in the two conditions. Both lesions consist essentially of foam-filled macrophages. In the case of malacoplakia, the cells contain a distinctive inclusion body called a Michaelis–Gutmann body, a lamellar structure which contains iron and stains prominently with the periodic Schiff stain.

References

1 Stamey TA. The role of introitial enterobacteria in recurrent urinary tract infections. *J Urol* 1973;**109**:467.
2 Guttman D. Follow-up of urinary tract infection in domiciliary patients. In: Brumfitt W, Asscher AW, eds. *Urinary Tract Infection.* Proceedings of the Second National Symposium, London, 1972. London: Oxford Univer-sity Press, 1973:62.
3 Fair WR, McClennan BL, Jost RG. Are excretory urograms necessary in evaluating women with urinary tract infection? *J Urol* 1979;**121**:131.
4 Mabeck CE. Treatment of uncomplicated urinary tract

infection in non-pregnant women. *Post Grad Med J* 1972; **48**:69.

5 Stamey TA, Condy M, Mihara G. Prophylactic effect of nitrofurantoin macrocrystals and trimethoprim-sulpha-methoxazole in urinary infections. *N Engl Med J* 1977; **296**:780.

6 Stamey TA. *The Pathogenesis and Treatment of Urinary Tract Infections*. Baltimore: Williams and Wilkins, 1980:156.

7 Kass EH. The role of asymptomatic bacteriuria in the patho-genesis of pyelonephritis. In: Quinn EL, Kass EH, eds. *Biology of Pyelonephritis*. Boston: Little, Brown, 1960:399.

8 Kass EH. Hormones and host resistance to infection. *Bacteriol Rev* 1960;**24**:177.

9 Kincaid-Smith P, Bullen M. Bacteriuria in pregnancy. *Lancet* 1965;**1**:395–9.

10 Kincaid-Smith P. Bacteriuria and urinary tract infection in pregnancy. *Clin Obst Gynecol* 2968;**11**:533–49.

11 Whaley PJ, Martin FG, Peters PC. Significance of asymp-tomatic bacteriuria detected during pregnancy. *J Am Med Assoc* 1965;**193**:897.

12 Fairley KF, Bond AG, Adey FD. The site of infection in pregnancy bacteriuria. *Lancet* 1966;**1**:939–41.

13 Fairley KF. The routine determination of the site of infection in the investigation of patients with urinary tract infection. In: Kincaid-Smith P, Fairley KF, eds. *Renal Infection and Renal Scarring*. Melbourne: Mercedes Publishing, 1971:107–16.

14 Asscher AW, Sussman M, Waters WE *et al*. The clinical signifi-cance of asymptomatic bacteriuria in the non-pregnant woman. *J Infect Dis* 1969;**120**:17.

15 Eykyn SJ, McFadyen IR. Supra-pubic aspiration of urine in pregnancy. In: O'Grady F, Brumfitt W, eds. *Urinary Tract Infection*. London: Oxford University Press, 1968:141.

16 Kincaid-Smith PO. Bacteriuria in pregnancy. In: Kass EH, ed. *Progress in Pyelonephritis*. Philadelphia: Davis, 1965:11–16.

17 Bullen, M, Kincaid-Smith P. Asymptomatic pregnancy bac-teriuria—a follow-up study 4–7 years after delivery. In: Kincaid-Smith P, Fairley KF, eds. *Renal Infection and Renal Scarring*. Melbourne: Mercedes Publishing, 1971:33–9.

18 Williams JD, Brumfitt W, Leigh D, Percival A. Eradication of bacteriuria by a short course of chemotherapy. *Lancet* 1965; **1**:831.

19 Fraser IR, Birch D, Fairley KF *et al*. A prospective study of cortical scarring in acute febrile pyelonephritis in adults: clinical and bacteriological characteristics. *Clin Nephrol* 1995;43:159–64.

20 Hodson CJ. The pathogenesis of reflux nephropathy. In: Margulis AR, Gooding CA, eds. *Diagnostic Radiology*. San Francisco: University of California, 1978:95–107.

21 Rosenfield AT, Glickman MG, Taylor JW, Crade M, Hodson J. Acute focal bacterial nephritis (acute lobar nephronia). *Radiology* 1979;**132**:553–61.

22 Meyrier A, Condamin M, Fernet M *et al*. Frequency of development of early cortical scarring in acute primary pyelonephritis. *Kidney Int* 1989;**35**:696–703.

23 Stamm W, McKevitt M, Counts G. Acute renal infection in women: treatment with trimethoprim-sulfamethoxazole or ampicillin for two or six weeks. *Ann Intern Med* 1987;**106**: 341–5.

24 Morgan W, Rand M, Nyberg L. Perinephric and intrarenal abscess. *Urology* 1985;**26**:529–33.

25 June CH, Browning MD, Smith P *et al*. Ultrasonography and computed tomography in severe urinary tract infection. *Arch Intern Med* 1985;**145**:841–5.

26 Smellie JM, Hodson J, Edwards D, Normand ICS. Clinical and radiological features of urinary infection in childhood. *Br Med J* 1964;**2**:1222–6.

27 Birmingham Reflux Study Group. A prospective trial of operative versus non operative treatment of severe vesico-ureteric reflux: 5 years observation. *Br Med J* 1987;**295**:237.

28 Weiss R, Duckett J, Spitzer A (on behalf of the International Reflux Study in Children). Results of a randomized clinical trial of medical versus surgical management of infants and children with grades III and IV primary vesicoureteric reflux. *J Urol* 1992;**148**:1667–73.

29 Stamey TA. *The Pathogenesis and Treatment of Urinary Tract Infections*. Baltimore: Williams and Wilkins, 1980.

30 Mulvaney WP. The clinical use of renacidin in urinary calcifications. *J Urol* 1960;**84**:206.

31 Nemoy NH, Stamey TA. Use of hemiacidrin in the manage-ment of infection stones. *J Urol* 1976;**116**:693.

32 Dawborn JK, Fairley KF, Kincaid-Smith P, King WE. The association of peptic ulceration, chronic renal disease and analgesic abuse. *Q J Med* 1966;**35**(137):69–83.

33 Bennett WE. General features of autosomal dominant polysystic disease of the kidney: evaluation and management of renal infection. In: Grantham JJ, Gardner KD, eds. *Problems in the Diagnosis*. Polycystic Kidney Research Foundation, 1985:98–105.

34 Ekstrom T, Engfeld B, Langergren C. *Medullary Sponge Kidney*. Stockholm: Almquist and Wiksill, 1959.

35 Arnold EP, Fukui J, Anthony A, Utley WLF. Bladder function following spinal cord injury: a urodynamic analysis of out-come. *Br J Urol* 1984;**56**:172–7.

36 Damanski M. Vesico-ureteric reflux in paraplegics. *Br J Surg* 1965;**52**:168–77.

37 Jacobson SA, Bors E. Spinal cord injury in Vietnamese combat. *Paraplegia* 1970;**7**:263.

38 Maizels M, Schaeffer AJ. Decreased incidence of bacteriuria associated with periodic instillations of hydrogen peroxide into the urethral catheter drainage bag. *J Urol* 1980;**123**:841–5.

39 Pearman JW, England EJ. *The Urological Management of the Patient Following Spinal Cord Injury*. Springfield: Charles C Thomas, 1973.

40 Douglas JF, Clarke S, Kennedy J. Late urinary tract infection after renal transplantation. *Lancet* 1974;**2**:1015.

41 Ramsay DE, Finch WT, Birch AG. Urinary tract infections in kidney transplant recipients. *Arch Surg* 1979;**114**:1022–5.

42 Clark AD, Crossley J. Closed system bladder irrigation and drainage afer major vaginal surgery. *Br J Obstet Gynaecol* 1973;**80**:271–3.

43 Richardson WP, Colvin RS, Cheesman SH *et al*. Glomerulo-pathy associated with cytomegalovirus viraemia in renal allografts. *N Engl J Med* 1981;**305**:57–63.

44 Luby JP, Ware A, Hull AR *et al*. Disease due to cytomegalovirus and its long term consequences in renal transplant recipients. *Arch Intern Med* 1983;**143**:1126–9.

45 Fassbinder W, Ernst W, Hanke P *et al*. Cytomegalovirus infections after renal transplantation. Effect of a prophylactic hyperimmunoglobulin. *Transplant Proc* 1986;**XVII**:1393–6.

45 Infections of the Kidney

G.A.Farrow

Introduction

Infections of the kidney are secondary to infections of the lower urinary tract. Because the normal adult kidney is remarkably resistant to infection, most cases of lower urinary infection or uncomplicated bacteriuria do not progress to upper tract infection, in part because of the abundant vascularity of the kidney and in part due to the effect of unobstructed urine output [1,2]. Also, the majority of those acute infections that do develop in the mature kidney resolve promptly with antimicrobial therapy leaving minimal or no residual scarring or functional impairment. However, several factors listed in Table 45.1 predispose the kidney to the development of bacterial infections. These factors also impair the resolution of established acute pyelonephritis leading to further complicated acute or chronic processes discussed below (Table 45.2).

Factors that predispose the kidney to infection

1 *Bacteriuria.* Bacteria must always be present to initiate acute pyelonephritis as an ascending infection. The nature and incidence of bacteriuria is discussed in Chapters 41 and 43 [3,4].
2 *Diabetes.* Diabetes particularly renders the kidney susceptible to infections and impedes the resolution of established infections. Multiple factors in the diabetic which predispose the kidney to the development and

Table 45.1 Factors predisposing to renal infection.

Bacteriuria
Diabetes
Urinary obstruction
Stone disease
Vesicoureteric reflux
Pregnancy
Analgesic nephropathy
Urate nephropathy
Immunosuppression
General debilitation

Table 45.2 Renal complications of acute pyelonephritis.

Chronic pyelonephritis
Perinephric abscess
Renal abscess
Renal papillary necrosis
Emphysematous pyelonephritis
Xanthogranulomatous pyelonephritis
Pyonephrosis

progression of infection are outlined in Table 45.3 [5,6]. Glucose is a nutrient for bacteria, and glycosuria promotes the concentration of bacteria within the urine and kidney. Diabetes causes dysfunction of inflammatory cells with impaired ability of leucocytes to neutralize and localize bacterial infection [7]. Small vessel disease with impairment of blood supply promotes ischaemia, affects the inflammatory process and inhibits the ability of antibiotics to penetrate the infection. Neuropathic vesical dysfunction in diabetes leads to poor bladder emptying and stasis.
3 *Urinary obstruction.* Urinary obstruction with impaired drainage leads to stasis and bacterial proliferation. Increased pressure within the calyces also promotes colonization of the collecting ducts with bacteria.
4 *Stone disease.* Urinary calculi in the presence or absence of obstruction lead to the inherent colonization of the stones by resistant organisms inaccessible to antibiotics despite high blood and urine concentration of these drugs.
5 *Vesicoureteric reflux.* The incidence of infections of the kidney is increased in patients with vesicoureteric reflux. The significance of intrarenal reflux of infected urine in the development of renal infection and renal scarring is discussed in Chapter 17.

Table 45.3 Factors in diabetes predisposing to renal infection.

Direct effect of glucose
Dysfunction of inflammatory cells
Small vessel disease
Neuropathic bladder function

6 *Pregnancy.* Although the incidence of bacteriuria is not increased in pregnancy in relation to the non-pregnant woman, the urinary stasis associated with pregnancy increases the incidence of pyelonephritis.

Other renal and general factors predisposing the kidney to the development or progression of infection are analgesic nephropathy, urate nephropathy, immunosuppression and general debilitation.

Acute pyelonephritis

Acute pyelonephritis is an acute bacterial tubulo-interstitial infection of the kidney and renal pelvis secondary to lower urinary tract infection or bacteriuria. It is a clinical diagnosis presenting with fever, flank pain and costovertebral angle tenderness.

Aetiology and pathogenesis

The bacteria responsible for pyelonephritis are of the same spectrum as organisms causing bacteriuria (Table 45.4). *Escherichia coli*, which normally colonizes the bowel, is the most common urinary tract pathogen making up 90% of non-hospital-acquired infections [8]. There are many hundreds of strains of *E. coli*. *Klebsiella* is also normally found in faecal flora, but in significantly lesser numbers than *E. coli*, and accounts for less than 10% of community-acquired infections. *Proteus* is present in approximately 25% of normal bowel flora and accounts for 5% of non-hospital-acquired infections. *P. mirabilis* is more common than *P. vulgaris* and is the most common organism associated with chronically infected stones [9]. Those infections acquired in the hospital setting or associated with chronic colonization of the urinary tract are caused by more resistant organisms.

Certain strains of *E. coli* contain pili or fimbriae on their surface, called adhesins, which promote binding to receptors on the host urothelial cell. These organisms appear to have a special propensity for infecting the kidney, with apparent increased bacterial virulence [10].

The organisms reach the renal pelvis as an ascending

Table 45.4 Bacteriology of urinary tract infections.

Escherichia coli
Klebsiella
Proteus mirabilis
Proteus vulgaris
Enterobacter aerogenes
Enterobacter cloacae
Providentia
Serratia
Pseudomonas
Staphylococcus aureus
Streptococcus faecalis

infection from the lower urinary tract. There is colonization of the renal pelvis, collecting ducts, tubules and interstitium of the renal parenchyma. Marked congestion and oedema results in enlargement of the kidney; however, the process is often patchy with intervening areas of uninvolved parenchyma. A polymorphonuclear infiltrate involves the tubules and interstitium of the medulla and rapidly affects the cortex of the involved medullary region. Tubules may contain large numbers of neutrophils, and local release of cytotoxins directly affects tubular epithelium. As the process progresses, microabscess formation develops. The glomeruli are usually spared unless there is extensive necrosis or complicated infection [11].

Immunological response to infection

Bacterial infections of the kidney stimulate both humeral and cellular immune responses. Antibodies are detected in both the serum and urine which react with bacteria-specific antigen [12]. Studies suggest there may be an increased level of antibody in the serum in infections of the kidney when compared to infections of the lower urinary tract [13,14]. In view of this immunological response, there is a great deal of interest in creating active immunization against *E. coli* for the prevention of pyelonephritis.

As previously discussed, the immune response is in part directed against the pili or adhesins on the surface of *E. coli* which have a propensity to infect the kidney. As a result, there has been considerable effort devoted to developing a pilus vaccine for immunization against pyelonephritis. [10,15]. This has been successful to a degree in animal experiments, however, at the present time is not clinically practical [16].

Immunological factors have also been implicated in the development of chronic pyelonephritis. It has been suggested that the renal scarring in chronic pyelonephritis may be related to a cell-mediated leucocyte response as opposed to a humeral response; however, this evidence is not convincing [11].

Diagnosis

Acute pyelonephritis presents classically in the female with fever, chills, flank pain and tenderness associated with lower urinary tract symptoms of urgency and dysuria. The spectrum of severity of clinical findings is variable, ranging from mild flank discomfort and progressing to symptoms and signs of Gram-negative sepsis. Bacteriuria, pyuria, white blood cell casts, leucocytosis and positive urine culture are present. White blood cell casts can develop with any parenchymal inflammation; however, if they are associated with positive urine culture they generally indicate kidney infection, and bacteria found within the casts are diagnositic of pyelonephritis. Renal function is generally normal unless the condition is bilateral. Bacteraemia is frequently present.

Radiology

Acute pyelonephritis is generally a clinical diagnosis, particularly in early and uncomplicated stages, and radiological investigation is usually normal. Imaging is helpful in patients who are unresponsive to initial treatment and are developing complications [17–19]. The intraveneous pyelogram is initially normal but may reveal an enlarged kidney with decreased contrast excretion as a result of impaired tubular function from inflammation or compression of collecting ducts. A non-obstructive dilatation of the collecting system develops which is related to the direct effect of bacterial toxins. Calyceal compression from congestion and oedema occurs infrequently.

Ultrasound is usually normal apart from enlargement. Patchy decreased echogenicity compared to the normal kidney is sometimes present. This becomes more evident as the severity of the condition progresses with micro-abscess formation. A computed tomography (CT) scan is usually also normal. Contrast-enhanced CT scans provide excellent resolution of the renal parenchyma and are very sensitive to inflammatory change. There may be renal enlargement and the involved tissue may demonstrate decreased enhancement which is disorganized and inhomogeneous in more advanced cases.

Localization of infection

Several special techniques which localize the site of infection to the upper urinary tract are listed in Table 45.5. The ureteric catheterization method described by Stamey and the bladder wash-out test described by Fairley, isolate positive cultures to the upper urinary tract but have very limited clinical significance and are useful primarily as research tools. Aside from the direct testing methods of Stamey and Fairley, these studies are either clinically unreliable or non-specific [13,20–22].

Management

Early diagnosis with immediate antimicrobial treatment reduces the severity and morbidity of the process. Urine and blood cultures are obtained before instituting therapy. Parenteral antibiotics and supportive measures including hydration, bed rest and analgesics generally lead to rapid resolution of symptoms in uncomplicated infections. Treatment is modified according to the results of cultures and the clinical response. Relief of any obstructive uropathy is essential. A combination of aminoglycoside and ampicillin is effective as an initial choice of drugs. In non-hospital-acquired infections, third-generation cephalo-

Table 45.5 Tests to localize the site of infection.

Stamey ureteric catheterization method
Fairley bladder wash-out method
Thomas antibody-coated bacteria test
Elevated serum antibody levels
Presence of antibodies to Tam–Horsfall protein
Impaired renal concentrating ability
Urinary lactate dehydrogenase
C-reactive protein

sporins are effective, and oral fluoroquinolones are useful for patients whose infections do not warrant hospitalization. Where blood cultures are positive, parenteral treatment should be maintained for 7–10 days. All cases of pyelonephritis should receive full doses of antimicrobial therapy for 1–2 weeks.

Most patients have a gradual clinical response after 2–3 days. If symptoms persist, complicating factors should be considered and appropriate investigation instituted. It is essential to monitor the infection with urine cultures 1 week after initiating treatment and 4–6 weeks after stopping treatment. Subsequent urinary infections are common in women who have had acute pyelonephritis.

Complications

Acute pyelonephritis associated with predisposing factors may be refractory to treatment. Particulary in the presence of obstructive uropathy and/or diabetes, pyelonephritis may progress to perirenal abscess, renal abscess, papillary necrosis, emphysematous pyelonephritis and xanthogranulomatous pyelonephritis. Each of these is discussed below. Rarely, acute pyelonephritis may develop into chronic atrophic pyelonephritis with coarse renal scarring.

Chronic pyelonephritis

Chronic pyelonephritis refers to the late effects of chronic tubulointerstitial infection producing focal coarse scarring or diffuse atrophic scarring of the kidney. The ambiguity and controversy surrounding this condition occurs because of two factors.

1 Pathologically the picture is similar to the end stage of other chronic interstitial conditions, including reflux nephropathy and interstitial nephritis.

2 Chronic pyelonephritis is frequently diagnosed radiologically with no previous history of infection and no evidence of active infection.

Pathology and pathogenesis

The classic morphological picture is that of coarse interstitial scarring overlying dilated calyces with atrophic papillae producing a deeply contracted renal surface. The scars are multiple, bilateral and asymmetrical, usually involving the upper and lower pole calyces [11]. Acute pyelonephritis rarely causes chronic renal scarring in the otherwise normal urinary system. The changes of chronic pyelonephritis usually, therefore, occur in infancy, presumably in the immature kidney or associated with vesicoureteral reflux (see Chapter 17).

Histologically there is interstitial fibrosis and chronic inflammation with lymphocytes and plasma cells. There is tubular atrophy with cystic dilatation of tubules containing casts creating the so-called thyroidization of chronic pyelonephritis. Sclerosis of vessels is present but the glomeruli are not affected. Periglomerular fibrosis may occur in advanced cases. Focal patchy disease overlying calyces with intervening normal parenchyma is characteristic of chronic pyelonephritis. Where the condition is more diffuse, creating a chronic atrophic kidney, it is impossible to differentiate it from other chronic end-stage diseases.

Presentation

Chronic renal scarring following acute pyelonephritis in the normal kidney occurs very infrequently and persistent bacteriuria is usually absent. Pyuria, proteinuria and occasional white blood cell casts are present. Impaired renal function with early loss of concentrating ability occurs and rarely, in advanced stages, renal failure develops [21].

Radiology

The kidneys are decreased in size and have coarse contracted scars overlying dilated or clubbed calyces with atrophic papillae. As described pathologically, these scars are multiple, asymmetrical, commonly involve the polar calyces and may be unilateral or bilateral. The intervening normal parenchyma may undergo compensatory hypertrophy creating a pseudo-tumour effect [18,23].

Management

Treatment is directed to eradicating residual infection and resolving underlying predisposing factors. When uncomplicated chronic pyelonephritis with focal or diffuse scarring is discovered in the adult, bacteriuria is usually absent and active urinary infection is not documented. These patients are susceptible to silent infection, however, and must be monitored on a regular basis. Further management depends on the degree of renal damage.

Perinephric abscess

Perinephric abscess is a collection of pus within the Gerota space between the renal capsule and the perirenal fascia.

Aetiology and pathogenesis

This localized infection characteristically occurs in susceptible hosts with predisposing conditions. Perinephric abscess progresses from a localized renal infection situated in the subcapsular parenchyma. Diabetes, stone or urinary obstruction in the presence of associated urinary infection are present in most cases of perinephric abscess. This condition rarely progresses from uncomplicated pyelonephritis [24,25]. Historically, perinephric abscess in the preantibiotic era was caused by *Staphylococcus aureus* bacteraemia from cutaneous or other sites. *E. coli* and *P. mirabilis* are the most common infecting agents while *S. aureus* rarely may be the cause in specific situations (such as intravenous drug abuse).

Diagnosis

Perinephric abscess usually presents with fever, chills and pain localized to the abdomen or flank. As opposed to the rapid course of acute pyelonephritis, this process often begins in a subacute fashion and may progress over a period of several weeks. General features of fatigue, malaise and loss of appetite and weight often complicate the clinical picture. Tenderness and mass may be present on palpation. Laboratory investigation reveals elevated white blood cell count, elevated sedimentation rate and positive urine culture. Positive blood culture is frequently present. Blood urea nitrogen may be elevated, but renal function is generally normal in the presence of a normal contralateral kidney.

Radiology

Ultrasound and CT scans have greatly improved the early diagnosis of perinephric abscesses [17,26]. Ultrasound reveals enlargement of the kidney with irregular complex collections of varying size containing internal debris and septations confined within the perirenal fascia. Gas is often present and is diagnostic of abscess formation. An adjacent subcapsular renal abscess may be present. Urinary calculi or obstructive uropathy may be demonstrated. A CT scan is generally diagnostic, outlining the location and extent of the abscess, the degree of loculation and the relation to kidney and surrounding tissue.

An intravenous pyelogram may be normal or may demonstrate impairment or non-function of the kidney, perirenal mass, perirenal gas and non-mobility of the kidney. Distortion or displacement of the collecting system occurs if there is an associated intrarenal abscess and pre-existing obstruction will be demonstrated.

A chest X-ray may demonstrate pleural effusion, an elevated diaphragm and atelectasis of the lower lobe of the lung. A plain film of the abdomen may reveal absent psoas margin, loss of renal outline, a mass and retroperitoneal gas formation. A radioopaque calculus may be seen.

Management

Treatment consists of antibiotic therapy and drainage of the abscess as soon as the diagnosis is made. Control of predisposing factors (i.e. diabetes, urinary obstruction or stone disease) is essential. Drainage is performed through a flank incision taking care to open and remove all loculations of pus with blunt finger dissection. Care must also be taken to avoid the pleural and peritoneal spaces.

If the abscess is suitably localized, ultrasound or CT-guided percutaneous drainage is now the treatment of choice. Positive culture may also be obtained percutaneously. Coexisting renal obstruction must be resolved either by percutaneous nephrostomy or ureteral stent. Subsequent definitive management of renal or ureteral stones is performed when the acute process has resolved.

Renal abscess

An intrarenal abscess or renal carbuncle is a localized collection of pus within the renal parenchyma.

Aetiology and pathogenesis

A renal abscess usually is a progression of acute pyelonephritis with necrosis and pus formation. Multiple small abscesses coalesce into a larger lesion. Diabetes and infected calculus disease generally are predisposing or underlying factors. Rarely, a renal abscess may develop from secondary infection of a renal cyst [27]. A subcapsular abscess may progress to a perinephric abscess, however, renal abscesses are much rarer than the latter as an isolated condition. The organism is usually a Gram-negative coliform. *S. aureus* abscesses can occur secondary to staphylococcal bacteraemia from other sites.

Diagnosis

The clinical picture is similar to that of a perinephric abscess, the patient presenting with unresolving acute pyelonephritis. The symptoms and findings are generally less severe than in a perinephric abscess; however, fever, leucocytosis and flank pain are present. Urine culture is usually positive for Gram-negative organisms (most commonly *E. coli* or *P. mirabilis*) unless the agent is a blood-borne *Staphylococcus*. The blood culture may be positive.

Radiology

Abdominal ultrasound demonstrates a spherical hypo-echoic mass with irregular thickened walls containing varying degress of echogenic necrotic debris and septations. Early small abscess formation associated with acute pyelonephritis may not be evident and differentiation from the latter may be difficult. The presence of air in the mass is diagnostic of an abscess and helps differentiate an abscess from a renal tumour with central necrosis. Necrotic tumours do not contain air unless secondarily infected, a condition which is extremely rare [17–19].

A CT scan clearly demonstrates the site and extent of intrarenal abscesses. Inhomogeneous enhancement of the wall occurs making differentiation from a tumour with central necrosis difficult, unless the abscess contains air. An intravenous pyelogram may demonstrate an enlarged kidney with abnormal renal outline, displaced or distorted calyces and impaired excretion of contrast, depending on the size and extent of the lesion. A renal angiogram reveals an avascular mass with irregular borders and displacement of the renal vessels. Although tumour vessels are absent, inflammatory neovascularity may be present and, accordingly, differentiation from a tumour may not be possible. A gallium scan can be employed to differentiate a tumour from an abscess; however, the result is usually ambiguous and unreliable [28]. Lymphomas also demonstrate increased uptake of gallium.

Management

Small lesions may respond to antibiotic treatment alone, however, drainage of the abscess is generally required. Drainage can be performed percutaneously with ultrasound or CT scan guidance [26,29]. This will often confirm the diagnosis and will allow culture and sensitivity studies of the organisms. A catheter is left in place for drainage and the lesion is monitored by serial ultrasound or CT scan. Needle biopsy may also help differentiate a renal tumour, although negative biopsy does not rule out tumours.

Exploration with open drainage is necessary if the lesion does not respond to conservative management. Nephrectomy is advised for extensive multiple abscesses and unresponsive lesions in acutely ill patients. Nephrectomy may also be required if a renal neoplasm cannot be excluded. The kidney is approached extrapleurally and extraperitoneally through a flank incision.

Renal papillary necrosis

Renal papillary necrosis occurs following ischaemia of the renal papilla. The blood supply to the papilla is supplied via the vasa recta of the long loops of Henle. Occlusion of these tiny vessels may occur in association with one or a combination of several predisposing factors, including pyelonephritis, diabetes, obstructive uropathy, sickle cell anaemia and analgesic abuse [30].

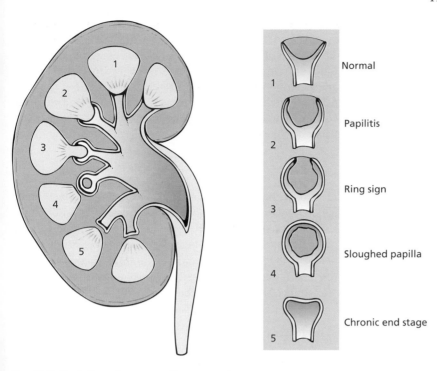

Fig. 45.1 Evolution of acute papilary necrosis.

Pathogenesis

Papillary necrosis is rarely associated with uncomplicated infections of the kidney. However, acute pyelonephritis may frequently precipitate acute papillary necrosis in patients with diabetes or obstructive uropathy. The ischaemic process depends on the precipitating condition. In diabetes the ischaemia is related to small vessel disease of the vasa recta; in chronic obstruction it is related to impaired renal perfusion; in sickle cell disease it is related to sludging in these small vessels; and in analgesic abuse, it is related to a local toxic effect of phenacetin concentrated in the renal medulla. Acute urinary infection potentiates each of these processes.

Renal papillary necrosis may present as either a chronic or an acute process. The chronic form is related to long-standing progressive ischaemia producing gradual fibrosis and erosion of the papillae. This is generally seen in sickle cell disease and analgesic abuse in the absence of acute infection. Acute papillary necrosis (or necrotizing papillitis) is usually precipitated in situations where acute pyelonephritis is superimposed on diabetes or obstructive uropathy. Ischaemia with necrosis of the pyramid occurs at the base of the papilla creating a sinus formation extending into the fornix. Eventual total slough of the papilla follows. The sloughed papilla may then act as a foreign body aggravating

obstruction and further sepsis. Adherent necrotic papillae may calcify and/or may form a nidus for chronic infection.

Diagnosis

The clinical features of renal papillary necrosis depend on the predisposing factors precipitating the disease, and range from chronic impairment of renal function, being diagnosed by an intravenous pyelogram, to an acute fulminating sepsis. The chronic indolent cases are generally asymptomatic and present with impaired renal function with loss of concentrating power, pyuria and proteinuria. Acute papillary necrosis may present as an acute progressive fulminating infection with acute renal failure and Gram-negative sepsis. One must be particularly aware of this possibility if acute urinary infection is superimposed on diabetes or chronic obstruction.

Radiology

A spectrum of X-ray changes occurs depending on the stage of the disease. The kidney may be enlarged and oedematous with impaired excretion of contrast when associated with acute infection. Figure 45.1 demonstrates the progressive degress of involvement of the medulla beginning with contrast extending into irregular sinuses in the medulla from the fornices at the base of the papillae. This sinus may progress to the classic ring sign about the papilla and may eventually lead to the irregular cavity that develops with total loss of the papilla. Dystrophic calcification may occur in an adherent papilla, however the sloughed papilla is usually a radiolucent body within the collecting system. Intravenous pyelogram or retrograde pyelogram are generally more diagnostic than ultrasound or a CT scan. Chronic renal papillary necrosis may be difficult to differentiate from other forms of end-stage chronic pyelonephritis, although chronic renal papillary necrosis tends to involve all papillae of both kidneys, except when associated with obstructive uropathy [31].

Management

The management of acute papillary necrosis requires controlling the acute infection and correcting the underlying predisposing factors. Obstructive uropathy must be immediately relieved, either by stenting, percutaneous nephrostomy or surgical repair. A sloughed papilla may produce acute ureteric obstruction requiring immediate relief. Early diagnosis with aggressive treatment of infection, obstruction and diabetes is critical to improving prognosis.

The restriction of the analgesic agent, along with treatment of the infection, may stabilize or even improve renal function in those cases associated with chronic analgesic abuse. Patients with chronic papillary necrosis related to analgesic abuse are susceptible to chronic urinary infection and have an increased incidence of urothelial malignancy. Accordingly, these cases should be monitored appropriately with urinalysis and urine cytology.

Emphysematous pyelonephritis

Emphysematous pyelonephritis occurs as a gas-forming necrotizing pyelonephritis, usually associated with diabetes with or without obstructive uropathy [32,33].

Aetiology and pathogenesis

Emphysematous pyelonephritis is a progression of acute pyelonephritis in the diabetic with impaired resistance to infection. Renal parenchymal ischaemia develops from the small vessel disease of diabetes, thrombosis of intrarenal vessels and oedema related to acute fulminating infection. Anaerobic metabolism of E. coli in the necrotic kidney produces hydrogen and nitrogen gases which form as patchy collections within the parenchyma. Renal abscess and perinephric abscess are frequently associated with emphysematous pyelonephritis. In some cases the process may progress to cause necrosis of the entire kidney [11].

Diagnosis

The clinical picture is one of unresolving infection following acute pyelonephritis. The acutely ill patients are usually diabetic and ureteric obstruction may be demonstrated. Flank pain, fever, malaise, positive urine culture usually for E. coli and leucocytosis are present. Bacteraemia is frequently demonstrated.

Radiology

Mottled collections of gas are present within the kidney parenchyma on plain film. Ultrasound reveals an enlarged kidney with intrarenal gas and patchy hypoechoic parenchyma. A CT scan best documents the extent of the necrotizing lesion with decreased inhomogeneous enhancement and patchy gas collections within the kidney allowing confirmation of the diagnosis [17–19].

Management

Treatment depends on the extent of the necrosis and gas-forming infection within the kidney. Immediate exploration with nephrectomy is usually necessary. Antibiotics to treat infection, control of diabetes and relief of obstructive uropathy are essential. Drainage of the necrotic area with preservation of the kidney is possible if the infection is localized to a segment of the kidney.

Xanthogranulomatous pyelonephritis

Xanthogranulomatous pyelonephritis is a chronic granulomatous inflammation involving one kidney, usually in response to chronic infection and obstruction related to stone disease. Although it may occur in diabetics, it does not bear the same direct relationship to diabetes as renal or perinephric abscess [34,35].

Pathogenesis

The specific precipitating factor of xanthogranulomatous pyelonephritis is not known; however, it is always related to chronic obstruction and infection, usually with stone disease. The granulomatous response to chronic infection begins in the calyces and adjacent parenchyma and progressively extends to involve major segments of the entire kidney.

The diagnostic features are large granulomas of lipid-filled histiocytes with plasma cells and lymphocytic infiltrate destroying and replacing the normal architecture. Central necrosis with abscess formation may coalesce to produce large necrotic areas within the kidney as well as within the perinephric space.

Grossly, the lesion is difficult to differentiate from tumour and perirenal or renal abscess formation. The kidney is enlarged and the tumour-like lesions are yellow coloured with central liquefaction. The process may be diffuse or segmental usually depending on the site of the associated obstruction or obstructing stone [11].

Diagnosis

The process generally follows chronic infection associated with stone disease. Pain, fever, leucocytosis and anaemia are related to chronic infection. Pyuria and haematuria are present and urine culture reveals *E. coli* or *P. mirabilis*. Most patients have had long-term antimicrobial treatment for infection and accordingly urine cultures may be sterile.

Radiology

Plain film reveals an enlarged kidney with indistinct margins and usually stone disease or calcification. An intravenous pyelogram demonstrates impaired function or non-functioning of the kidney with displacement and distortion of the collecting system, usually with a central obstructing stone. Ultrasound and CT scan best document the condition. Ultrasound reveals a complex mass with cystic and solid components. The diffuse condition involves a majority of the kidney with enlargement and patchy hypoechoic areas which are difficult to differentiate from tumour. CT provides the best imaging to demonstrate the extent of the renal and perirenal extension. There is loss of normal architecture with inhomogeneous enhancement along with central necrotic areas of decreased enhancement. Calyceal distortion and obstruction are related to stone disease. Differentiation from tumour is difficult when the process presents as a solid or complex mass infiltrating the kidney and perirenal space. Angiogram reveals a diffuse hypervascular mass but differentiation from a tumour is impossible.

The diagnosis is usually apparent on ultrasound and confirmed by CT scan, particularly with the presence of an associated obstructing stone [17–19]. Ultrasound or CT-guided needle biopsy of the lesion is frequently not helpful because of the extent of inflammation and necrosis.

Management

Xanthogranulomatous pyelonephritis is difficult to differentiate from a tumour. However, the presence of chronic infection and stone associated with a necrotic tumour mass raises the index of suspicion. Active infection is treated with antibiotics. Nephrectomy is the preferred treatment to clarify the diagnosis and treat the disease. Radical nephrectomy with early control of vessels along with removal of the perirenal fascia is recommended to eradicate all infiltrating granulomas. The condition is benign and clears promptly after removal of the affected kidney.

Malacoplakia

Malacoplakia is a rare focal chronic inflammatory disorder in patients with chronic illness, immunosuppression or immune deficiency [11,36]. The diagnosis is made pathologically by demonstrating the presence of characteristic large Von Hansemann histiocytes and the pathognomonic small basophilic Michaelis–Gutmann bodies. The Von Hansemann cells are large foamy macrophages and may be associated with multinucleated giant cells. Malacoplakia may involve any system including the urinary tract. Urinary malacoplakia usually involves the bladder, the site where it was first described; however, it occasionally involves the kidney. Urinary tract infection is usually present.

An intravenous pyelogram reveals an enlarged kidney with displacement or distortion of the collecting system. Urinary calculi are rare, a feature distinguishing it from xanthogranulomatous pyelonephritis. Ultrasound reveals a hypoechoic mass which may have complex cystic change. On CT scan, malacoplakia presents as a localized solid non-enhancing mass lesion. It may be multifocal and bilateral, and can cause distortion of the central renal complex.

Treatment is directed towards improvement of the patient's general health and control of the associated urinary infection.

Pyonephrosis

Pyonephrosis occurs when an infected hydronephrosis becomes purulent and the obstructed collecting system is filled with pus. Acute obstruction associated with acute pyonephritis may present as a fulminating illness with fever, chills and flank pain. This can rapidly develop into generalized sepsis. The infected hydronephrosis progresses to suppurative pyonephrosis and unless the condition is diagnosed and treated promptly, it may rapidly lead to progressive renal destruction.

Occasionally, a chronically obstructed kidney becomes infected in an indolent fashion with minimal clinical manifestations. Pyonephrosis develops and the patient presents with a mass, low-grade fever and vague general symptoms. Urine findings may be absent if the obstructive process is complete.

Radiology

An intravenous pyelogram reveals a non-functioning or poorly functioning hydronephrotic kidney associated with complete obstruction. The obstruction may occur at any level of the collecting system from an infundibulum to the ureterovesical junction. The plain film may demonstrate gas within the collecting system in acute cases [17–19]. Ultrasound confirms hydronephrosis to the level of obstruction. The dilated renal pelvis and ureter contain debris, suggesting a purulent-filled collecting system.

Management

The obstruction is relieved with either uteric catheterization or percutaneous nephrostomy and the diagnosis of pyonephrosis is confirmed. Suitable antimicrobial therapy is instituted and modified according to sensitivity studies. Further management depends on the underlying condition causing the obstruction and the degree of renal damage. In chronic cases where the renal parenchyma may be a thin atrophic fibrotic shell surrounding a dilated pus-filled collecting system, nephrectomy is indicated with removal of the ureter to the level of the obstruction.

References

1 Huland H, Busch R, Riebel TH. Renal scarring after symptomatic and asymptomatic upper urinary tract infection: a prospective study. *J Urol* 1982;**128**:682.

2 Kunin CM. *Detection, Prevention and Management of Urinary Tract Infections*, 4th edn. Philadelphia: Lea and Febiger, 1987: 309.

3 Kunin CM. *Detection, Prevention and Management of Urinary Tract Infections*, 4th edn. Philadelphia: Lea and Febiger, 1987: 57–60.

4 Fowler JE. *Urinary Tract Infection and Inflammation*. Chicago: Year Book Medical, 1989:42–55.

5 Kunin CM. *Detection, Prevention and Management of Urinary Tract Infections*, 4th edn. Philadelphia: Lea and Febiger, 1987:91–5.

6 Allen JC. The diabetic as a compromised host. In: *Infection and the Compromised Host: Clinical Correlations and Therapeutic Approaches*. Baltimore: Williams and Wilkins, 1981:229–70.

7 Mowat AG, Barcun J. Chemotaxis of polymorphonuclear leukocytes from patients with diabetes mellitus. *N Engl J Med* 1971;**284**:621.

8 Bryan CS, Reynolds KL. Community-acquired bacteremic urinary tract infection: epidemiology and outcome. *J Urol* 1984;**132**:490.

9 Bryan CS, Reynolds KL. Hospital-acquired bacteremic urinary tract infection: epidemiology and outcome *J Urol* 1984;**132**: 494.

10 Kunin CM. *Detection, Prevention and Management of Urinary Tract Infections*, 4th edn. Philadelphia: Lea and Febiger, 1987: 140–7.

11 Heptinstall RH. Pyelonephritis: pathologic features. In: *Pathology of the Kidney*, Vol. 3, 4th edn. Boston: Little, Brown, 1992.

12 Miller TE, Stewart E, North JDK. Immunobacteriological aspects of pyelonephritis. *Contrib Nephrol* 1979;**16**:11.

13 Thomas V, Shelokov A, Forland M. Antibody-coated bacteria in the urine and the site of urinary tract infection. *N Engl J Med* 1974;**290**:588.

14 Neter E. Estimation of *Escherichia coli* antibodies in urinary tract infection: a review and perspective. *Kidney Int Suppl* 1975;**4**:S23.

15 Roberts JA, Hardaway K, Kaack B *et al.* Prevention of pyelonephritis by immunization with P-fimbriae. *J Urol* 1984;**131**:602.

16 Kunin CM. Prospects of development of a pyelonephritis vaccine directed against *E. coli*. In: *Detection, Prevention and Management of Urinary Tract Infections*, 4th edn. Philadelphia: Lea and Febiger, 1987: 152–3.

17 Taveras JM, Ferrucci JT. In: *Radiology—Diagnosis—Imaging—Intervention*, Vol. IV. JB Lippincott, 1990:1–11.

18 Rumack CM, Wilson SR, Charbonneau JW. The urinary tract. In: *Diagnostic Ultrasound*. Mosby Year Book, 1991: 226–30.

19 Piceirillo M, Rigsby CM, Rosenfield AT. Sonography of renal inflammatory disease. *Urol Radiol* 1987;**9**(2):66–78.

20 Stamey TA, Govan DE, Palmer JM. The localization and treatment of urinary tract infections: the role of bactericidal urine levels as opposed to serum levels. *Medicine* 1965;**44**:1.

21 Stamey TA. *Pathogenesis and Treatment of Urinary Tract Infections*. Baltimore: Williams and Wilkins, 1980.

22 Kunin CM. *Detection, Prevention and Management of Urinary Tract Infections*, 4th edn. Philadelphia: Lea and Febiger, 1987:224–31.

23 Kay CJ, Rosenfield AT, Taylor KJW *et al.* Ultrasonic characteristics of chronic atrophic pyelonephritis. *Am J Radiol* 1979; **132**:47–9.

24 Sheinfeld J, Erturk C, Spataro RF *et al.* Perinephric abscess: current concepts. *J Urol* 1987;**137**:191.

25 Thorley JD, Jones SR, Sanford JP. Perinephric abscess. *Medicine* 1974;**53**:441.

26 Gerzoz SG, Gale ME. Computed tomography and ultrasonography for diagnosis and treatment of renal and retroperitoneal abscesses. *Urol Clin N Am* 1982;**9**:185.

27 Kinder PW, Rous SN. Infected renal cyst from hematogenous seeding: a case report and review of the literature. *J Urol* 1978; **120**:239.

28 Hampel N, Class RN, Persky L. Value of [67]gallium scintography in the diagnosis of localized renal and perirenal inflammation. *J Urol* 1980;**124**:311.

29 Costello AJ, Blandy JP, Hately W. Percutaneous aspiration of renal cortical abscess. *Urology* 1983;**21**:201.

30 Eknoyan G, Qunibi WY, Grisson RT *et al.* Renal papillary necrosis: an update. *Medicine* 1982;**61**:55.

31 Taveras JM, Ferrucci JT. Diffuse renal parenchymal diseases. In: *Radiology—Diagnosis—Imaging—Intervetion*, Vol. IV. JB Lippincott, 1990: 5–6.

32 Ahlering tE, Boyd SD, Hamilton CL *et al.* Emphysematous pyelonephritis: a 5-year experience with 13 patients. *J Urol* 1985;**134**:1086.

33 Michaeli J, Mogle S, Perlberg S *et al.* Emphysematous pyelonephritis. *J Urol* 1984;**131**:203.

34 Rosi P, Selli C, Carini M *et al.* Xanthogranulomatous pyelonephritis: clinical experience with 62 cases. *Eur Urol* 1986;**12**:96.

35 Tolia BM, Iloreta A, Freed SZ *et al.* Xanthogranulomatous pyelonephritis: detailed analysis of 29 cases and a brief discussion of atypical presentation. *J Urol* 1981;**126**:437.

36 Stanton MJ, Maxted W. Malacoplakia: a study of the literature and current concepts of pathogenesis, diagnosis and treatment. *J Urol* 1981;**125**:139.

46 Septicaemia Associated with the Genitourinary Tract

G.E.Griffin and H.P.Lambert

Epidemiology

Few patients under the care of an individual urologist will develop septicaemia, so it is easy for a clinician to underestimate the importance of infection in general, and especially of septicaemia and septicaemic shock in hospital patients. Epidemiological studies tell a different story. On one day in a large group of acute hospitals in England and Wales, 19.1% of patients were suffering from an infection; of those, 9.9% were community acquired and 9.2% were hospital acquired [1]. Of such hospital-acquired infections, the genitourinary tract is the most common source and its importance is reflected in studies of septicaemia and of septicaemic shock.

A 20-year study of septicaemia at St Thomas' Hospital in London [2] analysed 4000 cases of septicaemia, 60% of which were hospital acquired. Of these, 54% had their focus of origin in the urinary tract. Community-acquired septicaemia may be first encountered in general medical departments but here too the urinary tract is the most frequent source, in 62% of this series. Many of these patients have underlying conditions which will bring them under the care of urologists, or may already have done so.

A similar picture emerges from the USA. Gram-negative bacteraemia has been extensively studied for many years at the Boston City Hospital [3]. The largest single source, identified in 34% of 612 patients, is the genitourinary tract, followed by bacteraemia of unknown cause (30%) and the gastrointestinal tract (14%). If, however, the patients were classified according to the severity of their underlying clinical state, urinary tract sources were proportionately of even greater importance in patients with non-fatal underlying disease, accounting for 74% of the septicaemia.

Such studies give a valid picture of the importance of the genitourinary tract in the overall problem of hospital-acquired infection. The risk expressed as a proportion of urological procedures has been estimated in a district general hospital [4] in 433 procedures. Bacteraemic shock was suspected on clinical grounds in 52 patients, of whom 25 had positive blood cultures (0.58%). Urological proced-ures have long been known as a precursor of bacteraemia and this was confirmed in the same study in a group of 628 patients, of whom 12.7% developed positive blood cultures. The incidence after transurethral prostatectomy was 27%, after prostatic biopsy, 20% and after retropubic prostatectomy, 37%.

Infection, and sometimes septicaemia, has also come to be recognized as an important complication of extracorporeal shock wave lithotripsy (ESWL). Three patients in the group of 600 analysed by Coptcoat et al. [5] developed septicaemia in spite of antibiotic prophylaxis, a similar proportion to the six cases reported by Rao et al. [6] in the course of 500 endoscopic procedures for stones. These authors found, in contrast to some reports, a substantial incidence of postoperative bacteraemia, in 20 of 117 patients. A number of the patients, 38 of the 117, had infected urine preoperatively and 16 of them also had endotoxinaemia before their procedure. All this underlines the significance of preoperative infection and the importance of the precept, too often neglected, that preoperative infection requires, not prophylaxis, but whole-hearted treatment. The devastating effects of severe infection are shown in a case report of *Klebsiella* septicaemia with meningitis and endophthalmitis following ESWL [7]. The authors point out that, although the overall incidence of sepsis after this procedure is 0.3–0.8%, this rises to 2.7% when staghorn calculi are treated.

Other predisposing factors also contribute to an increased susceptibility to septicaemia and septicaemic shock. Old age and a background of serious illness are the most common. Patients with malignant disease, hepatic cirrhosis, diabetes or chronic renal disease are at special risk. Sometimes specific immunological defects can be involved, as in patients receiving corticosteroids or cytotoxic drugs, or those with neutropenia ($<0.5 \times 10^9/l$ polymorphonuclear leucocytes).

Aetiology

Aerobic Gram-negative bacilli are the predominant cause of

urinary infections and of septicaemia associated with the genitourinary tract. When these infections arise in a patient who has neither been in hospital nor experienced genitourinary manipulation or surgery, *Escherichia coli* is by far the most common pathogen, with smaller numbers caused by *Klebsiella* and *Proteus* species. This dominance of *E. coli* is is also found in hospital-acquired septicaemias, but a substantial minority of nosocomial infections are caused by other organisms, *Klebsiella*, other enterobacteria, *Pseudomonas*, *Enterococcus* and *Staphylococcus* species. These are of great importance because, as we shall see, they often exhibit resistance to a number of antimicrobial agents. Anaerobes such as *Bacteroides*, so important in infections related to the lower gut, are rarely involved in septicaemia from a urinary tract source.

So much interest has been engendered in recent years by Gram-negative septicaemia and its complications that Gram-positive pathogens are likely to be forgotten. Sepsis associated with urinary tract surgery may, however, be caused by *Staphylococcus* and *Streptococcus* species as well as by the more frequent Gram-negative bacilli.

Important changes in the incidence and resistance pattern of enterococci (*Enterococcus faecalis* and *E. faecium*, formerly grouped as streptococci) have been found in recent years. These organisms are found in clinical isolates most commonly in relation to the urinary tract, especially in nosocomial infections. A notable increase in their frequency has been seen in many countries. A record of all urinary isolates has been kept at University College Hospital in London since 1971; during this time the proportion of hospital isolates caused by enterococci rose from 4 to 12.6% in 1990 [8]. Similarly in a US hospital the proportion of nosocomial urinary tract infections caused by this organism rose from 5.3% in 1975 to 15.7% in 1984 [9]. The causes of this increase are not precisely known but are probably related to the remarkable capacity of the organism to develop antibiotic resistance by a variety of different mechanisms with consequent difficulties in establishing effective treatment.

Enterococci are also an important cause of bacterial endocarditis, and the urinary tract is the most common source of infection in enterococcal endocarditis. Polymicrobial septicaemias in association with the urinary tract are not uncommon.

Clinical presentation

The recent interest in Gram-negative septicaemia has also led to the idea that these infections can be differentiated on clinical grounds from those caused by other organisms such as Gram-positive cocci. This is not so, and with rare exceptions, such as meningococcal septicaemia, it is impossible to predict the causal organism from bedside observations.

Septicaemia arising in hospital, and especially in the postoperative period, may present with obvious features of infection, namely fever, rigors, malaise and neutrophil leucocytosis. But the presentation, especially in the elderly and in patients with severe underlying disease or associated metabolic disturbance, may vary greatly in pace and in character. Among common early features are otherwise unexplained vomiting, diarrhoea, hyperventilation, bleeding tendency and oliguria. Many of these features may precede or accompany the development of the bacterial shock syndrome. The pace of development varies between wide limits and at its most rapid, the condition may be as fulminating as acute meningococcal septicaemia, with a catastrophic decline in the patient's condition within a few hours. On the other hand, early clinical changes may be quite subtle and septicaemia should be considered, and blood cultures taken, in any otherwise unexplained deterioration in the postoperative patient. The peripheral blood film classically shows neutrophilia characteristic of pyogenic infections, but sometimes a transient leucopenia is observed, probably indicating sequestration of polymorphs into tissue sites such as the lung following their activation.

Bacterial shock syndrome

This syndrome poses a medical emergency. Even with appropriate antibiotic therapy and optimal support of failing organ systems, mortality remains within the region of 40–50%. The most characteristic form of this syndrome begins between 12 and 72 h after a surgical procedure or instrumentation. The patient has a rigor, the temperature rises quickly and nausea, vomiting and diarrhoea may develop. Within a few hours of these early symptoms the blood pressure falls rapidly and the signs of a low output state develop, rapid thready pulse, cold extremities with cyanosis of the hands, feet, nose and ear lobes. The urinary output diminishes rapidly. Less commonly, the patient when first seen may have a good pulse volume, warm extremities and pink skin associated with hypotension. At this stage hyperventilation can often be noted. Most commonly this phase is transient, and within a few hours the more familiar signs of shock will develop.

The haemodynamic changes corresponding to these clinical features have now been extensively studied. In the early phases, peripheral resistance falls, cardiac output increases and there is hyperventilation with a respiratory alkalosis. This last feature has been stressed as a common early sign of septicaemic shock. Later, cardiac output decreases, probably from a combination of poor filling from relative hypovolaemia and impaired myocardial function, and increasing lactic acidaemia rapidly produces a metabolic acidosis.

In many patients hypovolaemia, often severe, is present

from the earliest stages. This may result principally from fluid losses into the extravascular space, presumably resulting from early capillary damage or overt bleeding.

Unusual or additional features of bacterial shock

Cardiorespiratory features may develop so suddenly that the resulting syndrome may resemble that of pulmonary embolism or myocardial infarction, especially as the electrocardiogram may show changes suggestive of myocardial ischaemia, but the central venous pressure is initially low or normal. Often, however, a raised rectal temperature provides a corrective clue as poor perfusion and hyperventilation render oral and axillary readings unreliable. A few patients with bacterial shock have a normal or even subnormal temperature.

Several other features of septicaemic shock may provide helpful pointers to the diagnosis if their possible significance is recognized. Many patients show clouding of consciousness or confusion and a primary neurological syndrome may be wrongly diagnosed. Disturbance of liver function (classically raised plasma alkaline phosphatase) is common and jaundice sometimes develops and may be particularly seen in patients with pre-existing liver disease. An otherwise unexplained bleeding tendency may indicate thrombocytopenia, a common feature of septicaemia. A few patients develop more severe bleeding associated with the full syndrome of disseminated intravascular coagulation.

Vigorous treatment now enables many patients to recover from the initial stages of septicaemic shock. A few of these then develop the adult respiratory distress syndrome ('shock lung') characterized by tachypnoea, severe hypoxia and the development of diffuse pulmonary infiltrates.

Finally, although specific diagnostic features are rare, the necrotic erythematous lesions of erythema gangrenosum point strongly to a diagnosis of *Pseudomonas* septicaemia, although such skin lesions are also seen in other septicaemias, especially those caused by *Aeromonas hydrophila*. These common and uncommon features of bacterial shock are summarized in Table 46.1.

Table 46.1 Clinical features of sepsis syndrome.

Common	Uncommon
Fever	Bleeding, disseminated
Hypotension	intravascular coagulation
Hyperventilation	Jaundice
Oliguria	Adult respiratory distress syndrome
Mental clouding	Leucopenia
Leucocytosis	
Thrombocytopenia	

Pathogenesis of septic shock

The high mortality of the septic shock syndrome is related to tissue damage occurring early in the evolution of the disease, such as disseminated intravascular coagulation, respiratory distress syndrome, acute tubular necrosis and depressed myocardial function.

The syndrome of septic shock was originally known as endotoxic shock and the lipid A component of the endotoxin has been shown to be a potent stimulus causing a physiological change closely resembling this syndrome in humans and animals [10]. It is, however, now well established that lipid A is only one of many molecules acting on macrophages and endothelial cells to induce the cytokine cascade which is now thought to cause the syndrome. Cytokines are polypeptides which act as both local and systemic mediators in the response to infection. For example, tumour necrosis factor (TNF), interleukin-1 (IL-1) and IL-6 are pivotal in the evolution of fever, increased vascular permeability and induction of acute phase protein synthesis [11]. The detection of such cytokines in the plasma of humans and animal models of septic shock have unlocked fundamental mechanisms of sepsis and opened therapeutic avenues which will be discussed below.

Management

Choice of antimicrobial agent

Initial decisions about antibiotic treatment are made at the time of clinical diagnosis and most commonly before precise microbial diagnosis is available. They are therefore based on informed guesses about the bacteria likely to cause septicaemia in a particular setting. The main questions are: whether the septicaemia arose in or out of hospital; whether there is a known or presumed source such as the urinary tract; what preceding operation or manipulation may have induced the bacteraemia; what other general factors such as neutropenia may affect the likely causal organisms; whether there are relevant epidemiological factors such as the presence in the unit of a particular organism known to be causing cross-infection. By answering these questions, a short list of organisms likely to be causing the septicaemia can be constructed, and a suitable antibiotic policy devised. In the case of septicaemia associated with genitourinary surgery the main organism to be considered will be *E. coli*, other Gram-negative bacilli such as *Klebsiella* and *Proteus* species, and *Streptococcus* and *Staphylococcus* species.

The attempt to narrow the therapeutic target is much preferable to a blanket therapeutic approach based on attacking unspecified septicaemia of unknown origin. Such an approach leads to an unnecessarily complex therapeutic scheme; for example, it is common to see patients receiving antianaerobe antibiotics who have developed septicaemia not associated with any site of anaerobic colonization such as the lower bowel, and in whom, therefore, anaerobic septicaemia is most unlikely to occur.

Whatever the initial regimen, it is essential to obtain precise information as soon as possible about the aetiology of the septicaemia so that treatment can, if necessary, be modified accordingly. There is ample evidence that the patient's chances of survival are much improved if an antibiotic regimen is chosen which proves, in the event, to have been appropriate for the organism later isolated from blood culture.

The choice of therapy is bedevilled by rapid changes in antibiotic sensitivity of organisms from both community and hospital sources. For example, ampicillin and amoxycillin, to which most urinary tract organisms were once susceptible, are now unsuitable for initial use in septicaemia because about 50% of coliforms in urinary tract infections in the community and a higher proportion of hospital coliforms are resistant to their action. Likewise, resistance of coliform bacteria to trimethoprim is increasing. Gentamicin-resistant coliforms, too, are now common in many hospital environments and act as sources of dangerous cross-infection. These factors, together with local clinical and epidemiological data, and the rapid introduction of new agents make necessary a flexible policy for the treatment of septicaemia.

The main groups of agents applicable to 'best guess' initial treatment of septicaemia of urinary tract origin are the aminoglycosides, a number of β-lactam agents (penicillins, cephalosporins, monobactams and carbapenems) and the fluorinated quinolones. Each of these groups contains a considerable number of compounds, often with little to choose between them, and those selected for use need to conform to the antibiotic policy of the unit or hospital. Each of the main groups of agents has favourable and adverse features which can now be briefly outlined.

Aminoglycosides such as gentamicin, amikacin and netilmicin are still important options in the management of severe infections caused by Gram-negative pathogens, but their low therapeutic ratio makes them difficult to use. The estimation of plasma concentration is absolutely necessary in the clinical use of this group of antibiotics, but despite this, control is often less than perfect and the problem is compounded by the rapidly deteriorating renal function so common in septicaemia. The other disadvantage of aminoglycosides is their restricted range against some of the other causes of septicaemia associated with the urinary tract, as they are quite inactive against streptococci and are not agents of first choice in staphylococcal infections. In recent years the use of aminoglycosides has been improved in many centres by adopting a once daily regimen, as much pharmacokinetic

data has accumulated indicating that the therapeutic ratio can be increased using this method. The method requires a high initial dose, but it is often possible to review the necessity for continuing with an aminoglycoside after only one or two doses have been given, since microbiological results are then becoming available. The general principles are to give a high initial dose, at least 4–5 mg/kg, regardless of the state of renal function, to measure renal function during the next 24 h and amend subsequent doses as necessary, and to measure levels at a time agreed with the microbiology laboratory.

Extended-spectrum cephalosporins such as cefotaxime, ceftazidime and ceftiaxone now have a very important role in the treatment of septicaemia because of their high activity, wide spectrum of antibacterial activity and generally low toxicity. They are very active against *E. coli* and most of the other Gram-negative bacteria commonly isolated in community-acquired septicaemias, but some of the less common organisms involved in nosocomial infections are resistant. They are only moderately active against staphylococci, but streptococci (with the exception of *Enterococcus faecalis*) are very susceptible. A few cephalosporins, notably ceftazidime and cefsulodin, are active against *Pseudomonas aeruginosa*. There is some evidence that when this organism is identified or suspected as a cause of septicaemia, combined treatment with two agents is preferable to single drug therapy. One of these should be an aminoglycoside. The choices available for the other agent include the antipscudomonal cephalosporins just mentioned, and the antipseudomonal penicillins, carbenicillin, ticarcillin, mezlocillin and piperacillin.

Imipenem-cilastatin (Primaxin) a type of β-lactam agent distinct from the penicillins and the cephalosporins (a carbapenem) has a very wide spectrum of antibacterial activity and can be used both in the treatment of severe infections and in surgical prophylaxis.

The value of a much older drug combination, co-trimoxazole, should not be neglected in considering treatment options. Its disadvantages are the increasing incidence of resistant strains among urinary pathogens and the problem of drug reactions, especially frequent in patients with human immunodeficiency virus (HIV) infection. The frequency of resistance now makes it unsuitable for 'best guess' treatment, but it remains a valuable option once the pathogen has been identified as susceptible.

The fluorinated quinolones such as ciprofloxacin have established an important role in the treatment of urinary tract infections, although they are less commonly employed in septicaemia. They have generally low toxicity and several of them, notably ciprofloxacin and ofloxacin, are available in preparations for parenteral use. The antibacterial spectrum of this group is rapidly being extended but the presently available agents, while highly active against common Gram-negative bacteria, are inactive against *Pseudomonas*, and only moderately active against staphylococcal infections. Among the mainly hospital-based organisms, *Enterococcus* (formerly *Streptococcus*) *faecalis* presents a taxing problem because of its increasing range of resistance to many antibiotics. Definitive treatment must wait upon isolation and sensitivity testing of isolates since a 'best guess' policy which encompasses all the possible vagaries of this organism cannot be devised. If the organism is not penicillin resistant (i.e. does not produce a β-lactamase), ampicillin or one of its equivalents is the agent of choice, which in patients with septicaemia should, as in enterococcal endocarditis, be combined with an aminoglycoside. Options for penicillin-resistant strains include vancomycin and one of the penicillin-β-lactamase inhibitor combinations such as co-amoxiclav (Augmentin), clavulanic acid-ticarcillin (Timentin) or piperacillin-tazobactam (Tazocin). Aminoglycosides, even in combination, are ineffective in strains showing high-level resistance to this group. An increasing number of strains are resistant to vancomycin as well as to aminoglycocides, and these vancomycin-resistant enterococci, known as VRE, present a difficult and partly unsolved problem in chemotherapy.

The confusing variety of available antibiotics available, and the difficult task of identifying the most suitable agent, justifies reiteration of the central principles that agents should be chosen, within the general antibiotic policies of the unit or hospital, which are most likely to be active against the presumed or known infecting organism, and that their use should be carefully controlled with continuous review to ensure maximal effectiveness and minimal toxicity. The biggest factor in the successful treatment of septicaemia is the correct initial choice of treatment.

Table 46.2 gives general guidance on antibiotic choice before and after a specific organism has been identified. The agents are mainly listed as groups rather than as individual compounds to enable the reader to take into account different antibiotic purchasing policies in different centres.

Other aspects of management

Some patients with septicaemia have no apparent substantial local focus of infection but, if there is such a focus, its drainage or removal remains a dominant concern and should be achieved as soon as possible. This, together with appropriate antimicrobial therapy, constitute the most important aspects of management, to which must be added careful monitoring of the patient's renal function, fluid balance and nutritional state.

Even in patients with bacterial shock, drainage of purulent foci may lead to remarkable improvement, and should be done as soon as possible.

Circulatory, renal and respiratory support

Patients in impending or established bacterial shock usually have a normal or low venous pressure. Inadequate tissue perfusion should be quickly corrected through any suitable venous route, and a central venous line or, in some cases, a pulmonary artery catheter, should quickly be

Table 46.2 Initial choice of antibiotics in septicaemia associated with the urinary tract.

State of diagnosis	Organism	Treatment
Clinical diagnosis of septicaemia with no early information on the causal organism		
Community acquired		Cephalosporin*
Hospital acquired		Cephalosporin plus aminoglycoside†
Organism known, antibiotic susceptibility unknown	*Escherichia coli, Klebsiella*, etc.	As above
	Pseudomonas aeruginosa	Antipseudomonal β-lactam‡ aminoglycoside
	Staphylococcus aureus	Flucloxacillin
	Streptococcus pyogenes	Benzyl penicillin
	Enterococcus faecalis	Vancomycin
Organism known, antibiotic susceptibility known		Modify regimen if indicated

* Examples include cefotaxime, ceftazidime, ceftriaxone.
† Examples include gentamicin, netilmicin, tobramycin.
‡ Examples include azlocillin, piperacillin, carbenicillin, ticarcillin, ceftazidime, cefsulodin, aztreonam.

established. A plasma expander should be administered until clinical signs of good perfusion are achieved. It is usually safe to continue rapid intravenous infusion to a central venous pressure of 10–12 cmH$_2$O.

These measures may lead to notable improvement in circulatory performance within a few hours. If they do not, vasoactive drugs must be given. Methods currently used change rapidly as knowledge about the pathophysiology of shock increases. Adrenergic agonists are widely used—for instance, dopamine, in which this action is combined with non-β-adrenergic dilatation of the renal and splanchnic vessels. Low doses, using infusion rates of the order of 2–5 μg/kg min are used in shock since vasoconstrictor α-adrenergic effects tend to accompany the use of high doses. Dobutamine, another β-adrenergic agonist, has also recently been used widely in bacterial shock, usually in doses of 2.5–10 μg/kg/min. Both drugs act mainly on β 1-receptors, increasing myocardial contractility, and through this β-agonism also increase the heart rate which may be beneficial. Dopamine is thought to have specific renal effects in promoting renal blood flow at doses lower than that required for an inotropic effect and may be useful in the management of the oliguric patient.

Other aspects of treatment include the correction of hypoxia, chest physiotherapy and if respiratory failure develops, assisted ventilation. Renal failure almost invariably accompanies bacterial shock and often complicates septicaemia even when there is no evidence of circulatory failure, so the detection and management of this complication is an essential aspect of management, with necessary adjustment in the dosage of many drugs.

Steroids

Initial clinical studies using high-dose glucocorticosteroids in septic shock showed that this agent did not increase survival but did increase the incidence of a secondary infection [12]. At the time of these studies the potent effect of glucocorticoids on preventing cytokine release from macrophages *in vitro* or *in vivo* was not known. However, a detailed analysis of the mechanism of action of dexamethasone on TNF release from endotoxin-stimulated macrophages suggests that release is inhibited only if the steroid is given before the stimulus. Steroids, however, still have a place in the management of severe allergic reactions to antibiotics or other therapeutic agents.

Potential advances in therapy

A recent clinical trial [13] involved the use of monoclonal antibody (HAA) directed against endotoxin in patients in septic shock in intensive care units. This study involved the inclusion of all patients with a syndrome clinically resembling shock and therefore included patients with Gram-positive and fungal shock syndrome for whom the use of such an antibody would have no benefit. Indeed the results of this study reflected this problem of specificity. While this monoclonal antibody has now been withdrawn from clinical use in UK, there is a strong argument for its use in clinical shock syndromes where Gram-negative organisms are highly likely to be implicated, for example urinary tract infection or meningococcal septicaemia.

The pattern of plasma cytokines in human Gram-negative septicaemia is highly complex [14]. More recently, studies are in progress in which monoclonal antibodies directed against cytokines, such as TNF, have been given intravenously to patients with presumed septic shock and in animal models of sepsis. Antibodies directed against TNF protect against lethality in animal models of bacteraemia [15] and based on such studies great potential benefit was predicted in human sepsis. However, a recent trial of anti-TNF in humans was terminated when it was shown on interim analysis that patients receiving this monoclonal antibody had a higher rate of complications. Another specific way of blocking the action of cytokines is the use of cytokine receptor antagonists [16]. These molecules, which are found naturally in human plasma during infection, represent cell receptors for individual cytokines which become detached from their membrane site. The use of such recombinant molecules, therefore, potentially provides specific pharmacological competitive inhibition of cytokine molecules released into the circulation. Clinical studies are in progress using IL-1 receptor antagonist in humans suffering from septic shock. In addition non-specific pharmacological agents known to block TNF release both *in vivo* and *in vitro* such as oxypentifylline (Trental) and its derivatives provide another possible therapeutic approach which is currently being evaluated.

Management strategy

Management of septicaemic shock is thus a complex problem [17]. The treatment plan can, however, be simplified by considering it as a three-stage process, as

Table 46.3 Treatment of septic shock.

Stage 1	Take specimens for microscopy and culture Begin antimicrobial drugs Correct hypovolaemia Correct hypoxia
Stage 2	Review cardiac, pulmonary and renal function Consider the use of dopamine or other vasoactive drugs
Stage 3	Review microbiological data Adjust or change regimen if indicated
Throughout	Drainage or removal of infected foci whenever possible

summarized in Table 46.3. In the first stage, specimens are taken, hypovolaemia and hypoxia corrected and antibiotic therapy started. After a few hours, clear improvement is often achieved; if not, in the second stage, vasoactive drugs are introduced. In the third stage, all aspects of management are reviewed, including renal function, fluid balance, and pulmonary and cardiac function. The microbiological data are reviewed and any necessary changes or adjustments made in the treatment regimen. Septic foci are drained at any stage when the patient's condition permits.

Prevention

Septicaemia and sepsis syndrome arise in hospital from a background of cross-infection and colonization with a variety of bacteria, many of them resistant to antibiotics in common use. Some of these life-threatening illnesses could be prevented by greater attention to the well-studied techniques for the control of hospital cross-infection. These include the proper management of intravenous catheters and of equipment used in artificial ventilation, care of skin lesions of all kinds and isolation methods for the care of patients harbouring dangerous pathogens. In the context of genitourinary surgery, two aspects need special attention, the management of bladder catheters, and the role of perioperative chemoprophylaxis.

Catheter care

Catheters should be avoided whenever possible and, when used, there should be a high level of concern of all staff for their proper management, including sterility of technique on insertion, routine use of a closed drainage system and meticulous attention to sterility in specimen taking. The role of antibacterial drugs is still to some extent controversial but largely depends on whether the urinary tract is already infected, and on the expected duration of catheterization. If the urine is infected, there is no question of chemoprophylaxis, and full dosage of the appropriate antibiotic should be given. Antibiotics probably have no advantagefor a single catheterization in a low-risk patient, but chemoprophylaxis to cover short-term catheterization for periods of 3 or 4 days is often necessary in relation to gynaecological and urological surgery, and has been shown to diminish the incidence of postoperative infection; this aspect of chemoprophylaxis is discussed below. In long-term catheterization, antibiotics have no routine role, as they merely ensure that the inevitable infection is caused by drug-resistant organisms. They must be used, however, during episodes of bacteraemia.

Perioperative prophylaxis

Recent application of principles established many years ago in experimental studies have provided a rational basis for perioperative chemoprophylaxis for many operations formerly plagued by a high risk of postoperative infection and septicaemia. The principles are to use an agent or agents active against the likely pathogens or at least against a component of them and to achieve antibacterial activity in the blood and tissue during the actual operation and for a short time after it. This means beginning chemoprophylaxis at premedication or during the induction of anaesthesia and continuing for a period of no more than 24 h. The benefits of such procedures have been particularly well established for colonic and certain forms of gynaecological surgery and are now being defined also in urology. Urine should be cultured preoperatively if at all possible and, if infected, a full course of an appropriate agent, as judged by *in vitro* sensitivity testing, should be administered. Ideally infection is eradicated before the operation, but as an operation is often indicated for reasons (e.g. stone or obstructive uropathy) which themselves render infection impossible to eradicate, in practice antibiotics are often started immediately before the operation. Whether or not antibiotics should be given in the uninfected patient has for long been a matter of controversy, but there are now a number of trials showing a diminution of postoperative urinary infection and bacteraemia when a short course of perioperative chemoprophylaxis is given.

For example, in the well-studied and common operation of transurethral prostatectomy, it is now clear that postoperative bacteriuria and fever is significantly diminished by perioperative chemoprophylaxis. It is possible that perioperative contamination of the prostate itself is responsible for some infection, as positive prostatic chip cultures were found to be associated with postoperative infection although the preoperative urine specimen was usually sterile [18]. Among the agents used successfully for this purpose in prostatic surgery are co-trimoxazole and various cephalosporins including cefotaxime. The much greater rate of bacteraemia which follows transrectal prostatic biopsy as compared with cystoscopy alone indicates that this procedure too should be covered by antibiotic administration.

It is difficult to give a dogmatic choice of agent for chemoprophylaxis in urological surgery. Much depends on local factors such as the nature and drug resistance pattern of prevalent pathogens and on whether drugs can be administered orally immediately before surgery or instrumentation. 'Extended-spectrum' cephalosporins are at present the most generally suitable choices. In several reports, *Staphylococcus epidermidis* ranks as an important cause of postoperative urinary infection and the tendency of this organism to show trimethoprim resistance makes this a less suitable agent for perioperative chemoprophylaxis than co-trimoxazole. In surgery involving the lower bowel, metronidazole should be added to the drug regimen.

Patients with known heart disease or with prosthetic heart valves also need prophylaxis against the risk of endocarditis. The same general principles apply: administration should be begun immediately before surgery or instrumentation, and continued for a period of up to 24 h afterwards. Unfortunately the association between genitourinary instrumentation and *Streptococcus faecalis* endocarditis makes the relatively simple oral regimens now often used for dental prophylaxis unsuitable and parenteral methods of prophylaxis are necessary.

The scheme recommended by the British Society for Antimicrobial Chemotherapy [19] consists of amoxycillin 1 g with gentamicin 120 mg, both by intramuscular injection just before induction, with an additional 0.5 g of amoxycillin orally 6 h later. Patients allergic to penicillin or who have received penicillin more than once in the previous month are given vancomycin 1 g by slow intravenous infusion followed by gentamicin 120 mg intravenously just before induction or 15 min before surgery.

References

1 Meers P.D. Infection in hospitals. *Br Med J* 1981;**282**:1246.
2 Eykyn SJ, Gransden WR, Phillips I. The causative organisms of septicaemia and their epidemiology. *J Antimicrob Chemother* 1991;**146**:955–60.
3 Kreger BE, Craven DE, Carling PC, McCabe WR. Gram negative bacteremia III. Re-assessment of etiology, epidemiology and ecology in 612 patients. *Am J Med* 1980;**68**: 322–43.
4 Robinson MRG, Cross RJ, Shetty MB, Fittal B. Bacteraemia and bacteriogenic shock in a district hospital urological practice. *Br J Urol* 1980;**52**:10–14.
5 Coptcoat MJ, Webb DR, Kellett MJ et al. The complications of ESW lithotripsy: management and prevention. *Br J Urol* 1986;**58**:578–80.
6 Rao PN, Weightman NC, Oppenheim B, Morris J. Predictors of septicaemia following endourological manipulation for stones in the upper urinary tract. *J Urol* 1991;**146**:955–60.
7 Silber N, Kremer I, Gaton DD, Servadio C. Severe sepsis following extracorporeal shock wave lithotripsy. *J Urol* 1991;**145**:1045–6.
8 Felmingham D, Wilson APR, Quintana AL, Gruneberg RN. *Enterococcus* species in urinary tract infections. *Clin Infect Dis* 1992;**15**:295–301.
9 Morrison AJ, Wenzel RP. Nosocomial urinary tract infections due to *Enterococcus*. *Arch Intern Med* 1986;**146**:1549–51.
10 Rietschel ET, Seydel U, Zatiringer U et al. Bacterial endotoxin: molecular relationships between structure and activity. *Infect Dis Clin North Am* 1991;**5**:753–79.
11 Waage A, Halstenson A, Espevik T et al. Cytokines in meningococcal disease. *Clin Infect Dis* 1994;**1**:97–108.
12 Bone RC, Fisher CJ, Clemmer TP et al. A controlled trial of high dose methyl prednisolone in the treatment of severe sepsis and septic shock. *N Engl J Med* 1987;**317**:653–8.
13 Ziegler EJ, Fistier CJ, Sprung CL et al. Treatment of gram negative bacteraemia and septic shock with HA-IA human monoclonal antibody against endotoxin—a randomised double blind placebo controlled trial. *N Engl J Med* 1991;**324**:429–36.
14 Waage A, Brandtzaeg P, Halstenent et al. The complex pattern of cytokines in serum from patients with meningococcal septic shock. Association between IL-6, IL-1 and fatal outcome. *J Exp Med* 1989;**169**:333–8.
15 Tracey KJ, Bentler B, Lowry SF et al. Anti-cachexin/TNF monoclonal antibodies prevent septic shock during lethal bacteraemia. *Nature* 1987;**330**:662–4.
16 Fischer E, Marano MA, Van Zee KJ et al. Interleukin-1 receptor blockade improves survival and haemodynamic performance in *E. coli* septic shock but fails to alter host responses to sublethal endotoxaemia. *J Clin Invest* 1992;**89**:1551–7.
17 Bone RC, Balk RA, Cerra FB et al. Definitions for sepsis and organ failure and guidelines for the use of innovative therapies in sepsis. *ACCP/SCCM Consensus Conference Committee (American College of Chest Physicians/Society of Critical Care Medicine)*, Chest 1992;**101**:1644–55.
18 Prescott S, Hadi MA, Elton RA et al. Antibiotic compared with antiseptic prophylaxis for prostatic surgery. *Br J Urol* 1990;**66**: 509–14.
19 British Society for Antimicrobial Chemotherapy. Antibiotic prophylaxis of infective endocarditis. *Lancet* 1990;**1**:88–9.

47 Prostatitis

N. Blacklock

Introduction

The classification by Drach *et al.* [1] of the various ways in which prostatitis might present provided, at that time, welcome clarification of the clinical concept of this disease, its pathogenesis, pathophysiology and hence management. Previously ill-defined entities such as non-bacterial prostatitis and the painful prostate in the absence of evidence of inflammation became more clearly understood. The proper application in every instance of the diagnostic techniques described below should lead to a definitive diagnosis and avoid confusing terminology such as 'prostatosis' and 'prostatopathic syndrome'.

The classification by Drach *et al.* [1] defined three recognizable prostatic entities and one wherein symptoms may, in fact, originate from tissues in juxtaposition to the gland:
1 Acute bacterial prostatitis.
2 Chronic bacterial prostatitis.
3 Non-bacterial prostatitis.
4 Prostatodynia.

This classification depends upon the features observed in the examination, specifically, of the expressed prostatic secretion (EPS). This is an 'office' examination whose salient features, therefore, can be defined at the time the patient is first seen and allows the early use of antibiotic treatment if this is indicated.

Acute bacterial prostatitis is an illness in which there are usually general symptoms of infection (fever, chills and myalgia) and the EPS is purulent on microscopy, according to defined criteria, and there is significant growth of a microorganism on culture. In chronic bacterial prostatitis there are usually no generalized symptoms but the EPS is purulent and pathogenic bacteria are present. There is usually also a history of urinary symptoms of varying intensity and a tendency to relapse following treatment. Non-bacterial prostatitis is characterized by symptoms of variable degree which can be acute and the EPS is purulent but remains sterile or produces only insignificant numbers of bacteria on conventional culture. In prostatodynia,

symptoms are usually longstanding and include urgency, dysuria, poor urinary flow and — a prominent feature — prostatic pain (i.e. pain in the perineum, groins and suprapubic area and also the sacrum). Characteristically this pain is exacerbated by intercourse and ejaculation, by sitting for long periods and by physical activity. The EPS shows neither leucocytes nor bacteria in significant numbers.

Inflammatory prostatitis is the fundamental lesion in infections of the anatomically normal male urinary tract. The complications which may stem from this include chronicity, prostatic abscess (now rare), epididymitis and pyelonephritis. The original prostatic lesion should not be overlooked, therefore, in the management of either of the two latter conditions.

Pathogenesis

The mode of infection of the prostate is by ascent of infection from the urethra. This implies an earlier colonization of the urethra by the potential pathogen, the origin of which is sexual. This is supported by the observation that the age of onset is usually in the middle of the second decade at the time when sexual activity begins. Furthermore organisms identical to those found in the EPS have been observed concomitantly in the introitus and vagina of the spouse or consort [2,3]. The organism may have the potential to be pathogenic within the urethra itself, as in the case of *Chlamydia trachomatis*, whilst others do not excite a local reaction, for instance the coliform group. In the case of the former, a urethral discharge may be present whilst in the latter, and perhaps more common, instance it will not. Prostatitis occurred in approximately one-third of cases as a complication of a previous gonococcal urethritis [4,5] and in a quarter of cases with non-specific urethritis [6].

The further ascent of microorganisms from the urethra to the prostatic urethra may be by direct extension but also may result from turbulence in the urinary flow at the level of the external sphincter which can lift the microorganisms

633

from the bulbous to the prostatic urethra. Hinman [7] showed that any partial intrinsic obstruction to urine flow within the urethra resulted in increased turbulence and back-eddies of urine, promoting bacterial ascent. Mayo and Hinman [8] observed the obstructive component in lower urinary tract infection in women to be a high-pressure zone caused by spasticity of the external sphincter. Buck [9] postulated similar sphincter irritability and spasm in cases of prostatitis as accounting for the diminished peak flow rate (PFR) occurring as a concomitant event. Improvement in PFR usually followed effective treatment. The back-eddies accompanying turbulence produced at the level of the external sphincter (either from failure of complete sphincter relaxation at the time of micturition or by the greater anatomical rigidity of the urethra at this point even in the absence of sphincter contraction) lift the organisms from the bulbous to the prostatic urethra. The same mechanism conceivably results in raised pressure within the prostatic urethra to promote reflux from there into the prostatic ducts and acini. The most vulnerable ducts are, therefore, those whose mode of entry into the urethra is non-valvular (i.e. those whose line of entry into the urethra is perpendicular to/against the direction of flow). These are the ducts coming from the peripheral zone which McNeal [10] found to be the common location of prostatitis (Fig. 47.1). The ducts of the central zone of the prostate open obliquely into the prostatic urethra, in the direction of flow, and may be expected usually to be forced closed in the circumstances of increased prostatic urethral pressure.

Incomplete urethral sphincter relaxation may occur as an irritative phenomenon in prostatitis itself or as a feature of a prior urethritis; it may also occur spontaneously in a tense and anxious person [11] due to the stimulation of the noradrenergically innervated component of the sphincter by higher than normal circulating levels of noradrenaline or other similarly acting humoral agents. Tension within the external sphincter of the same type occurs also as a reflex with painful or irritative lesions in the anus and lower rectum and is the basis of the so-called anogenital syndrome [12,13]. In all cases there is a lower PFR and sometimes interrupted urination. It is important to recognize that, where this dynamic obstruction occurs at the level of the external sphincter, for whatever cause, there is the likelihood of turbulence and urinary reflux into the prostatic ducts and a predisposition to prostatitis if there is concomitant bacterial colonization of the urethra. Morphological obstruction, as by urethral valves and strictures, is accompanied by the same pressure–flow phenomena and these are therefore also predisposing lesions.

Microbiology

Bacterial isolation rates in prostatitis are low. These may be as much as 40–50% if *Staphylococcus albus* is accepted as a pathogen [14,15] but much less than this if these are excluded [16]. Coliform and other faecal organisms predominate. The pathogenicity of staphylococci isolated from EPS has been questioned, but when the organism is recovered in pure culture from a symptomatic patient, the wisest course is to assume that it is causal and to treat accordingly. Riedasch *et al.* [17], furthermore, found positive antibody coating of the bacteria in cases of prostatitis in whom *S. albus* was recovered. This organism should, therefore, be considered a potential pathogen.

One of the problems of prostatitis had been an inability to isolate a recognizable pathogen in a majority of cases. These therefore fell within the definition of non-bacterial prostatitis [1]. The number of such cases provoked scepticism about the significance of an inflammatory reaction in the EPS [18], but the study by Gray *et al.* [19] showed that the presence of leucocytes was invariably

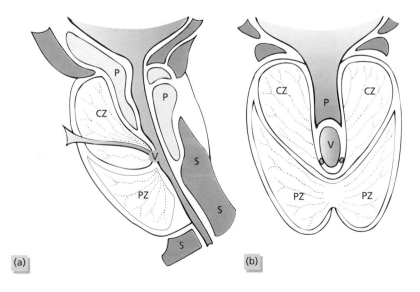

(a)   (b)

Fig. 47.1 (a) Midline sagittal and (b) coronal sections of the prostate showing the direction of ducts from the peripheral zone (PZ) as they enter the urethra. CZ, central zone; P, preprostatic sphincter; S, striated sphincter of the urethra; V, verumontanum.

accompanied by marked elevation of immunoglobulins IgG, IgA and IgM in prostatic fluid compared with normal subjects. Such a pattern in the serum would indicate exposure to a wide spectrum of antigens, similar to that arising from bacterial invasion. This evidence of antigenic stimulation, therefore, requires consideration of the presence of unidentified pathogens, including viruses, and perhaps biochemical irritants.

Non-gonococcal urethritis has been found to be due to *Chlamydia trachomatis* in approximately 50% of cases [20] and the prevalence of this infection suggested that the same organism was responsible in some cases of non-bacterial prostatitis. The isolation of this organism requires special cell culture procedures which are appropriate to specimens from the cervix, uterus and urethra. However, the chemical toxicity of prostatic fluid due to its zinc content interfered with attempts to isolate *C. trachomatis* from the EPS and modifications of the techniques were required. Furthermore, as any specimen of EPS was exposed within the milieu of the urethra prior to its isolation for culture, it was argued that any chlamydial organism isolated from it was likely to represent a urethral contaminant rather than a prostatic origin. Although Mardh *et al.* [21] observed the presence of chlamydial antibody in the serum of cases of non-acute prostatitis, this study and others thereafter were suspect for their inconclusiveness in defining with certainty a prostatic location for the infection. Brooman *et al.* [16] found evidence of *C. trachomatis* by either positive urethral culture or elevated antibody titre in 12% of cases of proven bacterial prostatitis and in 32% of cases of non-bacterial prostatitis. More recently Bruce and Reid [22], using tissue culture and immunofluorescence techniques found the organism within the prostatic fluid of six men with chronic prostatitis. Even more specifically, Brooman was the first to report from a series of nine patients with chronic prostatitis and positive urethral isolates of *C. trachomatis* that three of these had IgA specific against *C. trachomatis* in their EPS [23]. As IgA is an immunoglobulin which is secreted locally in response to infection this is almost conclusive of an intraprostatic location for the infecting organism. Thereafter there have been further reports of similar findings and, most recently, Tsunekawa *et al.* [24] found *C. trachomatis* specific IgA in the EPS of Japanese men with chronic prostatitis. Although there is still dispute over the conclusiveness of these and other studies on the prostatic location for chlamydial infection, Brooman [23] obtained a positive culture for *C. trachomatis* in a prostatic aspiration biopsy in one of four patients with positive EPS isolates.

If there is residual doubt as to the prostatic acinar location of *C. trachomatis*, clinical practicality suggests that it is to the patient's advantage if the existence of a *C. trachomatis* prostatitis is assumed. This means that specific treatment can be started for the putative infection,

especially in recurrence, and that the spouse or sexual partner of the patient can be investigated in case they have a reservoir of chlamydial infection.

Ureaplasma urealyticum, another organism requiring special culture techniques to define its presence, may also be involved in prostatitis. Quite apart from difficulties in culture it is known that a number of different species of *Myeoplasma* colonize the male reproductive tract without being pathogenic. Therefore, in spite of an isolate in inflammatory disease of the prostate, there is controversy as to its exact role in the individual case. Its main relevance appears to be its apparent association with male infertility.

The occurrence of viral infection, especially herpes simplex virus 2 (HSV2), in the female genital tract must indicate the possibility of virus transmission to the male and to the prostate. Virus isolation from the EPS, however, is again influenced, as in the case of *C. trachomatis* by the toxicity of the zinc content of the fluid for cell cultures. HSV2 and cytomegalovirus have, however, been isolated in several specimens and new techniques may make the investigation of a viral causation of prostatitis more feasible in the future [25].

Blacklock [3] postulated duct obstruction as leading to the peripheral isolation and loculation of the infecting organism whilst at the same time accounting for the presence of leucocytes in the EPS and therefore a 'non-bacterial' prostatitis. More recently it has been shown that the organisms within the prostatic acini and ducts can respond to an environment rendered hostile by antibiotics or an immune response by forming glycocalyx-enclosed microcolonies. This exopolysaccharide film can protect the bacteria from the effects of antibiotic and the host defence mechanism, so permitting their persistence within the gland [26]. This glycocalyx formation can explain the phenomenon of chronic prostatitis with recrudescence at intervals. The glycocalyx-enclosed bacteria are closely adherent to the acini and duct epithelium and are therefore difficult to dislodge by prostatic massage. This mechanical feature will encourage the persistence of infection and also account for the failure to culture microorganisms at the time of investigation, giving rise to an apparent non-infective or non-bacterial prostatitis. The intermittent release from these glycocalyx-enclosed colonies of small numbers of planktonic organisms may accompany flare-ups of infection at which time the organism in small numbers may be recoverable.

Whereas, before, the existence of a non-bacterial prostatitis was an enigma these more recent observations have shed light on the phenomenon.

Pathology

McNeal [10] observed the markedly greater frequency with which the peripheral zone of the prostate is involved in

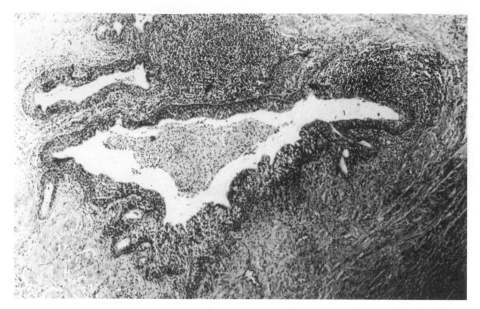

Fig. 47.2 Histological section of prostatic tissue in bacterial prostatitis showing an acinus containing leucocytes and infiltration of epithelium and peri-acinar tissues with leucocytes (H&E, ×48).

prostatitis. In 40 cases with histological evidence of prostatitis the inflammatory change was confined to the peripheral zone in 24 and to the central zone in only two. In 14 patients, the peripheral and central zones were involved, although in these the central zone was usually affected in continuity with the inflammation in the peripheral zone, suggesting that infection had extended from the peripheral into the central zone. The mechanism to account for this localization of prostatitis between these two zones has been described above.

Prostatitis, bacterial or non-bacterial, is an infection of the ducts and the acini of the gland with only secondary involvement of the stroma (Fig. 47.2). The course of the long ducts of the peripheral zone of the prostate are a predisposition to chronicity of infection, because at any point the duct may become obstructed by oedema, glyco-calyx material or calculi leading to stasis in its proximal part and the acini which it drains (Fig. 47.3). Chronic foci of

infection occur most often in the periphery of the gland (Fig. 47.4) and may be palpable digitally per rectum as nodular thickenings in chronic or longstanding disease. These are also obvious on transrectal ultrasound (TRUS) scanning. Local abscess formation in these positions may require surgical drainage under TRUS control.

Prostatic calculi may occur spontaneously from the prostatic secretion (intrinsic) and are usually formed of calcium phosphate [27]. These stones may be the natural progression for corpora amylacea which predominate in the central zone, the salts forming upon a fibrinous deposit within the acinus. The central zone appears homologous with the cranial lobe of the primate prostate which is known to contain a coagulase enzyme in its secretion causing a coagulum with seminal vesicular secretion [28]. About 50% of prostatic calculi are intrinsic whilst the remainder are formed from elements which can only have come from the urine (i.e. calcium oxalate and phosphate), and the implication from this is that there has been sufficiently frequent ingress of urine to ducts and acini over a period of time to allow crystallization, crystal aggregation and growth; these are therefore extrinsic in origin [27]. These calculi—either intrinsic or extrinsic—may provoke or complicate prostatitis and become reservoirs of organisms predisposing to recurrence and chronicity.

Clinical features

Prostatitis usually begins to be seen around the middle of the second decade, coinciding with the onset of sexual activity. In acute prostatitis there is frequently a history for several days of malaise before localizing features of dysuria, urinary frequency, and—variously—suprapubic, perineal and sacral pain. Terminal haematuria may occur and where infection is generalized within the gland there may be

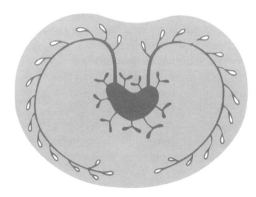

Fig. 47.3 Diagram of a transverse section through the prostate showing the course of the peripheral zone ducts through the parenchyma to the urethra.

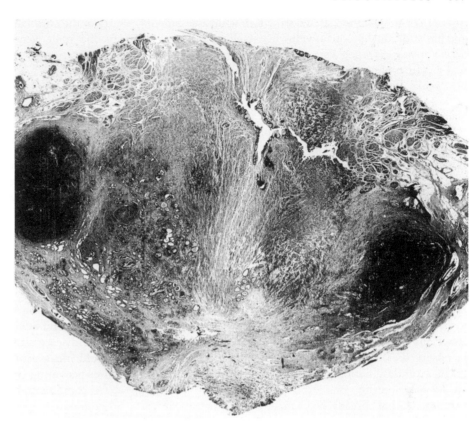

Fig. 47.4 Cross-section of the prostate showing the peripheral foci of infection (H&E, ×1).

fever. Generalized symptoms are uncommon in the chronic case and the history will usually extend over several months or several years either as recurrent minor episodes similar to that of acute prostatitis or more consistent micturitional disturbance and prostatic pain. In longstanding cases there may be partial impotence as a reactionary phenomenon and discomfort or actual pain with ejaculation.

The physical examination contributes little to the diagnosis. All prostates are sensitive (painful) to palpation, some more than others. A generalized acute prostatitis, however, renders the gland exquisitely tender and any attempt at prostatic massage to obtain secretion is strenuously resisted. Apart from this extreme state, 'tenderness' of the gland is not diagnostic. The more chronic the infection the greater the changes in consistency from homogeneity to nodularity on digital rectal examination. External examination should look for phimosis or meatal stenosis, both of which may be contributory to this condition by raising urethral pressure during micturition. The diagnosis of prostatitis depends entirely upon the examination of fractional urine and EPS specimens as described by Meares and Stamey [29]. Their technique and criteria are standard; neglect to use them in investigation as a routine renders diagnosis of 'prostatitis' spurious and suspect. Studies based on anything less than the application of this routine are difficult to accept as dealing with a series of cases of prostatitis.

The immediate microscopy of the wet film of the EPS is easily and quickly done as an 'office' procedure allowing rapid detection of prostatic inflammation. The secretion of the prostatic acinar cell is both apocrine and merocrine so that the prostatic fluid is representative of events within the acinar and duct cells. Changes in these produced by inflammation may be expected to influence the characteristics of the EPS. The detection of such changes provides a sensitive indicator of inflammation within the gland. For instance, Blacklock and Beavis [30] observed a profound change in the pH of EPS in prostatitis from a normal mean value of 6.6 to 7.4 or more. Anderson and Fair [31] confirmed its elevation in bacterial prostatitis, the mean value in their series being 8.3. White [32] found that there was a gradual return of the pH of the EPS to normal levels with resolution but this was often delayed until some time after the leucocytosis had disappeared. The factor responsible for the pH of the prostatic fluid is its citric acid content and this has been observed to fall significantly in inflammation from whatever cause [33]. This observation is so consistent that it is a reliable indicator of the presence of inflammation and, again, it is a test rapidly and effectively carried out at the time of the examination of the patient with the production of even a minute amount of EPS by using a pH paper (Duo test pH 5.0–8.0, Macherey Nagel GmbH & Co., Duren, Germany). Furthermore, it provides a sensitive measure of the rate and extent of resolution of the inflammation when repeated during follow-up assessments and has additional practical value in establishing a previous active prostatitis when a suspected case is seen after having had a course of antibiotics. If the patient is seen within a few weeks of taking antibiotics it is likely that the pH will still be elevated, although all other parameters have become normal.

The suspicion of prostatitis requires the utilization of these techniques for conclusive localization of inflammation within the prostate. Thereafter, classification of each case is possible into acute bacterial, chronic bacterial and non-bacterial forms of the disease and—the non-inflammatory type—prostatodynia. Rational management of the case is not possible unless this investigation is used and repeated throughout the course of the illness to evaluate resolution and its completeness.

TRUS is of some value in diagnosis—more so in the chronic or long established case, less so during the acute phase. Both hypo- and hyperechoic appearances occur, the former being more common in the acute condition, the latter more often seen in the chronic case. Calculi can also be observed. TRUS is, however, quite unable on its own to diagnose inflammation because the appearances are not sufficiently specific.

Reference has already been made to the disturbance of micturition patterns occurring in active prostatitis due to the tension and spasticity of the voluntary and involuntary components of the external urethral sphincter. Buck [9] observed a reduced PFR in prostatitis with abnormal flow curves. Significant improvement occurs following treatment where there is a clinically good response. Persistence of spasticity of the sphincter mechanism may provoke recurrence or perpetuate the course of the disease by causing reflux into the prostatic ducts.

Biochemical change in the EPS with inflammation is not just confined to a reduction in citric acid content. Kavanagh et al. [33,34] observed a profound fall in all of the secretory components of the prostate, including zinc, early in the onset of prostatitis and continuing long after the resolution of infection and even the disappearance of an inflammatory exudate. No other prostatic pathology is accompanied by such a profound and long-lasting effect. The recovery of secretory potential in its entirety is manifested by the reappearance of citric acid secretion (the 'marker' constituent) which is easily detectable by the returning acidity of the EPS on pH testing. Clearly, this secretory dysfunction is likely to have an effect upon the role of the prostatic secretion in male fertility. This may influence liquefaction but, perhaps of greater significance, has been the observation that infertility in some men is associated with diminished sperm chromatin stability and a lower zinc content of sperm nuclei as an accompaniment and sequel to inflammatory episodes [35]. The lowered content of nuclear zinc would impair the structural stabi-

lity of the chromatin and thereby increase the vulnerability of the male genome. This phenomenon awaits further investigation.

Complications

The availability of antibiotics has reduced the incidence of prostatic abscess which may otherwise occur as a complication of a bacterial prostatitis. When an abscess occurs the localization of the inflammation in the periphery of the gland may be followed by rupture and spontaneous drainage either into the urethra or rectum or via the perineum. A more common complication is the occurrence of chronicity of infection with the characteristic features already described; this usually follows either a failure to recognize and treat the earlier phase of the infection or the inadequacy of antibiotic treatment either in respect of duration of the course of the antibiotic or its inappropriateness as regards effective penetration into the acini and ducts. A greater understanding of the nature of the disease and the dynamics of antibiotic penetration should mean a progressive diminution in the number of cases becoming chronic.

A combination of infection within the prostate, and therefore the prostatic urethra, and a urethral high-pressure zone during micturition which may be secondary to the prostatitis fulfils the prerequisites for reflux of a bolus of microorganisms from the prostatic urethra along the vas to the epididymis. The frequently fulminating onset of acute epididymitis over a matter of hours suggests engulfment of the epididymis by a mass of organisms already established within the urinary tract. This sequence of events is supported by the clinical evidence. Some patients with epididymitis have premonitory symptoms of urinary frequency and some urethral discomfort before the onset of inflammation in the epididymis. Evidence of a coexistent prostatitis was observed in between 60 and 70% of cases of epididymitis [36]. The acute EPS changes (i.e. an increase in pH) is particularly helpful in differential diagnosis when there is the possibility of torsion; culture of the EPS may provide the identity of the organism and therefore help with the choice of antibiotic treatment. A corollary of the relationship between epididymitis and an underlying prostatitis is the necessity to ensure that the focus of infection within the prostate has responded to the antibiotic therapy as well as in the epididymis before cessation of treatment and/or surveillance of the patient. Failure to do so is one of the causes of recurrent epididymitis. It is noteworthy that one type of antibiotic may be superior in the management of the epididymitis whilst another may be more effective in the elimination of the infection in the prostate.

Auer and Seager [37] and Hanley [38,39] and others have provided both experimental and clinical evidence to support an ascending route of infection in pyelonephritis. This has been observed in females and children as reflux up the ureters from the focus of infection in the bladder. Whilst pyelonephritis rarely occurs in the adult male in the absence of structural abnormality of the urinary tract it has occurred as a complication of prostatitis [36]. The same mechanism of ascent of infection appears to apply in the male as in the female since oedema of the trigone and the intramural ureter has been observed in a number of cases urographically and confirmed endoscopically (Fig. 47.5). The sequence of events is that oedema of the trigone and intramural ureter from the underlying prostatitis interferes with the normal valvular closure of the intramural ureter during micturition, allowing reflux of infected urine. There is the same implication in management of pyelonephritis secondary to a prostatitis as in the management of secondary epididymitis—that resolution of the underlying prostatitis must be confirmed before treatment and surveillance is terminated.

Management

Acute bacterial prostatitis

Treatment is by an appropriate antibiotic in adequate dosage and for a sufficient length of time. The common coliform infection is perhaps now most effectively treated

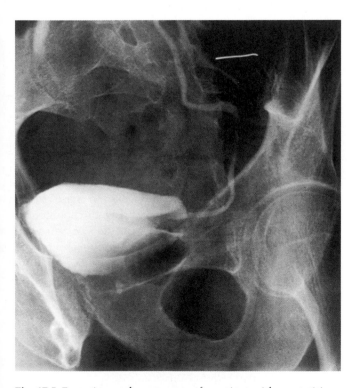

Fig. 47.5 Excretion pyelocystogram of a patient with prostatitis showing oedema of the trigone and intramural ureter.

using one of the second generation quinolones in conventional dosage. In order to achieve adequate penetration of the ducts and acini for a sufficient length of time to achieve elimination of the organism, the duration of the course should be not less than 2 weeks and, preferably, longer. It is in this situation that monitoring the progress of resolution by the Meares and Stamey routine [29] is important. Mixed Gram-positive and Gram-negative infection will require separate antibiotics. Erythromycin is usually effective against Gram-positive organisms and has the appropriate biochemical properties to achieve effective concentration within the acini and ducts [40]. If there is a satisfactory response to initial antibiotic treatment as manifested by the characteristics of fractional urines and EPS, consideration may be given to follow-on treatment with a urinary antiseptic such as nitrofurantoin. This achieves a high concentration in the urine and can maintain the lower urinary tract lumen free of pathogens while the prostate recovers its natural resistance to further bacterial invasion.

Bed-rest is advisable during the acute phase as this will alleviate symptoms rapidly even before the antibiotic has effect. The reason for this is considered to be the prompt relaxation of the pelvic floor and striated urethral sphincter which takes place in the supine position.

Where there has been no previous incidence of prostatitis and the patient responds satisfactorily to the treatment, there is not usually the necessity to carry out a full urological investigation. This, however, is advisable where resolution is prolonged or there is recurrence.

Chronic bacterial prostatitis

Long-standing prostatitis with exacerbation demands a complete urological evaluation including excretion urography, endoscopy, TRUS scan and urodynamic assessment. In addition, the spouse or consort should be interviewed and specimens for microbiological examination obtained from the vagina and cervix as this may provide the reasons for chronicity and recurrence (i.e. reinfection).

The choice of the antibiotic is again dependent upon bacterial sensitivity but the duration of the course should be additionally prolonged, perhaps for as long as 4–6 weeks. A lengthy period of surveillance with re-evaluation at each review is advisable.

The initial investigation of a case may reveal causal circumstances such as a urethral valve or cross-infection from the sexual partner and these should be managed appropriately. Persistent reduction in PFR suggesting a perpetuation of spasticity of the voluntary and/or involuntary external sphincter—and therefore the continuation of prostatic duct reflux—merits the use of a muscle relaxant either for voluntary (baclofen) or involuntary (indoramine or prazosin) muscles [41].

Non-bacterial prostatitis

Following investigation and confirmation of this condition, the case has been established earlier for regarding non-bacterial prostatitis as being due to *C. trachomatis* infection and management should be directed accordingly. *C. trachomatis* is effectively treated with a course of erythromycin, and its duration can usefully be for 28 days or until there is sign of resolution of the inflammatory reaction. Overall management must include adequate follow-up thereafter and it is essential that the spouse or sexual partner be investigated for the carriage of a similar organism and be treated and followed up concomitantly.

Prostatodynia

The patient with 'prostatic' pain and micturitional disturbances in the absence of any abnormal finding (i.e. absence of inflammatory reaction in fractional urines and EPS) is invariably difficult to manage. Although the probable mechanism whereby symptoms occur is now better perceived there are also neurotic and sometimes psychotic elements to be considered.

On referral there is the necessity for a complete review of the case from its beginning and for a full investigation of both the upper and lower urinary tracts even though the accompanying history suggests that a number of these investigations has already been done. Most of these patients will already have had some investigations and a multiplicity of antibiotic regimens and even bladder neck and prostatic surgery. If fractional urines and the EPS show no evidence of inflammation at this time, it is usually unnecessary to repeat antibiotic treatment.

A full urodynamic investigation is helpful. The PFR is usually reduced and, in the absence of organic urethral obstruction, is indicative of spasticity of the involuntary or voluntary sphincter or both. Osborn *et al.* [41] observed, in addition to a lowered PFR, a reduced voiding pressure and increased urethral closure pressures.

A patient with prostatodynia usually regards the likely outcome of the therapeutic attempts of the next medical attendant with cynicism, disbelief and despair. Considerable reassurance and attempts to uncover the cause of underlying anxiety or stress are necessary. Time is well spent in detailed enquiry of the circumstances accompanying exacerbation and remissions. These enable recommendations to be made on future lifestyle changes which will be necessary. Medicinal therapy is only supplementary to this. In a psychophysiological assessment, Reading *et al.* [42] found elevation of frontalis muscle electromyogram levels and raised pulse and respiration rates, suggesting the presence of functional, psychophysiological processes in these patients. This supports the concept that symptoms are generated by spastic musculature—either voluntary or involuntary—around the urethra.

In view of this, Osborn *et al.* [41], used baclofen (a striated muscle relaxant) and phenoxybenzamine (an α-adrenergic blocker) in a drug trial of 28 patients who were followed for a median interval of 10 months; eight patients improved with baclofen but only one patient remained symptom-free thereafter; 13 patients responded to phenoxybenzamine and of these, eight were cured and a further two claimed that they were much better. Six patients who had failed to respond to any treatment and one patient who had responded to a placebo alone were no better than before the therapeutic trial. This is perhaps a better response than might have been originally anticipated in patients so prone to anxiety and susceptibility to stress and stress-related phenomena. Psychophysiological testing and questionnaires designed to measure neurotic pathology were within normal limits in patients who responded to treatment, whereas in other groups the findings were similar to those in patients with an anxiety neurosis.

It appears from this study and others that α-adrenergic blocking drugs such as phenoxybenzamine or indoramine are specifically indicated in the management of prostatodynia and give a better chance of response than other supplementary therapy. However, Freixia *et al.* [43] have observed that prostaglandins of the E series (19-OH, PGE) are elevated in the seminal plasma in prostatitis and its aftermath which might provoke or aggravate spasm of the intrinsic prostatic musculature and therefore prostatic pain in these circumstances. If there is persistence of excess of E series prostaglandins as an irritative phenomenon after the inflammatory event, trial of treatment with a non-steroidal anti-inflammatory drug and even aspirin may have a specific indication.

The hot salt bath has for long been used in such cases—and in prostatitis in general—in continental Europe, but much less elsewhere. Such efficacy as it has is probably based on the diminution of α-adrenergic stimulation or its promoters in the circulation of tissue fluid, as a reflex from surface warming in the perineal area. Transurethral microwave thermotherapy is now able to raise tissue temperature at depth in the prostate and the sphincteric areas. There is a clear rationale for its use in well-conducted trials of a cohort, adequate in number, of proven cases of prostatodynia.

References

1 Drach GW, Fair WR, Meares EM, Stamey TA. Classification of benign diseases associated with prostatic pain; prostatitis or prostatodynia? *J Urol* 1978;**120**:266.

2 Stamey TA. The role of introital enterobacteria in recurrent urinary infection. *J Urol* 1973;**109**:467–72.

3 Blacklock NJ. Anatomical factors in prostatitis. *Br J Urol* 1974; **46**:47–54.

4 Thin RWT. Prostatitis after urethritis in Singapore. *Br Vener Dis* 1974;**50**:370–2.

5 Davis MJF. Urethritis and prostatitis in industry. *S Afr Med J* 1965;**39**:1101–5.

6 Chandiok S. Incidence of prostatitis as a complication of non-gonococcal urethritis. *Eur J STD* 1985;**2**:197–205.

7 Hinman F. Urethrovesical dysfunction and infection. *Ann Rev Med* 1973;**24**:83–8.

8 Mayo ME, Hinman F. Role of midurethral high pressure zone in spontaneous bacterial ascent. *J Urol* 1973;**109**:268–72.

9 Buck AC. Disorders of micturition in bacterial prostatitis. *Proc R Soc Med* 1975;**68**:508–11.

10 McNeal J. Regional morphology and pathology of the prostate. *Am J Clin Pathol* 1968;**49**:347–57.

11 George NJR, Slade N. Hesitancy and poor stream in neurologically normal younger men without outflow tract obstruction. *Br J Urol* 1979;**51**:506–10.

12 Muhrer KH, Weidner W, Filler D, Kaths T. Proctological findings in vegetative urogenital syndrome. In: Brunner H, Krause W, Rothauge CF, Weidner W, eds. *Chronic Prostatis*. Stuttgart: Schattauer Verlag, 1983:303–10.

13 Friesen A, Frank W, Streifinger W, Reichel U, Hofstetter A. Adnexitis and anogenital syndrome. In: Brunner H, Krause W, Rothauge CF, Weidner W, eds. *Chronic Prostatitis*. Stuttgart: Schattauer Verlag, 1983:311–18.

14 Smart CJ, Jenkins JD, Lloyd RS. The painful prostate *Br J Urol* 1976;**47**:861–8.

15 Drach GW. Problems in diagnosis of bacterial prostatitis: Gram negative, Gram positive and mixed infections. *J Urol* 1974;**111**:630–6.

16 Meares EM. Bacterial prostatitis versus 'prostatosis'. A clinical and bacteriological study. *J Am Med Assoc* 1973;**224**:1372–5.

17 Riedasch G, Ritz E, Mohring K, Ikinger U. Antibody coated bacteria in the ejaculate; a possible test for prostatitis. *J Urol* 1977;**118**:787–8.

18 O'Shaughnessy EJ, Parrino PS, White JD. Chronic prostatitis—fact or fiction? *J Am Med Assoc* 1956;**160**:540–2.

19 Gray SP, Billings J, Blacklock NJ. Distribution of immunoglobulins G, A and M in the prostatic fluid of patients with prostatitis. *Clin Chim Acta* 1974;**57**:163–9.

20 Oriel JD, Reeve P, Wright JT, Owen J. *Chlamydia* infection of the male urethra. *Br J Vener Dis* 1976;**52**:46–51.

21 Mardh PA, Ripa KT, Colleen S, Treharne JD, Darougar S. Role of *Chlamydia trachomatis* in non-acute prostatitis. *Br J Vener Dis* 1978;**54**:330–4.

22 Bruce AW, Reid G. Prostatitis associated with *C. trachomatis* in six patients. *J Urol* 1989;**142**:106–7.

23 Brooman PJC. Inflammatory prostatic disease. In: George NJR, Gosling JA, eds. *Sensory Disorders of the Bladder and Urethra*. New York: Springer Verlag, 1985:125–38.

24 Tsunekawa T, Kumanoto Y. *Chlamydia trachomatis* IgA. *J Jap Assoc Infect Dis* 1989;**63**:130–7.

25 Webber MM, Bouldin TR. Ultrastructure of human prostatic epithelium; secretion granules or virus particles? *Invest Urol* 1977;**14**:482–7.

26 Nickel JC, Olson ME, Barabas A *et al*. Pathogenesis of chronic bacterial prostatitis in an animal model. *Br J Urol* 1990;**66**:47.

27 Sutor DJ, Wooley SE. The crystalline composition of prostatic calculi. *Br J Urol* 1974;**46**:533–5.

28 Van Wagenen G. The coagulating function of the cranial lobe of the prostate gland in the monkey. *Anat Rec* 1936;**86**:411–21.

29 Meares EM, Stamey TA. Bacteriologic localisation patterns in bacterial prostatitis and urethritis. *Invest Urol* 1968;**5**:492–518.

30 Blacklock NJ, Beavis JP. The response of prostatic fluid pH in inflammation. *Br J Urol* 1974;**46**:537–42.

31 Anderson RW, Fair WR. Physical and chemical determinations of prostatic secretion in benign hyperplasia, prostatitis and adenocarcinoma. *Invest Urol* 1976;**14**:137–40.

32 White MA. Change in pH of expressed prostatic secretion during the course of prostatitis. *Proc R Soc Med* 1975;**68**: 511–13.

33 Kavanagh JP, Darby C, Costello CB. The response of seven prostate fluid components to prostatic disease. *Int J Androl* 1982;**5**:487–96.

34 Kavanagh JP, Darby C, Costello CB, Chowdhury SD. Zinc in post prostatic massage (VB3) urine samples: a marker of prostatic secretory function and indicator of bacterial infection. *Urol Res* 1983;**11**:1–4.

35 Kvist U, Kjelliberg S, Bjorndahl L, Hammar M, Doomans GM. Zinc in sperm chromatin and chromatin stability in fertile men and men in barren unions. *Scand J Urol Nephrol* 1988; **22**(1):1–6.

36 Blacklock NJ. Relation of prostatitis to urinary tract infection. In: Kass E, Brumfitt W, eds. *Infections of the Urinary Tract. Pyelonephritis*. Chicago: University of Chicago Press, 1978: 205–10.

37 Auer J, Seager LD. Experimental local bladder oedema causing reflux into ureters and kidneys. *Proc Soc Exp Biol Med* 1937;**35**:361–2.

38 Hanley, HG. Transient stasis and reflux into the lower ureter. *Br J Urol* 1962;**34**:283–5.

39 Hanley HG. Pyelonephritis and lower urinry tract inflammation. *Lancet* 1963;**1**:22–4.

40 Winningham DG, Nemoy NJ, Stamey TA. Diffusion of antibiotics from plasma into prostatic fluid. *Nature* 1968;**219**: 139–43.

41 Osborn DE, George NJR, Rao PN, Barnard RJ, Blacklock NJ. Prostatodynia: physiological characteristics and their rational management with muscle relaxants. *Br J Urol* 1981;**53**:621–3.

42 Reading C, Osborn D, George NJR, Marklow C, Blacklock NJ. Prostatodynia: a preliminary psychophysiological investigation. *Biol Psych* 1982;**9**:283.

43 Freixia R, Rosello J, Ramis I *et al*. Prostaglandin levels in infertile patients affected by astheno-zoosperma and prostatitis. *Prostaglandins Leukot Essent Fatty Acids* 1988;**31**(1): 41–4.

48 Parasitic Infections
A.G.A.Cowie

Introduction

Parasitic infections or infestations which can affect the genitourinary system in humans are mainly helminthic, but can be caused by protozoa or, rarely, to other organisms. Principal among these diseases are bilharzia, hydatid disease and filariasis. While none of these is endemic in the UK, with the present-day cosmopolitan nature of the population of the UK, widespread foreign travel and with visitors who may be tourists or long-stay residents, urologists need to be aware of the nature of these conditions and the treatments necessary to cure them. Table 48.1 summarizes the helminthic diseases.

Hydatid disease

Endemic areas for the pastoral forms of this disease are South America, the Near East, Africa, Australia and some parts of Europe. A reservoir of disease is maintained in these areas where dogs are allowed access to the raw offal of infected sheep or cattle, particularly where such animals are butchered at times of ritual sacrifice in farms or villages.

The sylvatic form of the disease involves the fox or wolf, with deer, moose or caribou as the secondary host. The causative organism is usually *Echinococcus granulosus* and rarely *E. multilocularis* which is much more invasive and has a high mortality [1]. When the carnivore ingests infective material, protoscolices—free in the cyst fluid or attached as buds of the internal cyst membrane—develop into hexacanth embryos which attach themselves to the upper small intestinal wall and there develop to maturity (Fig. 48.1). The short three-segment worms shed ova in large numbers which are passed out in faeces which contaminate vegetation or are transferred to the dog's tongue and fur, and which may then be accidentally ingested by sheep or humans.

The ova hatch in the stomach and soon penetrate to the portal circulation where the larval form usually encysts in the liver. Occasionally the larva may pass through to the lung or even to the general circulation and cysts may form anywhere in the body, including in the kidney. The life cycle is shown in Fig. 48.2.

Public health measures hold the promise of eradicating this disease by preventing the access of dogs to raw offal [2]. This may mean a rigorous policy of culling the population

Table 48.1 Helminthic parasitic diseases of the genitourinary system.

Type of organism	Species	Disease
Cestode (tapeworm)	*Echinococcus granulosus* *Echinococcus multilocularis*	Hydatid disease
	Taenia solium	Cysticercosis from encysted larval forms
Trematode (fluke)	*Schistosoma haematobium* *Schistosoma mansoni* *Schistosoma japonicum*	Bilharzia
Nematode (roundworm)	*Wuchereria bancroftii*	Filariasis
	Dracunculus medinensis	Dracunculosis
	Eustrongylus gigas	Strongylosis
	Onchocercus volvulus	Onchocerciasis
	Paragordius esavianus	Paragordiosis

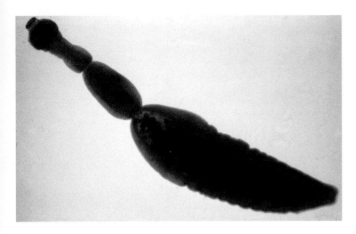

Fig. 48.1 Tapeworm of *Echinococcus granulosus* grown *in vitro*.

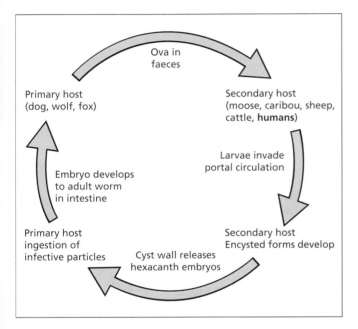

Fig. 48.2 The life cycle of *Echinococcus granulosus* and *E. multilocularis*.

of stray dogs, such as has been applied successfully in Cyprus, or by close supervision of farm dogs and worming procedures, such as in Scotland and Wales. However, measures such as these can be misunderstood and unpopular and the disease will continue to be troublesome.

In humans the disease causes problems because of the cysts which are composed of an inner lining of germinal epithelium capable of growing and releasing infective particles or developing into daughter cysts with a similar epithelium. This layer is supported by a laminated membrane of parasitic origin and then an ectocyst composed of compressed host tissue infiltrated with fibrous tissue formed as a host reaction to the infection. Cysts cause symptoms by taking up space and by applying pressure to nearby structures. The cysts are dangerous

because the contents are highly antigenic as well as infective and if such a cyst is ruptured either by accident or at surgery, the spilled fluid may provoke a severe allergic reaction, even anaphylaxis, or may seed into exposed tissues later to develop into multiple new cysts.

Most hydatid cysts are found in the liver, but in approximately 2% of patients with hydatid disease a cyst will be found in the kidney. A renal cyst lies within the parenchyma of the kidney as the larva will have arrived via the bloodstream. As it grows it will destroy renal parenchyma by pressure and it may eventually expand outwards, or rupture inwards into the renal pelvis (Fig. 48.3). Pelvic cysts lying low in the peritoneal cavity within the rectovesical pouch are found in approximately 5% of patients with hydatid disease [3,4]. Such cysts have grown as a result of the transcoelomic spread of a ruptured intra-abdominal cyst, usually from the liver. The enlarging pelvic cyst displaces and compresses the bladder (Fig. 48.4) to provoke frequency and may even result in urinary retention or obstructive azoospermia [5]. Haematospermia has been reported in a patient with a cyst involving the prostate and seminal vesicle. This must have been due to a haemato-genous infection [6] and cysts may appear anywhere in the body by this route, even in the testis [7].

It is possible for hydatid cysts to abort spontaneously and then to calcify progressively. Indeed, a degree of dystrophic calcification is often present even in live cysts. It is possible for the cysts to become secondarily infected, especially if there is contact with urine or bile. Whether the cyst is aborted, infected, alive or infective is often difficult to judge and in most cases it is best to assume that the cyst is alive and the cyst fluid is infective and that spillage is to be avoided at all costs. Blood tests may help in showing a raised white cell count with a rising eosinophilia. Serology by indirect haemagglutination, immunofluorescence and immunoelectrophoresis may also help but cross-reactions with other worm infestations are confusing and serology alone cannot be the sole criterion of infection [8]. The most reliable test would be the detection of circulating antigen but this test is available in only a very few centres. Imaging is very helpful and is usually performed initially by ultrasound. Further information from computed tomography (CT) scanning (Fig. 48.5) and more recently from magnetic resonance imaging (MRI) [9] is helpful in patients being followed up whilst on medical treatment and when planning surgery, especially in difficult cases where there are multiple cysts.

Management

Many clinical trials have shown that the benzimidazole compound albendazole is useful in treatment [10–14]. It has been possible to measure the levels of albendazole in cyst fluid after a period of treatment to assess penetration into

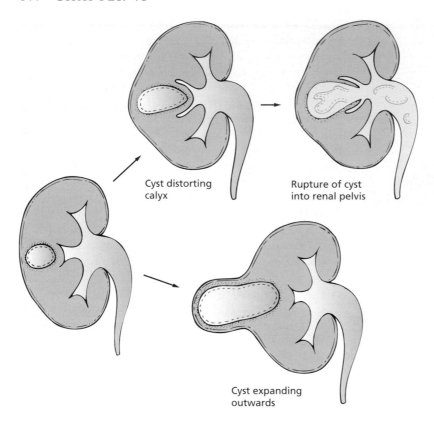

Cyst distorting
calyx

Rupture of cyst
into renal pelvis

Cyst expanding
outwards

Fig. 48.3 Development of the hydatid
cyst in the kidney.

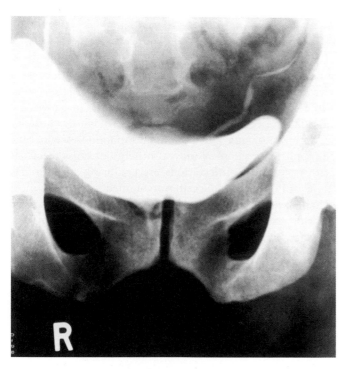

Fig. 48.4 A pelvic hydatid cyst displacing the bladder.

intact cysts, and therapeutic levels can be achieved. Cysts become smaller, osmotic pressure falls so the cyst becomes softer and floppy and the cyst membrane may separate

indicating that the cyst is dying. However, to achieve the best benefit, treatment may need to be continued for many months and the patient will need to be monitored for the possibility of hepatotoxicity. Albendazole is given in a dose of 10 mg/kg/day. Unfortunately, in some patients who have been treated for years and who appear to have had a good response, when treatment is discontinued there is evidence that the disease slowly regains its vigour and may eventually recur.

While albendazole can penetrate the intact cyst it is a relatively weak antihelminthic. A stronger agent is available which is useful at the time of surgery. Praziquantel in a dose of 40 mg/kg/day given for 1–2 weeks prior to the operation and continued for 1–2 weeks postoperatively will work well to eradicate infective particles spilled or released into the circulation. Unfortunately, it does not penetrate intact cysts. Even stronger still are chemical agents such as 0.5% silver nitrate [15] or 2.5% formalin which can be instilled directly into cysts after extraction of some of the fluid. Exposure of the germinal membrane to such an agent will sterilize the cyst in 1–2 min.

Ideally, therefore, patients should be treated with albendazole for at least 3 months and possibly longer, prior to evacuation of the cysts. Patients are brought to surgery with hydrocortisone cover to avoid serious allergic reactions and surgical evacuation is best done by using a method which avoids spillage, such as cryocone as advocated by Saidi [15,16] (Figs 48.6–48.8), and the

dissected [38]. Patients will often complain of episodes of fever and malaise with tenderness in the groin lymph nodes in attacks lasting 24 h or so.

Management

The worm responds to diethylcarbamazine 0.5–2 g/kg t.d.s. for 3 weeks. The lymphoedema that persists after treatment is often a problem especially in the penis or scrotum (Fig. 48.13). Initially treatment includes the use of antibiotics to eliminate secondary infection. A benzopyrone may help to reduce the high protein oedema as in other obstructive lymphoedemas [39]. Coumarin in a dose of 200 mg b.d. and continued for 6–12 months if benefit is achieved is useful [40]. The surgical excision of the hydrocele and the removal of excess lymphangiomatous tissue and skin may be required. It is virtually always possible to cover the genitalia with flaps of nearby skin to produce an acceptable cosmetic result (Fig. 48.14).

Chyluria

Collaterals and abnormal lymphatic routes may develop as a result of lymphangitis caused by the worms, and fistulas may develop between the lymphatics and the urinary tract—either into the bladder or into the renal pelvis, resulting in the development of milky urine. The patients lose considerable amounts of protein and fat and develop weight loss, oedema and possibly ureteric colic as proteinaceous plugs pass down the ureters. It may be possible to

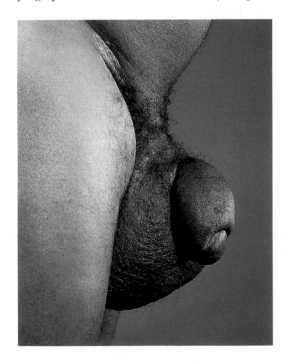

Fig. 48.13 Filarial lymphoedema of the scrotum and penis.

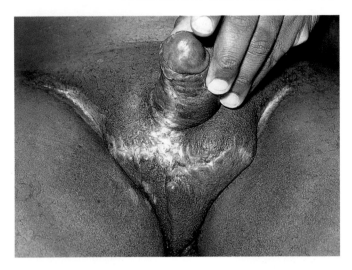

Fig. 48.14 The patient shown in Fig. 48.13 after surgery.

see the milky exudate at cystoscopy as it passes through the bladder wall, or after lymphangiography when the opportunity can be taken to continue the lymphangiogram infusion with a dye such as methylene blue which may become visible at cystoscopy (Fig. 48.15). Lymphangiography can demonstrate the abnormal lymphatic channels. In about 50% of patients the condition resolves itself and only in 2% can a filarial cause be identified positively.

Treatment, after management of the worm, is by fulguration of the area of visible abnormal lymphatic fistulas in the bladder, or by instillation of silver nitrate [41,42]. This may be by a catheter to the bladder or by a ureteric catheter to the renal pelvis. In treating the kidney 5–10 ml of 0.5% silver nitrate are instilled weekly for a period of 4 weeks or three times a day for 2 or 3 days. Such regimens have been reported to be 60–70% successful.

If the problem persists it is then possible to consider local surgery to strip the adventitia containing the lymphatics off the vessels of the renal pedicle to disrupt the lymphatic pathway [43]. It is helpful to use an intralymphatic infusion of methylene blue to colour the lymphatics at the time of surgery. The condition is bilateral in about 50% of cases and the second side may need a similar operation after 2–3 months if 24 h protein excretion rates remain high.

Other helminthic parasites affecting the genitourinary system

Adult worms

A few adult worms have been found in the tissues of the genitourinary tract. Gaining entry through wounds or by ingestion in the larval form or by injection at the time of an insect bite, an adult worm can migrate along tissue planes and some have a predilection for specific tissues. The patients suffer the noxious effect of the presence of an

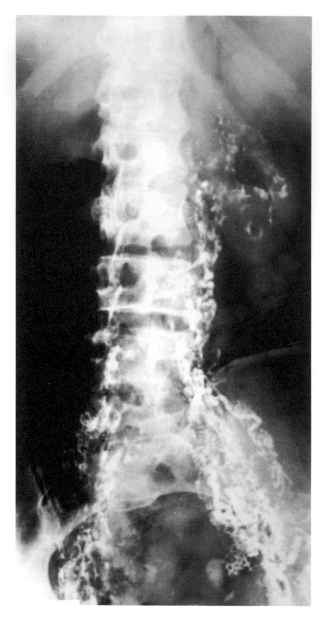

Fig. 48.15 Lymphangiogram of chyluria.

irritative or destructive foreign body with the possibility of additional secondary infection resulting in abscess formation. In some cases, the worm may encyst to form a nodular mass which may then calcify.

Ascaris lumbricoides

It is known that occasionally worms from the gastro-intestinal tract can be disseminated and can be the cause of a bladder problem. In a recent case report a perineal fistula following transurethral resection of the prostate was found to be related to a mass of worms in the bladder. The fistula closed spontaneously after removal of the worms [44].

Dracunculus medinensis

After ingestion the larva develops into a guinea worm which grows in the body in connective tissue planes and may reach 1 m in length. After copulation the male dies and the gravid female sooner or later seeks a skin surface in contact with water, usually in the feet or ankles, where she may discharge embryos through a blister into the water. Here they are taken up by a small crustacean (*Cyclops*) in which a larva develops. The new human host becomes infected by drinking infected water. Worms have been retrieved from, and were presumably the cause of, testicular [45] and scrotal [46] abscesses. It is also possible for such an abscess to result in a urethral fistula [47]. Treatment is by drainage of the abscess and, if possible, extraction of the worm. Medication with niridazole 25 mg/kg for 7 days appears to be effective.

Eustrongylus gigas

The giant kidney worm is primarily a parasite of the mink, racoon and wolf. Eggs are shed and later ingested by fish. It is the larval form in the fish which is infective to humans [48]. Only one or two worms survive to lodge in and gradually consume the renal parenchymal tissue over several years. Treatment is surgical.

Onchocercus volvulus

Transmitted by *Simulium*, the black fly, the microfilariae develop in humans until a male and one or two female worms coiled together, lodge in the subcutaneous tissue and become surrounded by fibrous tissue. The worms live for up to 15 years and release millions of microfilariae. Cutaneous oedema, especially in the groins, may result in wrinkled and hanging skin which may contain pendulous lymph nodes. Subsequently genital elephantiasis may develop.

Treatment is by the use of diethylcarbamazine in an initial dose of 30 mg daily for 3 days. This may be doubled and re-doubled if there is no untoward reaction to a normal dose of 150 mg daily which is continued for 12 days. Whilst this treatment is effective against the microfilariae, the adult worms may require treatment with suramin 1 g/week, but since this is nephrotoxic a test dose is essential and patients need close supervision.

Paragordius esavianus

There is a single report of a 15 cm worm passed through the urethra in a young woman thought to have been infested by urethral penetration when swimming [49].

Larval forms

Some worms are capable of producing larvae which may migrate around the body to produce a moving itchy eruption. Eventually the larvae settle into nodules which can develop especially in the scrotum, testis and epididymis. Examples of this infection in humans include:

1 Tinea soleum and tinea saginata.
2 Infection caused by *Ascaris lumbricoides*.
3 Infection caused by *Ancylostoma carnis*.
4 Infection caused by *Necator americanus*.
5 Infection caused by *Strongyloides stercoralis*.

Treatment may require surgical excision of the nodules or larval tracts. Disturbing the tissues may release antigens and evoke intense local reactions, but it is usually beneficial to eradicate the disease to avoid chronic infestation and ill health. Active disease may still be present 30 years after the initial infection, as has been reported for strongylosis [50]. Surgery usually achieves the best result in conjunction with suitable medication, according to the worm.

Non-helminthic parasitic genitourinary disease

Protozoa

Trichomonas vaginalis

This flagellate organism is commonly found in the secretions of inflamed genital surfaces such as vaginal or prepucial skin or the urethral mucosa. The disease is commonly transmitted sexually and may involve the Cowper or Skene glands. Rarely it is the cause of chronic prostatitis or seminal vesiculitis, and even more rarely it has been reported as a cause of cystitis or even pyelitis. The protozoa are easily recognized as actively motile organisms progressing through the fluid of a 'hanging drop' wet specimen without the need for special stains, and treatments with metronidazole by pessary or by mouth is effective.

Entamoeba histolytica

Transient haematuria followed by cystitis with bullous oedema and the development of inflammatory 'papillomas' can be due to infection with this amoeba, which is the only amoeba pathogenic to humans. Both vegetative and encysted forms exist and transmission is usually due to the ingestion of cysts, each of which is capable of developing into four amoebae in the intestine and can then penetrate into the portal venous system. Spread of disease to other areas may be by intestinal contamination as in balanitis [51], or by local penetration of the organism from the intestine to the retroperitoneum to produce periureteritis and perinephritis. Treatment of penile disease is by circumcision and local toilet hygiene, and for internal disease is by metronidazole which is very effective.

Plasmodium falciparum

The phenomenon of black water fever is the only urological manifestation of malaria. It is due to haemoglobinuria of considerable degree resulting from the lysis of large numbers of red blood cells by an immune mechanism involving complement, and is seen only in patients who have stayed 2–3 months in an endemic area and who have been treated with inadequate doses of quinine. The haemoglobinuria is of a sufficient degree to cause acute renal tubular necrosis in addition to other malarial symptoms, and uraemia may result. Treatment requires the use of appropriate antimalarials alongside the usual measures required to treat uraemia.

Rare parasites

Fly larvae

Cystitis due to the presence of *Anthomyia canicularis* larvae in the bladder is known as cystomyasis [51] and is due to the development of a larva within the bladder resulting from an egg laid near the urinary meatus. The condition resolves when the larva (up to 1 cm long) is passed per urethram.

Even the common housefly can be responsible for cystitis due to the development of a *Musca domestica* larva in the bladder [51].

Catfish

While normally surviving by attaching itself to the gills of other fish where a rich blood supply provides plenty of nourishment, *Vandellia cirrosa* is capable of sucking blood from the human mucosa. Apparently attracted by urine passed inadvertently by swimmers [52], the fish known as candiru (carnero) by the local Amazonian Indians, can enter the urethra and may die and later become encrusted with phosphate. This acts as a foreign body and treatment is by the evacuation of the foreign material.

References

1 Sammuels S, Fosmoe R. Alveolar hydatid disease with involvement of theinferior vena cava. *Am Surg* 1970;**6**: 698–701.
2 Dungal N. *Echinococcus* in Iceland. *Am J Med Sci* 1946;**212**: 12–17.
3 Borell JH, Barnes JM. Renal manifestations of hydatid disease. *NY J Med* 1933;**33**:1390–5.

4 Deklatz RJ. Echinococcal cyst involving the prostate and seminal vesicles: a case report. *J Urol* 1976;**115**:116–17.

5 Rar MS. Cyst causing obstructive azoospermia. Obstructive azoospermia due to retrovesical hydatid cyst. *Fertil Steril* 1979;**32**:706–7.

6 Whyman MR, Morris DC. Retrovesical hydatid causing haemospermia. *Br J Urol* 1991;**68**:100–101.

7 Kumar PV, Jahonshali S. Hydatid cyst of testis: a case report. *J Urol* 1987;**137**:511–2.

8 Kagan IG, Osimani JJ, Varela JC, Allain DS. Evaluation of intradermal and seriological tests for the diagnosis of hydatid disease. *Am J Trop Med Hyg* 1966;**15**:172–9.

9 Hoff FL, Aisen AM, Walden MW, Glazer GM. MR imaging in hydatid disease of liver. *Gastrointest Radiol* 1987;**12**:39–42.

10 Morris DL. Pre-operative albendazle therapy for hydatid cyst. *Br J Surg* 1987;**74**:805–6.

11 Rahentulla A, Bryceson AD, McManus DP, Ellis DS. Albendazole in the treatment of hydatid disease. *J R Soc Med* 1987;**80**:119–20.

12 Davidson RN, Bryceson AD, Cowie AGA, McManus DP. Pre-operative albendazole therapy and hydatid cysts. *Gastrointest Radiol* 1987;**12**:39–42.

13 Horton RJ. Chemotherapy for *Echinococcus* infection in man with albendazole. *Trans R Soc Trop Med Hyg* 1989;**83**:97–102.

14 Morris DL. Albendazole treatment of hydatid disease—follow-up at 5 years. *Trop Doct* 1989;**19**:178–80.

15 Saidi F. *Surgery of Hydatid Disease*. London: WB Saunders, 1976.

16 Shetty SD, Al-Saigh A, Ibrahim AI, Patil KM, Battachan CL. Management of hydatid cysts of the urinary tract. *Br J Urol* 1992;**70**:258–61.

17 Elem B. Spontaneous rupture of the bladder associated with *Schistosoma haematobium. Br J Urol* 1977;**49**:426.

18 Bret PM, Fond A, Bretognolle M *et al*. Percutaneous aspiration and drainage of hydatid cysts in the liver. *Radiology* 1988;**168**:617–20.

19 Rodstake HN. Bladder involvement in *Schistosoma mansoni. Trop Geogr Med* 1973;**25**:84–5.

20 Rocha H, Cruz T, Brito E, Susin M. Renal involvement in patients with hepatosplenic *Schistosoma mansoni. Trans R Soc Trop Med Hyg* 1976;**66**:505-7.

21 Muragasu R, Wang F, Dissanaike AS. *Schistosoma japonicum* type infection in Malaysia—report of the first living case. *Trans R Soc Trop Med Hyg* 1978;**72**:389–91.

22 Edington GM. Pathological effects of schistosomiasis in Ibadan, western state of Nigeria. 1. Incidence and intensity of infection, distribution and severity of lesions. *Am J Trop Med Hyg* 1970;**19**:982–9.

23 El Sebai J. Cancer of the bilharzial bladder. *Urol Res* 1978;**6**: 233–6.

24 Taylor MG, Denham DA, Nelson GS. Observations on the resistance to *Schistosoma* infection of neonatal mice born to immune mothers with a demonstration of increased resistance in lactating mice. *J Helminthol* 1971;**45**:223–8.

25 Sabour MS, El Said W, Abou-Gabal I. A clinical and pathological study of schistosomal nephritis. *Bull World Health Organ* 1972;**47**:549–57.

26 Von Lichtnburg F, Cheever AW, Erikson DG, Hickman RL. Experimental infection with *Schistosoma haematobium* in chimpanzees. Parasitological, clinical, serological and pathological observations. *Am J Trop Med Hyg* 1970;**19**:427–58.

27 Manson-Bahr PH. In: Wilcocks C, ed. *Manson's Tropical Diseases*, 16th edn. London: Ballière Tindall Cassells, 1966.

28 Mapilly J, Sunkwa-Mills HNO. Bilhariosis of the epididymis and spermatic cord. *Med J Zambia* 1976;**10**:58–9.

29 Joshi RA. Bilateral total infarction of the testis due to schistosomiasis of the spermatic cord. *Am J Trop Med Hyg* 1962;**11**:357–9.

30 Leslie TA, Goldsmith PC, Dowd PM. Valval schistosomiasis. *J R Soc Med* 1993;**86**:51.

31 Eustace D, Trehan A, Raju KS, Derias N. Abdominal pain and vaginal bleeding associated with schistosomiasis of the genital tract. *J Obstet Gynaecol* 1992;**12**:427–8.

32 Pugh RN, Gilles HM. Malumfashi endemic disease research project in urinary schistosomiasis, a longitudinal study. *Ann Trop Med Parasitol* 1978;**72**:471–82.

33 Fam A, Ramzy I. A clinical pathological study of carcinoma of the bladder in Egypt. *Int Surg* 1967;**47**:176–80.

34 Talib H. Problem of bilharzial bladder in Iraq. *Br J Urol* 1970;**42**:571–3.

35 Ravi G, Motalb MA. Surgical correction of bilharzial ureteric stricture by Boari flap technique. *Br J Urol* 1993;**71**:535–8.

36 Young SW, Farid Z, Bassily S, El Massy NA. Efficacy of medical treatment of schistosomal obstructive uropathy as determined by ^{131}I hippuron renography. *Trans R Soc Trop Med Hyg* 1978;**72**:627–30.

37 Cowie AG. Therapy for tropical urological diseases. In: Hendry WF, ed. *Recent Advances in Urology*. London: Churchill Livingstone, 1981:107–22.

38 Carbera Y, Caridad J. Filarial lymphatic cyst of the inguinal canal. *J Rev Kuba* 1967;**3**:111–14.

39 The conservative treatment of post mastectomy lymphoedema. In: Bartos V, Davidson JW, eds. *Advances in Lymphology*. Prague: Avicerium, 1982:471–4.

40 Casley-Smith JR, Wang CT, Cui Zi-hai. Treatment of filarial lymphoedema and elephantiasis with 5,6-benzo-α pyrone (coumarin). *Br Med J* 1993;**307**:1037–41.

41 Tan LB, Chiang CP, Chou CH, Wong CJ. Experiences in the treatment of chyluria in Taiwan. *J Urol* 1990;**114**:710–13.

42 Dalela D, Kramer A, Ahlawat R *et al*. Routine radioimaging in filarial chyluria—is it necessary in developing countries? *Br J Urol* 1992;**69**:291–3.

43 Yu HHY. Chyluria: results of surgical treatment in 50 cases. *J Urol* 1978;**199**:104–7.

44 Kesari D, Goralic U, Gantus I, Sibi Y. Ascoriosis of the urinary bladder. *B J Urol* 1994;**72**:984.

45 Raffii P, Dutz W. Urogenital dracunculosis. Review of the literature and report of three cases. *J Urol* 1967;**97**:542–3.

46 Pendse AK, Soni BM, Omprakash R, Gupta SP. Testicular dracunculosis — a distinct clinical entity. *Br J Urol* 1982;**54**: 56–8.

47 Shukla B, Singh H. Dracunculus causing urethral fistula. *Br J Urol* 1994;**73**:461–2.

48 Wong Hok Boon, Tan Kwan Hoh. Severe whipworm infestation in children. *Singapore Med J* 1961;**2**:34.

49 Burger R. *Paragordius esavianus* passed per urethram. *J Urol* 1972;**108**:469–70.

50 Gill GV, Bell DR. *Strongyloides stercoralis* infection in former Far East prisoners of war. *Br Med J* 1979;**2**:275–6.

51 Sanjurjo LA. Parasitic disease of the genito-urinary system. In: Campbell MF, Harrison JH, eds. *Urology*, Vol 1. Philadelphia: WB Saunders, 1970:480–511.

52 Herman JR. Candiru: urophilic catfish. *Urology* 1973;**1**:265.

49 Bilharziasis of the Genitourinary Tract

M.A.Ghoneim

Introduction

The larvae of *Schistosoma haematobium* continue to develop in the veins of the infected human host and, on reaching maturity, the coupled worms migrate to the veins of the vesical and pelvic plexuses where they mate and the female begins to lay eggs. Involvement of the various urogenital organs varies markedly and appears to correlate with the extent of their venous circulation. Thus, the urinary bladder, lower ends of the ureters and seminal vesicles are most commonly affected by the disease in view of their rich venous supply. Mohamed [1] reported the percentage distribution of the eggs of *S. haematobium* among the endopelvic organs as 90% in the urinary bladder, 80% in the seminal vesicles and 19% in the prostate. Furthermore, the intensity of egg deposition in the tissues bears a similar correlation. In a quantitative postmortem study, Smith *et al.* [2] noted a mean egg count of 4313/g of tissue in the urinary bladder, 19 929/g in the seminal vesicles and 8058/g in the prostate. There was a significant correlation between the egg burden and the histological severity of the tissue reaction.

Pathology and evolution of lesions

Initial response

The primary pathology represents a reaction of the host directed against the deposition of schistosomal eggs. Initially, a granulomatous lesion forms in the lamina propria (Fig. 49.1). The extent of this lesion and its subsequent evolution by healing, progression or complication depends on several factors, the relative importance of which are not yet clearly defined. These factors include the tissue egg load, the frequency of reinfestation, the efficiency of treatment and the onset of secondary infection.

Subsequent pathology

The secondary responses represent an epithelial reaction

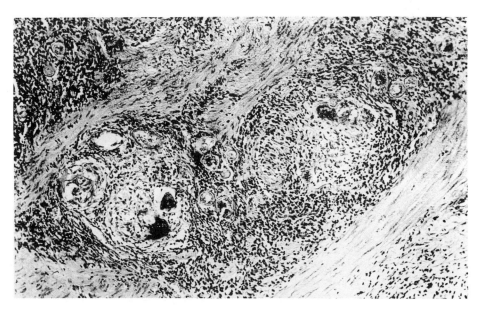

Fig. 49.1 The initial lesion is a bilharzial granuloma. The bilharzial ova are surrounded by inflammatory cells (×100).

resulting from events which started originally in the submucosa. The deposited eggs secrete a histiolytic antigen which is tissue fixed and evokes a cell-mediated immune response in surrounding host tissue. The cellular infiltrate is characterized by the presence of eosinophils and the overlying mucosa is raised into polypoid patches surrounded by hyperaemia. The pattern of the subsequent changes may be atrophic, proliferative or metaplastic.

Atrophic changes result from heavy submucous ova deposition with subsequent reduction of the blood supply to the overlying epithelium. The development of secondary bacterial infection may also play an aggravating part. Eventually, erosion of surface epithelium results in the formation of bilharzial ulcers.

In hyperplasia, the number of epithelial stratifications is increased beyond the normal value of six layers. In simple hyperplasia, there is no cellular atypia, whereas in dysplastic forms of hyperplasia, nuclear atypia is present but limited to the basal layers. The hyperplastic mucosa may be thrown into papillary surface projections, producing the lesion known as polypoid cystitis.

The transitional epithelium overlying and surrounding the lesion may undergo squamous or columnar metaplasic changes. Columnar metaplasia may be typified by predominant glandularis changes or cystica changes of epithelial enclosures. These are aetiologically related and represent columnar metaplasia of the urothelium rather than inflammatory epithelial inclusion. It is not unusual to find the concomitant association of cystitis cystica and cystitis glandularis in the same lesion (Fig. 49.2).

Secondary bacterial infection

The frequency of bacterial superinfection in urinary schistosomiasis appears to be related to the age of the patient and to the severity of infestation. In a survey of rural Egyptian children, *Escherichia coli* and *Salmonella* bacteriuria were detected in 5% of the studied cases. In patients with bilharzial cystitis, however, bacterial infection was invariably present, and 50% of these were due to *E. coli* [3].

In addition to aggravating the symptoms of bilharzial cystitis, secondary bacterial infection contributes greatly to morbidity of urinary bilharziasis by leading to ascending infection of the upper tract and serious deterioration of renal function. Furthermore, bacterial infection may have a significant role in the development of other urinary complications such as stricture, fistulas, calculi and malignancy.

Healing

The natural history of urinary schistosomiasis depends upon three main factors: the severity of infestation, frequency of reinfestation and adequacy of therapy. Thus, with occasional infestation and adequate treatment, favourable healing is the usual outcome. Active granulomatous lesions encountered in children and young adults are particularly reversible [4]. Favourable healing entails a reasonable amount of mural fibrosis and dystrophic calcification.

Chronicity and complications

Frequent reinfestation and inadequate treatment are usual among farmers living in endemic areas. The development of fixed and irreversible pathological states is not unlikely. These include the development of ureteric strictures, chronic cicatricial ulcers, bladder contraction, outflow obstruction, leucoplakia, carcinoma *in situ* and overt bladder malignancy.

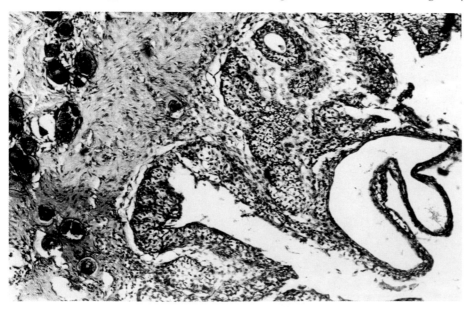

Fig. 49.2 Columnar metasplasia: cystitis cystica and cystitis glandularis (×100).

Bilharziasis of the ureters

The main site of involvement is the endopelvic part of the ureters. Less commonly, the lumbar portion of the ureter may also be affected [5]. Zahran *et al.* [6] suggested that ovideposition is mainly periureteral. Other studies have shown that the eggs are found in all layers, particularly suburothelially and between the muscle layers. The end result is healing with a variable degree of mural fibrosis, with the loss of muscle and periureteral adhesions. The sum of these changes is an obstructive uropathy due to stricture formation and/or atony and dilatation of the involved segment. Vesicoureteral reflux has also been reported in some 15% of cases [7]. Eventually, urinary stasis invites secondary bacterial infection and stone formation.

Clinical features and evaluation

Loin pain and renal colic with or without symptoms of pyelonephritis are the main presenting features. Patients may also present with a silent clinical hydronephrosis. Less commonly, the first presenting symptom is anuria [8]. Diagnosis is based on findings in urography and retrograde or antegrade studies (Fig. 49.3). Radioisotope renography has a definite place in the evaluation of renal function, determination of the degree of obstruction and follow-up after surgery [9].

Management

Antischistosomal therapy should be given for the early lesions. Some authors advise the administration of adjuvant corticosteroid therapy to reduce the intensity of the inflammatory and fibrotic reactions [10]. Endourological procedures may be also useful for early short segment strictures. Endoscopic dilatation visual internal ureterotomy with stenting were successful in 40–60% of such cases [11].

Open surgery is usually indicated for the more established lesions. Resection and reanastomosis is very suitable for the well-localized short segment stricture. Reimplantation of the ureter into the bladder is the procedure of choice for strictures of the lower ends of the ureter. Concomitant affection of the bladder and dilatation and thickening of the ureter above the strictured area may render adoption of an antireflux procedure extremely difficult. Under such circumstances anastomosis of the ureter to a sufficiently long Boari bladder tube flap provides an excellent alternative.

For long segment or multiple strictures of the ureter, replacement of the pathological segment by an isoperistaltic segment of ileum may be the only solution. Evidence has been provided that tailoring of the ileal ureter to reduce its cross-sectional diameter as well as the

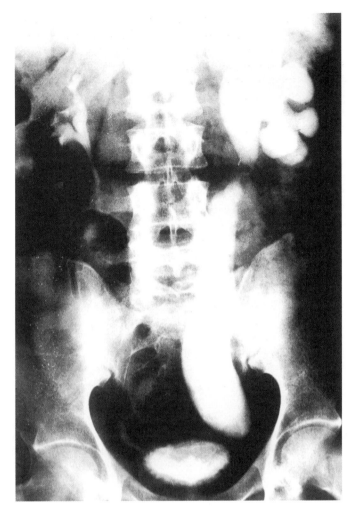

Fig. 49.3 Intravenous pyelogram of a stricture at the low end of the left ureter with significant back pressure changes.

creation of an intussuscepted nipple valve at its distal end for reflux prevention are followed by better functional results [12]. Nephrectomy is indicated for advanced cases with loss of renal function.

Bilharziasis of the bladder

Clinical features and evaluation

Patients suffering from bilharzial lesions of the lower tract present essentially with a common symptom complex: painful micturition, frequency, pyuria and haematuria. Pain is usually intense with bladder ulceration, and may be referred to the tip of the penis and to the perineum. In the active phase, there is invariably heavy excretion of viable eggs in the urine and, in addition, there may be bacteriuria. Anaemia and eosinophilia are commonly present.

The diagnosis is usually evident in patients from endemic areas and with the finding of schistosomal eggs in the urine. A plain X-ray may show bilharzial calcification, and cystography sometimes reveals filling defects of proliferative bladder lesions or may suggest the more chronic manifestation of contracted bladder or outlet obstruction. Critical evaluation of the bladder lesion, however, requires endoscopic examination and this remains the most important tool in the management of this group of patients.

Endoscopic features

Cystoscopy allows morphological indentification of the gross bladder lesion and, furthermore, permits histopathological verification of obtained biopsy material.

Bilharzial tubercles

These are characteristic of early and active infestation and appear as seed-like, yellowish specks, slightly prominent above the mucous membrane (Fig. 49.4). Initially, each tubercle is surrounded by a circle of hyperaemia but, later, these may fade out or disappear. Lesions which are distinctly larger and more prominent are sometimes described as bilharzial nodules.

Bilharzial polyps

El-Badawi [13] observed these lesions among 7.2% of bilharzial patients who underwent endoscopic examination, and described three types.

1 *Granulomatous polyps*. These were the most common finding (60.5%) and represented an active and dense granuloma in the submucosa. The preferential site is the bladder trigone, usually in the paraureteric region, and lesions may be pedunculated, red and occasional, multiple or clustered (Fig. 49.5).

2 *Fibrocalcific polyps*. These are usually encountered in older patients (over the age of 20 years) and are commonly single, pedunculated and bear a dull yellowish hue. Histological features are those of a healed granuloma covered by atrophic epithelium and there may be varying degrees of calcification.

3 *Villous polyps*. These are indistinguishable from vesical papillomas by cystoscopy. However, biopsy examination will reveal the characteristic bilharzial granulations at the pedicle of the polyp.

As already described, atrophy of the surface epithelium over bilharzial lesions results in a thinned-out covering, so that the old calcified bilharzia eggs buried immediately beneath the mucosa appear visually as sandy particles seen through shallow water. With repeated infestation, the bladder lining loses its healthy rosy colour and takes on a pale, dull, non-transparent lustre. The normal subepithelial branching of blood vessels is no longer seen; this is usually described as 'ground glass' mucosa. Less commonly, heavy deposition of eggs is localized and the calcific submucous granuloma appears as a raised white plateau usually known as the calcific plaque.

Bilharzial ulcers

Ulceration of surface epithelium is generally attributed to local ischaemia on account of bilharzial obliteration of deeper vessels and/or the onset of secondary bacterial infection. Shokeir *et al.* [14] reported the presence of bladder ulcers in 8% of 350 bilharzial patients subjected to cystoscopy. According to their appearance during endoscopy they may be classified into active or cicatricial ulcers.

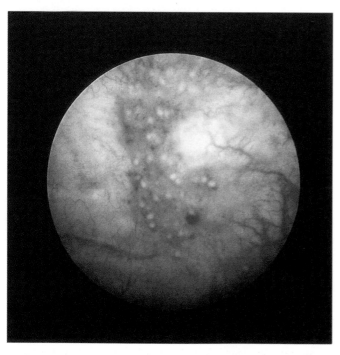

Fig. 49.4 Endoscopic picture of active bilharzial tubercles.

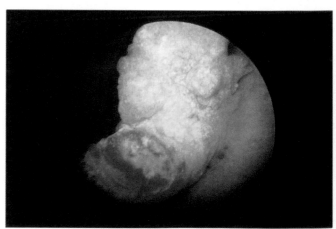

Fig. 49.5 A giant bilharzial polyp.

The active ulcer. These are seen in children and young adults and are overtly active granulomas located superfically in the bladder submucosa with a loss of surface epithelium. The surface bleeds readily on vesical distension during the course of diagnostic cystoscopy.

The cicatricial ulcer. These are characterized by dense fibrosis. Three morphological types were described: (i) stellate ulcers (Fig. 49.6) are shallow with thin margins and are surrounded by radial puckering; (ii) punctate ulcers appear as tiny bleeding spots with extensive circumferential fibrosis: and (iii) linear ulcers are flat with thick and raised indurated margins.

Cystitis cystica and cystitis glandularis

At cystoscopy, cystitis cystica appears either as tiny rounded transparent vesicles or as dark-brown well-defined structures (Fig. 49.7). The benign course of this lesions is undisputed. Cystitis glandularis, however, has a natural history that is believed to lead to subsequent development of adenocarcinoma. Nevertheless, hard-core evidence supporting this contention is lacking. The lesions of glandular cystitis appear at cystoscopy as velvety-red elevations of the mucous membrane. Biopsy and histopathological examination are essential for definitive diagnosis.

Leucoplakia

Chronic urosepsis, chronic epithelial irritation due to the presence or passage of schistosomal eggs, and vitamin A

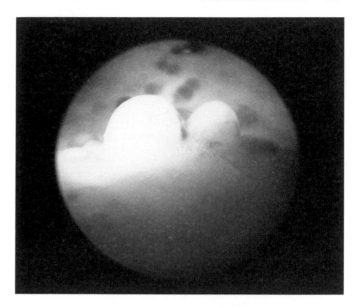

Fig. 49.7 Cystitis cystica and cystitis glandularis.

deficiency are all blamed for the evolution of squamous metaplastic changes. The endoscopic appearance is of well-defined, thick and raised white patches. The surface of these lesions may be covered with phosphatic encrustation and the surrounding mucosa is red and inflamed. Differentiation from other types of metaplasia and calcific plaques can only be made following biopsy resection and histological examination.

Carcinoma in situ

The incidence of this change in the bilharzial bladder is not yet known. There are no characteristic endoscopic findings and the bladder is generally noted to be inflamed, red and to bleed easily with overdistension. There may be areas of ulceration and phosphate encrustation. Biopsy is essential for definitive diagnosis.

Management

Benign superficial lesions

Active bilharzial bladder tubercles and polyps respond readily to specific antibilharzial therapy. Currently, the agent of choice is praziquantel. A single oral dose of 40 mg/kg is recommended. This can be repeated with minimal side effects. Antimicrobial agents will be required additionally for the treatment of secondary bacterial infection. Resection and biopsy may be indicated for residual lesions as many of these may be difficult to diagnose on the basis of morphological examination alone.

Active bilharzial ulcers may also respond satisfactorily to chemotherapy. The classic treatment of chronic ulcers, however, is total excision by partial cystectomy. Recur-

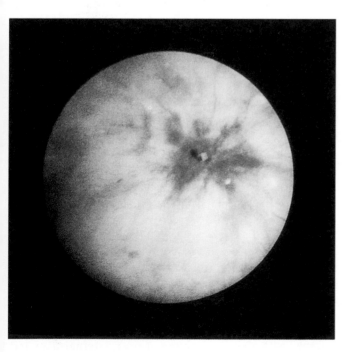

Fig. 49.6 A chronic stellate ulcer.

rence rate following this procedure is in the order of 5%. Excellent results have also been more recently reported following endoscopic resection of such lesions.

Contracted bilharzial bladder

Bilharzial contracted bladder is the outcome of severe and prolonged infection. Sayegh and Dimmette [15] recorded that this serious complication occurred in 0.6% of their urological admissions.

Clinical features and diagnosis

Patients are usually males and in the third or fourth decade of life. The presenting symptoms are intractable frequency, painful micturition and urge incontinence. The severity of these symptoms are directly related to the volume of the bladder. Urographic studies will demonstrate a small bladder in the cystographic phase. There is upper tract dilatation in one-third of cases and vesicoureteric reflux in two-thirds. Cystoscopy, performed under a general anaesthetic, will readily demonstrate the reduced bladder capacity.

Management

Surgery is indicated in cases where the bladder capacity is reduced to less than 100 ml. The procedure of choice is augmentation cystoplasty, using either ileum or colon [16,17].

Bladder outlet obstruction

Shokeir et al. [14] reported that bladder neck obstruction was a significant feature in 7.5% of patients with complicated bilharzial cystitis. Koraitim [18] stressed that three factors are largely responsible for the pathogenesis of outflow obstruction in the bilharzial bladder: muscle destruction, fibrosis of the trigone and bilharzial infestation of the first part of the urethra.

Clinical features and diagnosis

Patients, usually males between 20 and 40 years of age, present with symptoms of cystitis and difficulty on micturition. Calculus disease and secondary bacterial infection are sometimes coexisting findings. The diagnosis is based on urodynamic evaluation with simultaneous recording of the voiding pressure and flow rate.

Management

Endoscopic incision of the bladder neck provides the best functional results [19].

Carcinoma of the bilharzial bladder

Carcinoma of the urinary bladder is the most common solid tumour found amongst adult males in Egypt [20]. A causal relationship between urinary bilharziasis and cancer of the bladder was first reported by Fergusson [5] and has since been supported by other studies. Bilharzial bladder cancer may be initiated by exposure to an environmental or locally produced chemical carcinogen. Nitrates are present in human urine, particularly among individuals living in agricultural areas where nitrate fertilizers are liberally used. These compounds are readily reduced to carcinogenic nitrosamines as a result of secondary bacterial infection.

Clinicopathological features

The association of bladder cancer with urinary bilharziasis determines a distinct clinicopathological behaviour [21]. The peak age incidence is between the third and fifth decades. The male:females ratio is 4:1. Patients present with symptoms of cystitis, painful micturition, frequency and haematuria. Urography may reveal an irregular filling defect in its cystographic phase. The diagnosis depends upon cystoscopy, biopsy and careful bimanual examination under anaesthesia. Grossly, the tumours are generally of the nodular fungating type and occupy the vault, posterior or lateral walls of the bladder (Fig. 49.8). Histologically, two-thirds of cases show squamous cell features, the majority being of low-grade malignancy (Fig. 49.9).

Management

Endoscopic resection. In view of the bulk and advanced stage of these tumours, transurethral resection appears unfeasible for definitive treatment. Endoscopic resection is currently limited to obtaining biopsy material for histopathological diagnosis and evaluation.

Segmental resection. Local resection is only feasible in certain conditions: (i) if the tumour is solitary, does not involve the trigone and its size allows excision with adequate safety margin; and (ii) the rest of the bladder is free of any associated precancerous lesion. Very few patients with carcinoma of the bilharzial bladder satisfy these criteria.

Radical cystectomy. In view of the pathology and natural history of the disease, radical cystectomy and some form of urinary diversion provides the logical surgical approach to most cases with resectable tumours [20,21]. The extent of the excision includes the bladder with its perivesical fat, peritoneal covering, the prostate and the seminal vesicles, together with the distal common iliac, internal iliac and external iliac lymph nodes. In the female bladder the

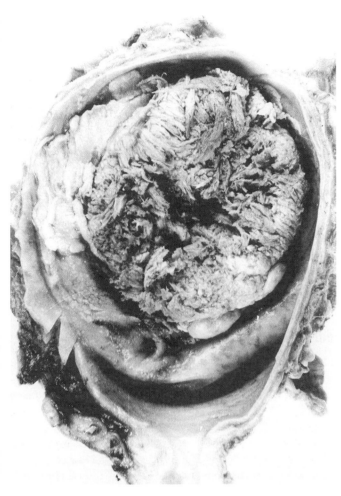

Fig. 49.8 A nodular fungating tumour that occupies the lateral wall.

urethra, uterus and upper two-thirds of the vagina, with pelvic cellular tissue and the aforementioned lymph nodes, are removed.

The reported 5-year survival rate following cystectomy is in the order of 48% [22]. Survival was significantly determined by the tumour P-stage, grade and nodal involvement. The 5-year disease-free survival was 73%, 65%, 46%, 31% and 19% for stage P1, P2, P3a, P3b and P4 respectively. Similarly, the 5-year disease free survival was 58% for grade I, 49% for grade II and 26% for grade III. The 5-year survival rate was 53% for cases with negative nodes and 23.4% for those with positive ones.

Radiation therapy. Early experience with external beam therapy for definitive control of these tumours showed disappointing results, particularly as many of these cases were already far advanced [23]. A randomized prospective trial was carried out at the Mansoura University Hospital comparing the results in 92 patients with carcinoma of the bilharzial bladder who underwent either radical cystectomy alone or in combination with 2000 rad preoperative radiation [24]. The postoperative mortality and morbidity were similar in both groups. Patients were followed for a minimum of 60 months. Overall, there was a marginal, statistically insignificant improvement in survival among patients receiving preoperative radiotherapy.

Chemotherapy. Several chemotherapeutic agents have been evaluated in bladder cancer patients at the Cancer Institute of Cairo University. All cases were unresectable T4 lesions. The most promising results were obtained with epidoxorubicin. Clinical trials with this agent in neo-adjuvant chemotherapy have also been started in patients with T3 lesions [25].

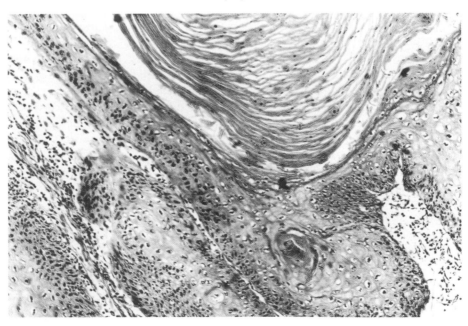

Fig. 49.9 A well-differentiated squamous cell carcinoma secondary to bilharzial cystitis (×100).

Bilharziasis of the urethra

Adult *Schistosoma haematobium* worms may gain access to the urethra via connections between the vesicoprostatic venous plexus, the urethral veins and the dorsal vein of the penis. In view of its rich venous network, the most common site of involvement is the roof of the bulbous urethra. Less commonly, the pathology involves the floor of the penile urethra [26].

Lesions usually develop in three successive phases. The initial phase of infiltration is characterized by the formation of bilharzial granulations in the submucosa. This is followed by atrophic changes in the overlying mucosa and the development of superficial ulcers. Mild ulcers may heal with a variable degree of scarring. If the disease is more extensive, and especially if there is superadded bacterial infection, the inflammatory process may invade the periurethral tissues and lead to the development of periurethral abscesses and fistulas ('watercan' perineum).

A recent, uncomplicated perineal fistula may undergo complete resolution with adequate antibilharzial and antibiotic drug therapy. In chronic cases, and where a large indurated mass is evident, temporary urinary diversion by suprapubic cystostomy is also necessary, and is maintained for an average of 2 weeks. Intermittent urethral dilatation may be indicated in the convalescent period so as to forestall the development of a urethral stricture. In advanced or recurrent cases complicated by stricture formation a two-staged skin-inlay urethroplasty may be necessary.

Bilharziasis of the male genital tract

Bilharzial seminal vesiculitis

Involvement of the seminal vesicles is usually bilateral. The pathological lesion evolves in three phases: the congestive, hyperplastic and fibrotic phases [27]. Microscopy invariably demonstrates bilharzial ova randomly deposited in all layers of tissue. There may be complete replacement of glandular tissue by calcified sheets of bilharzial infiltration.

Clinical features

Symptoms of seminal vesiculitis are often masked by those of concomitant bilharzial cystitis. Haematospermia is a characteristic feature and has been reported in 8% of cases with clinical evidence of bilharzial seminal vesiculitis [28]. Painful ejaculation, burning micturition and low back ache may also be encountered [29].

Rectal examination reveals bilaterally enlarged, firm and nodular or cystic seminal vesicles. The vesicular masses are characteristically 'date-shaped'. Examination of the seminal fluid will reveal bilharzial ova in 34% of cases [28]. Radiological examination may show calcification in the involved seminal vesicles and, characteristically, this shows a honeycomb appearance.

Studies by Aboul-Azm *et al.* [29], using the fructose test and seminal vesiculography in patients with bilharzial seminal vesiculitis, showed that the vesicular and ampullary canals, together with the ejaculatory ducts, remained patent. It seems unlikely, therefore, that bilharziasis has a direct role in the development of obstructive infertility in the male patient.

Management

Antibilharzial treatment, supported by antibiotic therapy, is the main line of management. In troublesome cases, with marked enlargement of the glands, seminal vesiculectomy may be indicated [29]. The procedure is performed through an extraperitoneal, retrovesical approach.

Bilharzial prostatitis

In a series of postmortem and surgical studies, bilharziasis was shown to involve the prostate in 18–47.3% of cases [1,28,30]. Grossly, the involved prostate is enlarged and granulomatous in the early stages, small and fibrous in the late stages. Bilharzial ova are distributed mainly in the stroma between acini. The latter are dilated and contain large, well-formed corpora amylaceae. In the late stages, the acini are compressed by stromal fibrosis and corpora amylaceae are no longer evident within their lumen. Secondary infection may cause a chronic bacterial prostatitis.

Clinical features

Early features are perineal heaviness, low back ache and painful micturition. With late fibrosis, the patient often complains of diminished sexual libido, weak erection or rapid ejaculation. Fibrous involvement of the bladder neck may result in frequency or difficulty in micturition and a poor urinary stream. These features are generally non-specific and are similar to those of chronic bacterial prostatitis. Diagnosis is based on the finding of bilharzia ova in tissue specimens obtained by needle biopsy or transurethral prostatic resection.

Conclusion

Bilharzial pathology of the genitourinary tract presents several interesting clinical models: obstructions, infections, stones and malignancy. Undoubtedly the severity of infestation and the relative incidence of complications will witness significant changes in the face of mass treatment using the new and safe orally administered antibilharzial agents. Hopefully, all that has been written in this chapter will soon be history.

References

1 Mohamed AS. Bilharziasis of the seminal vesicles. *J R Egyptian Med Assoc* 1952;**35**:613–26.

2 Smith JH, Kamel IA, Elwi A, Von Lichtenberg F. A quantitative post mortem analysis of urinary schistosomiasis in Egypt. *Am J Trop Med Hyg* 1974;**23**:1054–71.

3 El-Aaser AA, El-Merzabani MM, Abdel-Kader MM. A study on the aetiology factors of bilharzial bladder cancer in Egypt. 3. Urinary beta-glucorinidase. *Eur J Cancer* 1979;**15**:573–83.

4 Farid Z, Miner WF, Higashi GI, Hassan A. Reversibility of lesions in schistosomiasis: a brief review. *J Trop Med Hyg* 1976;**79**:161–6.

5 Fergusson AR. Associated bilharziasis and primary malignant diseases of the urinary bladder, with observations on a series of 40 cases. *J Pathol Bacteriol* 1911;**16**:76–94.

6 Zahran MM, Kamel M, Mooro H, Issa A. Bilharziasis of urinary and ureter. Comparative histopathologic study. *J Urol* 1976;**8**:73–9.

7 Lehman JS Jr, Farid Z, Smith JH, Bassily S, El-Masry NA. Urinary schistosomiasis in Egypt: clinical, radiological, bacteriological and parasitological correlations. *Trans R Soc Trop Med Hyg* 1973;**67**:384–99.

8 Ghoneim MA, Ashamallah A, Abdel-Khalik M. Bilharzial strictures of the ureter presenting with anuria. *Br J Urol* 1971;**43**:439–43.

9 Husain I, Ali IH, Kinare AS. Evaluating bilharzial ureteropathy for surgery. *Br J Urol* 1980;**52**:446–50.

10 Miller MJ, Reid EC. Steroid therapy in chronic urinary schistosomiasis. *Can Med Assoc J* 1967;**97**:594–9.

11 Ghoneim MA, Nabeeh A, El-Kappany A. Endourologic treatment of ureteral strictures. *J Endourol* 1988;**2**:263–70.

12 Shokeir AA, Gaballah MA, Ashamallah AA, Ghoneim MA. Optimization of replacement of the ureter by ileum. *J Urol* 1991;**146**:306–10.

13 El-Badawi AA. Bilharzial polypi of the urinary bladder. *Br J Urol* 1966;**38**:24–35.

14 Shokeir AA, Ibrahim AD, Hamid MY, Hussein HE, Badr M. Urinary bilharziasis in upper Egypt. IA. Clinicopathological study. *East Afr Med J* 1972;**49A**:298–311.

15 Sayegh ES, Dimmette RM. The fibrotic contracted urinary bladder associated with schistosomiasis and chronic ulceration. *J Urol* 1956;**75**:671–9.

16 Badr M, Zaher MF. The cystoplasty in the treatment of bilharzial contracted bladder. *J R Egyptian Med Assoc* 1959;**42**:33–5.

17 Ghoneim MA, Shoukry I. The use of ileum for correction of advanced or complicated lesions of the urinary tract. *Int J Urol Nephrol* 1972;**4**:25–33.

18 Koraitim M. A new concept of bilharzial bladder neck obstruction: the triple mechanism. *J Urol* 1973;**109**:393–6.

19 Ragi I. A new look at bladder neck obstruction syndrome with evaluation of different surgical corrections. Experience with 92 cases. *Egyptian J Urol* 1960;**4**:67–74.

20 El-Sebai I. Cancer of the bladder in Egypt. *Kasr El-Aini J Surg* 161;**2**:180–241.

21 El-Bolkainy NM, Ghoneim MA, Mansoura MA. Carcinoma of the bilharzial bladder in Egypt. Clinical and pathological features. *Br J Urol* 1972;**44**:561–70.

22 Ghoneim MA, Mohsen M, El-Mekresh MA et al. Radical cystectomy for carcinoma of the bladder: critical evaluation of the results in 1026 cases. *J Urol* 1997;**158**:393–399.

23 Awaad HK. Radiation therapy in bladder cancer. *Alexandria Med J* 1985;**4**:118–31.

24 Ghoneim MA, Ashamallah AK, Awaad HK, Whitmore WF. Randomized trial of cystectomy with or without preoperative radiotherapy for carcinoma of the bilharzial bladder. *J Urol* 1985;**134**:266–8.

25 Gad El-Mawla N, Hamza MR, Sikri Z et al. Chemotherapy in invasive carcinoma of the bladder. *Acta Oncol* 1989;**28**:73–6.

26 Maged A. A modern approach to the surgery of bilharzial perineal urinary fistulae with report of 122 cases. *Kars El-Aini J Surg* 1963;**4**:57–66.

27 Makar N. *Urologic Aspects of Bilharziasis in Egypt.* Cairo: SOP Press, 1955.

28 El-Sherbainy M. *Bilharziasis of the central genital tract in males.* MCh Thesis. University of Cairo, 1974.

29 Aboul-Azm TE, Saad SM, Arafa AE, Al-Ghorab MM. Can bilharziasis of the seminal vesicles be a cause of obstructive infertility? *Fertil Steril* 1977;**28**:775–6.

30 Zaher MF, Safwat MM, Fawzy RM, Badr MM. Bilharzial bladder neck obstruction, a neglected syndrome. *J R Egyptian Med Assoc* 1956;**39**:481–9.

50 Genitourinary Tuberculosis
S.A.H.Rizvi and S.A.A.Naqvi

Introduction

A third of the world's population carries the bacillus causing tuberculosis, although amongst healthy carriers only 10% are likely to develop the disease. The World Health Organization (WHO) has estimated that by the year 2000, tuberculosis will affect 10 million new patients every year [1]. These statistics should be seen against the backdrop of the rising incidence of acquired immune deficiency syndrome (AIDS) where the risk of developing tuberculosis in human immunodeficiency virus (HIV)-positive patients, mainly due to reactivation of an old focus, is greatly increased [2]. Genitourinary tuberculosis (GUTB) is the third most common extrapulmonary lesion.

Tuberculosis, known as consumption in the past, has been known to afflict humans since antiquity. Robert Koch in 1884 demonstrated that the organism could be grown in the laboratory and produce the disease in a susceptible host. Ekehorn, in 1908, proposed the haematogenous theory of disease spread, while Calmette and Guérin in 1925, by attenuating the organism, made the bacille Calmette–Guérin (BCG) vaccine. The term GUTB was given by Wildbolz in 1937 who pointed out that renal tuberculosis and tuberculous epididymitis were manifestations of the same disease.

Epidemiology

The epidemiology of tuberculosis is complex and knowledge of its natural history is important. The incidence of tuberculosis has a wide geographical variation. In the West there is an incidence of about 13–15 patients per 100 000 population [3], whereas in developing countries, the incidence can be as high as 1000 patients per 100 000 population. Of these, 8–10% in the West and 15–20% in developing countries will suffer from renal tuberculosis. Overall, there is male preponderance globally and the male to female ratio of the disease is about 2:1. An important regional difference is seen in the age incidence of the disease. In the affluent nations, tuberculosis affects the older population, whereas in developing countries, due to exposure early in life, children and young adults are the major sufferers.

The incidence of tuberculosis in the West had shown a gradual decline until the mid-1980s. However, with the growing infection rate of AIDS, tuberculosis has shown a resurgence not only in the West but in some African and Asian countries. Moreover, lack of compliance and inappropriate treatment have produced a high incidence of multiple drug-resistant tuberculosis (MDRTB) which has transformed a treatable disease into one that is life threatening. Therefore, the annual infection rate of the disease remains the most important epidemiological indicator [3]. Unless concerted efforts are made to control the disease, almost 4 million persons, most of them in their prime, will perish annually, which has been declared by WHO to be a global emergency.

There is generally a lag period of between 10 and 40 years following a primary infection, usually in the lungs [4]. Unlike the pulmonary disease, there has been little change in the reported incidence of GUTB. Modern chemotherapy can render the patients non-infectious in a very short time, yet in resource-poor developing countries, lack of effective measures frustrate the efforts of disease control. The present trends therefore indicate a higher incidence of genitourinary manifestation in the twenty-first century.

Immunology

The immunological response associated with the mycobacterial infection is a hypersensitivity reaction and is of a cell-mediated type, activated by lymphokines. The first infection with the tubercle bacillus leads to the development of allergy to protein tuberculin. This has become the basis of testing the allergy (not the immunity) against tuberculosis. Tuberculin is injected intradermally as a protein-purified derivative (PPD) [2]. If an induration of more than 10 mm develops after 48–72 h, the test is positive. Tuberculin testing does not indicate the presence or extent of disease but is sometimes helpful in diagnosis, permitting the physician to proceed to further investigations.

BCG, an avirulent strain of *Mycobacterium tuberculosis*, had been employed for the induction of immunity against tuberculosis. The degree of protection after immunization is highly variable, from negligible to 80%. The reason for this is poorly understood and seems to be differing mechanisms of cell-mediated responses. The status of BCG in adults has been controversial. In the West, due to limited protection in adults who are the main sufferers, it has been discontinued in many countries [3]. However, BCG vaccination is effective in protecting children and is very useful in countries with a high prevalence for tuberculosis [1], but the effect does not last more than 15 years [3] and unless the vaccine is given to infants, many children will die before attaining their teens.

Pathology and pathogenesis

Mycobacterium tuberculosis, the organism responsible for causing the disease, is the most virulent of all mycobacteria. The mycobacterium, classified as typical and atypical or according to its propensity to divide and grow, varies considerably. *M. tuberculosis* is 2.4 µm long and has a thick cell wall and no flagellum. The organism is non-motile and is strictly aerobic. It is extremely slow growing, dividing once in 24 h. It can also remain dormant, even up to the lifetime of a patient.

Mycobacterium bovis is an uncommon organism occasionally causing disease in industrialized countries in less than 1% of patients. In developing countries, due to the lack of milk pasteurization, the incidence may be higher. *M. bovis* causes primary lesions in the intestines which then spread to other parts by the haematogenous route.

The hallmark of tuberculosis is a tubercle. Microscopic examination shows central caseation necrosis surrounded by epithelial cells, Langhans giant cells and, more peripherally, lymphocytes and plasma cells. Characteristic caseating necrosis with cavitation, abscess formation and ensuing fibrosis and calcification are typical of the disease (Fig. 50.1).

The primary infection usually starts from the lungs. Depending on the infecting dose, the virulence of the organism and host resistance, either the organism may be destroyed by normal tissue resistance or an infection sets in. A latent period varying from months to over 40 years has been described in the clinical manifestation of the disease [4]. GUTB is an example of secondary tuberculosis caused by metastatic spread of organisms through the haematogenous route. The other routes are descent via the urinary tract, lymphatic spread, retrocanalicular dissemination or by direct extension [5]. All structures of the urinary system and genital tract may become involved later on. The disease can occur either by reactivation of old infection or reinfection from an active case. Reactivation involves multiplication of dormant bacilli because of changed circumstances such as diabetes mellitus, immunosuppressive therapy, trauma or debilitating diseases.

Kidney

Renal tuberculosis is slow to progress and may take 15–20 years to destroy a kidney. Although both kidneys are seeded, the clinically apparent disease is usually unilateral. The initial lesion involves the renal cortex with several

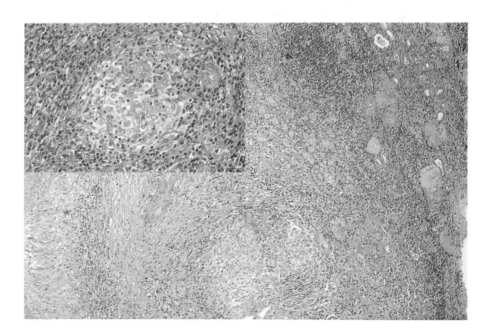

Fig. 50.1 Tubercular granulomata in kidney (mag×60). Inset: a granuloma in kidney consisting of epitheloid cells, histiocytes and lymphocytes (mag ×300).

small granulomas involving the glomeruli and the surrounding area. No clinical symptoms develop until the calyces or the pelvis are involved, when organisms may be intermittently discharged into the urine.

On gross appearance, the kidney may appear normal on the outer surface accompanied by marked perinephritis. In more advanced cases, the parenchyma is destroyed with areas of caseation and abscess formation (Figs 50.2 and 50.3). There is thickening of the wall of the pelvis, calyces

and ureter. In very advanced cases, the whole parenchyma is replaced by caseous material or fibrous tissue.

Ureter

The ureter may be involved by a seeding process from above, causing inflammation which heals by fibrosis. This results in multiple strictures, particularly in the upper and vesical ends causing hydronephrosis. Extensive fibrosis can

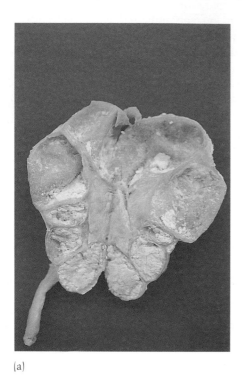

(a)

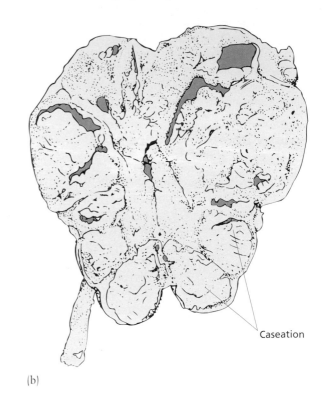

(b)

Fig. 50.2 Caseation in tuberculous kidney.

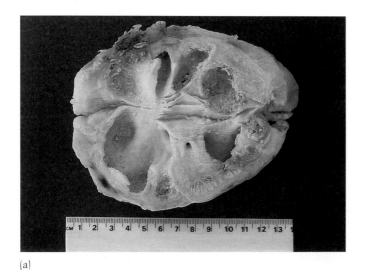

(a)

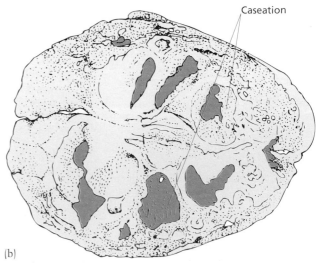

(b)

Fig. 50.3 Renal parenchymal destruction in tuberculosis.

shorten the length of the ureter, pulling up the orifice as a gaping hole—the so-called 'golf hole'.

Bladder

Once the bladder is bathed in infected material, the mucosa becomes inflamed and vesical irritability develops. Tubercles form in the area close to the orifice and may coalesce and ulcerate, causing bleeding. If the disease progresses, the lesions in the bladder form deep ragged ulcers penetrating into the muscle wall. The healing causes fibrosis resulting in reduced bladder capacity. This induces marked frequency in the patient, while stenosis of the orifice due to fibrosis causes hydronephrosis.

Urethra

Urethral tuberculosis is very rare. It occurs in association with upper urinary tract tuberculosis or occasionally following female genital involvement. In the acute form the patient presents with urethritis whereas in the chronic stage strictures result, causing obstructive symptoms.

Prostate and seminal vesicles

The prostate is invaded by the passage of infected urine through the urethra. However, the prostate may also be involved through the haematogenous route. The prostate shows nodules and areas of induration and fibrosis, giving a craggy feel on digital examination. The seminal vesicles are secondarily infected from the prostate and appear indurated, enlarged and fixed. Healing may result in calcification.

Testis and epididymis

The testis is fairly resistant to tubercular infection and is generally not involved except by an extension of an epididymal abscess. The epididymis may be enlarged and is affected from the prostate along the vas or through the perivasal lymphatics. The vas appears thickened or often 'beaded' because of fusiform swellings. If the epididymal infection is extensive, an abscess may develop which may rupture through the skin leaving a sinus.

External genitalia

Tuberculosis of the penis is very rare but in developing countries occasional cases are seen after sexual contact with partners harbouring genital lesions. The lesion appears as an ulcer which can progress to the corpora and urethra and the diagnosis is made on biopsy.

Genital tuberculosis in females is rare in the West, but can be diagnosed in a significant proportion of infertile patients in India [6]. It is commonly transmitted through the haematogenous route, although sexual transmission has been reported. Sometimes inguinal lymphadenopathy in females may be the only presentation. The fallopian tubes may be affected causing infertility. Granulomatous lesions of the vaginal canal and vulva are uncommon, yet in developing countries biopsy of non-healing lesions will often prove the diagnosis.

Clinical features

Because of the slow progression and variable course of the disease, the presentation of patients with tuberculosis sometimes poses a difficult clinical problem. A high index of suspicion is required as the symptoms are vague and the physical examination is unrewarding in the majority of patients. The family history of the patient and their contacts is of paramount importance. This is particularly true in developing countries where large families live in cramped, ill-ventilated and unhygienic surroundings.

Renal tuberculosis generally lacks classic clinical features. Malaise, fatiguability, low grade fever and night sweats may be non-specific complaints in patients; although they may be absent until the disease is far advanced. The affected kidney is usually asymptomatic and occasionally there is only a vague flank pain. Renal and ureteric colic may be a manifestation of the passage of clots or sloughed debris. The symptoms are usually vesical because of the irritation of the bladder from infected material shed off from the kidney. Burning, frequency and nocturia are common. Haematuria and suprapubic pain results from ulceration in the bladder.

There are no specific symptoms of tuberculosis of the prostate and seminal vesicles, and often a painless, non-tender swelling of the epididymis gives the clue to genital tuberculosis. Haemospermia may be an occasional complaint [7]. Not uncommonly, an abscess may burst through the scrotal wall.

On examination, the prostate and seminal vesicle feel nodular and indurated. The vas may be thickened and beaded. In advanced disease, the epididymis cannot be differentiated from the testis, which may be involved by extension as an epididymo-orchitis. Sometimes hydrocele accompanies tuberculous epididymitis which needs to be tapped to obtain material for culture or occasionally to unmask a testicular tumour.

Patients with neglected disease may present with complications which include perinephric abscess or renal stones. Some patients may have uncontrolled hypertension or renal failure. Others may present with sinuses in the flank or scrotum or seek a clinician's help due to infertility.

There is a higher incidence of tuberculosis in patients on dialysis compared to the normal population. Furthermore, patients receiving renal allografts show a still higher incidence of tuberculosis because of reactivation of old foci following chemical immunosuppression. In developing countries, reinfection may be an additional cause. The majority of recipients develop pulmonary disease, but extrapulmonary tuberculosis has been reported in over one-third of patients. However, renal tuberculosis following transplantation is very uncommon.

Investigation

The diagnosis of tuberculosis is based upon an unequivocal demonstration of tubercle bacilli. Due to sealing off of cavities in the kidney, cultures can continue to be negative whereas the disease continues to progress, delaying the diagnosis considerably. The diagnosis of GUTB can be challenging, more so in resource-poor countries where the incidence is unfortunately very high. An approach for the diagnosis in varying situations is given in Fig. 50.4.

Laboratory findings

Urine examination

The urinalysis is invariably abnormal, containing proteins,

pus cells and red blood cells, and the pH is usually acidic. Acid-fast smear from urinary concentrate is helpful but can be misleading due to the likelihood of a positive result in the presence of saprophytes such as *M. smegmatis*. Sterile pyuria (i.e. absence of positive culture for the pathogen) warrants serious consideration. Secondary bacterial infection is present in about one-third of patients and the organism is usually *Escherichia coli*.

Undoubtedly the most important laboratory test is urine culture for *M. tuberculosis*, which can be positive in almost 90% of patients. Three to five early morning specimens should be cultured irrespective of the presence or absence of pus cells. Two culture media are used—plain Lowenstein–Jensen culture medium for *M. tuberculosis* and pyruvic egg medium to identify *M. bovis* which is partially anaerobic. Sensitivity tests are mandatory to select the most appropriate chemotherapy. Guinea pig inoculation has largely been given up due to excellent results of cultures.

Blood examination

Blood haemoglobin should be examined to check for anaemia along with a complete blood count. The erythro-

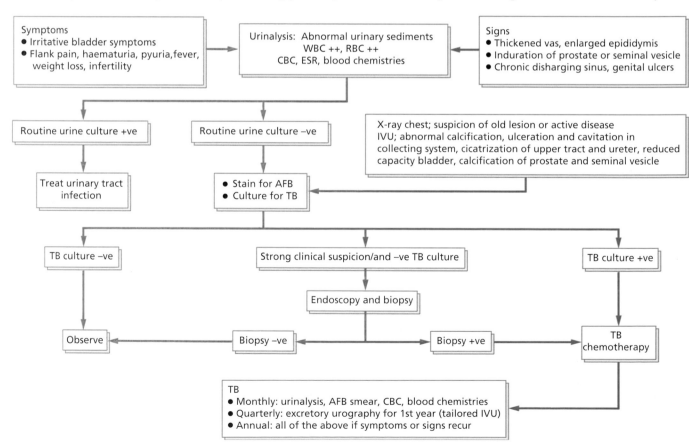

Fig. 50.4 Diagnosis and management of genitourinary tuberculosis.

cyte sedimentation rate is non-specific for diagnosis but is a good guide to monitor the progress of the disease. In the presence of calcification in the renal tract, serum calcium, phosphorus and plasma proteins should be estimated preferably on three occasions. A 24 h urinary excretion of calcium, uric acid and oxalate should also be done to investigate calcification.

Widespread damage of kidneys from tuberculosis may compromise renal function. Blood urea nitrogen, serum creatinine and electrolyte estimation can demonstrate evidence of renal impairment which may be caused by ureteric stricture or secondary amyloidosis and should always be considered and investigated. Tuberculous interstitial nephritis as a cause of renal failure has also been reported [8]. Renal function tests are also essential in adjusting the dosages of antitubercular drugs.

Special laboratory tests

Enzyme-linked immunosorbent assay (ELISA) has been used for the serological diagnosis of disease, including GUTB [9,10]. The test has the advantage of providing results within hours but as yet lacks the differentiation between recent and older sensitization.

A highly reliable test employing DNA technology (i.e. genetic 'fingerprinting') of mycobacteria has also been reported [11]. From being a research tool, this technology has rapidly acquired potential in clinical laboratories. Furthermore, amplification of mycobacterial DNA, using the polymerase chain reaction (PCR), has shown promise for a rapid diagnosis of tuberculosis. PCR is likely to become an exciting investigation for epidemiological work as well as for diagnosis of mycobacterial infection [11,12]. Furthermore, identification of mutations responsible for drug resistance by PCR techniques, especially isoniazid (INH), offers a new means for rapid detection of drug resistance.

Radiological findings

A chest film showing evidence of active or healed tuberculosis should make the physician aware of coexisting urogenital involvement in the presence of urinary symptoms. A plain film of the abdomen may show enlargement of one kidney or obliteration of psoas shadows due to perinephric extension of the renal lesion. Discreet or punctate calcification in the renal area may be due to tuberculosis. Renal stones may be seen in the region of the kidney or ureter. Large calcified bodies in the area of the prostate may also be indicative of the disease.

Excretory urogram

Intravenous urography (IVU) is mandatory, being the gold standard for visualization of the pelvicalyceal system [13].

High-dose urography is excellent for early identification of renal lesions and has largely obviated the use of retrograde pyelography. Radiological changes of early lesions of tuberculosis may be difficult to find but IVU can be employed to follow-up patients in various stages of disease progression (Fig. 50.5).

The typical changes include ulceration of calyces, appearing as a slight irregularity or a 'moth-eaten' lesion due to ulcerated calyces. Occasionally one or more calyces may be obliterated. Abscess cavities may show connections with calyces or parenchymal destruction. Sometimes, hydronephrosis or ureteric dilatation occurs due to strictures of the ureter. In others, single or multiple strictures in the ureter can cause secondary dilatation or shortening. The kidney may appear non-functioning due to complete ureteric occlusion. Renal destruction can appear as a calcified mass (autonephrectomy).

Retrograde pyelography

The place of retrograde pyelography is in the delineation of strictures and the amount of obstruction above the ureteric lesion (Fig. 50.6). The study can be combined with dynamic examination of ureteric function by the visualization of peristalsis on the image intensifier to see abnormalities. The other indication for retrograde pyelography is catheterization of the ureter to obtain urine samples for culture from the affected renal unit.

Percutaneous antegrade pyelography

The ease with which percutaneous antegrade studies can be performed has made it a frequently used procedure. This is indicated in a radiologically non-functioning kidney where visualization of the tract above the obstruction is not possible. The other indication is aspiration of the content of the renal pelvis for culture or the estimation of the drug level in a tuberculous cavity.

Angiography

Angiography, being an invasive test, is not employed for routine evaluation. The indications for arteriography are either for planning of surgery for partial nephrectomy or more importantly, the diagnosis of coincidental renal tumours. Renal vein sampling may sometimes be required to assess renin levels from the affected kidney for some patients with uncontrollable hypertension following renal tuberculosis. This may be helpful in evaluating a patient who may benefit from nephrectomy [14].

Ultrasound examination

Ultrasound is relatively inaccurate in demonstrating early

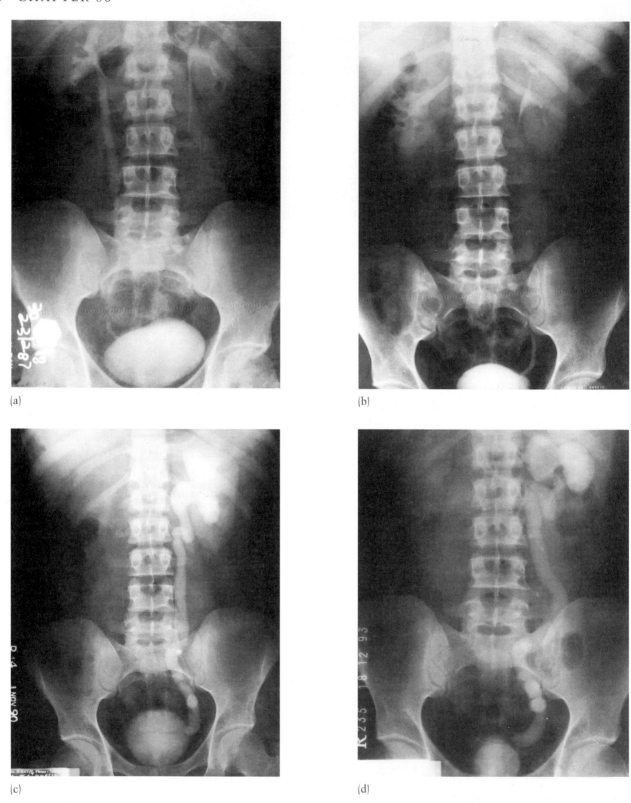

(a)

(b)

(c)

(d)

Fig. 50.5 Serial intravenous urograms of same patient showing progressive radiological changes. (a) *First presentation*: Slight fullness of right pelvicalyceal system and ureter without any obstruction. The left system and bladder being unremarkable. (b) *One year later*: There is further deterioration of functions with delayed opacification of pelvicalyceal system. (c) *Three years later*: At this stage the kidney is almost completely non-fuctional with slight diminution of bladder volume. There is moderate hydronephrosis and hydroureter on the left side due to partial obstruction at left uterovesical junction. (d) *Six years later*: There has been further deterioration with small volume thimble-shaped bladder and severe hydronephrosis and hydroureter on the left side. The right kidney is non-functional showing faint curvilinear calcifications.

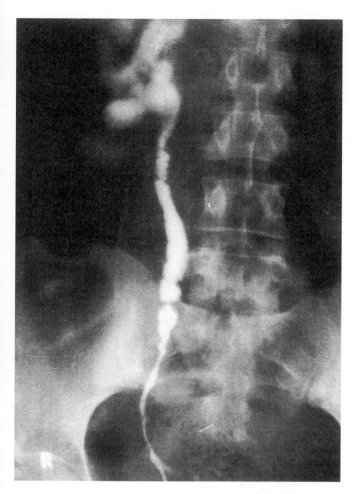

Fig. 50.6 Retrograde ureterogram showing irregularly beaded ureter with multiple strictures.

changes in renal tuberculosis but when the kidney cannot be seen on excretory urography, it permits visualization of calyceal dilatation and hydronephrosis. Moreover, renal mass lesions, sometimes associated with tuberculosis or other causes, are easily seen [15] so that further investigations to confirm the diagnosis are carried out.

Radioisotope studies

Isotope studies are of little diagnostic help but may aid during the treatment period for evaluation of ureteric scarring resulting in hydronephrosis. It is also a useful test to monitor the differential function of the affected renal unit.

Computed tomography and magnetic resonance imaging

Neither of these modalities have the spatial resolution capable of demonstrating the fine erosive damage that affects the urothelium. However, single or multiple abscesses can be seen well (Fig. 50.7). Computed

tomography (CT) scanning is extremely useful in detecting mass lesions, even in the non-visualized kidney, and is the investigation of choice for evaluating adjacent retroperitoneal areas to look for extension of the disease [4].

Instrumental examination

Cystourethroscopy should be done to visualize the urethra for suspicious areas or strictures and is indicated to see the extent of disease in the bladder, revealing the size of the viscus as well as visualization of the tubercles. Ulcers and changes in ureteric orifice can be seen very well on cystoscopy (Fig. 50.8). A biopsy can be taken for tissue diagnosis, and reflux, if present, could be demonstrated on cystography.

Ureteroscopy, employing modern instruments, permits direct examination of the ureter and provides the capability of taking tissue for histology. Fine needle aspiration cytology is another promising tool for diagnosing tuberculosis [16]. It is accurate, inexpensive and minimally invasive and can be used for suspected renal and epididymal lesions. Diagnostic laparoscopy is performed in infertile patients where tuberculosis is an important aetiological factor [17]. This is accompanied by culture for *M. tuberculosis* from endometrial samples.

Differential diagnosis

In the absence of classic signs and symptoms, the diagnosis of tuberculosis may become difficult. Though not infallible, the tuberculin test and chest X-rays are valuable in the diagnosis of patients. However, up to 50% of patients may have normal X-ray films and between 6 and 8% of tuberculin tests may be negative in culture-proved GUTB.

Radiology plays an important part in the differential diagnosis particularly where urine cultures are negative. A host of conditions need to be considered in the differential diagnosis (Table 50.1). Medullary sponge kidneys, pyelonephritis, renal stones and transitional cell cancer of the pelvis are important clinical conditions. Epididymitis and non-healing sinuses and ulcers are some other conditions worth considering in the diagnosis [4,18].

Medullary sponge kidney shows an accumulation of contrast outside the calyces but parenchymal calcification is not common. Ring calcification near a sloughed papilla is suggestive of papillary necrosis. Pyelonephritis may show distortion of the cortex and collecting system but calyceal, pelvic and ureteric strictures usually seen in tuberculosis are not common.

Transitional cell carcinoma of the pelvis may show calyceal amputation or infundibular narrowing but it is not associated with parenchymal calcification or cavity formation. Similarly, schistosomial infection causes calcification of the ureter and bladder but is not associated with

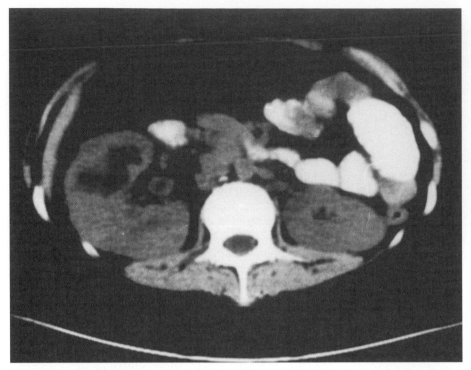

(a)

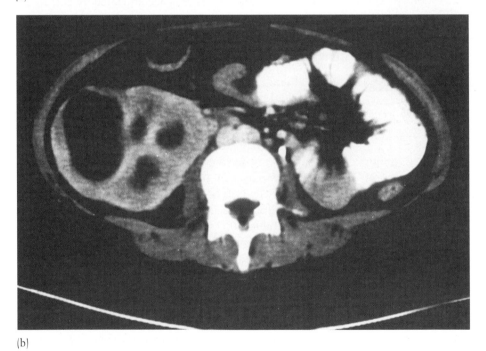

(b)

Fig 50.7 (a) Pre and (b) postcontrast enhanced axial sections of renal areas at different levels showing thick walled multiple abscesses in enlarged right kidney with oedematous thick walled ureter.

renal calcification. Renal stones may be an important diagnosis worth differentiating. Stones are seen in the collecting system whereas calcification in tuberculosis is generally seen in the parenchyma. Secondary stones, however, may be seen in tuberculosis due to strictures causing urinary tract obstruction.

Acute and chronic non-specific epididymitis may require

differentiating from tuberculosis which may also show palpable changes in the seminal vesicle. Sometimes the diagnosis is only made on the histology of surgically removed epididymis. Similarly, non-healing sinuses or ulcers, particularly in the lower abdomen and external genitalia, must make the physician aware of the possibility of tuberculosis in the differential diagnosis.

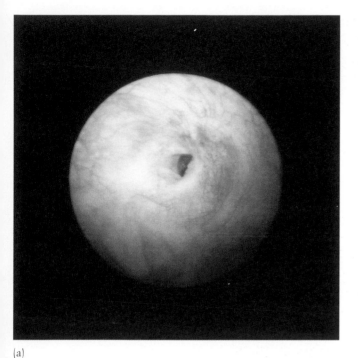
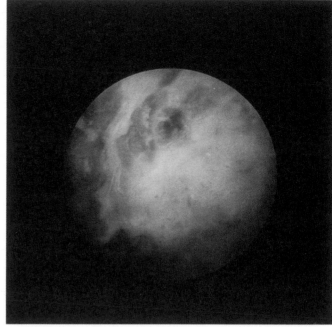

(a)   (b)

Fig 50.8 Cystoscopic appearance. (a) Coalescing tubercles around the ureteric orifice causing shortening of the ureter, making the orifice a 'golf hole'. (b) Tuberculous ulcer, penetrating deep into the muscle with ragged margins and areas of haemorrhage.

Table 50.1 Differential diagnoses of GUTB.

Suspected urinary tuberculosis	Suspected genital tuberculosis
Pyelonephritis	Epididymitis
Medullary sponge kidney	Prostatitis seminal vesiculitis
Renal stones	Haemospermia
Transitional cell carcinoma of the pelvis	Genital sinuses or ulcers
Schistosomiasis	Infertility

Management

Tuberculosis should be considered a generalized disease, and in the presence of urogenital manifestation the possibility of disease activity elsewhere in the body should not be discounted. The aim of management is to treat the active disease aggressively so as to make the patient non-infectious in the shortest possible time. Hospitalization is generally not required unless complications of the disease are present or surgical intervention is contemplated. At the same time, preservation of renal function should be given the highest priority in planning the management strategy.

In the developed world, management poses little difficulty other than ensuring drug compliance. The problems of management in poorer countries are multifarious. The living conditions and nutrition of the patients is generally unsatisfactory. Moreover, pulmonary infections can coexist with the urogenital form of disease. Therefore, hospitalization to render the patients non-infectious is of paramount importance but lack of hospital beds and health facilities make it a daunting task. Furthermore, illiteracy and lack of health education promote non-compliance, responsible for the development of MDRTB.

Chemotherapy

There is a lack of consensus on the chemotherapeutic programme for tuberculosis, including GUTB, because of the protean nature of the disease and the various stages at which the patient may present. Aggressive treatment with bacteriocidal drugs is the regimen of choice and the place of bacteriostatic drugs should be reserved for the problem of drug resistance. Patients with positive urine culture for tuberculosis and yet no abnormality on urinalysis or IVU may need a two-drug regimen of isoniazid and rifampicin. However, patients with clinically manifest disease should be managed by three drugs such as isoniazid, pyrazinamide and rifampicin. Table 50.2 gives the commonly used drugs, their doses and adverse effects.

Gow has convincingly argued for adopting a short-term 4-month therapy [19,20]. The rationale for this is first, renal tuberculosis involves fewer organisms than the pulmonary form; secondly, the blood supply of the kidney is excellent; and thirdly, the urinary concentration of primary drugs are good and isoniazid and rifampicin can penetrate diseased cavities very well. The cost of drugs and maintenance of infrastructure and personnel involved in the control of the disease can all be benefited by the shorter regimen.

There is no doubt that chemotherapy should be aggressive and comprise of three bacteriocidal drugs in order to achieve good sterilization of diseased organs or tissue. However, a 6-month chemotherapy regimen for GUTB is preferred in developing countries rather than the 4-month therapy (Fig. 50.9). Because of adverse environmental factors, such as unhygienic and cramped living areas, there is an increased risk of a relapse in a regimen shorter than 6 months. Moreover, the nutritional state of the patients in these countries is generally poor. A year of chemotherapy is recommended when the disease is advanced or has complications. Streptomycin injections may be needed in addition to the three-drug regimen for a period of between 2 and 3 months in such patients.

Some exceptions to short-term therapy are patients following a transplantation where immunosuppression is likely to cause reactivation of the disease and these patients need 1 year or more of therapy. Also, patients on

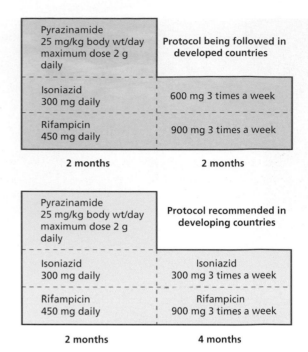

Fig. 50.9 Treatment protocol.

dialysis have lowered immunity and require longer treatment. As most antitubercular drugs are dialysable, they should therefore be given after a dialysis session.

The dosages of antitubercular drugs have to be adjusted according to renal function. Instead of making the dosage smaller, the same effect can be achieved by increasing the time interval between doses according to creatinine clearance; for example when creatinine clearance is 50 ml/min, the dose of streptomycin 1 g is repeated every 72 h instead of the usual once-a-day regimen.

The use of steroids has not met with general agreement

Table 50.2 Commonly used agents in the treatment of tuberculosis.

Drug*	Usual dose	Adverse effects
Primary drugs		
Isoniazid	300 mg/day	Hepatotoxicity, peripheral neuritis
Rifampicin	600 mg/day	Hepatotoxicity, thrombocytopenia
Pyrazinamide	1000 mg/day	Hepatotoxicity, dose/duration related
Streptomycin	750–1000 mg/day	Ototoxicity, rash and fever
Secondary drugs		
Ethambutol	15–25 mg/kg/day	Retrobulbar neuritis
Ethionamide	750–1000 mg/day	Nausea, vomiting, anorexia, abdominal pain
Cycloserine	750–1000 mg/day	Headache, drowsiness, convulsions, psychotic disturbance
Para-amino salicylic acid	10–12 g/day	Genitointestinal irritation, rash and fever, haemolysis in G6PD deficiency

*Minor agents: kanamycin and thiacetazone.
G6PD, glucose-6-phosphate dehydrogenase.

among physicians. Steroids in doses of up to 20 mg three times a day have been used in patients undergoing stricture formation in the ureter or in patients with severe cystitis [3]. Higher steroid doses are necessary when rifampicin interacts with steroids whose bioavailability is cut down appreciably.

Patients should be followed up regularly after a full course of chemotherapy. On the follow-up visits three consecutive early morning urine specimens are examined and ultrasound examination is performed to see the affected renal unit. A limited IVU is a useful and important investigation to check the progress of the disease. If the results are satisfactory, the patient, after 1 year of follow-up chemotherapy, is discharged and instructed to report whenever there is any recurrence of previous symptoms.

Surgical management

The place of surgery has become more focused and targeted after the natural history and pathogenesis of the disease became better understood. Surgery is performed earlier nowadays, after a good chemotherapeutic cover of 2 months is given which precludes dissemination. Surgery is no longer reserved for salvaging burnt-out lesions as in the past.

Endoscopic management

Surgical intervention has undergone changes both in its indications as well as its spectrum. Minimally invasive techniques have been employed with great success in the diagnosis as well as treatment of GUTB. Percutaneous access, the use of stents and ureterorenoscopy are some of the procedures used in the management of the disease which have demonstrated efficacy and minimal morbidity. Infundibular stenosis, non-draining calyces and pelvic obstruction can be manipulated percutaneously with encouraging results [4]. Ureterorenoscopy is now able to provide access to the kidney for diagnosing lesions, obtaining tissue for examination as well as for bypassing obstructions by placement of stents.

Ablative surgery

Nephrectomy

As the frequency of late complications of non-functioning kidneys on long-term chemotherapy are less than 5%, nephrectomy is not required for all such patients. The major indication for nephrectomy is a non-functioning kidney with a growing calcification. However, intractable pain, uncontrollable fever, refractory hypertension and life-threatening haematuria may be other important indications to remove the affected kidney. Suspicion of a coexisting cancer is one other important indication for nephrectomy. The previous practice of removing the whole of the ureter and a cuff of bladder (nephroureterectomy) has been largely given up. The affected kidney is removed along with as much of the ureter as is possible through a single incision.

Partial nephrectomy

With modern chemotherapy, this procedure is being performed far less frequently. One indication is a localized lesion of the poles with calcification which has failed to respond to 12 weeks of chemotherapy. The other important indication is an area of calcification that is slowly expanding in size and is likely to affect normal renal tissue.

Cavernostomy

With modern imaging techniques, aspiration of abscesses have become less invasive, leaving very few indications for this procedure.

Percutaneous access of cavities not only permits draining of the lesion but is useful in obtaining culture material or allows one to monitor levels of antitubercular drugs. It may also permit instillation of drugs. A solution of 5% rifampacin and 1% INH is generally recommended.

Epididymectomy

The most important indication is a caseating abscess not responding to chemotherapy. The other indication is a swelling not responding to drug treatment. As tuberculosis of the testis is very rare, there is invariably no need to perform orchidectomy unless epididymo-orchitis produces a suspicious mass.

Reconstructive surgery

Reconstruction of the renal tract may be required due to the destruction from the disease but equally from the ill effects of cicatrization. The procedure involves the kidney, ureter and bladder.

Ureteric stricture

In clinical practice strictures at the pelviureteric junction are uncommon because sufficient destruction of the renal parenchyma has already occurred for any reconstructive procedure to be meaningful. A double-J ureteric silicone stent can bypass a stricture and dilate it and can be kept in for up to 6 months. Children can also be treated by the use of paediatric size stents [21]. The progress of the affected kidney is monitored by ultrasound, limited IVU or radio-isotope renography on a monthly basis. Failure to relieve obstruction after chemotherapy or obstruction which is getting worse during drug treatment is an indication for open surgery. Both the Anderson–Hynes and Culp technique could be employed depending on the choice of the surgeon.

Stricture in the middle third of the ureter could be dealt with by stenting the ureter or by using a Davis intubated ureterostomy. The strictures at the lower end should be managed by a combination of chemotherapy and surgery. Steroids have been used together with antitubercular drugs to reduce oedema. To follow-up, short IVU or renography is employed to assess progress at intervals of 2–4 weeks. Short stricture at the ureterovesical junction would require the excision of the diseased segment and the employment of antirefluxing ureteroneocystostomy through a submucosal tunnel. A stricture longer than 5 cm would require the construction of a Boari flap or a psoas hitch. Alternatively, pancalyceal ileoneocystostomy is a promising procedure for the replacement of the ureter in the presence of a reasonably functioning kidney [22].

Augmentation cystoplasty

The procedure of choice is one that is able to increase the bladder capacity, yet retain the healthy portion. Ileum was the first to be used for augmentation but it suffered from loop stagnation and narrowing of anastomosis. The colon was the next to be employed for augmentation. The advantages are a long mesentery and complete extraperitoneal vesicocolic anastomosis. The caecum has the advantages of diminished mucus discharge and infection. Moreover, the emptying of the reservoir is better and residual urine is acceptably low. Both the segments are satisfactory but the caecum has an advantage of accompanying ileum for the antireflux procedure which can be reconstructed more effectively. With this procedure, the absorption of solutes is much less and the incidence of hyperchloraemic acidosis is acceptably low.

Follow-up

Up until the 1980s patients were recommended to have lifelong follow-up with yearly bacteriological and radiological tests. It is now believed that with better understanding of the natural history of the disease, effective chemotherapy and minimally invasive surgical options, the outlook has changed for the better. A 1-year follow-up after an effective short-term chemotherapy course appears to be safe and achieves good compliance from the patients [19]. However, in the presence of calcification, patients are required to be followed up indefinitely until it has been demonstrated convincingly that the disease is not progressing. This is necessary because it has been shown that calcification may enlarge insidiously to destroy the kidney [20].

On follow-up visits, pyuria is suggestive of recurrence, and necessitates cultures. Excretory urography should be performed at 6 months and 1 year. Radioisotope scans are useful to see differential renal function, particularly in the affected renal unit. After 1 year, the patient should be discharged but told to return if symptoms recur. Notwithstanding the current advances, tuberculosis has shown a resurgence globally, whereas GUTB has not lost the spectre of destruction of various organs of the urinary and genital tracts and remains a disease warranting a high index of suspicion.

References

1 Shears P. Introduction. In: *Tuberculosis Control Programmes in Developing Countries*, 2nd edn. Oxfam Practical Health Guide No. 4 Oxford: Oxfam, 1988:1.

2 Crofton J. General background to clinical tuberculosis. In: Crofton J, Horne N, Miller F, eds. *Clinical Tuberculosis*. London: 1992:1–27.

3 Gow JG. Genito-urinary tuberculosis. In: Walsh PC, Retik AB, Stamey TA, Vaughan ED Jr, eds. *Campbell's Urology*, 6th edn. Philadelphia: WB Saunders, 1992:951–81.

4 Schaeffer AJ. Renal infection. In: Gillenwater JY, Grayhack JT, Howards SS, Duckett JW, eds. *Adult and Paediatric Urology*, 2nd edn. St Louis: Mosby Year Book, 1987:767–74.

5 Wolf JS Jr, McAninch JW. Tuberculous epididymo-orchitis: diagnosis by fine needle aspiration. *J Urol* 1991;**145**:836–8.

6 Varma TR. Genital tuberculosis and subsequent fertility. *Int J Gynecol Obstet* 1991;**35**:1–11.

7 Marshall BF, Fuller NL. Hemospermia. *J Urol* 1983;**129**: 377–8.

8 Morgan SH, Eastwood JB, Baker LRI. Tuberculosis interstitial nephritis—the tip of an iceberg? *Tubercle* 1990;**71**:5–6.

9 Eduardo SD, Ferguson LE, Daniel TM. An ELISA for the serodiagnosis of tuberculosis using a 30,000-Da native antigen of *Mycobacterium tuberculosis*. *J Infect Dis* 1990;**162**: 928–31.

10 Maniar P, Joshi L. ELISA–an aid in rapid diagnosis of genito-urinary tuberculosis. *J Postgrad Med* 1988;**34**:158–64.

11 Pao CC, Benedict Yen TS, You JB, *et al*. Detection and identification of *Mycobacterium tuberculosis* by DNA amplification. *J Clin Microbiol* 1990;**28**:1877–80.

12 Sjobring U, Mecklenburg M, Anderson AB, Miorner H. Polymerase chain reaction for detection of *Mycobacterium tuberculosis*. *J Clin Microbiol* 1990;**28**:2200–4.

13 Becker JA. Renal tuberculosis. *Urol Radiol* 1988;**10**:25–30.

14 Kelley JF, Atkinson AB, Adgey AAJ. Renal tuberculosis and accelerated hypertension: the use of renal vein renin sampling to predict the outcome after nephrectomy. *Int J Cardiol* 1987; **16**:318–20.

15 Das KM, Indudhara R, Vaidyanathan S. Sonographic features of genito-urinary tuberculosis *Am J Radiol* 1992;**158**:327–9.

16 Baniel J, Manning A, Leiman G. Fine needle cytodiagnosis of renal tuberculosis. *J Urol* 1991;**146**:689–91.

17 Marana R, Muzzi L, Lucisano A *et al*. Incidence of genital tuberculosis in infertile patients submitted to diagnostic laparoscopy: recent experience in an Italian university hospital *Int J Fertil* 1991;**36**:104–7.

18 Tanagho EM. Specific infections of the genito-urinary tract. In: Tanagho EM, McAninch JW, eds. *Smith's General Urology*, 13th edn. London: Prentice Hall, 1992:240–7.

19 Gow JG, Barbosa S. Genito-urinary tuberculosis. A study of 1,117 cases over a period of 34 years. *Br J Urol*; 1984;**56**: 449–55.

20 Weinberg AC, Boyd SD. Short-course chemotherapy and role of surgery in adult and pediatric genito-urinary tuberculosis. *Urology* 1988;**31**:95–102.

21 Hill DE, Kramer SA. Specific infections of the genito-urinary tract. In: Kelalis PP, King LR, Belman AB. *Clinical Paediatric Urology*, 3rd edn. Philadelphia:WB Saunders, 1992:331–5.

22 Wong SH, Lau WY. Pan-caliceal ileoneocystostomy: indications, modifications and further evaluation. *J Urol* 1984;**132**: 668–9.

51 Interstitial Cystitis

T.J.Christmas

Introduction

Interstitial cystitis (IC) is a rare chronic inflammatory disease of the bladder that predominantly affects middle-aged females. The aetiology of IC is unknown and remains as one of the great enigmas of urology. It has been suggested that the number and variety of aetiological theories and treatment modalities for a particular condition is inversely related to the degree of certainty regarding its aetiology. This maxim seems to apply in the case of IC. It is also theoretically possible that IC may have more than one aetiology and that it is a pooled diagnosis. Once the diagnosis of IC is established it is important to explain the clinical implications to the patient and to concentrate on treating the particular symptoms that cause the individual most trouble.

There are several references in medical literature from the Victorian era to individual patients who almost certainly had IC. However, the descriptive term 'interstitial cystitis' was not used until 1887 when the condition was described by Skene [1]. The first person to describe the clinical condition comprehensively, including his eponymous ulcer and the histological features of IC, was Guy Hunner [2]. Since the 1920s there have been numerous publications describing the clinical features and natural history of IC. An incredible number of hypotheses for the aetiology of IC have been published ranging from bacterial infection in the early days to allergy, psychosomatic disturbance, autoimmune antibodies, antibiotics, leaking urothelium and aggressive sexual intercourse. The most plausible of the aetiological theories will be described in detail later in the chapter.

Diagnosis

The diagnosis of IC is confirmed by systematic exclusion of other disorders that may mimic the disease. An important first step is to exclude urinary tract infection by urine culture. However, secondary infection is a not uncommon feature in IC. Persistent symptoms after antibiotic therapy and sterile urine should alert the urologist to the possibility of underlying IC. Cystoscopy and bladder biopsy are mandatory for the exclusion of other conditions that may mimic IC and to confirm the diagnosis. The conditions that may mimic IC are listed in Table 51.1 — all these can be excluded by urine culture, cystoscopy and bladder biopsy. The classic findings in IC are outlined below.

Symptoms

There is often a considerable delay between the onset of symptoms and the diagnosis of IC. This is due to a lack of awareness of the condition amongst general practitioners as well as amongst the patients themselves. It is not uncommon for women with IC to give a history of having received several courses of antibiotics for presumed bacterial cystitis without resolution of symptoms. The classic symptoms of IC are suprapubic pain partially or completely relieved by voiding and urinary frequency. Other less common symptoms are listed in Table 51.2.

Cystoscopic findings

Cystoscopy and bladder biopsy under general anaesthesia is essential to confirm the diagnosis in IC. The cystoscopic appearances of the bladder vary according to the severity of the disease. The bladder capacity is usually less than 300 ml. Urothelial erythema is a common feature but Hunner ulcers are found in only about one-third of IC patients. Glomerulation of suburothelial blood vessels is commonly seen. Cystodistension under light general anaesthesia (named ECDULGA by Richard Turner-Warwick) generally leads to tachycardia and tachypnoea. Also, cystodistension usually brings about petechial haemorrhages beneath the urothelium. In some cases this leads to haemorrhage within the irrigant solution on bladder drainage. Bladder biopsies should be taken from erythematous areas or randomly from the lateral wall of the bladder if no macroscopic abnormality is evident. When taking bladder biopsies it is important to ensure that the biopsy is

Table 51.1 Differential diagnosis of IC.

Infective*	Inflammatory	Neoplastic
Bacteria	Radiation cystitis	Endometriosis
Mycobacteria	Cyclophosphamide cystitis	Carcinoma *in situ*
Syphilis	Chemical cystitis	Leucoplakia
Viruses	Amyloidosis	Leukaemia
Yeasts	Eosinophilic cystitis	Lymphoma
Chlamydia	Pemphigus vulgaris	Carcinoma
Mycoplasma	Progressive systemic sclerosis	
Ureaplasma	Xanthogranulomatous cystitis	
Trichomonas	Malacoplakia	
Schistosomiasis	Lichen planus	
	Psoriasis	
	Epidermolysis bullosa acquisita	
	Chronic granulomatous disease	
	Polyarteritis nodosa	
	Behçet syndrome	

*Enterovesical fistula due to diverticular disease, colonic carcinoma or Crohn's disease should also be excluded.

Table 51.2 Diagnostic features of IC.

Symptoms	Cystoscopic findings	Bladder biopsy
Frequency	Reduced bladder capacity	Chronic inflammatory cell infiltrate within the submucosa
Suprapubic pain relieved by voiding	Glomerulations of suburothelial vessels	Urothelial ulceration and fissures
Perineal pain	Erythema	Lymphoid follicles
Urgency	Ulcers	Mast cells (especially within the detrusor muscle)
Dysuria	Fissures	Vascular ectasia
Dyspareunia	Petechial haemorrhage after cystodistension	Nerve fibre proliferation
Haematuria	ECDULGA leading to tachycardia and tachypnoea	Aberrant urothelial HLA-DR expression

ECDULGA, cystodistension under light general anaesthesia; HLA, human leucocyte antigen.

sufficiently deep to include some detrusor muscle. The areas that are biopsied may require application of cauterization to prevent haemorrhage and it is prudent to leave a urethral catheter *in situ* for approximately 24 h after biopsy.

Bladder biopsy

Histological examination of bladder wall biopsies is an important step in confirmation of the diagnosis of IC. The presence of a chronic inflammatory cell infiltrate within the bladder wall in IC was first recognized by Hunner [2] although at that time it was thought to be a response to active infection. The inflammatory cell infiltrate in IC is mainly located within the submucosa and is composed predominantly of lymphocytes and plasma cells. There is also infiltration by macrophages, neutrophils, mast cells and a few eosinophils. Denudation of the urothelium, submucosal vascular ectasia, detrusor myopathy and fibrosis are features in more chronic cases [3]. It is important to emphasize that there are no pathognomonic histological characteristics of IC. The diagnosis of IC is made by correlating symptoms, cystoscopic features and bladder biopsy findings.

Epidemiology and genetic predisposition

There have been few epidemiological studies of IC and these have been hampered by the rarity of the condition and inconsistencies in the diagnostic criteria between different countries. A study from Finland reported a prevalence of 10.6 cases of IC per 100 000 people with a female: male ratio of 12:1 [4]. Epidemiological studies suggest that there is a higher prevalence of IC in the USA than in the UK and continental Europe [5,6], but this finding may merely reflect local differences in diagnostic criteria. IC is rarely found in black people [7] and hence few reports have emanated from the African continent. There have been descriptions of IC occurring in a mother and daughter and also almost synchronously in a pair of monozygotic female twins [8]. It is impossible to ascertain if such familial association is due to a genetic factor, common exposure to an environmental agent or indeed a combination of the two.

Several studies have examined the possibility that there may be a genetic predisposition for IC. Comparison between ABO blood groups in 34 IC cases and 100 normal controls failed to show an association with any of the ABO antigens [9]. The first study in which human leucocyte antigen (HLA) tissue types were analysed in IC tested 20 loci (A and B antigens only) in 28 IC cases and 600 normal controls. There was a weakly significant association ($P = 0.038$) between IC and HLA-A10 and HLA-B17 [10]. In a small study of nine IC cases no HLA associations were found [8]. The most recent study of 31 white female IC patients and 140 white female normal controls, residing in the same geographical area, examined a total of 102 HLA tissue types (A, B, C, DQ, DR) and demonstrated a significant association between the HLA-DR6 allele and IC but no other associations. The relative risk factor for IC with HLA-DR6 was 4.91 [11]. The low relative risk of having an HLA-DR6 tissue type makes it unlikely that this specific gene is responsible for the development of IC, but raises the question of whether HLA-DR6 is associated by linkage disequilibrium with a specific gene for IC or whether individuals with the HLA-DR6 are genetically predisposed to develop IC when exposed to a specific environmental aetiological factor. However, such a genetic association could explain the familial association in IC as well as the variable geographical distribution. Further multicentre genetic studies would be needed to confirm this hypothesis.

Associated diseases

A number of conditions have been shown to be associated with IC. There is a high incidence of allergy in IC patients—26% in one series [8]. Other conditions sometimes found in IC patients include thyroiditis (7%) and rheumatoid arthritis (12%) [12]. IC has also been described in patients with systemic lupus erythematosus (SLE), however, it is most likely that this represents bladder involvement with SLE and hence it is a separate disorder from IC [13]. The association between IC and disorders of the immune system has led to the suggestion that the pathogenesis of IC is somehow mediated by the immune system.

Natural history

One of the most interesting features of IC is the variability in its severity and natural history. There is a broad spectrum of symptomatic severity in the disorder that has led to the suggestion that there might be multiple different aetiologies for IC. In order to reflect this some workers have renamed IC the 'painful bladder syndrome'.

In mild or early forms of IC the bladder capacity may be normal and there is often a good and maintained therapeutic response to cystodistension or intravesical dimethyl sulphoxide therapy. However, in more severe cases the bladder becomes contracted and the patients are resistant to conservative measures. These patients may ultimately require bladder replacement if their symptoms are sufficiently severe. The reason why some cases progress to bladder contracture while others maintain their capacity is not understood. However, histological examination of the detrusor muscle in some cases of IC may reveal evidence of detrusor myopathy—small muscle cells, vacuolation of detrusor cytoplasm and an increase in connective tissue between muscle cells [14]. It has recently been shown that IC patients with detrusor myopathy are more likely to progress to bladder contracture, necessitating enterocystoplasty, than those with normal detrusor biopsies [15].

Aetiological theories

The precise aetiology of IC remains obscure but there has been no shortage of hypotheses. In the 1920s and 1930s it was thought that IC was a chronic bacterial infection and some still believe this to be the case [16]. However, secondary infection is common in IC and it is difficult to be sure that any organism isolated from the urine is the primary pathogen. It has recently been proposed that Crohn's disease, a disorder that is in many ways similar to IC, results from infection with atypical mycobacteria [17]. However, a search for such fastidious organisms in IC bladder tissue using mycobacteria-specific DNA probes with signal amplification by polymerase chain reaction has not demonstrated any evidence of mycobacterial involvement [18].

The bladder urothelium is lined by a surface layer of glycosaminoglycans (GAG), the so-called glycocalyx, and this is thought to be important in preventing reabsorption of urinary constituents into the bladder wall. It has been suggested that in IC there is a primary deficiency of the glycocalyx which leads to reabsorption of solutes and that this is the aetiology of IC [19]. However, electron microscopic study of the glycocalyx has shown it to be intact in early cases of IC [20] and radioisotope experiments have revealed no significant difference in the bladder's absorptive capacity between IC and normal controls [21].

The possible role of the nervous system in the pathogenesis of IC was first proposed in 1949 when large numbers of nerve fibres were observed within the submucosa in IC biopsies [22]. The proliferation of nerve fibres in IC was later quantified in comparison with normal bladder and bacterial cystitis [23]. Further study of these nerves has shown that many contain neuropeptide Y and vasoactive intestinal peptides (VIP) [24]. Similar proliferation of such nerves is found in other chronic inflammatory conditions such as rheumatoid arthritis. The pathophysiological significance of the proliferating nerve fibres is not yet understood.

There are numerous other aetiological theories for IC including antibiotics, diet, sympathetic dystrophy and allergy. However, all these remain controversial. The presence of large amounts of immunoglobulins and chronic inflammatory cell infiltrate within the bladder wall in IC leads one to conclude that the immune system must play a part in the pathogenesis of IC. The evidence supporting the role of the immune system in the aetiology of IC is presented below.

Role of the immune system

Humoral immunology

Circulating antibodies capable of binding to bladder tissue were first identified within the serum of IC patients in 1970. Indirect immunofluorescence techniques were used to identify binding of bladder-specific autoantibodies to normal bladder. Antibody binding was seen in 45% of IC cases whilst normal control groups were all negative [12]. However, other similar studies have failed to detect bladder-specific autoantibodies in IC [25,26]. All the above three studies failed to recognize the potential artefact arising from the use of ABO mismatched bladder tissue and serum. A recent report of experiments using indirect immunofluorescence to examine antibody binding to blood group O normal bladder has shown binding to the bladder

of immunoglobulin G (IgG) class in 75% of IC cases and in 40% of normal controls. IgM class antibody binding to the normal bladder were detected in 63% of IC cases and 30% of controls [27]. Therefore, although the binding of antibodies to the bladder wall is a feature in IC there is currently no evidence to suggest that IC, unlike conditions such as juvenile onset diabetes mellitus (with islet cell-specific autoantibodies), is caused by an organ-specific autoantibody.

Cellular immunology

The presence of chronic inflammatory cells within the bladder wall has been recognized for many years [2]. The majority of the infiltrate of lymphocytes, plasma cells, neutrophils, mast cells and macrophages is found within the submucosa and urothelium [3,26]. Particular attention has been paid to the mast cell and its potential role in the pathogenesis of IC. The presence of mast cells within the bladder wall in IC patients was first recognized in 1958. Treatment with the antihistamine pyribenzamine, which inhibits the effects of histamine released from mast cell granules, was shown to be of short-term benefit in IC patients [28]. The presence of mast cells in bladder biopsies has been proposed as a diagnostic criterion for IC [29]. However, large numbers of mast cells are also evident within bladder biopsies in bacterial cystitis [30]. It is now apparent that a high density of mast cells within the detrusor muscle layer is a more specific finding for IC. A density of >20 mast cells/mm^2 of detrusor muscle has a specificity of 88% and a sensitivity of 95% for IC when compared to normal bladder and bacterial cystitis [30,31]. Therefore, it can be concluded that the presence of mast cells in bladder biopsies, especially within the detrusor layer, can be used to support the diagnosis of IC but is not absolutely diagnostic in isolation.

The presence of lymphocytes within the bladder wall in IC was first recognized by Hunner [32]. The normal bladder contains a few CD8+ T cells within the urothelium and lamina propria/submucosa and a few CD4+ T cells within the lamina propria/submucosa (Fig. 51.1). There are even less lymphocytes within the detrusor muscle layer [33]. In IC the urothelium and submucosa are infiltrated by increased numbers of CD8+ and CD4+ T cells, B lymphocytes and plasma cells, but few of these cells are found within the detrusor layer [27,34]. Plasma cells manufacturing IgG, IgA and IgM are found in large numbers within the submucosa in IC (Fig. 51.2) and it is thought that the immunoglobulins (especially IgA) produced by these cells are a protective mechanism for the denuded urothelium. A recent study of lymphocyte subpopulations within the bladder has demonstrated a significant increase in the number of γδ T cells in IC compared to normal bladder and bacterial cystitis [35]. These cells are attracted

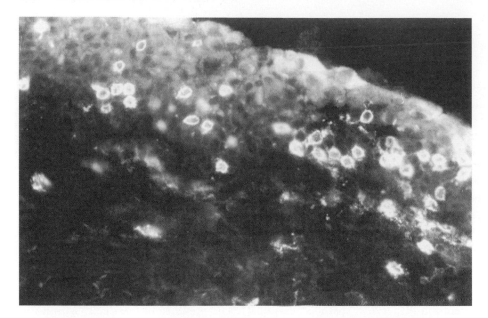

Fig. 51.1 CD3+ T cells within the urothelium/submucosa in a bladder biopsy from a patient with IC.

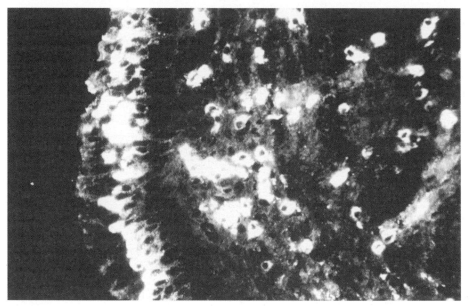

Fig. 51.2 IgA + plasma cells within the urothelium/submucosa in a bladder biopsy from a patient with IC.

towards epithelial surfaces in chronic inflammatory disorders and have also been seen within the synovium in rheumatoid arthritis and the mucosa in inflammatory bowel disease. The precise role of these cells is not yet understood.

The factor or factors activating T cells within the bladder wall in IC has, until recently, been uncertain. An immunohistochemical study of bladder biopsies from 22 cases of IC and 14 controls has shown that in IC, but not in the normal bladder or bacterial cystitis, there is abnormal HLA-DR molecule expression by the urothelium (Fig. 51.3). This aberrant HLA-DR expression by the urothelium in IC could induce activation of helper T cells and hence ultimately destruction of the urothelium through immune pathways [36].

In IC the bladder wall is also infiltrated by macrophages/monocytes, neutrophils and eosinophils. These cells are particularly concentrated within areas of urothelial ulceration where they phagocytose cellular debris and are thought to be attracted by the release of chemotactic factors from mast cells [37].

Management

The bewildering array of aetiological theories for IC is matched by an equally varied assortment of treatment options. It should be emphasized that none of the currently available treatments, except cystectomy, is curative. The management options can be broadly divided into four different approaches: (i) systemic medical therapy; (ii)

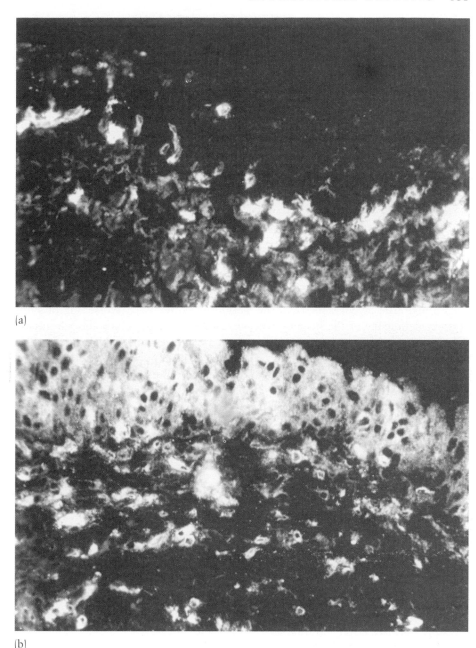

Fig. 51.3 HLA-DR expression in biopsies of (a) normal and (b) in a patient with IC.

(a)

(b)

intravesical drug instillation; (iii) interventional local bladder treatments; and (iv) open surgical operations (including neurosurgical procedures). The contemporary treatment options are listed in full in Table 51.3.

Systemic medical treatment

A wide variety of agents have been used as systemic therapy for IC. The first anti-inflammatory agent to be used as systemic therapy for IC was sodium gold thiosulphate although the reported results were uncontrolled [38]. More recently other anti-inflammatory and immunosuppressive agents such as chloroquine derivatives, adrenocortico-

trophic hormone (ACTH), corticosteroids and azathioprine have been used to treat IC producing symptomatic relief [39].

The presence of large numbers of mast cells within the bladder wall in IC has stimulated interest in treating the condition with systemic agents that inhibit the stimulation and degranulation of mast cells. Amitriptyline, hydroxyzine and nalmefene stabilize mast cells and also have other variable, potentially advantageous actions in IC: anticholinergic properties (inhibiting detrusor contraction and neuronal mast cell stimulation), sedative and anxiolytic effects and histamine receptor antagonism. Trials treating IC patients with amitriptyline [40], hydroxyzine

Table 51.3 Contemporary treatments options for IC.

Intravesical drug treatment	Systemic drug treatment	Surgical and interventional treatments
Dimethyl sulphoxide	Sodium pentosanpolysulphate	Cystodistension
		Local ulcer treatments
Oxychlorosene	Corticosteroids	Laser
Heparin	Azathioprine	Denervation
Corticosteroids	Amitriptyline	Supratrigonal cystectomy and cystoplasty
Silver nitrate	Hydroxyzine	Subtotal cystectomy and substitution cystoplasty
	Nalmefene	Total cystectomy and urinary diversion

[41] and nalmefene [42] have shown symptomatic improvement.

Although the hypothesis that the aetiology of IC is primary deficiency of the bladder urothelial GAG layer is dubious, it would be of potential therapeutic advantage to reconstitute this layer, particularly in ulcerative IC. The orally administered polysaccharide compound sodium pentosanpolysulphate (Elmiron) is brought to exert its effect by lining the bladder urothelium with a synthetic GAG layer. Placebo-controlled trials have shown that sodium pentosanpolysulphate therapy can lead to a statistically significant improvement in symptoms in patients with IC [43].

Intravesical instillation treatment

Intravesical pharmacotherapy for IC has certain advantages over systemic therapy. High concentrations of drug can be achieved locally within the bladder without significant systemic side effects, assuming that there is minimal drug absorption. However, there are disadvantages such as painful catheterization, the cost and inconvenience of multiple hospital visits and the risk of introducing urinary tract infection.

The first non-surgical treatment recommended for ulcerative IC was instillation of silver nitrate [44]. Although painful at the initial instillation, silver nitrate and other similar caustic agents such as phenol, argyrol and aniline dyes did lead to at least short-term symptomatic relief in some IC patients. Silver nitrate has now been superseded by dimethyl sulphoxide (DMSO) as first choice intravesical treatment for IC. Controlled trials of courses of intravesical DMSO in IC patients have shown significant improvement in symptoms with repeat administrations [45]. A course of DMSO can be administered at 1–2-week intervals given four to eight times. The overall response rate is 50–90% and is greater in patients without ulcers. Relapse will occur in 35–40% of patients but 60–80% of

these will respond to further DMSO treatment. DMSO instillation may cause a chemical cystitis and an initial worsening of symptoms in 10–15% of cases, DMSO may also be administered intravesically in combination with other agents such as corticosteroids and heparin [46].

Patients that fail to respond to DMSO should be considered for a course of intravesical sodium oxychlorosene (Clorpactin). This chemical should be inserted under general anaesthesia or careful regional anaesthesia because it usually induces bladder pain. Approximately 50% of IC patients will achieve symptomatic benefit from a course of four Clorpactin instillations [46].

Interventional treatments

A wide variety of local non-surgical treatment modalities have been used in IC. The first cystoscopic treatment for IC was local debridement of ulcers which was shown to be of short-term therapeutic benefit [47]. More recent technological advances have enabled surgeons to achieve similar local ulcer destruction by fulguration [48], resection using the cautery loop [49] and laser ablation [50].

Although focused therapy toward areas of ulceration may prove beneficial in particular cases it is more likely in IC that treatment of the entire bladder would prove to be of more lasting benefit. To this end Bumpus [51] was the first to advocate cystodistension under general anaesthesia. Such hydrodistension is thought to improve the bladder capacity by stretching the detrusor muscle and collagen fibres and to decrease bladder pain by ischaemic necrosis of sensory nerve fibres. The therapeutic response and its duration after hydrodistension are unpredictable [51,52].

Other minimally invasive techniques have been developed in an attempt to interrupt or destroy sensory nerve fibres subserving pain transmission from the bladder. Subtrigonal phenol injection therapy is rarely of long-term benefit in this aim as the nerves may regenerate. Furthermore, subtrigonal phenol injection can cause tissue necrosis leading to formation of vesicovaginal fistulas as well as sciatic nerve palsy and is no longer recommended [53]. An exciting new treatment for bladder pain in IC, which is in the early stages of development, is laparoscopic laser ablation of the ganglia and pain fibres at the base of the bladder [54]. Destruction of ganglia rather than the nerve fibres is theoretically less likely to enable sensory nerve fibres to regenerate.

Bladder pain in IC has been treated with success in some patients using transcutaneous electrical nerve stimulation (TENS) with the electrodes applied suprapubically.

Open surgical treatments

Neurosurgical and denervation operations

Many different neurosurgical procedures have been devised to attempt to interrupt pain fibres arising from the bladder. Presacral neurectomy [55], cordotomy [56], excision of the superior hypogastric plexus [57], sacral root rhizotomy [58] and sacral root neurectomy [59] have all been suggested but have all fallen out of favour because of limited efficacy and unacceptable side effects, including detrusor hypocontractility and sexual dysfunction in males. It has been suggested that visceral sensory and pain fibres arising from the bladder follow the sympathetic nerve fibres. However, division of the sympathetic fibres within the hypogastric plexus [57] and more locally [60] does not reliably lead to long-term symptomatic relief in IC. This finding also casts doubt upon the hypothesis that the aetiology of IC is some sort of reflex sympathetic dystrophy.

Local bladder denervation operations have been developed as a treatment for IC patients with severe pain but without reduction of bladder capacity. The first surgical procedure of this type, named cystocystoplasty, entailed supratrigonal bladder transection and reanastamosis [61]. This was subsequently modified to supratrigonal cystolysis, a more radical operation that involves division of the superior and inferior neurovascular pedicles [62,63]. Although in the short term this procedure leads to relief of pain and frequency [64], in the long term symptoms will recur in most cases after 5 years [65]. Furthermore, extravesical denervation procedures may exacerbate bladder contracture to the extent that about one third of cases require augmentation or substitution cystoplasty within 8 years [66]. With advances in conservative treatments there are very few IC patients in whom it is now appropriate to perform open bladder denervation surgery.

Urinary diversion

The irritative effects of urine upon the ulcerated bladder in IC are now well known and this was first recognized as long ago as 1870 when Tait reported relief of bladder pain in 'ulcerative cystitis' after surgical construction of a vesicovaginal fistula [44]. Urinary diversion by bilateral ureterosigmoidostomy was later also shown to relieve bladder pain without removal of the bladder [67].

Urinary diversion is rarely necessary for intractable IC. However, in the most severe cases of IC that have become refractory to conservative therapies, have urethral involvement or urethral incompetence leading to incontinence, it is on occasion necessary to perform total cystectomy and urinary diversion. In such cases the traditional technique for urinary diversion has been ileal conduit formation [68]. However, incontinent urinary stomas lead to more social restrictions and psychosexual problems than continent urinary stomas [69]. A number of different techniques are now available for the construction of continent urinary stomas. The cutaneous Kock pouch is the method of choice because it protects the upper tracts by virtue of an antireflux nipple and has the lowest reported complication and reoperation rate [70].

Augmentation cystoplasty

The end stage in some severe IC cases is fibrotic contracture of the bladder. The capacity of the bladder in such cases may be as little as 50 ml. It is tempting in such circumstances simply to augment the bladder without removing the diseased bladder tissue. However, although augmentation of the bladder may reduce the frequency of micturition the remaining diseased bladder usually leads to persistence of pain and urgency postoperatively. Therefore augmentation alone is not sufficient to relieve the symptoms of IC.

Supratrigonal cystectomy and enterocystoplasty

The most widely practised surgical procedure worldwide for severe IC refractory to other treatments has been supratrigonal cystectomy and enterocystoplasty [61]. The bowel segment used for the cystoplasty can be caecum, caecum with ascending colon, caecum with terminal ileum, sigmoid colon, ileum or even part of the stomach. The aim of such cystoplasties is to create a low-pressure reservoir with a reasonable capacity (>500 ml) that can empty efficiently leaving small residual urine volumes (<50 ml). When non-detubularized segments of bowel, particularly caecum/colon, are utilized peristaltic contractions within the cystoplasty can lead to frequency, urgency and incontinence in some cases. However, detubularization of the bowel segment produces a low-pressure reservoir that may not empty efficiently necessitating intermittent clean self-catheterization to drain the residual urine and hence prevent urinary tract infection. Also supratrigonal cystectomy and enterocystoplasty can lead to an hour-glass neobladder configuration which precludes efficient empty-

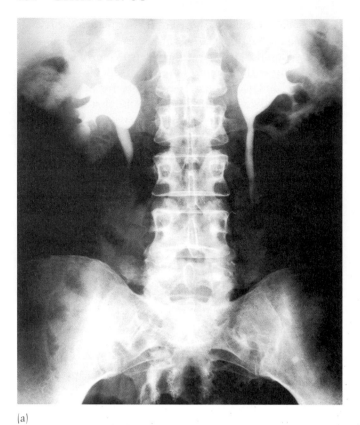

(a)

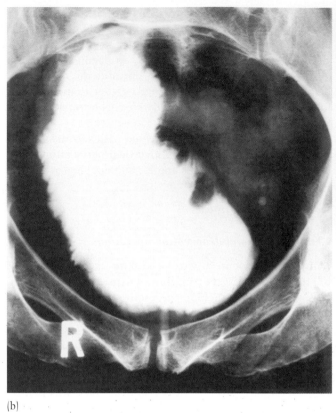

(b)

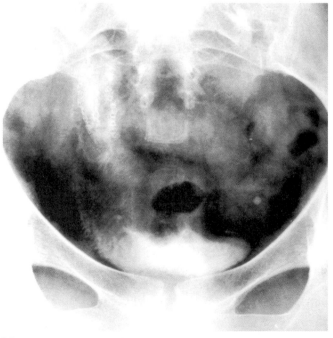

(c)

Fig. 51.4 Intravenous urogram with compression (a) in a female patient with IC previously treated by bladder replacement using a Kock pouch. The bladder is (b) shown to be of good capacity and (c) empties almost completely.

ing. Preservation of the natural antireflux mechanism of the ureterovesical junction in supratrigonal cystectomy is advantageous in most cases. However, in some IC patients trigonal disease can lead to loss of the antireflux property of the ureterovesical junction leading to vesicoureteric reflux (VUR). VUR in association with high-pressure peristaltic contractions within a non-detubularized cystoplasty is particularly likely to cause recurrent urinary tract infection and in some circumstances chronic pyelonephritis and impairment of renal function. Another problem with supratrigonal cystectomy in IC is the persistence of symptoms due to disease within the bladder remnant. When severe, trigonal disease may ultimately necessitate total cystectomy and urinary diversion [71].

Total bladder replacement (substitution enterocystoplasy)

Residual disease within the trigone in IC leads to problems such as pain and frequency after supratrigonal cystectomy and cystoplasty. Preservation of the trigone can result in an hour-glass configuration neobladder which may not empty efficiently. Recurrent urinary tract infections may follow, necessitating intermittent clean self-catheterization to drain the residual urine. When IC involves the trigone, inflammation and subsequent scarring can compromise the antireflux property of the ureterovesical junction and hence lead to VUR. VUR may also lead to recurrent urinary tract infection and this may be exacerbated by high-pressure peristaltic contractions when non-detubularized bowel segments are used for the cystoplasty.

The potential problems of supratrigonal cystectomy for IC outlined above can be overcome by removing the entire bladder apart from a 1–2 cm cuff around the bladder neck (subtotal cystectomy). Although there have been reports of persistent pain following cystectomy in IC [72], the author has not encountered this phenomenon in 38 IC cases treated by subtotal or total cystectomy. After subtotal cystectomy the bladder can be replaced by a segment of bowel and the ureters implanted into the bowel segment. A variety of ureteric reimplantation techniques have been used but all these carry a risk of stenosis and reflux. Historically, the most commonly used bowel segment for total bladder replacement in IC has been the caecum and ascending colon [72]. The ureters can be implanted into the terminal ileum or into the taeniae by the Leadbetter–Clarke method; the latter has a stenosis rate of about 14%. Unfortunately caecal segments do not always empty completely and therefore intermittent self-catheterization is often indicated.

Many of the potential postoperative problems outlined above can be overcome by performing subtotal cystectomy and bladder replacement with the Kock pouch. The bladder is removed leaving a 1–2 cm cuff of tissue around the bladder neck. The neobladder is constructed from 72 cm of terminal ileum detubularized to form a Kock pouch which also incorporates an antireflux nipple created by intussusception of the distal afferent limb of the pouch into the pouch itself. The nipple is kept in position within the pouch by three rows of Autosuture TA55 linear staples. The ureters are anastomosed to the afferent limb proximal to the antireflux nipple. This technique has been described in detail as a treatment for bladder cancer in males [73]. We have performed this operation in 24 IC patients (22 females, two males) with complete relief of pain in each case. Although four female patients leak slightly at night the remainder are now completely continent with a mean bladder capacity of 420 ml. One patient developed severe incontinence and was converted to an ileal conduit. Since the Kock pouch is virtually spherical it empties more efficiently than some other cystoplasties. The mean post-micturition residual volume in these patients is less than 70 ml and only two of them need to perform intermittent catheterization. Cystography performed at 3 months post-operatively has not demonstrated evidence of VUR. Thus the Kock pouch bladder replacement appears to be the best currently available surgical treatment for severe IC [74] (Fig. 51.4).

Conclusion

IC is a rare, chronic, debilitating condition predominantly affecting middle-aged females. The diagnosis, made by a combination of symptoms, cystoscopic findings and bladder biopsies, is often delayed due to a lack of awareness among general practitioners. The precise aetiology remains obscure but there is an apparent genetic predisposition and the immune and neurological systems appear to have a role in the pathogenesis of IC. A wide assortment of therapies are available, all of which offer palliation of symptoms in some patients. Severe cases, in whom more conservative measures fail to relieve symptoms, can be offered a potential cure in the form of surgical replacement of the bladder by enterocystoplasty.

The non-steroidal anti-inflammatory drug Tiaprofenic Acid (Surgam) has been shown to induce a form of chronic abacterial cystitis that may mimic IC. The symptoms and cystoscopic appearance are similar to IC. However, it is usual for the symptoms to improve soon after discontinuation of drug therapy [75].

References

1 Skene AJC. *Diseases of the Bladder and Urethra in Women*. New York: William Wood, 1887:167.
2 Hunner GL. A rare type of bladder ulcer in women. *Trans South Surg Gynecol Assoc* 1915;**27**:247–92.
3 Lynes WL, Flynn SD, Shortliffe LD, Stamey TA. The

histology of interstitial cystitis. *Am J Surg Pathol* 1990;**14**: 969–76.

4 Oravisto KJ. Epidemiology of interstitial cystitis. *Ann Chir Gynaecol Finnae* 1975;**64**:75–7.

5 Somerset JB. Chronic interstitial cystitis. *West J Surg* 1960;**68**: 235–7.

6 Weyeneth R, Rohner A. Simple ulcer of the bladder. Interstitial ulcerous cystitis, Fenwick–Hunner ulcer. *Schweiz Med Weischrift* 1961;**91**:1042.

7 de Juana CP, Everett JC. Interstitial cystitis, experience and review of recent literature. *Urology* 1977;**10**:325–9.

8 Oravisto KJ. Interstitial cystitis as an autoimmune disease, a review. *Eur Urol* 1980;**6**:10–13.

9 Christmas TJ. Interstitial cystitis: immunological aspects and progress in treatment. In: Hendry WF, ed. *Recent Advances in Urology/ Andrology*, Vol. 5. Edinburgh: Churchill Livingstone, 1991:103–17.

10 Rosin RD, Griffiths T, Sofras F, James DCO, Edwards L. Interstitial cystitis. *Br J Urol* 1979;**51**:524–7.

11 Christmas TJ, Bottazzo GF, Milroy EJG. Interstitial cystitis; an hereditary autoimmune disease? *Eur Urol* 1990;**18**:415.

12 Silk MR. Bladder antibodies in interstitial cystitis. *J Urol* 1970;**103**:307–9.

13 Boye E, Morse M. Huttner I *et al*. Immune complex-mediated interstitial cystitis as a major manifestation of systemic lupus erythematosus. *Clin Immunol Immunopathol* 1979;**13**:67–76.

14 Holm-Bentzen M, Larsen S, Hainau B, Hald TT. Non-obstructive detrusor myopathy in group of patients with chronic abacterial cystitis. *Scand J Urol Nephrol* 1985;**19**: 21–26.

15 Christmas TJ, Rode J. Detrusor myopathy: an accurate predictor of bladder contracture in interstitial cystitis. *J Urol* 1993;**149**:506A.

16 Wilkins EGL, Payne SR, Read PJ, Moss ST, Maskell RM. Interstitial cystitis and the urethral syndrome: a possible answer. *Br J Urol* 1989;**64**:39–44.

17 Hampson SJ, MacFadden JJ, Hermon-Taylor J. Mycobacteria and Crohn's disese. *Gut* 1989;**29**:1017–19.

18 Hampson SJ, Christmas TJ, Moss MT. Search for mycobacteria in interstitial cystitis using mycobacteria-specific DNA probes with signal amplification by polymerase chain reaction. *Br J Urol* 1993;**72**:303–6.

19 Parsons CL, Schmidt JD, Pollen JJ. Sucessful treatment of interstitial cystitis with sodium pentosanpolysulfate. *J Urol* 1983;**130**:51–3.

20 Dixon JS, Holm-Bentzen M, Gilpin CJ *et al*. Electron microscopic investigation of the bladder urothelium and glycocalyx in patients with interstitial cystitis. *J Urol* 1986;**135**:621–5.

21 Chelsky MJ, Rosen SI, Knight LC *et al*. Bladder permeability in interstitial cystitis is similar to that of normal volunteers: direct measurement by transvesical absorption of technetium diethylenetriaminepenta-acetic acid. *J Urol* 1994;**151**:346–9.

22 Hand JR. Interstitial cystitis: report of 223 cases (204 women and 19 men). *J Urol* 1949;**61**:291–310.

23 Christmas TJ, Rode J, Chapple CR, Milroy EJG, Turner-Warwick RT. Nerve fibre proliferation in interstitial cystitis. *Virchows Archiv [A]* 1990;**416**:447–51.

24 Hohenfellner M, Nunes L, Schmidt RA *et al*. Interstitial cystitis: increased sympathetic innervation and related neuropeptide synthesis. *J Urol* 1992;**147**:587–91.

25 Jokinen EJ, Alfthan OS, Oravisto KJ. Anti-tissue antibodies in interstitial cystitis. *Clin Exp Immunol* 1972;**11**:333–9.

26 Skoluda D, Wegner K, Lemmel EM. Kritische benerkungen zur immunopathogenese der interstitiellen cystitis. *Urologe [A]* 1974;**13**:15–23.

27 Anderson JB, Parivar F, Lee G *et al*. The enigma of interstitial cystitis—an autoimmune disease? *Br J Urol* 1989;**63**:270–5.

28 Simmons JL. Interstitial cystitis: an explanation for the beneficial effect of an anti-histamine. *J Urol* 1961;**85**:149–55.

29 Larsen S, Thompson SA, Hald T *et al*. Mast cells in interstitial cystitis. *Br J Urol* 1982;**54**:283–6.

30 Christmas TJ, Rode J. Characteristics of mast cells in normal bladder, bacterial cystitis and interstitial cystitis. *Br J Urol* 1991;**68**:473–8.

31 Kastrup J, Hald T, Larsen S, Nielsen VG. Histamine content and mast cell count of detrusor muscle in patients with interstitial cystitis and other types of chronic cystitis. *Br J Urol* 1983;**55**:495–500.

32 Hunner GL. A rare type of bladder ulcer; further notes and a report of 18 cases. *J Am Med Assoc* 1918;**70**:203–12.

33 Gardiner RA, Seymour GJ, Lavin MF *et al*. Immunohisto-chemical analysis of the human bladder. *Br J Urol* 1986;**58**: 19–25.

34 MacDermott JP, Stone AR, Miller CH, Levy N. Cellular immunity in interstitial cystitis. *J Urol* 1991;**145**:274–8.

35 Christmas TJ. Lymphocyte sub-populations in the bladder wall in normal bladder, bacterial cystitis and interstitial cystitis. *Br J Urol* 1994;**73**:508–15.

36 Christmas TJ, Bottazzo GF. Abnormal urothelial HLA-DR expression in interstitial cystitis. *Clin Exp Immunol*, 1992;**87**:450–4.

37 Dixon JS, Hald T. Morphological studies of the bladder wall in interstitial cystitis. In: George NJR, Gosling JA, eds. *Sensory Disorders of the Bladder and Urethra*. Berlin: Springer Verlag, 1986:63–71.

38 Fister GM. Similarity of interstitial cystitis (Hunner ulcer) to lupus erythematosus. *J Urol* 1938;**40**:37–51.

39 Oravisto KJ, Alfthan OS. Treatment of interstitial cystitis with immunosuppressive and chloroquine derivatives. *Eur Urol* 1976;**2**:82–4.

40 Hanno PM, Buehler J, Wein AJ. Use of amitriptyline in the treatment of interstitial cystitis. *J Urol* 1989;**141**:846–8.

41 Theoharides TC. Hydroxyzine in the treatment of interstitial cystitis. *Urol Clin North Am* 1994;**21**:113–19.

42 Stone NN. Nalmefene in the treatment of interstitial cystitis. *Urol Clin North Am* 1994;**21**:101–6.

43 Parsons CL, Mulholland S. Successful treatment of interstitial cystitis with sodium pentosanpolysulfate. *J Urol* 1987;**138**: 153–5.

44 Tait L. Cure of chronic perforating ulcer of the bladder by the formation of an artificial vesico-vaginal fistula. *Lancet* 1870;**2**:738.

45 Perez-Marrero R, Emerson LE, Feltis JT. A controlled study of dimethyl sulfoxide in interstitial cystitis. *J Urol* 1988;**140**: 36–9.

46 Sant GR, LaRock DR. Standard intra-vesical therapies for interstitial cystitis. *Urol Clin North Am* 1994;**21**:73–83.

47 Fenwick EH. The clinical significance of the simple solitary ulcer of the urinary bladder. *Br Med J* 1896;**1**:1133–5.

48 Kreutzmann HAR. The treatment of Hunner's ulcer of the bladder by fulguration. *Califor State Med J* 1992;**20**:128–30.

49 Sears NP. Elusive ulcer of the bladder with special reference to its treatment with phenol. *N Y State J Med* 1936;**36**:724–8.

50 Shanberg AM, Malloy T. Treatment of interstitial cystitis with neodymium: YAG laser. *Urology* 1987;**29**:31–3.

51 Bumpus HC. Interstitial cystitis: its treatment by over-distension of the bladder. *Med Clin North Am* 1930;**13**:1495–8.

52 Dunn M, Ramsden PD, Roberts JBM, Smith JC, Smith PJB. Interstitial cystitis treated by prolonged bladder distention. *Br J Urol* 1977;**49**:641–5.

53 Chapple CR, Hampson SJ, Turner-Warwick RT, Worth PHL. Subtrigonal phenol injection. How safe and effective is it? *Br J Urol* 1991;**68**:483–6.

54 Gillespie L. Destruction of the vesico-ureteric plexus for the treatment of hypersensitive bladder disorders. *Br J Urol* 1994;**74**:40–3.

55 Pieri G. Clinical contributions on the surgery of the sympathetic nervous system. The treatment of tuberculous cystitis. *Arch Ital Chir* 1930;**27**:454–82.

56 Grant FC. Cordotomy for relief of pain in the genito-urinary tract. *J Urol* 1931;**25**:551–8.

57 Douglass HL. Excision of the superior hypogastric plexus in the treatment of intractable interstitial cystitis, report of five cases. *Am J Surg* 1934;**25**:249–57.

58 Franksson C. Interstitial cystitis: a clinical study of fifty-nine cases. *Acta Chir Scand* 1957;**113**:51–62.

59 Milner WA, Garlick WB. Selective sacral neurectomy in interstitial cystitis. *J Urol* 1957;**78**:600–4.

60 Scott WJM, Schroeder CF. Denervation of the bladder for relief of intractable pain. *Ann Surg* 1938;**108**:730–40.

61 Turner-Warwick RT, Ashken MH. The functional results of partial, subtotal and total cystoplasty with special reference to ureterocaecocystoplasty, selective sphincterotomy and cystocystoplasty. *Br J Urol* 1967;**39**:3–12.

62 Worth PHL, Turner-Warwick RT. The treatment of interstitial cystitis by cystolysis with observations on cystoplasty. *Br J Urol* 1973;**45**:65–71.

63 Worth PHL. The treatment of interstitial cystitis by cystolysis with observations on cystoplasty. A review after 7 years. *Br J Urol* 1980;**52**:232.

64 Freiha FS, Stamey TA. Cystolysis: a procedure for the selective denervation of the bladder. *J Urol* 1980;**123**:360–3.

65 Albers DD, Geyer JR. Long-term results of cystolysis (supra-trigonal denervation) of the bladder for intractable interstitial cystitis. *J Urol* 1988;**139**:1205–6.

66 Christmas TJ, Worth PHL, Turner-Warwick RT. The management of bladder hypersensitivity due to interstitial cystitis by supra-trigonal denervation. In: *Proceedings of the British Association of Urological Surgeons Annual Meeting*, Scarborough, June 1990, p. 23.

67 Counsellor VS. Bilateral transplantation of the ureters in the female. *Am J Obstet Gynecol* 1937;**33**:24–9.

68 Jacobo E, Stamler FW, Culp DA. Interstitial cystitis followed by total cystectomy. *Urology* 1974;**3**:481–5.

69 Boyd SD, Feinberg SM, Skinner DG *et al.* Quality of life survey of urinary diversion patients: comparison of ileal conduits versus continent Kock ileal reservoirs. *J Urol* 1987;**138**:1386–7.

70 Skinner DG, Lieskovsky G, Boyd S. Continent urinary diversion. *J Urol* 1989;**141**:1323–7.

71 Webster GD, Maggio MI. The management of chronic interstitial cystitis by substitution cystoplasty. *J Urol* 1989; **141**:287–91.

72 Baskins LS, Tanagho EA. Pelvic pain without pelvic organs. *J Urol* 1992;**147**:683–6.

73 Skinner DG, Boyd SD, Lieskovsky G, Bennett C, Hopwood B. Lower urinary tract reconstruction following cystectomy: experience and results in 126 patients using the Kock ileal reservoir with bilateral ureteroileal urethrostomy. *J Urol* 1991;**146**:756–60.

74 Christmas TJ, Holmes SAV, Hendry WF. Bladder replacement using the Kock pouch; the final treatment for interstitial cystitis? *Br J Urol* 1996;**78**:69–73.

75 Bramble FJ, Morley R. Drug-induced cystitis: the need for vigilance. *Br J Urol* 1997;**79**:3–7.

**Epididymo-orchitis
and Scrotal Infections**
S. J. Eykyn

Introduction

Infection may involve the epididymis alone (epididymitis), the testis alone (orchitis) or both organs (epididymo-orchitis), but in clinical practice the term epididymo-orchitis tends to be used indiscriminately, indeed it may not always be possible to define the extent of the infection. Epididymitis is much more common than orchitis but most patients with clinical evidence of epididymitis usually have some testicular involvement although the epididymis is the predominant site of pathology. As the microbial aetiology and pathogenesis of epididymitis (and epididymo-orchitis) differ from those of orchitis, the conditions will be considered separately. Patients with these infections present to general practitioners and genitourinary physicians as well as to urologists. These specialists do not always have the same approach to the problem.

Epididymitis

Epididymitis is common and causes considerable morbidity. It has been reported to account for more days lost from military service in the USA than any other disease [1]. Although previously many cases were considered 'idiopathic' and attributed to the reflux of sterile urine or to straining, since the late 1970s several studies [2–6] that have employed improved diagnostic techniques have shown that the majority of cases of epididymitis have an infectious aetiology, and that the initial infection arises in the urethra, prostate or bladder. Infected urine or secretions are thought to enter the ejaculatory ducts by reflux or direct extension and ascend the vas deferens to colonize and infect the epididymis. Most cases of epididymitis begin in the tail of the epididymis; there is an acute polymorphonuclear intraluminal exudate, tubal epithelial damage and sometimes microabscess formation. The infection is usually unilateral and a hydrocele is often present. Epididymitis can be acquired by sexual transmission as a result of antecedent urethritis, it can also result from bacteriuria usually associated with underlying urological pathology, from systemic infection and, rarely, from other causes. These different types of epididymitis are most conveniently considered separately.

Types of epididymitis

Sexually transmitted epididymitis

Sexually transmitted epididymitis is the commonest type of epididymitis seen in men under the age of 35. In the pre-antibiotic era gonococcal epididymitis was common; it was reported to occur in 10–30% of cases of gonococcal urethritis. The commonest pathogen in the developed world is now *Chlamydia trachomatis*; *Neisseria gonorrhoeae* is less common than previously, and when it does occur, it is sometimes associated with concomitant *C. trachomatis* infection. Berger [1] reported nine cases (21%) of *N. gonorrhoeae* but 18 cases (43%) of *C. trachomatis* amongst 42 men with epididymitis aged less than 35 years. In a further case both organisms were present. Prevalence of *C. trachomatis* epididymal infection in this age group has also been reported from the UK [7,8] and elsewhere in the developed world [4] as well as the USA. However, in the developing world, at least in South Africa, *N. gonorrhoeae* may still be the predominant sexually transmitted epididymal pathogen; it was the commonest organism isolated from 134 men under 35 years with epididymitis seen in a sexually transmitted diseases (STD) clinic in Durban [6]. *N. gonorrhoeae* alone was isolated in 59 cases (44%) and *N. gonorrhoeae* plus *C. trachomatis* in 17 cases (13%); *C. trachomatis* alone accounted for 29 cases (22%). It was also the commonest isolate in a study of epididymitis in migrant mineworkers (ages not stated) reported from Johannesburg [5], although 17% of patients with gonorrhoea also had *C. trachomatis* isolated and a further 39% had serological evidence of chlamydial infection. In these South African series some 15% of gonococci were penicillinase-producing *Neisseria gonorrhoeae* strains (PPNG); these organisms are more likely to be encountered in the developing world. Although sexually transmitted epididymitis is most likely to occur in men under 35 years, it may occur in older men, and either *C. trachomatis* or *N. gonorrhoeae*, or both, may be involved.

Other organisms have occasionally been reported from cases of sexually transmitted epididymitis. In 1977, Harnisch *et al.* [2] isolated *Ureaplasma urealyticum* from the urethra of five of 17 men with epididymitis under 32 years in whom specific cultures were set up, and in two of these patients it was the only isolate. *U. urealyticum* was also isolated from the urethra and epididymal aspirate of a man of 24 years with acute epididymitis reported by Jalil *et al.* [9], from whom no other pathogens were isolated and who had no serological evidence of chlamydial infection. As few studies have specifically sought *U. urealyticum* its role in epididymitis remains to be defined. The case for *Trichomonas vaginalis* is even less convincing. Syphilitic epididymitis was also reported in the pre-antibiotic era.

Not all patients with epididymitis caused by sexually transmitted organisms will have symptoms of urethritis, but even in those who deny such symptoms a urethral discharge can sometimes be expressed and polymorphs detected on a Gram stain of an endourethral swab or in the first few millilitres of urine passed. Hence all patients should be investigated regardless of symptoms or the lack of them.

Epididymitis associated with bacteriuria

Epididymitis can be caused by urinary pathogens in patients with bacteriuria. This is most likely to occur in men over 35 years, but can occur at any age if there is an underlying urological abnormality, and has been reported in pre-pubertal boys. It may also be associated with urethral catheterization or instrumentation. In Berger's series of 17 men with epididymitis aged over 35 years, 12 infections (70%) were caused by urinary tract pathogens (coliforms or *Pseudomonas aeruginosa*) and only one by *C. trachomatis* [1]. He also reported seven men aged less than 35 years with epididymitis caused by Gram-negative bacilli (six by coliforms and one by *Haemophilus influenzae*); all were homosexuals who regularly practised anal-insertive intercourse. In two additional homosexual men in this study no urethral pathogen was identified. All nine homosexual men had numerous polymorphs in a midstream specimen of urine. Symptomatic bacteriuria (almost always *Escherichia coli*), sometimes with urethral discharge, has been reported to be more common in homosexual or bisexual men than in heterosexual men amongst those attending an STD clinic [10], and anal intercourse is thought also to predispose to bacterial prostatitis [11].

Epididymitis associated with systemic infection

These infections usually occur as a result of haematogenous dissemination, but also occasionally by direct extension from a genitourinary tract focus; they are uncommon. *Mycobacterium tuberculosis* can cause epididymitis [12]. Mittemeyer [13] reported five (0.8%) cases of tuberculous infection associated with epididymitis amongst 610 cases seen in the US army between 1958 and 1964, and Berger [1] detected one (1.5%) amongst his 68 cases of epididymitis. Such patients invariably have coincidental tuberculous infection of the seminal vesicle, prostate or kidney. In contrast to epididymitis caused by sexually transmitted organisms or urinary pathogens, tuberculous epididymitis is often bilateral.

According to Christie [14], epididymo-orchitis occurs in between at least 2 and 5% of adult males with brucellosis, but higher rates have been recorded. In a large study from Kuwait [15] 22 (9.5%) of the 231 male patients with brucellosis presented with epididymo-orchitis. Although brucellosis is now only rarely encountered in the UK (usually imported), worldwide it remains an important zoonotic disease. There have been occasional reports of epididymitis in patients with bacteraemia caused by a variety of organisms including *Streptococcus pneumoniae* [16] and *H. influenzae* [17,18]. It has also been reported in meningococcal infection [19,20], although in the series of 706 consecutive cases of 'meningococcosis' reported by Banks [21] there was no case of orchitis or epididymitis. *Neisseria meningitidis* has been known to mimic the gonococcus and cause (presumably sexually acquired) urethritis and this has been associated with epididymitis [22]. It is likely that other bacteria are also capable of producing epididymitis by blood-borne dissemination. Systemic fungal diseases can, though rarely do, cause epididymitis, and it has also been reported in association with parasitic disease including filariasis, schistosomiasis and amoebiasis [23].

Other causes of epididymitis

Although straining with reflux of sterile urine was a previous popular explanation for 'idiopathic' epididymitis it is probably seldom if ever implicated and the role of trauma in the disease remains to be defined. In 1985, epididymitis was reported in five of 56 men taking the anti-arrhythmic drug amiodarone [24]. Epididymal biopsy showed lymphocytic infiltration and fibrosis.

Diagnosis

In boys and young men the main differential diagnosis of epididymitis (and orchitis) is torsion of the testis which requires emergency surgery. Torsion of the testis is most common between 12 and 18 years though it may occur at other ages. Microscopic examination of the urine and or urethral discharge may be helpful in differentiating epididymitis from torsion since pyuria or bacteriuria is frequently present in epididymitis but is not found with torsion. Doppler ultrasonography has been used to evaluate bloodflow to the affected scrotum; epididymitis is associated with increased bloodflow whereas torsion results in decreased bloodflow. But as Krieger [23] points out the results of such studies do not always correlate with surgical findings. Nuclear medicine techniques can also be used to evaluate bloodflow. Holder *et al.* [25] reported the correct diagnosis of epididymitis in all of 22 patients so investigated and Abu-Sleiman *et al.* [26] reported a correct diagnosis in 86% of cases. The diagnostic difficulty in such cases is emphasized by Berger's report of a patient with simultaneous epididymitis and torsion [1].

Some patients with epididymitis will complain of a urethral discharge, but whether this is present or not, all should ideally have two endourethral swabs taken: one for microscopic examination by Gram stain to detect pus cells and Gram-negative diplococci (presumptive gonococci), which should then be cultured on both selective and non-selective media for the isolation of *N. gonorrhoeae* (not all strains of gonococci will grow on selective medium); the second endourethral swab is for the detection of *C. trachomatis* either by the demonstration of antigen by immunofluorescence or enzyme-linked immunosorbent assay (ELISA) techniques or by isolation in an appropriate cell culture. It must be said that laboratories vary in the service (or lack of it) that they offer clinicians for the detection of *Chlamydia*, and also that not all clinicians are as enthusiastic in their quest for *Chlamydia* as those who have published reports on this infection. If a chlamydial service is available, it should be used. Few laboratories offer cell culture facilities for *Chlamydia*, but commercial kits are available for antigen detection by immunofluorescent and ELISA techniques. Chlamydial serology (which is not generally available) requires the demonstration of a rising antibody titre as the positive predictive power of a single antibody determination is poor and patients seldom return for such investigations to be done even if available. In addition to endourethral swabs, urine (preferably first voided and midstream specimens) should be examined microscopically for pus cells and organisms and cultured. STD clinicians are more likely than urologists to perform both chlamydial investigations and differential urine tests.

Epididymal aspirates have been obtained in some studies on epididymitis and have yielded the causative pathogen on culture. They cannot be recommended routinely as the pathogen can nearly always be detected on endourethral swabs or urine analysis. Other investigations have included culture of semen, prostatic secretion and endourethral swabs after prostatic massage, some or all of which may yield the pathogen. None of them are necessary.

Management

In addition to symptomatic treatment such as bed rest, scrotal elevation and analgesia, antibiotics should always be given as the majority of cases have a microbial aetiology. Since the routine use of antibiotics in these patients the incidence of subsequent abscess formation and testicular infarction has decreased. Such complications are more common with coliform infections. If presumptive gonococci are seen on the Gram-stained endourethral smear or if *N. gonorrhoeae* is later isolated on culture, then specific treatment for gonorrhoea should be given. When treatment is initiated on the result of the Gram stain (i.e. before the sensitivity of the gonococcus is known) the choice of antibiotic will be guided by local STD experience concerning the incidence of PPNG, but ampicillin, a cephalosporin or ciprofloxacin are possible agents.

If there is clinical or microscopical evidence of ure-thritis, treatment for chlamydial infection (whether *C. trachomatis* is demonstrated or not) should be given with oral oxytetracycline (500 mg qds) or oral doxycycline (100 mg bid) for 10–14 days for both gonococcal and non-gonococcal infection. As these infections are sexually acquired, it is important to examine and treat the patient's sex partner(s) as well. If there is bacteriuria, or if epididymitis occurs in men over 35 years without urethritis, a urinary source for the pathogen should be assumed. Local information on urinary isolates will determine the most appropriate initial therapy before sensitivities are available, but oral trimethoprin (200 mg b.i.d.) or oral ciprofloxacin (500 mg b.i.d.) are reasonable choices. Parenteral antibiotics are rarely indicated. It is likely that the newer quinolones will prove to be the drugs of choice for epididymitis whether this is caused by gonococci, *Chlamydia* or urinary organisms. Although clinical experience of ciprofloxacin in men with chlamydial urethritis has been disappointing, the drug was only given for 7 days in two reported studies [27,28], but the quinolone ofloxacin (200 mg b.i.d. for 14–21 days) has been shown to be highly effective [4].

Although it is known that the inflammation in acute epididymitis is not confined to the epididymis but also involves the testis, it is not known to what extent such testicular involvement affects fertility, but in bilateral involvement this is likely to be reduced.

Orchitis

As has already been discussed, in most cases of epididymi-tis the infection also involves the testis, hence the universal clinical use of the term epididymo-orchitis.

Orchitis is much less common and is associated with certain viral infections particularly mumps. Mumps virus has been isolated from fine-needle biopsy specimens of the testis in cases of mumps orchitis. Testicular involvement in patients with mumps was first noted by Hippocrates, and orchitis is the most common complication of mumps in pubertal and post-pubertal patients. In their population-based study over a 40-year period (1935–1974). Beard *et al.* [29] found a 10% incidence of mumps orchitis amongst 1310 cases of males with the disease, but this was a retrospective study and others have reported higher rates. The median age of the patients with orchitis was 28 years (range 11–64 years). In two-thirds of the cases parotitis preceded the appearance of orchitis by about 7 days. Orchitis was bilateral in 17% of cases. Some degree of testicular atrophy is common after mumps but atrophy does not necessarily imply sterility, in fact it is likely that in the past the incidence of sterility after mumps has been grossly exaggerated and much anecdotal evidence exists to suggest that it is rare. Coxsackie B viruses can also cause orchitis and this complication has been reported in Bornholm disease; Coxsackie virus B5 has been isolated from testicular tissue [30].

Scrotal infections

Scrotal abscess

Scrotal abscesses can arise spontaneously but they can also occur after intrascrotal surgery and as an unusual complication of epididymo-orchitis when there is usually testicular infarction. Abscesses that result from epididymo-orchitis are invariably caused by urinary pathogens, usually *E. coli*, and the original epididymal infection will have been associated with bacteriuria with the same microbe. Other scrotal abscesses, whether spontaneous or related to scrotal surgery are usually caused by anaerobes, although mixed cultures with aerobes are quite common. In a series of 41 scrotal abscesses that were not secondary to epididymo-orchitis studied at St Thomas' Hospital [31], anaerobes alone were isolated in 14 cases, anaerobes with aerobes in 25 cases and aerobes alone in only two cases. The commonest anaerobes isolated were *Peptostreptococcus* spp., *Porphyromonas asaccharolytica*, *Bacteroides ureolyticus* and *Prevotella* spp. Interestingly the anaerobes perhaps best known to clinicians, *Bacteroides fragilis* and related organisms of the 'fragilis' type, were seldom isolated; they are the least technically demanding anaerobes, and thus the easiest to isolate.

Spontaneous scrotal abscesses are often recurrent, and one of the patients in the study [31] had suffered from recurrent abscesses for 9 years. They are also more common in black people than white people and this may be related to the fact that apocrine glands are three times more common in black skin than white skin. Obesity, poor hygiene and diabetes are possibly relevant to the development of scrotal abscesses, but it seems likely that the basic defect that predisposes to anaerobic scrotal abscess is apocrine blockage and the resultant infection is secondary to this [32]. Apocrine blockage has been shown to underlie anaerobic breast and axillary abscesses that are caused by similar anaerobes [33,34]. Most anaerobic infection is secondary to other pathology rather than a primary infection. Some patients with recurrent scrotal abscesses have, or give a history of, recurrent infections at other sites that are rich in apocrine glands. One patient in the St Thomas' series with an anaerobic scrotal abscess had coincidental bilateral hidradenitis of the axilla, and the same anaerobic species were recovered from the axillae and scrotum. It is possible, though unproven, that the anaerobic bacteria causing scrotal abscesses gain access to the blocked apocrine glands via the skin.

Scrotal abscesses after surgery (for hydrocele, scrotal reduction and hypospadias, for example) probably result from infected haematoma. Postoperative infections can be severe: in one patient a scrotal abscess that occurred after the excision of epididymal cysts resulted in infarction of the testis. The source of the anaerobes in such cases is unknown, but the normal commensal flora of the urethra contains small numbers of similar anaerobes and it may be relevant. Scrotal abscesses require surgical drainage, whatever their aetiology. Antibiotics are often given but it is doubtful if they confer any benefit. At least they should be appropriate for the pathogens involved. More logical is the giving of prophylactic antibiotics such as metronidazole for scrotal surgery but no trial has shown efficacy.

Necrotizing fasciitis of the genitalia (Fournier's gangrene)

This uncommon but devastating condition is still eponymously linked with the name of the French venereologist Fournier, yet his description of the disease (*gangrène foudroyante de la verge*) differs in many respects from what we now recognize as Fournier's gangrene [35,36]. His original papers which were published over a century ago can be commended to the reader with plenty of time and the ability to read French. The florid prose spares no clinical detail. Fournier described five previously healthy men aged 25–30 years with no antecedent local cause or lesion who developed sudden penile pain, swelling and redness that rapidly progressed to penoscrotal gangrene.

> La maladie a toujours débuté par une sensation de cuisson, de brûlure, de chatouillement de la verge, douleur d'abord légère, mais qui ne tarde pas à s'exaspérer … Mais au bout de peu d'heures, la scène change de face, et les événements se précipitent avec une effrayante rapidité. Tout d'abord, la verge,

devenue assez douloureuse se tuméfie dans son ensemble, elle devient oedémateuse et sa coloration change: elle se transforme en une sorte de gros boudin rose, puis rouge, puis livide ...

Remarkably, when the gangrenous tissue had sloughed off, the testes were spared. All five patients survived. Fournier attributed the disease he described to infection and reported that cultures were set up from his cases but no results for these are given. It is also of interest that despite such detailed clinical description of the cases, there is no mention of the smell of the gangrenous tissues; this has been a feature of later reports of the condition, even when no bacteriology was undertaken.

Fournier's original papers were followed by reports of genital gangrene mostly in the French and German literature, and the gangrene was variously attributed to many organisms including anaerobes. In 1920, nearly 40 years after Fournier's work was published, the American urologist Randall [37] reported 16 cases of 'idiopathic gangrene of the scrotum'. In contrast to Fournier's cases, those described by Randall were 'past middle life' and five of them died. They too had been previously healthy. Although six had penoscrotal gangrene, in the other 10 cases the gangrenous process only involved the scrotum. Six cases had local genital lesions including phimosis, chancroidal infection and urethritis, that may have initiated the infection. He commented on the 'repulsive fetid odor' of the tissue and predicted that anaerobes were responsible for the infection, although bateriological studies were 'unproductive'. He described the progression of the infection thus:

> About 3 days from the time that the line of demarcation shows the limits of the gangrenous process, a massive, stinking, slough separates. Where the scrotum is involved the skin, subcutaneous tissues, fascia, and all the structures of its wall, come away in a stringy, fetid mass. The testes, bared to their tunica vaginales, hang suspended by their cords, shamefully exposed, though remarkably free of gangrene, inured and oblivious to their new surroundings (or possibly I should say lack of surroundings) and can be handled freely without causing the slightest discomfort.

Randall observed that once the gangrenous scrotal tissue had sloughed off and the wound was clean, a new scrotum regenerated. Ten years later in 1930, Gibson, another American urologist, [38] reviewed over 200 reported cases (including Randall's 16 cases and one of his own) of what was now known as 'idiopathic gangrene of the scrotum'. Although most cases were aged 20–50 years, the range was 5 weeks to 80 years. The mortality rate was 27%, similar to that reported by Randall. In over half the patients the infection was penoscrotal, in a third it only involved the scrotum and in about a tenth it only involved the penis. A portal of entry, usually urogenital, was detected in 40% of cases. Gibson also commented on the smell ('nauseating gangrenous odor') and speculated that these infections were anaerobic.

Since these classic descriptions of 'idiopathic' peno-scrotal gangrene, cases continue to be reported, but as the condition is uncommon it is difficult for any single clinician to have extensive experience of it and surgeons other than urologists tend to be involved in the management of these patients. Although the disease still tends to be referred to as Fournier's gangrene, it is now known to be a necrotizing fasciitis of soft tissues involving subcutaneous fat and superficial fascia with thrombosis of the small subcutaneous arteries. Some authors also describe myonecrosis in addition. Although the earlier descriptions of the disease were all in men, it is clear that necrotizing fasciitis can involve not only the female genitalia, but sites other than the genitalia in both sexes. While eponymous descriptions should not be readily be abandoned, particularly when they have existed for over a century, Fournier's gangrene is clearly only one manifestation of necrotizing fasciitis and this latter term is really preferred and indeed has already been adopted by several authors.

For many years little attempt was made to define the bacterial cause of these devastating infections as such investigations are technically demanding. It is now clear that they are caused by a combination of anaerobic and aerobic bacteria, usually colonic or urogenital commensals; they are synergistic infections, but why what is initially a localized cryptoglandular or periurethral infection becomes a necrotizing destructive process remains a mystery. Although earlier series focused on the urogenital tract as the portal of entry for the infection, the source of these infections can be anorectal or cutaneous as well as genitourinary. Obviously the specialty of the reporting clinician will largely dictate the source of the infection in the cases in many series and case reports. A series of 57 male patients with necrotizing fasciitis of the genitalia was reported by urologists and colorectal surgeons in 1990 [39] and this probably gives a realistic assessment of the incidence of the different types of infection: in 26 cases there was a genitourinary source (urethral stricture with documented urinary extravasation, 18; recent traumatic urethral catheterization, 1; chronic indwelling urethral catheter, 1; chronic condom catheter, 2; preceding epididymo-orchitis 3; penile trauma, 1). In 19 cases the infection resulted from an anorectal source and 14 of these patients had anorectal abscesses, seven of which were ischiorectal. Twelve infections were preceded by cutaneous infections of the penile or scrotal skin and two patients had used the superficial penile vein to inject drugs.

A variety of anaerobes and aerobes have been isolated from these infections. The predominant anaerobe is

B. fragilis but many other species are usually present if the laboratory has the expertise and the time to identify them. Although *Clostridium perfringens* and other clostridia are sometimes isolated from these infections and they are characterized by the formation of gas in the affected tissues, the clostridia are never found as sole pathogens and the disease is quite different from clostridial gas gangrene. Coliforms, especially *E. coli* are the commonest aerobes but many other species are also isolated. It is clear now that in contrast to the previously healthy individuals in the original reports of Fournier's gangrene, necrotizing fasciitis, and particularly the more extensive infections, are more likely to occur in patients with diabetes and a history of alcohol abuse [39–41].

Whatever the source of the infection in necrotizing fasciitis, the mainstay of the successful treatment of the condition remains early recognition and aggressive surgical debridement. All non-viable tissue must be removed to arrest the progress of the infection. If this is done the patient should survive. Antibiotics are entirely secondary to adequate debridement and it is doubtful whether they contribute to the patient's recovery. They are nevertheless always given and a broad-spectrum combination including metronidazole is generally recommended. They should be stopped as soon as possible or the granulating tissue will become colonized with resistant bacteria and yeasts; these organisms seldom cause harm but their presence tends to worry clinicians. Hyperbaric oxygen is of no value and merely serves to delay essential surgery.

References

1 Berger RE. Acute epididymitis. In: Holmes KK, Mardh PA, Sparling PF *et al.* eds. *Sexually Transmitted Diseases*. New York: McGraw Hill, 1990:641–51.

2 Harnisch JP, Berger RE, Alexander ER *et al.* Aetiology of acute epididymitis. *Lancet* 1977;**1**:819–21.

3 Berger RE, Alexander ER, Harnisch JP *et al.* Etiology, manifestations and therapy of acute epididymitis: prospective study of 50 cases. *J Urol* 1979;**121**:750–4.

4 Melekos MD, Asbach HW. Epididymitis: aspects concerning etiology and treatment. *J Urol* 1987;**138**:83–6.

5 Fehler HG, Ballard RC, Dangor Y *et al.* Sexually acquired acute epididymitis. *S African J Epid Infect* 1989;**4**:23–4.

6 Hoosen AA, O'Farrell N, van den Ende J. Microbiology of acute epididymitis in a developing community. *Genitourin Med* 1993;**69**:361–3.

7 Hawkins DA, Taylor-Robinson D, Thomas BJ, Harris JRW. Microbiological survey of acute epididymitis. *Genitourin Med* 1986;**62**:342–4.

8 Mulcahy FM, Bignell CJ, Rajakumar R *et al.* Prevalence of chlamydial infection in acute epididymo-orchitis. *Genitourin Med* 1987;**63**:16–18.

9 Jalil N, Doble A, Gilchrist C, Taylor-Robinson D. Infection of the epididymis by *Ureaplasma urealyticum. Genitourin Med* 1988;**64**:367–8.

10 Barnes RC, Daifuku R, Roddy RE, Stamm WE. Urinary-tract infection in sexually active homosexual men. *Lancet* 1986;**1**: 171–3.

11 Drach GW. Sexuality and prostatitis: a hypothesis. *J Am Vener Dis* 1976;**3**:87.

12 Ross JC, Gow JG, St Hill CA. Tuberculous epididymitis: a review of 170 patients. *Br J Surg* 1961;**48**:663–6.

13 Mittemeyer BT, Lennox KW, Borski AA. Epididymitis: a review of 610 cases. *J Urol* 1966;**95**:390–2.

14 Christie AB. *Infectious Diseases: Epidemiology and Clinical Practice*, 4th edn. London: Churchill Livingstone, 1987: 1143–4.

15 Mousa ARM, Elhag KM, Khogali M, Marafie AA. The nature of human brucellosis in Kuwait: a study of 379 cases. *Rev Infect Dis* 1988;**10**:211–17.

16 McDonald JH, Heckel NJ. Acute pneumococcal epididymitis. *Illinois Med J* 1949;**95**:304–6.

17 Waldman LS, Kosloske AM, Parsons DW. Acute epididymo-orchitis as the presenting manifestation of *Haemophilus influenzae* septicaemia. *J Pediatr* 1977;**90**:87–9.

18 Thomas D, Simpson K, Ostojic H, Kaul A. Bacteremic epididymo-orchitis due to *Haemophilus influenzae* type B. *J Urol* 1981;**126**:832–3.

19 Laird SM. Meningococcal epididymitis. *Lancet* 1944;**i**:469–70.

20 Davis WH, Scardino P. Meningitis presenting as epididymitis. *South Med J* 1972;**65**:936.

21 Banks HS. Meningococcosis: a protean disease. *Lancet* 1948;**ii**: 677–81.

22 William DC, Felman YM, Corsaro MC. *Neisseria meningitidis*: probable pathogen in two related cases of urethritis, epididymitis and acute pelvic inflammatory disease. *J Am Med Assoc* 1979;**242**:1653–4.

23 Krieger JN. Epididymitis, orchitis and related conditions. *Sex Transm Dis* 1984;**11**:173–81.

24 Gasparich JP, Mason JT, Greene HL *et al.* Amiodarone-associated epididymitis in the absence of infection. *J Urol* 1985;**133**:971–2.

25 Holder LE, Martire JR, Holmes ER, Wagner HN. Testicular radionuclide angiography and static imaging: anatomy, scintigraphic interpretation, and clinical indications. *Radiology* 1977;**125**:739–52.

26 Abu-Sleiman R, Ho JE, Gregory JG. Scrotal scanning: present value and limits of interpretation. *Urology* 1979;**13**:326–30.

27 Arya OP, Hobson D, Hart CA *et al.* Evaluation of ciprofloxacin 500 mg twice daily for one week in treating uncomplicated gonococcal, chlamydial and non-specific urethritis in men. *Genitourin Med* 1986;**62**:170–4.

28 Fong IW, Linton W, Simbul M *et al.* Treatment of non-gonococcal urethritis with ciprofloxacin. *Am J Med* 1987;**82**(Suppl. 4A):311–16.

29 Beard CM, Benson RC, Kelalis PP *et al.* The incidence and outcome of mumps orchitis in Rochester, Minnesota, 1935 to 1974. *Mayo Clin Proc* 1977;**52**:3–7.

30 Craighead JE, Mohoney EH, Carver DH *et al.* Orchitis due to Coxsackie virus Group B type 5. *N Engl J Med* 1962;**267**: 498–500.

31 Eykyn SJ. Anaerobic infection in urological practice. In: Hendry WF, Kirby RS, eds. *Recent Advances in Urology/Andrology*. London: Churchill Livingstone, 1993:36–7.

32 Whitehead SM, Leach RD, Eykyn SJ *et al.* The aetiology of scrotal sepsis. *Br J Surg* 1982;**69**:729–30.

33 Leach RD, Eykyn SJ, Phillips I *et al.* Anaerobic subareolar breast abscess. *Lancet* 1979;**1**:35–7.

34 Leach RD, Eykyn SJ, Phillips I *et al.* Anaerobic axillary abscess. *Br Med J* 1979;**2**:5–7.

35 Fournier AJ, Gangrène foudroyante de la verge. *Sem Med* 1883;**3**:345–47.

36 Fournier AJ. Etude clinique de la gangrène foudroyante de la verge. *Sem Med* 1884;**4**:69–70.

37 Randall A. Idiopathic gangrene of the scrotum. *J Urol* 1920;**4**: 219–35.

38 Gibson TE. Idiopathic gangrene of the scrotum. With report of case and review of the literature. *J Urol* 1930;**23**:125–53.

39 Clayton MD, Fowler JE, Sharifi R, Pearl RK. Causes, presentation and survival of fifty-seven patients with necrotizing fasciitis of the male genitalia. *Surg Gynecol Obstet* 1990; **170**:49–55.

40 Spirnak JP, Resnick MI, Hampel N, Persky L. Fournier's gangrene: report of 20 patients. *J Urol* 1984;**131**:290–1.

41 Enriquez JM, Moreno S, Devesa M *et al.* Fournier's syndrome of urogenital and anorectal origin. A retrospective comparative study. *Dis Colon Rect* 1987;**30**:33–7.

53 Sexually Transmitted Diseases

R.N.Thin

Introduction

Worldwide most sexually transmitted diseases (STDs) are increasing, including genital herpes simplex virus infection, genital warts, human immunodeficiency virus (HIV) infection, chlamydial and non-gonococcal infection and trichomoniasis. Gonorrhoea is common, but syphilis is rare in some countries. Genital ulceration is frequent in tropical countries where it may be chronic and called genital ulcer disease. Genital ulcer disease, gonorrhoea, chlamydial infection and trichomoniasis may enhance transmission of HIV infection [1,2].

Clinical examination

Patients who suspect an STD are anxious; staff should be friendly, reassuring, sympathetic and explain that treatment is confidential. Clinical examination follows the usual pattern of history, physical examination and investigation.

The history covers genital symptoms including in both sexes genital ulceration, rash, itch, pain, swelling and urinary symptoms specially burning on micturition. Men should be asked about urethral discharge and women about vaginal discharge. General health is covered including menstruation and recent treatment, especially antimicrobials and antivirals. The sexual history is important and should include the number of sexual partners, dates, casual or regular relationship, partners' symptoms and form of contact—genital to genital, anogenital and orogenital. Contraception is important, especially condom use including contact without condoms. Drug and other hypersensitivities must be noted. Past and family history should include treatment for STD and obstetric history.

The genitals must be examined; in females this includes passing a bivalve speculum with the patient in the lithotomy position which gives the best view of the internal genitalia. The history will indicate other systems requiring examination; ideally all patients should have a complete physical examination.

Several infections may be present at the same time, so if possible patients should have all the investigations in Table 53.1 at their first visit.

Epidemiology and control

Spread

Fundamental to the spread of STD is the acquisition of infection from one partner and transmission to another. Partner change depends on the numbers available; this increases with migration from rural to urban areas and travel. Social factors influencing spread include affluence, alcohol consumption, leisure time, personal freedom, prostitution and ignorance. Other factors include asymptomatic infection—more common in women than in men—antimicrobial resistance and contraception. Unlike condoms and to a lesser extent the cap, oral contraceptives and the intrauterine device provide no barrier to transmission. All socioeconomic groups acquire STDs. People at special risk include those aged 16–24 years, those who travel, including members of the armed forces and merchant seamen, entertainers and prostitutes. The probability of sexual activity and the possibility of partner change should be remembered among patients in these groups.

Control

Control of STD requires rapid accurate diagnosis, effective treatment, partner notification (the identification and treatment of partners), education and clinical and laboratory screening. The aim in specialist clinics is to screen all patients for all the common STDs, and ideally all the relevant investigations in Table 53.1 should be undertaken. Sexual health and STD education should be part of general health education and reinforced when patients are at risk. Screening and management are important control measures and should be undertaken in urology departments if there are no nearby specialist facilities.

Table 53.1 Investigations for different groups of patients with STD.

Patient group	Site	Investigations
Males	Urethra	Swab for Gram stain and culture for gonococci Sample for microscopy and culture for trichomonads Sample for *Chlamydia* detection
Females	Vagina	Swab for Gram stain and culture for *Candida* Sample for microscopy of wet film and culture for trichomonads Microscopy of both samples to include search for evidence of anaerobic/bacterial vaginosis
	Cervical os	Swab for Gram stain and culture for gonococci Swab for *Chlamydia* detection Smear for cytological examination
	Urethra	Meatal swab for Gram stain and culture for gonococci
All patients		Blood for serological tests for syphilis (Offer HIV antibody tests after counselling according to local policy) Urinalysis according to local policy

Males and females
    when indicated
	Genital ulcers	Scraping for herpes simplex virus identification
		Scraping for dark ground microscopy for treponemas
		Swab for bacterial culture if secondarily infected
		Microscopy of scraping for *Haemophilus ducreyi* and *Calymobacterium granulomatis*
		    when indicated

Contacts of gonorrhoea	Rectum Throat	Swab for Gram stain and culture for gonococci Swab for gonococci
Drug misusers Homosexual and bisexual men	Blood Blood Rectum Throat	Sample for hepatitis B and C markers and HIV antibodies (after counselling) Sample for hepatitis B markers and HIV antibodies (after counselling) Swabs for Gram stain and culture for gonococci Swab or culture for gonococci

HIV, human immunodeficiency virus.

Bacterial sexually transmitted disease

Syphilis

Syphilis is due to *Treponema pallidum* and is chronic, infectious and systemic from the beginning; florid features may alternate with long periods of latency. Syphilis responds to penicillin—the drug of choice—tetracyclines and erythromycin. It may be transmitted to the fetus. Table 53.2 summarizes the classification of syphilis. Some classifications include cardiovascular and neurosyphilis in the tertiary stage, but there are advantages in separating the benign from the serious forms. The division between early and late syphilis is 2 years after infection.

Acquired syphilis

Early stage

Primary syphilis. The primary lesion or chancre develops at the site of infection, usually on the genitals, after an incubation period which is commonly 14–28 days with extremes of 9–90 days. A small pink macule appears,

Table 53.2 Classification of syphilis.

Acquired syphilis	Congenital syphilis
Early	*Early*
Primary	Clinical and latent
Secondary	
Latent	*Late*
	Clinical and latent
Late	Stigmas (or scars)
Latent	
Tertiary (benign gummatous)	
Quarternary	
Cardiovascular	
Neurosyphilis	

becomes papular and ulcerates. A typical ulcer has a well-defined margin, an indurated base and is less tender than genital ulcers due to other causes. When traumatized it produces less blood and more serum than other types of ulcers. The regional lymph nodes may be moderately enlarged, mobile, discrete, rubbery, painless and non-tender. The diagnosis is established by identifying *T. pallidum* on dark ground microscopy (available in specialist clinics) of exudate from the chancre.

Antimicrobial treatment is summarized in Table 53.3. After treatment patients must be followed up carefully with clinical examination and serological tests (see below) to ensure that a cure has been achieved.

Primary syphilis must be considered in the differential diagnosis of genital ulceration with includes herpes simplex virus infection, erosive balanitis, trauma with secondary infection and, less commonly, secondary syphilis, scabies, Reiter's disease, Stevens–Johnson syndrome and Behçet's syndrome.

Secondary syphilis. Six to 8 weeks after the chancre appears, secondary syphilis starts with mild fever, malaise and headache. The common features are a rash in 75% of cases, lymphadenopathy, often generalized, in 50% and mucosal ulceration in 30%; less common features found in 10% or less of cases include bone and visceral disease and central nervous system and eye involvement. The rash starts with faint macules on the trunk and proximal limbs; it becomes generalized, papular, is dull red, polymorphic and symmetrical, it does not itch and turns scaly. Characteristically, the palms and soles are affected. In warm moist areas such as the anus, scrotum and labia majora, the rash is modified to form large flat papules called condylomata lata. Enlarged lymph nodes have the same characteristics as in primary syphilis. Mucosal ulcers affect the genitals, mouth, pharynx and larynx. Early lesions are superficial and may be difficult to see; later they develop a white base, a red margin and coalesce to form 'snail track ulcers'.

The diagnosis is made from the clinical features supported by identifying *T. pallidum* by dark ground examination of fluid expressed from the papules or mucosal ulcers, or by positive results to serological tests (see below).

Antimicrobial treatment is as outlined in Table 53.3. After treatment patients must be followed up carefully clinically, with repeated serological tests to ensure cure. Secondary syphilis must be differentiated from various conditions. For example the macular rash must be identified from drug eruptions, rubella and pityriasis rosea, the papular rash from drug eruptions, scabies and acne vulgaris, and condylomata lata from viral warts. Genital ulcers must be differentiated from herpes simplex, erosive balanitis and primary syphilis, while the lymphadenopathy must not be confused with mononucleosis and lymphoma.

Without treatment resolution occurs after several months and the disease enters the latent phase. Two years after infection the disease passes into the late stage.

Late stage

Latency may persist for many years and can only be detected by means of serological tests (see below). Many cases are found in the latent stage following serological screening. The serological tests for syphilis include:
1 Non-specific or lipoidal antigen tests:
  (a) the Venereal Disease Research Laboratory (VDRL) test;
  (b) the rapid plasma reagin (RPR) test.
2 Specific treponemal antigen tests:
  (a) *T. pallidum* haemagglutination assay (TPHA);
  (b) fluorescent treponemal antibody-absorbed (FTA-abs) test;
  (c) treponemal enzyme assay (enzyme-linked immunosorbent assay, ELISA).

These tests are positive from the fourth week of acquired syphilis and at birth in congenital syphilis. False-positive results occur occasionally in the VDRL and RPR tests with other infections and connective tissue diseases, so positive results to these tests results must be confirmed with specific tests. When syphilis is suspected lipoidal antigen and specific tests are used together.

Table 53.3 Management of acquired syphilis.

Stage	Drug*	Treatment regimen
Primary	Procaine penicillin	600–1200 mg i.m. once daily for 12 days
	Oxytetracycline	500 mg orally four times daily for 15 days
	Doxycycline	100 mg orally three times daily for 15 days
Secondary, tertiary and latent	Procaine penicillin	600–1200 mg i.m. once daily for 15 days
	Oxytetracycline	500 mg orally four times daily for 15 days
	Doxycycline	100 mg orally three times daily for 15 days
Quarternary cardiovascular neurosyphilis	Procaine penicillin	900–1200 mg i.m. once daily for 21 days
	Oxytetracycline	500 mg orally four times daily for 28 days
	Doxycycline	100 mg orally three times daily for 28 days

*Procaine penicillin is the treatment of choice when possible. Tetracyclines are for patients who are hypersensitive to penicillin, except for pregnant women who should have erythromycin stearate in the same dose. Erythromycin crosses the placenta poorly so after this treatment for the mother, the baby should be carefully monitored. All patients must be followed up to ensure satisfactory response; partner notification is important.

Tertiary stage. This stage is rare and takes at least 10 years to develop. It affects the skin, mucosa and bones. The characteristic feature is a granuloma called a gumma which occasionally affects the genitalia, causing a flat granuloma or an ulcer.

Quaternary stage. Cardiovascular syphilis and neuro-syphilis take longer to develop and may progress to death. When these conditions are suspected the patient should be referred to a specialist.

Congenital syphilis

Congenital syphilis is rare where antenatal serological screening is practised. Treatment during pregnancy usually produces a healthy baby. Again, when congenital syphilis is suspected the mother and baby should be referred to a specialist.

Gonorrhoea

Gonorrhoea is due to the Gram-negative diplococcus *Neisseria gonorrhoeae* which infects the columnar epithelium in the lower genital tract, rectum, pharynx and eyes. Anterior urethritis in men is the most common form of gonorrhoea seen in surgical practice and has an incubation period of 2–10 days. There is burning on micturition and a purulent discharge, but symptoms are absent in 5–10% of cases.

In women the lower cervical canal is infected in 80% of cases with the urethra and rectum involved in 50%. There may be vaginal discharge and dysuria, but many women with uncomplicated infection are symptom free.

Homosexual men may have asymptomatic rectal infection. Symptomless pharyngeal gonorrhoea occasionally affects males and females.

Investigations

Diagnosis depends on the investigations being undertaken. Whenever possible, swabs of infected secretions should be sent to a laboratory with experience of culturing gonococci. Gram-negative intracellular diplococci may be seen on microscopy of infected secretions but must be confirmed by culture (see Table 53.1).

Course

Symptoms gradually resolve without treatment but it is not known how long the patient remains infectious. Delay in treatment can lead to complications which include:

1 Epididymo-orchitis—pain and tender swelling (see pp. 688 and 689).

2 Salpingitis and pelvic infection—pain and vaginal tenderness.
3 Perihepatitis—rare, right hypochondral pain and tenderness.
4 Bacteraemia—rare, fever, joint pains and sparse peripheral pustular rash.
5 Acute gonococcal arthritis and septicaemia—rare in developed countries.
6 Acute purulent conjunctivitis (ophthalmia neonatorum) in infants born to infected mothers—rare in developed countries.

Management

Uncomplicated gonorrhoea responds to a single adequate dose of a suitable antimicrobial. In the UK infections are usually sensitive to penicillin. Up to 50% of infections elsewhere, such as in the Far East and West Africa, are totally resistant to penicillin. Occasional strains of *N. gonorrhoeae* isolated in Europe and more in the Far East have diminished sensitivity to ciprofloxacin.

Antimicrobial regimens for uncomplicated infection are shown in Table 53.4. Complications such as epididymitis require a course of antimicrobials such as ampicillin 500 mg four times daily or ciprofloxacin 500 mg twice daily for 10 days. Partners should be notified quickly.

Uncomplicated gonorrhoea must be differentiated from various conditions. Gonococcal urethritis in men must be identified from non-gonococcal urethritis (NGU) and, less often, from bacteruria. In females gonorrhoea must be differentiated from bacteruria, trichomoniasis, candidiasis and bacterial vaginosis. In males and females gonorrhoea may need to be considered as a cause of proctitis and pharyngitis.

Non-gonococcal infection; including non-gonococcal urethritis in men

NGU resembles gonococcal urethritis and in many countries, including the UK, NGU is the more common. The incubation period varies from a few days to a few weeks and the symptoms are milder. Approximately 50% of cases are due to *Chlamydia trachomatis* (serotypes D–K), a few cases may be due to *Ureaplasma urealyticum*, *Trichomonas vaginalis*, herpes simplex virus, bacteruria or trauma, but in the remainder the cause is obscure. Features include urethral discharge which may be mucoid or mucopurulent and dysuria, but they may be mild or absent.

Investigations

When possible a swab should be sent to the laboratory. Urethritis is confirmed by finding polymorphonuclear leucocytes in a Gram stain of urethral secretions;

Table 53.4 Treatment of uncomplicated gonorrhoea.

Drug	Route	Treatment regimen
Penicillin sensitive		
Ampicillin plus probenicid	Oral	2–3.5 g ampicillin plus 1 g probenicid together as a single dose
Co-trimoxazole	Oral	8 × 480 mg tabs as a single dose
Dispersible tabs	Oral	4 × 480 mg tabs 12-hourly in three doses
Penicillin resistant		
Ciprofloxacin	Oral	250–500 mg as a single dose
Cefotaxime	i.m.	0.5–1.0 g as a single dose
Spectinomycin	i.m.	2–4 g as a single dose
Pharyngeal gonorrhoea		
Co-trimoxazole dispersible tabs	Oral	5 × 480 mg tabs 12-hourly for three doses
Ciprofloxacin	Oral	500 mg as a single dose

Repeat positive cultures to ensure a satisfactory response; notify partners promptly

gonorrhoea is excluded by the absence of organisms on Gram stain and culture. An additional urethral swab or first catch urine sample [3] should be taken to identify *Chlamydia*. A wet preparation in saline will show *T. vaginalis*. A simple additional investigation is the two glass urine test. In the presence of anterior urethritis, macroscopic examination of a first catch urine sample shows specks or threads while a midstream urine sample is clear.

Management

Antimicrobial treatment of *Chlamydia*-positive or -negative NGU is summarized in Table 53.5. The tetracyclines and erythromycin should be given for at least 7 days and often for 14 days. Positive response to a single course of therapy is 80%. Non-response should be retreated with an alternative regimen. Epididymo-orchitis should be treated with oxytetracycline or erythromycin 500 mg 6-hourly for 14 days or doxycycline 100 mg 12-hourly for 14 days. Whether or not a causative agent is identified, partner notification is important as untreated female partners may develop pelvic inflammatory disease.

Course

Untreated NGU runs a prolonged low grade course and

Table 53.5 Treatment of non-gonococcal infection. Tetracyclines and erythromycin are given for 7 – 14 days.

Drug	Treatment regimen
Oxytetracycline	250 mg 6-hourly *or* 500 mg 12-hourly
Doxycycline	100 mg 12-hourly
Erythromycin	250 mg 6-hourly *or* 500 mg 12-hourly
Azithromycin	1 g as a single dose

may be complicated by epididymo-orchitis. In the UK and some other countries, epididymo-orchitis is more common with NGU than with gonorrhoea. NGU also occurs in Reiter's disease.

Non-gonococcal infection in women

This is due to *C. trachomatis* in 50% of cases and no other cause has been identified. *C. trachomatis* infects the lower cervical canal and rarely the urethra.

Clinical features

Uncomplicated lower genital tract *Chlamydia*-positive or -negative infection causes no symptoms or signs. Untreated *Chlamydia*-positive or -negative cases progress to pelvic inflammatory disease which may recur, become chronic and lead to tubal pregnancy or infertility. A rare complication is perihepatitis. A woman with cervical infection may infect her baby's eyes at birth.

Investigations

These should be carried out as in Table 53.1; many women have additional infections so all patients require full investigation.

Management

The antimicrobial treatment of uncomplicated and complicated *Chlamydia*-positive and -negative infection is the same as for men, (see Table 53.5).

Lymphogranuloma venereum

Lymphogranuloma venereum is due to *C. trachomatis* (serotypes LI–III); it is mainly a tropical condition but is found worldwide. The incubation period is 1–5 weeks to the appearance of the genital lesion, a small papule which may ulcerate but is often not recognized or may not appear. There is marked inguinal node enlargement taking a maximum of 3 months to develop; nodes are unilateral, matted, adherent, suppurative and multilocular. There may be mild erythema of the overlying skin, and systemic features including malaise, fever, variable rash, generalized lymphadenopathy and hepatosplenomegaly. The diagnosis can be strongly suspected from the clinical features, supported by culture or antigen identification and raised titres of circulating microimmunofluorescent antibodies. The treatment is with oxytetracycline or erythromycin 500 mg given four times daily for a minimum of 2 weeks or doxycycline 100 mg twice daily for the same period. Suppurating nodes should be aspirated not incised. Energetic treatment of this early stage is important to avoid chronic sinuses which may occur later and and cause grave surgical problems with fistulas.

Chancroid or soft sores

Chancroid is a common cause of genital ulceratiaon in the tropics. It is due to the small Gram-negative bacillus *Haemophilus ducreyi*. There is an incubation period of 1–8 days. The genital lesions comprise multiple, small, irregular, painful, tender ulcers. There is tender unilateral matted inguinal lymph node enlargement; nodes suppurate but tend to be unilocular. Diagnosis can be suspected from the clinical appearance supported by microscopy and culture (on freshly prepared special medium) of scrapings from the margin of ulcers. Treatment is with erythromycin 500 mg four times daily for 7 days or co-trimoxazole 2 × 480 mg tablets twice daily for 7 days. Suppurating nodes should be aspirated not incised. Chancroid should be differentiated from other causes of genital ulceration, especially herpes simplex infection and primary syphilis.

Granuloma inguinale or donovanosis

This is found in the tropics among people with pigmented skin. It is due to the coccobacillus *Calymobacterium granulomatis*. This can be identified in Wright- or Giemsa-stained scrapings from the margin of lesions as pleomorphic organisms within mononuclear cells, classically showing a bipolar appearance. There is an incubation period from a few days to 3 months. Small or spreading genital granulomas appear with a pink to red velvety appearance. As lesions spread peripherally they may heal centrally. Granulomas may also develop in the inguinal regions where they resemble enlarged lymph nodes. True lymphadenopathy only develops when there is secondary bacterial infection. Diagnosis is suspected from the appearance, supported by identifying the organism in scrapings as above. Treatment is with oxytetracycline or erythromycin 500 mg four times daily for 14–21 days. Differentiation is from other causes of genital ulceration especially primary syphillis. Chronic genital ulceration or genital ulcer disease may be due to mixed infection with *H. ducreyi* and *C. granulomatis* and usually responds to erythromycin 500 mg four times daily for 2 weeks.

Viral sexually transmitted diseases

Viral diseases are more serious than bacterial diseases, because viruses cannot be eradicated so infection is for life, and serious complications may occur.

Anogenital herpes simplex

This is due to herpes simplex virus spread by sexual contact.

Course

There is a severe first episode followed by milder recurrences which resemble labial herpes simplex (cold sores).

First episode

This starts with malaise, fever and local irritation followed by widespread, painful, tender vesicles affecting the genitals and rarely the anorectum. The vesicles rupture leaving painful tender erosions followed by further crops of lesions. Regional lymph nodes enlarge, men may have a urethral discharge and dysuria, and women may have a vaginal discharge. There may be root pains in the second and third sacral dermatomes and rarely retention of urine. First episodes heal in 2–3 weeks and are often followed by recurrence.

Recurrence

Recurrences resemble first episodes but there is one cluster of lesions covering an area of about 1 cm^2 which heals in 7–10 days.

Investigations

The virus can be identified in vesicular fluid or scrapings from fresh erosions.

Management

Lesions always heal and local saline bathing may be all that is necessary. Aciclovir 200 mg five times daily for 5 days by mouth, inhibits viral replication so if given early shortens the first episode Aciclovir is not prescribed for mild or infrequent recurrences. A few patients suffer frequent recurrence which may be suppressed by continuous oral aciclovir 400 mg twice daily.

Few other conditions cause vesicles on the genitals. Erosions should be identified from primary syphilis, chancroid and the other conditions mentioned under the differential diagnosis of primary syphilis.

Genital warts

Warts are due to human papilloma virus and are common on the genitals and anus. Human papilloma virus may be one factor predisposing to carcinoma, especially of the cervix. It is unclear if the virus influences subsequent penile carcinoma. Exophytic warts can be recognized from their appearance but flat warts are more difficult to diagnose. Atypical and persistent lesions should be biopsied.

Treatment is with 10–25% podophyllin applied weekly, or 0.5% podophyllotoxin applied twice daily for 3 consecutive days in a week for a maximum of 5 weeks. Alternative methods are destruction by cryotherapy, electrocautery or laser. Warts tend to recur so patients should be carefully followed up to ensure cure. Meatal warts in men may extend into the fossa navicularis causing treatment problems for non-urologists. The use of an auroscope to examine the distal urethra allows more rational treatment [4]. Partners must be notified.

Molluscum contagiosum

Molluscum contagiosum virus produces little shiny pink papules with a central depression which differentiates them from warts. Treatment is with cryotherapy or electrocautery.

Hepatitis

Hepatitis B is transmitted between homosexual men, and less often between heterosexuals. The infection is usually subclinical but occasionally progresses to cirrhosis. Hepatitis A and C are rarely sexually transmitted. Vaccines are available against hepatitis A and B.

Miscellaneous conditions

Balanitis and balanoposthitis

Balanitis is inflammation of the glans penis; balanoposthitis involves the glans and undersurface of the prepuce. These conditions are common in men with a long tight prepuce whose hygiene is poor. Causal agents include *Candida* species, *T. vaginalis*, some streptococci and

anaerobes; but sometimes no cause is identified. Immune deficiency conditions, diabetes mellitus, broad-spectrum antimicrobials, corticosteroids and antimitotic drugs predispose to candidiasis.

There is general or patchy erythema with erosions when severe and a white or purulent exudate. Circinate balanitis occurs in Reiter disease with erosions which coalesce. Balanitis xerotica obliterans is the genital manifestation of the skin condition lichen sclerosis et atrophicus; initial patchy erythema progresses to atrophy with a white appearance, meatal stenosis and phimosis. Diagnosis is from the clinical appearance. Swabs are taken to identify *Candida* and bacteria.

Management

Local saline bathing is always advised and is sufficient in mild to moderate cases and when no cause is found. Candidiasis should be treated with twice daily applications of 1% clotrimazole cream. If anaerobic bacteria are isolated and saline bathing is insufficient then metronidazole 200 mg three times daily for 7 days should be prescribed. Streptococcal infection should respond to amoxycillin 250 mg three times daily for 5 days. Saline may suffice for circinate balanitis and balantitis xerotica obliterans but hydrocortisone cream 1% is recommended in severe cases; these patients should be followed up so meatal stenosis may be recognized early. Erosive lesions should be identified from other ulcerative conditions especially herpes simplex. Partner notification is indicated in trichomoniasis and recurrent candidiasis.

Vulvovaginal conditions

Vaginal discharge is a frequent complaint. A common cause is bacterial vaginosis due to *Gardenerella vaginalis* and anaerobic bacteria. This produces an odorous off-white discharge but no inflammation. Accurate diagnosis needs microscopic examination of the discharge, and treatment is with metronidazole 200 mg three times daily for 7 days. The second most common cause of discharge is vaginal candidiasis characterized by a white discharge and itch. Diagnosis is by clinical features and microscopic examination and culture of *Candida* species. Treatment is with one clotrimazole 500 mg pessary at night for one night plus clotrimazole cream twice daily to the vulva, or in resistant cases fluconazole 150 mg in one dose by mouth. A less common cause of vaginal discharge is trichomoniasis, often found in association with gonorrhoea. Trichomoniasis causes a yellow-white discharge, irritation and erythema. Diagnosis is by microscopic, cultural or cytological recognition of the flagellate parasite *T. vaginalis*. Treatment is with metronidazole 200 mg three times daily for 7 days. In post-menopausal women, senile vaginitis may cause irritation and discharge even in association with hormonal replacement therapy. Treatment is with dienoestrol cream. All the organisms may occur without symptoms but treatment is indicated as symptomatic disease may develop. Partner notification is required in trichomoniasis and recurrent candidiasis. The possibility of other STDs being present with vaginal conditions should always be remembered.

Parasitic conditions

Scabies and pediculosis can be sexually transmitted and this must be considered in their management.

References

1 Cameron DW, Simonsen JN, D'Costa LJ *et al*. Female to male transmission of human immunodeficiency virus type 1: risk factors for seroconversion in men. *Lancet* 1989;**2**: 403–7.
2 Laga M, Manoka A, Kivuvu M *et al*. Non-ulcerative sexually transmitted diseases as risk factors for HIV 1 transmission in women: results from a cohort study. *AIDS* 1993;**7**:95–102.
3 Taylor Robinson D. Laboratory methods for chlamydial infection. *J Infect* 1992;**25**(Suppl. 1):61–7.
4 Thin RN. Meatoscopy; an important technique for assessing meatal warts in men. *Int J STD AIDS* 1994;**5**:18–20.

54 Opportunist (Nosocomial) Urinary Tract Infections

A. Simpson and S. Tabaqchali

Introduction

Although almost any infection involves a degree of opportunism on the part of the infecting organism, the term opportunist infection is usually applied to those infections where there is a major defect or breach of host defences, such that organisms of normally low virulence may cause infection. There are a number of differences in predisposing factors and the spectrum of organisms involved compared to uncomplicated infections. As a result, different management is required.

Predisposing factors

Endogenous factors (defects in host defences)

A patient's age or general debility due to other pathology will predispose them to many infections, including urinary tract infection (UTI). However, some specific factors are of importance and will be discussed further.

Length of urethra

Urine is normally sterile. UTIs are usually caused by bacteria reaching the bladder by ascending the urethra (which itself is normally colonized with bacteria), although haematogenous spread can occur. The length of the structurally intact urethra is therefore important and there is a higher incidence of UTI in females. Bypassing this defence mechanism by a urinary diversion procedure such as ileal conduit or through a congenital abnormality such as hypospadia, may predispose to infection.

Urinary flow

Bacteriuria is not an automatic result of bacteria entering the bladder, as they must both persist and multiply. The flow of urine through the bladder both dilutes the organism count, and allows for flushing of the bladder (and spontaneous clearance of bacteria) on voiding [1]. Defects in this flushing action are very important with regard to opportunistic infection. These defects include both anatomical abnormalities (congenital such as a urethral valve, or acquired such as prostatic hypertrophy) and neurological defects such as occur with myelomeningocele, multiple sclerosis or traumatic paraplegia. Any factor which leads to urinary stasis predisposes to infection. In addition to the above factors, urinary flow may be obstructed by a variety of mechanisms, such as calculi, urethral stricture, extrinsic ureteric obstruction or polycystic kidneys [2]. Calculi may in addition provide a continuing nidus of infection. Ureteric reflux also predisposes to infection, probably by maintaining a residual pool of urine after voiding.

Local defences

Several local factors help to prevent infection [3]. Urine appears to have some antibacterial activity itself, probably related to low pH and high urea concentrations [4]. This effect may be inhibited, for instance by raised glucose concentrations in diabetes mellitus. This antibacterial activity is of limited effect and, generally speaking, urine provides a good culture medium for bacteria, which is why urinary stasis is an important predisposing factor [5]. Prostatic secretions may also have a protective effect [6]. The bladder mucosa has some intrinsic resistance to bacterial adherence, which may be an important prerequisite for establishment of infection [7]. This can be overcome—uropathogenic bacteria show an increased ability to bind to the bladder epithelium (see below). The significance of local defences is difficult to assess, but defects in these mechanisms alone are probably not sufficient to produce opportunistic infections.

Host immunity

The onset of infection results in other defence mechanisms coming into play, particularly involving leucocytes to phagocytose and destroy bacteria [8]. The role of serum or local antibody remains unclear [9]. There is little evidence of increased incidence of UTI associated with defects of humoral immunity.

Exogenous factors (bypass of host defences)

Bacteria can be introduced directly into the urinary tract (thus avoiding the host defence mechanisms) in a variety of ways. The most important of these is urethral catheterization [10] or instrumentation, but other procedures include prostatectomy, suprapubic catheterization or nephrostomy.

Causative organisms

There is a very significant difference in the spectrum of organisms causing uncomplicated UTIs compared with those found in opportunist infections.

Bacteria

Bacteria are the commonest organisms causing UTI. In uncomplicated UTI, *Escherichia coli* is the most common organism isolated, but is less prominent in opportunist infection, especially in hospitals [11] (Table 54.1). Organisms such as *Klebsiella*, *Pseudomonas*, enterococci and staphylococci are more prominent. A very wide range of bacteria can occasionally cause opportunistic UTI. Tuberculosis, although relatively rare in the UK, is a very common cause of renal infection worldwide.

Fungi

Candida species are often isolated from urine specimens, but in non-catheterized patients this often represents specimen contamination, especially in patients with thrush (usually female). True candiduria, usually due to *C. albicans*, is uncommon; it is more common in hospital patients [12]. Predisposing factors include urinary catheterization, diabetes mellitus and antibiotic therapy. Renal infection is usually a result of haematogenous spread (fungaemia) in disseminated candidiasis rather than ascending infection.

Viruses

Most viral infections of the urinary tract arise via haematogenous spread, such as cytomegalovirus. This latter virus may be a problem in immunosuppressed patients, who are at risk of both primary infection or reactivation from previous infection prior to the period of immunosuppression.

Parasites

Several parasites can cause genitourinary tract infection. The most well known of these is *Schistosoma haematobium* (bilharzia). Parasitic infection is covered in Chapters 48 and 49.

Factors determining the infecting organisms

In acute uncomplicated UTIs, the spectrum of organisms is determined by their virulence, that is, their relative ability to cause disease (or their degree of pathogenicity). These organisms need to overcome normal host defences, as discussed above. The most important virulence factor may be fimbrial structures responsible for adhesion to uroepithelial cells. Even amongst *E. coli*, there is a wide variation in capacity to cause infection, which appears to relate to their capacity to bind to the uroepithelium [13]. If host defences are bypassed or impaired, other relatively avirulent organisms may cause infection.

Most UTIs arise from the patient's own flora, but, particularly in hospitals, may originate from the environment or from other patients or staff via cross-infection. In the latter case, organisms such as *Klebsiella* appear more prominent than *E. coli*. With environmental sources, *Pseudomonas aeruginosa* or other *Pseudomonas* species are often implicated. These organisms are widespread in the environment, but are often resistant to commonly used antibiotics. This favours their survival over other organisms if a patient is receiving antibiotic therapy. It is perhaps surprising how relatively avirulent *P. aeruginosa* appears, considering the comprehensive array of virulence factors it possesses, although it can occasionally cause devastating opportunistic infection, usually outside the urinary tract.

The nature of any compromise of host defences affects to some extent the type of infecting organism. Bacteria vary in their capacity to bind to urethral catheters, but those found in nosocomial UTI cases adhere strongly to many types of catheter tubing [14].

Table 54.1 Comparison of organisms isolated in urinary tract infections (UTIs) in hopital and general practice. Modified from [11].

Organism	Organisms causing UTI (%)	
	General practice	Hospital
Escherichia coli	7.25	48.3
Proteus mirabilis	5.0	5.7
Klebsiella and *Enterobacter* spp.	5.5	9.2
Enterococci	4.7	13.0
Staphylococci	3.4	7.4
Pseudomonas aeruginosa	–	7.3
Others	8.9	9.1

Antibiotic resistance

Prior antibiotic therapy will influence the organisms which make up the patient's resident flora. Thus organisms which are relatively resistant to antibiotics, such as *P. aeruginosa*, enterococci or yeasts, are important in opportunistic infection. They are likely to become an increasingly difficult problem. Hospital-acquired organisms are often resistant to one or more classes of antibiotic (Table 54.2). The avoidance of unnecessary antibiotic use is of great importance in reducing the level of infection with these resistant organisms, both at the individual patient level and, perhaps more importantly, in a hospital as a whole, by keeping the selective pressure which gives them a survival advantage to a minimum.

Mixed infections

Another feature of the microbiology of opportunist UTIs is that mixed infection is more common, in contrast with its rarity in uncomplicated infections. In patients with grossly abnormal urinary tracts, it is often possible to show that even when there appears to be only one infecting organism, others are present in small numbers.

Clinical significance

Acute infections

Opportunistic infection may be associated with symptoms identical to those found in uncomplicated UTI. Bacteriuria in this context is associated with little or no morbidity. The major concern, acutely, is of complications such as pyelonephritis, epididymitis or septicaemia. In hospital,

Table 54.2 The sensitivity patterns of organisms isolated from UTIs in hospital and general practice patients. Modified from [11].

	Strains fully sensitive to antibiotics (%)	
	General practice	Hospital
Antibiotic	(n = 2129)	(n = 8763)
Ampicillin	61.9	51.3
Cephaloridine	86.3	64.6
Ciprofloxacin	94.7	86.6
Co-trimoxazole	83.7	72.2
Nitrofurantoin	87.8	76.7
Sulphonamide	66.8	52.7
Tetracycline	66.1	55.6
Trimethoprim	82.5	69.7

the most common source for Gram-negative septicaemia is the urinary tract [15].

Chronic infections

The two main long-term complications of opportunistic UTI are renal damage and calculus formation. However, in the absence of obstruction or renal calculi, chronic infection rarely leads to renal damage.

Management

Indications for therapy

The detection of bacteriuria is not an automatic indication for antimicrobial therapy, whether it occurs in an uncomplicated case or otherwise. It is important to assess all patients, and consider the likelihood of infection and its natural history (Fig. 54.1).

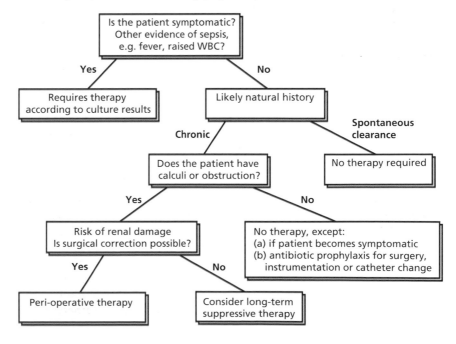

Fig. 54.1 Scheme for the management of opportunist UTIs. WBC, white blood cell count.

Symptomatic infection clearly requires treatment. Pyuria is usually present in true infection, but may also occur in the presence of a urethral catheter, or urethral or vaginal discharge. Opportunistic infections, particularly those associated with catheters, may be asymptomatic so a different approach is required. Correction of the deficit in the host immune response may be all that is required, for example removing the urethral catheter under appropriate antibiotic cover if indicated. However, chronic infections may be very difficult to eradicate. Treatment of an infected long-term catheter is likely to lead merely to the replacement of the original infecting organism with another more resistant organism. These infections may also be 'mixed', with several organisms involved, and treatment may lead to the predominance of a single organism. Treatment is not indicated in such patients unless the infection becomes symptomatic, or if catheter change or surgery involving the urinary tract is proposed.

Corrective treatment is required for stones or obstruction. The eradication of infection is unlikely unless the underlying cause can be removed. Long-term suppressive therapy may be needed.

When *Candida* species are isolated from urine, sample contamination must first be excluded, as must systemic candidiasis. For those with true local UTI the best treatment is still unclear, but removing factors such as a urethral catheter or the use of broad spectrum antibiotics may lead to resolution in many cases. Some patients will require treatment for symptomatic candidasis. Oral agents such as fluconazole are very useful [16]. Bladder irrigation with amphotericin B has also been used successfully [17].

Antimicrobial therapy

Treatment of uncomplicated infection on an empirical basis, even with single-dose regimens, is often successful [18]. In opportunistic infection it is vital to obtain specimens for culture before therapy is started.

The drug selected (Table 54.3) must have activity against the infecting organism, but must have appropriate pharmacokinetic properties, to achieve adequate concentration at the target site. In male patients, failure of therapy may relate to an infective focus within the prostate and penetration of the drug into prostatic tissue may be important. Trimethoprim and ciprofloxacin both penetrate the prostatic tissue well [19]. Many patients with opportunistic infections will have impaired renal function, which limits the use of agents such as nitrofurantoin or nalidixic acid. The aminoglycosides and vancomycin require monitoring of serum levels to avoid nephrotoxicity and hence must be used very carefully. Impaired renal function also results in poor concentrations of any agent in the urine, which will compound the difficulties of treatment.

Prevention

Considerable effort should be expended in attempts to prevent opportunistic UTI. Correction of any deficit in host immunity should always be the first aim.

Surgery

Surgical correction of anatomical abnormalities should be considered. Stones may need surgical removal if lithotripsy is ineffective.

Infection control

Many opportunistic infections are of nosocomial origin, and attention to infection control procedures is vital in keeping numbers to a minimum.

Alternative strategies

In patients with a neurogenic bladder, the technique of clean intermittent self-catheterization may avoid long-term catheterization and its consequent infective problems [20,21]. This is particularly important in young patients with a neurogenic bladder. The technique has many advantages over other approaches such as urinary diversion.

Antimicrobial prophylaxis

Uncontrolled antibiotic prophylaxis can cause problems itself, for example with resistant organisms. There are certain circumstances where it is undoubtedly of use. Single-dose prophylaxis is indicated whenever a urethral catheter is inserted in a patient with bacteriuria, to prevent bacteraemia. Used perioperatively in patients at high risk of significant infection or for prosthetic surgery (where infection could be disastrous), short-course prophylaxis is useful. Long-term suppressive therapy in patients with recurrent infections may limit renal damage in those at risk.

Hospital-acquired infection

Infections acquired in hospital differ from those in the community for several reasons. Hospital patients may be at increased risk of infection as a result of operations, or because of the presence of urinary catheters. The organisms involved in hospital infections also differ, principally in their patterns of resistance to antibiotics. Organisms causing hospital infections are more likely to show antibiotic resistance, mainly due to the selection pressure exerted by the widespread use of these agents in any hospital.

Table 54.3 Antibiotics used in urinary tract infections (UTIs).

Group	Oral (O) Parenteral (P)	Remarks	Group	Oral (O) Parenteral (P)	Remarks
Pencillins			Amikacin	P	Active against many gentamicin-resistant strains—reserved for this purpose
Amoxycillin Ampicillin Pivampicillin	O/P	Up to 50% of enterobacteriaceae may be resistant			
Co-amoxiclav (Augmentin: amoxycillin plus clavulanic acid)	O/P	Active against many β-lactamase-producing organisms, including some amoxycillin-resistant strains	Netilmicin	P	Possibly less toxic than gentamicin. Active against some gentamicin-resistant strains, but less active against *Pseudomonas*
Piperacillin Ticarcillin Carbenicillin Azlocillin	P	Broader spectrum than amoxycillin; useful antipseudomonal activity	Tobramycin	P	Similar to gentamicin
			Trimethoprim		
Tazocin (piperacillin and tazobactam)	P	Combination with β-lactamase inhibitor broadens spectrum	Co-trimoxazole (sulphamethoxazole and trimethoprim)	O/P	Useful first-line drug for UTIs
Timentin (ticarcillin and clavulanic acid)	P	As for Tazocin	Trimethoprim	O/P	Probably as effective as co-trimoxazole; avoids sulphonamide-related toxicity and hypersensitivity
Flucloxacillin Cloxacillin	O/P	Antistaphylococcal agents			
Cephalosporins			*Quinolones*		
Cephradine Cefadroxil Cephalexin	O/P O O	Active against some amoxycillin-resistant enterobacteriaceae	Ciprofloxacin	O/P	Good activity against enterobacteriaceae and *Pseudomonas*
Cefuroxime	O/P	Broader spectrum than earlier cephalosporins	Nalidixic acid	O	Moderately useful first-line agent for UTIs. Inadequate blood levels for renal infections
Cefotaxime	P	Better anti-Gram-negative activity, but reduced activity against Gram-positive organisms	Norfloxacin Ofloxacin	O	As for ciprofloxacin but oral formulations only
Ceftazidime	P	As for cefotaxime but with good anti-pseudomonal activity	*Glycopeptides*		
			Vancomycin	P	Gram-positive organisms only. Used for strains resistant to other antibiotics. Monitoring of levels required
Other β-lactams					
Imipenem	P	Very broad-spectrum antibiotic, often reserved for organisms resistant to other agents	Teicoplanin	P	As for vancomycin. Monitoring of levels not usually required
Aminoglycosides			*Nitrofurans*		
Gentamicin	P	Broad spectrum against enterobacteriaceae and *Pseudomonas*. Ototoxic and nephrotoxic; monitoring of plasma concentrations required (for all aminoglycosides). Resistant strains occur	Nitrofurantoin	O	Low blood levels; not suitable for renal infection. Suitable for uncomplicated UTI
			Antifungals		
			Fluconazole	O/P	Useful for *Candida* infections
			Amphotericin B	P	Active against a wide range of fungi; toxic

Significance

Hospital-acquired infections fall into two broad epidemiological categories: endemic infections and outbreaks of infection. Whilst the latter may attract considerable attention and expenditure, the former category is much larger. Many studies have looked at hospital-acquired infection rates. Nosocomial infections occurred in 9% of patients in a study in the UK in 1980 [22], with UTI the most common. This study was repeated in 1993–1994 with similar findings [23]. Studies in other countries have shown similar results [24–27]. In the USA, UTIs account for about 40% of nosocomial infections, with about 80% of these following urinary tract instrumentation or catheterization [28]. Good infection control practices can reduce the rates of all types of nosocomial infection [29] and such practice should be the concern of all who work in hospitals. This very large number of infections on a national scale represents a significant number of patients suffering excess morbidity and mortality. Thus Jepson *et al.* showed that the prevalence of hospital-acquired bacteraemia in patients with UTI was five times higher than in those without a UTI [30]. The probability of a further nosocomial infection is also much increased after a first episode [31]. Hence there is a considerable cost in terms of lengthened hospital stay and expenditure on treatment in addition to extra morbidity and mortality, and nosocomial UTIs alone consume considerable resources [32,33].

The lesser risk of an outbreak of infection cannot be ignored. Outbreaks may become apparent if an organism with an unusual sensitivity pattern is isolated on several occasions, or through the frequent isolation of an uncommon organism. Outbreaks usually involve single strains which may be resistant to a number of commonly used antibiotics. Many patients may become infected if control measures are not instituted early.

Predisposing factors

Several factors will predispose to cross-infection and outbreaks. First, the activity of present-day hospitals results in the clustering of large numbers of patients susceptible to urinary infection, either because of urinary catheterization or because of urinary tract abnormality, within single wards, rooms, bays or units. The second major factor is the widespread use and even misuse of antibiotics. This has two interdependent effects. First, antibiotics tend to eliminate the normal sensitive enterobacteriaceae and alter the ecological balance in the patient's gut microflora. This will select for organisms which are resistant to that antibiotic and, additionally, by virtue of the carriage and spread of bacterial plasmids possessing antibiotic-resistance genes, for organisms which are resistant to other structurally unrelated antibiotics.

Secondly, the factor known as colonization resistance will be affected. The normal microflora of healthy individuals, who have not received recent antibiotics, appears to offer protection against colonization of the gut by more potentially pathogenic or virulent organisms, such as *Salmonella* or *Pseudomonas* species or yeasts, by mechanisms which are poorly understood. This colonization resistance may involve the inhibition of growth by various factors, such as volatile fatty acids and the production of bacteriocins, as well as by direct competition for nutrients and mucosal binding, in addition to host factors such as secretory immunoglobulin A (IgA), gastric acid and digestive enzymes [34]. The normal flora, predominantly composed of obligate anaerobes, will be suppressed by antibiotic therapy, leading to impairment of colonization resistance. Once an organism has colonized the bowel, it may subsequently cause UTI in that patient, or act as a source of cross-infection.

The final factor leading to outbreaks is a breakdown in normal infection control practices, such as handwashing between patients or wearing gloves when handling body fluids (e.g. emptying urinary catheter bags) [35], or a failure to sterilize equipment properly.

An example demonstrating the different factors involved in an outbreak of opportunistic infection in a urological ward is outlined here [36]. During 2 weeks in the late summer of 1979 a multiresistant strain of *Acinetobacter calcoaceticus* was isolated from the urine samples of eight patients in a male urological ward. Two of the patients required treatment for symptomatic infection. The common factors preceding isolation of this organism were urological surgery, catheterization and the prophylactic use of co-trimoxazole to prevent infection.

Operating theatre practice was reviewed but no source of infection was identified. An environmental study revealed the organism was widely distributed in pools of water in the ward sluice area and was present on the inside of the bedpan washer/pasteurizer used to disinfect the jugs into which urinary catheter bags were emptied. Subsequent investigation revealed that the water heater and steam generator in the pasteurizer, which were supposed to heat bedpans to a temperature of 80°C for 1 min, were not working at all. The organism was also present in the urine jugs just processed by this equipment, and even the jugs used for patients not involved in the outbreak were contaminated. Unfortunately, these jugs were stored upright before re-use and failed to dry completely.

Care of urinary catheters by the nursing staff was by closed-system drainage. The procedure incorporated all the then recommended methods of preventing infection with the exception of adding disinfectant to the catheter bag. The weak point appeared to be the bedpan washer, which contaminated the collecting jugs. Contamination of the gloved hand when a jug was picked up could have led to subsequent contamination of the catheter bag valve, with possible retrograde infection in the urine collection system.

The widespread use of co-trimoxazole prophylactically was probably responsible for the selection of an organism in which co-trimoxazole resistance was linked to resistance to several other antibiotics, including gentamicin.

Disinfection of the urine-collecting equipment in the bedpan pasteurizer was discontinued. Instead a system was introduced of emptying the urine collecting jugs, rinsing with water and soaking in 1% hypochlorite solution followed by drainage. Nursing staff were reminded of the importance of eliminating residual pools of water in the sluice. These measures, together with probable improvement in catheter care technique, brought the outbreak to a close.

Sources of infection

Outbreaks can be subdivided into those due to a common source, such as is outlined above and those due to cross-infection. The latter is more common, although less easy to control—a common source outbreak can be abruptly halted if the source can be removed. An epidemiological link between the putative environmental source and patient infection must be demonstrated in the case of a common-source outbreak; it is possible for the environment to become contaminated with the outbreak organism too!

Cross-infection outbreaks may be transmitted in a variety of ways, such as air-borne transmission, direct contact between patients or via surgical instruments such as cystoscopes if these are not adequately decontaminated between patients. The most likely route of transmission in a nosocomial UTI outbreak is via the hands of staff, particularly if they fail to wash their hands between visiting patients.

Control of infection

It can be seen that many nosocomial infections are likely to be due to a failure to adhere to standard infection control measures, and that the best way of preventing them is staff education. All staff have a responsibility to help prevent cross-infection. Considerable resources are needed to provide a satisfactory continuing education for all staff. It is also essential to have an infection control team, usually consisting of a microbiologist and at least one infection control nurse, to coordinate outbreak investigation and, more importantly, produce infection control policies covering all aspects of hospital activity [37].

Control of hospital-acquired UTI affects many areas. Antibiotic usage can be controlled by implementation of local antibiotic policies, in order to limit the range of agents used. This not only has cost implications but aids in limiting the appearance of resistance due to selection pressures, as well as reducing inappropriate or unnecessary prescribing. This is most apparent in the use of antibiotics for prophylaxis [38]. Prophylaxis in urology has recently been reviewed [39]. Often prophylaxis is not needed and in cases where it is appropriate, is often given for too long. Short courses, or even single doses, are preferred.

Considerable attention needs to be paid to areas such as catheter insertion and catheter care. The importance of hand-washing, an extremely basic infection control measure, cannot be overemphasized. In most areas of hospital practice, thorough washing with soap and water is as effective as more expensive antiseptic preparations.

The role of surveillance of infection must be considered on its merits for each individual unit. This is usually best managed by members of the infection control team, but can be time consuming. Computer software to 'flag' particular organisms of interest being reported by a laboratory may make this easier. The intention is to reduce levels of endemic infection and detect potential problems before outbreaks occur.

Catheter-associated bacteriuria

In dealing with catheter-associated urinary infections a clear distinction must be drawn between short-term catheterization in postoperative or acutely ill patients, and long-term catheterization of patients for urinary retention or severe incontinence.

Short-term catheterization

The incidence of bacteriuria in patients with short-term urethral catheters is 10–20% [40]. In patients who have a catheter for over 1 month it is 100% [10]. Urinary catheterization is such a common procedure that even if the complication rate is low, significant numbers of patients will develop problems, such as prostatitis, pyelonephritis or septicaemia.

Until the 1960s, even short-term catheterization resulted in inevitable bacteriuria, as open systems were used, allowing free entry of bacteria to the urinary tract. As early as the 1920s it had been shown that a closed system of drainage could dramatically reduce infection rates [41]. This was not confirmed until work was done in the 1960s [42], and since then closed systems have been in common use.

Bacteria may enter the bladder when a catheter is inserted, may migrate up the outside of the catheter or may migrate up its internal surface. The latter is limited by the use of a closed drainage system, but drainage bags may become colonized with bacteria if good infection control practice is not maintained. Migration up the outside of a catheter is probably the most important route, particularly in female patients [10].

Prevention of catheter-associated urinary infection

Many strategies have been proposed for preventing catheter-associated urinary infection, not all of them successful. Guidelines from the Centers for Disease Control in the USA and from Great Britain and Ireland have been published [43,44]. These concentrate on several areas. Catheters should only be used when necessary, and removed as soon as possible. Alternative methods such as condom catheters should be considered. Catheter insertion should be carried out using aseptic technique and sterile equipment, by trained staff. Adequate cleansing of the periurethral area with an antiseptic should be ensured. After insertion using a sterile lubricant, the catheter should be connected to a sterile drainage system with a bag which can be emptied by a tap. The catheter should be adequately secured.

Good catheter care is vital. Staff should be educated in proper care techniques, and should always wash their hands or change gloves between patients, even if only emptying drainage bags. Urine samples should be obtained aseptically using ports in the tubing. Unobstructed urine flow should be maintained at all times, with the bag regularly emptied and kept below the level of the patient's bladder. Drainage bags should not touch the floor.

Antibiotics have been used in several studies [45] and generally are of little use, but their use in patients with indwelling catheters for between 3–14 days remains controversial. Some studies have shown a benefit in this group [45,46]. Routine use risks the appearance of resistant organisms. The use of antiseptics for meatal care, bladder irrigation or to prevent colonization of drainage bags has been shown to be both ineffective and costly [10].

Various methods to prevent bacterial adherence to catheters have been tested, such as silicone, silver-coated or antibiotic-impregnated catheters. Results of trials have been inconsistent. Further trials using hydrophilic-coated or electrically charged catheters are awaited.

Microbiological examination of catheter urine specimens is of limited value, but is indicated if the patient has evidence of systemic infection, or is to undergo catheter manipulation or urinary tract surgery or instrumentation so that appropriate treatment or prophylaxis may be given. Treatment should be started if the patient develops systemic infection or if symptoms of frequency or dysuria develop after the catheter is removed. Antibiotics should be withheld from patients with asymptomatic catheter-associated bacteriuria.

Long-term catheterization

Problems with blockage and infection make long-term use of indwelling catheters unsatisfactory. Intermittent catheterization is to be preferred, but is not suitable for many elderly or disabled patients.

The same principles for preventing infection apply as for short-term catheterization. Antibiotics may have a temporary effect, but are unlikely to eliminate an organism entirely, although they may facilitate replacement with resistant organisms. Bladder wash-outs with sterile saline rather than antiseptics are preferable if needed to maintain catheter viability [44].

The significance of bacteriuria in these patients is unclear. One study in geriatric patients showed bacteriuria to be well tolerated [47]. As a result, microbiological examination of urine is rarely required, unless systemic infection occurs and antibiotic treatment is required.

Other special problems

Urinary tract instrumentation

Instrumentation in patients with previously sterile urine does not require antibiotic prophylaxis [48]. Infection may be introduced in several ways, such as on inadequately cleaned cystoscopes or via contaminated irrigation fluid, but these problems should be kept to a minimum by normal surgical practice.

Patients with infected urine or bacteriuria undergoing cystoscopy are at risk of bacteraemia and septicaemia. Ideally, infection should be treated prior to instrumentation, but if this is not possible, therapy should be started prior to the procedure and continued for a full course postoperatively. Microbiological examination of urine is obviously mandatory in this respect if an appropriate antibiotic is to be prescribed.

Prostatectomy

In addition to the potential for infection described above and the presence of a postoperative irrigation catheter after transurethral resection of the prostate, patients are also at risk of catheter-associated bacteriuria. The use of prophylaxis is still controversial, but there is no evidence of clinically significant benefit from its use [48]. It should be used when patients have bacteriuria or an indwelling catheter at the time of operation. Infected patients should be treated as for urinary tract instrumentation (see above).

Urinary diversion procedures

Bacteriuria in patients with a urinary diversion, such as an ileal conduit, is a common finding [49]. Urine is able to reflux freely along the ureters, with consequent susceptibility to pyelonephritis and renal damage. However, unless bacteriuria is causing symptomatic infection, antibiotic therapy is not indicated, as the reappearance of bacteriuria is likely.

Prophylaxis for the operative diversion procedure should cover bowel flora, with antibiotics such as gentamicin or cefuroxime, plus metronidazole.

References

1 O'Grady F, Cattell WR. Kinetics of urinary tract infection. II. The bladder. *Br J Urol* 1966;**38**:156–62.

2 Sobel JD, Kaye D. Urinary tract infections. In: Mandell GL, Douglas RG Jr, Bennett JE, eds. *Principles and Practice of Infectious Diseases*, 3rd edn. New York: Churchill Livingstone, 1990:582–611.

3 Measley RE Jr, Levison ME. Host defense mechanisms in the pathogenesis of urinary tract infection. *Med Clin North Am* 1991;**75**:275–86.

4 Kaye D. Antibacterial activity of urine. *J Clin Invest* 1968;**47**:2374–90.

5 Mims CA. *The Pathogenesis of Infectious Disease*, 3rd edn. London: Academic Press, 1987.

6 Levy BJ, Fair WR. Localization of antibacterial activity in rat prostatic secretions. *Invest Urol* 1973;**11**:123–77.

7 Parsons CL, Schrom SH, Hanno P *et al*. Bladder surface mucin: examination of possible mechanism for its antibacterial effect. *Invest Urol* 1978;**6**:196–200.

8 Bryant RE, Sutcliffe MC, McGee FA. Human polymorpho-nuclear leukocyte function in urine. *Yale J Biol Med* 1973;**43**:113–24.

9 Rene P, Dinolfo M, Silverblatt FJ. Serum and urogenital antibody response to *Escherichia coli* pili in cystitis. *Infect Immun* 1982;**38**:542–7.

10 Garibaldi RA. Catheter-associated urinary tract infection. *Curr Opin Infect Dis* 1992;**5**:517–23.

11 Grüneberg RN. Changes in the antibiotic sensitivities of urinary pathogens, 1971–1989. *J Antimicrob Chemother* 1990;**26**(Suppl. F):3–11.

12 Ang BSP, Telenti A, King B, Steckelberg JM, Wilson WR. Candidemia from a urinary tract source: microbiological aspects and clinical significance. *Clin Infect Dis* 1993;**17**:662–6.

13 Schoolink GK. How *Escherichia coli* infects the urinary tract. *N Engl J Med* 1989;**320**:804–5.

14 Roberts JA, Fussel EN, Kaack MB. Bacterial adherence to urethral catheters. *J Urol* 1990;**144**:264–9.

15 Muder RR, Brennen C, Wagener MM, Goetz AM. Bacteremia in a long-term-care facility: a five-year prospective study of 163 consecutive episodes. *Clin Infect Dis* 1992;**14**:647–54.

16 Gubbins PO, Piscitelli SC, Danziger LH. Candidal urinary tract infections: a comprehensive review of their diagnosis and management. *Pharmacotherapy* 1993;**13**:110–27.

17 Sanford JP. The enigma of candiduria: evolution of bladder irrigation with amphotericin B for management—from anecdote to dogma and a lesson from Machiavelli. *Clin Infect Dis* 1993;**16**:145–7.

18 Neu HC. Urinary tract infections. *Am J Med* 1992;**92**(Suppl. 4A):63–70S.

19 British Medical Association/Royal Pharmaceutical Society of Great Britain. *British National Formulary*. London: BMA/Royal Pharmaceutical Society of Great Britain, 1994:27.

20 Perkash I, Giroux J. Clean intermittent catheterization in spinal cord injury patients: a followup study. *J Urol* 1993:**149**:1068–71.

21 Hunt GM, Oakeshott P, Whitaker RH. Intermittent catheterisation: simple, safe and effective but underused. *Br Med J* 1996;**312**:103–7.

22 Meers PD, Ayliffe GAJ, Emmerson AM *et al*. Report on the National Survey of Infection in Hospitals, 1980. *J Hosp Infect* 1981;**2**(Suppl.):23–8.

23 Emmerson AM, Enstone JE, Griffin M *et al*. The second national prevalence survey of infection in hospitals—overview of the results. 1996;**32**:175–90.

24 Aavitsland P, Stormark M, Lystad A. Hospital-acquired infections in Norway: a national prevalence survey in 1991. *Scand J Infect Dis* 1992;**24**:477–83.

25 Jarvis WR, Edwards JR, Culver DH *et al*. Nosocomial infection rates in adult and pediatric intensive care units in the United States. National Nosocomial Infections Surveillance System. *Am J Med* 1991;**91**(Suppl. 3B):185–91S.

26 Horan TC, Culver DH, Gaynes RP *et al*. Nosocomial infections in surgical patients in the United States, January 1986–June 1992. National Nosocomial Infections Surveillance (NNIS) System. *Infect Control Hosp Epidemiol* 1993;**14**:73–80.

27 Campins M, Vaque J, Rossello J *et al*. Nosocomial infections in pediatric patients: a prevalence study in Spanish hospitals. EPINE Working Group. *Am J Infect Control* 1993;**21**:58–63.

28 Meares EM Jr. Current patterns in nosocomial urinary tract infections. *Urology* 1991;**37**(Suppl. 3):9–12.

29 French GL, Cheng AF, Wong SL, Donnan S. Repeated prevalence surveys for monitoring effectiveness of hospital infection control. *Lancet* 1989;**2**:1021–3.

30 Jepson OB, Larsen SO, Dankert J *et al*. Urinary tract infection and bacteraemia in hospitalised medical patients — a European multi-centre prevalence survey on nosocomial infection. *J Hosp Infect* 1982;**3**:241–52.

31 Brawley RL, Weber DJ, Samsa GP, Rutala WA. Multiple nosocomial infections. An incidence study. *Am J Epidemiol* 1989;**130**:769–80.

32 Patton JP, Nash DB, Abrutyn E. Urinary tract infection: economic considerations. *Med Clin North Am* 1991;**75**:495–513.

33 Coello R, Glenister H, Fereres J *et al*. The cost of infection in surgical patients: a case-control study. *J Hosp Infect* 1993;**25**:239–50.

34 Guiot HFL. Colonisation resistance and the use of antimicrobial agents for prophylaxis and therapy. *Rev Med Microbiol* 1991;**2**:194–9.

35 Ayliffe GAJ, Lowbury EJL, Geddes AM Williams JD, eds. *Control of Hospital Infection—a Practical Handbook*, 3rd edn. London: Chapman and Hall 1991:115–39.

36 Lowes JA, Smith J, Tabaqchali S, Shaw EJ. Outbreak of infection in a urological ward. *Br Med J* 1980;**1**:722.

37 Joint DOH/PHLS Hospital Infection Working Group. *Hospital Infection Control. Guidance on the Control of Infection in Hospitals*. London: Department of Health and Social Services, 1988.

38 Moss F, McNichol MW, McSwiggan DA, Miller DL. Survey of antibiotic prescribing in a district general hospital (1): pattern of use. *Lancet* 1981;**2**:349–52.

39 Amin M. Antibacterial prophylaxis in urology: a review. *Am J Med* 1992;**92**(Suppl. 4A):114–17S.

40 Stamm WE. Catheter-associated urinary tract infections: epidemiology, pathogenesis, and prevention. *Am J Med* 1991;**91**(Supply. 3B):65–71S.

41 Dukes C. Urinary infections after excision of the rectum: their cause and prevention: *Proc R Soc Med* 1928;**22**:259–67.

42 Kunin CM, McCormack RC. Prevention of catheter-induced urinary tract infections by sterile closed drainage. *N Engl J Med* 1966;**274**:1156–61.

43 Wong ES, Hooton TM. Guidelines for prevention of catheter-associated urinary tract infections. *Infect Control* 1981;**2**: 126–30.

44 Falkiner FR. The insertion and management of indwelling urethral catheters — minimising the risk of infection. *J Hosp Infect* 1993;**25**:79–90.

45 Anon. Catheter-acquired urinary tract infection. *Lancet* 1991; **338**:857–8.

46 van der Wall E, Verkooyen RP, Mintjes de-Groot J *et al*. Prophylactic ciprofloxacin for catheter-associated urinary tract infection. *Lancet* 1992;**339**:946–51.

47 Reid RI, Webster O, Read PJ, Maskell R. Comparison of urine bag-changing regimens in elderly catheterized patients. *Lancet* 1982, **2**:754–6.

48 Christensen MM. Antimicrobial prophylaxis in transurethral resection of the prostate. With special reference to preoperatively sterile urine. *Scand J Urol Neprhol* 1991;**25**:169–74.

49 Schmidt JD, Hawtrey CE, Flocks RH, Culp DA. Complications, results and problems of ileal conduit diversions. *J Urol* 1973; **109**:210–16.

55 Human Immunodeficiency Virus Infection and the Urologist

J.M.Zelin and J.Anderson

Introduction

Acquired immune deficiency syndrome (AIDS) and its causative organism human immunodeficiency virus (HIV) have been the focus of intense publicity and investigation. Although up to 16% patients may experience urinary symptoms [1] the emphasis of many writers has been on the renal rather than the urological aspects of the disease. AIDS was first described in 1981 when clusters of cases of Kaposi sarcoma and *Pneumocystis carinii* pneumonia (PCP) were reported in previously healthy young homosexual men in Los Angeles [2,3] and New York City [4]. In 1983 the retrovirus HIV was discovered and shown to be the aetiological agent. Although HIV can be isolated from all body fluids the majority of infections are transmitted via semen, cervical secretions and blood. Infection is via sexual intercourse, contaminated blood, blood products and organ donations, contaminated needles and vertically from mother to child. In the USA and UK the majority of the infections have occurred in homosexual men, but the commonest route of infection worldwide is through heterosexual intercourse. The World Health Organization (WHO) estimates that by the year 2000, 30–40 million people will have been infected worldwide [5].

Immunopathogenesis

HIV-1 and -2 are retrovirus belonging to the lentivirus group. Retroviruses contain viral RNA and the enzyme reverse transcriptase which allows RNA to be transcribed into DNA. This can then be incorporated into host cell genetic material. HIV-2 was identified in 1986 and is largely confined to West Africa where it is associated with AIDS. This chapter is restricted to HIV-1. The viral structure is shown in Fig. 55.1.

HIV infection leads to defects in cell-mediated immunity

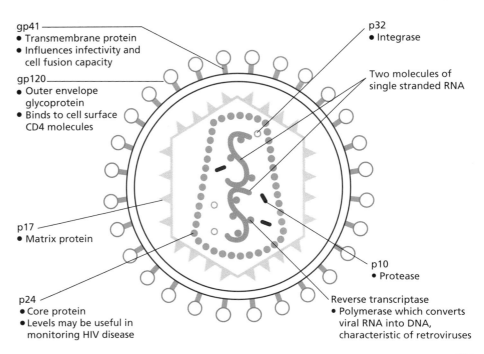

Fig. 55.1 Human immunodeficiency virus. Redrawn with permission from Mr Cedric Gilson, EMIS and Dr Jacqueline Parkin, Department of Immunology, St Bartholomew's Hospital, London.

gp41
- Transmembrane protein
- Influences infectivity and cell fusion capacity

gp120
- Outer envelope glycoprotein
- Binds to cell surface CD4 molecules

p17
- Matrix protein

p24
- Core protein
- Levels may be useful in monitoring HIV disease

p32
- Integrase

Two molecules of single stranded RNA

p10
- Protease

Reverse transcriptase
- Polymerase which converts viral RNA into DNA, characteristic of retroviruses

with progressive immunosuppression. The virus is tropic for cells carrying the CD4 molecule on their surface, which include T helper lymphocytes, monocytes, macrophages and a range of antigen-presenting cells. T helper lymphocytes, which have a pivotal role in the immune response, are the most affected. HIV infection produces progressive depletion of both their absolute numbers and functional ability with resulting widespread immune dysfunction. Direct infection and impaired functioning of macrophages occurs. Envelope proteins of HIV are able to activate B lymphocytes, leading to an increase in spontaneous antibody production and hypergammaglobulinaemia. However, humoral responses to new agents may be impaired, and granulocytes have reduced bacterial killing capacity secondary to impaired chemotaxis and phagocytosis. This combination of factors lays the host open to a range of infections and tumours.

Diagnosis

Antibodies formed to components of gp120 on the envelope of HIV are used as a marker of infection. Routine laboratory tests are enzyme-linked immunosorbent assay (ELISA) techniques and Western blot assays.

Testing for HIV may be done at the request of the patient or may be undertaken in the course of clinical investigation. It is a test that carries many implications and it is important that these are rehearsed with individuals prior to testing and permission to carry out HIV testing should be specifically sought. It is critical that issues surrounding HIV status are not allowed to obscure the need for proper clinical management of patients. It is rare that HIV testing is required within a timeframe that precludes full and fitting discussion of the test. In the case of sick patients proper diagnostic and therapeutic interventions can be made in ignorance of the patient's HIV status.

HIV antibody crosses the placenta, thus all babies born to HIV-infected women will carry maternal antibody which may take up to 18 months to disappear from uninfected infants. HIV antibody testing is therefore not an indicator of infection in this situation.

Antibodies may take as long as 3 months to be produced after initial exposure to infection, leaving a 'window period' when antibody testing is not diagnostic. p24 Antigen from the core of the virus may be detected shortly after infection but is short lived, disappearing by 8–10 weeks after exposure. It may reappear as infection progresses and if so can be useful as a surrogate marker of viral activity. Anti-p24 can be detected in the first few weeks of infection and persists throughout the asymptomatic period. As the disease progresses it is lost. Other techniques, available include viral cultivation and the use of polymerase chain reaction technology.

Surrogate markers of disease progression

The most commonly used laboratory marker of disease progression in HIV infection is the CD4+ lymphocyte count, the normal range for which is $450-1200\times10^6/l$. As immune function deteriorates, the absolute numbers and percentage of CD4+ cells progressively fall and the risk of opportunistic infections and other conditions which fulfil the criteria for AIDS increases (see Tables 55.2 and 55.3). The measurement of viral load is a useful prognostic indicator. It is expressed as the number of copies of viral RNA per ml. In asymptomatic HIV infection, a viral load above 100 000 copies is considered high and below 10 000 copies low. Viral load monitoring is a useful way to measure the effectiveness of antiretroviral treatment and an increasing viral load may indicate the need to change medication. Other markers of immune deterioration are a raised serum β2-microglobulin and a raised serum neopterin.

Antiretroviral therapy

Intensive study of the structure and lifecycle of HIV has highlighted potential areas for therapeutic intervention. Although a number of agents have been shown to slow viral replication and reduce the viral load thus slowing disease progression, none are curative. A range of compounds that antagonize the action of the viral enzyme reverse transcriptase have been identified. The first to enter clinical practice was the nucleoside analogue zidovudine (AZT). Early studies demonstrated a survival advantage in people with AIDS treated with AZT versus placebo. Until recently AZT was widely used alone for patients with either symptomatic HIV or AIDS. The benefit of therapy in early or asymptomatic diereses is less clear. It is now clear that dual and triple therapy regimes are superior to AZT monotherapy in terms of improved survival and delayed progression to AIDS. Suggested combinations are AZT plus one or two other nucleoside analogues such as didanosine (ddI), zalcitabine (ddC) lamivudine (3TC) or stavudine (d4T); two nucleoside analogues plus either a non-nucleoside reverse transcriptase inhibitor such as nevaripine or a protease inhibitor such as saquinavir, ritonavir or indinavir or two protease inhibitors [6].

Adverse reactions to AZT include headache, abdominal pain, nausea, disturbance of sleep patterns, haematological toxicity and inflammatory myopathy. Important side effects of other antiretrovirals include pancreatitis (ddI, lamivudine, stavudine), peripheral neuropathy (ddI, stavudine, lamivudine, saquinavir), peripheral parasthesiae (ritonavir), raised liver function tests (stavudine) and renal stone formation (indinavir).

Table 55.1 CDC classification for HIV infection in adults [7].

Category A	Asymptomatic HIV infection Persistent generalized lymphadenopathy Acute (primary) seroconversion illness or history of acute infection
Category B	Symptomatic conditions • conditions that are attributed to HIV or defective cell-mediated immunity or • conditions that are considered to have a clinical course and/or require management that is complicated by HIV infection
Category C	Clinical conditions listed in 1993 AIDS surveillance case definition (see Table 55.2)

Natural history of HIV infection

The clinical spectrum associated with HIV infection is broad. A commonly used classification system is that of the Centres for Disease Control (CDC) [7], shown in Table 55.1. Since 1993 the definition of AIDS has differed between the USA and Europe, with the USA including individuals with CD4 counts of less than 200/mm^3 in the AIDS category. In Europe AIDS remains a clinical diagnosis made on the basis of specific opportunistic infections or tumours, as shown in Table 55.2. These must be diagnosed in the absence of other causes of immunosuppression.

Although seroconversion to HIV is usually subclinical, an acute, self-limiting mononucleosis-like syndrome occurring 3–6 weeks after exposure is experienced by up to 10% of patients (CDC category A). The illness is characterized by lymphadenopathy, arthralgia, myalgia, sore throat, fever and malaise. A transient generalized maculopapular rash may occur. Aseptic meningitis, encephalitis and transverse myelitis have been associated [8]. Severe genital ulceration has been reported [9]. Lymphopenia, thrombocytopenia and abnormal liver function tests occur [10]. During this stage of infection antibodies to HIV may not yet have been formed but p24 antigen from the core of the virus may be identified in the circulation.

An asymptomatic phase of variable duration follows seroconversion. A mean of 7–9 years has been reported from seroconversion to development of AIDS [11]. Viral replication continues and the individual remains infectious. A subgroup have persistent generalized lymphadenopathy (PGL). PGL is defined as lymphadenopathy of at least 3 months' duration with nodes 1 cm or more in size in at least two extrainguinal sites. Splenomegaly may be associated. Disease progression is similar in patients with or without PGL [12].

Symptomatic infection (CDC categories B and C) is associated with a wide range of manifestations reflecting underlying immunosuppression and chronic infection with HIV. Constitutional symptoms such as fever, malaise,

Table 55.2 AIDS defining conditions, opportunistic infections and tumours included in the 1993 AIDS Surveillance Case Definition [7].

Candidiasis of bronchi, trachea or lungs
Candidiasis of oesophagus
Cervical carcinoma, invasive
Coccidioidomycosis disseminated or extrapulmonary
Cryptococcus, extrapulmonary
Cryptosporidiosis, chronic intestinal (> 1 month's duration)
Cytomegalovirus disease (other than liver, spleen or nodes)
Cytomegalovirus retinitis (with loss of vision)
Encephalopathy, HIV-related
Herpes simplex, chronic ulcers (> 1 month's duration); or bronchitis, pneumonitis or oesophagitis
Histoplasmosis, disseminated or extrapulmonary
Isopsoriasis, chronic intestinal (> 1 month's duration)
Kaposi's sarcoma
Lymphoma, Burkitt's (or equivalent term)
Lymphoma, immunoblastic (or equivalent term)
Lymphoma, non-Hodgkin's (or equivalent term)
Lymphoma, primary of brain
Mycobacterium avium intracellulare or *M. kansaii*, disseminated or extrapulmonary
Mycobacterium tuberculosis, any site
Mycobacterium other species or unidentified species, disseminated or extrapulmonary
Pneumocystis carinii pneumonia
Pneumonia, recurrent bacterial
Progressive multifocal leucoencephalopathy
Salmonella septicaemia, recurrent
Toxoplasmosis of brain
Wasting syndrome due to HIV

weight loss, diarrhoea and drenching night sweats occur. Skin and mucous membranes of the mouth and genital tract are frequently the site of viral and fungal infections with herpes simplex, varicella zoster and *Candida*. Human papilloma virus causes genital warts which are typically more florid and more resistant to therapy than in HIV-negative patients. Candidiasis affecting the oropharynx is common and in women candidal vulvovaginitis may become increasingly severe and recurrent.

Neurological disease results either from direct HIV infection of glial cells or the effects of HIV proteins on neuronal function. The clinical manifestations include peripheral neuropathy, usually sensory, in the lower limbs and a vacuolar myelopathy producing lower limb signs and sphincter disturbance. Cognitive impairment incorporating memory deficit, poor concentration and personality change may occur; depression is common. Computed tomography (CT) scans of the brain show atrophic changes of varying degree.

Haematological complications of advanced HIV infection are common [13]. Normochromic, normocytic anaemia and mild neutropenia are frequently seen and may be iatrogenically exacerbated. Thrombocytopenia may be isolated and be the only manifestation of HIV infection. Although the aetiology is unclear, both reduced production and increased peripheral destruction of platelets via circulating antiplatelet antibodies are implicated. Gastrointestinal problems such as chronic diarrhoea and weight loss become more common as disease progresses. These are often associated with underlying opportunistic infections or malignancies which need full investigation.

Opportunistic disease in HIV infection

As immunosuppression becomes more profound the patient will become susceptible to a range of infections and malignancies. Three interrelated factors determine the profile of pathology for each individual.

1 The microbial repertoire to which the patient has been exposed during life is important as many episodes of illness are reactivation of previously acquired infection. The geographical origins of the patient will have an influence on this. Organisms controlled largely by cell-mediated immunity such as *Mycobacterium* and *Salmonella* species will have the greatest impact.

2 The pathogenicity of organisms will determine when particular problems may occur. The more virulent organisms such as *Streptococcus pneumoniae* and herpes viruses will give problems at earlier stages of immuno-suppression than less virulent organisms such as *Pneumocystis carinii* or *Toxoplasmosis gondii*. The latter two are uncommon until the CD4 lymphocyte count is consistently below 200/mm³.

3 The degree of immunosuppression of the individual will determine whether organisms of very low pathogenicity are able to become disseminated. Atypical mycobacteria which are of very low pathogenicity are able to colonize profoundly immunosuppressed patients. The lack of immune response is one of the factors that makes therapy of this organism so difficult.

Knowledge of these factors allows for rational diagnostic algorithms and also for appropriate intervention with prophylaxis. In practice, immunodeficiency leads to multiple pathology with a lack of the typical signs which a normal immune response permits. Consequently tissue is frequently required to identify the organisms responsible or to provide histological evidence to explain a particular clinical picture. The major opportunistic pathogens associated with HIV are shown in Table 55.3.

Protozoa

Pneumocystis carinii most commonly causes pneumonia (PCP) but may present as disseminated infection which can include the kidneys where it is a cause of nephrocalcinosis [14] leading to hypocalcaemia and acute renal failure. PCP characteristically presents with persistent non-productive

Table 55.3 Major pathogens and tumours associated with HIV infection.

Protozoa	*Pneumocystis carinii*
	Toxoplasma gondii
	Cryptosporidium parvum
	Isospora belli
	Microsporidia spp.
Viruses	Herpes simplex
	Varicella zoster
	Cytomegalovirus
	Papovavirus
Fungi and yeasts	*Candida* spp.
	Cryptococcus neoformans
	Histoplasma capsulatum
	Coccidioides immitis
Bacteria	*Streptococcus pneumoniae*
	Staphylococcus aureus
	Haemophilus influenzae
	Moraxella catarrhalis
	Salmonella spp.
	Rhodococcus equi
	Rochalimaea quintana
	Nocardia
	Mycobacterium tuberculosis
	Mycobacterium avium intracellulare
Tumours	Kaposi's sarcoma (HHV8 related)
	Non-Hodgkin's lymphoma (EBV related)

cough and shortness of breath. Fever, tachycardia, tachypnoea and hypoxia are the common signs and the diagnosis is made by detection of oocysts on bronchoalveolar lavage. Renal biopsy and direct tissue examination is necessary to make the diagnosis of renal pneumocystis. Preferred therapy is with intravenous high-dose co-trimoxazole for 21 days. A significant proportion of HIV-infected patients are sensitive to sulphur-containing drugs and up to 50% may need to be changed to second line agents such as pentamidine or a combination of dapsone and trimethoprim. Recurrence is common, hence secondary prophylaxis with co-trimoxazole 960 mg three times per week is offered to patients who have had an episode of PCP. Primary prophylaxis in those HIV-infected individuals with CD4+ counts below 200 cells/mm³, has reduced the incidence of PCP from about 60 to 5% in the UK. Aerosolized pentamidine may be used as prophylaxis in people intolerant of co-trimoxazole [15]. Such an approach can only protect the lungs and pneumocystis can develop in other organs such as the kidney.

Toxoplasma gondii in the context of HIV infection most commonly leads to encephalitis and cerebral abscesses. This is usually a reactivation of previously acquired infection as immunosuppression deepens. Primary symptomatic infection in those previously unexposed to *Toxoplasma* is rare, although it may present with febrile illness and lymphadenopathy. Orchitis due to *Toxoplasma gondii* is rare in the immunocompetent and has been reported in only a few cases of generalized acute toxoplasmosis [16], but has been reported in AIDS patients [17]. In general, subclinical testicular involvement occurs as a part of the systemic nature of the infection, but clinically significant symptoms have been reported [18]. Treatment of toxoplasmosis is with sulphadiazine and pyrimethamine with folinic acid support for 6 weeks after which maintenance therapy is instituted.

A limiting side effect of sulphadiazine therapy is crystalluria which was well recognized in the past and has now been reported in patients with AIDS [19,20]. It can lead to acute renal failure due to crystal deposition in the urinary tract. The condition is dose related and is associated with dehydration (an important consideration in patients with AIDS as diarrhoea and fever are very common). Treatment of sulphadiazine-induced crystalluria consists of the rapid administration of fluids and sodium bicarbonate to increase the urine output to over 2 l/day and to elevate the urinary pH to over 7.5. Recovery of renal function usually occurs rapidly with minimal residual damage to the kidney. Should the patient remains anuric, urological intervention may be required including ureteric catheterization or nephrostomy tube placement, followed by lavage with warm 5% bicarbonate solution.

Cryptosporidium parvum is a frequent cause of profuse watery diarrhoea in those with HIV infection. Involvement of other organs, including the bladder, by way of an enterovesical fistula has been reported [21]. Treatment is largely supportive due to the lack of effective anticryptosporidial agents, although the non-absorbable aminoglycoside paromomycin may help control diarrhoea.

Penile amoebiasis can occur and may be misdiagnosed as carcinoma [22].

Viruses

Cytomegalovirus

Cytomegalovirus (CMV) causes considerable morbidity and mortality in HIV infection, especially in the later stages of disease. The commonest presentation is with retinitis which occurs in up to 30% of AIDS patients and can cause blindness. In addition colitis, oesophagitis, encephalitis, pneumonitis, adrenalitis and polyradiculopathy are caused by CMV. CMV inclusions are commonly seen in the renal tissues of patients with AIDS [23,24] at postmortem, but this represents the multiorgan nature of the infection rather than primary local infection of the kidneys. The testis and prostate may also be infected with CMV [25–28]. Although the epididymis is rarely involved in AIDS-related illness, it may be infected with CMV [27] and CMV epididymitis can occur [29].

CMV has been isolated from the bladder and urine of AIDS patients with disseminated CMV infection [1]. Symptomatic CMV cystitis has also been reported [30] and may be the presenting AIDS-defining diagnosis in some patients [31]. The presentation is with frequency, strangury, dysuria and haematuria which is unresponsive to conventional antibiotic treatment. Intravenous urography may show a thickened bladder wall with erythematous and oedematous mucosa noted on cystoscopy. CMV inclusions are found on biopsy. Treatment is with high-dose intravenous aciclovir [1], the success of which is attributed to the high urinary concentration of aciclovir which is primarily excreted in the urine. CMV can also cause a polyradiculopathy leading to urinary retention which may occur in up to 2% of AIDS patients who have neurological problems [32]. Both ganciclovir and foscarnet are effective agents. However, CMV infection in the context of HIV requires long-term suppressive therapy to reduce recurrence. Both of these drugs must be given intravenously necessitating the insertion of an indwelling central venous catheter. The use of an indwelling central venous catheter may now be avoided in some patients as an oral formulation of ganciclovir has recently been licensed for use as maintenance therapy in CMV retinitis. Although oral ganciclovir has the disadvantage of slightly reduced efficacy, this may be outweighed by the fact that it is less toxic than the intravenous drug and is much easier to administer.

Herpes

Herpes simplex virus (HSV), types I and II and varicella zoster virus (VZV) are causes of morbidity and occasional mortality in HIV-infected individuals. Both remain in latent form in the nervous tissue with potential for reactivation and clinical recurrence as immunosuppression supervenes. Serological surveys show that there is a very high prevalence of prior HSV infection in homosexual men with AIDS. The commonest areas to be involved are the mouth, lips, genitalia and perianal region. Recurrence may be more frequent and severe, with more extensive tissue destruction than in HIV-negative patients. In addition, viral shedding persists for a longer period than in immunocompetent patients with HSV infection. Treatment with aciclovir is usually effective and may need to be given long term to suppress frequent recurrences. The emergence of aciclovir-resistant strains of HSV in HIV-infected patients has become clinically important. Most are thymidine kinase-deficient mutations which do not usually produce symptoms in the immunocompetent but can lead to devastating infection in immunosuppressed people. These viral strains typically lead to chronic mucocutaneous ulceration. Disseminated disease, although rare, has been described. Foscarnet, which does not require phosphorylation for its activity, is a useful alternative therapy in this situation.

VZV is commonly seen in HIV-infected patients, often with an atypical presentation. Being a reasonably pathogenic organism it may appear early in the course of HIV disease. More than one dermatome can be involved and attacks may be more frequent than in immunocompetent individuals. VZV can involve the genitalia causing extensive ulceration. High-dose acyclovir speeds healing and reduces the duration of viral shedding. Aciclovir-resistant VZV has also been reported.

Bacteria

Many bacteria are important pathogens in the context of HIV immunosuppression. Those that are intracellular pathogens such as *Mycobacteria*, or which are capsulated such as *Streptococcus pneumoniae* or *Haemophilus influenzae*, are poorly handled in HIV-infected hosts. In general, infection is more often disseminated in HIV-infected patients. Common bacteria may be found in atypical sites (e.g. renal salmonellosis) or uncommon organisms isolated (e.g. *Rochlimaea quintana* in cat scratch disease). Non-typhoidal *Salmonella* infections, particularly bacteraemia, are frequently seen. This organism requires intact macrophage activity for its elimination. *Pseudomonas* can cause challenging clinical problems.

Mycobacterial infection

Mycobacteria are intracellular organisms requiring intact cell-mediated immunity for their control. Early in the AIDS epidemic, an association was noted with *Mycobacterium tuberculosis*. In areas of the world where tuberculosis is endemic a substantial increase in the incidence of tuberculosis has been reported. In the USA where cases of tuberculosis had been falling steadily there has been a marked shift with the incidence rising over the past 10 years. Although it was initially assumed that HIV-associated tuberculosis represented the reactivation of latent *M. tuberculosis*, there is clear evidence for new infection and nosocomial spread in HIV-infected populations. At least 50% of HIV-related tuberculosis is extrapulmonary and disseminated infection is common. *M. tuberculosis* has been isolated from blood, urine and other sites. Twenty-four to 40% of HIV-infected patients with tuberculosis are bacteraemic, a presentation that used to be rare prior to the advent of HIV. In consequence, as well as renal infection, genitourinary tuberculosis and its potential urological complications can be expected to be seen more often. It is important to remember that the response to tuberculin testing is blunted in patients with HIV and is an unreliable test in this context. Sputum examination may be negative even in those with proven pulmonary infection and

the diagnosis rests on culture results. Any tissue specimens taken during surgery must be sent for culture to ensure that the diagnosis is not missed. Mycobacterial tuberculosis usually responds well to standard antituberculous chemotherapy, but reports of multidrug-resistant strains in association with HIV infection are becoming more common. It is therefore recommended that HIV-infected patients with tuberculosis be treated with a four-drug regimen.

Atypical mycobacterial infections, especially with disseminated *Mycobacterium avium intracellulare*, are commonly seen in advanced immunosuppression. *M. avium intracellulare* is a saprophytic organism of very low pathogenicity, which is common in soil and water. It is thought to enter the body through the macrophages of gastrointestinal tract or lungs and become disseminated. Testicular infection with *M. avium intracellulare* has been reported [26]. Symptoms are weight loss, fever and malaise. Associated anaemia is commonly found. Diagnosis is best made by culture of blood or bone marrow. Treatment is problematical as not only is the organism resistant *in vitro* to most antituberculous drugs but patients are usually so profoundly immunosuppressed that there is no way of eliminating the organism. None the less, symptomatic improvement can be gained using multidrug combinations based on newer drugs such as rifabutin and clarithromycin.

Fungi

In the context of HIV, *Cryptococcus* usually causes meningitis or pulmonary infection. Infection of the kidney [33] and prostate [34] have been reported. The prostate gland may act as a reservoir of cryptococci once meningitis has been treated [35]. It is a widely distributed pathogen and infection is thought to be due to inhalation of unencapsulated yeasts which then become disseminated. Typical features of meningitis such as neck stiffness and photophobia are often absent as the necessary immune response is lacking. Diagnosis is made on examination of cerebrospinal fluid and the culture of blood and cerebrospinal fluid. Serum cryptococcal antigen will be positive. Treatment is with amphotericin B. In some milder cases fluconazole may be used. Long-term secondary prophylaxis, usually with fluconazole, is required to prevent relapse.

More unusual fungi such as *Mucor* species may be found causing renal mucormycosis, an aggressive infection with a mortality of 75–100% [36]. Renal coccidiomycosis has also been documented [37]. Isolated renal aspergilloma has also been described [38] presenting with renal colic, dysuria and haematuria. Early aggressive treatment with surgery and high-dose intravenous amphotericin B is advocated for these conditions with the addition of itraconazole (in doses of 200 mg b.i.d.) if the patients do not respond.

Malignancies

HIV infection is associated with an increase in Kaposi's sarcoma and high grade B cell non-Hodgkin's lymphoma. Additional neoplastic conditions such as cervical intra-epithelial neoplasia and anal intraepithelial neoplasia are also reported with increasing frequency.

Kaposi's sarcoma

Kaposi's sarcoma, first described in 1827, is a tumour which was rare in the UK before the advent of HIV and AIDS, the annual incidence ranging from 0.02 to 0.06 per 100000 people. The classic form of the disease affects elderly men of predominantly Jewish or eastern European origin and presents as an indolent tumour of the lower limbs. A more aggressive form of the disease has been recognized in Africa which affects young adults [39]. In 1981 an increased incidence of very aggressive Kaposi's sarcoma was noted in homosexual men in New York and California which in part lead to the recognition of AIDS [2]. In the UK, HIV-related Kaposi's sarcoma is most frequently seen in homosexual men and is unusual in those infected non-sexually. In studies of people with AIDS, Kaposi's sarcoma has been found in 26% of homosexual men but only 3% of heterosexual intravenous drug users and 1% of haemophiliacs. This led to the hypothesis that a second, sexually transmitted factor is implicated in the pathogenesis of the condition [40] and indeed, the aetiological agent for Kaposi's sarcoma is now known to be Herpes hominis virus type 8 (HHV8). Kaposi's sarcoma causes considerable morbidity, both psychological and physical, and can be a direct cause of death in its more aggressive visceral form.

Kaposi's sarcoma is a multicentric tumour occurring as red/purple nodular plaques in the skin and mucous membranes, including the genitalia. The glans penis is commonly involved [41]. Kaposi's sarcoma infiltrates lymph nodes and viscera, including the bladder and prostate [1]. Bladder involvement may lead to symptoms of cystitis, and cytoscopy may be needed to make the diagnosis. Kaposi's sarcoma is rarely found in the testes and epididymis [27]. Although there are no reports of isolated clinically significant renal Kaposi's sarcoma, it is a common postmortem finding in disseminated disease [33]. Lymphoedema is common in Kaposi's sarcoma resulting both from regional lymph node involvement and also diffuse lymphatic spread. Scrotal, penile and lower limb oedema are commonly seen in the later stages. Superficial plaques are generally non-tender unless affecting weight-bearing or pressure areas.

Kaposi's sarcoma lesions consist of widely dilated vascular spaces that are lined by irregular spindle-shaped cells. A plasma cell infiltrate is seen together with proliferating vascular structures. The cell of origin of the spindle cells is not clear but they express endothelial cell markers.

Treatment of Kaposi's sarcoma is influenced by the severity of symptoms associated with the condition and the ability of the patient to tolerate therapy. Local therapy can be helpful in the control of oedema, pain if present and in improving cosmetic appearance. Cutaneous lesions respond well to local radiotherapy and good cosmetic results can be obtained. Care must be taken to control the dose of radiation when mucous membranes are involved as local postradiation complications are common [42]. Surgical excision, cautery and cryosurgery may all have a place in the management of individual lesions. Isolated lesions on the genitalia may be suitable for treatment with intralesional vinblastine. Systemic chemotherapy may be necessary for control of visceral disease with regimens containing bleomycin, vinca alkaloids and anthracyclines being the most widely used. Combinations of vincristine and bleomycin are usually reasonably well tolerated and are relatively marrow sparing. More recently, liposomal preparations of doxorubicin and daunorubicin have been introduced with encouraging early results [43]. Interferon α also has some activity against Kaposi's sarcoma, particularly when used in combination with AZT.

Non-Hodgkin's lymphoma

As therapy for HIV and many of the associated infections improve, survival is prolonged and the incidence of lymphomas increases. Large cell immunoblastic lymphoma is the commonest histological type found in association with HIV. The pathogenesis is not clear although there is likely to be a multifactorial basis including uncontrolled B cell proliferation, Epstein–Barr virus infection of cells and aberrant genetic trans-formations to induce tumour formation. Extranodal involvement at presentation is characteristic in this setting and in consequence only a minority of cases will be diagnosed on lymph node biopsy. This means that the diagnosis must be considered and appropriate biopsies taken in patients with unusual mass lesions or those with systemic 'B' symptoms. Common sites are the gastro-intestinal tract, lung, bone marrow and central nervous system. Involvement of the testes may be the presenting AIDS diagnosis [44–46]. Six to 11% of patients with lymphomas may have renal involvement demonstrable on a CT scan as either multiple renal masses or as a direct extension of retroperitoneal nodes [47]. A case of primary urethral T cell lymphoma presenting with bloodstained urethral discharge in a patient who was HIV positive has also been described [48].

Therapy is based on variations of standard chemother-apeutic regimens, but these are frequently complicated by intercurrent infection and bone marrow suppression. Use of steroids serves to immunosuppress patients further and may result in additional complications. Anaemia and neutropenia are frequently encountered as a direct effect of HIV infection and may be disastrously exacerbated by chemotherapy; the use of colony-stimulating factors (especially granulocyte colony-stimulating factors) which may limit cytopenias could lead to advances in the use of chemotherapy.

Other malignancies

Testicular seminoma can occur in patients with HIV [37,49,50] and although non-seminoma testicular tumours are thought to be more common than seminoma by some authors [51], an association between HIV infection and seminoma has been suggested by others [49,50]. One group found the incidence of seminoma in an HIV clinic (136 per 100000) to be 68 times that expected (0.4 per 50000) [49]. Secreting adrenal cell carcinoma [52] and renal cell adenocarcinoma [53] have both been reported in patients with AIDS.

Organs/syndromes

Testes and epididymis

Arrest of spermatogenesis and testicular atrophy have been consistently demonstrated in postmortem studies of patients with AIDS [1,26,27,33,54,55]. Maturation arrest is usually at the spermatocyte stage. In one study spermatozoa were seen in only five of 31 patients and then only in low numbers [27]. The low sperm count found in AIDS patients may be due to underlying factors such as chronic debility, fevers, weight loss or drug toxicity. However, these factors alone cannot explain the severity of the changes [26]. Homosexual men both with and without AIDS often have elevated serum antisperm antibody titre which has led to the hypothesis that testicular atrophy may be autoimmune in origin [27,54]. Such atrophy is, however, found in both heterosexual and homosexual men with HIV which is contradictory [56]. Human spermatogenesis can be impaired following viral infection of the genital tract (e.g. CMV). HIV has been detected in the testes, and it may be that testicular atrophy in AIDS results from a direct viral effect of HIV on the testes although the exact mechanism remains to be elucidated [55]. A reduction in Leydig cell numbers has been found in some, but not all, studies [26,27,33]. Other abnormal findings include interstitial fibrosis with basement membrane thickening [26] and chronic inflammatory infiltrate [27,55].

Voiding dysfunction

Neurological abnormalities due either to the direct effects

of HIV or to opportunist infections and tumours occur in a substantial proportion of patients with AIDS [57]. Lumbar and sacral radiculopathy may be caused by CMV, HSV and VZV. HIV is associated with both a vacuolar myelopathy in established infection and transient transverse myelitis during acute seroconversion. Central changes may be associated with HIV encephalopathy or with progressive multifocal leucencephalopathy, caused by a papovavirus infection of white matter. Such lesions may result in voiding difficulties.

In a small study, neurogenic bladder was diagnosed in nine of 11 patients with HIV referred for urodynamic studies [57]. The remaining two had benign prostatic hyperplasia. Urinary retention was the most common presenting symptom, although urinary frequency and poor urinary flow were reported. Neurological pathology included toxoplasmosis, HIV encephalopathy, myelopathy, cauda equina syndrome and cerebral lymphoma. The authors conclude that urodynamic evaluation is useful in the evaluation and proper management of voiding dysfunction in AIDS patients.

Urinary tract infection

The range of other pathological processes seen in the context of HIV (e.g. immunosuppression, voiding dysfunction and malignancy) are all potential predisposing factors for urinary tract infection (UTI). However, there are few reports dealing specifically with UTI or bacteriuria in HIV-positive individuals. Some studies have shown UTIs to be more common among sexually active homosexual men than heterosexuals [58], but this has not been confirmed [59]. Overt UTI appears to be uncommon in men with asymptomatic HIV infection although bacteriuria has been reported in up to 8% [60]. In patients with more advanced HIV infection the picture is rather different. Pyuria has been described in 52% of AIDS patients admitted to hospital with associated UTI in 20% [61]. Most were young men with no obvious predisposition to UTI. The commonest infecting organisms were *Pseudomonas* (33.3%), *E. coli* (25%) and *Klebsiella* (16%). Unusual organisms such as *Candida*, CMV and *Salmonella* were also isolated. An uncontrolled prospective study of 57 patients with symptomatic HIV infection with no other risk factors for, or history of, UTI found bacteriuria in 14% [62]. The organisms found were *E. coli*, *Enterobacter* species, *Klebsiella* species and *Pseudomonas* species (one of each). The same group carried out a controlled cross-section study of inpatients with AIDS [63] and found bacteriuria and UTI to be significantly more frequent in patients with AIDS (13.3%) than in HIV-negative inpatients (1.8%) or asymptomatic HIV-positive individuals (3%). Symptomatic UTI was seen in 6% of the AIDS patients, but in none of the other groups. *E. coli* was the predominant pathogen found. A retrospective study of 355 AIDS patients [62] found 48 *Pseudomonas* infections of which 20 were UTIs. All the patients had indwelling urinary catheters and not all were symptomatic. *Pseudomonas* and *E. coli* have both been documented as important urinary pathogens in this context [24,61,64]. Another retrospective study [1] found that 14% of 120 hospital inpatients with AIDS or AIDS-related complex had culture-proven UTI. Organisms isolated included CMV, *Cryptococcus*, *Streptococcus*, *Enterococcus* and *Gonococcus*, as well as *E. coli*. These studies have failed to find any significant difference in the incidence of urinary tract infection between homosexual and heterosexual men, confirming previous findings that the significant increase in the frequency of bacteriuria and in symptomatic UTI observed in patients with AIDS does not seem to be related to sexual orientation but rather to immune suppression [60,65].

Genital ulceration

Genital ulceration is an important clinical syndrome in HIV infection. It is increasingly clear than an association exists between the presence of genital ulcers and the transmission of HIV during sexual intercourse. Particular culprits include chancroid and early syphilis in African and Asian countries. The control of these conditions is crucial in reducing the spread of HIV infection. Whether HIV infection alters the clinical presentation or natural history of these infections is still under scrutiny.

Genital ulceration has been noted during acute primary HIV infection. Ulcers may be solitary or few in number with an irregular edge. They are tender and last for up to 10 days before healing completely. HSV and VZV (see p. 717) both cause genital ulceration with increased frequency and severity.

Iatrogenic ulceration may be seen secondarily to radiotherapy for penile Kaposi's sarcoma. Foscarnet, used for the treatment of CMV infections, may cause florid, thin-walled bullae which break down to form ulcers on the glans penis. It is a strongly alkaline drug excreted mainly through the renal tract and is also associated with chemical urethritis. Increasing fluid intake may reduce urethritis, although the dose needs to be lowered to manage penile ulceration. .

Kidney

Proteinuria may occur in up to 82% of patients with AIDS, with 10% reaching the nephrotic range [23,61,66]. It may be the presenting symptom of HIV infection in a few patients and in some cities AIDS is the most frequent cause of nephrotic syndrome in adults aged 20–50 [67]. Microscopic haematuria may occur in 15–25% [23,61] independent of other predisposing conditions. Although a variety of renal lesions have been described, attention has focused on a syndrome first recognized in patients with AIDS by Rao and associates in 1984 [68] and now referred to as HIV-associated nephropathy (HIVAN). It is characterized by a nephrotic range of proteinuria and rapidly advancing renal failure. Histologically there is focal and segmental glomerulosclerosis. The incidence of HIVAN varies widely both geographically and genetically from 10% in Brooklyn, New York to 2% at San Francisco General Hospital [66,69], possibly reflecting the different populations with HIV in those cities. Both HIVAN and heroin-associated nephropathy occur chiefly in black male patients and it has been suggested that HIVAN is a form of heroin-related nephropathy. However, the severity of renal failure in patients with HIVAN is far greater than that associated with heroin use [70] and it may occur in the absence of intravenous drug use. In one series only 49% of patients with HIVAN were intravenous drug users, the rest of the patients had other risk factors for HIV. Even in this series, however, 90% of the cases were black and 70% of them were men [71]. The cause of HIVAN has still to be elucidated; however, proviral HIV DNA has been found using *in vitro* DNA hybridization techniques in the tubular and glomerular epithelial cells of patients with HIVAN [72]. Whether HIV alone can cause HIVAN or whether other viruses (e.g. CMV), drug misuse, genetic factors, or a combination of all these are also necessary remains to be elucidated. The prognosis of HIVAN, particularly in patients who already have AIDS is unfavourable, with rapid deterioration in renal function mostly resulting in end-stage renal disease within a few weeks [68]. Treatment of HIVAN has not been established. There is no evidence that treatment with steroids or cyclosporin are of any benefit [73], but successful treatment with AZT has been reported [74].

Occupational exposure

As the incidence of HIV infection rises so urologists will become increasingly involved in the management of the condition, either directly in the urogenital tract manifestations or indirectly as coincidental HIV infection in the general urological setting. The majority of the latter group of patients may be unaware of their HIV status. HIV has been isolated from blood, semen, cervical secretions, cerebrospinal fluid, saliva, tears, breast milk and urine [75]. The concentration of virus in each of these body fluids is variable and not all are known to transmit infection. Occupational transmission of HIV to health care workers has been documented [76,77]. Parenteral and mucous membrane exposure to infected blood are the commonest risks.

Occupational exposure as a possible cause for sero-conversion has been reported in four cases in surgeons in the USA [78]. A study from San Francisco reported that the knowledge of a patient's HIV status did not alter the rate at which surgeons contaminated themselves with blood, or sustained penetrating injuries during operations [79]. Studies coordinated by the CDC in the USA [80] have provided an estimate of the risk of acquiring HIV infection following substantial parenteral exposure to HIV-infected material. Seroconversion was recorded for six of 1962 individuals who had a total of 2008 needlestick injuries producing a risk of one in 320 exposures. Needlestick injury to the finger pulp is considered to be low risk [80]. Although HIV has been cultured in low titre from urine samples [81], no cases of seroconversion after exposure to urine have been reported [79]. A study of 61 health care workers who performed or assisted in procedures involving exposure to the urine of HIV-positive patients found none to be HIV positive [82]. In the USA the CDC does not consider urine, unless it is bloodstained, to be a fluid against which full universal precautions are necessary [75].

Policies should be instituted to minimize the opportunity for nosocomial transmission and direct contact with potentially infected body substances should be avoided. In urology this means preventing parenteral and mucous membrane exposures to blood, semen and urine. The splashing of blood, urine and irrigation solutions over the face and eyes have all been reported [83,84] and occur commonly, accounting for 46% of contaminations during endoscopic procedures [84]. Impervious gowns and boots should be worn where substantial exposure to infected body fluids is anticipated [85].

The prevention of needlestick injuries, particularly from hollow needles, is important in reducing the risk of occupational transmission of HIV. No cases of seroconversion after injury from suture or other solid needles has been reported [86,87]. The passing of sharp instruments should be done with care and the practice of resheathing needles be stopped. All sharps should be placed safely into approved containers as soon as possible. Double gloving reduces the risk of contamination of the hands with blood and may reduce the incidence of needlestick injuries [79]. Any cuts or abrasions should be covered with waterproof dressings [88]. In cases of needlestick or other 'high risk' injury from a patient known to be HIV positive, antiretroviral postexposure prophylaxis should be offered after appropriate counselling in accordance with local guidelines. A four-week course of AZT in combination with lamivudine and also a protease inhibitor such as indinavir is usual and is best started within 1–2 hours of the injury. Starter packs should be available at all times to avoid delay in commencing postexposure prophylaxis.

There is one reported incident of documented patient-to-patient transmission [89] among patients operated upon by a surgeon on the same day. The exact mode of transmission

is not known, but the case emphasizes the need for rigorous infection control procedures and the proper sterilization of equipment between patients.

The potential risks of infection of a patient by an infected surgeon also merit some discussion. Other than one case of a Florida dentist with AIDS transmitting HIV to five patients, there have been no documented cases of transmission of HIV from an infected surgeon to a patient [90,91]. Patients who have been found to be HIV positive after being operated on by HIV-positive surgeons were all found to have other non-hospital-associated risks for HIV.

In the UK, the Department of Health does not consider compulsory testing for surgeons to be justified [91,92]. Such a policy is regarded as discriminatory, an infringement of individuals' rights and to deter those in most need from seeking counselling, education and advice. In addition, the organization, administration and costs of such a screening programme would be enormous, especially as testing would have to be repeated every 3 months. Guidelines for health care workers infected with HIV were issued by the Department of Health [92] which re-emphasizes the ethical, legal and professional obligation of health care workers who believe that they have been exposed to HIV in seeking testing and advice.

Conclusion

Although it acts as a significant vector for its transmission, the urinary tract seems to be relatively spared from symptomatic involvement in HIV infection. Nevertheless, urologists must be aware of the various issues surrounding HIV: patients may require urological consultation or intervention because of the urinary tract manifestations of HIV, or HIV-positive patients may have coincident urological problems. In addition, many people are unaware that they are HIV positive or may choose to withhold this information from the urologist. Most HIV-related conditions affect the urinary tract only as a manifestation of disseminated disease, but there are some notable exceptions and urologists should be alert to some of the clinical presentations of conditions that can cause urinary symptoms in HIV and AIDS.

References

1 Miles BJ, Melser M, Farah R, Markowitz N, Fisher E. The urological manifestations of the acquired immunodeficiency syndrome. *J Urol* 1989;**142**:771–3.
2 Weekly Epidemiological Record, Centres for Disease Control. *Pneumocystis* pneumonia—Los Angeles. *Morbid Mortal Weekly Rep* 1981;**30**:250.
3 Centres for Disease Control. Kaposi's sarcoma and *Pneumocystis* pneumonia among homosexual men. *Morbid Mortal Weekly Rep* 1981;**30**:305.
4 Gottlieb MS, Schroff R, Schranker HM *et al. Pneumocystis*

carinii pneumonia and mucosal candidiasis in previously healthy homosexual men. *N Engl J Med* 1981;**305**:1425.

5 World Health Organization Global Program on AIDS: Mertens TE, Belsey E, Stoneburner RL *et al.* Global estimates and epidemiology of HIV-1 infections and AIDS: further heterogeneity of spread and impact. *AIDS* 1995;**9**(Suppl. A):S252–72.

6 BHIVA Guidelines Coordinating Committee: Gazzard BG, Moyle GJ, Weber J *et al.* British HIV Association guidelines for antiretroviral treatment of HIV seropositive individuals. *Lancet* 1997;**349**:1086–92.

7 National Center for Infectious Diseases Division of HIV/AIDS: Castro KG, Ward JW, Slutsker L *et al.* Revised classification system for HIV infection and expanded case definition for AIDS among adolescents and adults. *Morbid Mortal Weekly Rep* 1992;**41**(RR-17):1–19.

8 Cooper DA, Maclean P, Finlayson R *et al.* Acute AIDS retrovirus infection. Definition of a clinical illness associated with seroconversion. *Lancet* 1985;**1**:537.

9 Biggar RJ, Johnson BK, Musoke SS *et al.* Severe illness associated with the appearance of antibody to human immunodeficiency virus in an African. *Br Med J* 1986;**293**: 1210–11.

10 Tindall B, Barker S, Donovan B *et al.* Characterization of the acute clinical illness associated with human immunodeficiency virus infection. *Arch Intern Med* 1988;**148**:945–9.

11 Curran JW, Jaffe H, Hardy A *et al.* Epidemiology of HIV infection and AIDS in the United States. *Science* 1988;**239**:610.

12 Melbye M, Goedert JJ, Blattner WA. The natural history of human immunodeficiency virus infection. In: Gottlieb MS, Jeffries DJ, Mildvan D *et al. Current Topics in AIDS*, Vol. 1. Chichester: John Wiley, 1987:57–93.

13 Doweiko JP. Haematologic aspects of HIV infection. *AIDS* 1993;**7**:753–7.

14 Bargman JM, Wagner C, Cameron R. Renal cortical nephrocalcinosis: a manifestation of extra pulmonary *Pneumocystis carinii* in the acquired immune deficiency syndrome. *Am J Kidney Dis* 1991;**17**:712–15.

15 Montgomery AB, Luce JM, Turner J *et al.* Aerosolised pentamidine as sole therapy for *Pneumocystis carinii* pneumonia in patients with acquired immunodeficiency syndrome. *Lancet* 1987;**2**:480–3.

16 Krick JA, Remington JS. Toxoplasmosis in the adult: an overview. *N Engl J Med* 1978;**298**:550–3.

17 Nistal M, Santana A, Paniagua R, Palacios J. Testicular toxoplasmosis in two men with the acquired immunodeficiency syndrome (AIDS). *Arch Pathol Lab Med* 1986;**110**: 744–6.

18 Haskell L, Fusco MJ, Ares L, Sublay B. Case report; disseminated toxoplasmosis presenting as symptomatic orchitis and nephrotic syndrome. *Am J Med Sci* 1989;**298**: 185–90.

19 Molina J-M, Belenfant X, Doco-Lecompt T, Idatte J-M, Modai J. Sulphadiazine-induced crystalluria in AIDS patients with *Toxoplasma* encephalitis. *AIDS* 1991;**5**:587–9.

20 Simon DI, Brosius FC III, Rothstein DM. Sulphadiazine crystalluria revisited: the treatment of *Toxoplasma* encephalitis in patients with acquired immune deficiency syndrome. *Arch Intern Med* 1990;**150**:2379–84.

21 Meyers SA, Kuhlman JE, Fishman EK. Entero vesical fistula in a patient with cryptosporidiosis and AIDS—CT demonstration. *Clin Imaging* 1990;**14**:143–5.

22 Thomas JA, Antony AJ. Amoebiasis of the penis. *Br J Urol* 1976;**48**:269–73.

23 Gardenswartz MH, Lerner CW, Seligson GR *et al.* Renal disease in patients with AIDS: a clinicopathological study. *Clin Nephrol* 1984;**21**:197–204.

24 O'Regan S, Russo P, Lapointe N, Rousseau E. AIDS and the urinary tract. *J Acquir Immune Defic Syndr* 1990;**3**:244–51.

25 Reiser IW, Shapiro WB, Porush JG. The incidence and epidemiology of human immunodeficiency virus infection in 320 patients treated in an inner city haemodialysis centre. *Am J Kidney Dis* 1990;**16**:26–31.

26 De Paepe ME, Waxman M. Testicular atrophy in AIDS: a study of 57 autopsy cases. *Human Pathol* 1989;**20**:210–14.

27 Dalton ADA, Harcourt-Webster JN. The histopathology of the testes and epididymis in AIDS—a post mortem study. *J Pathol* 1991;**163**:47–52.

28 Da Silva M, Chevchuk MM, Cronin WJ *et al.* Detection of HIV related protein in testes and prostates of patients with AIDS. *Am J Clin Pathol* 1990;**93**:196–201.

29 Randazzo RF, Hulette CM, Gottleib MS *et al.* Cytomegalovirus epididymitis in a patient with acquired immune deficiency syndrome. *J Urol* 1986;**136**:1095–7.

30 Benson MC, Kaplan MS, O'Toole K, Romagnoli M. A report of cytomegalovirus cystitis and a review of other genito-urinary manifestations of the acquired immune deficiency syndrome. *J Urol* 1987;**140**:153–4.

31 Lucas SB, Parr DC, Wright E, Papadaki L, Patou G. AIDS presenting as cytomegalovirus cystitis. *Br J Urol* 1989;**64**: 429–30.

32 De Gans J, Portegies P. Neurological complications of infection with the human immunodeficiency virus type 1: a review. *Clin Neurol Neurosurg* 1989;**91**:197–217.

33 Welch, Finkbeiner W, Alpers CE *et al.* Autopsy findings in acquired immune deficiency syndrome. *J Am Med Assoc* 1984;**252**:1152–9.

34 Lief M, Sarfarazi F. Prostatic cryptococcosis in acquired immune deficiency syndrome. *Urology* 1986;**28**:318–19.

35 Larsen RA, Bozzette S, McCutchan JA *et al.* Persistent *Cryptococcus neoformans* infection of the prostate after successful treatment of meningitis. *Ann Intern Med* 1989;**111**: 125.

36 Vesa J, Bielsa O, Arango O, Llado C, Gelabert A. Massive renal infarction due to mucormycosis in an AIDS patient. *Infection* 1992;**20**:234–6.

37 Green ST, Nathwani D, Goldberg DJ, Paterson PJ, Kennedy DH. Urological manifestations of HIV related disease. *Br J Urol* 1991;**67**:188–90.

38 Halpern M, Szabo S, Hochberg E *et al.* Renal aspergilloma: an unusual cause of infection in a patient with the acquired immunodeficiency syndrome. *Am J Med* 1992;**92**:437–40.

39 Bayley AC. Occurrence, clinical behaviour and management of Kaposi's sarcoma in Zambia. *Cancer Surv* 1991;**10**:53–71.

40 Beral V, Petermann TA, Berkelman RL, Jaffe HW. Kaposi's sarcoma among persons with AIDS: a sexually transmitted infection? *Lancet* 1990;**335**:123–8.

41 Seftel AD, Sadick NS, Waldbaum RS. Kaposi's sarcoma of the penis in a patient with the acquired immunodeficiency syndrome. *J Urol* 1986;**136**:673–5.

42 Chak LY, Gill PS, Levine AM *et al.* Radiation therapy for acquired immunodeficiency syndrome related Kaposi's sarcoma. *J Clin Oncol* 1988;**6**:863–7.

43 Milliken S, Boyle MJ. Update on HIV and neoplastic disease. *AIDS* 1993;7(Suppl. 1):S203–9.

44 Rogers C, Klatt EC. Pathology of the testes in acquired immunodeficiency syndrome. *Histopathology* 1988;12:659–65.

45 Tirelli U, Rezza G, Lazzarin A *et al*. Malignant lymphoma related HIV infection in Italy: a report of 46 cases. *J Am Med Assoc* 1987;258:2064.

46 Levine AM, Gill PS, Meyer PR *et al*. Retrovirus and malignant lymphoma in homosexual men. *J Am Med Assoc* 1985;254:1921.

47 Kuhlman JE, Browne D, Shermak M *et al*. Retroperitoneal and pelvic CT of patients with AIDS: primary and secondary involvement of the genito-urinary tract. *RadioGraphics* 1991;11:473–83.

48 Khan DG, Rothman PJ, Weismann JD. Urethral T-cell lymphoma as the initial manifestation of the acquired immune deficiency syndrome. *Arch Pathol Lab Med* 1991;115:1169–70.

49 Moyle G, Hawkins DA, Gazzard BG. Seminoma and HIV infections. *Int J STD AIDS* 1991;2:293–4.

50 Palmer MC, Mador DR, Venner PM. Testicular seminoma associated with the acquired immunodeficiency syndrome (AIDS) and acquired immunodeficiency syndrome related complex: two cases. *J Urol* 1989;142:128–30.

51 Tessler AN, Cantanese A. AIDS and germ cell tumours of testes. *Urology* 1987;30:203–4.

52 Pedretti G, Magnani G, Guazzi AM, Nizzoli R, Fiaccadori R. Secreting adrenal carcinoma in an HIV infected patient. *AIDS* 1993;7:594.

53 Azon-Masoliver A, Moreno A, Gatell JM, Mascaro JM. Renal cell adenocarcinoma associated with AIDS related Kaposi's sarcoma. *AIDS* 1990;4:818–19.

54 Chabon AB, Stenger RJ, Grabstald H. Histopathology of testes in acquired immune deficiency syndrome. *Urology* 1987;29:658–63.

55 Pudney J, Anderson D. Orchitis and human immunodeficiency virus type 1 infected cells in reproductive tissues from men with the acquired immune deficiency syndrome. *Am J Pathol* 1991;139:149–60.

56 De Paepe ME, Vuletin JC, Lee MH, Rojas-Corona RR, Waxman M. Testicular atrophy in homosexual patients: an immune mediated phenomenon? *Human Pathol* 1989;20:572–8.

57 Khan Z, Singh VK, Yang WC. Neurogenic bladder in acquired immune deficiency syndrome (AIDS). *Urology* 1992;40:289–91.

58 Barnes RC, Roddy RE, Daifuku R, Stamm WE. Urinary tract infection in sexually active homosexual men *Lancet* 1986;1:171–3.

59 Wilson AP, Tovey SJ, Adler MW, Gruneberg RN. Prevalence of urinary tract infection in homosexual and heterosexual men. *Genitourin Med* 1986;62:189–90.

60 Welch J, Pilkington H, Bradbeer C. Urinary tract infections in men. *Br Med J* 1989;229:184.

61 Kaplan MS, Wechsler M, Benson MC. Urologic manifestations of AIDS. *Urology* 1987;30(5):441–3.

62 De Pinho AMF, Maranconi DV, Moreira BM *et al*. Bacteria in patients with CDC group IV manifestations: a prospective study. *AIDS* 1991;5(3):342.

63 De Pinho AMF, Lopes GS, Ramos-Filho CF *et al*. Urinary tract infection in men with AIDS. *Genitourin Med* 1994;70:30–4.

64 Franzetti F, Cernuschi M, Eposito R, Moroni M. *Pseudomonas* infections in patients with AIDS and AIDS-related complex. *J Int Med* 1992;231:437–43.

65 Hoepelman AIM, van Buren NM, van den Broek J, Borleffs JCC. Bacteriuria in men with HIV 1 is related to the their immune status (CD4+ cell count). *AIDS* 1992;6:179–84.

66 Schoenfeld P, Feduska NJ. Acquired immunodeficiency syndrome and renal disease: report of the National Kidney Foundation—National Instititutes of Health task force on AIDS and kidney disease. *Am J Kidney Dis* 1990;16:14–25.

67 Bourgoignie JJ, Meneses R, Ortiz C *et al*. The clinical spectrum of renal disease associated with human immunodeficiency virus. *Am J Kidney Dis* 1988;12:131–7.

68 Rao TK, Filippone EJ, Nicastri AD *et al*. Associated focal and segmental glomerulosclerosis in the acquired immunodeficiency syndrome. *N Engl J Med* 1984;310:669–73.

69 Humphries MH. Human immunodeficiency virus associated nephropathy—east is east and west is west? *Arch Intern Med* 1990;150:253–4.

70 Langs C, Gallow GR, Schacht RG, Sidhu G, Baldwin DS. Rapid renal failure in acquired immunodeficiency syndrome associated focal glomerulosclerosis. *Arch Intern Med* 1990;150:287–92.

71 Glassock RJ, Cohen AH, Danovich G, Parser KP. Human immunodeficiency virus (HIV) infection and the kidney. *Ann Intern Med* 1990;112:35–49.

72 Cohen AH, Sun NCJ, Shapshak P, Imagawa DT. Demonstration of human immunodeficiency virus in renal epithelium in HIV associated nephropathy. *Mod Pathol* 1989;2:125–8.

73 Seney FD J, Burns DK, Silva FG. Acquired immunodeficiency syndrome and the kidney. *Am J Kidney Dis* 1990;16:1–13.

74 Harrer T, Hunzelmann N, Stoll R, Baur A, Kalden J-R. Therapy for HIV 1 related nephritis with zidovudine. *AIDS* 1990;4:815–16.

75 McMahon Casey K. Safety precautions for health care workers. In: DeVita VT Jr, Hellman S, Rosenberg S, eds. *AIDS: Etiology, Diagnosis, Treatment and Prevention*. Philadelphia: JB Lipincott, 1992:517–26.

76 Editorial. Needlestick transmission of HTLV III from a patient infected in Africa. *Lancet* 1984;2:1376.

77 Neisson-Vernant C, Arfi S, Mathez D, Leibowitch J, Monplaisir N. Needlestick HIV seroconversion in a nurse. *Lancet* 1986;2:814.

78 Centres for Disease Control. 1989 guidelines for prevention of transmission of human immunodeficiency virus and hepatitis B virus to health care and public safety workers. *Morbid Mortal Weekly Rep* 1989;38(Suppl. S6).

79 Gerberding JL, Littell C, Tarkington T, Brown A, Schecter WP. Risk of exposure of surgical personnel to patient's blood during surgery at San Francisco General Hospital. *N Engl J Med* 1990;322:1788–93.

80 Centres for Disease Control Co-operative Needlestick Surveillance Group. Surveillance of health care workers exposed to blood from patients infected with HIV. *N Engl J Med* 1988;319:1118–23.

81 Levy JA, Kaminsky LS, Morrow WJ. Infection by the retrovirus associated with the acquired immunodeficiency syndrome. Clinical, biological and molecular features. *Ann Intern Med* 1983;103:694.

82 Gerberding JL, Bryant-LeBlanc CE, Nelson K *et al*. Risk of transmitting the human immunodeficiency virus, cytomegalovirus and hepatitis B virus to health care workers exposed to patients with AIDS and AIDS-related conditions. *J Infect Dis* 1987;156:1–8.

83 Hagen MD, Klemens B, Meyer MD, Paukar SG. Routine preoperative screening for HIV. Does the risk to the surgeon outweigh the risk to the patient? *J Am Med Assoc* 1988;**259**: 1357–9.

84 Davis JH, Harrison GSM. Should urologists wear spectacles for transurethral resection of the prostate? *Br J Urol* 1991;**67**: 182–3.

85 Kreiger JN. The acquired immunodeficiency syndrome: prudent precautions for the practising urologist. *J Urol* 1988; **139**:801–2.

86 Joint Working Party for the Hospital Infection Society and the Surgeon Infection Study Group. Risk to surgeons and patients from HIV and hepatitis: guidelines on precautions and management of exposure to blood, or body fluids. *Br Med J* 1992;**305**:1337–42.

87 Working Group of the Royal College of Pathologists. HIV Infection: *Hazards of Transmission to Patients and Health Care Workers during Invasive Procedures.* London: London Royal College of Pathologists, 1992.

88 Centres for Disease Control. Update: human immunodeficiency virus infections in health care workers exposed to blood of infected patients. *Morbid Mortal Weekly Rep* 1987;**36**: 285–9.

89 Chant K, Lowe D, Rubin G *et al.* Patient-to-patient transmission of HIV in private surgical consulting rooms. *Lancet* 1993;**342**:1548–9.

90 Mishu B, Schaffner W, Horan JM *et al.* A surgeon with AIDS: lack of evidence of transmission to patients. *J Am Med Assoc* 1990;**264**:467–70.

91 Cockcroft A. Compulsory HIV testing for surgeons? *Br J Hosp Med* 1992;**47**:602–4.

92 Department of Health. *AIDS–HIV Infected Health Care Workers: Guidance on the Management of Infected Health Care Workers.* London: Department of Health, 1994.

Section 5
Calculous Disease

56   The History of Stone Disease
P. Alken and C. Dawson

Historical perspective of the treatment of urinary calculi

C. DAWSON

The oldest stone so far discovered is a 7000-year-old bladder calculus found among the pelvic bones of a teenage boy in a prehistoric tomb at El Amara. It is doubtful that treatment for stones was available at this time, and there is no evidence for the practice of lithotomy in Ancient Egypt. Later Egyptian surgical treatments were described by the Italian physician, Prospero Alpino, in the sixteenth century.

Medicine in India was first described in the *Ayurveda*. This sacred book was said to have been handed down by Buddha, and then passed to mankind through Susruta. Susruta is thought to have been the author of the *Ayurveda* and also the *Susruta Samhita*. Although his understanding of anatomy and physiology was rather vague, he describes well the symptoms of renal colic, said to be due to stones formed from 'phlegm, bile, air or semen'. Hindu treatments for stones relied mostly on a vegetarian diet, and exercise was recommended. Charaka (first century AD), physician to the King of Indo-Scythia, described the extraction of urethral calculi using a hook. Susruta advised lithotomy for stones failing to respond to medical treatments, although he was quick to point out the dangers. He advised caution, and suggested a sacrifice and the surgeon's prayer to Isvara before the operation commenced. His account of lithotomy is very similar to that of Celsus (see below), and it is highly likely that the operation was introduced into Asia by the conquering armies of Alexander the Great.

Primitive medicine was greatly advanced by the Greek and Roman physicians. The most famous of these is Hippocrates, born in 460 BC, the son of a physician, on the island of Cos. He had remarkable powers of observation and, despite a lack of detailed anatomical knowledge, was the author of many learned works. Hippocrates was aware of the existence of urinary stones and wrote about various kidney disorders. His works contain a description of the incision of a perinephric abscess which resulted from stone disease. Hippocrates appears to have been aware of the existence of lithotomy, for in his famous *Oath* he stated 'I will not cut persons labouring under the stone but will leave this to be done by practitioners of this work'. It is not clear why Hippocrates objected to lithotomy, although it may have been in an attempt to keep the reputation of physicians untarnished from the association with a procedure with so poor a success rate and with so many complications. It has also been suggested that difficulties in translating his words may have led to a misunderstanding, and that in actual fact he was banning *castration*, a practice which was strongly opposed by Greek culture. This view has been challenged. Whatever the case, and because of his undoubted eminence, his words were heeded by physicians for centuries, with the result that stone surgery was left to itinerant surgeons.

The term lithotomy was first used by the Greek surgeon Ammonius (276 BC) to describe his technique of cutting or breaking the stone (*lithotomus*) to facilitate its removal. The technique of lithotomy was first properly described by the Roman physician Celsus (25 BC to 25 AD). The description below, from his book *De Re Medicina*, was handed down virtually unchanged for the next 1500 years, such was the lack of further progress in this area.

> The surgeon, whose nails should be carefully pared, dips the index and middle fingers of the left hand in oil and introduces them gently into the anus....He presses the fingers of the right hand on the lower abdomen....The stone must be sought near the neck of the bladder....If it is not at the bladder neck or if it is situated further back, the fingers must be passed more deeply into the anus....To this purpose, one must push forwards with the fingers of the left hand whilst the right hand, placed on the abdomen, prevents it from falling back, until it reaches the bladder neck....Once the stone is engaged, an incision is made in the skin over the bladder, near the anus, down to the bladder neck....Then in the deepest and most narrow part of this incision a second transverse opening is made, opening the bladder neck, so that a hole

allowing urine to escape is made and the hole is larger than the stone.

Celsus recommended that this procedure be performed only in patients between the ages of 9 and 14 years, and only in the springtime. Persistent haemorrhage after the operation was treated by sitting the patient in strong vinegar and salt. Damage to the rectum sometimes occurred and postoperative incontinence of urine was common. Later names for this procedure were 'cutting on the gripe' and the 'petit appareil' (or 'apparatus minor'), due to the small number of instruments required.

The technique of lithotomy described by Celsus continued to be practised with little alteration until the eighteenth century, but at the beginning of the sixteenth century a new technique was developed which eventually superseded the former. The operation was devised by Giovanni de Romanis of Cremona, but became known through the writings of his student Marianus Sanctus de Barletta (1490-1550), in his book *Libellus aureus*, from whence if coined the name 'Marian operation'. The dissection in this new procedure was similar to that for the *petit appareil* of Celsus, but the innovative step was the use of a urethral sound to act as a guide to the urethra. This allowed the lithotomist to be sure that his incision would enter the bladder neck, and gave rise to the later name of 'cutting on the staff'.

Having passed the grooved sound to identify the urethra, the surgeon cut down onto the sound with a knife known as the novacula, dividing the tissues down to the bladder neck. The description by Marianus suggests that the bladder neck was not incised for fear of subsequent incontinence, but this point was modified by later surgeons. A gorget was passed into the wound along the groove of the urethral sound and was followed by two conductores which served to open up the wound to allow the passage of the dilator (aperiens). If the wound was still too small then other retractors (latera) were available. Finally the stone was grasped with forceps and removed, after crushing if necessary, although Marianus advised against this. The *grand appareil* (so-called because of the larger number of instruments required) was adopted by many lithotomists including Pierre Franco, Ambroise Paré and the Colot family.

The need for a procedure with greater success and fewer complications was always in the forefront of the lithotomist's mind but it was eventually revealed from the least likely source. Jacques de Beaulieu was born at Beaufort in Burgundy in 1651. His parents were poor and his education was meagre as a result. He served for 5 years as a trooper in the French cavalry, and on his discharge became apprenticed to Pauloni, an itinerant Italian lithotomist. It was from Pauloni that he learnt the techniques of the *petit appareil* and the *grand appareil*, after which

he travelled throughout Provence as an itinerant lithotomist. Between 1688 and 1690 he adopted monk-like clothes and began to call himself Frère Jacques. It was about this time that he began to use a lateral incision for his lithotomy. In 1697 he went to Paris to show off his new technique of cutting for the stone. Armed with 'certificates of cure' he applied for permission to cut at the Charité and the Hôtel Dieu. The surgeons at these two hospitals demanded first a demonstration on a cadaver, in the presence of Méry, the First Surgeon of the Hôtel Dieu. Although Méry was very impressed with Frère Jacques' technique his favourable opinion changed after two further demonstrations by Jacques, who subsequently left Paris and went to Fontainebleu. After a successful stay of 3–4 months he returned to Paris to apply again for permission to cut at the Hôtel Dieu. Further failures hailed a downturn in his popularity. In a 4-month period he cut 60 patients, curing only 13 of them. Twenty-five patients died and the remainder were left with crippling injuries. The final insult to Jacques' reputation was the death of the Maréchal de Lorges following surgery by Frére Jacques.

The difficulties experienced by surgeons performing perineal lithotomy have already been mentioned, but none were so great as to overcome the apprehension felt by all of opening the bladder from above. Indeed, the first recorded suprapubic lithotomy, performed by Pierre Franco in 1556, was only done so in a moment of severe difficulty encountered while performing a lithotomy in a child of 2 years. Finding it impossible to bring the stone down, and at the request of the parents, he agreed to cut above the symphysis pubis. In Franco's words:

I shall relate what once happened to me in trying to remove a stone from a child aged two or thereabouts, in whom, finding a stone as big as a hen's egg, more or less, I did all that I could to bring it down, and seeing that with all my efforts I made no progress, and that the patient was marvellously tormented and that the parents hoped that he might die rather than live in such agony, and also that I should not be reproached for not having been able to extract it (which was very foolish of me), I decided in view of the importunity of the father, mother and friends, to cut the child above the pubic bone, in as much as the stone would not come down, and made the incision a little to one side over the stone, for I lifted this with my fingers pressed on the fundament, and on the other side, holding it steady with the hands of an assistant who compressed the little stomach above the stone, from which it was removed by this means, and afterwards the patient was cured (notwithstanding he was extremely sick), and the wound healed. However, I advise men not to do this but rather to use the method invented by us (the *grand appareil*) in two stages.

Although discarded by Franco, the high operation (which

also became known as the *haut appareil*) was used with success by John Douglas (brother of James Douglas, who described the retrovesical pouch). His experience was recorded in a book titled *Lithotomia Douglassiana* published in 1722.

Complications of surgery were common, particularly haemorrhage, infection and incontinence. Damage to the bladder and rectum happened not infrequently and patients were left in hospital to die an undignified death. Their willingness to submit to such operations is almost beyond belief but the pain of a bladder stone was known to be intense, and patients would often prefer to die at the surgeon's hands than to continue to suffer the pain. Perhaps the most interesting case in the literature concerns that of Jan de Doot, a Dutch blacksmith, who in 1651 removed his own bladder stone with a kitchen knife while his wife was away at the market.

The beginning of the nineteenth century saw the introduction of yet another method of dealing with bladder stones. Lithotrity was first introduced by Jean Civiale in Paris in 1823, using an instrument called a trilabe which he designed himself while a medical student. This consisted of two straight coaxial tubes which ended in three spreading arms designed to grip and hold a stone in the bladder. The stone was then crushed by an iron rod passed up the instrument. Civiale is said to have operated on 1600 patients using this technique. The first lithotrity in the UK was performed by Baron Heurteloup, a Frenchman, in 1829.

The earliest instrument (such as those of Civiale) were drilling lithotrites, where the stone was grasped by forceps and drilled by an instrument passed up the centre. Advances in design quickly followed and lithotrites relying on percussion, or a screw, were developed. The modern lithotrite, consisting of two parallel blades closed by a screw thread, was probably designed by Charrière.

Perhaps the most famous advocate of this technique was Sir Henry Thompson, who in 1858, at the age of 38, travelled to Paris to learn lithotrity from Civiale. He rose to fame following his treatment of two patients in particular. The first of these, King Leopold I of Belgium, had previously received treatment from Civiale himself, although this had failed. Thompson was summoned and two treatments were all that were required to rid the king of his bladder stone. Thompson returned to England richer for this experience, and was knighted in 1867. His second distinguished patient was Charles Louis Napoleon Bonaparte who in 1852, after a *coup d'état*, became Emperor Napoleon III of France. His first symptoms appeared about 4 years after seizing power and over the next few years became more frequent and more intense. His symptoms worsened just before the outbreak of the Franco-Prussian war which was declared on 19 July 1870. On 2 September the emperor had reached Sedan where his army became surrounded by a quarter of a million German troops. Such

was the intensity of his symptoms that he is reputed to have exposed himself to the enemy fire. Surrender followed, and the emperor was exiled to England. On 26 December Thompson performed a bladder sounding which confirmed the diagnosis of a bladder stone. Lithority was performed on 2 January 1873 and stone and debris were removed. Over the next few days the emperor's symptoms worsened until a second lithotrity was performed to remove a fragment of stone impacted at the bladder neck. Following this the condition of the emperor continued to decline until on 9 January 1873 he lapsed into a coma and died. Autopsy showed gross pyonephrosis, with a large stone still present in the bladder.

The reader will be aware that the preceding account concentrates on the treatment of bladder stone, and this reflects in no small measure the great majority of bladder stones which existed during the periods described.

Kidney surgery was opposed by Hippocrates, Celsus and Galen because it was felt to lead to fatal complications. Although it is known that stones were removed from a renal abscess or sinus during the fifteenth century, the first recorded nephrolithotomy was in 1474 on a French archer in the town of Bagnolet. The operation was a success and the man survived for many years.

In the early sixteenth century, Cardan of Milan opened a lumbar abscess and described in detail the removal of 18 stones. In the latter part of the seventeenth century experiments on dogs showed that unilateral nephrectomy was not fatal, but despite this nephrectomy in humans was derided. The situation remained the same until the mid-nineteenth century when a number of discoveries occurred which made safe operating possible — in particular the discovery of the anaesthetic properties of ether and the development of antisepsis by Lister.

It fell to Gustave Simon of Heidelberg to perform the first nephrectomy for stone in 1869, using both antisepsis and anaesthesia. Unhappily the patient died 3 weeks later of septicaemia. Sir Henry Morris, Surgeon to the Middlesex Hospital, performed the first recorded nephrolithotomy and also showed that the risk of haemorrhage was less if the renal pelvis was incised posteriorly.

Further reading

1 Murphy LJT. Urology in ancient times in the Orient. In: *The History of Urology*. Springfield, Illinois: Charles C Thomas, 1972:5–17.

2 Riches E. The history of lithotomy and lithotrity. *Ann R Coll Surg Engl* 1968;**43**:185.

3 Goldman IL, Resnick MI, Buck AC. The history of urinary lithiasis and its treatment. In: Wickham JEA, Buck AC, eds. *Renal Tract Stone. Metabolic Basis and Clinical Practice*. Edinburgh: Churchill Livingstone, 1990:3–18.

4 Hippocrates. *The Genuine Works of Hippocrates*. Sydenham Society, 1849.

5 Thomalla JV. The myth of stone. Lithotomy history and the Hippocratic oath. *Indiana Med* 1989;**82**:434–9.
6 Ellis H. *A History of Bladder Stone*. Oxford: Blackwell Scientific Publications, 1969:1–77.
7 Murphy LJT. Urology in Greece and Rome. In: *The History of Urology*. Springfield, Illinois: Charles C Thomas, 1972:18–33.
8 Murphy LJT. Lithotomy and lithotomists. In: *The History of Urology*. Springfield, Illinois: Charles C Thomas, 1972:90–123.
9 Lin JI. Vesical calculus, lithotrity, and Napoleon III. *N Y State J Med* 1989;**89**:472–5.

Modern history of stone disease

P. ALKEN

Experimental and clinical work on urolithiasis has always covered two different fields: stone formation and prevention, (i.e. the physicochemical and metabolic part of urolithiasis) and stone removal, (i.e. the surgical part). Between the 1960s and early 1980s, when urological surgeons concentrated on the small but difficult area of staghorn stone removal, a wealth of information on stone formation and prevention was imparted, mostly by non-urological researchers. A series of international symposia on urolithiasis and related clinical research started in Leeds in 1968 and continued at 4-yearly intervals in Madrid, Davos, Williamsburg, Garmisch-Partenkirchen and finally in Cairns in 1992. The proceedings of these conferences and those of the international conferences in Perth 1979 and Singapore 1983 still serve as the most important guidelines for metabolic and related problems of urolithiasis. Participation in these conferences rapidly expanded and the steadily increasing number of abstracts led to the typical change in style of large meetings with parallel poster sessions. Up to the late 1970s, surgical topics were not usually included or were only found in the 'plumber's corner', attracting only a limited interest by the 'metabolists'.

The first World Congress on Percutaneous Renal Surgery [1], organized by Wickham in 1983 in London, marked a historical change, because it was the first international meeting exclusively devoted to stone removal. Annual meetings followed worldwide with changing titles and topics. The Annual Symposium on Extracorpeal Shock Wave Lithotripsy (ESWL) began in 1985 in Indianapolis and the International Society of Urologic Endoscopy joined the World Congress on Endourology and ESWL in 1990.

Currently, the World Congress on Endourology and ESWL is the most important and heavily sponsored international meeting on urolithiasis, although today it covers many other aspects of urology. Unfortunately, the urologists have not yet reserved a corner for the 'metabolists' who are reverting back to workshop-type meetings again. Thus there is still a gap between the two important topics of urolithiasis.

The present situation is best described in the preface of the special issue of the *Journal of Urology* [2] on the Consensus Development Conference on the prevention and treatment of kidney stones.

Those of us who have devoted our working lives to the study of kidney stones may hardly be surprised that the National Institutes of Health chose to convene a Consensus Development Conference on our subject, nor be in doubt about why. The ESWL technique has simplified the treatment of kidney and ureteral stones so much, that some authorities have questioned the value of medical stone prevention…[3].

ESWL and endourology have taken the lead in the work on urolithiasis, but, at a time of reduced resources in medicine, it has been realized that these techniques have a tremendous impact on costs. Stones that were simply observed some 10 years ago are now treated by non-invasive techniques. Hospital statistics in Germany already showed in 1988 that the new techniques have not only replaced old procedures but were widely applied (Fig. 56.1), thus leading to increased costs in the health system. ESWL and the currently available medical therapy are only symptomatic forms of therapy and neither is treating the cause of stone formation since the mechanism of most stone formation is not known. The detection of metabolic abnormalities, effective medical therapy and medical means of stone prevention would be more cost effective. There are several reasons why this is difficult to achieve.

Stone formation and prevention

There was, and still is, a general agreement that the four main mechanisms leading to stone formation are: (i)

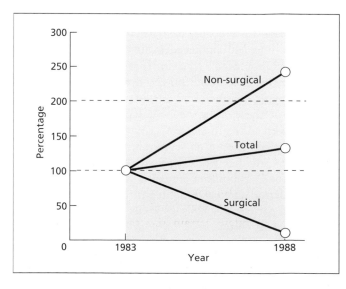

Fig. 56.1 Development of surgical, non-surgical (endourology and ESWL) and total procedures for stone removal in Germany between 1983, when the first lithotripters were installed, and 1988. Data are based on insurance statistics.

saturation of urine with crystal formation; (ii) promotion and (iii) inhibition of crystal formation, growth and aggregation; and (iv) crystal or microlith fixation. But these conditions are influenced by the concentrations of at least the stones-forming ions, various inhibitors and promoters in the urine. Their respective concentrations change with time of day, food intake, season, occupation and genetic inheritance, and so far only theories based on the saturation of urine and the inhibition of stone formation have gained clinical relevance. Historically idiopathic hypercalciuria has long been regarded as the main factor leading to formation of calcium-containing stones seen in 70–80% of all stone patients. The term idiopathic hypercalciuria was replaced by expressions such as absorptive hypercalciuria, renal hypercalciuria or renal phosphate leak absorptive hypercalciuria which seemed to describe the precise conditions leading to stone formation. In 1975, Pak and co-workers presented a simple clinically applicable test to differentiate between these causes of hypercalciuria enabling subsequent, appropriate specific therapy [4]. Twenty years later, this test is still regarded as a cornerstone of metabolic evaluation of stone patients. Absorptive hypercalciuria is most frequently seen and an adequate therapy is dietary reduction of calcium or, more effectively, intake of the ion exchange resin sodium cellulose phosphate [5], whereby thiazide therapy is necessary for the minority of patients with renal hypercalciuria.

However, there are some problems with the conversion of diagnostic findings into therapy. Successful prevention of stone recurrence had already been described for thiazides [6] and orthophosphate [7] in large, not specifically classified, patient groups. At the same time it was shown that variations of urinary oxalic acid concentration had a more pronounced impact on urinary supersaturation than calcium [8]. Consequently the term 'mild hyperoxaluria' was forwarded by Robertson et al. [9] as one of the main factors leading to calcium stone formation. But we have no proper medical therapy for hyperoxaluria and some authors think that most patients with oxalate stones have no disease but a metabolic disturbance with a slight variation from normal.

Single factor analysis was subsequently regarded insufficient to differentiate between normal persons, single stone formers and recurrent stone formers. Therefore, Robertson et al. [10] (Fig. 56.2) and many other authors introduced formulae that combined several diagnostic findings to calculate certain risk factors. Unfortunately, they only served to discriminate between normal persons and stone formers in a retrospective manner and these calculations have never been applied in a prospective manner to document their predictive power.

The more sophisticated evaluations and classifications are valuable only for a small subset of patients with metabolically active stone disease and frequent recur-

$$P_{SF} = \frac{\alpha_{Ca}\alpha_{Ox}\alpha_{pH}\alpha_{AMPS}\alpha_{UA}}{(1 + \alpha_{Ca}\alpha_{Ox}\alpha_{pH}\alpha_{AMPS}\alpha_{UA})}$$

Fig. 56.2 Equation developed by Robertson et al. [10] to measure the overall relative probability of forming stones (P_{SF}). By measuring the different factors in a 24-hour urine it should be possible to measure the risk of forming a calcium-containing stone.

rences. These patients usually follow the physician's advice and impressive graphs on the effects of a selective therapy on stone recurrence are produced by devoted physicians and patients. In the majority of patients, the risk of stone recurrence is less than 20% in 10 years and thus this majority does not profit from the knowledge gained from many years of research. In these patients, simple analysis of 24-hour urine is a decisive step in the diagnosis of such metabolic disorders as mild hyperoxaluria, which cannot be treated by anything else but the reduction of food rich in oxalate. Then again, hardly anyone eats excessive amounts of this type of food and the low compliance of stone patients to dietary or medical advice is historically well documented in every urologist's records. Hypercalciuria may also be diagnosed and treated by at least the advice to keep a low dietary calcium intake. But a recent prospective study on 45 619 men followed for 4 years showed an inverse relationship between the dietary calcium intake and the actual stone-formation rate. This can be explained by an increased intestinal oxalate absorption and increased urinary oxalic acid concentration under a low calcium diet [11]. Then we are again where we started.

Finally, medical therapy seems to follow not only scientific progress but sometimes becomes a matter of trends. Already in the 1940s hypocitraturia was regarded as an important factor leading to stone formation, and it was suggested that the urinary concentration of this low molecular inhibitor should be increased by specific therapy to prevent recurrent stone formation [12]. This concept was not well followed until the late 1950s. Today oral citrate therapy is probably the most widely performed kind of therapy that seems to be effective also in patients that could be classified into one of the several subgroups of hypercalciuria [13].

Most of what has been published on urinary stone disease up to the present compiles a book with many contradictory statements and a lot of white pages. Consequently, only a few paragraphs of this book can be taken as a sound basis for conservative treatment of stone disease. My personal illusions on the importance of a thorough investigation of stone patients were destroyed by lectures held by Bill Robertson and a few other experts during a stone conference in Saudi Arabia. The question whether an increase in fluid intake does not influence stone recurrence because the concentration of the stone-forming solutes *and* the inhibiting substances in the urine were equally lowered, remained unanswered. At that time, a graph published by Finlayson *et al.* in 1990 [14] depicting an essential, if not most important, parameter of stone formation 'bad luck' was to be published (Fig. 56.3). To get a better insight into what 'bad luck' exactly is, the interested reader is referred to the article by Ryall and Marshall [15] which clearly describes all the problems gained with all the research so far and leaves a lot of precise question marks behind a lot of classic statements.

Surgery

Surgery for staghorn stones was the most difficult, demanding and controversial urological procedure in the 1960s and 1970s. But quotations such as 'medical therapy is the treatment of choice for asymptomatic staghorn calculi' [16] or 'our patients and colleagues still need to be convinced that it is safer to remove a [staghorn] stone than to leave it *in situ*, the traditional concept of the silent [staghorn] stone being by no means extinct' [17] not only marked a disparity of opinions but also reflected the problems of a sometimes extremely complicated surgical procedure. Anatrophic nephrolithotomy [18], extended pyelocalycotomy [19] and multiple small radial nephrotomies [20] were the terms that described the principal procedures and Boyce, Gil-Vernet and Wickham were the urologists who popularized them. Perfectly performed, these techniques even concurred with the ultimate procedure: workbench surgery for staghorn stone removal [21].

Anatrophic nephrolithotomy was performed with a longitudinal incision after identification of the border between the posterior and anterior renal segments by intravenous or intra-aortal injection of methylene blue. Local hypothermia with slush ice allowed removal of staghorn stones and plastic repair of strictured calyceal infundibula by calyrrhaphy or calycoplasty in an average renal ischaemia time of 2–3 hours or more. This approach was popular in the USA up to the early 1980s. The interested reader will find a thorough description of this technique in the *AUA Courses in Urology* [22] and a vivid discussion of how to do it properly in the section letters to the editor in the *Journal of Urology* [23]. This technique never became really popular in Europe, where the extended pyelocalycotomy was initially favoured. With this approach, frequently cumbersome intraoperative pyeloscopy was required to remove stones from remote calyces. When the technique of multiple small radial nephrotomies was added, this combined approach through the pyelon and the parenchyma could definitely concur with the sometimes difficult and finally 'atrophic' longitudinal nephrotomy.

However, clamping of the renal artery and cooling of the kidney was still necessary and although a wealth of literature described many methods of optimal hypothermia techniques, troublesome bleeding, partial renal infarction, prolonged procedural times and residual stones were not infrequent, at least in the hands of some urologists.

A last but essential progress in staghorn stone surgery blossomed only for a short period: intraoperative localization of intraparenchymal renal arterial branches with Doppler sonography and of stones with B-mode sonography [24]. The precise localization of these structures obviated the need for renal ischaemia in most cases and the added

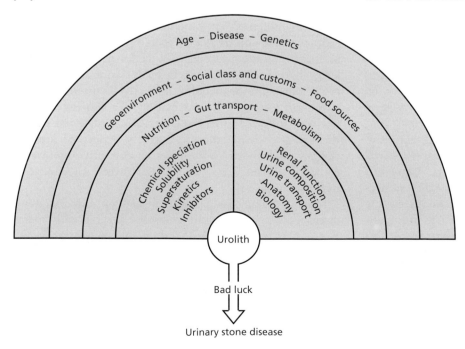

Fig. 56.3 'The big picture': the variety of considerations that influence the development of urolithiasis and urinary stone disease. (Reproduced from Finlayson *et al.* [14].)

technology turned the sometimes breathtaking adventure of staghorn surgery—both Wickham and Boyce knew why it was still necessary to describe the applied anatomy of their respective accesses in 1980 [25] and 1981 [26]—into a precise objective manoeuvre [27].

But at that time, the first easy staghorn stones were already being removed by percutaneous nephrolithotomy (PNL). With the broadening indication of ESWL which initially excluded patients with urinary tract infections, the minimal invasive combined treatment of staghorn stones with PNL and ESWL soon replaced surgery, even in complicated cases. Percutaneous electrosurgical incision of scarred infundibula was also later described [28] although the need to do such plastic revisions seems to have vanished in recent years. Today, open surgery for staghorn stones is an extremely rare event and only a few principles of staghorn stone surgery, such as hypothermia or the extended intrasinusidal approach, have survived in conservative surgery for renal tumours.

Endourology

The term endourology was coined by Smith *et al.* in 1979 [29] when they described the possible future application of percutaneous nephrostomy. Nowadays, endourology includes percutaneous and transurethral procedures and stone therapy is only a minor aspect of this continuously expanding field.

Ureterorenoscopy

By 1964 Marshall had already described the inspection of a stone in the lower ureter with a flexible fibrescope [30]. Using a similar instrument, Takayasu *et al.* reported on the first transurethral inspection of the renal collecting system in 1971 [31]. But flexible endoscopy of the upper urinary tract, even today, has not become clinically routine and ureterorenoscopy (URS) evolved slowly with causal reports on endoscopic inspections of dilated ureters through gaping orifices with conventional cystoscopes. A conventional paediatric cystoscope was used by Goodmann [32] and Lyon *et al.* [33] to inspect and treat tumours and stones in the lower ureter. In a subsequent paper, Lyon *et al.* presented a paediatric cystoscope of standard adult length to compensate for the urethral length in male patients and to facilitate routine inspection of the lower ureter in this particular patient group [34]. Adding another 20 cm to such an instrument does not seem to be that significant at first glance. But it was Perez-Castro Ellendt's idea that this rigid instrument, designed by himself, could be used for the inspection and therapy of the whole upper urinary tract [35,36].

The design of different small-calibre scopes, instruments to be used through them and the formation of ultrasonic

lasers or electrohydraulic probes for stone disintegration all followed Perez-Castro Ellendt's basic idea. Today URS is the only endoscopic technique that still competes with ESWL. With the steadily increasing number of ureteric stones treated, the question whether ESWL or URS is the most efficient and economic form of therapy is still controversial. Nowadays, it is not a staghorn stone but the single case of an impacted ureteric stone that can cause significant problems and complications during multi-modal, multisession treatment. It is not surprising that lumboscopic ureterolithotomy celebrates a small, albeit significant, revival as a 'laparoscopic' procedure.

Percutaneous nephrolithotomy

The description of radiologically controlled percutaneous stone removal by Fernström and Johansson in 1976 [37] and a few casual reports on percutaneous stone manipulation via operatively established tracts stimulated the development of a systematic approach to percutaneous nephrolithotomy in the departments of radiology and urology at Mainz University. Nearly 20 years later, the author learned that the German urologist von Rohr [38] had already described many aspects of percutaneous transrenal procedures, including studies on animals and corpses in 1958 in the East German urological journal. For unknown reasons, he never performed any clinical procedures, but it was obviously still too early for such a technique.

Our first report of a case treated by percutaneous ultrasound lithotripsy [39] was followed by presentations with increasing patient numbers and refinement of the technique at the 1979 annual meeting of the European Intrarenal Surgery Society in Bern and the meeting of the German Urological Society in the same year [40]. Our 1980 presentation at the 75th American Urological Association (AUA) annual meeting in San Francisco is contained in the abstract section of the programme book which turned out to be a truly historically important document (see below).

The manuscript on PNL that was submitted to the *Journal of Urology* at the AUA meeting in San Francisco was accepted with minor modifications. One of the referees disliked some concluding remarks in the last three paragraphs of the discussion:

'With a set of instruments currently being developed, we expect to reduce the time for the whole procedure to two ambulant sessions for dilation and a 1-week hospital stay for stone removal....Percutaneous stone manipulation has to compete with the techniques for operative stone removal established over the past 100 years. Its specific place among the various techniques of stone therapy will be defined on the basis of further experience'.

We respected his comment 'the *Journal of Urology* is

not a medicine man's paper' by slightly changing these statements, but without changing our ideas [41].

The use of PNL quickly expanded. After personal experience with PNL, Marberger *et al.* designed a purpose-built nephroscope and ultrasound lithotrite for percutaneous use [42]. Clayman and Castaneda-Zuniga were the first to publish a book on almost every aspect of percutaneous renal surgery [43]. Wickham was probably the first person to reintroduce a pelvic stone into the kidney to demonstrate the ease of the procedure to the patient and the first to try not to insert a nephrostomy after a percutaneous procedure, as no bleeding from the tract was observed (JEA Wickham, personal communication). But he was also the one who realized the potential of PNL and organized the first world meeting on this topic [1]. One-stage PNL was initiated by the design of telescope dilators [44] and the Amplatz dilators and sheath became the most popular access instruments [45]. Segura *et al.* were the first to publish a series of 1000 procedures [46]. Many other urologists have contributed to this technique and they, like Clayman *et al.* in 1984 [47], reported in the early 1980s that PNL had replaced 90% or more of their surgical procedures for renal stone removal. But at that time minimal invasive PNL was being continuously replaced by a non-invasive technique.

Extracorporeal shock wave lithotripsy

In vitro studies on ESWL had started in 1972 in Munich [48] and the actual revolution of stone therapy was already standing on the doorstep in 1980: Abstract No. 386 of the San Francisco AUA meeting entitled 'Contact-free break-up of kidney stones by shockwaves'. Again, it was probably a medicine man that refused acceptance and the authors Chaussy, Fried, Forssmann, Brendel and Jocham found their abstract, describing successful ESWL in 60 animals, under the rubric of rejected papers. In the time between the deadline of abstract submission in 1979 and the 1980 AUA meeting, they successfully treated their first 20 patients (Fig. 56.4). In December 1980 this clinical experience was published in the *Lancet* [49]. The AUA honoured the merits of Chaussy, Eisenberger and Schmiedt by the Distinguished Contribution Award at the 1989 AUA meeting in Dallas. Several other international rewards more than compensated the authors for the rejection of their paper in 1980.

A very careful approach to the clinical application of ESWL led to unsurpassed high success and low complication rates in their first series. A careful selection of patients initially excluded cases with urinary tract infection, stones larger than a cherry and ureteric stones. Another reason for the high success rates was the availability of the subsequently marketed ESWL unit HM3 from Dornier Medical Systems which was, for many years, the most powerful and effective machine on the market. Today, this machine is considered to be one of the first-generation lithotripters that set the golden standards of ESWL.

All machines produced later by other companies were subsequently called second-generation lithotripters. They differed from the HM3 in many aspects—no water bath, different shock wave sources, ultrasound focusing and multipurpose use. Another major difference was the lower performance of most of these lithotripters, with retreatment rates of up to 60% depending on the type of lithotripter. Many of those who had to change from the HM3 to other machines for different reasons regretted this

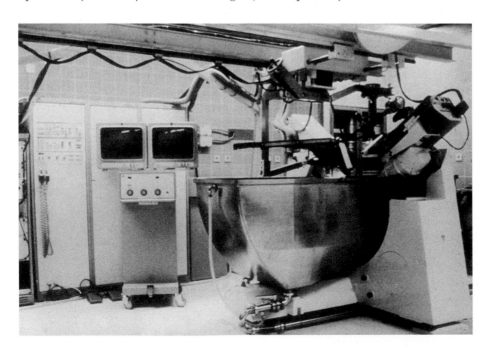

Fig. 56.4 First clinical ESWL prototype machine—the Dornier HM1 installed in the Department of Urology, University of Munich, in 1980.

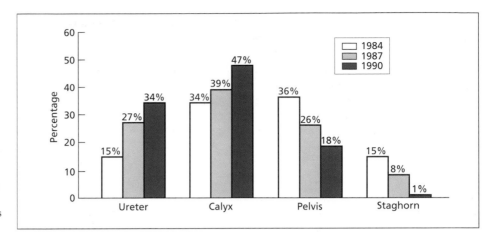

Fig. 56.5 Change of frequency of stones seen between 1984 and 1990 based on hospital statistics from the Departments of Urology in Mainz and Mannheim.

step back. But modern lithotripters are cheaper to run and easier to use and a few of them do reach the efficacy of the HM3. A true second-generation lithotripter that converts stones into fine dust and not just fragments—that may cause problems during their passage—and that makes focusing obsolete must still become established. Nevertheless, the impact of ESWL on urolithiasis with currently available machines is tremendous.

In 1984, Chaussy *et al.* published a paper entitled 'ESWL—beginning of change in therapy of urinary calculi?' [50]. Based on their experience of 852 treatments in 3.5 years and the significant expansion of the indications for ESWL, the authors anticipated a permanent decrease of surgical stone removal. In fact, not only surgery, but also PNL, was replaced by ESWL and in 1984 the frequency of PNL was already down to 10% in the author's experience. Today PNL is performed in 5% of cases, ESWL in 85% and surgery for stones has become an extremely rare procedure. This change in therapy had other consequences. In 1984, the author realized that the patient material was also changing: the frequency of large stones was decreasing. This change reflected an earlier and aggressive therapy of stones encouraged by physicians and accepted by patients because of the minimal invasiveness of ESWL. The trend continued parallel to the increasing installation of lithotripters in Germany. Their number quickly surpassed the calculated requirements and as early as 1987 the waiting lists for ESWL in Germany declined. The 1987 prospective calculation for 1990, based on the relative change of our patient material between 1984 and 1987, exactly matched the actual 1990 data (Fig. 56.5). Since then the trend has stabilized and today approximately 80% of the patients treated in Germany have small calyceal or ureteric calculi. From a purely medical point of view, this secondary ESWL effect is probably the most important impact that any form of therapy has had on urolithiasis. Today, at least in the USA, funding for research on the metabolic and physicochemical aspects of urolithiasis is

slowly increasing. Renewed efforts will allow a second revolution in stone therapy.

References

1 Wickham JEA, Miller R, eds. Percutaneous renal surgery. *Br J Urol* 1983; Special Supplement.
2 Various articles. *J Urol* 1989;**141**:705–808.
3 Coe LF, Gillenwater JY. The time of our lives. *J Urol* 1989;**141**:706.
4 Pak CYC, Kaplan RA, Bone H *et al.* A simple test for the diagnosis of absorptive, resorptive and renal hypercalciurias. *N Engl J Med* 1975;**292**:497–500.
5 Pak CYC, Delea CS, Bartter FC. Successful treatment of recurrent nephrolithiasis (calcium stones) with cellulose phosphate. *N Engl J Med* 1974;**290**:175–80.
6 Yendt ER, Cohanim M. Ten years' experience with the use of thiazides in the prevention of kidney stones. *Trans Am Clin Climatol Assoc* 1973;**85**:65–73.
7 Smith LH, Thomas WC, Arnaud CD. Orthophosphate therapy in calcium renal lithiasis. In: Cifuentes Delatte A, Rapado A, Hodgkinson A, eds. *Urinary Calculi: Recent Advances in Aetiology, Stone Structure and Treatment.* Basel: Karger, 1973:188–97.
8 Finlayson B. Renal lithiasis in review. *Urol Clin North Am* 1974;**1**:181–212.
9 Robertson WG, Peacock M, Ouimet D, Heyburn PJ, Rutherford A. The main risk for calcium oxalate stone disease in man: hypercalciuria or mild hyperoxaluria? In: Smith LH, Robertson WG, Finlayson B, eds. *Urolithiasis: Clinical and Basic Research.* New York: Plenum Press, 1981:3–12.
10 Robertson WG, Peacock M, Heyburn PJ. Risk factors in calcium stone disease of the urinary tract. *Br J Urol* 1978;**50**:449–54.
11 Curhan GC, Willet WC, Rimm EB, Stampfer MJ. A prospective study of dietary calcium and other nutrients and the risk of symptomatic kidney stones. *N Engl J Med* 1993;**328**:833–8.
12 Shorr E, Almay TP, Sloan MH, Taussky H, Toscani V. The relation between the urinary excretion of citric acid and calcium: its implications for urinary calcium stone formation. *Science* 1942;**96**:587–8,
13 Pak CYC, Skurla C, Sakhaee K, Preminger GM, Britton F. Long-

term treatment of calcium nephrolithiasis with potassium citrate. *J Urol* 1985;**134**:11–19.

14 Finlayson B, Khan SR, Hacket RL. Theoretical chemical models of urinary stones. In: Wickham JEA, Buck AC, eds. *Renal Tract Stone*. Edinburgh: Churchill Livingstone, 1990:133–47.

15 Ryall RL, Marshall VR. The investigation and management of idiopathic urolithiasis. In: Wickham JEA, Buck C, eds. *Renal Tract Stone*. Edinburgh: Churchill Livingstone, 1990:307–31.

16 Libertino JA, Newman Hr, Lytton B, Weiss RM. Staghorn calculi in solitary kidneys. *J Urol* 1971;**105**:753–7.

17 Blandy JP, Singh M. The case for a more aggressive approach to staghorn stones. *J Urol* 1976;**115**:505–6.

18 Boyce WH, Smith MJV. Anatrophic nephrotomy and plastic calyrrhaphy. *Trans Am Assoc Genito-urin Surg* 1967;**59**:18–24.

19 Gil-Vernet J. New surgical concepts in removing renal calculi. *Urol Int* 1965;**20**:255–88.

20 Wickham JEA, Coe N, Ward JP. 100 cases of nephrolithotomy under hyperthermia. *Eurol Int* 1975;**1**:71–4.

21 Sullivan MJ, Joseph E, Taylor JC. Extracorporeal renal parenchymal surgery with continuous perfusion. *J Am Med Assoc* 1974;**229**:1780.

22 Harrison LH. Anatrophic nephrolithotomy: update 1978. In: Bonney WW, Weems WL, Donohue JP, eds. *AUA Courses in Urology*, Vol. 1. Baltimore: Williams and Wilkins, 1978:1–23.

23 Boyce WH. Letter to the editor. *J Urol* 1980;**123**:604.

24 Thüroff JW, Frohneberg D, Riedmiller R *et al.* Localization of segmental arteries in renal surgery by doppler sonography. *J Urol* 1982;**127**:863–6.

25 Sleight MW, Gower RL, Wickham JEA. Intrarenal access. *Urology* 1980;**15**:475–7.

26 Resnick MI, Pounds DM, Boyce WH. Surgical anatomy of the human kidney and its application. *Urology* 1981;**17**:367–9.

27 Alken P, Thüroff JW, Riedmiller H, Hohenfellner R. Doppler sonography and B-mode ultrasound scanning in renal stone surgery. *Urology* 1984;**23**:455–60.

28 Clayman RC, Hunter D, Surya V *et al.* Percutaneous intrarenal electrosurgery. *J Urol* 1984;**131**:864–7.

29 Smith AD, Lange PH, Fraley EE. Applications of percutaneous nephrostomy. New challenges and opportunities in endo-urology. *J Urol* 1979;**121**:382.

30 Marshall VF. Fiber optics in urology. *J Urol* 1964;**91**:110–14.

31 Takayasu H, Aso Y, Takagi T, Go T. Clinical application of fiber-optic pyeloureteroscope. *Urol Int* 1971;**26**:97–104.

32 Goodman TM. Ureteroscopy with pediatric cystoscope in adults. *Urology* 1977;**9**:394.

33 Lyon ES, Kyker JS, Schoenberg HW. Transurethral ureteroscopy in women: a ready addition to the urological armamentarium. *J Urol* 1978;**119**:35–6.

34 Lyon ES, Banno JJ, Schoenberg HW. Transurethral ureteroscopy in men using juvenile cystoscopy equipment. *J Urol* 1979;**122**: 152–3.

35 Perez-Castro Ellendt E, Martinez-Pinneiro JA. La uretero-renoscopia transuretral. Un actual proceder urologico. *Arch Esp Urol* 1980;**33**:3–18.

36 Perez-Castro Ellendt E, Martinez-Pinneiro JA. Ureteral and renal endoscopy. A new approach. *Eur Urol*, 1982;**8**:117–20.

37 Fernström I, Johannson B. Percutaneous pyelolithotomy: a new extraction technique. *Scand J Urol Nephrol* 1976;**10**: 257–9.

38 Von Rohr H. Die endoskopische Pyeloskopie: Neues Verfahren der Nierenbeckendiagnostik und Grundlage der vereinfachten Entfernung von Nierenbeckensteinen. *Z Urol Nephrol* 1958;**12**: 697–712.

39 Alken P, Kurth KH, Günter R. Die perkutane Instrumentation bei Nierensteinen. In: Gasser G, Vahlensieck W, eds. *Fortschritte der Urologie und Nephrologie*. Darmstadt: Steinkopf Verlag, 1977:393–7.

40 Alken P, Altwein J. Die perkutane Nephrolitholapaxie. In: *Verhandlungsbericht der Deutschen Ges f Urol*. Berlin: Springer, Verlag, 1979:109–12.

41 Alken P, Hutchenreiter G, Günter R, Marberger M. Percutaneous stone manipulation. *J Urol* 1981;**125**:463–6.

42 Marberger M, Stackl W, Hruby W. Percutaneous litholapaxy of renal calculi with ultrasound. *Eur Urol* 1982;**8**:236–42.

43 Clayman RV, Castaneda-Zuniga W. Techniques in endourology: a guide to the percutaneous removal of renal and ureteral calculi. 1984.

44 Seemann O, Alken P. Use of metal dilators. In: Smith AD, ed. *Controversies in Endourology*. Philadelphia: WB Saunders, 1995:42–9.

45 Rusnak B, Castaneda-Zuniga W, Kotula F, Herrera M, Amplatz K. An improved dilator system for percutaneous nephro-stomies. *Radiology* 1982;**144**:174.

46 Segura W, Patterson DE, Le Roy AJ *et al.* Percutaneous removal of kidney stones: review of 1000 cases. *J Urol* 1985;**134**:1077–81.

47 Clayman RV, Surya V, Miller RP *et al.* Percutaneous nephrolithotomy: extraction of renal and ureteral calculi from 100 patients. *J Urol* 1984;**131**:868–71.

48 Chaussy C, Eisenberger F, Wanner K *et al.* The use of shock waves for the destruction of renal calculi without direct contact. *Urol Res* 1976;**4**:175.

49 Chaussy C, Brendel W, Schmiedt E. Extracorporeally induced destruction of kidney stones by shock waves. *Lancet* 1980;**2**: 1265–8.

50 Chaussy C, Schmiedt E, Jocham D, Schüller J, Brandl H. Extrakorporale Stoßwellenlithotripsie—Beginn einer Um-strukturierung in der Behandlung des Harsteinleidens? *Urologe [A]* 1984;**23**:25–9.

57 Epidemiology of Stone Disease

J.Hofbauer and M.Marberger

Introduction

There is general agreement among epidemiologists that by the end of the nineteenth century the incidence of upper tract urinary stones in industrialized countries was rising. Simultaneously bladder stones, which until then had been endemic in the very same areas, became significantly less common. This development is confirmed by numerous studies, and it is consistent with the fact that less developed areas of the world tend to be characterized by a high percentage of bladder calculi even today. Between 1900 and 1940, substantial amounts of data had been collected that paved the way for a surge of investigations, beginning in the 1950s, into the pathogenesis of urolithiasis and possible prophylactic measures. Vast amounts of epidemiological data were compiled in the following decades until in the 1980s the focus of interest moved to new developments in the area of minimally invasive therapy.

With all the possibilities that they offer for treating urinary tract stones, extracorporeal shock wave lithotripsy (ESWL) and sophisticated endourological options have greatly reduced the morbidity of urinary stone disease. However, these innovations have also shifted the emphasis away from the disorder itself and its underlying problems. Meanwhile the incidence of urolithiasis has continued to rise, largely because of the high incidence of recurrent stones. With these considerations in mind, it is important to take a fresh look at the currently available knowledge of the epidemiology of this disease and to try to encourage new studies in this field.

The wide variety of possible epidemiological factors were categorized into two fundamental groups by Andersen [1], namely intrinsic factors that comprise age, sex, heredity, race and ethnic determinants, as well as what he referred to as extrinsic factors, which could equally well be termed environmental factors and include aspects such as climate, drinking and eating habits, occupation and standard of living. These classifications will be largely maintained in this chapter.

Rate of occurrence, age and sex

Studies of the prevalence and incidence of a disease provide the basis for epidemiological investigations aimed at establishing its course and possible risk factors, in order eventually to institute prophylactic measures.

There are a considerable number of possible epidemiological factors, all of which have been the subject of thorough investigations, but their interactions are still poorly understood. The situation is additionally complicated by the fact that the incidence and prevalence figures reported rest upon criteria as diverse as hospital statistics, radiographic data, surgical admissions or population studies. A review of the literature of the past two decades shows that the prevalence figures vary considerably from country to country (Table 57.1), but it also becomes evident that the basis for comparison is sometimes poor.

Despite their shortcomings, however, these studies make clear that the problem of urolithiasis is of worldwide importance. Since Kneise and Beyer in 1933 [12] and Bibus in 1939 [13] presented an oscillating incidence curve, there has been consensus that over recent decades the rate of occurrence has been progressively rising [14–16]. Vahlensieck et al. demonstrated an increase in stone incidence from 0.54% in 1979 to 0.88% in 1984, including both first episodes and recurrences [17], and similar results were obtained by Frangos and Rous [18]. In real figures 510 000 citizens of former West Germany suffered at least one stone episode during 1984, and so do an average of 720 000 US citizens per year. More impressively still it means that 2.4 million West Germans or 12 million Americans have experienced one or more stone episodes.

All relevant reports also single out the age factor as crucial [7,15,19,20]. A study conducted by Larsen and Philip in 1962 involved 5710 Danish physicians and showed an age-dependent increase of stone incidence from 2.5% among men aged 26–30 years up to 18.7% among those over 70 years [20]. This tendency has been confirmed by numerous more recent studies [15,21–23].

Several studies have shown that the peak incidence of

Table 57.1 Occurrence rate of stones in selected countries.

Reference	Year	Country	Occurrence rate (%)
Hüttner [2]	1972	Former German Democratic Republic	3.6
Takasaki & Maeda [3]	1977	Japan	1.0
Scott et al. [4]	1977	Scotland	3.8
Ljunghall et al. [5]	1977	Sweden	9.0
Pavone-Macaluso & Miano [6]	1979	Italy	13.0
Joost et al. [7]	1980	Austria	4.8
Boer et al. [8]	1979	Netherlands	4.7
Vahlensieck et al. [9]	1980	Former Federal Republic of Germany	5.0
Robertson et al. [10]	1984	UK	3.8
Yoshida & Okada [11]	1990	Japan	5.4

urolithiasis is between the ages of 30 and 50 [24,25]. However, in most of these patients the onset of the disease was detected in their late twenties [15,26]. Given the fact that the prevalence is highest among patients in their fifties and sixties, this illustrates that many of them have to cope with the disease for a long time.

Stones containing calcium, particularly when presenting as idiopathic disease, are usually reported to be much more common in men than in women. There are two to three men to every woman with the disease, based on the reported incidence. Distribution patterns to this effect have been shown consistently, regardless of study design [27–29], with only a few exceptions such as that of a group of gypsies in which the ratio was shown to be reversed [30]. This difference between the sexes has been attributed to the higher excretion of calcium, oxalate and uric acid in men and less to their lower citrate excretion [31,32]. Testosterone levels have also been held responsible [33]. From this it would appear that the increase in western societies of upper tract stones throughout the twentieth century has affected men more than women [34]. By contrast, however, there seems to be no such difference in terms of stone prevalence [17,35,36]. One explanation for these seemingly irreconcilable results would be that the long-term prevalence pattern neutralizes year-to-year variations in incidence. Autopsy studies also failed to demonstrate a sex-specific difference in stone prevalence [37], which would suggest that the increased incidence among male patients is primarily one of symptomatic stones.

Hereditary and familial disposition

Cystinuria, xanthinuria and congenital hyperoxaluria are known to be caused by a genetically determined error of metabolism with a mainly autosomal recessive hereditary pattern. It has been suggested that there is some genetic heterogeneity in the inheritance pattern (homozygous or heterozygous, complete or incomplete) [38,39]. Renal tubular acidosis is known to be dominantly transmitted [40]. However, these are the only genetic disorders known to be accompanied by increased urinary stone formation, and they only account for a small percentage of cases.

Resnik et al. and McGeown, in their reports on a genetic predisposition to calcium oxalate stones, excluded a monogenetic inheritance pattern but hypothesized a polygenetic defect associated with reduced penetrance [41,42]. In other words, the genetic disposition is transmitted but the disease does not manifest itself in every generation. This was confirmed by Churchill and colleagues [43]. Immunological studies suggested the existence of a link between human leucocyte antigen (HLA) polymorphism and renal stone formation, but the association detected was weak, and the authors could not rule out the possibility that it was purely adventitious [44,45].

It is conceivable that certain risk factors are genetically transmitted. For example, there are reports of a familial link in certain forms of hypercalciuria, with first-degree relatives of hypercalciuric children exhibiting a higher urinary calcium excretion than controls [46,47].

One observation that has been reported consistently for a long time is that urinary stones are uncommon among groups as racially distinct as North American Indians, black Africans or Afro-Americans. Findings like those by Goetze, Eickenberg or Schey et al. [48–50] of a differential incidence of calcium urolithiasis in black as compared with white people would indeed suggest a genetic role. As an argument against genetic factors, factors such as the standard of living and eating and drinking habits have been postulated as being of importance [51–54].

Several publications also reported different stone frequencies depending on ethnicity. In one of the more recent studies, Zaidman showed that Israelis with a Georgian background are more likely to develop stones than indigenous Israelis [55,56]. Ethnocultural differences were also demonstrated in India, with the tendency of stone formation decreasing from Hindus through Muslims down to tribes in northeastern India [57].

Increased familial stone rates have been reported by various authors [58–61]. A striking correlation has been demonstrated between fathers and sons and between brothers [59,62]. According to White *et al.*, however, phenomena of this type should be attributed to household diet and other specific family habits rather than to an underlying genetic disposition [63]. This opinion is supported by the observation that stone incidence is also higher among wives of stone formers than among wives of other men (58). It was also reported that male relatives of stone patients are more frequently affected than female relatives; this too has to be brought into perspective given the overall difference between men and women in terms of stone incidence.

Geography and climate

The frequencies of stone occurrence varies widely throughout the world. Areas with a high rate of stone disease have been studied for many years, including the UK, the Scandinavian countries, northern India and Pakistan, northern Australia, central Europe, China and the east coast of the USA. Other areas of the world have a relatively low rate of idiopathic urolithiasis. They are usually characterized by a high proportion of indigenous inhabitants, such as Central and South America, large stretches of Africa and aboriginal Australia. There is evidence of an increased stone incidence in hot countries such as the United Arab Emirates, Kuwait and Saudi Arabia as well as in certain parts of the USA, Australia and Europe [64,65] although Esho and Mbonu *et al.* demonstrated a very low stone incidence among Nigerians and black South Africans [66–68].

Urinary stones in various regions of the world differ not only in their incidence but also in their composition. Sharma *et al.* demonstrated a low incidence of struvite stones among Indians, who mainly develop calcium oxalate and calcium phosphate stones [69]. By contrast, Pantanowitz *et al.* reported a very high percentage of struvite stones among South Africans [70]. Citizens of former Czechoslovakia and Israel seem to be at an increased risk of developing uric acid stones [71].

Several investigations point to seasonal variations in stone formation. Studies by Prince and Scardiño and Rivera indicate that stone incidence is highest during the summer months [72,73]. Reasons given for this remain speculative, although an explanation would be that higher temperatures, via dehydration, promote stone formation [74]. Hallson *et al.* attributed this finding to a different excretion pattern of calcium and oxalate in summer, with a possible role of dietary factors or of elevated 25-hydroxyvitamin D_2 — an active metabolic of vitamin D_3 — levels due to increased exposure to sunlight [75,76]. Other authors deny the existence of seasonal variations [77–79].

Drinking habits and diet

There is general consensus that urinary stones arise because of oversaturation of urine with stone-forming substances. It was repeatedly shown that increased fluid intake significantly counteracts urinary stone formation in high-risk patients [80–83]. Likewise, Frank and DeVries and Blacklock demonstrated a markedly lower stone incidence if the urinary volume was increased [84,85]. Hodgkinson reported that following an average diuresis increase of 500 ml, 60% of idiopathic calcium stone formers remained recurrence free [86].

However, a low urine output is caused not only by low fluid intake but also by extensive perspiration. This, of course, would readily suggest itself as an explanation for the higher stone incidence in hot areas like the Middle East. Occupations performed in high environmental temperatures were shown to result in chronic dehydration associated with an increased risk of stone formation [87]. An impressive example of this relationship was reported by Blacklock, who demonstrated an increased stone incidence among British troops stationed in the Middle and Far East [85]. Marathon runners have a three- to five-fold higher stone incidence than age- and sex-matched individuals, presumably also owing to chronic dehydration [88].

Embon *et al.* showed that 62% of 818 patients with stones were chronically dehydrated due to hot climate, high temperatures at the workplace, or low water intake, and concluded that these were instrumental factors in the causation of urolithiasis [89]. Although this notion is generally accepted, Ljunghall *et al.* showed that the recurrence rate of 115 recurrent stone formers amounted to 23% irrespective of urinary volume [90], concluding that fluid intake had no appreciable effect on stone formation. A possible explanation of these contradictions is provided by Finlayson, who calculated that it would theoretically require a urine output of more than 3600 ml/day for the reduction of urinary oxalate concentrations to be effective [81]. In practice such volumes would be scarcely achievable even in highly motivated patients. Similarly, Goldfarb showed that although the likelihood of nucleation of stone-forming substances rose significantly as the urinary volume fell below 1 l/day, adequate dilution with successful reduction of oversaturation did not effectively stop crystal formation [91,92]. This might have been because of a non-stoichiometric decline in the activity of stone inhibitors [93].

There has been a longstanding belief that the softness of drinking water is a promoter of urinary stone formation. Churchill *et al.* and Barker and Donnan demonstrated an increased incidence of urinary stones associated with soft drinking water [94,95], and childhood bladder stones were shown to be completely absent in areas with very hard water [96]. In contrast, population studies in Newfoundland and Sweden showed no apparent relationship between the hardness of drinking water and stone prevalence [97–100]. Insufficient data are yet available on the possible usefulness of mineral water solubles in dealing with urolithiasis. When restricted to regular tap water intake, the incidence of urinary stones rises as the ratio of magnesium to calcium falls [101].

Substantial efforts have also been devoted to determining the role of eating habits in the pathogenesis of urinary stones. Numerous investigators have observed the effects of changing dietary constituents. As with other factors, however, the complexities involved are such that many of the results are hard to reconcile.

One effect of food on urinary stone formation was clearly demonstrated by Robertson et al., that is, an increased risk of stone formation associated with high animal protein intake [102–105]. Such an eating habit enhances the excretion of calcium, oxalate and uric acid, which are considered to be promoters of stone formation [106]. They also showed that the incidence of stones was markedly lower among vegetarians [107]. Trinchieri et al. demonstrated that stone formers tended to consume significantly more protein and purine than normal individuals [108]. A recent prospective study of 45 000 men by Curhan et al. confirmed the adverse effect of a protein-rich diet [109]. In addition, however, they also noted that a calcium-rich diet reduced the risk of stone formation. This was indeed revolutionary considering the fact that avoidance of milk and dairy products used to be an established dietary recommendation. Other authors failed to show that the dietary habits of stone formers differ significantly from those of other individuals [110–113].

The substantial difficulties in addressing the question of nutrition were comprehensively dealt with in a recent article by Schwille and Herrmann [114]. They elaborated on the pros and cons of all major food constituents such as fat, protein, sugar, fibres and minerals with respect to urinary stone formation, concluding that while a wide array of questions remained unanswered, it was safe to assume that upper tract stone formation in western industrialized countries was causally related to hypernutrition.

Socioeconomic factors and occupation

While there exists no definite proof of a marked difference between the eating habits of stone formers and those of other individuals, it appears clear that the daily calorie intake of the average western person is too high. The per capita expenditure based on monthly income for foodstuffs correlates with the rate of stone occurrence [115].

Asper [116] evaluated the socioeconomic aspects of stone frequency through a meta-analysis. He reviewed 200 publications containing pertinent epidemiological data on a total of 250 000 urinary stone patients in 50 countries. Disregarding the drawbacks of retrospective data pooling, the study revealed that populations with similar socioeconomic conditions showed similar patterns of urolithiasis. The authors also pointed out distinct similarities of stone characteristics in nineteenth century Europe and today's developing countries and inferred a correlation between socioeconomic development and urinary stone disease.

A negative effect on stone occurrence is also seen with excessive intake of certain affluence-related products such as coffee, black tea and alcohol [117,118]. Urinary stones were significantly more rare following the worldwide economic depression up to and following World War II. Today, there are significant differences between western industrialized countries and developing countries in South America, Africa and parts of Asia. Within countries urolithiasis is more prevalent among the well-to-do than among the poor. A low standard of living, in most instances, will be accompanied not only by a restricted diet but also by poorer sanitary conditions, poorer quality of medical care, as well as by a lower level of education motivating fewer people to seek medical advice. These are just some of the factors that not only are liable to influence the risk of recurrent stone formation but also add up to a vast number of pitfalls when trying to illuminate the disease in terms of racial, ethnic, geographical or even dietary influences.

Firmly connected to socioeconomic factors is the role of occupation. People with higher incomes tend to consume more protein-rich food and, therefore, show a higher urinary excretion of calcium, oxalate and uric acid. Lonsdale showed that urinary stones were more common among people with a sedentary occupation [119]. This was confirmed by Mates [120]. Chief executives, pilots and doctors count among those with an elevated risk of stone formation [121]. Arguably, however, the standard of living in this group has a greater bearing on the likelihood of developing stones than their occupation. A purely occupation-related tendency towards stone formation is demonstrable only in people who work in high environmental temperatures [122].

Endemic bladder stones

Another of the few generally accepted notions about epidemiological factors in urolithiasis is that bladder stone formation is causally related to monotonous, low-protein diets. An impressive example of this relationship is found in the UK county of Norfolk. In the nineteenth century, the incidence of bladder stones was almost five times higher in its eastern than in its western part. This discrepancy was due to the fact that eastern Norfolk at that time was predominantly a wheat-growing area, with the people subsisting chiefly on bread, water, tea and some milk. By contrast, the western part of the county predominantly relied on a mixed agriculture that yielded a more varied diet. When, early in the twentieth century, western Norfolk diversified its agriculture, this resulted in a drastic reduction of bladder stones, and by around 1938 the disease was effectively contained [123].

A massive reduction of childhood bladder stones after changing a low-protein diet was also observed in Sicily [124] and in Thailand [125]. In the latter country, the northeastern parts are predominantly affected. Compared with city dwellers, who showed significantly lower stone frequencies, people in rural areas tended to be on a very low-fat diet of rice, vegetables and raw meat. Srivastava demonstrated that among 132 Afghan children with bladder stones observed over the period of 1 year, the predominant diet consisted of wheatbread and oxalate-rich food, while intake of milk and dairy products, as well as eggs and meat, was very low [126].

Teotia and Teotia, in their analysis of the geographical distribution of bladder stones in India, demonstrated that the incidence was highest in areas with low-protein diets and lower in areas with higher protein intake [127]. Another useful finding was that bladder stones were absent in areas with adequate fluoride intake. Similar observations were made for Thailand by Valyasevi et al. [128]. On the other hand, it has not been possible up to now to verify previous assumptions of a causal role of vitamin deficiencies in bladder stones [129,130].

The geographical distribution of bladder stones has changed considerably over the course of time. They have practically vanished in affluent societies but continue to be endemic in rural, agricultural areas of developing countries [131]. There still exists a bladder stone belt extending from southern Russia and the Balkans through Egypt, Turkey, Israel, Lebanon, Syria and Iran to Pakistan, India, China, Thailand and Indonesia [132–136]. The example of Turkey illustrates how the incidence of bladder stones continuously falls as the socioeconomic situation improves [137].

One puzzling aspect about endemic bladder stones is that they appear to affect boys of around 5 years of age almost exclusively. All of them not only show similarities with respect to diet but also share the characteristic of a low standard of living. In areas with endemic bladder stones, hygienic conditions are usually bad and gastrointestinal infections accompanied by diarrhoea and dehydration are common. Increased uric acid excretion promotes ammonium production, and urine is oversaturated with stone-forming substances. Calcium, oxalate, uric acid and ammonium acid urate have been found to be the chief constituents of endemic childhood bladder stones in several countries. More often than not, however, these were mixed stones, with the relative percentages of constituents varying in different studies.

Bladder stones are virtually non-existent in western industrialized countries. Wherever they do occur, especially in children, they tend to be associated with hydronephrosis or infection.

Conclusion

The substantial body of research into the epidemiology of urolithiasis does not provide a clear picture. The relative importance of any single epidemiological factor remains undecided, and some of the opinions put forward continue to be contradictory. Interest in epidemiological studies is decreasing, which becomes all the more evident when comparing the number of relevant publications before and after the late 1980s. In the 1990s, there have been more good, yet repetitive, summaries of data previously collected. With the demonstration that people on a calcium-rich diet show a lower urinary stone incidence, Curhan et al. really offer the only new and interesting aspect [109].

This loss of interest has been due to the revolutionary progress that has occurred in minimally invasive treatment options. However, from broad economic and health care considerations it is essential that further epidemiological data are gathered and research into the pathogenesis of urolithiasis continues. Every year US$47.3 million are reportedly spent on treating urinary stones in the USA alone [138].

It is also evident that the methodologies used in previous studies are no longer good enough; this is particularly true of incidence and prevalence calculations. Most of these studies were based on hospital statistics or X-ray studies, and only few were drawn from population statistics. None the less, the figures offered in these studies do bring home the dimensions of urinary stone disease. Although the best data available are 10 years old, they seem to support the currently dominant notion that calcium stone disease is multifactorial—that is that any single underlying metabolic or environmental factor does not make a significant difference. Epidemiological factors may aggravate the situation by favouring an altered composition of urine which contributes to a greater risk of crystalluria. Factors with this potential include excessive protein and fat intake, inadequate fibre intake, a high ratio of oxalate to calcium, a low ratio of magnesium to calcium, high environmental temperatures, excessive exposure to sunlight or to other sources of ultraviolet rays, and low fluid intake.

It is interesting how various epidemiological factors have been interpreted in completely different ways, as illustrated by diverging dietary trends and recommendations towards high-protein or low-protein intake. Bladder stones are apparently caused by a continuous low-protein and low-calcium diet. A higher standard of living and dietary guidelines have virtually eradicated this disease and, at the same time, have resulted in a sharply rising incidence of nephrolithiasis. This development reflects the gradual shift from one extreme lifestyle to the opposite; from monotonous diets to the excessive consumer behaviour observed in western societies. This notion would also be consistent with the different prevalence figures for various countries and areas, which cannot be explained exhaustively in terms of climatic factors and genetic determinants. The lesson to be drawn from this once more appears to be that a balanced diet is the best choice.

The task of evaluating the relative importance of individual epidemiological factors is complicated by a host of possible interactions. It is logical, but also difficult, if the assessment of one set of factors comes into conflict with previous studies when factors that have not been previously analysed are introduced. The study of the aetiology and pathophysiology of urolithiasis clearly needs a new impetus in order to help resolve this major worldwide problem. Randomized studies would be necessary to unravel its intricacies systematically. With the possibilities of modern data processing, many of the problems that used to detract from the value of previous epidemiological work should be easily overcome. It would, however, require a concerted effort of urologists worldwide to standardize selection criteria and basic treatment strategies to obtain meaningful results.

References

1 Andersen DA. Environmental factors in the etiology of urolithiasis in urinary calculi. In: Cifuentes L, Rapado A, Hodgkinson A, eds. *Urinary Calculi. International Symposium on Renal Stone Research.* New York: S Karger, 1973: 130–44.

2 Hüttner I. Soziologische Merkmale und Gesundheitsverhalten des Harnsteinträgers. II. Jenaer Harnsteinsymposium. In: *Wissenschaftliche Beiträge der Freidrich-Schiller-Universität.* Jena: 1972:144–51.

3 Takasaki E, Maeda K. A population study of urolithiasis. *Dokkyo J Med Sci* 1977;4:88–92.

4 Scott R, Freeland R, Mowat W *et al.* The prevalence of calcified upper urinary tract stone disease in a random population—Cumbernauld Health Survey. *Br J Urol* 1977;49: 589–95.

5 Ljunghall S, Christensson T, Wengle B. Prevalence and incidence of renal stone disease in a health screening programme. *Scand J Urol Nephrol Suppl* 1977;41:39–54.

6 Pavone-Macaluso M, Miano L. Epidemiology of urolithiasis in Italy. *Proc XVIII Congr Soc Int Urol* 1979;1:113–37.

7 Joost J, Egger G, Hohlbrugger G, Marberger M. Epidemiologie des Nierensteinleidens in Tirol. *Österr Ärztetagung* 1980;35: 1016–20.

8 Boer PW, Van Geuns H, Van der Hem GK, Blickman JR. Population survey in a community on the occurrence of stone disease. *Proc VIII Congr Soc Int Urol* 1979;2:64–5.

9 Vahlensieck W, Hesse A, Bach D. Zur Prävalenz des Harnsteinleidens in der Bundesrepublik Deutschland. *Urologe[B]* 1980;20:273–6.

10 Robertson WG, Peacock M, Baker M. Epidemiological studies on urinary stone disease in men in Leeds. In: Vahlensieck W, Gasser G, eds. *Pathogenese und Klinik der Harnsteine X.* Darmstadt: Steinkopff, 1984:15–22.

11 Yoshida O, Okada Y. Epidemiology of urolithiasis in Japan: a chronological and geographical study. *Urol Int* 1990;45: 104–11.

12 Kneise O, Beyer G. Die Harnsteinwelle in Mitteldeutschland. *Z Urol* 1933;27:1–20.

13 Bibus B. Zur Frage der Harnsteinwelle. *Z Urol* 1939;33:37–43.

14 Norlin A, Lindell B, Granberg PO, Lindvall N. Urolithiasis: a study of its frequency. *Scand J Urol Nephrol* 1976;10:150–3.

15 Ljunghall S. Incidence of upper urinary tract stones. *Mineral Electrolyte Metab* 1987;13:220–7.

16 Robertson WG, Peacock M. The pattern of urinary stone disease in Leeds and in the United Kingdom in relation to animal protein intake during the period 1960–80. *Urol Int* 1982;30:394–9.

17 Vahlensieck W, Hesse A, Schaefer RM. Epidemiologische Studien zur Inzidenz, Prävalenz und Mortalität des Harnsteinleidens in der Bundesrepublik Deutschland 1979 und 1984. In: Vahlensieck W, Gasser G, eds. *Pathogenese und Klinik der Harnsteine XII.* Darmstadt: Steinkopff, 1986:1–4.

18 Frangos DN, Rous SN. Incidence and economic factors in urolithiasis. In: Orlando FL, ed. *Stone Disease: Diagnosis and Management.* 1987:3–10.

19 Ljunghall S, Hedstrand H. Epidemiology of renal stones in a middle aged male population. *Act Med Scand* 1975;197: 439–45.

20 Larsen JF, Philip J. Studies on the incidence of urolithiasis. *Urol Int* 1962;13:53–64.

21 Hiatt RA, Friedman GD. The frequency of kidney and urinary tract disease in a defined population. *Kidney Int* 1982;22:63–8.

22 Hiatt RA, Dales LG, Friedman GD, Hunkeler EM. Frequency of urolithiasis in a prepaid medical care program. *Am J Epidemiol* 1982;115:255–65.

23 Pak CYC. *Renal Stone Disease.* Boston: Martinus Nijhoff Publishing, 1987.

24 Bailey RR, Dann E, Greenslade NF *et al.* Urinary stones: a prospective study of 350 patients. *N Z Med J* 1974;79: 961–5.

25 Fetter TL, Zimskind PD. Statistical analysis of patients with ureteral calculi. *J Am Med Assoc* 1961;186:21–3.

26 Johnson CM, Wilson DM, O'Fallon WM, Malek RS, Kurland LT. Renal stone epidemiology: a 25 year-study in Rochester, Minnesota. *Kidney Int* 1979;16:624–31.

27 Vahlensieck EW, Bach D, Hesse A. Incidence, prevalence and mortality of urolithiasis in the German Federal Republic. *Urol Res* 1982;10:161–4.

28 Almby B, Meirik O, Schönebeck J. Incidence, morbidity and complications of renal and ureteral calculi in a well defined geographical area. *Scand J Urol Nephrol* 1975;9:249–53.

29 Juuti M, Heinonen OP. Incidence of urolithiasis and composition of household water in southern Finland. *Scand J Urol Nephrol* 1980;14:181–7.

30 Torres Ramirez C, Fernández Morales E, Zuluaga Gómez A, Gálvez Alcaraz L, Del Rio Samper S. An epidemiological study of renal lithiasis in gypsies and others in Spain. *J Urol* 1984;131:853–6.

31 Robertson WG. Epidemiology of urinary stone disease. *Urol Res* 1990;**18**(Suppl. 13):3–8.

32 Welshman SG, McGeown MG. Urinary citrate excretion in stone formers and normal controls. *Br J Urol* 1976;**48**:7–11.

33 Liao LL, Richardson KE. The metabolic of oxalate precursors in isolated perfused rat livers. *Arch Biochem Biophys* 1972;**153**:438–48.

34 Ahlgren SA, Lorstad M. Renal and ureteric calculi in a Swedish district I. *Acta Chir Scand* 1965;**130**:344–53.

35 Scott R. Epidemiology of stone disease. *Br J Urol* 1985;**57**: 491–7.

36 Scott R. Prevalence of calcified upper urinary tract stone disease in a random population survey. *Br J Urol* 1987;**59**: 111–17.

37 Schumann HJ. Die Häufigkeit der Urolithiasis im Sektionsgut des pathologischen Instituts St Georg, Leipzig. *Zentralbl Allg Pathol* 1963;**105**:88–94.

38 Thier SO, Segal S. Cystinuria. In: Stanbury JB, Wyngaarden JB, Frederickson DS, eds. *The Metabolic Basis of Inherited Disease.* New York: McGraw Hill, 1978:1578–92.

39 Watts RWE. Xantinuria and xanthine stone formation. In: Williams DI, Chisholm GD, eds. *Scientific Foundations of Urology I.* London: Heinemann, 1976:310–15.

40 Feest TG, Wrong OM. Inherited defects in distal tubule acidification. *Ann Intern Med* 1975;**82**:584–5.

41 Resnick M, Pridgen DB, Goodman HO. Genetic predisposition to formation of calcium oxalate stones. *N Engl J Med* 1968;**278**:1313–18.

42 McGeown MG. Heredity in renal stone disease. *Clin Sci* 1960;**19**:645–71.

43 Churchill DN, Maloney CM, Bear J *et al.* Urolithiasis—a study of drinking water hardness and genetic factors. *J Chron Dis* 1980;**33**:727–31.

44 Bear JC, Churchill DN, Morgan J, Marshall WH, Gault MH. HLA and urolithiasis. *Tissue Antigens* 1984;**23**:181–4.

45 Säfwenberg J, Backman V, Danielson BG, Johansson G, Ljunghall S. HLA and kidney stone disease. *Scand J Urol Nephrol* 1978;**12**:151–4.

46 Coe FL, Parks JH, Moore ES. Familial idiopathic hypercalciuria. *N Engl J Med* 1979;**100**:337–40.

47 Weinberger A, Schechter J, Pinkhas J, Sperling O. Hereditary hypercalciuric urolithiasis: a study of a family. *J Urol* 1981;**53**: 285–9.

48 Goetze T. Urinary calculi in the Indian and African in Natal. *S Afr Med J* 1963;**18**:1092–5.

49 Eickenberg H. Urolithiasis bei Negern. In: Vahlensieck W, Gasser G, eds. *Pathogenese und Klinik der Harnsteine VI.* Darmstadt: Steinkopff, 1978:75–6.

50 Schey HM, Corbett WT, Resnick MI. Prevalence rate of renal stone disease in Forsyth Country, North Carolina during 1977. *J Urol* 1979;**122**:288–91.

51 Modlin M. The aetiology of renal stone. A new concept arising from studies of a stone free population. *Ann R Coll Surg Engl* 1967;**40**:155–77.

52 Modlin M. Renal calculus in the Republic of South Africa. In: Hodgkinson A, Nordin BEC, eds. *Proceedings of the Renal Stone Research Symposium, Leeds 1968.* London: Churchill Livingstone, 1969:49–58.

53 Mason JC, Miles BJ, Belville WD. Urolithiasis and race: another viewpoint. *J Urol* 1985;**134**:501–2.

54 Tshipeta N, Lufuma L. Urolithiasis in black Africans. *Urology* 1983;**22**:517–20.

55 Zaidman JL, Eidelman A, Pinto N, Negelev S, Assa S. Trends in urolithiasis in various ethnic groups and by age in Israel. *Clin Chem Acta* 1986;**160**:87–92.

56 Zaidman JL, Pinto N. Studies of urolithiasis in Israel. *J Urol* 1976;**115**:626–7.

57 Singh PP, Singh LBK, Prasad SN, Singh MG. Urolithiasis in Manipur (north eastern region of India). Incidence and chemical composition of stone. *Am J Clin Nutr* 1978;**34**: 1519–23.

58 Ljunghall S. Family history of renal stones in a population study of stone formers and healthy subjects. *Br J Urol* 1979;**51**: 249–52.

59 Ljunghall S, Danielson BG, Fellström B *et al.* Family history of renal stones in recurrent stone patients. *Br J Urol* 1985;**57**: 370–4.

60 Robertson WG, Peacock M, Baker M *et al.* Studies on the prevalence and epidemiology of urinary stone disease in men in Leeds. *Br J Urol* 1983;**55**:595–8.

61 Boyce WH. Epidemiology of lithiasis in the United States. *Proc XVIII Congr Soc Int Urol* 1979;**1**:79–86.

62 Marya RK, Dadoo RC, Sharma NK. Genetic predisposition to renal stone disease in the first-degree relatives of stone-formers. *Urol Int* 1981;**36**:245–7.

63 White RW, Cohen AD, Vince FP *et al.* Minerals in urine of stone formers and their spouses. In: Hodgkinson A, Nordin BEC, eds. *Proceedings of the Renal Stone Research Symposium, Leeds 1968.* London: Churchill Livingstone, 1969:289–96.

64 Bateson EM. Renal tract calculi and climate. *Med J Aust* 1973; **2**:111–13.

65 Sierakowski R, Finlayson B, Landes RR, Finlayson C, Sierakowski N. The frequency of urolithiasis in hospital discharge diagnoses in the United States. *Invest Urol* 1978; **15**:438–41.

66 Esho JU. The rarity of urinary calculus in Nigeria. *Trop Geogr Med* 1978;**30**:477–81.

67 Esho JU. Analysis of urinary calculi formed by Nigerians. *Eur Urol* 1978;**4**:288–91.

68 Mbonu O, Attah C, Ikeakor I. Urolithiasis in an African population. *Int Urol Nephrol* 1984;**16**:291.

69 Sharma RN, Shah I, Gupta S, Sharma P, Beigh AA. Thermogravimetric analysis of urinary stones. *Br J Urol* 1989;**64**: 564–6.

70 Pantanowitz D, Pollen JJ, Politzer WM, Van Blerk PJP. Urinary calculi. *S Afr Med J* 1973;**47**:128.

71 Herbstein FH, Kleeberg J, Shalitin Y *et al.* Chemical and x-ray diffraction analysis of urinary stones in Israel. *Isr J Med Sci* 1974;**10**:1493.

72 Prince CL, Scardiño PL. A statistical analysis of ureteral calculi. *J Urol* 1960;**83**:561.

73 Rivera JV. Urinary calculi in Puerto Rico. II. Seasonal incidence. *Bull Assoc Med Puerto Rico* 1973;**65**:28.

74 Prince CL, Scardiño PL, Wolan CT. The effect of tem-perature, humidity and dehydration on the formation of renal calculi. *J Urol* 1956;**75**:209–14.

75 Hallson PC, Kasidas GP, Rose GA. Seasonal variations in urinary excretion of calcium and oxalate in normal subjects and in patients with idiopathic hypercalciuria. *Br J Urol* 1977; **49**:1–10.

76 Elliot JP, Gordon JO, Evans JW, Platt L. A stone season. A 10-year retrospective study of 768 surgical stone cases with respect to seasonal variation. *J Urol* 1975;**114**:574–7.

77 Ahlstrand C, Tiselius HG. Renal stone disease in a Swedish district during one year. *Scand J Urol Nephrol* 1981;**15**:143–6.

78 Rose AG, Westbury EJ. Seasonal and geographic variations in urinary composition in England, Scotland and Wales. *Urol Res* 1979;**7**:235–40.

79 Al-Dabbagh TQ, Fahadi K. Seasonal variations in the incidence of ureteric colic. *Br J Urol* 1977;**49**:269–75.

80 Smith LH. Medical aspects of urolithiasis: an overview. *J Urol* 1989;**141**:707–10.

81 Finlayson B. Symposium on renal lithiasis. Renal lithiasis in review. *Urol Clin North Am* 1974;**1**:181.

82 Thomas WC. Symposium on renal lithiasis. Medical aspects of renal calculous disease. Treatment and prophylaxis. *Urol Clin North Am* 1974;**1**:261.

83 Seftel A, Resnick MI. Metabolic evaluation of urolithiasis. *Urol Clin North Am* 1990;**17**:159.

84 Frank M, DeVries A. Prevention of urolithiasis. *Arch Environ Health* 1966;**13**:625.

85 Blacklock NJ. The pattern of urolithiasis in the Royal Navy. In: Hodgkinson A, Nordin BEC, eds. *Proceedings of the Renal Stone Research Symposium, Leeds 1968*. London: Churchill Livingstone, 1969:33–47.

86 Hodgkinson A. Composition of urinary tract calculi from some developing countries. *Urol Int* 1979;**34**:26–35.

87 Borghi L, Meschi T, Amato F *et al*. Hot occupation and nephrolithiasis. *J Urol* 1993;**150**:1757–60.

88 Milvy P, Colt E, Thornton J. A high incidence of urolithiasis in male marathon runners. *J Sports Med Phys Fitness* 1981;**3**:295–8.

89 Embon OM, Rose GA, Rosenbaum T. Chronic dehydration stone disease. *Br J Urol* 1990;**66**:357–62.

90 Ljunghall S, Fellström B, Johansson G. Prevention of renal stones by a high fluid intake? *Eur Urol* 1988;**14**:381–5.

91 Goldfarb S. Dietary factors in the pathogenesis and prophylaxis of calcium nephrolithiasis. *Kidney Int* 1988;**34**:544–55.

92 Goldfarb S. The role of diet in the pathogenesis and therapy of nephrolithiasis. *Endocrinol Metab Clin North Am* 1990;**19**:805.

93 Fleisch H. Role of inhibitors and promoters of crystal nucleation, growth and aggregation in the formation of calcium stones. In: Wickham JEA, Buck AC, eds. *Renal Tract Stone. Metabolic Basis and Clinical Practice*. New York: Churchill Livingstone, 1990:295–9.

94 Churchill D, Bryant D, Fodor G, Gault MH. Drinking water hardness and urolithiasis. *Ann Intern Med* 1978;**88**:513–14.

95 Barker DJP, Donnan SPB. Regional variations in the incidence of upper kidney tract stones in England and Wales. *Br Med J* 1978;**1**:67–70.

96 Gaches CGC, Gordon IRS, Shore DF, Roberts JBM. Urolithiasis in childhood in the Bristol clinical area. *Br J Urol* 1975;**47**:109–10.

97 Shuster J, Finlayson B, Scheaffer R *et al*. Water hardness and urinary stone disease. *J Urol* 1982;**128**:422–5.

98 Churchill DN, Maloney CM, Nolan R, Gault MH, Winsor G. Pediatric urolithiasis in the 1970s. *J Urol* 1980;**123**:237–8.

99 Ljunghall S. Regional variations in the incidence of urinary stones. *Br Med J* 1978;**1**:439.

100 Donaldson D, Pryce JD, Rose AG, Torey JE. Tap water calcium and its relationship to renal calculi and 24 h urinary calcium in Great Britan. *Urol Res* 1979;**7**:273–6.

101 Kohri K, Kodama M, Ihikawa Y *et al*. Magnesium-to-calcium ratio in tap water, and its relationship to geological features and the incidence of calcium-containing urinary stones. *J Urol* 1989;**142**:1272–5.

102 Robertson WG, Peacock M, Hodgkinson A. Dietary changes and the incidence of urinary calculi in the UK between 1958 and 1976. *J Chron Dis* 1979;**32**:469–76.

103 Robertson WG, Peacock M, Heyburn PJ, Marshall DH, Clark PB. Risk factors in calcium stone disease of the urinary tract. *Br J Urol* 1978;**50**:449–54.

104 Robertson WG, Heyburn PJ, Peacock M, Hanes FA, Swaminathan R. The effect of high animal protein intake in the risk of calcium stone-formation in the urinary tract. *Clin Sci* 1979;**57**:285–8.

105 Robertson WG, Peacock M. The pattern of urinary stone disease in the United Kingdom in relation to animal protein intake during the period 1960–1980. *Urol Int* 1982;**37**:393–9.

106 Robertson WG, Peacock M, Marshall RW, Speed R, Nordin BEC. Seasonal variations in the composition of urine in relation to calcium stone-formation. *Clin Sci Mol Med* 1975;**49**:597–602.

107 Robertson WG, Peacock M, Heyburn PH *et al*. Should recurrent calcium oxalate stone-formers become vegetarians? *Br J Urol* 1979;**51**:427–31.

108 Trinchieri A, Mandressi A, Luongo P, Longo G, Pisani E. The influence of diet on urinary risk factors for stones in healthy subjects and idiopathic renal calcium stone formers. *Br J Urol* 1991;**67**:230–6.

109 Curhan GC, Willett WC, Rimm EB, Stampfer MJ. A prospective study of dietary calcium and other nutrients and the risk of symptomatic kidney stones. *N Engl J Med* 1993;**328**:833–8.

110 Rao PN, Gordon C, Davies D, Blacklock NJ. Are stone formers maladapted to refined carbohydrates? *Br J Urol* 1982;**54**:575–7.

111 Fellström B, Danielson BG, Karlström B *et al*. Dietary habits in renal stone patients compared with healthy subjects. *Br J Urol* 1989;**63**:575–80.

112 Breslau NA, Brinkley L, Hill KD, Pak CYC. Relationship of animal protein-rich diet to kidney stone formation and calcium metabolism. *J Endocrinol Metab* 1988;**66**:140–6.

113 Griffith HM, O'Shea B, Kevany JP, McCormick JS. A control study of dietary factors in renal stone formation. *Br J Urol* 1981;**53**:416–20.

114 Schwille PO, Herrmann U. Environmental factors in the pathophysiology of recurrent idiopathic calcium urolithiasis (RCU), with emphasis on nutrition. *Urol Res* 1992;**20**:72–83.

115 Zechner O, Latal D, Pflueger H, Scheiber V. Nutritional risk factors in urinary stone disease. *J Urol* 1981;**125**:51–4.

116 Asper R. Epidemiology and socioeconomic aspects of urolithiasis. *Urol Res* 1984;**12**:1–5.

117 Vahlensieck W, Bach D, Hesse A, Strenge A. Epidemiology, pathogenesis and diagnosis of calcium oxalate urolithiasis. *Int Urol Nephrol* 1982;**14**:333.

118 Zechner O, Scheiber V. Alcohol as an epidemiological risk in urolithiasis. In: Smith LH, Robertson WG, Finlayson B, eds. *Urolithiasis: Clinical and Basic Research*. New York: Plenum Press, 1981;319–20.

119 Lonsdale K. Human stones. *Science* 1968;**159**:1199–207.

120 Mates J. External factors in the genesis of urolithiasis. In: Hodgkinson A, Nordin BEC, eds. *Proceedings of the Renal*

Stone Research Symposium, Leeds 1968. London: Churchill Livingstone, 1969;59–64.

121 Scott R. Prevalence of calcified upper urinary tract stone disease in a random population survey. Report of a combined study of general practitioners and hospital staff. *Br J Urol* 1987;**59**:111–17.

122 Ferrie BG, Scott R. Occupation and urinary tract stone disease. *Urology* 1984;**24**:443–5.

123 Thomas JMR. Vesical calculus in Norfolk. *Br J Urol* 1949;**21**: 20–3.

124 Andersen DA. The nutritional significance of primary bladder stones. *Br J Urol* 1973;**45**:160–77.

125 Halstead SB, Valyasevi A. Current epidemiology of bladder stone disease. Studies in the Thailand endemic area. In: Van Reen P, ed. *Proceedings of the WHO Regional Symposium in Vesical Calculus Disease.* Washington: US Dept of Health, Education and Welfare, 1972:17.

126 Srivastava RN, Hussainy MAA, Goel RG, Rose GA. Bladder stone disease in children in Afghanistan. *Br J Urol* 1986;**54**: 374–7.

127 Teotia M, Teotia SPS. Urinary tract stone disease. *J Assoc Phys India* 1984;**32**:731–9.

128 Valyasevi A, Halstead B, Dhanamitta S. Studies of bladder stone disease in Thailand. *Am J Nutr* 1967;**20**:1362–8.

129 Vermooten V. The occurrence of renal calculi and the possible relation to diet. *J Am Med Assoc* 1937;**109**:857–9.

130 Gershoff SN, Prien EL, Chandraparond A. Bladder stones in Thailand. *J Urol* 1967;**90**:285–8.

131 Van Reen R. Idiopathic urinary bladder stone disease. In: Fleisch H, Robertson WG, Smith LH, Vahlensieck W, eds. *Urolithiasis Research.* New York: Plenum Press, 1976: 569–72.

132 Sadre M, Bastenfar M, Ziai M. The urinary calculus in Iran. *Trans R Soc Trop Med Hyg* 1973;**67**:374–8.

133 Shahjahan S, Rahman MA. Studies on the etiology of urolithiasis in Karachi. *Am J Clin Nutr* 1970;**24**:32–7.

134 Teotia M, Teotia SPS. Kidney and bladder stones in India. *Postgrad Med J* 1977;**53**:41–8.

135 Thomson JO. Urinary calculus at the Canton hospital, Canton, China, based on 3500 operations. *Surg Gynecol Obstet* 1921;**32**:44–55.

136 Halstead SB, Valyasevi A. Studies of bladder stone disease in Thailand III. Epidemiological studies in Ubol Province. *Am J Clin Nutr* 1967;**20**:1329.

137 Remzi D, Cakmak F, Erkan I. A study of the urolithiasis incidence in Turkish schoolchildren. *J Urol* 1980;**123**: 608.

138 Malek RS. Urolithiasis. *Arch Int Med* 1989;**142**:1089.

58 Biochemical Aspects and Investigation of Urinary Stone Disease

V.R.Marshall

Introduction

Urinary stone disease has been reported to affect as many as one in 10 men in western communities [1]. By far the most common are stones composed primarily of calcium oxalate, but up to 20% will contain some phosphate. Of the remainder, uric acid stones are the next most common, followed by struvite and cystine stones. While the steps in the initial investigation of urinary stone disease are similar for all stones, the biochemical aspects vary considerably and these have been considered by stone type.

Biochemical aspects

Calcium oxalate calculi

Given that in western societies approximately 85% of renal stones are composed primarily of calcium oxalate, it should be a simple matter to establish the biochemical determinants and hence devise a simple protocol for the investigation of individuals with these stones. In simple terms, calcium oxalate urolithiasis can be regarded as in imbalance between the opposing influences of urinary saturation and inhibitory activity. It is only when one starts to look at these two factors in more detail that it becomes apparent that there are a significant number of components to each of these factors and they can all have a potential impact on the process of supersaturation and crystal nucleation. If one looks initially at supersaturation in detail, it is evident that the concentrations of calcium and oxalate are of fundamental importance, but Finlayson et al. [2] have pointed out that consideration also has to be given to the total sodium, potassium, magnesium, ammonium, phosphate, sulphate, citrate and chloride concentrations, as well as the pH. This complex series of interactions have been taken into account using a computer program which was developed by Werness et al. [3], which allowed for the calculation of Gibbs-free energy—the energy available for driving stone formation. This program did not take into account, initially, the effect of urate nor does it take into account the potential role of urinary macromolecules. Evidence suggests that the macromolecules do not have an important influence on supersaturation, but have a potentially important role in the inhibition of both crystal growth and aggregation once nucleation has occurred. Therefore, it would appear that urinary stone formation is a complex process with many factors involved in the key steps.

In spite of the potentially complex nature of stone formation, there has been a considerable preoccupation with the measurement of calcium and oxalate. Often these two substances have been examined in isolation, which has made it difficult to interpret the relevance of various reports and the application of their findings to clinical practice. Perhaps the most important observation is the dominance of the urinary oxalate concentration [4] over that of calcium in determining the likelihood of precipitation of calcium oxalate from the urine. This being the case, there appears little doubt that high oxalate concentrations in the urine pose the most significant threat to the formation of crystalluria and subsequently stones. Therefore, it is particularly important to understand the way in which oxalate is handled by the body.

It has long been recognized that high urinary oxalate levels can result from either an increased absorption from the gut or enhanced endogenous production. While considerable research has been undertaken regarding oxalate transport across the intestinal mucosa and also its removal by the kidney, important biochemical reactions may also occur within the gut which can either have a protective or promotory effect on the potential for stone formation. In the past, there has been enthusiasm for encouraging stone-forming patients to follow a low calcium diet; however, Robertson and Hughes [5], recognizing the dominance of urinary oxalate concentration over that of calcium in determining the probability of calcium oxalate precipitating in urine, advocated a high calcium diet to reduce stone recurrence in patients with mild hyperoxaluria. This observation was further supported by the study of Curhan et al. [6]. In a large prospective epidemiological study involving 45 619 men, they showed that the risk of developing a symptomatic kidney stone was inversely related to dietary calcium intake. They proposed that calcium had the ability to bind oxalate in the gut, thus preventing its absorption and hence reducing the load of oxalate that ultimately was excreted by the kidney.

It has been suggested that there is an increased absorption of oxalate from the upper alimentary tract in some stone formers. However, it has not been possible to establish any structural defect to explain this, and indeed the observation may simply have reflected the experimental protocols used and the bioavailability of oxalate in these individuals. It has now been generally agreed that oxalate is freely filtered by the glomerulus and, in contrast to most other substances, is handled primarily in the proximal tubule where transport occurs along the full length of the proximal tubule. In the proximal tubule, secretion exceeds reabsorption and there appears to be little change in the amount of oxalate in the urine after it leaves that area. In a rat model, both urate and thiazides impair oxalate secretion, but relatively little is known about the mechanisms by which the secretion of oxalate is controlled. However, in a detailed review of oxalate transport across intestinal and renal epithelia, Hatch and Freel [7] have highlighted the fact that there is conflicting information as to whether the net effect of this bidirectional transport of oxalate results in either tubular secretion or reabsorption. From their evidence they suggest that oxalate handling varies across species and, indeed, varies quite significantly within the kidney of certain individual species.

With regard to the metabolism of oxalate, Bais et al. [8] were able to show in rat liver homogenates that sulphhydryl compounds could inhibit carbon dioxide and oxalate formation. They proposed that the decrease in production of oxalate was a result of the formation of a cysteine glyoxalate adduct, carboxy-4-thiazolydine carboxylate, which prevents the glyoxalate from undergoing further oxidation. This raises the possibility that cysteine or similar sulphhydryl compounds may have the potential to lower oxalate excretion and prevent renal stones. In a novel approach to developing new methods for lowering the excretion of oxalate, Lung et al. [9] have cloned the coenzyme A (CoA) decarboxylase gene from Oxalobacta formigenes, with the ultimate possibility that gene therapy could be an option, albeit well into the future, for reducing oxalate excretion. This, of course, may have important ramifications in individuals suffering from primary hyperoxaluria, which often runs an unremitting course and ends in renal failure.

Calcium handling

The level of calcium in the urine will have an influence on the propensity of an individual to form calcium oxalate crystals. This level is influenced by numerous factors, including dietary intake, the rate of absorption from the gut, the concomitant sodium intake, serum protein concentrations, vitamin D levels and the levels of both parathyroid hormone and thyroid hormone [10,11].

More recently, Holmes et al. [12] have shown that a pair of codominant alleles exert a major influence on calcium excretion. They have also proposed that the locus most probably responsible for the genetic influence on calcium excretion is one associated with the synthesis of 1,25-dihydroxyvitamin D_3. The potential significance of this observation is that if the genetic locus responsible for controlling calcium excretion could be identified, it may be possible to determine the calcium excretory class for an individual (high, intermediate or low) from the DNA sequence, thus obviating the need to rely on measurements of the 24 h excretion of calcium. This would also avoid the problems of multiple urine measurements and the effect of diet.

Under normal physiological conditions, the kidney filters approximately 200–250 mmol of calcium in 24 h. Of this amount, only 1–2% is finally excreted in the urine. Approximately two-thirds of the filtered calcium is absorbed in the proximal tubule, with 20% being absorbed in the loop of Henle and the remainder in the distal convolute tubule. In the proximal tubule, calcium is absorbed at a rate similar to both sodium and water, which is consistent with reabsorption by a passive transport mechanism. While there is broad agreement that the majority of the calcium is absorbed passively, it has been proposed that there may be a small active component [13]. As with the proximal tubule, the absorption of calcium, which takes place primarily in the thick ascending limb of the loop of Henle, is a passive process occurring as a result of a positive voltage in the lumen [14]. As with most ions, the amount of calcium absorbed from the distal tubule and collecting duct is small compared with the amounts absorbed from the other parts of the tubule. However, the absorption from this segment has a vital role in the final regulation of calcium excretion [15]. Contrary to the process that occurs in the proximal tubule and the loop of Henle, this appears to be an active process, as adjudged by the fact that calcium is absorbed against high chemical gradients as well as high electrical potential gradients. The precise molecular events have not been elucidated, but one proposed mechanism depends on the presence of a vitamin D-dependent calcium-binding protein in the cytozol of the distal tubular cells. The other possible transport mechanism depends on the presence of a high affinity calcium–magnesium–adenosine triphosphatase (ATPase) which provides the basis for a calcium pump.

While the initial part of this section provides a brief outline of the normal physiological mechanisms involved in calcium excretion, it is more germane to focus on factors that may influence calcium excretion. While there has been considerable interest in the role of growth hormone, gluca-gon, insulin, prolactin, glucocorticoids and, in particular, parathormone and calcitonin, there is no convincing evidence that any of these hormonal agents has a signi-ficant regulatory role in the renal handling of calcium [13].

The presumed role of parathormone is to enhance intestinal absorption of calcium and bone resorption. Its known ability to enhance renal calcium reabsorption is overwhelmed by its ability to increase the filtered load by the former mechanisms. Buck et al. [16] were the first to examine the possible role of prostaglandins in the renal handling of calcium. Studies by Hirayama et al. [17] and Henriquez-La-Roche et al. [18] have also supported a relationship between prostaglandin activity and calcium excretion. In animal studies, Buck [19] was able to show that cyclo-oxygenase inhibition prevented nephrocal-cinosis. This has not been further extended in human studies, but it is possible that prostaglandins may be able to be used to influence calcium excretion.

Another piece of information important to the under-standing of calcium excretion has been provided by studies on the role of thiazide diuretics. These drugs have been used since the early 1970s [20]. While shedding light on the handling of calcium, their precise mechanism of action has not been established. A number of theories have been proposed. Calcium may be resorbed coincidentally as a result of changes in the renal handling of sodium, there may be a direct effect on distal tubular cells or there may be alterations in parathormone activity. It is evident that the renal handling of calcium is complex and a multitude of factors can influence the level of calcium in the different parts of the nephron. Hence, fluctuations in different parts of the nephron may facilitate the presence of supersatura-tion and crystal formation for short periods of time. Considerable work still needs to be performed to under-stand how the renal handling of calcium may influence stone formation.

Urate

The handling of urate in the kidney is complex; it involves bidirectional transport, with the vast majority of the filtered urate being absorbed and the fraction which appears in the urine being secreted from the proximal nephrons. It is also evident that large numbers of factors can influence the renal handling of urate. They range from work to alcohol; Lang [21] has listed some 130 factors. However, it would seem in essence from this extensive list that anything that enhances luminal flow will lead to raised levels of urate in the urine. It is also well documented that there is a circadian pattern to the excretion of urate with peak levels in the afternoon and low levels at night. Lang et al. [22] showed that this pattern coupled with urine flow rates may afford some protection from stone formation. In

examining the list of substances that influence the supersaturation of urine with calcium oxalate, urate appears to be something of a misfit. It was only in the late 1960s when Gutman and Yu [23] indicated that there may be a 'suspicion' of a higher incidence of calcium oxalate stone disease in gouty individuals that attention began to be focused on urate in calcium oxalate disease. Since then, three theories have been proposed to explain the role of urate in calcium oxalate stone disease. The first, by Coe et al. [24], proposed that crystals of sodium urate in the urine induce heterogeneous nucleation of calcium oxalate. The second was proposed by Robertson et al. [25] who believed that urate could have a promotory effect by binding glycosaminoglycans. The rationale behind this was that glycosaminoglycans had been proposed to be inhibitors and the binding by urate would nullify this property.

The third theory was based on the concept that urine can salt out calcium, which was first demonstrated by Kallistratos and Timmermann [26]; this work was further developed by Grover et al. [27]. In a detailed review of the evidence available to support the various theories [28], it is argued that salting out is the most likely mechanism by which urate can influence the saturation of urine with calcium oxalate.

Citrate

Like most substances, the majority of filtered citrate is reabsorbed in the nephron. As with urate, bidirectional absorption occurs in the proximal tubule and there is little evidence to support any substantial transport in the distal tubule. The renal handling of citrate is influenced greatly by the luminal pH. A more acid urine enhances citrate absorption, hence the rates of citrate absorption and excretion are strongly influenced by acid–base balance [29]. For example, the low level of citrate in the urine in distal renal tubular acidosis is a direct result of the influence of the pH on the renal handling of citrate. Calcium may also influence citrate excretion as high calcium levels will complex the citrate and this will result in increased renal excretion of citrate [30].

Magnesium

Magnesium is handled quite differently from calcium in the kidney: only about 20–30% of the filtered load of magnesium is reabsorbed in the proximal tubule. The majority is absorbed in the ascending limb of the loop of Henle under the influence of the parathyroid hormone, while the distal nephron is capable of absorbing up to 10% of the filtered magnesium. It is also of interest to note that while thiazide diuretics reduce calcium excretion, they have the reverse effect on magnesium. Magnesium has the ability to form a soluble complex with oxalate, making it unavailable to calcium. There is also evidence to suggest that magnesium may bind citrate and by this means enhance the excretion of that ion. Rudman *et al.* [31] have proposed that a deficiency of magnesium could lead to a reduced excretion of citrate and this in turn may promote calcium oxalate stone formation.

pH

The maintenance of the acid–base balance, and hence the urine pH, is a complex process and beyond the scope of this chapter. However, it is well established that the solubility of calcium oxalate is pH dependent and, as already indicated, the excretion of citrate is also highly influenced by the acid–base status. Consequently, the pH does have the potential to have an important bearing on urinary stone formation.

Urinary volume

The ability of the kidney to concentrate or dilute urine is vital to the maintenance of the constant osmolality of the tissue fluid. The kidney also has a vital role in the regulation of the excretion of water, particularly in relation to the solute load. The kidney dilutes the urine by removing sodium chloride primarily from the thick ascending limb of the loop of Henle, but also from the distal tubule, the connecting tubule and the collecting duct. This can be achieved because these parts of the nephron are impermeable to water. The countercurrent system is vital for this process and depends for its operation on a number of factors: the anatomical arrangement of the nephrons, the active transport of sodium from the ascending limb of the loop of Henle, countercurrent multiplication by the loop of Henle, the ability of the collecting ducts to respond to antidiuretic hormone and the ability of the papillae to maintain a concentration gradient. While this is a complex process, there is little to suggest that aberrations in the handling of water by the kidney are significant in the formation of renal stones.

Macromolecules

The prime focus of most studies to date has been on the mineral component of urine. However, it is well known that in many instances urine will become saturated with respect to calcium oxalate with the likely formation of crystals and stones, but these last two steps do not invariably occur. It has, therefore, been proposed that there are substances in the urine which inhibit the nucleation, growth and aggregation of calcium oxalate crystals. These inhibitors fall into two broad groups: the low and high molecular weight substances. Two of the low molecular weight substances—magnesium and citrate—have already

been examined earlier in this chapter. It is the macromolecular group, however, that has recently attracted the greater attention.

The concentration of most of the proteins, which make up a significant proportion of these macromolecules, depends upon their plasma concentration and their filtration ratio. However, some of these macromolecules, such as Tamm–Horsfall glycoprotein (THG), are secreted by the tubular cells and are not derived from the plasma. THG is a particularly interesting protein in that it has been shown in highly concentrated urines [32] to be a promoter of crystallization, but in more dilute urine it has been shown to inhibit this process [33].

In 1983, Nakagawa *et al.* [34] published studies describing the isolation of what they termed 'the principal inhibitor of calcium oxalate crystal growth in human urine'. Subsequently, Shiraga *et al.* [35] published data showing that an aspartic acid-rich protein which they named uropontin was a potent inhibitor of calcium oxalate crystal growth. At virtually the same time, Doyle *et al.* [36] described a protein that had been included in calcium oxalate crystals, which they named crystal matrix protein, which was subsequently shown and demonstrated [37] to have potent inhibitory activity [38] and to be related to the human prothrombin. Also, Atmani *et al.* [39] isolated another protein with inhibitory activity which they named uronic acid-rich protein and which was subsequently shown to have structural homology with the inter-α-trypsin inhibitor and with α₁-microglobulin. Studies by Ebisuno *et al.* [40] have identified yet another macromolecule with a molecular weight in the 10–30 kDa range which inhibited calcium oxalate aggregation in inorganic solutions, and whose activity for this substance in the urine of stone formers compared with healthy controls.

Therefore, there has been a substantial increase in the number of macromolecules with inhibitory activity described in the last 5–10 years. While all have been shown to have an effect in a variety of test systems, most have either not been evaluated in whole urine systems or have not been shown to be deficient in stone formers. While these agents may well have an important bearing on stone formation, further clinical studies are required to determine how significant any one, or any combination, of these macromolecules may be in the prevention of calcium oxalate lithiasis. It is a promising field for further study.

Uric acid stones

Uric acid is a trioxypurine and a weak acid. As in the case of calcium oxalate, urine is frequently supersaturated with sodium urate; however, the spontaneous crystallization of sodium urate is a long, slow process and this provides an important protective effect. It would also appear that urine inhibits sodium urate precipitation, and early studies [41] identified a substance that was similar to THG. Whereas there has been considerable interest in inhibitors of calcium oxalate crystallization, this area has not been pursued to any great extent for uric acid stones. High levels of uric acid in the urine can result from numerous factors; however, a common cause of hyperuricosuria is a diet rich in purines, usually derived from animal protein. Not surprisingly, there is a high incidence of uric acid stone formation in patients with gout and it is anticipated that in patients with uric acid stones, 50% will already have been known to have gout or will be found to have gout as a result of investigation of the stone episode.

Urinary pH also has an extremely important role in both the formation and dissolution of these stones. Sodium urate is far less soluble in acid urine. In gouty patients and those with normal serum and urinary uric acid levels who had stones, the only consistent finding in both groups was a low urinary pH [42]. While the cause of the low pH may be dietary in origin, the basis for the low urine pH in both groups of patients is not well established.

Struvite stones

Struvite is a geological expression for magnesium ammonium phosphate [43]. The presence of microorganisms with the ability to split urea is vital to this process. As a result of the urealysis, there is a significant increase in the urine pH with an associated rise in the concentration of both ammonia and bicarbonate. Under these conditions it is possible for crystals of magnesium ammonium phosphate to form. These stones are often associated with a profuse gelatinous matrix. The source of this matrix is not clear; however, it is known that elevated ammonia levels have a toxic effect on the mucosa and may be a source of the matrix. It is also possible that the amount of this gelatinous material is further increased by the presence of bacteria. As a result of the damage to epithelial cells by the ammonia, the protective glycosaminoglycan layer is removed, and the bacteria can adhere to these cells and produce an inflammatory response, the resultant exudate contributing to the matrix.

Cystine stones

Cystine stones result from an inborn error of metabolism in which there is a transport defect in the renal tubule which results in an excessive excretion of a number of dibasic amino acids. A similar defect is also observed in the intestine. Of these amino acids, cystine is the least soluble—hence the reason for the formation of stones of this composition.

Investigation of urinary stone disease

In the investigation of urinary stone disease, controversy still exists as to the extent of the metabolic evaluation, particularly of a calcium oxalate stone former. Most would agree that patients presenting with their first stone episode require assessment of overall renal function with a serum creatinine measurement, as well as microscopy and culture of the urine and visualization of the urinary tract, usually with an intravenous urogram. For individuals with conditions where irradiation needs to be avoided, or there is poor renal function, the intravenous urogram may be replaced by ultrasonographic studies. Depending on whether the stone is radio-opaque or radiolucent, then serum calcium or uric acid measurements are required. Also, in the case of lucent or faintly opacified stones, particularly in young people with a family history of stones, the nitroprusside test needs to be performed to exclude cystinuria. This series of investigations, coupled with a detailed medical history, should be able to identify hyperparathyroidism, structural abnormalities such as medullary sponge disease, urinary infection, recumbency, sarcoidosis or small bowel surgery as possible aetiological factors. These initial investigations should also confirm if the stones are cystine or uric acid in nature, and these require little further evaluation.

Analysis of the stone should also be performed, if possible, as it may negate the need for detailed metabolic evaluation. Having excluded the above possible aetiological factors, the remaining stones can be broadly classified as idiopathic and these will account for approximately three-quarters of all renal stones composed of calcium oxalate, calcium phosphate or a combination or both. A vexed question has been whether any further investigations are required. Uribarri et al. [44] reviewed six large retrospective studies and found stone recurrence rates of 14% at 1 year, 35% at 5 years and 52% at 10 years. From their analysis of randomized trials published at that time, using either thiazides or allopurinol, they estimated a benefit of 35% over placebo. Taking into account the risk of the therapy, they reasoned that therapy was not needed for patients presenting with their first stone and therefore extensive metabolic investigation was unnecessary. Whilst this is disputed by some, there appears to be a belief that detailed metabolic evaluation is not necessary for individuals presenting with their first stone. Most, however, would still support the notion that even if detailed metabolic studies are not performed, then an analysis of a 24 h urine specimen should be performed to determine the daily volume and levels of calcium, uric acid, oxalate, phosphorus, citrate and creatinine excretion.

Whether one undertakes detailed metabolic evaluation or limited metabolic studies, the question that needs to be answered is whether it is worthwhile even undertaking such an evaluation, as it assumes that the information will be of value in determining the need and nature of further treatment to prevent recurrence. In this regard, those who have a nihilist approach to investigation can point to recurrence rates as low as 5% [45], whereas those who support early investigation can point to recurrence rates as high as 50% [46]. One of the difficulties in assessing recurrence rates is that often data are drawn from referral centres, which may only reflect the pattern for patients with persistent problems, where the population is not balanced by stone sufferers who pass a single stone and have no further problems. Undoubtedly, more prospective long-term studies are required to ascertain recurrence rates in unselected populations to determine what proportion of patients with idiopathic stones will have a recurrence. The other important information which is lacking is whether the results of these 24 h urine measurements can be used to predict accurately the likelihood of response to treatment. For example, this is highlighted with hypercalciuria where thiazides have been equally beneficial in both normocalciuric and hypercalciuric individuals [47].

Failure over the last two to three decades to find a simple single cause for idiopathic calcium oxalate stones clearly supports the intuitive belief that a number of factors must contribute to the formation of the stone. The other problem, of course, is that stones tend to form episodically and are often only unilateral. Therefore, we may simply be undertaking detailed examination of the urine at a time when the relevant factors are not active. Returning to the value of the 24 h urine collection, it is perhaps important to examine the potential benefit by looking in detail at each of the parameters that are frequently measured; namely, calcium, oxalate, urate and citrate concentrations, and pH and volume.

Calcium

Measurement of 24 h urinary calcium excretion has been described as the 'sacred cow of stone investigation' [48], and Ryall and Marshall go on to say 'No other urinary parameter has been subjected to such scrutiny or dietary manipulation or has so consistently borne the blame for the disease.' The interest in calcium measurement was first generated by Flocks [49] when he was able to show that stone formers had higher urinary calcium levels than normal controls. This was extended by Albright et al. [50] when they too found a raised a calcium output and they were the first to use the term idiopathic hypercalciuria to account for this observation. Hypercalciuria may be defined as the excretion of abnormally high amounts of calcium in the urine; however, this is, of course, dependent on what is defined as the upper limit of normal. Ryall and Marshall [48] in reviewing some 15 studies in which the 24 h calcium excretion had been measured in men with no history of stone disease, found that if one took the upper limit to be that which encompassed 95% of all normal values, then the upper limit for normal men could range from 4.9 mmol/day [51] to 13.64 mmol/day [52]. Thus it is

imperative that an appropriate reference range is used for the population being studied, not one that has been established by other workers for populations coming from other regions. The other aspect which diminishes the value of this measurement has been the failure to obtain uniform agreement linking a raised calcium with subsequent recurrence rate. Ljunghall and Danielson [46] and Marickar and Rose [53] all reported increased recurrence rates in patients with elevated calcium. However, Ryall and Marshall [48] and Ettinger [54] could not find such an association.

Another important practical problem associated with a 24 h urine collection is the wide day to day variation. Laerum and Palmer [55] found that by taking two values and determining the mean of both, they had a higher likelihood of finding elevated calcium than if only one or other of the values had been used. In a more detailed study, Ryall and Marshall [48] found that on a free diet, it may take as many as six consecutive 24 h urine specimens before a person could be categorized as being hypercalciuric.

Oxalate

On theoretical grounds, one might expect that variation in oxalate levels might be readily observed in stone formers. As has already been indicated, oxalate has a far more powerful effect on the degree of supersaturation of the urine with calcium oxalate than does calcium. Again, wide daily fluctuations [56] and the inability to show consistently significant differences between stone formers and normals has made it difficult to place reliance on such measurements when deciding on long-term therapy.

Other parameters

The same problems arise for all of the other parameters measured, including 24 h volume, urate, pH, citrate, pyrophosphate and magnesium [48]. It therefore seems that while abnormalities will be found from the measurement of these parameters in a single 24 h urine collection, the scientific data currently available do not strongly support this approach, as there is consistent overlap of values with individuals who have not formed a stone, and it has not been possible to find consistent correlations between altered levels of these parameters and stone recurrence rates. Detailed metabolic studies therefore seem best restricted to those individuals who have had more than one stone episode.

Investigation protocols

If such studies are undertaken, then protocols similar to those recommended by Pak et al. [57] seem to be the most appropriate. Their protocol entails the collection of 24 h urine specimens on two occasions with patients taking their normal diet. From the data presented earlier in this chapter, it seems that if reliable information is to be obtained to categorize individuals, then two measurements may not be sufficient. The parameters they recommend being measured are: volume, the amounts of calcium, urate, oxalate and citrate, and the pH. In their protocol, the patient is then placed on a calcium- and sodium-restricted diet for 1 week (400 g of calcium and 100 mg sodium per day) and a further 24 h specimen collected and analysed for calcium, phosphate, uric acid and creatinine. Blood levels of calcium, phosphorus, uric acid and creatinine are also determined while the patient is on both a free and restricted diet. The protocol is also extended, if necessary, to exclude renal tubular acidosis by means of the ammonium chloride loading test. Further studies are performed to determine whether the elevated calcium levels are due to disturbances of absorption from the gut or due to altered renal handling. It has been estimated that by undertaking this pattern of investigation, some 90% of individuals will be found to have abnormal results, thus affording a basis for the selection of appropriate therapy.

Management

While a detailed study of treatment outcomes is beyond the scope of this chapter, it is useful to review briefly how successful this strategy has been. Thomson [58] reviewed the stone literature of the preceding 28 years, looking for the results of controlled studies. In this review he was able to find a number of studies in which thiazides had been used to treat stone formers. Although he showed that the thiazides reduced the incidence of stones, he found two studies [47,59] in which the thiazides seemed to be equally effective irrespective of whether the patients were normocalciuric or hypercalciuric. Similarly, in examining the effect of trials of allopurinol therapy in preventing recurrences, uncertainty exists as to how effective this agent is. More importantly, there is no unequivocal evidence from Smith's study [60] that allopurinol might be equally effective in patients with normal urinary uric acid excretion as in those with hyperuricosuria. The other commonly used agent has been citrate, and whilst Barcelo et al. [61] in a randomized trial showed there is a protective effect of potassium citrate in hypocitraturic calcium stone formers, this agent may be equally as effective in individuals who are normocitraturic. Therefore, the practical value of extensive metabolic investigations in the tailoring of treatment still requires a review of a wide range of parameters. There is no doubt that although elevated levels may be identified, as yet it has not been possible to show that treatment will only be of benefit in reducing recurrences in these individuals. Undoubtedly, more carefully controlled randomized trials are necessary before

we can unequivocally show that this pattern of investigation greatly assists us in the management of stone disease.

The other important question that must also be considered results from the introduction of relatively non-invasive techniques of managing stones. Is anything to be gained from early detailed investigation, with a view to starting treatment, rather than waiting to determine whether further stones will form? We know that at least 50% of individuals will apparently never get a second stone. There is, therefore, an important place for appropriate cost–benefit studies to also be performed to assist in this decision-making process.

While urinary stone disease is one of the most common problems encountered by a urologist, a rational basis for investigation and management still remains elusive.

References

1 Sierakowski R, Finlayson B, Landes RR, Finalyston CD, Sierakowski N. The frequency of urolithiasis in hospital discharge diagnoses in the United States. *Invest Urol* 1978; **15**:438–41.
2 Finlayson B, Khan S-R, Hackett RL. Theoretical chemical models of urinary stones. In: Wickham JEA, Buck AC, eds. *Renal Tract Stone; Metabolic Basis and Clinical Practice.* Edinburgh: Churchill Livingstone, 1990:133–47.
3 Werness P, Brown C, Smith LH, Finlayson B. EQUIL2: a BASIC computer program for the calculation of urinary saturation. *J Urol* 1985;**134**:1242–4.
4 Finlayson B. Renal lithiasis in review. *Urol Clin North Am* 1974;**1**:181–212.
5 Robertson WG, Hughes H. Importance of mild hyperoxaluria in the pathogenesis of urolithiasis—new evidence from studies in the Arabian peninsula. *Scanning Microsc* 1993;**7**:391–402.
6 Curhan GC, Willett WC, Rimm EB, Stampfer MJ. A prospective study of dietary calcium and other nutrients and the risk of symptomatic kidney stones. *N Engl J Med* 1993;**328**: 833–8.
7 Hatch M, Freel RW. Oxalate transport across intestinal and renal epithelia. In: Khan S-R, ed. *Calcium Oxalate in Biological Systems.* New York: CRC Press, 1995:217–38.
8 Bais R, Rofe AM, Conyers RA. The inhibition of metabolic oxalate production by sulphydryl compounds. *J Urol* 1991; **145**:1302–5.
9 Lung HY, Cornelius JG, Peck AB. Cloning and expression of the oxalyl-CoA decarboxylase gene from the bacterium, *Oxalobacter formigenes*: prospects for gene therapy to control Ca-oxalate kidney stones formation. *Am J Kidney Dis* 1991;**17**: 381–5.
10 Lemann J, Gray RW. Idiopathic hypercalciuria. *J Urol* 1989;**141**: 715.
11 Pak CYC, Ohata M, Lawrence EC, Snyder W. The hypercalciurias: causes, parathyroid functions and diagnostic criteria. *J Clin Invest* 1974;**43**:387.
12 Holmes RP, Goodman HO, Assimos DG. Genetic influences on urinary calcium excretion. In: Ryall R, Bais R, Marshall VR, Rofe A, Smith LH, Walker VR, eds. *Urolithiasis*, Vol. 2. New York: Plenum Press, 1994:3–8.
13 Buck AC, Lote CJ. The renal handling of calcium. In: Wickham

JEA, Buck AC, eds. *Renal Tract Stone: Metabolic Basis and Clinical Practice*. Edinburgh: Churchill Livingstone, 1990: 165–82.

14 Burg MB. Thick ascending limb of Henle's loop. *Kidney Int* 1982;**22**:454.

15 Rouse D, Suki WN. Calcium and the kidney. *Semin Nephrol* 1981;**1**:295–305.

16 Buck AC, Sampson WF, Lote CJ, Blacklock NJ. The influence of renal prostaglandins on glomerular filtration rate (GFR) and calcium excretion in urolithiasis. *Br J Urol* 1981;**53**:485–91.

17 Hirayama H, Ikegami K, Shimomura T, Yamamoto T. The possible role of prostaglandin E2 in urinary stone formation. In: *Proceedings of the XX Congres de la Société International d'Urologie*, Vienna, 1985:354–62.

18 Henriquez-La-Roche C, Rodriquez-Iturbe B, Herrera J, Parra G. Patients with idiopathic hypercalciuria have increased prostaglandin excretion. In: *Proceedings of the Tenth Congress of Nephrology*, 1987:abstr. 428.

19 Buck AC. *The influence of renal prostaglandins on calcium metabolism in relation to the pathogenesis of idiopathic urolithiasis*. PhD thesis, University of Wales, 1987.

20 Yendt ER, Guay GF, Garcia DA. The use of thiazides in the prevention of renal calculi. *Can Med Assoc J* 1970;**102**:614–20.

21 Lang F. Renal handling of oxalate, urate, citrate, phosphate and sulphate. In: Wickham JEA, Buck AC, eds. *Renal Tract Stone: Metabolic Basis and Clinical Practice*. Edinburgh: Churchill Livingstone, 1990:183–213.

22 Lang R, Geger R, Sporer H, Oberleithner H, Deetjen P. Renal handling of urate and oxalate: possible implications for urolithiasis. *Urol Res* 1979;**7**:143–8.

23 Gutman AB, Yu T-F. Uric acid nephrolithiasis. *Am J Med* 1968;**45**:756–79.

24 Coe FL, Lawton RL, Goldstein RB, Tember V. Sodium urate accelerates precipitation of calcium oxalate *in vitro*. *Proc Exp Biol Med* 1975;**149**:926–9.

25 Robertson WG, Knowles F, Peacock M. Urinary mucopolysaccharide inhibitors of calcium oxalate crystallisation. In: Fleisch H, Robertson WG, Smith LH, Vahlensieck W, eds. *Urolithiasis Research*. New York: Plenum Press, 1976:331–4.

26 Kallistratos G, Timmermann A. The 'salting-out' effect as a possible causative factor for the formation of calcium oxalate crystals in human urine. Presented to the 66th Annual Meeting of the American Urology Association, Chicago, 17 May 1971.

27 Grover PK, Ryall RL, Marshall VR. Effect of urate on calcium oxalate crystallization in human urine: evidence for a promotory role of hyperuricosuria in urolithiasis. *Clin Sci* 1990;**79**:9.

28 Grover PK, Ryall RL. Urate and calcium oxalate stones: from repute to rhetoric to reality. *Miner Electrolyte Metab* 1994;**20**:361–70.

29 Crawford MA, Milne MD, Scribner BH. The effects of changes in acid–base balance on urinary citrate in the rat. *J Physiol (Lond)* 1959;**149**:413–23.

30 Crawford MA, Loughbridge L, Milne MD, Scribner BH. Organic acid excretion after calcium gluconate infusions. *J Clin Path* 1959;**2**:524–9.

31 Rudman D, Dedonis JL, Fountain MT *et al*. Hypocitraturia in patients with gastrointestinal malabsorption. *N Engl J Med* 1980;**303**:657–61.

32 Rose GA, Sulaiman S. Tamm–Horsfall mucoprotein promotes calcium phosphate crystal formation in whole urine: quantitative studies. *Urol Res* 1984;**12**:217.

33 Grover PK, Ryall RL, Marshall VR. Does Tamm–Horsfall mucoprotein inhibit or promote CaOx crystallization in human urine? *Clin Chim Acta* 1990;**190**:223–8.

34 Nakagawa Y, Abram V, Kézdy FJ, Kaiser ET, Coe FL. Purification and characterization of the principal inhibitor of calcium oxalate monohydrate crystal growth in human urine. *J Biol Chem* 1983;**258**:12594.

35 Shiraga H, Min W, Vandusen WJ *et al*. Inhibition of calcium oxalate crystal growth *in vitro* by uropontin: another member of the aspartic acid-rich protein superfamily. *Proc Natl Acad Sci* 1992;**89**:426–30.

36 Doyle IR, Ryall RL, Marshall VR. Inclusion of proteins into calcium oxalate crystals precipitated from human urine: a highly selective phenomenon. *Clin Chem* 1991;**37**: 1589–94.

37 Stapleton AMF, Simpson RJ, Ryall RL. Crystal matrix protein is related to human prothrombin. *Biochem Biophys Res Commun* 1993;**195**:1199–203.

38 Ryall RL, Grover PK, Stapleton AMF *et al*. The urinary F1 activation peptide of human prothrombin is a potent inhibitor of calcium oxalate crystallization in undiluted human urine *in vitro*. *Clin Sci* 1995;**89**:533–41.

39 Atmani F, Lacour B, Drueke T, Daudon M. Isolation and purification of a new glycoprotein from human urine inhibiting calcium oxalate crystallization. *Urol Res* 1993;**21**:61–6.

40 Ebisuno S, Kohjimoto Y, Yoshida T, Ohkawa. Effect of urinary macromolecules on aggregation of calcium oxalate in recurrent calcium stone formers and healthy subjects. *Urol Res* 1993;**21**:265–8.

41 Sperling O, De Vries A, Kedem O. Studies on the etiology of uric acid lithiasis. IV. Urinary nondialyzable substances in idiopathic uric acid lithiasis. *J Urol* 1965;**94**:286.

42 Pak CY, Skurla C, Harvey J. Graphic display of urinary risk factors for renal stone formation. *J Urol* 1985;**134**:867.

43 Goldstone L, Griffith DP. Infection calculi. In: Wickham JEA, Buck AC, eds. *Renal Tract Stone: Metabolic Basis and Clinical Practice*. Edinburgh: Churchill Livingstone, 1990:367–85.

44 Uribarri J, Man SO, Carroll HJ. The first kidney stone. *Ann Intern Med* 1989;**12**:1006–9.

45 Joost J, Putz A. Calcium oxalate stone formers—five years later. In: Schwille PO, Smith LH, Robertson WG, Vahlensieck W, eds. *Urolithiasis and Related Clinical Research*. New York: Plenum Press, 1985:557–60.

46 Ljunghall S, Danielson BG. A prospective study of renal stone recurrence. *Br J Urol* 1984;**56**:122–4.

47 Laerum I, Larsen S. Thiazide prophylaxis of urolithiasis. A double-blind study in general practice. *Acta Med Scand* 1984;**215**:383–9.

48 Ryall RL, Marshall VR. The investigation and management of idiopathic urolithiasis. In: Wickham JEA, Buck AC, eds. *Renal Tract Stone: Metabolic Basis and Clinical Practice*. Edinburgh: Churchill Livingstone, 1990:307–31.

49 Flocks RH. Calcium and phosphorus excretion in the urine of patients with renal or ureteral calculi. *J Am Med Assoc* 1939;**113**:1466–71.

50 Albright F, Henneman R, Benedict PH, Forbes AP. Idiopathic hypercalciuria (a preliminary report). *Proc R Soc Med* 1953;**46**:1077–81.

51 Baumann JM, Bisaz S, Felix R *et al*. The role of inhibitors and other factors in the pathogenesis of recurrent calcium-containing renal stones. *Clin Sci Molec Med* 1977;**53**: 141–8.

52 Jorgensen FS. The urinary excretion and serum concentration of calcium, magnesium, sodium and phosphate in male patients with recurring renal stone formation. *Scand J Urol Nephrol* 1975;**9**:243–8.

53 Marickar YMF, Rose GA. Relationship of stone growth and urinary biochemistry in long-term follow-up of stone patients with idiopathic hypercalciuria. *Br J Urol* 1985;**57**: 613–17.

54 Ettinger B. Recurrence of urolithiasis. A six year prospective study. *Am J Med* 1979;**67**:245–8.

55 Laerum E, Palmer H. Methodological aspects of examination of 24 h urinary excretions in outpatients with recurrent urolithiasis. *Scand J Urol Nephrol* 1983;**17**:321–4.

56 Zarembski PM, Hodgkinson A. Some factors influencing the urinary excretion of oxalic acid in man. *Clin Chim Acta* 1969;**25**:1–10.

57 Pak CYC, Sakhaee K, Crowther C, Brinkley L. Evidence justifying a high fluid intake in treatment of nephrolithiasis. *Ann Intern Med* 1980;**93**:36–9.

58 Thomson CRV. Prevention of recurrent calcium stones: a rational approach. *Br J Urol* 1995;**76**:419–24.

59 Yendt ER, Cohanim M. Prevention of calcium stones with thiazides. *Kidney Int* 1978;**13**:397–409.

60 Smith MJV. Placebo versus allopurinol for renal calculi. *J Urol* 1977;**117**:690–2.

61 Barcelo P, Wuhl O, Servitge E, Rousaud A, Pak CY. Randomized double-blind study of potassium citrate in idiopathic hypocitraturic calcium nephrolithiasis. *J Urol* 1993;**150**:1761–4.

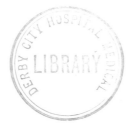

59 Inherited Metabolic Stone Disease
O. Sperling

Introduction

By definition, inherited metabolic stone disease relates to inherited metabolic abnormalities associated with stone formation. Most of these disorders are rare, and such stone patients constitute a minority in any general stone clinic. Nevertheless, special attention should be given to the diagnosis of these abnormalities, as in some of them the treatment should differ from that given to regular stone patients. In inherited metabolic stone diseases, the metabolic abnormalities are associated with overexcretion of the stone component, reflecting either overproduction of the substance, as for uric acid in the Lesch–Nyhan syndrome and in most of the other inherited disorders of purine metabolism associated with urolithiasis, or renal transport disorders, as for cystine in cystinuria or uric acid in hereditary renal hypouricaemia.

In all the inherited metabolic stone diseases, the aetiology of stone formation is associated with supersaturation of the urine with the insoluble metabolite. However, although in the genetic defects supersaturation occurs from birth, stone formation in the affected subjects may start later in life, sometimes only at adulthood. This phenomenon indicates that urinary supersaturation, important as it is as a single aetiological factor, may require additional supporting conditions for stone formation.

Another point of interest is that at least in two of the inherited metabolic stone diseases, cystinuria and uric acid lithiasis, the stones extracted from patients led to the first identification of the relevant stone-forming metabolite, that is cystine and uric acid.

Stone disease associated with inborn errors of purine metabolism

Hereditary disorders in purine metabolism constitute the largest group of inborn metabolic stone diseases. Gout is the most common metabolic disorder in this group, associated with uric acid lithiasis [1], but as such, it does not represent a single, well-defined genetic metabolic defect. On the other hand, a small proportion of the gouty patients are affected with well-defined, although very rare, inborn errors in purine metabolism causing uric acid overproduction and urolithiasis. Two such abnormalities are well established: partial deficiency of hypoxanthine-guanine phosphoribosyltransferase (HGPRT) [2] and superactivity of 5-phosphoribosyl-1-pyrophosphate (PRPP) synthetase [3]. Complete deficiency of HGPRT causes the paediatric Lesch–Nyhan syndrome [4,5], associated with severe and untreatable neurological manifestations. Affected subjects produce uric acid stones and are prone to develop nephropathy but probably do not live long enough to become gouty. Uric acid lithiasis, occasionally associated with calcium stones, is relatively common among subjects with the renal urate transport (reabsorption) disorder hereditary renal hypouricaemia [6]. Three inborn errors in purine metabolism are associated with non-uric acid stone disease. These disorders are deficiency of adenine phosphoribosyltransferase (APRT), associated with 2,8-dihydroxyadenine (2,8-DHA) lithiasis [7], and xanthine oxidase deficiency [8] and combined xanthine oxidase and sulphite oxidase deficiency [9], associated with xanthine stone formation.

The discussion of each of these metabolic abnormalities will be preceded by a general description of purine metabolism in humans.

Purine metabolism in humans

Purine nucleotides have an important role in nearly all biochemical processes [10–12]. Adenosine triphosphate (ATP) is the universal currency of energy in biological systems. In addition, the purine nucleotides are the activated precursors of DNA and RNA and participate as structural units in several low molecular weight compounds, such as histidine and certain vitamins. Adenine nucleotides are components of three major coenzymes: NAD+, FAD and CoA, and of the important methyl donor, 5'-adenosylmethionine. Other important functions of the nucleotides are the carrying of a wide variety of groups, and their transfer to appropriate acceptors, mediation of hormone messages (regulatory signals) by cyclic adenosine monophosphate (AMP) and cyclic guanosine monophosphate (GMP), and the regulation of many metabolic pathways through an allosteric effect on the enzymes and through the energy charge of the cells.

The pathways of purine nucleotide metabolism (Fig. 59.1) operate to maintain an optimal level of the various nucleotides in the tissues. The nucleotides are produced either from small non-purine molecules, by the relatively energetically costly *de novo* pathway or from preformed purines by the relatively economical salvage pathways. There are interconversions between the nucleotides and excess nucleotides are degraded to uric acid [10–12].

De novo *biosynthesis of purine nucleotides*

The purine ring is assembled from glycine (C_4, C_5 and N_7), from the amino nitrogen of aspartate (N_1), from the amide nitrogen of glutamine (N_3 and N_9), from activated derivatives of tetrahydrofolate (C_2 and C_8) and from carbon dioxide (C_6) (Fig. 59.2). The purine ring structure is assembled in 10 steps on a ribosyl moiety and when completed it is the nucleotide inosine monophosphate (IMP). The first committed step in the *de novo* pathway is the formation of 5'-phosphoribosylamine from PRPP and glutamine, catalysed by glutamine-PRPP amidotransferase. The other components of the purine skeleton are introduced in nine additional reactions, finally yielding IMP (Fig. 59.2). IMP is the parent purine nucleotide molecule, but as a nucleotide it has no role in metabolism,

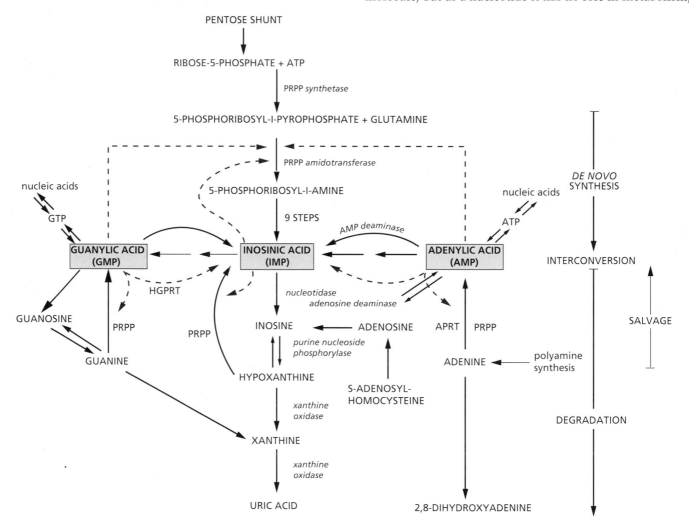

Fig. 59.1 Pathways of purine metabolism in humans. Dashed lines represent regulation by feedback inhibition. APRT, adenine phosphoribosyltransferase; ATP, adenosine triphosphate; GTP, guanosine triphosphate; HGPRT, hypoxanthine-guanine phosphoribosyltransferase; PRPP, 5-phosphoribosyl-1-pyrophosphate. (Redrawn from [12] with permission.)

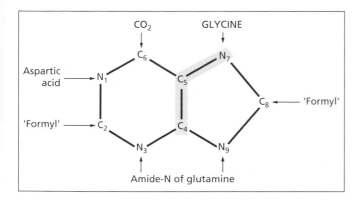

Fig. 59.2 The source of the carbon and nitrogen atoms of the purine ring. CO_2, carbon dioxide. (Redrawn from [12] with permission.)

except for being the precursor of AMP and GMP. AMP and GMP are synthesized from IMP, each in two steps. They can be converted to each other through IMP. The conversion of GMP and AMP to their respective di- and triphosphates occurs in two successive steps, catalysed by respective kinases and requiring ATP.

Salvage nucleotide synthesis

De novo synthesis of AMP or GMP is energetically very costly. The synthesis of IMP consumes the equivalent of six high energy phosphodiester bonds (by ATP hydrolysis). Additional two high energy bonds are consumed for IMP conversion to GMP, and one bond for the conversion of IMP to AMP. Therefore, not surprisingly, once formed the purine ring is recycled many times between the base (or nucleoside) and the nucleotide forms, before being further degraded to uric acid, the waste end-product of purine nucleotide metabolism excreted in the urine.

Two general mechanisms perform salvage of the preformed purine compounds: the phosphoribosylation of bases and the phosphorylation of adenosine. Two enzymes in human tissues can phosphoribosylate purine bases. HGPRT (EC 2.4.2.8) phosphoribosylates hypoxanthine and guanine with PRPP to yield IMP and GMP, respectively. Another enzyme, APRT (EC 2.4.2.7), phosphoribosylates similarly adenine to AMP.

Physiologically, the salvage of hypoxanthine and guanine is much more important than that of adenine. This is indicated by the finding of PRPP accumulation in HGPRT-deficient tissues [13], but not in APRT deficiency [14]. However, the recent finding of 2,8-dihydroxyadenine urolithiasis in APRT deficiency [7], furnishes evidence that some adenine is formed in the human, probably as a by-product of the synthesis of polyamines from 5'-adenosyl-methionine [15], and that it is rapidly salvaged to AMP. The salvage of adenosine, catalysed by adenosine kinase, is probably the main salvage pathway operating in erythro-

cytes [16], the heart [17] and skeletal muscle [18]. The main source of adenosine is probably the transmethylation reactions (from 5'-adenosylmethionine). In some tissues, such as heart muscle, adenosine may also be generated from AMP when this substrate accumulates during enhanced ATP degradation [17].

Regulation of purine biosynthesis

Substrate PRPP is the most important regulator of purine synthesis. PRPP synthetase (EC 2.7.6.1) catalyses its formation from ribose-5-phosphate and ATP. Ribose-5-phosphate is generated by the pentose phosphate pathway, as well as from ribose-1-phosphate, produced by degradation of the purine nucleosides inosine and guanosine. There is evidence suggesting that in many tissues the availability of ribose-5-phosphate is saturating for PRPP synthesis and, therefore, also for purine synthesis [19]. However, this is not the case in skeletal and heart muscle, in which tissues, probably due to low activity of the oxidative pentose phosphate pathway, ribose-5-phosphate availability is limiting for PRPP synthesis and therefore also for purine synthesis [17,20].

In accord with the main purpose of the various pathways of purine nucleotide synthesis, which is the maintenance of optimal nucleotide concentration, the nucleotide end-products regulate purine synthesis. The rate of the *de novo* pathway is controlled by feedback inhibition at several sites. The first committed step in the pathway, catalysed by glutamine-PRPP amidotransferase, is sensitive to inhibition by the various purine nucleotides in a synergistic (cooperative) manner. These inhibitors are competitive with substrate PRPP, whose concentration is a major regulator of the amidotransferase activity. The activity of PRPP synthetase, which is therefore regulating the activity of the amidotransferase is also subjected to feedback inhibition by the nucleotides, particularly AMP, adenosine diphosphate (ADP), GMP and guanosine diphosphate (GDP) [21,22]. The most conclusive indication for the important role of the activity of this enzyme in the regulation of purine synthesis is the flamboyant purine synthesis in the patients with the hereditary (X-linked) superactivity of PRPP synthetase, due to resistance to feedback inhibition by nucleotides [3,23–25] or other molecular alterations [26]. The branching point in the synthesis of AMP and GMP from IMP is also regulated by the respective nucleotides. Another level at which the nucleotides control their biosynthesis is the product inhibition of the salvage pathways. IMP and GMP inhibit HGPRT, whereas AMP inhibits adenosine kinase.

Degradation of purine nucleotides

ATP constitutes the largest nucleotide pool. The main

pathway for ATP degradation, following its conversion to AMP, is probably through deamination of AMP to IMP. This has been demonstrated in the liver [27], erythrocytes [28] and in skeletal [18] and heart muscle [17]. IMP is the main nucleotide substrate for degradation to non-nucleotide purines. Surplus IMP, formed from AMP, or from excessive *de novo* production (see p. 758) is degraded by 5'-nucleotidase (EC 3.1.3.5) to inosine. GMP can be similarly dephosphorylated to guanosine. The extent of this reaction is not known, but xanthine production in xanthinuria indicates that it may have quantitative significance (see p. 762). Inosine and guanosine are degraded by purine nucleoside phosphorylase (EC 2.4.2.1) to hypoxanthine and guanine, respectively. Guanine is deaminated by guanase (EC 3.5.4.3) to xanthine, and hypoxanthine and xanthine are degraded by xanthine oxidase (EC 1.3.2.3) to uric acid, which is the waste end-product of purine metabolism in humans (see Fig. 59.1).

Uric acid is not an ideal end-product because it is hardly soluble in body fluids. Excess uric acid in blood or urine tends to precipitate, as sodium hydrogen urate in joints or other tissues (tophi formation) or as uric acid, sodium urate or ammonium urate in calculi in the urinary tract [27,28]. Interestingly, the renal handling of urate is also very complicated unlike that of classic end-products (see p. 763).

PRPP synthetase superactivity

About 20 families have been reported with excessive purine production due to hereditary superactivity of PRPP synthetase. In the first case reported in 1972 [3,23–25], the enzyme superactivity was characterized to reflect resistance to feedback inhibition by nucleotides. In the other cases, the enzyme superactivity was found to reflect increased specific activity (increase V_{max}), increased affinity (low K_m) for substrate ribose 5'-phosphate or combinations of such abnormalities [26]. The pattern of inheritance is X-linked recessive [29]. The defect is manifested in the affected males in uric acid lithiasis and juvenile gout. Treatment with allopurinol is very effective.

The patient reported by Sperling *et al.* [3,23–25], is described here as an illustrative case. He started to suffer clinically at the age of 14, when he voided a few reddish concrements. At the age of 18 he started to suffer from recurrent renal colic and at the age of 20 he had an attack of gouty arthritis; shortly afterwards he became totally anuric and was hospitalized. Catheters were passed into both renal pelvises and subsequently the right kidney started to excrete, but the left kidney did not excrete and retrograde pyelography showed three filling defects in the left ureter. Shortly afterwards the patient became drowsy and his urea concentration rose to 386 mg/100 ml. Surgery was performed on the left ureter and several stones, proved to be pure uric acid, were removed. After the operation, the

patient was treated with a low purine diet, forced fluid intake, oral alkalinization and probenecid, and he remained well for several years, until uric acid crystalluria and renal colic reappeared. In the following 7 years he expelled a total of 34 stones, all pure uric acid except one which was mixed with calcium salt. Since 1965 he has been on allopurinol 600 mg/day and alkalinization. His serum concentration of uric acid and urinary uric acid excretion became and remained normal at below 4 mg/100 ml and 600 mg/day, respectively. He did not form new stones and his creatinine clearance remained normal. In 1969 allopurinol was discontinued for a short period for the purpose of investigation. After 6 days his serum uric acid had risen to 13.6 mg/100 ml, his 24 h urinary uric acid excretion had risen to 2400 mg and both remained stable around these levels.

The excessive purine production characteristic to all mutants of superactive PRPP synthetase emphasizes the role of both the enzyme PRPP synthetase and product PRPP in the regulation of purine synthesis.

Complete HGPRT deficiency

Complete HGPRT deficiency causes the X-linked (recessive) Lesch–Nyhan syndrome. The clinical syndrome was first reported in 1964 [4]. It is characterized by cerebral palsy with choreoathetosis and spasticity, self-mutilation, mental and physical retardation and severe purine over-production. HGPRT deficiency, underlying the Lesch–Nyhan syndrome, was revealed in 1967 [5]. The purine overproduction is attributed to the accumulation of PRPP, due to the absence of salvage nucleotide synthesis from hypoxanthine and guanine. Allopurinol effectively reduces uric acid level in the blood and urine and thereby prolongs the life of these patients, who otherwise are prone to develop severe renal insufficiency (gouty nephropathy). Nevertheless, allopurinol treatment in HGPRT deficiency may be associated with the formation of xanthine stones (see below). No specific treatment is available for the neurological manifestations, the aetiology of which is not yet clarified.

Partial HGPRT deficiency

Partial deficiency of HGPRT, first reported in 1967 [2], causes excessive purine production resulting in uric acid lithiasis and juvenile gout, but apparently does not cause significant neurological abnormalities [30]. The affected subjects in one family, studied by Sperling *et al.* [31,32], are described here as illustrative cases. The propositus, a 56-year-old male, was admitted because of gouty arthritis dating back to the age of 21 years, and bilateral uric acid lithiasis dating back to the age of 31. Physical examination revealed severe deformation of the joints of the hands and feet and huge, multiple tophi. Neurological examination was normal. His serum uric acid was 7.3 mg/100 ml and his 24 h urinary uric acid excretion was 2040 mg. The urine contained numerous uric acid crystals and the creatinine clearance was 75 ml/min. He was treated with allopurinol, which reduced his blood and urinary uric acid to normal values, but was associated with xanthine lithiasis (see below). His 19-year-old nephew was admitted because of gouty arthritis starting at the age of 16 and renal colic 5 months earlier. His serum uric acid was 11 mg/100 ml and his 24 h urinary uric acid excretion was 1670 mg; his creatinine clearance was 115 ml/min. There was massive uric acid crystalluria. The physical and neurological examination was normal. The patient was allergic to allopurinol and his treatment was aimed at lowering the serum urate level by uricosuric drugs and preventing stone formation by high fluid intake and alkalinization.

As in the Lesch–Nyhan syndrome and in partial HGPRT deficiency, allopurinol is the treatment of choice for reducing uric acid production. However, allopurinol administration to HGPRT-deficient subjects may be associated with xanthine stone formation. Allopurinol, an xanthine oxidase inhibitor, reduces uric acid formation by two mechanisms: through the inhibition of xanthine oxidase and by the reduction of total purine production *de novo*. The first effect is associated with accumulation of hypoxanthine and xanthine. The conversion of the accumulating hypoxanthine and of allopurinol into their nucleotidic forms, catalysed by the purine salvage enzyme HGPRT, is associated with consumption of PRPP, a substrate whose availability regulates also the activity of the first committed, rate-limiting enzyme in the pathway of *de novo* purine synthesis (PRPP amidotransferase). A decelerated rate of purine production is caused by the reduced availability of PRPP, and probably the feedback inhibition exerted on the PRPP amidotransferase by the increased concentration of the nucleotides IMP and allopurinol ribonucleotide. Xanthine is less soluble in urine than uric acid, but in the vast majority of hyperuricaemic patients (those with normal HGPRT activity), its accumulation associated with allopurinol administration does not reach the concentration product of crystal formation. However, in absence of HGPRT activity, whether partial or virtually complete (as in the Lesch–Nyhan syndrome), total purine production is not inhibited by allopurinol and the accumulation of xanthine reaches high levels conducive to xanthine stone formation [32–35].

In the patient with partial HGPRT deficiency studied by Sperling *et al.* [31], xanthine stone formation started following several years of treatment with allopurinol and continued despite trials in which the dosage of allopurinol was decreased or increased [32]. In contrast, in several cases of Lesch–Nyhan syndrome under our observation, allopurinol treatment has not been associated as yet with

xanthine stone formation despite the high urinary xanthine concentrations. One of the Lesch–Nyhan syndrome patients in our clinic has been treated with allopurinol for 16 years.

APRT deficiency: 2,8-DHA lithiasis

Hereditary APRT deficiency is associated with an inability to salvage the purine base adenine to its nucleotide form AMP. The main source of endogenous adenine is probably the polyamine pathway, of which adenine is a metabolic by-product. Adenine-rich foods may be a precipitating factor in the expression of the more severe clinical manifestations of the defect. In the absence of any other significant pathway of adenine metabolism in humans, it is oxidized by xanthine oxidase to insoluble 2,8-DHA (see Fig. 59.1), resulting in crystalluria and the possible formation of kidney stones [7,15]. The clinical symptoms include colic, haematuria, urinary tract infection and dysuria. The defect is inherited in an autosomal recessive manner [36]. A relatively high frequency of heterozygosity has been noted in several Caucasian population studies (0.4–1.1%), suggesting that homozygosity for the defect may be more prevalent than is currently thought. Approximately 15% of homozygotes are completely symptomless. On the other hand, a minority present with acute renal failure, some of whom have suffered permanent and severe renal damage requiring dialysis.

2,8-DHA is protein bound. Adenine and 2,8-DHA are secreted by the human kidney. Both factors tend to minimize toxicity in tissues other than the kidney *in vivo*. 2,8-DHA is nephrotoxic due to its insolubility at any pH. Its solubility in human urine ranges from about 2.7 mg/l at pH 5.0 to about 5.0 mg/l at pH 7.8. Nevertheless, in urine it can remain in supersaturation for hours even at 40 mg/l (37°C *in vitro*) or 96 mg/l (*in vivo*). 2,8-DHA crystals are yellow-brown and round, resembling leucine crystals. Being a uric acid analogue, 2,8-DHA is indistinguishable from uric acid by chemical analysis, alkaline ultraviolet (UV) spectrum or thermogravimetric analysis. Both stones are radiolucent. This similarity caused many 2,8-DHA stones to be diagnosed as uric acid stones. Correct diagnosis may, however, be obtained by subjecting the stones to infrared spectrometry, mass spectrometry, X-ray crystallography and UV spectroscopy in acid and alkali. In addition, the 2,8-DHA stone material is resistant to uricase. 2,8-DHA can be diagnosed in urine by high-performance liquid chromatography (HPLC) or isotachophoresis. Determination of APRT activity in red cell lysates will furnish a conclusive diagnosis.

Allopurinol does not affect the total excretion of adenine compounds in the urine, but reduces its oxidation to 2,8-DHA (by inhibition of xanthine oxidase); 10 mg/kg/day will eliminate all 2,8-DHA from urine in most cases. This amount should be decreased in children and in patients with permanent renal damage. High fluid intake is recommended.

Xanthinuria

Xanthinuria is a rare autosomal recessive disorder characterized by a gross deficiency of xanthine oxidase [37]. The absence of the last enzyme in the pathway of purine nucleotide degradation (see Fig. 59.1) has the result that uric acid is almost absent from blood and urine, and that hypoxanthine and xanthine are the end-products of purine degradation. Some of the hypoxanthine is salvaged to IMP, catalysed by HGPRT, with the result that xanthine is the main excreted purine (four times the amount of hypoxanthine) and that there is a diminution in the amount of total purines produced (due to the increased consumption of PRPP by the augmented salvage of hypoxanthine). Xanthine is almost insoluble in acid solutions. Normal urine at 26°C dissolves 6.7 mg at pH 5.8 and 16.5 mg at pH 8.1. The xanthinuric patients excrete about 250 mg of xanthine in 24 h (normal excretion is about 6.1 mg/24 h), an amount which in most cases markedly exceeds the solubility of xanthine in the urine. This results in the development of xanthine calculi in the urinary tract in about one-third of xanthinuric subjects.

The patient studied by Sperling et al. [38,39] is described as an illustrative case. The patient, a 32-year-old female, was admitted for metabolic investigation of hypouricaemia (0.2–0.42 mg/100 ml) and hypouricosuria (8.5–22.5 mg/24 h). Her blood oxypurine (hypoxanthine plus xanthine) level was 0.298 mg/100 ml (in equivalents of uric acid) and urinary oxypurine excretion 346–359 mg/24 h (437–567 mg/24 h in equivalents of uric acid), of which xanthine constituted 70–87.5%. The activity of xanthine oxidase in a biopsy of jejunal mucosa was 5.7% of normal [38] and in her colostrum 0–3.2 u, in comparison to 37–125 u in control women [39]. Her sister and two brothers were normo-uricaemic. The propositus did not have clinical manifestations related to the disorder (xanthine urolithiasis or precipitation of xanthine in tissues). Xanthine stones are rare among general stone collections (one pure stone and three mixed in 10 000 calculi) [40]. The stones are brownish or brown-yellow, smooth, round or oval. They are non-opaque to X-rays, unless they contain calcium. Xanthine stones can be identified by differential spectrophotometry, paper and column chromatography, HPLC and X-ray crystallography.

Treatment is aimed at decreasing xanthine excretion and increasing its solubility in the urine. This is achieved mainly by a high fluid intake, alkalinization and a low purine diet. Allopurinol may be used in cases with residual xanthine oxidase activity, in whom its administration may reverse the hypoxanthine:xanthine ratio, increasing the amount of highly soluble hypoxanthine and decreasing the amount of the almost insoluble xanthine.

Combined deficiency of xanthine oxidase and sulphate oxidase

This relatively new subtype of xanthinuria [9] is much more rare (15 documented cases) than xanthinuria. The primary defect is in molybdenum metabolism. These subjects suffer mainly from neurological symptoms, which are attributable to the sulphate oxidase deficiency. Treatment with ammonium molybdate may correct in some of the patients the disorder of both purine and sulphur metabolism.

Hereditary renal hypouricaemia

Hereditary renal hypouricaemia is a rare hereditary condition of increased renal urate clearance, caused by a specific (isolated) inborn error of membrane transport for urate in the renal proximal tubule and manifested in hypouricaemia [6]. This defect is inherited in an autosomal recessive mode. Twenty-eight cases are well documented. In homozygotes the defect is fully manifested in hypouricaemia and an increased renal urate clearance, whereas heterozygosity may be detected by moderately decreased serum urate levels and a moderately but significantly increased renal urate clearance.

The present understanding of the renal handling of urate in humans includes four components: glomerular filtration, early proximal reabsorption, secretion and post-secretory reabsorption, which could occur at the same location as the secretion, or separate and distal to it [41] (Fig. 59.3). Recently, a similar model was proposed, including the same four components, but according to which, reabsorption and secretion of urate occur simultaneously along all the proximal tubule, each at different intensities at the different segments of the tubule [42]. Studying the effect of drugs inhibiting urate reabsorption or secretion, revealed that in most patients with the hereditary isolated abnormality the defect appears to be in the presecretory urate reabsorption site [6].

The clinical consequences in renal hypouricaemia are the manifestations of hyperuricosuria, which appears to be a constant feature of this syndrome [6,43]. The hyperuricosuria reflects the diversion of intestinal urate elimination to urinary urate excretion, consequent to the hypouricaemia. Uricolysis by intestinal bacteria is responsible for the elimination of about 33% of the uric acid turnover each day [44]. The uric acid enters the alimentary tract from the blood in saliva, gastic juice and bile. Accordingly, the blood urate level influences the amount of uric acid secreted into the gut. Therefore, in hypouricaemia, as this fraction is markedly smaller, a

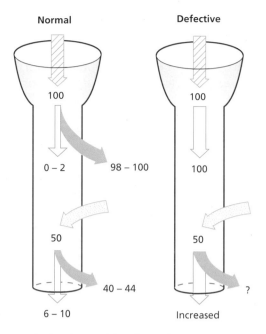

Normal **Defective**

Fig. 59.3 Model for the renal handling of urate in normal humans and the possible defect that may cause renal hypouricaemia. The size and direction of arrows indicate the intensity and direction of urate transport. The hatched arrows represent filtered urate; the solid arrows, urate reabsorption; the dotted arrows, urate secretion; and the open arrows, urate remaining in the tubular fluid after reabsorption. Numerical values indicate the hypothetical order of magnitude of the transport process. The normal model is based on the model suggested by Rieselbach and Steele [41].

greater fraction of the uric acid produced leaves the body intact via the kidneys, manifested in hyperuricosuria. There is no evidence in hypouricaemic hyperuricosuric subjects for purine overproduction [45,46]. The hyperuricosuria may be associated with uric acid lithiasis or uric

acid nephropathy. Five out of the 28 propositi with inborn isolated renal hypouricaemia had urinary calculi [6]: three had uric acid stones, one a calcium oxalate stone and one a stone of unidentified composition. In four other propositi [47], urolithiasis was present in other family members. Acute uric acid nephropathy in this syndrome was reported in four cases. In one patient requiring haemodialysis due to oliguric renal failure, renal biopsy showed amorphous uric acid crystals in some of the tubular lumina and mild to moderate interstitial inflammation [48]. Mild acute renal failure induced by exercise was reported in three subjects with renal hypouricaemia [49].

Stone disease associated with inborn errors of pyrimidine metabolism

Pyrimidine metabolism

The body requirement for pyrimidines is equal to that of purines. Like purine nucleotides, pyrimidine nucleotides can be synthesized *de novo* from small molecules or by salvage of preformed pyrimidines, available from body cell turnover or dietary sources. They can interconvert and finally undergo degradation to β-alanine and β-amino-isobutyric acid [50] (Fig. 59.4). The rate-limiting step of the *de novo* synthesis is catalysed by carbamyl phosphate synthase (CPS), but under conditions of increased ATP, at a time when uridine nucleotides and PRPP levels are low, the orotate phosphoribosyltransferase (OPRT) catalysed reaction is the rate-limiting one. Uridine 5′-monophosphate (UMP) synthesis is regulated by feedback inhibition of CPS by the pyrimidine nucleotides. Altogether, UMP synthesis *de novo* requires five ATP, whereas the salvage synthesis of pyrimidine nucleotides requires only one energy-rich bond. The main salvage enzymes are uridine kinase

Fig. 59.4 Pathways of pyrimidine metabolism in humans. The deficiency of uridine 5′-monophosphate (UMP) synthase is associated with accumulation of orotic acid. ATC, aspartate transcarbamylase; ATP, adenosine triphosphate; CPS, carbamyl phosphate synthetase; ODC, orotidine 5′-monophosphate decarboxylase; OMP, orotidine monophosphate; OPRT, orotate phosphoribosyltransferase; PRPP, 5-phosphoribosyl-1-pyrophosphate.

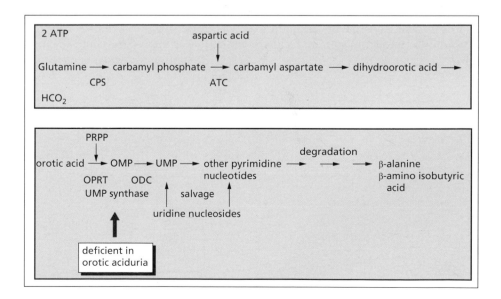

(phosphorylates both uridine and cytidine), deoxycytidine kinase and thymidine kinase.

Orotic aciduria

Orotic aciduria is a very rare (13 documented cases) autosomal recessive disorder in the *de novo* pathway of pyrimidine nucleotide synthesis, caused by the deficiency of two enzyme activities, that of OPRT and orotidine 5'-monophosphate decarboxylase (ODC), residing in a single polypeptide, bifunctional protein, UMP synthase [50]. In one of the 13 documented cases, ODC activity was barely detectable but OPRT activity was normal (orotic aciduria type II). All patients have macrocytic hypochromic megaloblastic anaemia, reflecting pyrimidine nucleotide deficiency, and orotic acid crystalluria, reflecting the overproduction of pyrimidines and the enzymatic block preventing the metabolism of accumulating orotic acid. The excessive production of orotic acid in orotic aciduria is attributed to the decreased cellular levels of pyrimidine nucleotides, resulting in decreased feedback inhibition of the CPS. The quantities of orotic acid excreted by the affected patients is enough to cause crystalluria in the urine specimens and frequently also in the urinary tract. This crystalluria has been of diagnostic importance in six of the 13 cases. Some of the patients developed episodes of urethral obstruction, requiring catheterization or meatotomy. One patient developed blockage of the collecting tubules by the orotic acid crystals. Other patients exhibited crystal-induced damage to the renal tract and one patient presented with intermittent partial obstruction of the upper urinary tract.

The treatment of choice is uridine (50–300 mg/kg/day), which bypasses the enzymatic block following its salvage conversion by the specific kinase to UMP. Its administration produced haematological and clinical remission in all treated cases, including the deceleration of pyrimidine synthesis and consequent disappearance of orotic acid crystalluria (through resuming feedback inhibition of the CPS).

Diagnosis is made in patients with the above described clinical manifestations by measurement of orotic acid in urine and by the assay of OPRT and ODC in red blood cells. Orotic acid may also be excessive in other inborn disorders, including urea cycle defects and lysinuric protein intolerance.

Primary hyperoxaluria

Primary hyperoxaluria is a general term for two rare genetic disorders, manifested by an excessive production of oxalic acid, leading to recurrent calcium oxalate nephrolithiasis and nephrocalcinosis, frequently associated with progressive renal insufficiency [51]. Renal stones may appear in childhood and progression of the disease may lead to death before the age of 20 years. Calcium oxalate was recognized in normal urine in 1838 [52]. Primary hyperoxaluria was first described in 1925 [53]. However, the first detailed study of a case diagnosed following postmortem examination was reported in 1950 [54] and the first case diagnosed during life was reported in 1953 [55].

Oxalic acid metabolism in humans is not yet fully clarified. Oxalic acid is probably an end-product of metabolism, and like uric acid may cause disease due to its insolubility. The free acid is soluble in water at 8.7 g/100 g, but its calcium salt is soluble in neutral or alkaline pH at only 0.67 mg/100 g. The solubility of the salt is greatly affected by its ionic environment as well as the pH of the solution.

It has been estimated that in normal subjects about 33% of urinary oxalate is derived from glycine via glyoxalate [56,57]; about 40% arises from the cleavage of carbon atoms 1 and 2 from ascorbate catabolism (this does not involve glyoxalate as the intermediate) and the rest (about 25%) derives from dietary sources [58]. Glyoxalate is metabolized in peroxisomes, mitochondria and cytosol (Fig. 59.5). The normal excretion of anhydrous oxalic acid is about 45 mg/24 h in adults of both sexes [59]. Children excrete less, but the normal upper values are not yet assessed. The oxalate ion is freely filtrable at the glomerulus and its

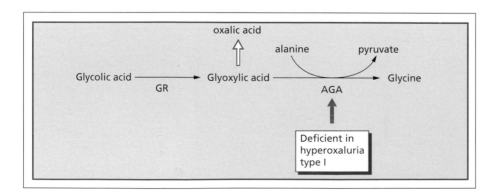

Fig. 59.5 The peroxisomal pathway from glycolic acid to glycine (the glycolate pathway). The deficiency of AGA (primary hyperoxaluria type I) is associated with the accumulation of glyoxylic acid, which is shunted to oxalic acid synthesis, and with the accumulation of glycolic acid. AGA, alanine-glyoxalate-aminotransferase; GR, glycolate reductase.

clearance is greater than the glomerular filtration rate (GFR), indicating net tubular secretion. There is some degree of passive reabsorption.

Primary hyperoxaluria type I

Primary hyperoxaluria type I is a rare, autosomal recessive inborn error of metabolism due to the deficiency of peroxisomal alanine:glyoxalate aminotransferase (AGA) [60]. Patients excrete equimolar amounts of oxalate (about 90–360 mg/day) and glycolate (about 76–304 mg/day) together with increased amounts of glyoxalate.

In most cases the disease appears during childhood (juvenile type), with symptoms of urinary stones or infections. The stones usually recur and there is progressive loss of renal function due to developing nephrocalcinosis. Parallel to the decrease in renal function there is an increased risk of precipitation of calcium oxalate in many organs (oxalosis). Pyridoxal phosphate is a co-factor for the AGA and about 30–50% of the affected patients respond well to pharmacological doses of pyridoxine. This phenomenon suggests that in the responding patients, the deficient activity of the enzyme is due to decreased affinity to the co-factor.

The infantile type presents with the passage of grit and stones, urinary infections, obstructive uropathy or advanced renal failure in the neonatal period or later in infancy. It is characterized by very extensive oxalosis, especially in the brain. The adult type presents with stones during the third decade or later.

The treatment of the stone disease in primary hyperoxaluria type I is aimed at: (i) lowering oxalate excretion by controlling the diet (low in oxalate, vitamin C, vitamin D and calcium) and by decelerating oxalate synthesis (administration of pyridoxine to responsive patients, 800 mg/day for an adult); (ii) lowering oxalate concentration in the urine by increased fluid intake (to obtain a urine volume of at least 3 l/day); and (iii) inhibition of calcium oxalate crystallization by the addition of inhibitors of crystallization (oral administration of sufficient magnesium oxide or magnesium hydroxide to increase urinary magnesium excretion, and orthophosphate to increase the excretion of inorganic phosphate). Surgical treatment is complicated because of the need for multiple procedures. Fragmentation of the stones by extracorporeal shockwave lithotripsy is of value, but special precautions should be taken to allow the complete passage of all stone fragments, which otherwise remain as foci for new stone formation. Renal transplantation should be performed when the GFR is about 25 ml/min/1.73 m^2, and not lower than that, as the transplanted kidney may not cope with the mass of accumulated oxalate. Even so, the prognosis for pyridoxine-resistant hyperoxaluria type I is not very good. The future treatment of choice may be a combined renal orthopic hepatic transplantation, anticipating that the liver tissue will furnish the normal activity of the deficient enzyme.

Primary hyperoxaluria type II

Primary hyperoxaluria type II is a second hereditary (autosomal recessive) metabolic disorder leading to excessive production and excretion of oxalic acid. This very rare disease (four patients documented in two pedigrees) is caused by the deficiency of D-glycerate dehydrogenase (DGD) [61] (Fig. 59.6). The pathogenesis of the excessive oxalate production in type II hyperoxaluria is not yet conclusively clarified. It is possible that direct linkage exists between the glycolate and glycerate pathways (see Figs 59.5 and 59.6) in such a way that accumulation of hydroxypyruvate, due to the deficiency of DGD, prevents the normal metabolism of glyoxalate, shunting it to oxalate [51]. The amount of oxalate excreted is similar to that in primary hyperoxaluria type I. The amount of L-glycerate is also increased, but the excretion of glycolate and glyoxalate is normal. The disease is first manifested in later childhood and is less severe in comparison to hyperoxaluria type I. Treatment is as for type I, except that pyridoxine is not effective.

Cystinuria

Cystinuria is an inherited specific transport defect for the amino acids cystine, lysine, arginine and ornithine, which is expressed in two organs, the kidney and the intestine [62]. Were it not for the insolubility of cystine, causing

Fig. 59.6 Pathway from glyceric acid to serine (the glycerate pathway). The deficiency of DGD (primary hyperoxaluria type II) is associated with the accumulation of hydroxypyruvic acid accelerating, in an as yet unclarified mechanism, the synthesis of oxalic acid. AHT, alanine:hydroxypyruvate transaminase; DGD, D-glyceric dehydrogenase.

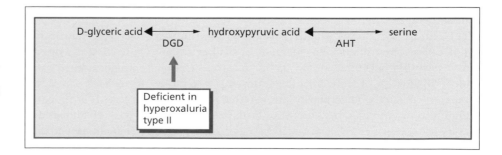

cystine lithiasis, cystinuria would be of no clinical significance. Cystine was first found in 1810 in stones removed from the urinary bladder, named cystic oxide stones [63]. In 1833, the name cystic oxide was changed to cystine [64] and only in 1902 was the chemical structure of cystine defined. In 1908, cystinuria was thought to be an inborn error of metabolism [65], and only in 1951 was the nature of the common transport defect for cystine and the dibasic amino acids established [66]. Apparently there are two transport systems for cystine, one with a high affinity shared with the dibasic amino acids and one with a low affinity specific to cystine only. The intestinal defect in cystinuria was established only in 1961 [67].

Based on newborn screening, the overall prevalence of homozygous cystinuria is estimated to be one in 700 [68], which makes cystinuria one of the most common inherited disorders. It is inherited in an autosomal recessive pattern, occurring equally in both sexes, but the males are more severely affected, probably related to urinary tract anatomy. Cystinuria is a classic disorder of renal tubular function, affecting the transepithelial transport mechanism shared by cystine and the dibasic amino acids. Study of the intestinal mucosal transport patterns of the dibasic amino acids in homozygous cystinuric subjects allowed their differentiation into three groups: type I, which includes the majority of the patients, lacks the intestinal transport mechanism for cystine, lysine and arginine; type II exhibits no transport of lysine and markedly reduced cystine transport; and type III, exhibiting variable reduction in the transport of cystine and lysine. Homozygotes for the three types exhibit the same pattern of urinary excretion of amino acids. Cystine has a low solubility in acid solutions. At urinary pH 5.0 the solubility of cystine is about 300 mg/l and at pH 7.0, about 400 mg/l. Most cystinuric subjects excrete in the range of 1 g of cystine per day, which is much above the solubility capacity of the urine.

The diagnosis of cystinuria is relatively simple. Microscopic crystalluria is present in between 26 and 83% of the patients. The cyanide nitroprusside test is a good screening procedure, sensitive enough to detect most homozygote stone formers and some of the heterozygotes (false positive results can occur in homocystinuria and in the presence of urinary ketones). Cystine excretion may be quantified colorimetrically, by thin layer chromatography, high voltage electrophoresis or, best, by ion exchange chromatography.

The clinical symptoms usually develop within the first two decades, often due to development of bladder calculi [69]. Cystinuria accounts for up to 3% of stone-forming adults [70] and 6% of stone-forming children [71]. Cystine stones are partially radio-dense, due to the presence of sulphur atoms, and may be difficult to visualize on a plain X-ray.

The treatment is aimed at reducing cystine excretion (dietary restriction of precursor methionine and of sodium to less than 100 mg/day) and increasing cystine solubility (high fluid intake, during the day and night, alkalinization to pH 7.5 and pharmacological conversion of cystine to more soluble compounds).

The use of drugs which convert cystine to more soluble compounds deserves more detailed discussion. Several drugs are available, which through a disulphide exchange reaction produce the mixed disulphide of cysteine with the drug, which is significantly more soluble than cystine. The first such drug to be introduced was D-penicillamine. Later, a related compound, N-acetyl-D-penicillamine, was developed and, more recently, mercaptopropionylglycine. D-penicillamine (1–2 g/day) has been proved to reduce free cystine excretion effectively to amounts which may be soluble in the urine (below 200 mg/g creatinine). The administration of this drug to cystinurics, but not to normal subjects, is associated in addition with a reduction of total cystine excretion (free cystine plus cysteine penicillamine disulphide). Nevertheless, D-penicillamine has many undesirable and even severe side effects, such as allergic reactions, including the nephrotic syndrome and pancytopenia, proteinuria, epidermolysis, thrombocytosis, hypogeusia and others. Thus, this treatment is advocated only in cases which do not respond well to more conservative therapy, and should always be initiated under strict medical supervision and followed-up carefully. The other drugs developed for the same purpose are reported to have the same therapeutic effectiveness with lower toxicity, but some of these drugs are not yet available on the market.

As for the surgical approaches, irrigation with alkaline solutions of N-acetylpenicillamine, D-penicillamine and tromethamine appears to be successful [72–74] and should be preferred over surgery. Extracorporeal lithotripsy is not very effective as cystine stones are among the most resistant stones to disintegration. Percutaneous lithotripsy is more effective. Surgical removal of obstructing stones should be nearly eliminated by the above procedures, but still may be necessary in some patients. Transplantation, which may occasionally be needed, should be effective as, if the donor is normal, the transplanted kidney will remain disease free [75].

Hereditary hypercalciuric stone disease

Hypercalciuria is a well-established aetiological factor in renal stone disease [76]. Hypercalciuria can reflect many abnormalities, such as hyperparathyroidism, renal tubular acidosis, sarcoidosis and malignancy, but in the majority of cases it is idiopathic [77]. A certain proportion, not assessed yet, of idiopathic hypercalciuric subjects present with a hereditary pattern. Hereditary hypercalciuric stone disease includes the following conditions: familial (idiopathic) hypercalciuric urolithiasis; renal tubular acidosis with nephrolithiasis; and hypophosphataesia, manifested in some patients with the infantile type in hypercalcaemia, hypercalciuria and nephrocalcinosis. An additional condition, that of hereditary hypophosphataemic rickets with hypercalciuria is also discussed, although for reasons as yet unknown the hypercalciuria in this condition is not associated with stone disease.

Familial hypercalciuric (idiopathic) urolithiasis

Studies of large series of patients affected with hypercalciuric (idiopathic) urolithiasis revealed that a substantial proportion of the patients could be classified as affected with familial idiopathic hypercalciuria [78,79]. Detailed investigation of some of these families revealed a dominant autosomal pattern of inheritance. In the family with hereditary (idiopathic) hypercalciuric urolithiasis studied by Weinberger et al. [80], 39 family members of the propositus, over three generations, were studied. Four male subjects were found to have hypercalciuric urolithiasis, two additional relatives were found to have hypercalciuria without urolithiasis and four others were found to have urolithiasis without hypercalciuria. This family is similar to the eight families studied by Coe et al. [81] and by others [82]. In another study of 22 families with idiopathic hypercalciuria [79], a familial pattern of the condition was confirmed, but attributed to environmental (excessive ingestion of electrolytes) rather than to genetic factors.

Primary type I renal tubular acidosis
(inherited classic hypokalaemic distal renal tubular acidosis)

Renal tubular acidosis (RTA), is characterized by hyperchloraemic metabolic acidosis secondary to an abnormality in renal acidification [83]. There are several types of RTA: classic distal RTA (type I), proximal RTA (type II) and generalized distal nephron dysfunction (type IV). Of the various types of RTA, only the classic (hypokalaemic) type I is associated with nephrocalcinosis and stone disease. The mechanisms involved in the pathogenesis of this disease are not yet fully clarified. Probably there is some type of lesion in the medullary collecting duct or a selective lesion of the cortical collecting tubule [83]. There is an inability to acidify the urine to below pH 5.5 during spontaneous or chemically induced metabolic acidosis [84]. As a result there is a positive acid balance, hyperchloraemic metabolic acidosis and volume depletion. The disorder is often accompanied by hypokalaemia and hypercalciuria [85]. The hypercalciuria reflects the acidosis-induced bone dissolution. Chronic metabolic acidosis also decreases renal excretion of citrate [85,86]. The combination of hypercalciuria and hypocitraturia results in nephrocalcinosis and stone

formation [85,87–89]. Nephrocalcinosis is a typical marker for RTA type I, as it does not occur in the other types.

The primary (hereditary) disease is rare. About 200 affected individuals in approximately 30 families have been reported [83]. In some families an autosomal dominant mode of inheritance was documented, in others it was X-linked, and in some the mode of inheritance is unclear [83].

Hypercalciuria, nephrocalcinosis and stone disease are common in most cases of the genetic classic type I RTA, but not in all of them. Without therapy, nephrocalcinosis may be evident as early as the age of 5 years. However, high-dose alkali therapy, initiated early enough, has been reported to avoid nephrocalcinosis and nephrolithiasis for 20 years of follow-up [90]. Apparently, high-dose alkali therapy corrects both the hypercalciuria and hypocitraturia and decreases or avoids nephrocalcinosis and nephrolithiasis. Therapy is aimed at correction of the metabolic acidosis by administration of alkali in the amount necessary to neutralize the production of metabolic acids derived from the diet (in adults, 1–1.5 mEq/kg/day; in growing children, 2–3 mEq/kg/day or more). Shohl solution is tolerated well by children.

Hypophosphataesia

This hereditary metabolic bone disease is caused by some defect in the gene coding for tissue-non-specific alkaline phosphatase [91]. The affected patients exhibit subnormal activity of this enzyme in serum. There is defective skeletal mineralization manifested as rickets in infants and children and as osteomalacia in adults. Hypercalcaemia and hypercalciuria develop in some of the patients with the infantile type, resulting in nephrocalcinosis which is often fatal. There is no effective treatment.

Hereditary hypophosphataemic rickets with hypercalciuria

This is a relatively new disorder reported to occur in closely related members of a single Bedouin tribe in Israel [92,93]. The major clinical manifestations in the presumed homozygotes are bone pain, skeletal deformities, short stature and muscle weakness with X-ray signs of rickets and osteomalacia. The primary defect in this disorder is renal leakage of phosphate (low TmP/GFR), resulting in hypophosphataemia and hyperphosphaturia. There is increased synthesis of 1,25-dihydroxyvitamin D_3, resulting in hyperabsorption of phosphate and calcium from the intestinal tract and suppression of parathyroid hormone secretion. The persistent hypophosphataemia is sufficient to lead to a reduction in the rate of bone mineralization and growth. The patients respond very well to oral phosphate therapy. The hyperabsorption of calcium from the intestinal tract leads to marked hypercalciuria, which disappears with phosphate treatment. For an as yet unknown reason, the hypercalciuria in this syndrome is not associated with urolithiasis.

References

1 Gutman AB. Urate urolithiasis in primary and secondary gout. *Ann Intern Med* 1963;**58**:741–2.
2 Kelly WN, Rosenbloom FM, Henderson JF, Seegmiller JE. A specific enzyme defect in gout associated with overproduction of uric acid. *Proc Natl Acad Sci USA* 1967;**57**:1735–9.
3 Sperling O, Boer P, Persky-Brosh S, Kanarek E, de Vries A. Altered kinetic property of erythrocyte phosphoribosylpyrophosphate synthetase in excessive purine production. *Eur J Clin Biol Res* 1972;**17**:703–6.
4 Lesch M, Nyhan WN. A familial disorder of uric acid metabolism and central nervous system function. *Am J Med* 1964;**36**: 561–70.
5 Seegmiller JE, Rosenbloom FM, Kelly WN. Enzyme defect associated with a sex-linked human neurological disorder and excessive purine synthesis. *Science* 1967;**155**:1682–4.
6 Sperling O. Hereditary hypouricemia. In: Scriver CR, Beaudet AC, Sly WS, Valle D, eds. *The Metabolic Basis of Inherited Disease*, 7th edn. New York: McGraw Hill 1995:3747–62.
7 Cartier MP, Hamet M. A new metabolic disease: the complete deficit of adenine phosphoribosyltransferase and lithiasis of 2,8-dihydroxyadenine. *C R Acad Sci [111]* 1974;**279**:883–6.
8 Dent CE, Philpot GR. Xanthinuria, an inborn error (or deviation) of metabolism. *Lancet* 1954;**1**:182–5.
9 Duran M, Beemer FA, Heiden CVD *et al.* Combined deficiency of xanthine oxidase and sulfite oxidase: a defect of molybdenum metabolism or transport. *J Inherited Metab Dis* 1978;**1**:175–8.
10 Henderson JF, Paterson ARP. *Nucleotide Metabolism. An Introduction.* New York: Academic Press, 1973.
11 Kelley WN, Weiner IM, eds. *Uric Acid.* Berlin: Springer Verlag, 1978.
12 Sperling O. Human purine metabolism. In: De Jong WN, ed. *Myocardial Energy Metabolism.* Dordrecht: Martinus Nijhoff, 1988: 225–36.
13 Rosenbloom FM, Henderson JF, Caldwell IC, Kelley WN, Seegmiller JE. Biochemical bases of accelerated purine biosynthesis *de novo* in human fibroblasts lacking hypoxanthine-guanine phosphoribosyltransferase. *J Biol Chem* 1968;**243**:1166–73.
14 Spector EB, Hershfield MS, Seegmiller JE. Purine reutilization and synthesis *de novo* in long term human lymphocyte cell lines deficient in adenine phosphoribosyltransferase activity. *Somat Cell Mol Genet* 1978;**4**:253–8.
15 Simmonds HA, Van Acker KJ. Adenine phosphoribosyltransferase deficiency: 2,8-dihydroxyadenine lithiasis. In: Stanbury JB, Wyngaarden JB, Fredrickson DS, Goldstein JL, Brown MS, eds. *The Metabolic Basis of Inherited Disease*, 5th edn. New York: McGraw Hill 1983:1144–56.
16 Plageman PGW, Wohlhueter RM, Kraupp M. Adenine nucleotide metabolism and nucleoside transport in human erythrocytes under ATP depletion conditions. *Biochim Biophys Acta* 1985;**817**:51–60.
17 Zoref-Shani E, Kessler Icekeson G, Sperling O. Pathways of adenine nucleotide catabolism in primary rat cardiomyocytes. *J Mol Cell Cardiol* 1988;**20**:23–33.
18 Zoref-Shani E, Shainberg A, Sperling O. Pathways of adenine nucleotide catabolism in primary rat muscle cultures. *Biochim Biophys Acta* 1987;**926**:287–95.
19 Sperling O. Ribose-5-phosphate and the oxidative pentose shunt in the regulation of purine synthesis *de novo*. In: Elliot K, Fitzsimons DW, eds. *Purine and Pyrimidine Metabolism.* Ciba Foundation Symposium 48. Amsterdam: Elsevier, 1977: 347–55.
20 Zoref-Shani E, Shainberg A, Sperling O. Characterization of purine nucleotide metabolism in primary rat muscle cultures. *Biochim Biophys Acta* 1982;**716**:324–30.
21 Hershko A, Razin A, Mager J. Regulation of the synthesis of 5-phosphoribosylpyrophosphate in intact red blood cells and in cell free preparations. *Biochim Biophys Acta* 1969;**184**:64–76.
22 Switzer RL. Regulation and mechanism of phosphoribosylpyrophosphate synthetase. III. Kinetics studies of the reaction mechanisms. *J Biol Chem* 1971;**246**:2447–58.
23 Sperling O, Eilam G, Persky-Brosh S, de Vries A. Accelerated erythrocyte 5-phosphoribosyl-1-pyrophosphate synthesis. A familial abnormality associated with excessive uric acid production and gout. *Biochem Med* 1972;**6**:310–16.
24 Sperling O, Persky-Brosh S, Boer P, de Vries A. Human erythrocyte PRPP synthetase mutationally altered in regulatory properties. *Biochem Med* 1973;**7**:389–95.
25 Zoref E, de Vries A, Sperling O. Mutant feedback-resistant phosphoribosyl-pyrophosphate synthetase associated with purine overproduction and gout. Phosphoribosylpyrophosphate and purine metabolism in cultured fibroblasts. *J Clin Invest* 1975;**56**:1093–9.
26 Becker MA, Losman MJ, Simmonds HA. Inherited phosphoribosylpyrophosphate synthetase superactivity due to aberrant inhibitor and activator responsiveness. *Adv Exp Med Biol* 1986;**195A**:59–66.
27 De Vries A, Sperling O. Uric acid stone formation: concepts of etiology and treatment. In: Chisolm GD, Williams DI, eds: *Scientific Foundations of Urology*, 2nd edn. London: William Heinemann Medical Books, 1982: 308–14.
28 Sperling O. Uric acid nephrolithiasis. In: Wickham JEA, Buck AC, eds. *Renal Tract Stone: Metabolic Basis and Clinical Practice.* London: Churchill Livingstone, 1990:349–65.
29 Zoref E, de Vries A, Sperling O. Evidence for X-linkage of phosphoribosyl-pyrophosphate synthetase in man: studies with cultured fibroblasts from a gouty family with mutant feedback resistance enzyme. *Hum Hered* 1977;**27**:73–80.
30 Kelley WN, Greene ML, Rosenbloom FM, Henderson JF, Seegmiller JE. Hypoxanthine-guanine phosphoribosyltransferase deficiency in gout: a review. *Ann Intern Med* 1969; **70**:155–206.
31 Sperling O, Frank M, Ophir R *et al.* Partial deficiency of hypoxanthine-guanine phosphoribosyltransferase associated with gout and uric acid lithiasis. *Europ J Clin Biol Res* 1970; **15**:942–7.
32 Sperling O, Brosh S, Boer P, Liberman UA, de Vries A. Urinary xanthine stones in an allopurinol treated gouty patient with partial deficiency of hypoxanthine-guanine phosphoribosyltransferase. *Israel J Med Sci* 1978;**14**:288–92.
33 Greene ML, Fujimoto WY, Seegmiller JE. Urinary xanthine stones: a rare complication of allopurinol therapy. *N Engl J Med* 1969;**280**:426–7.
34 Ogawa A, Watanabe K, Minejima N. Renal xanthine stone in Lesch–Nyhan syndrome treated with allopurinol. *Urology* 1985;**26**:56–8.

35 Oka T, Utsunomiya M, Ichikawa Y *et al*. Xanthine calculi in a patient with the Lesch–Nyhan syndrome associated with urinary tract infection. *Urol Intern* 1985;**40**:138–40.

36 Van Acker KJ, Simmonds HA, Potter CF, Sahota A. Inheritance of adenine phosphoribosyltransferase deficiency. *Adv Exp Med Biol* 1980;**122A**:349–53.

37 Holmes EW, Wyngaarden JB. Hereditary xanthinuria. In; Stanbury JB, Wyngaarden JB, Fredrickson DS, Goldstein JL, Brown MS, eds. *The Metabolic Basis of Inherited Disease*, 5th edn. New York: McGraw Hill, 1983:1192–201.

38 Sperling O, Liberman UA, Frank M, De Vries A. Xanthinuria: an additional case with demonstration of xanthine oxidase deficiency. *Am J Clin Pathol* 1971;**55**:351–4.

39 Oliver I, Sperling O, Liberman UA, Frank M, De Vries A. Deficiency of xanthine oxidase activity in colostrum of a xanthinuric female. *Biochem Med* 1971;**5**:279–80.

40 Herring LC. Observations on the analysis of ten thousand urinary calculi. *J Urol* 1962;**88**:545–62.

41 Rieselbach RE, Steele TH. Influence of the kidney upon urate homeostasis in health and disease. *Am J Med* 1974;**56**:665–75.

42 Grantham JJ, Chonko AM. Renal handling of organic anions and cations; metabolism and excretion of uric acid. In: Brenner BM, ed. *The Kidney*, 3rd edn. Philadelphia: WB Saunders, 1986:663–700.

43 Sperling O. Urate deposition and stone formation in renal hypouricemia. In: Zollner N, Gresser U, eds. *Urate Deposition in Man and its Clinical Consequences*. Berlin: Springer Verlag, 1991:65–77.

44 Sorensen LB. Degradation of uric acid in man. *Metabolism* 1959;**8**:687–703.

45 Akaoka I, Nishizawa T, Yano E *et al*. Renal urate excretion in five cases of hypouricemia with an isolated renal defect of urate transport. *J Rheumatol* 1977;**4**:86–94.

46 Kawabe K, Muryama T, Akaoka I. A case of uric acid renal stone with hypouricemia caused by tubular reabsorption defect of uric acid. *J Urol* 1976;**116**:690–2.

47 Takeda E, Kuroda T, Ito M *et al*. Hereditary renal hypouricemia in children. *J Pediatr* 1985;**107**:71–4.

48 Erley ChMM, Hirshberg RR, Hoefer W, Schaefer K. Acute renal failure due to uric acid nephropathy in a patient with renal hypouricemia. *Klin Wochenschr* 1989;**67**:308–12.

49 Ishikawa I, Sakurai Y, Masuzaki S *et al*. Exercise-induced acute renal failure in 3 patients with renal hypouricemia. *Jpn J Nephrol* 1990;**32**:923–8.

50 Suttle DP, Becroft DMO, Welester DR. Hereditary orotic aciduria and other disorders of pyrimidine metabolism. In: Scriver CR, Beaudet AL, Sly WS, Valle D, eds. *The Metabolic Basis of Inherited Disease*, 6th edn. New York: McGraw Hill, 1989:1095–126.

51 Hillmon RE. Primary hyperoxaluria. In: Scriver CR, Beaudet AL, Sly WS, Valle D, eds. *The Metabolic Basis of Inherited Disease*, 6th edn. New York: McGraw Hill, 1989:933–44.

52 Donne MA. Tableau de differents depots de matieres salines et de substance organiees qui se font dans les urines, presentatant les caracteres propre a les distinguer entre eux et a reconnaitre leure nature. *C R Acad Sci [D]* 1838;**6**:19–21.

53 Lepoutre C. Calculus multiples chez un enfant. Infiltration du parenchyme renal par des crystaux. *J Urol* 1925;**20**:424–5.

54 Davis JS, Klingberg WG, Stowell RE. Nephrolithiasis and nephrocalcinosis with calcium oxalate crystals in kidneys and bones. *J Pediatr* 1950;**36**:323–34.

55 Newns GH, Black JA. A case of calcium oxalate nephrocalcinosis. *Great Ormond St J* 1953;**5**:40–4.

56 Crawhall JC, Scowen EF, Watts RWE. Conversion of glycine to oxalate in primary hyperoxaluria. *Lancet* 1959;**2**:806–9.

57 Crawhall JC, De Mowbray RR, Scowen EF, Watts RWE. Conversion of glycine to oxalate in a normal subject. *Lancet* 1959;**2**:810.

58 Atkins GL, Dean BM, Griffin WJ, Watts RWE. Quantitative aspects of ascorbic acid metabolism in man. *J Biol Chem* 1964;**239**:2975–80.

59 Watts RWE. Hyperoxaluric states. In: Wickham JEA, Colin Buck A, eds. *Renal Tract Stone. Metabolic Basis and Clinical Practice*. Edinburgh: Churchill Livingstone, 1990:384–400.

60 Danpure CJ, Purkiss P, Jennings PR, Watts RWE. Mitochondrial damage and the subcellular distribution of 2-oxoglutarate: glyoxalate carboligase in normal human and rat liver and the liver of a patient with primary hyperoxaluria type I. *Clin Sci* 1986;**74**:417–25.

61 Williams HE, Smith LH. L-glyceric aciduria, a new genetic variant of primary hyperoxaluria. *N Engl J Med* 1968;**278**:233–9.

62 Segal S, Thier SO. Cystinuria. In: Scriver CR, Beaudet AL, Sly WS, Valle D, eds. *The Metabolic Basis of Inherited Disease*, 6th edn. New York: McGraw Hill, 1989:2479–96.

63 Wollaston WH. On cystic oxide: a new species of urinary calculus. *Philos Trans R Soc Lond* 1810;**100**:223–30.

64 Berzelius JJ. Calculus urinaries. *Traite Chem* 1833;**7**:424–8.

65 Garrod AE. Inborn errors of metabolism [Lectures I–IV]. *Lancet* 2 1908;**2**:1, 73, 142, 214.

66 Dent CE, Rose GA. Amino acid metabolism in cystinuria. *Q J Med* 1951;**20**:205–19.

67 Milne MD, Asatoor AM, Edwards KDG, Loughridge LW. The intestinal absorption defect in cystinuria. *Gut* 1961;**2**:323–7.

68 Segal S, Thier SO. Cystinuria. In: Stanbury JB, Wyngaarden JB, Fredrickson DS, eds. *The Metabolic Basis of Inherited Disease*, 4th edn. New York: McGraw Hill, 1983;1774–91.

69 Pruszanski W. Cystinuria and cystine urolithiasis in childhood. *Acta Paediatr Scand* 1966;**55**:97–106.

70 Caldwell FP, Townsend JI, Smith MJV. Genetics of cystinuria in an inbred population. *J Urol* 1978;**119**:531–3.

71 Piel CF, Roof BS, Renal calculi. In: Ruben MI, Barratt TM, eds. *Pediatric Nephrology*. Baltimore: Williams and Wilkins, 1975:760–6.

72 Smith AD, Lange PH, Miller RP, Reinke DB. Dissolution of cystine calculi by irrigation with acetylcysteine through percutaneous nephrostomy. *Urology* 1979;**13**:422–3.

73 Crissey MM, Gittes RF. Dissolution of cystine ureteral calculus by irrigation with tromethamine. *J Urol* 1979;**121**:811–12.

74 Stark H, Savir A. Dissolution of cystine calculi by pelviocaliceal irrigation with D-penicillamine. *J Urol* 1980;**124**:895–8.

75 Kelly S, Nolan DP. Postscript on excretion rates in post-transplant cystinuric patient. *J Am Med Assoc* 1980; **243**:1897.

76 Hodgkinson A, Pyrah LN. The urinary excretion of calcium and inorganic phosphate in 344 patients with calcium stone of renal origin. *Br J Surg* 1958;**46**:10–18.

77 Pak CYC, Ohata M, Lawrence EC, Snyder W. The hypercalciuria causes, parathyroid functions and diagnostic criteria. *J Clin Invest* 1974;**54**:387–400.

78 Weinberger A, Sperling O, Schachter J *et al*. Idiopathic hypercalciuria. A series of 50 patients. *Intern Urol Nephrol* 1977;**9**:213–16.

79 Aladjem M, Modan M, Lusky A. Idiopathic hypercalciuria: a familial generalized renal hyperexcretory state. *Kidney Int* 1983;**24**:549–54.

80 Weinberger A, Schechter J, Pinkhas J, Sperling O. Hereditary hypercalciuric urolithiasis: a study of a family. *Br J Urol* 1981;**53**:285–6.

81 Coe FL, Parks JH, Moore ES. Familial idiopathic hypercalciuria. *N Engl J Med* 1979;**300**:337–40.

82 De Luca R, Guzetta F. Hipercaliuria idiopatica infantile. *La Pediatria* 1965;**73**:613–15.

83 Du Bose TD, Alpern RJ. Renal tubular acidosis. In: Scriver CR, Beaudet AL, Sly WS, Valle D, eds. *The Metabolic Basis of Inherited Disease*, 6th edn. New York: McGraw Hill, 1989:2539–68.

84 Wrong O, Davies HE. The excretion of acid in renal disease. *Q J Med* 1959;**28**:259–313.

85 Coe FL, Parks JH. Stone disease in hereditary distal renal tubular acidosis. *Ann Intern Med* 1980;**93**:60–1.

86 Simpson DP. Influence of plasma bicarbonate concentration and pH on citrate excretion. *Am J Physiol* 1964;**206**:875–82.

87 Buckalew VM Jr, McCurdy DK, Ludwig GD, Chaykin LB, Elkinton JR. The syndrome of incomplete renal tubular acidosis. *Am J Med* 1968;**45**:32–42.

88 Dedmon RE, Wrong O. The excretion of organic anion in renal tubular acidosis with particular reference to citrate. *Clin Sci* 1962;**22**:19–32.

89 Morrissey JF, Ochoa M, Lotspeich WD, Waterhouse C. Citrate excretion in renal tubular acidosis. *Ann Intern Med* 1963;**58**:159–66.

90 Mcsherry EM, Pokroy MV. The absence of nephrocalcinosis in children with type 1 RTA on high dose alkali therapy since infancy. *Clin Res* 1978;**26**:470A.

91 Whyte MP. Hypophosphatasia. In: Scriver CR, Beaudet AL, Sly WS, Valle D, eds. *The Metabolic Basis of Inherited Disease* 6th edn. New York: McGraw Hill, 1989:2843–56.

92 Tieder M, Modai D, Samuel R *et al.* Hereditary hypophosphatemic rickets with hypercalciuria. *N Engl J Med* 1985;**312**:611–17.

93 Tieder M, Modai D, Shaked U *et al.* 'Idiopathic' hypercalciuria and hereditary hypophosphatemic rickets. *N Engl J Med* 1987;**316**:125–9.

60 Management of Disorders of Calcium Metabolism

P.O.Schwille, A.S.Schmiedl and G.Rümenapf

Introduction

In retrospect, the literature on disorders of calcium metabolism in calcium stone disease and their medical treatment has grown enormously. All information of relevance to the subject cannot be incorporated in a chapter of restricted length aimed at serving the needs of the postgraduate student. We have, therefore, here confined ourselves to presenting facts arising from clinical and laboratory work, and identifying unsolved questions. Among the major sources of information to which the reader is referred is the earlier edition of this textbook [1], and the proceedings of a number of meetings dealing with basic and clinical research work in urolithiasis, such as the International Urolithiasis Symposium [2–8]. The proceedings of the Bonn–Vienna symposia (between 1972 and 1987) and the European Urolithiasis Symposium (starting from 1989) may not be contained in international databases, but information may be obtained from the publishers (Steinkopff, Darmstadt, Germany and Springer, Heidelberg, Germany, respectively).

A number of excellent monographs contain in-depth information on pathophysiology, including such topics as the pathogenesis of idiopathic hypercalciuria and nephrolithiasis [9], primary hyperparathyroidism as a cause of calcium nephrolithiasis [10], calcium nephrolithiasis and forms of renal tubular acidosis (RTA) [11], intestinal calcium absorption and vitamin D metabolism in idiopathic hypercalciuria [12] and bone as a source of urinary calcium [13]. Other international literature focusing on treatment regimens includes articles on the physical and clinical aspects associated with calcium stones [14], orthophosphate therapy in renal calcium lithiasis [15], physiochemical action and extrarenal manifestations of alkali therapy [16], the prevention of calcium stones with thiazides [17], idiopathic calcium lithiasis [18], the origin of hypocitraturia [19], and the stone clinic effect in patients with idiopathic calcium urolithiasis [20]. This list is of course merely a selection, for there are

also specialized review articles and data collections, for example on stone analysis procedures, methods of calculating supersaturation of urine, etc., that are often contained in non-medical journals and books.

In this chapter, we present an overview of the more frequent disorders of calcium metabolism with which calcium urolithiasis may be associated. These include hypercalcaemia, but also idiopathic recurrent calcium urolithiasis (RCU), a disorder which is always normocalcaemic but often hypercalciuric. The degree of calciuria in RCU varies considerably, with the normocalciuria subset being more frequent (about 50–60%), and the subset with hypercalciuria of various types (absorptive, fasting, renal hypercalciuria) accounting for the rest. There is no agreement among physicians and researchers as to whether the aetiology of hypercalciuria has to be known in cases where there is a need to institute anti-stone treatment, but it is agreed that importance should be attached to reducing calciuria and oxaluria, the well-documented risk factors and stone promoters. Calcium-related factors in RCU pathophysiology are discussed separately under extrinsic and intrinsic factors. As used here, 'intrinsic' means that, despite a normal lifestyle and nutrition, RCU patients can often be distinguished from non-stone-forming individuals on the basis of differences in their metabolic response to such challenges as oral loading with calcium, other nutrients, etc., due to 'intrinsic' abnormalities. One section of the chapter is devoted to the way we carry out the laboratory examination of patients with disorders of minerals, another deals with the modes of treatment of RCU currently considered to be effective.

Forms of RTA and medullary sponge kidney—the latter named for the underlying anatomical irregularity, namely dilatation of collecting ducts—are not properly addressed (for literature see above), although there are reports on associated calcium and acid–base disorders [21–24]. Given that these latter need medication, the effective principle of treatment may be identified among those of relevance for idiopathic calcium urolithiasis (see p. 784).

Calcium-related factors in idiopathic renal calcium urolithiasis

An impressive body of basic and clinical research data on such factors is contained in the literature cited above. In accordance with current terminology, many of these factors can be classified as either promoters or inhibitors of crystal- and stone-forming processes (Fig. 60.1), and they are active either *per se* or via metabolic pathways requiring their presence; there are two important exceptions, drinking water (see below) and urinary proteins (see p. 776), which deserve a special comment.

Extrinsic factors

These are summarized under the subheadings climate, stress and nutrients (see Fig. 60.1). Among the nutrients, domestic drinking water, supplied by public water utilities, probably has a dual role. Although water hardness and its effect on stone frequency in a given geographical region has been a subject of research for decades [25], its significance for RCU remains uncertain. Often, a high level of calcium is associated with low magnesium, and vice versa. In terms of stone-forming processes these two factors may cancel each other out, i.e. high calcium can inhibit stones [26], probably via precipitation of calcium oxalate and calcium phosphate in the gut lumen, thereby reducing oxaluria and phosphaturia; whereas low magnesium can contribute to a low inhibitory potential of urine [27,28] or deinhibit oxalate biosynthesis through its various interactions with enzymes [29] and thereby increase oxaluria and the frequency of stones. However, some geographical areas with low calcium but high magnesium levels in drinking water, have a significantly increased occurrence of magnesium-ammonium phosphate (struvite) stones, apparently unaccompanied by urinary tract infection [30]. Thus, the actual significance of the composition of tap water in the aetiology of RCU is still inadequately known, and awaits final clarification.

Among the common beverages, bottled mineral water needs commenting on because of the heterogeneous spectrum of minerals contained in the various brands. An examination of 165 commercial mineral waters in Germany [31] showed that the sodium chloride content is below 2 g/l in only about two-thirds, while in the other third sodium chloride, a determinant of urinary calcium excretion in humans [32] and animals [33], is the dominating salt [31]. The quantitative relationship between

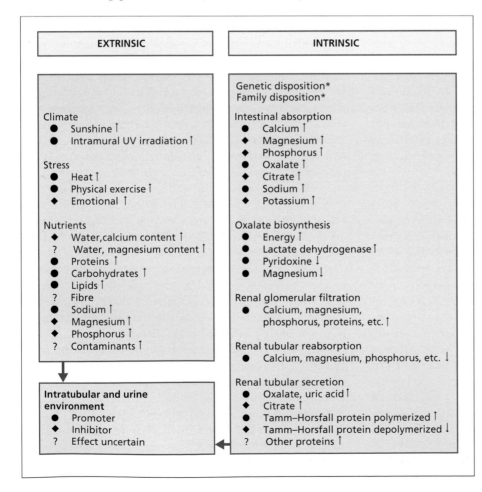

Fig. 60.1 Overview of calcium-related extrinsic and intrinsic factors in the pathophysiology of idiopathic renal calcium stones. Their mode of activity in the tubular fluid and urine is either as a promoter or an inhibitor, but in several cases it may be dual or is unknown. The direction of arrow indicates the change in activity. * Site of primary manifestation unknown. UV, ultraviolet.

the two ions in healthy males and females is illustrated in Fig. 60.2. In view of the frequently high urinary sodium excretion per day (>250 mmol) in stone patients, the associated high calcium excretion in these patients is not surprising.

The body's vitamin D stores are increased by enhanced ultraviolet (UV) irradiation of the skin and subsequent hepatic 25-hydroxylation of the native vitamin. There are numerous older reports of higher stone incidence in areas with prolonged periods of sunshine [25], and during seasons with many hours of sunshine the average 25-hydroxyvitamin D (25-OHD) serum levels are higher too [34]. However, a causal role of this vitamin D metabolite in RCU, for instance via enhancement of intestinal calcium absorption and calciuria, has not been established. Heat stress increases transpiration and leads to reduced urinary volume, which accelerates urine supersaturation; in addition, heat stress produces unduly high urine acidity — for a number of reasons [35]. Low urine pH ensures that undissociated uric acid predominates over the urate, which favours the precipitation of uric acid and the subsequent heterogeneous precipitation of calcium salts, especially calcium oxalate. This sequence of events has been well documented by investigations in native and artificial urine.

Emotional stress in humans has been found to stimulate calciuria [36], but in rats acutely stressed by restraint undersaturation of urine with respect to the major stone substances was achieved [37]. Extreme physical exercise, such as marathon running, leads to a spectrum of urine crystals, predominantly calcium oxalate [38]. The role of the major calorie carriers among the nutrients and their mode of contribution to stone processes when taken in excessive amounts, are described in detail elsewhere

[39–41]. Several lipids, some of which stimulate oxalogenesis [42], attract the interest of researchers and physicians because in animal models hyperlipidaemia and hypercholesterolaemia lead to nephrocalcinosis and calcium phosphate renal stones [43,44], while others prevent hypercalciuria [45]. It has long been known that urinary sodium and urinary calcium are directly correlated [46], but not until the 1980s was it recognized that the restriction of dietary salt could be a means of reducing calciuria [47,48], and that increasing salt intake can have a negative influence on systemic mineral metabolism [49] and urine composition [50]. The role of phosphorus has not yet been settled; some investigators feel that phosphorus intake is declining, but others assume that there is no threat from exogenous phosphorus deficit [51]. The impact of phosphorus deficit on the homeostasis of calcium and the urinary environment is enormous. After all, a phosphorus deficiency inside cells drives enhanced synthesis of 1,25-dihydroxyvitamin D (1,25(OH)$_2$D), and high serum levels of the latter are the most potent stimulus to intestinal calcium absorption [12]. As a result of calcium hyperabsorption, the calcium concentration in the intestinal lumen is thought to decline, whereas hyperabsorption of oxalate appears to be turned on [52,53]; the two risk factors, hypercalciuria and hyperoxaluria, make it likely that calcium oxalate will precipitate out of the urine. This wide field of ionic interactions at transporting epithelia, in which a number of questions are still unanswered, deserves consideration when selecting a treatment regimen for stone metaphylaxis in RCU (see p. 784), a disorder involving various intrinsic abnormalities.

In affluent societies a deficiency of dietary fibre is considered a key factor in the development of a number of diseases [54] including calcium urolithiasis [55]. Many physicians, therefore, advocate the use of bran in treatment regimens. Dietary fibre and phytate, constituents of cereal bran, are able to bind intestinal calcium [56], and for that reason both substances were long considered to be anti-stone agents. More recent work has shown that phytate also binds zinc and iron, in addition to calcium, and that the human organism does not adapt to a high intake of phytate [57]. These changes affect skeletal minerals directly, and indirectly via parathyroid gland stimulation. We speculate that the majority of fibre preparations induce hyperabsorption of oxalate and oxaluria. These facts reveal a clear need to investigate conventional foodstuffs with regard to their fibre content, if bone and other mineral disorders, renal stones included, are to be prevented. In a study done by our laboratory, inadequate consumption of fibre was not a feature of RCU patients [58] but, unfortunately, we did not pay specific attention to phytic acid in their fibre. When ingested in amounts of up to 350 mg, contained in 10 g of fibre in a single meal, phytic acid has adverse effects on calcium metabolism [59].

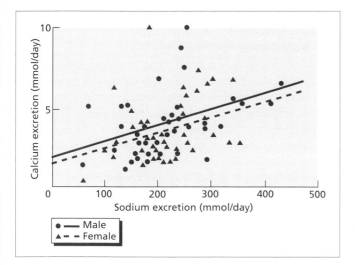

Fig. 60.2 Relationship between urinary sodium excretion and calcium excretion. ——, regression line for males ($Y = 0.010\,X + 1.915$); -----, regression line for females ($Y = 0.010\,X + 1.641$). (Redrawn from [32])

Toxic contaminants are ubiquitous in the air, soil, water and food, and the heavy metal cadmium is found in abundance. The damaging effect of cadmium on tissues, especially the kidney, has been proven [60] and an effector role of cadmium in calcium metabolism shown [61]. At present, the role of cadmium in renal stones is unclear, although there have been studies on the frequency of stone disease as influenced by exposure to cadmium, and on changes of the renal epithelial morphology observed after long-term exposure to the metal [62], which are intriguingly reminiscent of the early cellular events seen in animal models on nephrocalcinosis and calcium phosphate stone formation [43,44].

Intrinsic factors

Genetic and family disposition

Suspicion is growing that renal calcium stone formation reflects a genetic predisposition, and there are well-described examples in humans and animals [63]. Moreover, the fact that it is possible to breed animals with genetically determined hypercalciuria [64], supports the view that a genetic defect underlies hypercalciuric RCU. On this point, however, no evidence has yet been provided by population studies. In contrast, a defined genetic disorder is under discussion as the cause of the impaired transmembrane transport of ions, recognized in the gene coding for a proteinaceous constituent of the cellular membrane [65]. Many of the intrinsic factors exhibited by RCU may merely reflect acquired abnormalities that themselves can lead to calcium stones, or facilitate their development. It should be remembered that the incidence of, for example, hypercalciuria in the general population is about 10% and that the majority of cases do not form stones; this means that simple calcium excess in the urine does not suffice for stone development. This is in accord with the fact that large amounts of calcium (approximately 40 mmol/l) need to be added to precipitate calcium phosphate [66]. From this, it may be inferred that under normal conditions additional factors must be involved, possibly high levels of oxalate, an inhibitor deficit, or a combination of the two. It is worth noting that the increased incidence of stones in certain families is no proof of a genetic trait necessarily leading to stones in the descendents in accordance with the Mendel law; in most instances the presence of stones may simply reflect a certain dietary habit which, in the long-term, favours their formation [67,68]. Therefore, the diagnosis 'hereditary calcium lithiasis' should be made only after a careful prior check of dietary factors. Once the factors responsible for stones, whether genetic or non-genetic, have been identified with the aid of appropriate examination of patients in the stone clinic and laboratory (see p. 776), the majority can be managed by experienced physicians.

Intestinal absorption and oxalate biosynthesis

Intestinal mineral absorption (calcium, magnesium, phosphorus) is normally finely tuned by serum $1,25(OH)_2D$ which, when high, suppresses the activity of 1α-hydroxylase (positive–negative feedback regulation), thereby resetting the serum hormone level to normal. With regard to activity of the enzyme it is important to know that parathyroid hormone (PTH) plays an interactive and stimulating, but not primary, part, as is also true for primary hyperparathyroidism (see p. 778). In the majority of RCU patients, serum PTH is normal to low, yet $1,25(OH)_2D$ is high [53,69,70], suggesting the existence of additional factors in the regulation of this hormone. A number of hypotheses have been put forward to explain the low levels of PTH and high levels of $1,25(OH)_2D$ in subsets of RCU patients, such as those showing absorptive or renal hypercalciuria [9,71–74]. Among other causes, increased bone calcium efflux due to enhanced bone resorption—suppressing parathyroid gland function—and increased renal phosphate losses due to diminished tubular phosphate reabsorption—creating an intracellular phosphorus deficiency and a PTH-independent stimulation of 1α-hydroxylase—are discussed.

Preliminary data obtained at our laboratory indicate that much credence should be given to the phosphate loss theory, as postprandial hyperphosphaturia appears characteristic for RCU as a whole, i.e. unclassified by calciuria [53,70], and it can adequately explain the majority of additional abnormalities exhibited by RCU. These include high levels of $1,25(OH)_2D$, some degree of enhanced bone resorption mediated by this vitamin D metabolite, and high levels of fasting and postprandial calciuria. The high basal serum level of $1,25(OH)_2D$, however, cannot account for increased jejunal, that is segmental, calcium uptake [75], nor increased in vitro uptake of calcium by jejunal mucosa found in biopsies from hypercalciuric stone-forming individuals [76]. Thus, the combination of mineral metabolic changes suggests that some other intrinsic defect must exist, possibly in transmembrane calcium transport [77].

Intestinal oxalate absorption is normal when in the order of 8–10% of dietary oxalate [78]. It may be fine-tuned by the concomitant intestinal concentration and absorption of calcium and magnesium, which is best illustrated by the fact that oxaluria may be markedly decreased by increased dietary uptake of calcium or magnesium [79,80]. The underlying mechanism may be sought in intraluminal oxalate precipitation by these cations. Oxalate absorption in RCU is probably normal [78], and the mild hyperoxaluria in RCU subsets not explainable by high dietary oxalate

[53,79–81] should therefore have a different aetiology—it should result from peroxisomal overproduction of oxalate from oxalate precursors, or from exaggerated renal oxalate losses. The oxalate production rate in RCU is largely unknown. Circumstantial evidence of increased oxalate production is provided by a consideration of the total energy consumed by RCU patients [82]. Also, *in vitro* studies suggest that the activity of one isoform of lactate dehydrogenase is a major determinant of oxalate production [83]. It may, therefore, be speculated that the portion of oxaluria contributed by oxalate from endogenous sources differs between people with or without stones. To elucidate this situation further, a greater knowledge of the state of pyridoxine and magnesium, both documented modulators of oxalate production via the diminution of the glyoxylate precursor pool size [29,84], is mandatory. Alternative interpretations may, however, exist. One is that, intraintestinally, crystals formed may adhere to superficial structures of enterocytes [85]; in the acidic microclimate of these anatomical regions crystals may be dissolved and oxalate or calcium ions absorbed or released into the lumen, as dictated by the need for homeostasis. This possible route of influence on the urinary excretion rate awaits further clarification. Another possible cause of hyperoxaluria is the non-enzymatic conversion of ascorbic acid to oxalate, which has plagued research work on the true state of oxaluria in RCU for many years. Currently the situation in RCU appears to have been clarified, as plasma and urinary ascorbic acid levels proved to be normal when both substances were measured reliably; this also applies to the associated oxalate [86].

Intestinal malabsorption of citrate in RCU has been reported, and has been explained by a predominance of hyperabsorption of other carboxylic acids such as ascorbate [87]. More recently, urinary citrate, which is sensitive to acid–base changes, was found to be determined by the intestinal absorption of alkali [88]. This would explain the hypocitraturia associated with metabolic acidosis, such as RTA, in which intestinal alkali absorption is probably also impaired [88]; however, in RCU with its high frequency of hypocitraturia, reliable information on the intracellular acid–base status is not available. Alternatively, hypocitraturia in RCU may originate in renal sites (see below).

Renal function

In RCU, the contribution of renal glomerular filtration and tubular reabsorption of calcium to the urinary excretion of calcium was first assessed by Lemann and co-workers in a series of impressive publications beginning in 1969. The origin of increased calciuria was long considered to be diminished tubular reabsorption of calcium ions, and this view is still held by many investigators. More recently, it

has been assumed, on the basis of studies into the defective exchange mechanism of anions such as oxalate [89] that in RCU there is enhanced calcium complexation by oxalate in the thick ascending limb of Henle's loop. These authors have postulated that hypercalciuria and hyperoxaluria should ensue, but did not mention whether they found any crystals. However, hyperoxaluria in RCU is restricted to some subset(s), whereas hypercalciuria is widespread. Interestingly, the recalculation and plotting by the Lemann group [9] of the individual data from an earlier work of their own [90], shows that for a given calcium excretion there was a higher underlying glomerular filtration rate and higher ultrafiltrable serum calcium, both of which are consistent with a markedly higher rate of calcium filtered by the glomeruli. This important finding of a possible non-tubular renal origin of hypercalciuria has not so far been investigated in more recent studies, all favouring the view that hypercalciuria reflects diminished tubular reabsorption [91]. If higher than normal creatinine clearance is more common in RCU, it may explain not only hypercalciuria but also hyperphosphaturia and the somewhat elevated glycosuria and proteinuria (P.O. Schwille, unpublished observations). Thus, the concept of a generalized tubulopathy covering several abnormalities needs to be reappraised, as has already been attempted [24]. Such studies should involve participants meticulously matched for sex, age and anthropometric criteria (body weight, height, body mass index, etc.); these regulations appear mandatory because obesity is frequently encountered in RCU [92], and obesity increases the fraction serum calcium filterable by glomeruli [93].

With respect to renal tubular citrate and oxalate handling in RCU, there are still large gaps in our understanding. Both anions chelate calcium, and therefore a knowledge of the residual intratubular ion concentration would be desirable. In other words, the intratubular calcium oxalate product in terms of the free ions may differ from that in urine, and may be dictated by the actual citrate rather than oxalate. Whether calciuria or oxaluria is more important for the initiation of RCU [94,95] is unclear, but citrate may be of similar importance. In fact, unpublished data in RCU patients at our laboratory show 'ionic' hypocitraturia, 'ionic' hypercalciuria and 'ionic' normo-oxaluria. Citrate clearance is often low in RCU, as is the ratio of citrate : creatinine clearance. While the low citrate clearance is mainly an expression of somewhat higher serum citrate, the latter reflects increased net tubular reabsorption of citrate [96]. For this intriguing situation to occur, some backdiffusion of incompletely deprotonated luminal citrate has been postulated [19]; this would fit in with the unduly low pH of urine often observed in subsets of RCU. It is not known whether impaired tubular citrate secretion contributes to hypocitraturia. In contrast to citrate, the oxalate clearance and the fractional oxalate clearance were found to be elevated; the high clearance is due to low plasma oxalate, not high oxalate excretion [97]. This situation leaves unanswered the question as to whether there is diminished reabsorption of filtered oxalate or increased oxalate secretion; both variations can lead to low plasma oxalate. A consideration of both citrate and oxalate shows that expressing urinary excretion in terms of their clearance alone may be misleading. The question arises as to what happens with the two substances, and what interplay do they have with calcium, in the various parts of the nephron of RCU subjects?

Urate handling by the kidneys in health and various disorders with renal calcium and non-calcium stones is described in current textbooks on nephrology. The formation of calcium urate in biological fluids, tubular fluid and urine included, should theoretically be possible, but so far this substance has not aroused the interest of stone physicians and researchers.

At present, proteins in urine are considered to be stone promoters, because they intensify crystallization stages (in particular nucleation) of calcium oxalate [98]. However, many proteins behave like calcium 'scavengers' and remove calcium ions from urine [99]; it is not yet clear whether this property of proteins means binding of calcium to form an organic calcium-containing stone matrix accumulating more and more stone-forming calcium salts until a microstone is formed (promoter activity), or whether the decrease in supersaturation (resulting from protein–calcium interaction) means the inhibition of crystallization (inhibitor activity). One example of a possible dual action appears to be the Tamm–Horsfall protein. In urine of non-stone-forming individuals it behaves as an inhibitor, in that of RCU patients as a promoter [100]. When calcium is removed from solution by calcium-chelating agents such as citrate, the molecular conformation of the protein, as isolated from the urine of stone patients, shifts from the previously folded and polymerized state to an unfolded and depolymerized state, and in this form the protein no longer acts as a promoter but as an inhibitor [100].

Retention of particles

It is not known whether some, as yet unknown, intrinsic calcium-related factor predisposes the kidney of RCU patients to retain crystalline particles. However, the fact that the Tamm–Horsfall protein is able to inhibit crystal aggregation only after chelation of calcium [100] suggests that abnormal interaction between calcium and urinary proteins contributes indirectly to particle retention. This phenomenon, interpreted under the term 'free or fixed particle theory of stone formation', was first addressed by Finlayson and Reid [101]. On the basis of the anatomical construction and geometry of tubules, and giving consideration to the necessary physicochemical reactions

during crystallization, they concluded that for a stone to develop, crystal retention must take place at some tubular site (fixed particle), because even fast-growing crystals (free particle) will be swept away and are therefore unable to form a stone inside the kidney. More recently, it has become evident that oxalate and calcium oxalate crystals can damage tubular epithelium [102,103] and that this interaction may lead to crystal adhesion to, and crystal incorporation by, tissue [104,105]. Also, an evaluation of particle size must take into account the fact that crystals regularly form aggregates, and that the much larger diameter of aggregates facilitates their intratubular accretion. Enhanced aggregation of crystals in urine is characteristic of stone patients [106,107], and in animal models with calcium oxalate crystalluria it was found that nucleation, growth and aggregation allow formation of cyrstalline particles which are big enough to be retained intrarenally [108]. Clinically, in RCU, calcium oxalate crystalluria may be the exception rather than the rule [109] and retention should therefore be substantial.

Laboratory assessment

The diagnosis and treatment of patients with calcium stones (normocalcaemic RCU, hypercalcaemic disorders) requires access to the minimum of laboratory facilities needed to characterize the metabolic state. In RCU, preference should be given to outpatient evaluation, which in our experience ensures that the external conditions during which the stones develop will be reflected by the laboratory data. The necessary organization comprises four points.

1 Provision of detailed written information to the patient about the date and purpose of the visit, and what preparations are needed for this (details of urine collection, etc.).

2 Procurement of a stone analysis, obtained by the use of a reliable method (infrared spectroscopy, X-ray diffractometry, polarization microscopy).

3 Careful documentation of the history of the stone disease, pinpointing the extrinsic factors listed in Fig. 60.1 and discussed above, with emphasis on whether any familial or hereditary disposition is present.

4 Assessment of the calcium metabolic and associated parameters in the blood and urine; this should permit not only reliable differentiation between abnormal and normal values, but also the identification of borderline values that necessitate repeated follow-up.

To achieve a reliable diagnosis of the state of calcium and related parameters of metabolism, a standardized laboratory procedure would appear indispensable if unspecific confounding factors, such as diurnal rhythmicity of variables, etc., are to be avoided. The extent of the procedure itself may vary, depending on what can be afforded by a given institution, and the literature contains a number of workable proposals on how to minimize the laboratory work-up. Minimum prerequisites for the establishment of the diagnosis may be fasting venous blood drawn without stasis, reliable analysis of calcium and other minerals, etc., collection of untimed ('spot') fasting urine and the measurement of pH and a number of substances (Fig. 60.3). Cases of RTA (incomplete or complete forms) can be identified by a urinary pH > 6.10, measured on two different occasions [110], and stone analysis (pure calcium phosphate is predominant). Most critical to the further procedure is the calcium : creatinine ratio, which should be not higher than 0.12 mg calcium : 1 mg creatinine. In idiopathic calcium stone patients this ratio allows one to separate fasting hypercalciuria from intestinal absorptive and bone resorptive hypercalciuria [111]. In questionable situations repeat measurements after a prolonged nocturnal fast, or after prior intake of calcium-binding agents [112,113], will assist in decision making. An example of a tentative abridged laboratory programme is shown in Fig. 60.3. In practice, it begins with stone analysis, and then proceeds to bladder voiding and measurement of urinary pH, calcium, creatinine and other substances. With regard to idiopathic lithiasis, including patients with pure uric acid stones in addition to patients with RCU, the majority of metabolic abnormalities in fasting urine can be identified and serve as a basis for treatment strategies.

In our institution we have gradually improved on a previously communicated laboratory programme [40,63, 114], the basic constituents of which were originally proposed by Pak and co-workers [111]. Among other things, it entails collection of 24 h urine, a baseline fasting urine period of 2 h and the intake of a calcium-rich test meal followed by collection of a postprandial urine sample over 3 h. Optional procedures are several samplings of blood,

alternative composition of the meal, prolongation of the postprandial period, etc. An overview is presented in Fig. 60.4. The programme can be practiced as dictated by the needs prevailing, that is either as a whole package or only parts of it undertaken. Provided the various stages are sufficiently standardized in terms of both timing and environmental conditions, the results obtained are highly reproducible. Classification into the various types of calciuria (normocalciuria, fasting, absorptive, resorptive hypercalciuria) is readily feasible, provided the overnight fasting period which preceeds the first urine collected in the morning in the laboratory (so-called fasting urine) was of sufficient duration (no less than 12 h). Calculation of all the clinical chemistry data and other variables, and of the supersaturation products (propensity to form crystals) is done on a computer. Determination of the total oxalate concentration tolerated by urine at the stage of nucleation is a valuable step and is carried out by us in postprandial urine [115], in which there is a high content of calcium and a low content of phosphate, as an expression of parathyroid gland suppression by the calcium-rich test meal ingested. Such a urinary environment minimizes the co-precipitation of calcium phosphate. Preliminary results suggest that an evaluation of growth and aggregation of calcium oxalate crystals is also possible with the same urine that is used for determination of tolerable oxalate [116]. Identification of increased tolerable oxalate and aggregation inhibition in response to treatment, for example with citrate, appears to be a useful feature of this test [117]. Disadvantages of the full programme are the need for trained personnel and the considerable size of the workload. On the other hand, the complete programme is embedded in a user-friendly software which can be run on standard PC hardware.

Fig. 60.3 Example of an abridged laboratory programme for ambulatory examination of patients with idiopathic urolithiasis (uric acid, calcium-containing stones). Note that the basic elements of the programme are stone analysis, collection of fasting urine with immediate measurement of pH, analysis of creatinine, calcium, oxalate, phosphate and citrate, calculation of the substance : creatinine ratio in this urine and a critical comparison with the laboratory's own normal range.
* Defined disorders with associated urolithiasis are excluded (e.g. primary hyperparathyroidism, sarcoidosis, RTA, medullary sponge kidney, oxalosis, urinary tract infection); [a] no differentiation made between the stone core and shell; [b] in fasting urine. IR, infrared spectometry; X-RD, X-ray diffractometry; PM, polarization microscopy.

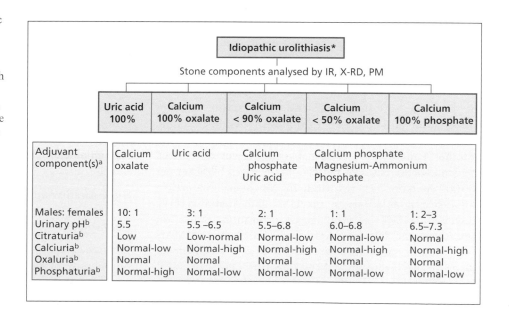

Idiopathic urolithiasis*				
Stone components analysed by IR, X-RD, PM				
Uric acid 100%	Calcium 100% oxalate	Calcium < 90% oxalate	Calcium < 50% oxalate	Calcium 100% phosphate
Adjuvant component(s)[a]	Calcium oxalate	Uric acid	Calcium phosphate Uric acid	Calcium phosphate Magnesium-Ammonium Phosphate	
Males: females	10: 1	3: 1	2: 1	1: 1	1: 2–3
Urinary pH[b]	5.5	5.5 –6.5	5.5–6.8	6.0–6.8	6.5–7.3
Citraturia[b]	Low	Low-normal	Normal-low	Normal-low	Normal
Calciuria[b]	Normal-low	Normal-high	Normal-high	Normal-high	Normal-high
Oxaluria[b]	Normal	Normal	Normal	Normal	Normal
Phosphaturia[b]	Normal-high	Normal-low	Normal-low	Normal-low	Normal-low

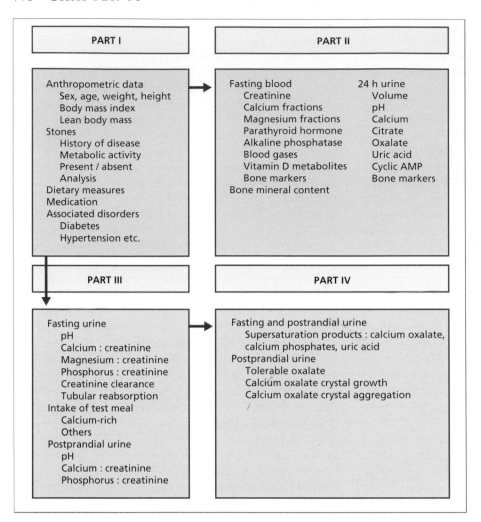

Fig. 60.4 Overview of the steps (parts I–IV) of the standardized ambulatory laboratory programme regularly practiced for identifying disturbances of mineral metabolism, including the various categories of renal stone patients. AMP, adenosine monophosphate.

Hypercalcaemia and renal stones

In earlier reports, 70% of hypercalcaemic patients had malignoma-associated hypercalcaemia (MAH), and only 20% suffered from primary hyperparathyroidism (pHPT) [118]. Since reliable routine serum calcium determinations became available, increasing numbers of patients with asymptomatic pHPT have been detected, so that the above percentages have undergone a change. Currently, 35% of the patients with hypercalcaemia (i.e. serum calcium corrected for protein above 2.7 mmol/l) attending a clinic have MAH, 55% have pHPT and 10% have hypercalcaemia of other causes [119]. These figures reflect an annual incidence of 25 cases of pHPT and 15 cases of MAH per 100 000 persons as reported in an overview article comprising populations in the USA and Australia [119]. However, pHPT is the most common cause of hypercalcaemic calcium urolithiasis [120], while in MAH renal calcium stones are a very rare finding [121]. The major reason for this discrepancy is the slow time course of pHPT. Thus, pHPT is usually diagnosed years after its onset, as the patient adapts to the slowly rising serum calcium levels that cause no clinical symptoms. Accordingly, hypercalciuria persisted for years in pHPT patients, giving renal stones time to develop. MAH often signals generalized disease with osteolytic metastases (70%), develops within a short period of time and causes clinical symptoms early, as the patient has no opportunity to adapt to the rapidly rising serum calcium. Nevertheless, calcium urolithiasis may sometimes be the first clinical symptom of a hitherto unknown malignant tumour and urologists, especially those working in a stone laboratory, should keep these diseases in mind so as to identify MAH patients early enough to treat them.

Hyperparathyroidism

Definition

Primary hyperparathyroidism is a result of hyperfunctioning of the parathyroid tissue which has lost its normal set-point of feedback inhibition by serum calcium.

Of the 160 pHPT patients treated in our surgical department between 1975 and 1994, 85% had developed adenomatous growth of one of the four existing parathyroid glands (solitary adenoma); in 4% more than one adenoma was found, and in 10% pHPT was due to hyperplasia of all four parathyroid glands. Only two patients had parathyroid carcinoma. While the aetiology of pHPT remains hypothetical, the pathogenesis of pHPT-related clinical symptoms ('stones, bones and abdominal groans') is clearly related to excessive secretion of PTH. PTH accelerates bone resorption, increases renal calcium reabsorption and enhances intestinal calcium absorption via stimulation of the renal synthesis of 1,25(OH)$_2$D. These metabolic changes result in hypercalcaemia, which is responsible for most of the clinical symptoms of pHPT. In 2–25% of cases, pHPT is accompanied by enteropancreatic neuroendocrine (32–75%), as well as anterior pituitary tumours (16–40%), the so-called multiple endocrine neoplasia type I (MEN-I) [122]. In MEN-I, overt pHPT is almost obligatory. In MEN-II, which is characterized by medullary thyroid carcinoma, pheochromocytoma and pHPT, the latter develops clinical relevance in less than 10%, although four-gland parathyroid hyperplasia is present in 40–60% of the patients [123]. As the present article will focus on pHPT-related nephrolithiasis, we refer to recent reviews covering all aspects of this multisymptomatic disease [118]. Tertiary hyperparathyroidism will not be discussed.

Epidemiology of urolithiasis in pHPT

The incidence of pHPT in western societies approaches that of colorectal cancer. However, in Germany the frequency of surgical interventions for pHPT is about one-third of this incidence, indicating that a large number of pHPT cases go undetected or are asymptomatic.

Two to 13% of all urolithiasis patients have pHPT [10], with an average of 7% [124]. In contrast to RCU, the pathophysiology of pHPT-related stone disease is less enigmatic, the diagnosis is relatively easy to establish and the disease can be cured by surgery, as was first demonstrated by Mandl in 1926 [125]. In the early twentieth century, the clinical presentation of pHPT was dominated by bone disease. HPT-related urolithiasis was first described in 1930 [126], in combination with bone disease. In 1937, Albright [127] identified urolithiasis as the predominant clinical symptom of pHPT. Today, calcium urolithiasis is the most common clinical manifestation of pHPT, while severe bone disease has become a rarity. This may be due to the fact that calcium intake was once lower than it now is [127], and that vitamin D deficiency was more frequent. pHPT patients, in whom bone disease predominates, were reported to have higher PTH levels, lower 1,25(OH)$_2$D and low intestinal calcium absorption as compared with those with nephrolithiasis. Owing to

excessive bone resorption, their calcium balance is negative. In contrast, pHPT patients with urolithiasis have high levels of 1,25(OH)$_2$D, high intestinal calcium absorption, relatively low PTH, less active bone resorption, and for long periods a neutral external calcium balance [128,129]. However, with subtle radiological methods minimal changes in bone structure are detectable in most pHPT patients [130], indicating that the classification of pHPT patients into the two categories of bone disease and nephrolithiasis may be too rough.

In a recent review of 2585 pHPT cases since 1961, the prevalence of renal stones was 41% [120]. In our institution, 52% of pHPT patients had urolithiasis (Table 60.1), which is therefore the most important clinical symptom of pHPT. Thanks to a more widespread determination of serum calcium, increasing numbers of asymptomatic pHPT patients are detected, and in some reports fewer than 10% of the patients have nephrolithiasis [131]. Only 6% of our pHPT patients had (mostly mild) nephrocalcinosis (see Table 60.1). Among 80 pHPT patients seen in our institution between 1985 and 1994, 13 were normocalcaemic with a serum calcium ≤2.7 mmol/l. Of these, eight patients (62%) had urolithiasis.

The composition of calculi in pHPT is similar to that in RCU. The predominant stone phase is calcium oxalate, followed by a mixture of calcium oxalate and calcium phosphate, and pure calcium phosphate. Mixtures of calcium oxalate and uric acid are frequent, while struvite or uric acid stones are rare.

Pathogenesis of urolithiasis in pHPT

Hypercalciuria (males >300 mg calcium/24 h, females >250 mg/24 h) is frequently found in pHPT (see above). Hypercalciuria is undoubtedly the major driving force in the development of calcium-containing renal stones in pHPT patients. Owing to hypercalcaemia, the filtered load of calcium in pHPT exceeds the distal tubular reabsorptive

Table 60.1 Renal and skeletal manifestations as well as accompanying diseases and metabolic disturbances in 160 pHPT patients treated at the surgical department of the University Erlangen-Nürnberg between 1975 and 1994.

Disturbances	Cases (%)
Urolithiasis	52
Nephrocalcinosis	6
Bone disease	20
Hyperuricaemia	52
Goitre	30
Arterial hypertension	30
Diabetes mellitus type II	22
Hypercholesterolaemia	23
Pancreatitis	7.6

capacity, and hypercalciuria ensues. As hypercalciuria is found even in normocalcaemic pHPT patients, despite the anticalciuric action of their elevated serum PTH levels, regulation of the renal reabsorption capacity for calcium appears to be the major determinant of the degree of hypercalciuria as compared with the filtered calcium load, unless hypercalcaemia is excessive [132]. Also, excess PTH gives rise to hyperphosphaturia, which again makes the urine more lithogenic. Additionally, pHPT may enhance the urinary concentration of promoters of stone formation [133], and decrease the activity of inhibitors or complexors, such as citrate, chondroitin sulphate and magnesium [134]. Uric acid is known to promote calcium oxalate stone formation by inducing epitaxial growth of calcium oxalate crystals as well as by adsorbing inhibitors of stone formation. However, the urinary uric acid concentration is normal in pHPT, although serum levels are elevated [135].

Among the pHPT patients seen at our institution, 22% had type II diabetes mellitus (see Table 60.1). Patients with pHPT were found to have glucose intolerance and elevated plasma insulin levels, indicating peripheral insulin resistance [136], which was explained by their hypophosphataemia [137]. As insulin can stimulate small intestinal calcium absorption [138] and has a calciuretic action [139], these factors may be important in the pathogenesis of pHPT-related hypercalciuria [10].

Malignoma-associated hypercalcaemia and nephrolithiasis

Pathophysiology

Formerly, three separate tumour-associated hypercalcaemia syndromes were differentiated [119]: (i) humoral hypercalcaemia of malignancy (pseudohyperparathyroidism); (ii) hypercalcaemia due to osteolytic bone metastases; and (iii) hypercalcaemia associated with haematological malignancies. In recent years, much has been learned about humoral and local factors that can induce hypercalcaemia, and the above classification is no longer valid as local and humoral mechanisms may be operative at the same time [140]. In the present overview, therefore, the more general term MAH is used.

Several cancer types may be complicated by MAH, and hypercalcaemia may be the most common systemic metabolic aberration in malignancy. As noted above, a major percentage of hypercalcaemic patients have a malignant tumour. MAH is due mainly to excessive bone resorption and, to a smaller degree, to extracellular volume contraction or impaired renal calcium excretion [119]. Hypercalciuria—often accompanied by hyperphosphaturia—arises because of the phosphaturetic action of malignoma-associated humoral factors that mimic the action of PTH. The urine may become supersaturated with respect to calcium-containing stone phases, and calcium urolithiasis may ensue. This is often favoured by the hyperuricosuria caused by the rapid turnover of tumour cells, as in multiple myeloma. Hyperuricosuria is a known risk factor of renal stone formation.

Tumour types and humoral and local factors

The most common tumour inducing MAH is squamous cell cancer of the lung or other organs, such as the head, neck and oesophagus, where MAH can occur in up to 40% of cases [140]. The second most frequent tumour inducing MAH is breast cancer, where MAH can occur in 25–75% of cases, depending on the stage of the disease [140]. In renal cortical carcinoma, MAH is seen in 3–13% of cases [141], and MAH has been described in cancer of the liver, pancreas, prostate, bladder, melanoma and haematological malignancies (frequency 5–20%), such as multiple myeloma (20–40% of cases) or adult T cell lymphoma (approximately 100% [121]).

In 80–90% of unselected MAH cases, irrespective of whether bone metastases are present or not, the mechanism for MAH is mainly humoral [140]. Local mechanisms are most important for haematological malignancies. Several humoral factors have been identified, the most important being PTH-related peptide (PTHrP) [140,142,143], which accounts for more than 80% of all MAH cases [144]. Thus, detectable or elevated PTHrP was found in 100% of patients with MAH without bone metastases and in 75% of patients with bone metastases, but was detectable in only 2.6% of normal controls [140]. Other tumour-associated factors may induce MAH, such as transforming growth factor-α (TGF-α), cytokines such as interleukins (IL-1α, IL-1β, IL-6) and tumour necrosis factor-α (TNF-α; cachectin), TNF-β (lymphotoxin), prostaglandins of the E family, as well as other arachidonic acid metabolites such as the leucotrienes. In rare cases vitamin D metabolites may be involved in the development of MAH, and ectopic PTH secretion is a rarity (see review in [144]).

Clinical features of urolithiasis in MAH

In urolithiasis research, this interesting aspect has been somewhat neglected, and few systematic statistical data have been published in the urolithiasis literature. One of the main differences between MAH and pHPT concerns nephrolithiasis (Table 60.2). In pHPT, calcium urolithiasis is still by far the most common clinical symptom. Ten to 50% of all pHPT patients have renal stones, while the stone incidence is much lower in MAH [119,140]. If a stone occurs in an MAH patient, it is not possible to determine whether it has been newly formed or is pre-existing, or whether the patient had been suffering from RCU

Table 60.2 Clinical and biochemical differences between malignoma-associated hypercalcaemia (MAH) and primary hyperthyroidism (pHPT).

Variables	MAH	pHPT
Time course of disease	Fast	Slow
Loss of body weight	Frequent	Rare
Nephrolithiasis	Rare	Frequent
Clinical relevance of nephrolithiasis	Low	High
Serum-PTH	Low	High
Serum-PTHrP	High	Low
Serum-1,25-dihydroxyvitamin D	Low to normal	High
Serum total calcium	High	High
Serum phosphorus	Low	Low
Serum chloride	Low	High
Capillary blood bicarbonate	High	Low
Nephrogenous cyclic AMP	High	High
Bone resorption	High	High
Bone formation	Low	High
Intestinal calcium absorption	Low or normal	High

AMP, adenosine monophosphate; PTH, parathyroid hormone; PTHrP, parathyroid hormone-related peptide.

beforehand. Also, the patient might have some coexisting tumour-linked renal dysfunction, e.g. RTA or uric acid nephropathy, such as is seen in multiple myeloma (see above). The clinical symptoms of urolithiasis are similar in MAH and pHPT patients. Typically, hypercalcaemia is more symptomatic (weakness, anorexia, nausea, vomiting, mental changes such as lethargy, confusion, stupor) than in pHPT, owing to the relatively higher serum calcium levels in these patients and the shorter time course of the disease. Often, signs of hypercalcaemia are wrongly interpreted to be symptoms of progressive tumour stage or sequelae of concomitant cytotoxic drug therapy or irradiation.

Urolithiasis in renal cortical carcinoma and enteropancreatic neuroendocrine tumours

As examples of MAH-related calcium urolithiasis, we present some details on renal cell carcinoma as well as enteropancreatic neuroendocrine tumours. Albright was the first to describe a renal cancer patient with MAH in whom hypercalcaemia and hypophosphataemia resolved following irradiation of a bone metastasis; he concluded that the tumour produced ectopic PTH [145]. Typically, renal cell carcinoma is accompanied by osteolytic bone metastases when MAH becomes apparent. However, the degree of MAH is not correlated with the histological tumour grade or with the degree of bone destruction, and MAH without bone metastases is also a frequent finding in renal cancer patients. Hypercalcaemia is thought to result from increased bone resorption, caused by the bone metastases directly, or by humoral mechanisms [119,146]. Calcium urolithiasis is seen in 8% of these patients [141].

Among the enteropancreatic neuroendocrine tumours, the VIPoma (vasoactive intestinal polypeptide (VIP)-producing adenoma) deserves more comment. VIP is a 28-amino acid peptide which is located mainly within neural structures. It functions as a neurotransmitter, neuromodulator or a paracrine factor. An endocrine role for VIP is unlikely. VIP causes relaxation of vascular and non-vascular smooth muscle cells, thereby inducing overall vasodilatation. VIP stimulates secretion of hormones by the endocrine pancreas, and secretion of water and bicarbonate by the exocrine pancreas [147]. Acting on specific membrane receptors, it increases net fluid and electrolyte secretion in the small and large bowel by increasing cellular cyclic adenosine monophosphate (AMP), in similar manner to choleratoxin [148]. VIPomas are VIP-secreting tumours leading to elevated levels of VIP in the plasma. The tumours are usually located within the pancreas and are responsible for the Verner–Morrison or WDHA syndrome [149]—characterized by watery diarrhoea (> 700 ml/day), hypokalaemia and hypo- or achlohydria. Ninety eight per cent of the tumours are solitary and are usually larger than 3 cm. More than 60% are malignant, two-thirds of the patients (30–50 years old) presenting with metastases at the time of presentation. Less than 2% of VIPomas are associated with MEN-I, the vast majority arising spontaneously [122]. Hypercalcaemia is seen in 25–75% of VIPoma patients [150–153]. In a series of 62 VIPoma patients [151], 60% had hypophosphataemia and 41% hypercalcaemia. In contrast to other tumour-associated hypercalcaemias, the natural history of VIPoma is long, and the diagnosis is not established until years after the onset of clinical symptoms, so that renal calcium stones may be expected. In fact, two of the above 62 patients [151] had urolithiasis.

The reasons for the VIPoma-associated disturbances in calcium metabolism are unclear. Intestinal hyperabsorption of calcium is unlikely, as VIP has been shown to decrease intestinal calcium absorption independently of the calciotropic hormones [154]. In sporadic VIPoma, nothing is known about the circulating PTH levels. Presumably they are suppressed, possibly by efflux of calcium from the bone owing to enhanced osteolytic activity (see below). The association of hypercalcaemia and hypophosphataemia makes some PTH-like bioactivity likely, but as yet nothing has been reported on PTHrP or other agents known to induce MAH. Only a few (<2%) VIPoma patients have pHPT in association with MEN-I. Elevated serum calcium levels have been observed in dogs during VIP infusion [155], and VIP has been shown to stimulate bone resorption via a cyclic AMP-dependent mechanism [156]. Also, VIPoma patients suffer from metabolic hypokalaemic, hyperchloraemic acidosis of greater severity than that seen in pHPT. Metabolic acidosis is known to induce decalcification of the skeleton [157], which, if high enough, may result in hypercalcaemia. Additionally, mild hypercalcaemia may ensue from hypophosphataemia, for example through the intake of phosphate-binding agents or by malabsorption of phosphorus due to diarrhoea (such as in the VIPoma syndrome). In these cases $1,25(OH)_2D$ levels are usually elevated. However, nothing is known about the serum levels of the hydroxylated vitamin D metabolites in VIPoma patients, nor are any data available on their intestinal calcium and phosphorus absorption.

In patients with the MEN-I syndrome, which is characterized by pHPT, enteropancreatic endocrine tumours and tumours of the anterior pituitary, 87–97% develop pHPT first, which has the same clinical picture and the same symptoms as sporadic pHPT. By the time these patients present with enteropancreatic endocrine tumours (gastrinoma, insulinoma, VIPoma) more than 95% will already have developed pHPT. Hypercalcaemia and calcium urolithiasis in these patients will therefore usually reflect coexisting pHPT.

Diagnosis and differential diagnosis of primary hyperparathyroidism and malignoma-associated hypercalcaemia

The early stages in the development of our clinical laboratory to one specializing in kidney stones and other disturbances of minerals dates from a time when open stone surgery was frequently inevitable, and identifying pHPT stone patients was therefore crucial and a main task. Until the late 1960s, the diagnosis of pHPT was not easy to establish, due to the lack of PTH assays and difficulties in obtaining accurate serum calcium measurements. Also, procedures for identifying enlarged parathyroid glands were lacking. With the advent of radioimmunoassays for the intact PTH molecule, these difficulties have now been largely overcome.

A detailed search for pHPT is indicated, and now performed, in most patients forming calcium-containing renal stones. In hypercalcaemic stone patients, intact PTH is indispensable. If PTH is elevated, the diagnosis of pHPT is almost certain. The serum phosphorus levels are of little diagnostic value, while determination of the urinary excretion of cyclic AMP may be useful. In hypercalcaemic patients with low or undetectable PTH, a meticulous search for malignancy should be instituted. PTHrP should be determined, because more than 80% of MAH patients have elevated values. The acid–base status should be evaluated, tumour markers such as CEA, CA 19-9, CA 15-3, AFP, etc. should be determined, and radiographs of the thorax and the skeleton obtained, as well as a bone scintigram. Rare causes of hypercalcaemia, such as vitamin D intoxication and sarcoidosis (see below), immobilization etc., should be excluded by a thorough medical history and physical examination of the patient. VIPoma-associated disturbances of calcium metabolism may constitute a rare cause of calcium urolithiasis, and can easily be differentiated from pHPT by the typical clinical symptoms of VIPoma, the presence of a pancreatic tumour, elevated plasma VIP levels and the absence of high PTH levels in the blood. If both VIP and PTH are elevated, the patient is likely to have MEN-I, which must prompt screening of the whole family. In general, MAH differs from pHPT, the main disease with which it may be confounded, in a number of respects (see Table 60.2).

Management

Primary hyperparathyroidism

While conservative measures may be justified to lower excessively high serum calcium levels of a pHPT patient preoperatively (see below), there is no effective medical treatment for the associated urolithiasis [136]. Thanks to advances in anaesthesia and intensive care medicine, the risks of parathyroidectomy have become negligible even in very elderly patients. Therefore, any symptomatic patient in whom the diagnosis of pHPT is confirmed should undergo neck exploration. A skilled parathyroid surgeon will cure the disease in 95% of cases without the need for prior localization procedures. The only preoperative localization procedure which is reasonable and economic is the ultrasonographic examination of the thyroid region. Skilled specialists can localize more than 80% of enlarged parathyroid glands. An advantage of preoperative ultrasound is that the operating time may be shortened as a result. In the case of positive preoperative localization, the surgeon will start neck exploration on the side on which the parathyroid tumour is presumed to be. In the case of an adenoma, and when the ipsilateral second parathyroid gland is normal, the surgeon should leave the contralateral side unexplored, and in this way achieve success in 95% of pHPT patients. In cases of doubt, where there is identification of none or more than one ipsilateral parathyroid tumour, the surgeon must extend the exploration to the other side. In the case of four-gland hypertrophy, subtotal (3.5) parathyroidectomy or total parathyroidectomy with autotransplantation of small parathyroid fragments to a forearm is recommended. In any such situation, some of the removed parathyroid tissue should be cryoconserved for autotransplantation in the event of permanent postoperative hypoparathyroidism [118,120]. Administration of bisphosphonates (e.g. clodronate) may be a therapeutic alternative for pHPT patients refusing surgery.

Malignoma-associated hypercalcaemia

Removal of the tumour is the main therapeutic aim in

MAH. Depending on the stage (metastases?) and type of the tumour, this may be achieved by surgery or conservative treatment (chemotherapy, irradiation). Symptomatic antihypercalcaemic therapy should be restricted to a highly hypercalcaemic patient awaiting surgery or receiving conservative anti-cancer treatment, or in whom the disease is very advanced, such as in metastatic breast cancer. In the former patients, sodium chloride infusions, concurrently with frusemide administration, are of major importance, while the latter patients are best treated by glucocorticoids and osteoclast-inactivating agents such as clodronate. Curative surgery is the treatment of choice in VIPoma. If the VIPoma has metastasized, radical tumour debulking must be performed because it can ameliorate or even eliminate the patient's symptoms for long periods. As a conservative approach, administration of the synthetic somatostatin analogue octreotide (Sandostatin) has proved useful. Chemotherapy using streptozotocin or chlorozotocin, alone or in combination with 5-fluorouracil, has also been recommended.

Hypervitaminosis D

Regulatory aspects and extrarenal production of 1,25(OH)$_2$D

Vitamin D$_3$ is formed from its precursor, the lipophilic 7-dehydrocholesterol, in the skin during exposure to sunlight, or is absorbed in the small bowel and carried by transport proteins to the liver. There it is hydroxylated by a liver-specific hydroxylase at position 25 to 25-OHD, and is further hydroxylated in the mitochondria of the renal proximal tubules by a 1α-hydroxylase, to produce the most active form, namely 1,25(OH)$_2$D. Renal hydroxylation is regulated by PTH, phosphate and calcium, and appears to downregulate the formation of 24,25-dihydroxyvitamin D [158,159]. The most important physiological action of 1,25(OH)$_2$D is to increase active intestinal transcellular calcium transport, mainly by stimulating the production of a calcium-binding protein in the enterocyte. In the distal renal tubule, 1,25(OH)$_2$D inhibits the 1α-hydroxylase activity, which is accompanied by stimulation of the 25-(OH)D-24-hydroxylase; presumably, the metabolite 24,25-dihydroxyvitamin D$_3$ (24,25(OH)$_2$D) enhances the reabsorption of phosphate as well as PTH-dependent calcium reabsorption, although this is debated [160,161]. Degradation of 1,25(OH)$_2$D occurs in several ways, one of which is via hydroxylation at position 24, to the 1,24,25-trihydroxyvitamin D$_3$ that shows weaker activity in the regulation of renal calcium and phosphate handling [162]. In pHPT, the excess of PTH augments 1,25(OH)$_2$D by stimulating the 1α-hydroxylase. It is felt that high serum levels of the metabolite are one cause of the high levels of calcium in serum and urine in pHPT [163].

Extrarenal production of 1,25(OH)$_2$D is a feature of granulomatous diseases. In 1939, Harrell and Fisher [164] were the first to describe hypervitaminosis D in sarcoidosis. In 1983, Adams et al. [165] reported the rapid conversion of 25-OHD to 1,25(OH)$_2$D by alveolar macrophages cultured from sarcoidotic tissue. At present it is widely agreed that the activity of the 1α-hydroxylase is increased in sarcoidosis. As PTH is low, and in this situation the activity of the enzyme cannot have been stimulated by this hormone, the level of 1,25(OH)$_2$D should depend exclusively on the prevailing levels of either the native vitamin D or the precursor metabolite 25-OHD [166]. In contrast to pHPT, in sarcoidosis, hypercalcaemia is present in only about 20% and hypercalciuria in 62% [167,168], but nephrolithiasis in only 10% [168,169].

There is a lack of feedback control in the production of 1,25(OH)$_2$D (an absence of product-enzyme inhibition) not only in sarcoidosis, but also in other granulomatous states such as Wegener's granulomatosis [170], tuberculosis, histoplasmosis [158,159], and in lymphoma [171], Hodgkin's lymphoma [172] and granulomas associated with silicone implantation [173]. The putative mechanism in the production of 1,25(OH)$_2$D is as in sarcoidosis, except in lymphoma, where proof is wanting. These non-sarcoid disorders are extremely rare causes of renal stone formation. Recently, a case of increased 1,25(OH)$_2$D that developed in granulomas arising after the implantation of silicone and accompanied by nephrolithiasis, has been reported [173]. Other tissues with the potency for producing 1,25(OH)$_2$D include the human decidua and placenta [174]. Also, hypercalciuria in the last 3 months of pregnancy is not a rare finding [13,159], but to date there has been no investigation into a possible aetiological link between this type of hypercalciuria and the simultaneously increased 1,25(OH)$_2$D levels. In addition, a possible linkage of the former with urolithiasis is not clear, as renal calcium stones occur in only one out of 1500 pregnancies, a figure no different from that of age-matched, non-pregnant females [175].

In individuals with normal calcium metabolism, both the intake of nutrients rich in vitamin D (fish, veal, mushrooms) and exposure to sunlight may lead to high-normal 25-OHD levels; but these factors do not result in an overproduction of 1,25(OH)$_2$D because of the close positive–negative feedback regulation of the 1α-hydroxylase by its product, the biologically active hormone. However, an aetiological role of the 25-OHD precursor, and the intermediate product 24,25(OH)$_2$D, in the cause of hypercalciuria and stone disease has not been sufficiently investigated. There are those who attribute to 25-OHD a potency for affecting calcium metabolism [176], and we [69,70] and others [177] found high levels of this metabolite in the blood of RCU patients. There is evidence that a high level of 1,25(OH)$_2$D is one of the calcium homeostatic factors that is disturbed in hypercalciuria RCU [12], and probably in RCU as a whole [53,69,70], but the nature of overproduction of this D metabolite is not sought in elevated native vitamin D (see p. 774).

Principles of management

To prevent calcium urolithiasis, any form of therapy should aim at restoring normal serum levels of vitamin D and its hydroxylated metabolites, and hence normal serum and urinary calcium, and to keep the degree of supersaturation of urine with stone-forming calcium salts within normal limits. Hypervitaminosis D in pHPT is eradicated by parathyroid surgery (see above). In all other situations with hypervitaminosis D, the first step should be to check oral vitamin D intake carefully especially in countries with government-licensed vitamin D supplementation of food such as milk, and where there might be self-medication with vitamin D; stone patients are often not aware of the risk of vitamin D intoxication. The dietary intake of vitamin D can be adapted to the prevailing calcium metabolic needs by restricting such vitamin D-rich foods as fish and mushrooms; in addition, patients at risk of disorders of calcium control should avoid excessive UV irradiation of the skin [178]. In sarcoidosis and other granulomatous diseases, inhibition of the 1α-hydroxylase in the macrophages of the granulomas can be achieved by the administration of prednisone at an initial dose of 50–60 mg/day [179]. The antimalarial agent chloroquine, at doses of up to 4 mg/kg body weight, is also reliably effective [180], but the mechanism of $1,25(OH)_2D$ reduction achieved by this compound is not clear; an example of the course of treatment of such a patient is illustrated in Fig. 60.5. Because antimalaria drugs can cause retinopathy and dermal pigmentation changes, their administration should be closely monitored by the physician. In contrast to these situations with treatable extrarenal production of $1,25(OH)_2D$, the treatment of renal overproduction of this hormone in RCU is still a problem and the subject of research.

Treatment with potent calcaemic agents, such as dihydrotachysterol and vitamin D or its hydroxylated metabolites, is often necessary following complete removal of the parathyroid glands during the course of surgery for adenoma, hyperplasia or malignancy, or in cases developing surgical complications during total or subtotal thyroidectomy, all leading to hypocalcaemia from hypoparathyroidism. The widely used dihydrotachysterol analogue of vitamin D is not capable of maintaining normal reabsorption of calcium by the renal tubules, and patients receiving this type of replacement therapy are therefore permanently at risk of developing hypercalciuria, renal calcifications and stones [181]. A similar situation is seen with the D metabolites. In these situations careful maintenance of serum calcium at the lower limit of normalcy is mandatory, as otherwise there is an increased likelihood that the drug dose will be too high relative to the calciuria.

Management of idiopathic calcium urolithiasis

On the basis of the information available to us in the 1990s, we will focus on two topics: (i) the stone clinic effect; and (ii) the various drugs and substances with actions on calciuria or oxaluria or which are capable of increasing the inhibitory activity of urine. Generally speaking, the therapeutic efforts should aim at reducing supersaturation and crystallization in urine.

Stone clinic effect

The term, initially coined in the Mayo Clinic [182], refers to the fact that calcium stone patients do not show further stone growth or new stone formation during the follow-up period, despite the absence of any specific antistone drug therapy [20]. In more than 50% of patients with so-called indeterminate metabolic activity [183], there was cessation of stone growth, new stone formation and spontaneous stone passage, and similar percentages of patients with risk factors such as hypercalciuria or hyperuricosuria became metabolically inactive [20]. These impressive results were ascribed to the higher mean 24 h urine volume shown at follow-up, and support the view that increased fluid intake should be recommended [20]. The control of supersaturation dictates that a minimum urine volume per day—we recommend 20–25 ml/kg body weight—should be maintained; this is achieved by drinking beverages 'neutral' to calcium stone-forming processes. There is controversy, however, as to what fluids, apart from low-sodium water (see below), meet this criterion. There is also controversy as to methods of treatment involving the manipulation of dietary factors other than fluids. As a number of reports revealed that the dietary habits, especially with respect to the major calorie carriers and minerals, of the average calcium stone patient are not different from those of the average non-stone-forming individual of identical sex, age and body weight [39,41,184], there may in fact be little room for further dietary modification. Thus, in order for dietary advice to be effective, it is necessary to scrutinize each patient's dietary habits and to construct a diet plan which, when practiced by the patient, will afford protection from existing risk factors for stones or help to prevent their expression.

As already mentioned, intrinsic factors may modulate a stone-former's response to a normal diet. For example, calciuria, which is often severe, became the subject of treatment regimens, including a diet low in calcium. Today,

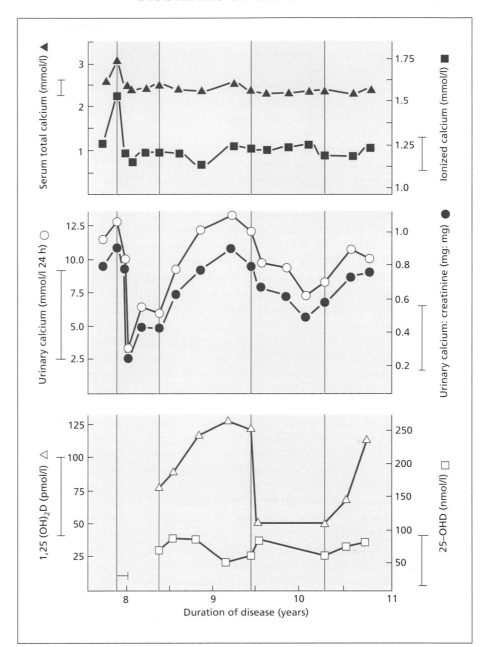

Fig. 60.5 Serum urinary calcium and vitamin D metabolites of a patient (aged 65 years) with an 8-year history of sarcoidosis, mononeuropathy, renal calculi and inflammatory arthritis. The pink areas indicate periods of administration of chloroquine phosphate (500 mg/day) and Prednisolone (40 mg/day instead of 15 mg/day). The vertical brackets indicate the normal ranges. (Redrawn from [180].)

however, most authors feel that dietary calcium restriction is ultimately useless, for a number of reasons. First, patient compliance is poor, as over the long term only 14% adhere to this recommendation [185]. Secondly, only patients whose stones are due to excessive consumption of calcium are likely to benefit, but these are in a minority [185]. Thirdly, factors other than dietary calcium *per se* may be important for the determination of calciuria, when the intake of fluid is high and that of calcium low [185–187]. Fourthly, urine volume and urinary calcium oxalate supersaturation are not simply inversely correlated; rather the latter appears to reach a lower limit, irrespective of the urine volume [188,189]. One contributory factor to this

latter situation may be that there is some dependency of oxalate and calcium excretion upon urine flow [190,191]. On augmenting fluid intake some degree of extracellular volume expansion, mediating an increase of both natriuresis and calciuria, is an inevitable sequela [192]. In response to the associated drop of serum ionized calcium, the parathyroid glands are activated and enhance phosphaturia and bicarbonaturia [46], thereby compensating for the decrease in calcium phosphate supersaturation expected from urine dilution. In general, measures preventing dietary or intestinal calcium from reaching the urine introduces the risk of regulatory hyperparathyroidism, and ultimately calcium and oxalate hyperabsorption and hyperoxaluria. Finally, with increasing urine dilution, a number of inhibitors of crystallization show a disproportionate decrease, or even total loss, of efficacy, unrelated to the underlying stoichiometry [106]. Thus, given these serious restrictions, Coe and co-workers feel that 'supersaturations of urine seem a part of human life not easily prevented, nearly universal, and more marked in stone-formers than in normals' [71].

In contrast to extreme fluid intake and dietary calcium restriction, dietary sodium restriction is a simple yet powerful means of reducing supersaturation, mainly via a reduction in calciuria, and the resulting state of mineral homeostasis is probably not compromised by altered regulatory effectors such as hormones, enzymes, etc. This fact has been neglected by the above authors [71] and, unfortunately, it is not known to many physicians caring for stone patients today, although RCU patients often exhibit both hypercalciuria and hypernatriuria [48,193]. A marked decrease in calciuria occurs upon dietary salt (sodium chloride) restriction. The calciuria equivalent of sodium varies in several reports, with a mean value of approximately 20, i.e. a reduction of calciuria by 2 mmol (80 mg) necessitates a decrease in dietary sodium of about 80 mmol (1800 mg) [47–49,194]. Salt intake in economically developed countries worldwide ranges between 5 and 15 g (approximately 2000–6000 mg sodium) per day, although less than 5 g [187] or even a minimum of 2 g (approximately 800 mg sodium) would be sufficient to maintain good health. On this basis, in patients with calciuria of >250 mg/day (females) or >300 mg/day (males), a reduction of 150–200 mg would be possible [47,48,187]. Also, the observation of lowered calciuria [48], stimulated citraturia [194] and increased inhibition of crystal growth and agglomeration [49], in response to sodium restriction in humans, supports the idea that in stone patients this mode of treatment should be considered first before offering drug treatment. Moreover, calcium conservation via sodium restriction is about to become a valuable principle in the

population-wide prevention and treatment of exaggerated bone mineral loss [32]. Notably, low bone mineral content is a feature of subsets of renal calcium stone patients characterized by low calcium but high protein and sodium intake [195], and these individuals in particular may benefit from a salt-restricted diet.

Drugs and substances in the treatment of calcium stones

For many years, a number of medications have been used to treat RCU patients forming either calcium oxalate, calcium phosphate or mixed stones. The more important substances are listed in Table 60.3. Several of these are able to reduce calciuria, such as thiazide and phosphate, whereas others mainly inhibit crystallization, such as citrates. Sulphate and cimetidine are mentioned, because unpublished work suggests that they may be able to lower urinary pH, although they do not directly contribute exogenous acid. After decades of searching, antioxaluric drugs are now being used, namely the alkaline earth (magnesium, calcium) citrates (see below) and pyridoxine.

Regarding pyridoxine, dramatic reduction of oxaluria (from 72 to 27 mg/day and from 63 to 20 mg/day) and blunting of stone formation has been achieved in two patients with RCU receiving 200 mg pyridoxine twice daily alone (patient 1) or pyridoxine in combination with thiazide (patient 2); both patients exhibited increased glycolate excretion but none of the known causes for endogenous overproduction of oxalate (oxalosis, pyridoxine deficiency, exogenous glycine load, ethylene glycol intoxication), suggesting that there exists a new and not yet sufficiently characterized cause of hyperoxaluria in RCU [219]. Even smaller doses of pyridoxine (10 mg/day) were found to act beneficially in RCU with mild hyperoxaluria [220,221], despite the fact that increased calciuria (from PTH suppression) develops when pyridoxine is administered together with magnesium [221], which like pyri-

Table 60.3 The effects of various drugs in the treatment of idiopathic calcium urolithiasis.

	Urine supersaturation		Crystallization* and stone recurrence	References (selection)
	Promoters	Inhibitors		
Thiazide(s)	Ca↓↓, Ox↑	Cit↓, Mg↑	C↓, S↓	[14,17,72, 196–204]
Phosphate(s)	Ca↓↓, Pi↑↑	Cit↑, PPi↑↑	C↓↓, S↓	[14,15,205–207]
Cellulose phosphate	Ca↓, Ox↑, Pi↑	PPi?	C?, S↓	[14,206,208–210]
Citrate(s)	Ca?, Ox?, Pi?	Cit↑↑↑	C↓↓↓, S↓↓	[211–215]
Magnesium	Ca↑, Ox↓, Pi↓	Cit↑, Mg↑↑	C↓, S?	[14,27,28,80,117,216]
Calcium	Ca↑↑, Ox↓, Pi↓	Cit↑↑, Mg↑	S↓, C?	[71,79,217,218]

* Crystallization of calcium oxalate or calcium phosphate.
Abbreviations relate to urinary concentration and excretion of calcium (Ca), oxalate (Ox), citrate (Cit), phosphate (Pi), pyrophosphate (PPi) and magnesium (Mg), and to crystallization (C) and stone recurrence (S). Arrows indicate the direction of change; the number of arrows the degree of action. ?, effect uncertain.

doxine inhibits oxalate production [222]. However, there are other reports which cannot confirm these optimistic results. It appears definite that endogenous pyridoxine deficiency in animals leads to oxalate overproduction [223], but the question as to whether there is some pyridoxine deficiency in RCU, accounting for mild hyperoxaluria, is unanswered, because in humans with known pyridoxine-deficiency states hyperoxaluria was not detectable [224]. Others found that pyridoxine levels in blood and urine do not differ between RCU patients and non-stone-forming healthy controls [225], and that long-term pyridoxine administration in doses of 25–200 mg/day was ineffective on urinary oxalate [196].

We are not dealing with allopurinol here, because its usefulness in RCU is seen in the reduction of urinary uric acid and its sodium salt, thereby indirectly reducing the calcium oxalate supersaturation, whereas a direct interference of allopurinol with calcium metabolism has never been proved and inhibition of calcium oxalate crystallization is merely indirect too [71].

Thiazides

This group of diuretics has long been known; they reduce calciuria by enhancing calcium reabsorption in the distal tubule [46]. By 1977, Finlayson had already pointed out the desired effects of thiazides as well as their unwanted side effects [14]. Thiazides may reduce the likelihood of crystal and stone formation, but they have both enthusiastic protagonists [17,72] and others, ourselves included, who have certain reservations [14,198,203] about them. Interestingly, since the 1970s, the well-documented serious side effects of the thiazides, such as glucose intolerance, hyperlipidaemia, gout, hypokalaemia, hypotension and, in our experience, a possible risk of cardiac arrest (serum potassium < 3.5 mmol/l), as observed even at the customary dose of 50 mg twice a day, has only occasionally stimulated the interest of stone physicians. Moreover, the hypocalciuric effect is most expressed when serum potassium is already low — and many stone patients have low-normal values [14]. We recommend thiazide intake over a period of several months in cases with high fasting calciuria and borderline increased parathyroid gland function, in order to 'unmask' the presence of autonomous calcium regulation, due to a small parathyroid adenoma. If the latter is present, serum calcium, PTH and urinary cyclic AMP clearly rise to abnormal levels. During this diagnostic period, and during long-term metaphylaxis with thiazides, there is a need to substitute serum potassium. It appears that with the advent of safer drugs in metaphylaxis, thiazide may be removed from the list of antistone agents. This is all the more likely, as in two adequately controlled trials, the recurrence rate of stones in patients on thiazide is probably not substantially decreased [198,203].

Orthophosphate

Phosphate replacement therapy was proposed by Nordin and co-workers in 1967, on the basis of the hypercalciuria observed in response to diet-induced phosphate deficiency [14,227]. Later, phosphate deficit-induced hypercalciuria was confirmed, as was the associated enormous change in the vitamin D metabolism (turnover of 25-OHD is increased by more than 100% both in males and females) [226]; this combination is suspected to underlie the high serum levels of $1,25(OH)_2D$ in RCU patients with absorptive hypercalciuria [12,70]. The safety of phosphate therapy in RCU was proven by Smith and co-workers [15], in that serum PTH remained unchanged, despite the rise of serum phosphate and the fall in serum calcium.

Orthophosphate (potassium, sodium, potassium-sodium form) dramatically reduces urinary calcium oxalate supersaturation [14,15,205] and crystallization [206], and lowers serum $1,25(OH)_2D$ [228]. In healthy humans, oral intake of phosphorus determines the production rate of $1,25(OH)_2D$ [229]. Thus, the phosphorus-induced decrease of $1,25(OH)_2D$ in RCU patients presumably is the result of elimination of some pre-existing phosphate deficiency caused by renal phosphate losses [70]. At the same time, patient tolerance of orthophosphate is quite good at the recommended doses (1–2 g elemental phosphorus per day), with diarrhoea occurring only in a few cases [15]. Interestingly, oxaluria does not change under orthophosphate, whereas calciuria and stone recurrence are markedly reduced [207]. The failure of oxaluria to increase is surprising, as hyperabsorption of oxalate is thought to follow the reduction of intestinal calcium absorption [208], in the case of phosphate administration as a sequela of intraintestinal calcium phosphate precipitation. It is likely that the key effect elicited by orthophosphates is the lowering of $1,25(OH)_2D$ levels. Unfortunately, orthophosphates have increasingly been neglected during the last decade. It would appear that orthophosphate therapy of RCU needs reviving, because it may be able to compete successfully with the more modern citrate drugs (see below) in terms of the prevention of stone recurrence. So far, no comparative studies on phosphate and citrate have been reported. Unfortunately, in many European countries, including Germany, the preferred potassium phosphate is not approved for use in humans.

Cellulose phosphate (calcium-exchange resins)

Developed for use as a cation-exchange resin, sodium cellulose phosphate was early shown to be anticalciuric when given as an acute load [112] or over the short term [113] as a result of effective inhibition of intestinal calcium absorption by the drug. When a calcium-binding resin, chemically different from cellulose phosphate, was administered in RCU patients over 6, 13 and 24 weeks, calciuria and oxaluria were unchanged, although in acute load tests the intestinal calcium absorption was reduced by approximately 50% [210]. Both drugs have in common that after treatment over 24 months the urinary calcium oxalate and calcium phosphate activity product remained unchanged [210] or above the formation product [205]. These findings suggest that resin-based calcium exchange drugs cannot prevent stones, but ultimately favour their formation (see below), especially due to the body's overcompensation of the drug-induced initial inhibition of intestinal calcium absorption [210]. There have been no specific studies on calcium oxalate crystallization under cellulose phosphate, and it appears that the concomitant urinary pyrophosphate excretion is unchanged [230]. With regard to the inhibition of calcium phosphate precipitation, Finlayson [14] has challenged Pak's theory that brushite is the nidus for stone formation [231] and his assumption that this process will be delayed by an increase in the brushite formation product [206]. In the light of our present knowledge of precipitation processes, some objection may be raised against the sodium moiety, because this ion is calciuretic (see above) and may offset the fall of calciuria in response to increased intraintestinal calcium binding to cellulose. A contribution of pyrophosphate to calcium complexation is unrealistic, as the pyrophosphate concentration in urine is only 10–100 µmol/l [232]; also, in the long term, unchanged calciuria and the elevation in the associated phosphaturia would not decrease, but rather enhance calcium phosphate supersaturation. Thus, the value of sodium cellulose phosphate may be seen in its ability to reduce calciuria over the short term, thereby helping to distinguish between true fasting calciuria and overspill of dietary calcium to urine, in individuals with an insufficiently long prior nocturnal fast [112].

For the purpose of broadening the spectrum of anti-stone drugs, it would be interesting to investigate the effects of potassium cellulose phosphate on, for example, the intraintestinal formation of an insoluble cellulose–phosphate–calcium complex. Such a phosphate drug may combine an effective reduction of calciuria, with urine alkalinization, increased phosphaturia, pyrophosphaturia and citraturia, and normalization of serum 1,25(OH)$_2$D. It may be speculated that the crucial end-points of such trials should be the development of oxaluria, decreased bone mineral content and no restoration, or loss of restoration, of the previously enhanced calcium oxalate and calcium phosphate crystallization.

Citrates

Urinary citrate deficiency most probably has a key role in the pathogenesis of calcium-containing renal stones [16,19]. Therefore, management of such disorders by citrate should have a solid basis. In the form of alkali citrate, especially potassium citrate, these substances have moved to the top of the list of anti-stone drugs since the 1980s. Although known for decades as a calcium-complexing agent in biological fluids, citrate has been used in stone therapy only since the pioneering work done about 15 years ago in Berlin [211,233] and Dallas [212,234]. With respect to the beneficial physicochemical effects (calcium complexation, direct inhibition of calcium oxalate, calcium phosphate crystallization) and the mostly stabile calciuria and oxaluria, as observed with potassium, sodium or potassium–sodium citrates, reference is made to more detailed overviews [16,19,213,235]. It is worth noting that at the dosage recommended (up to 60 mEq bases and cations, respectively), alkali citrate is virtually free of unwanted side effects. For a long time there was a lack of adequately controlled trials with citrate, but one double-blind study that clearly shows that potassium citrate prevents stone recurrence is now available [214]. Thus, the powerful actions of this drug, often documented in acute load or short-term studies in both healthy volunteers [215,236] and stone patients [237,238], also appear to be operative in the long-term treatment of the latter. Several authors are less optimistic regarding the long-term effectiveness of citrate in the treatment of RCU, and they anticipate that the stone clinic effect (see above) would be superior in terms of new stone formation [239].

Magnesium

Several early investigators considered that magnesium was able to reduce calcium oxalate stones in animals and humans, probably via a reduction of oxalate in urine [14,27,28]. Despite this, no final decision has been reached about the value of magnesium in the metaphylaxis of stones in RCU. The reasons should be sought, at least in part, in the rather contradictory biochemical findings in RCU patients, in whom the separation of those subsets with and without manifest magnesium deficiency has not readily been possible with the tools available; also, there is ongoing uncertainty about the chemical nature of the magnesium salt to be preferred (oxide, hydroxide, carbonate, phosphate, citrate, etc.) [71]. Neutral magnesium citrate (containing 12 mmol (292 mg) magnesium), when given orally together with a continental breakfast, decreases oxaluria and increases magnesiuria and citraturia, by about 75, 200 and 200%, respectively, as compared with breakfast alone; calculation of the accompanying supersaturation by EQUIL-II revealed a decrease in calcium oxalate, but an increase in brushite and hydroxyapatite [80,117].

Additional preliminary data from our laboratory in healthy individuals showed that the intake of an alkalinizing mixture of magnesium, potassium and sodium citrate effectively inhibited calcium oxalate nucleation, growth and aggregation, despite the fact that there is increased calciuria (due to parathyroid gland inhibition) and deprotonation of phosphate (due to urine alkalinization) [117]. We ascribe the inhibition of crystallization to the combined actions of high urinary magnesium and deprotonated citrate (due to urine alkalinization), as well as to the decrease in urinary oxalate. The situation has been illustrated in Fig. 60.6 for three volunteers. Other investigators made similar observations when magnesium (as citrate or oxide) was given together with meals, but failed to demonstrate anti-stone effects when magnesium was taken on an empty stomach [216]. Thus, comparative clinical trials with magnesium are clearly needed, especially in subsets of stone patients with mild hyperoxaluria, proven magnesium deficiency or some combination of the two.

Calcium

For the treatment of enteric hyperoxaluria, a disorder arising from intestinal oxalate hyperabsorption due to various intestinal abnormalities, the use of oral calcium is firmly established [217]. As mentioned previously, more intense study of calcium therapy in RCU patients may be considered worthwhile because the consumption of calcium-rich food may not stimulate, but rather inhibit, stone formation [240]. This exciting finding is at variance with the findings by others, showing that a low calcium diet protects against stone recurrence [72]; however, none of the studies cited in that review article were controlled with regard to the stone clinic effect [20,182]. Although the cause underlying the anti-stone effect of the high calcium diet is not fully clear, the association of high urinary

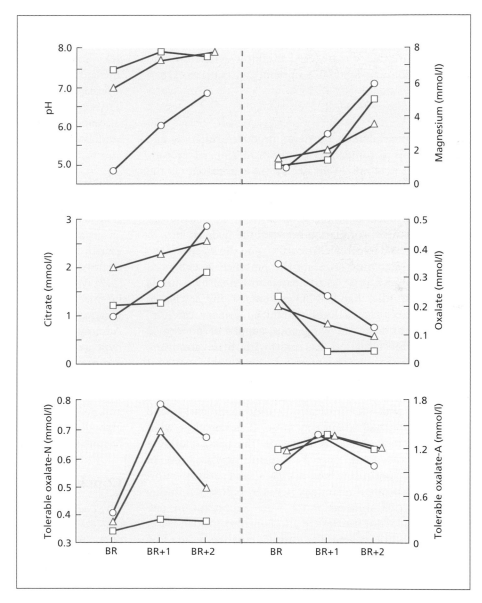

Fig. 60.6 Effect of a continental breakfast, with and without supplementation of 150 ml of a drink containing anti-stone substances (a salt mixture containing magnesium, potassium, sodium and citrate in the molar ratio of 1.5:4.5:1.5:3.0). Depicted are pH, the concentration of magnesium, citrate, oxalate and calcium oxalate crystallization, all in the first 2 h post-load urine collected from three healthy volunteers. For technical details see references [115,116]. Tolerable oxalate-A, total oxalate concentration in urine at the stage of crystal aggregation (on addition of 0.2 mmol/l sodium oxalate at nucleation); tolerable oxalate-N, total oxalate concentration in undiluted urine at the stage of nucleation (calcium oxalate crystals are visible under the microscope; note the difference in scales). BR, breakfast alone; BR+1, breakfast and 1 dose (5.14 g) of anti-stone drink; BR+2, breakfast and two doses (10.3 g) of anti-stone drink.

calcium and high urinary citrate with a high intake of, for example, milk and dairy products, suggests that much of the urinary calcium is complexed with citrate or phosphate, and that the citrate moiety of milk may ultimately be responsible for the inhibition of crystallization [71]. In addition, oxaluria is reduced with increasing dietary calcium [79], and the same is true with supplementation of normal food by an alkalinizing calcium–sodium citrate preparation [80]. Moreover, when bone calcium content is diminished, the same drug achieves normalization of both bone mineral quantity and bone quality [241]; others found that in females, suffering from both RCU and osteoporosis, the treatment of the latter disorder with the non-alkalinizing oral calcium citrate does not increase the lithogenicity of urine [218]. Finally, in a subset of children with idiopathic hypercalciuria a high dietary calcium load (1000 mg/day) was able to reduce serum $1,25(OH)_2D$ [242]. Thus, ironically, calcium in the form of an organic acid salt such as calcium citrate should be considered a useful candidate for an anti-stone drug, especially in subsets with normocalciuria but documented inhibitor deficiency, and low-normal or decreased bone mineral content [195, 218].

Sulphate

Oxidation of sulphur in nutrients produces sulphate, and the process is accompanied by the formation of protons ('endogenous acid rain') that need to be eliminated via the urine. These events stimulate calcium release from bone and hypercalciuria [157]. Calciuria is further increased by the chelating effect of sulphate on calcium; in fact there is a significant direct correlation between the two variables in both normo- and hypercalciuric RCU, and the steeper slope of the regression line suggests the presence of enhanced 'calcium complex-uria', as compared with healthy controls [40]. On the other hand, RCU patients, being at risk of developing too high a level of ionized urinary calcium, would benefit from an exogenous supply of preformed sulphate. This situation has met with little attention, although increased formation of the soluble calcium sulphate complex in the urine of RCU patients would be desirable. Thus, two advantages may arise from sulphate (but not sulphur) administration: urine acidification and removal of ionized calcium in urine. It is not clear what type of sulphate should be used. In the past, efforts to achieve an adequate degree of urine acidification in unclassified (according to calciuria and other abnormalities) renal calcium stone patients by enforced drinking of sulphate-rich mineral water were successful in one laboratory [243] but fruitless in another [244]. In such water the concentration of free (i.e. ionized) sulphate is too low [31], whereas the calciuric effect may be substantial due to the high amount of preformed calcium sulphate complex in these waters.

Another trial investigated the effect of ammonium sulphate on systemic acid–base status and urine acidification in patients with phosphate stones, including infected (struvite) stones and non-infected calcium oxalate, calcium phosphate and mixed stones [245]. In this work, all the study groups initially exhibited urinary pH >6.0; in response to ammonium sulphate the rate of stone formation was reduced when treatment was maintained for 1–12 years, the urine pH was lowered, as were the supersaturation products of octacalcium phosphate and brushite, while systemic acidosis and hypercalciuria did not develop and oxaluria was even slightly increased. This cohort study thus demonstrates the usefulness of urine acidification in patients with predominantly non-infected (i.e. metabolically developed) calcium stones, in the aetiology of which a weakly acidic urine has a crucial role. The intriguing question is whether the sulphate effect resides in the anion itself, which, for example, may interfere with renal acid–base regulation, or whether it reflects the fact that sulphate was combined with a metabolizable cation ($(NH_4)_2SO_4 \rightarrow 2\ NH_3 + SO_4^{2-} + 2\ H^+$). As there is a clear need for anti-stone drugs in the management of calcium stones not originating from RTA but still presenting with a urine pH between 6 and 7—possibly due to a tubular damage secondary to nephrolithiasis [246]—the present lack of studies on sulphate is regrettable.

Cimetidine

Originally, the idea of looking for a link between gastric acid secretion and urine acidification was born of our observation of a negative correlation between serum gastrin and pH in fasting urine of RCU patients, which contrasts with a positive correlation in healthy controls [247]. We reasoned that the greater the amount of gastrin produced, the more protons may be generated extra-gastrically and possibly eliminated by the kidney. Administration of cimetidine is reportedly followed by hypergastrinaemia; in our preliminary work there was, in addition to hypergastrinaemia, also a marked fall of urinary pH and increase of net acid secretion, whereas urinary calcium and oxalate remained unchanged [248]. Another, and even more surprising result was that calcium oxalate crystallization was inhibited, presumably by cimetidine degradation products in urine [249].

Conclusion

The past decade, which roughly spans the period since the appearance of the first edition of this textbook, was characterized by major advances in our understanding of renal stone chemistry and physicochemistry, pathophysiology and the treatment of patients. During this time we also had to learn a number of bitter lessons, including the fact that elevated immunoassayable PTH in the serum of patients with RCU is not necessarily identical with elevated biological activity of the hormone, that measurement of oxalate in urine and plasma can turn out to be a herculean task, that calcium deprivation by whatever means can have a variety of unwanted effects on the composition of urine, that without an evaluation of the physicochemical state and crystallization of stone substances in urine interpretation of treatment effects may be difficult, that alkalinization of urine is not straightforward, but also requires the consideration of overall metabolism, and that the deleterious long-term effects of exogenous acid loads upon the state of mineral metabolism may be elegantly circumvented by one or other drug used in the treatment of disorders apparently unrelated to kidney stones. It would appear that we have now arrived at a level of understanding of the role of calcium in patients with stones that enables us to manage these disorders better, but the gaps in our knowledge of cellular metabolism in RCU are still considerable. We need more, carefully designed clinical trials on the efficacy of drug treatment of calcium urolithiasis. This situation has already been alluded to in terms of the lack of trials meeting the necessary criteria [250]. Our hope is that the forthcoming decade will see intelligent approaches to the deranged processes of stone disease at the cellular level, along lines already indicated [65,77]; this should be possible with the technical tools now available for unravelling them. In 1982, Peacock felt that 'urinary calcium is not the only and not the major risk factor in calcium stone formation' [251], and this challenging proposition needs to be proved.

References

1 Whitfield HN, Hendry WF. *Textbook of Genito-Urinary Surgery.* 1st edn. Edinburgh: Churchill Livingstone, 1985.

2 Hodgkinson A, Nordin BEC. *Renal Stone Research Symposium.* London: J and A Churchill, 1969.

3 Cifuentes DeLatte L, Rapado A, Hodgkinson A. *Urinary Calculi.* Basel: S Karger, 1973.

4 Fleisch H, Robertson WG, Smith LH, Vahlensieck W. *Urolithiasis Research.* New York: Plenum Press, 1976.

5 Smith LH, Robertson WG, Finlayson B. *Urolithiasis: Clinical and Basic Research.* New York: Plenum Press, 1981.

6 Schwille PO, Smith LH, Robertson WG, Vahlensieck W. *Urolithiasis and Related Clinical Research.* New York: Plenum Press, 1985.

7 Walker VR, Sutton RAL, Cameron BEC, Pak CYC, Robertson WG. *Urolithiasis.* New York: Plenum Press, 1989.

8 Ryall R. *Urolithiasis and Related Clinical Research.* New York: Plenum Press, 1994.

9 Lemann J Jr. Pathogenesis of idiopathic hypercalciuria and nephrolithiasis. In: Coe FL, Favus MJ, eds. *Disorders of Bone and Mineral Metabolism.* New York: Raven Press, 1992: 685–706.

10 Halabe A, Sutton RAL. Primary hyperparathyroidism as a cause of calcium nephrolithiasis. In: Coe FL, Favus MJ, eds. *Disorders of Bone and Mineral Metabolism.* New York: Raven Press, 1992:671–84.

11 Buckalew VM Jr. Calcium nephrolithiasis and renal tubular acidosis. In: Coe FL, Favus MJ, eds. *Disorders of Bone and Mineral Metabolism.* New York: Raven Press, 1992:729–56.

12 Favus MJ, Favus LH. Intestinal calcium absorption and vitamin D metabolism in idiopathic hypercalciuria. In: Wickham JEA, Buck AC, eds. *Renal Tract Stone. Metabolic Basis and Clinical Practice.* Edinburgh: Churchill Living-stone, 1990:253–70.

13 Parfitt AM. Bone as a source of urinary calcium — osseous hypercalciuria. In: Coe FL, ed. *Hypercalciuric States. Pathogenesis, Consequences and Treatment.* Orlando: Grune and Stratton, 1984:313–78.

14 Finlayson B. Calcium stones: some physical and clinical aspects. In: David DS, ed. *Calcium Metabolism in Renal Failure and Nephrolithiasis.* New York: John Wiley and Sons, 1977:337–82.

15 Smith LH, Thomas WC Jr, Arnaud CD. Orthophosphate therapy in calcium renal lithiasis. In: Cifuentes DeLatte L, Rapado A, Hodgkinson A, eds. *Urinary Calculi.* Basel: S Karger, 1973: 188–97.

16 Pak CYC. Physico-chemical action and extrarenal manifestations of alkali therapy. In: Walker VR, Sutton RAL, Cameron ECB, Pak CYC, Robertson WG, eds. *Urolithiasis.* New York: Plenum Press, 1989:511–16.

17 Yendt EG, Cohanim M. The prevention of calcium stones with thiazides. In: Schwille PO, Smith LH, Robertson WG, Vahlensieck W, eds. *Urolithiasis and Related Clinical Research.* New York: Plenum Press, 1985:463–70.

18 Sutton RAL, Dirks JH. Idiopathic calcium lithiasis. In: Coe FL, ed. *Nephrolithiasis.* Contemporary Issues in Nephrology, Vol. 5. New York: Churchill Livingstone, 1980:165–87.

19 Schwille PO. Citrate and idiopathic recurrent calcium urolithiasis: an approach to the origin of hypocitraturia and correction by two oral alkali citrates. In: Walker VR, Sutton RAL, Cameron ECB, Pak CYC, Robertson WG, eds. *Urolithiasis.* Plenum Press: 1989:517–22.

20 Hosking DH, Erickson SB, Van den Berg CJ, Wilson DM, Smith LH. The stone clinic effect in patients with idiopathic calcium urolithiasis. In: Schwille PO, Smith LH, Robertson WG, Vahlensieck W, eds. *Urolithiasis and Related Clinical Research.* New York: Plenum Press, 1985:453–6.

21 Rose GA. Disturbances of calcium metabolism. In: Whitfield HN, Hendry WF, eds. *Textbook of Genito-Urinary Surgery.* 1st edn. Vols 1 and 2. Edinburgh: Churchill Livingstone, 1985: 639–58.

22 Higashihara E, Munakata A, Hara M et al. Medullary sponge kidney and hyperparathyroidism. *Urology* 1988;**31**:155–8.

23 Higashihara E, Nutahara K, Tago K, Keno A, Niijima T. Unilateral and segmental medullary sponge kidney: renal function and calcium excretion. *J Urol* 1984;**132**:743–5.

24 Jaeger P, Portmann L, Ginalski JM et al. Tubulopathy in nephrolithiasis: consequence rather than cause. *Kidney Int* 1986;**29**:563–71.

25 Soucie MJ, Thum MJ, Coates RJ, McClellan W, Austin H. Demographic and geographic variability of kidney stones in the United States. *Kidney Int* 1994;**46**:893–9.

26 Shuster F, Finlayson B, Schaeffer R et al. Water hardness and urinary stones. *J Urol* 1982;**128**:422–5.

27 Hammarsten G. On calcium oxalate and its solubility in the presence of inorganic salts with special reference to the occurrence of oxaluria. *C R Lab Carlsberg* 1929;**17**:1–85.

28 Desmars JF, Tawashi R. Dissolution and growth of calcium oxalate monohydrate. I. Effect of magnesium and pH. *Biochim Biophys Acta* 1973;**313**:256–67.

29 Sidhu H. *Biochemical mechanisms of hyperoxaluria and the role of urinary inhibitors of calcium oxalate crystallization in pyridoxine and thiamine deficient rats.* PhD Thesis Postgraduate Institute for Medical Education and Research, Chandigarh, India, 1985.

30 Kohri K, Kodama M, Ishikawa Y *et al.* Magnesium-to-calcium ratio in tap water, and its relationship to geological features and the incidence of calcium-containing urinary stones. *J Urol* 1989;**142**:1272–5.

31 Oberstein T, Schwille PO, Köberlein M. Composition of German mineral waters reexamined—implications for renal stone metaphylaxis. In: Tiselius HG, ed. *Renal Stones— Aspects of their Formation, Removal and Prevention.* Edsbrük: Academitryck, 1996:174–75.

32 Itoh R, Oka J, Echizen H *et al.* The interrelation of urinary calcium and sodium intake in healthy elderly Japanese. *Int J Vitam Nutr Res* 1991;**61**:159–65.

33 Blaustein MP. The interrelationship between sodium and calcium fluxes across cell membranes. *Rev Physiol Biochem Pharmacol* 1974;**70**:34–82.

34 Berlin T, Holmberg I, Björkhem I. High circulating levels of 25-hydroxyvitamin D_3 in renal stone formers with hyperabsorptive hypercalciuria. *Scand J Clin Lab Invest* 1986;**46**:367–74.

35 Berghi L, Meschi T, Amato F *et al.* Hot occupation and nephrolithiasis. *J Urol* 1993;**150**:1757–60.

36 Brundig P, Berg W, Schneider HJ. Untersuchungen zum Bildungsrisiko von Calciumoxalat unter besonderer Berücksichtigung von Stressmomenten. *Urol Int* 1979;**34**:105–13.

37 Bonakdar S, Schwille PO, Kissler H, Manoharan M. Immobilisation stress in the rat—reduction of urinary supersaturation and inhibitors. In: Rao PN, Kavanagh J, Tiselius HG, eds. *Urolithiasis Consensus and Controversies.* Proceedings of the Fifth European Urolithiasis Symposium, Manchester, 21–23 April 1994. South Manchester University Hospitals, Manchester, 1995:257–9.

38 Irving RA, Noakes TD, Rodgers AL, Swartz L. Crystalluria in marathon runners. I. Standard marathon—males. *Urol Res* 1986;**14**:289–94.

39 Schwille PO, Herrmann U. Environmental factors in the pathophysiology of recurrent idiopathic calcium urolithiasis (RCU), with emphasis on nutrition. *Urol Res* 1992;**20**:70–81.

40 Schwille PO, Rümenapf G. Idiopathic recurrent calcium urolithiasis—clinical problems and suggested approaches in an ambulatory stone clinic. In: Wickham JEA, Buck CA, eds. *Renal Tract Stone. Metabolic Basis and Clinical Practice.* Edinburgh: Churchill Livingstone, 1990:217–38.

41 Buck CE. Hypercalciuria in idiopathic calcium oxalate urolithiasis In: Wickham JEA, Buck CA, eds. *Renal Tract Stone. Metabolic Basis and Clinical Practice.* Edinburgh: Churchill Livingstone, 1990:239–51.

42 Nath R, Thind SK, Murthy MSR, Talwar HS, Farooqui S. Molecular aspects of idiopathic urolithiasis. *Mol Aspects Med* 1984;**7**:107–125.

43 Schwille PO, Brandt P, Ulbrich D, Kömpf W. Pankreasinseln, Plasmaglucagon und renale Verkalkungen unter verschiedener Grunddiät bei der Ratte. *Urologe* [A] 1975;**14**:306–14.

44 Nelde HJ, Bichler KH, Strohmaier WL, Kriz W. Nephrocalcinosis in the kidney of the rat on atherogenic diet and the effect of calcium antagonists (nifedipine). In: Bichler KH, Strohmaier WL, eds. *Nephrocalcinosis, Calcium Antagonists and Kidney.* Berlin: Springer Verlag, 1988:113–33.

45 Tulloch I, Smellic WSA, Buck AC. Evening primrose oil reduces urinary calcium excretion in both normal and hypercalciuric rats. *Urol Res* 1994;**22**:227–30.

46 Walser M. Divalent cations: physico-chemical state in glomerular filtrate and urine and renal excretion. In: Orloff J, Berliner RW, eds. *Handbook of Physiology. Section 8, Renal Physiology.* Washington DC: American Physiological Society, 1973:555–86.

47 McCarron DA, Rankin LI, Bennett WM *et al.* Urinary calcium excretion at extremes of sodium intake in normal man. *Am J Nephrol* 1981;**1**:84–90.

48 Silver J, Friedländer MM, Rubinger D, Popovtzer MM. Sodium-dependent idiopathic hypercalciuria in renal-stone formers. *Lancet* 1983;**2**:484–6.

49 Kok D, Iestra JA, Doerenbos CJ, Papapoulos SE. The effects of dietary excess in animal protein and in sodium on the composition and the crystallization kinetics of calcium oxalate monohydrate in urines of healthy men. *J Clin Endocrinol Metab* 1990;**71**:861–7.

50 Breslau NA, McGuire JL, Zerwekh JE, Pak CYC. The role of dietary sodium on renal excretion and intestinal absorption of calcium and vitamin D metabolism. *J Clin Endocrinol Metab* 1982;**55**:369–73.

51 Knochel J. Renal handling of phosphorus, clinical hypophosphatemia and phosphorus deficiency. In: Brenner BM, Rector FC, eds. *The Kidney.* Philadelphia: WB Saunders, 1986:619–62.

52 Erickson SB, Cooper K, Broadus AE. Oxalate absorption and postprandial urine supersaturation in an experimental human model of absorptive hypercalciuria. *Clin Sci* 1984;**67**:131–8.

53 Giannini S, Nobile M, Castrignano R *et al.* Possible link between vitamin D and hyperoxaluria in patients with renal stone disease. *Clin Sci* 1993;**84**:51–4.

54 Sandstead HH. Fiber, phytates, and mineral nutrition. *Nutr Rev* 1994;**50**:30–1.

55 Griffith HM, O'Shea B, Kevany JP, McCornick JS. A control study of dietary factors in renal stone formation. *Br J Urol* 1981;**53**:416–22.

56 James WPT, Branch WJ, Southgate DAT. Calcium binding by dietary fibre. *Lancet* 1978;**25 March**:638–9.

57 Brune M, Rossander L, Halberg L. Iron absorption: no intestinal adaptation to a high-phytate diet. *Am J Clin Nutr* 1989;**49**:542–5.

58 Spiess U. *Fasern in der Nahrung von Patienten mit calciumhaltigen Nierensteinen - Eine Pilotstudie mit Kontrollgruppe.* PhD Thesis, University of Erlangen, 1987.

59 Knos T, Kassarjiian Z, Dawson-Hughes B. Calcium absorption in elderly subjects on high and low fiber diets: effects of gastric acidity. *Am J Clin Nutr* 1991;**53**:1480–92.

60 Hong Bin Q, Gerfinkel D. The cadmium toxicity hypothesis of aging: a possible explanation for the zinc deficiency hypothesis of aging. *Med Hypoth* 1994;**42**:380–4.

61 Piscator M. The nephropathy of chronic cadmium poisoning. In: Foulkes EC, ed. *Cadmium.* Handbook of Experimental

Pharmacology Vol. 80. Heidelberg: Springer Verlag, 1986: 179–94.

62 Scott R, Cunningham C, McLelland A *et al.* The importance of cadmium as a factor in calcified upper urinary tract stone disease—a prospective 7 year study. *Br J Urol* 1982;**54**:584–9.

63 Schwille PO, Scholz D. Role of calcium metabolism in renal stone formation. In: Anghileri LJ, Tuffet-Anghileri AM, eds. *The Role of Calcium in Biological Systems*, Vol. III. Boca Raton: CRC Press, 1982:103–22.

64 Bushinsky DA, Favus MJ. Mechanism of hypercalciuria in genetic hypercalciuric rats. Inherited defect in intestinal calcium transport. *J Clin Invest* 1988;**82**:1585–91.

65 Baggio B, Gambaro G, Marchini F *et al.* An inheritable anomaly of red cell oxalate transport in 'primary' nephrolithiasis correctable with diuretics. *N Engl J Med* 1986;**314**:599–604.

66 Nicar MJ, Hill K, Pak CYC. A simple technique for assessing the propensity of crystallization of calcium oxalate and brushite precipitation. *Metabolism* 1983;**32**:906–10.

67 Andersen DA. Environmental factors in the aetiology of urolithiasis. In: Cifuentes DeLatte L, Rapado A, Hodgkinson A, eds. *Urinary Calculi. Recent Advances in Aetiology, Stone Structure and Treatment.* Basel: S Karger, 1973:130–44.

68 Trinchieri A, Mandressi A, Luongo P, Coppi F, Pisani E. Familial aggregation of renal calcium stone disease. *J Urol* 1988;**139**:478–81.

69 Schwille PO, Töpper K, Schwille K, Herrmann U. Recurrent idiopathic calcium urolithiasis (RCU)—blood levels of two vitamin D metabolites in males. In: Norman AW, Bouillon R, Thomasset M, eds. *Vitamin D. Gene Regulation, Structure–Function Analysis, and Clinical Application.* Berlin: Walter de Gruyter, 1991:932–3.

70 Schwille PO, Herrmann U, Kissler H. Phosphate and glucose metabolism in idiopathic recurrent calcium urolithiasis (RCU) of males. Association of postprandial urinary hyperexcretion of phosphate, glucose, protein, with high blood levels of 1,25(OH)$_2$ vitamin D. In: Norman AW, Bouillon R, Thomasset M, eds. *Vitamin D.* Berlin: Walter de Gruyter, 1994:908–9.

71 Coe FL, Parks JH, Nakagawa Y. Inhibitors and promoters of calcium oxalate crystallization. Their relationship to the pathogenesis and treatment of nephrolithiasis, In: Coe FL, Favus ML, eds. *Disorders of Bone and Mineral Metabolism.* New York: Raven Press, 1992:757–99.

72 Coe FL, Parks JH, Asplin JR. The pathogenesis and treatment of kidney stones. *N Engl J Med* 1992;**327**:1141–52.

73 Lemann J Jr, Gray RW, Maierhofer WJ. The role of serum 1,25(OH)$_2$-vitamin D concentration in determining urinary calcium excretion. In: Frame B, Potts JT Jr, eds. *Clinical Disorders of Bone and Mineral Metabolism.* Amsterdam: Excerpta Medica, 1983:411–15.

74 Broadus AE, Insogna KL, Lang R *et al.* A consideration of the hormonal basis and phosphate leak hypothesis of absorptive hypercalciuria. *J Clin Endocrinol Metab* 1984:**58**:161–9.

75 Braman PG, Morawski S, Pak CYC, Fordtran JS. Selective jejunal hyperabsorption of calcium in absorptive hypercalciuria. *Am J Med* 1979;**66**:425–8.

76 Duncombe VM, Watts RWE, Peters TJ. *In vitro* calcium uptake by jejunal biopsy specimens from patients with idiopathic hypercalciuria, *Lancet* 1980;**2**:1334–6.

77 Bianchi G, Vezzoli G, Cusi D *et al.* Abnormal red-cell calcium

pump in patients with idiopathic hypercalciuria. *N Engl J Med* 1988;**319**:897–901.

78 Schwille PO, Hanisch E, Scholz D. Postprandial hyperoxaluria and intestinal oxalate absorption in idiopathic renal stone disease. *J Urol* 1984;**132**:650–5.

79 Lemann J Jr, Pleuss JA, Gray RW. Increased dietary calcium intake reduces urinary oxalate excretion in healthy adults. In: Walker VR, Sutton RAL, Cameron ECB, Pak CYC, Robertson WG, eds. *Urolithiasis.* New York: Plenum Press, 1989:435–8.

80 Schwille PO, Herrmann U, Fan J *et al.* Acute effects of alkali and alkaline earth citrates in humans—a synopsis of preliminary data in urine. In: Ryall R, Bais R, Marshall VR, Rofe AM, Smith LH, Walker VR, eds. *Urolithiasis and Related Clinical Research.* New York: Plenum Press, 1994:77–8.

81 Laminski NA, Meyers AM, Krüger M, Sonnekus MI, Margolius RP. Hyperoxaluria in patients with recurrent calcium oxalate calculi. Dietary and other risk factors. *Br J Urol* 1991;**68**:454–8.

82 Conyers RAJ, Fazzalari N, Rofe AM, Bais R. Nutrient energy intake, fasting serum insulin and urinary oxalate excretion. In: Walker VR, Sutton RAL, Cameron ECB, Pak CYC, Robertson WG, eds. *Urolithiasis.* New York: Plenum Press, 1989:643.

83 Sharma V, Schwille PO. Oxalate production from glyoxylate by lactate dehydrogenase *in vitro*: inhibition by reduced glutathione, cysteine, cysteamine. *Biochem Int* 1992;**27**: 431–8.

84 Nath R, Thind SK, Murthy MSR *et al.* Role of pyridoxine in oxalate metabolism. *Ann NY Acad Sci* 1990;**585**:274–84.

85 Sharma V, Schwille PO. Effect of calcium on oxalate uptake and transport by the rat intestine. *Scand J Clin Lab Invest* 1992;**52**:339–46.

86 Manoharan M, Schwille PO. Measurement of ascorbic acid in human plasma and urine by high-performance liquid chromatography. Results in healthy subjects and patients with idiopathic calcium urolithiasis. *J Chromatogr* 1994;**654**: 134–9.

87 Cowley DM, McWhinney C, Brown JM. Chemical factors important to calcium nephrolithiasis: evidence for impaired hydroxy-carboxylic acid absorption causing hyperoxaluria. *Clin Chem* 1987;**33**:243–7.

88 Pak CYC. Citrate and renal calculi: new insights and future directions. *Am J Kidney Dis* 1991;**17**:420–5.

89 Baggio B, Gambaro G, Marchini F *et al.* Abnormal erythrocyte and renal furosemide-sensitive sodium transport in idiopathic calcium nephrolithiasis. *Clin Sci* 1994;**86**:239–43.

90 Lemann J Jr, Piering WF, Lennon EJ. Possible role of carbohydrate-induced calciuria in calcium oxalate kidney-stone formation. *N Engl J Med* 1969;**280**:232–6.

91 Kai Lau Y, Wasserstein A, Westby GR *et al.* Proximal tubular defects in idiopathic hypercalciuria: resistance to phosphate administration. *Miner Electrol Metab* 1982;**7**:237–49.

92 Ljunghall S, Hedstrand H. Glucose metabolism in renal stone formers. *Urol Int* 1978;**33**:417–21.

93 Andersen T, McNair P, Fogh-Andersen NH *et al.* Increased parathyroid hormone as a consequence of changed complex binding of plasma in morbid obesity. *Metabolism* 1986;**35**: 147–51.

94 Robertson WG, Peacock M. The cause of idiopathic calcium stone disease, hypercalciuria or hyperoxaluria. *Nephron* 1980;**26**:105–9.

95 Smith LH, Baggio B. Oxalate. In: Walker VR, Sutton RAL,

Cameron ECB, Pak CYC, Robertson WG, eds. *Urolithiasis.* New York: Plenum Press, 1989:417–20.

96 Schwille PO, Scholz D, Schwille K *et al.* Citrate in urine and serum and associated variables in subgroups of urolithiasis. Results from an outpatient stone clinic. *Nephron* 1982;**31**: 194–202.

97 Schwille PO, Manoharan M, Rümenapf G, Wölfel G, Berens H. Oxalate measurement in the picomol range by ion chromatography: values in fasting plasma and urine of controls and patients with idiopathic calcium urolithiasis. *J Clin Chem Clin Biochem* 1989;**27**:87–96.

98 Rodgers AL, Ball D, Harper W. Urinary macromolecules are promoters of calcium oxalate nucleation in human urine: turbidimetric studies. *Clin Chim Acta* 1993;**220**:125–34.

99 Resnick MI, Gammon CW, Sorell MB, Boyce WH. Calcium binding proteins and renal lithiasis. *Surgery* 1980;**88**:239–43.

100 Hess B, Zipperle L, Jaeger P. Citrate and calcium effects on Tamm–Horsfall glycoprotein as a modifier of calcium oxalate crystal aggregation. *Am J Physiol* 1993;**265**:F784–91.

101 Finlayson B, Reid F. The expectation of free and fixed particle in urinary stone disease. *Invest Urol* 1978:**15**:442–8.

102 Menon M, Strzelecky T, McGraw B, Scheid C. Effect of oxalate on kidney mitochondrial function. In: Walker VR, Sutton RAL, Cameron ECB, Pak CYC, Robertson WG, eds. *Urolithiasis.* New York: Plenum Press, 1989:429–30.

103 Khan SR, Hackett RL. Retention of calcium oxalate crystals in renal tubules. *Scanning Microsc* 1991;**5**:707–12.

104 Hackett RL, Shevock PN, Khan SR. Madin–Darby canine kidney cells are injured by exposure to oxalate and to calcium oxalate crystals. *Urol Res* 1994;**22**:197–204.

105 Wiessner JH, Mandel GS, Mandel NS. Membrane interactions with calcium oxalate crystals: variation in hemolytic potential with crystal morphology. *J Urol* 1986;**135**:835–9.

106 Fleisch H. Mechanisms of stone formation: role of promoters and inhibitors. *Scand J Urol Nephrol Suppl* 1980;**53**:53–74.

107 Kok DJ, Papapoulos SE, Bijvoet OLM. Excessive crystal agglomeration with low citrate excretion in recurrent stone formers. *Lancet* 1986;**1**:1056–8.

108 Kok DJ, Khan SR. Calcium oxalate nephrolithiasis, a free or fixed particle disease. *Kidney Int* 1994;**46**:847–54.

109 Herrmann U, Schwille PO, Kuch P. Crystalluria determined by polarization microscopy. Technique and results in healthy control subjects and patients with idiopathic recurrent calcium urolithiasis classified in accordance with calciuria. *Urol Res* 1991;**19**:151–60.

110 Chafe L, Gault MH. First morning pH in the diagnosis of renal tubular acidosis with nephrolithiasis. *Clin Nephrol* 1994;**41**: 159–62.

111 Pak CYC, Kaplan R, Bone H, Townsend J, Waters O. A simple test for the diagnosis of absorptive, resorptive and renal hypercalciurias. *N Engl J Med* 1975;**292**:497–500.

112 Knebel L, Tschöpe W, Ritz E. A one day cellulose phosphate (CP) test discriminates non-absorptive from absorptive hypercalciuria. In: Schwille PO, Smith LH, Robertson WG, Vahlensieck W, eds. *Urolithiasis and Related Clinical Research.* New York: Plenum Press, 1985:303–6.

113 Preminger GM, Peterson R, Pak CYC. Differentiation of unclassified hypercalciuria utilizing a sodium cellulose phosphate trial. In: Walker VR, Sutton RAL, Cameron ECB, Pak CYC, Robertson WG, eds. *Urolithiasis.* New York: Plenum Press, 1989:325–8.

114 Scholz D, Schwille PO. Klinische Laboratoriumsdiagnostik der Urolithiasis. *Dtsch Med Wochenschr* 1981;**106**:999–1002.

115 Schmiedl A, Schwille PO. Tolerables Oxalate im Urin — Grundlagen, Verbesserung der Messmethode und Bewertung bei idiopathischer Calcium-Urolithiasis. *Klin Lab* 1994;**40**: 757–65.

116 Fan J, Schwille PO, Manoharan M, Schmiedl A. Crystallization of calcium oxalate evaluated by microscopy and image analysis. Preliminary results in undiluted urine of controls and renal calcium stone patients [Abstract] *Urol Res* 1993: **21**:146.

117 Herrmann U, Schwille PO, Fan J, Manoharan M. Oral magnesium citrate load in healthy males — acute effects of three preparations on acid–base and mineral homeostasis, and urine parameters of renal stone formation [Abstract]. *Urol Res* 1993;**21**:159.

118 Rothmund M. *Hyperparathyreoidismus.* Stuttgart: Thieme, 1991.

119 Mundy GR, Martin TJ. The hypercalcaemia of cancer: pathogenesis and management. *Metabolism* 1982;**31**:1247–77.

120 Klugman VA, Favus MJ, Pak CYC. Nephrolithiasis in primary hyperparathyroidism. In: Bilezikian JP, Marcus R, Levine MA, eds. *The Parathyroids. Basic and Clinical Concepts.* New York: Raven Press, 1994:505–17.

121 Mundy G. Hypercalcaemia of malignancy. In: Avioli LV, Krane SM, eds. *Metabolic Bone Disease and Clinically Related Disorders.* Philadelphia: WB Saunders, 1990:793–803.

122 Metz DC, Jensen RT, Bale AE *et al.* Multiple endocrine neoplasia type I. Clinical features and management. In: Bilezikian JP, Marcus R, Levine MA, eds. *The Parathyroids. Basic and Clinical Concepts.* New York: Raven Press, 1994:591–646.

123 Gagel RF. Multiple endocrine neoplasia type II. In: Bilezikian JP, Marcus R, Levine MA, eds. *The Parathyroids. Basic and Clinical Concepts.* New York: Raven Press, 1994:681–98.

124 Broadus A. Nephrolithiasis in primary hyperparathyroidism. In: Coe FL, Brenner B, Stein J, eds. *Nephrolithiasis.* New York: Churchill Livingstone, 1980:59–85.

125 Mandl F. Therapeutischer Versuch bei einem Falle von Ostitis fibrosa generalisata mittels Exstirpation eines Epithelkörperchentumours. *Zentralbl Chir* 1926;**53**:260–4.

126 Barr DP, Bulger HA. The clinical syndrome of hyperparathyroidism. *Am J Med Sci* 1930;**179**:471–3.

127 Albright F, Sulkowitch HW, Bloomberg E. Further experience in diagnosis of hyperparathyroidism, including discussion of cases with minimal degree of hyperparathyroidism. *Am J Med Sci* 1937;**193**:800–12.

128 Peacock M. Bone and renal stone disease in patients with primary hyperparathyroidism. In: Talmage RV, Owen M, Parsons IT, eds. *Calcium Regulating Hormones.* Amsterdam: Excerpta Medica, 1975:78–103.

129 Patron P, Gardin JP, Paillard M. Renal mass and reserve of vitamin D: determinants in primary hyperparathyroidism. *Kidney Int* 1987;**31**:1174–80.

130 Silverberg SJ, Shane E, de la Cruz L. Skeletal disease in primary hyperparathyroidism. *J Bone Miner Res* 1989;**4**:321–5.

131 Heath H III, Hodgson SF, Kennedy MA. Primary hyperparathyroidism: incidence, morbidity and potential economic impact on the community. *N Engl J Med* 1980;**302**: 189–93.

132 Gardin JP, Paillard M. Normocalcemic primary hyperpara-

thyroidism: resistence to PTH effect on tubular reabsorption of calcium. *Miner Electrol Metab* 1984;**10**:301–8.

133 Pak CYC, Holt K. Nucleation and growth of brushite and calcium oxalate in urine of stone formers. *Metabolism* 1976;**25**:665–73.

134 Zerwekh JE, Hwang TIS, Poindexter J *et al*. Modulation by calcium of the inhibitor activity of naturally occurring urinary inhibitors. *Kidney Int* 1988;**149**:1005–8.

135 Broulik PD, Stepán JJ, Pacovsky V. Primary hyperparathyroidism and hyperuricaemia are associated but not correlated with indicators of bone turnover. *Clin Chim Acta* 1987;**170**:195–200.

136 Kim H, Kalkhoff RK, Costrini NV, Cerletty JM, Jacobson M. Plasma insulin disturbances in primary hyperparathyroidism. *J Clin Invest* 1971;**50**:2596–605.

137 DeFronzo RA, Lang R. Hypophosphataemia and glucose intolerance: evidence for tissue insensitivity to insulin. *N Engl J Med* 1980;**303**:1259–63.

138 Rümenapf G, Issa S, Schwille PO. The influence of progressive hyperinsulinaemia on duodenal calcium absorption in the rat. *Metabolism* 1987;**36**:60–5.

139 DeFronzo RA, Cooke CR, Andres R, Faloona GR, Davis PJ. The effect of insulin on renal handling of sodium, potassium, calcium, and phosphate in man. *J Clin Invest* 1975;**55**: 845–55.

140 Grill V, Martin TJ. Parathyroid hormone-related protein as a cause of hypercalcaemia in malignancy. In: Bilezikian JP, Marcus R, Levine MA, eds. *The Parathyroids. Basic and Clinical Concepts*. New York: Raven Press, 1994:295–310.

141 DeKernion JB, Pavone-Macaluso M, eds. *Tumours of the Kidney*. Baltimore: Williams and Wilkins, 1986.

142 Strewler GJ, Williams RD, Nissenson RA. Human renal carcinoma cells produce hypercalcaemia in the nude mouse and a novel protein recognized by parathyroid hormone receptors. *J Clin Invest* 1983;**71**:769–74.

143 Suva LJ, Winslow GA, Wettenhall REH *et al*. A parathyroid hormone-related protein implicated in malignant hypercalcaemia: cloning and expression. *Science* 1987;**2153**:893–6.

144 Black KS, Mundy GR. Other causes of hypercalcaemia. Local and ectopic secretion syndromes. In: Bilezikian JP, Marcus R, Levine MA, eds. *The Parathyroids. Basic and Clinical Concepts*. New York: Raven Press, 1994:341–57.

145 Albright F. Case records of the Massachusetts General Hospital (Case 11575061). *N Engl J Med* 1941;**225**:789–91.

146 Cook SA, Tarar RA, Lalli AF. Bony metastasis in renal cell carcinoma. *Cleveland Clin Q* 1975;**42**:263.

147 Said SI. VIP overview. In: Bloom SR, Polak JM, eds. *Gut Hormones*. Edinburgh: Churchill Livingstone, 1981:379–84.

148 Playford RJ, Calam J, Bloom SR. Pathophysiological aspects of gut peptide hormones. In: Brown DR, ed. *Gastrointestinal Regulatory Peptides*. Berlin: Springer Verlag, 1993;387–416.

149 Verner JV, Morrison AB. Islet cell tumour and a syndrome of refractory watery diarrhea and hypokalaemia. *Am J Med* 1958;**29**:529–35.

150 Mekhjian H, O'Dorisio TM. VIPoma syndrome. *Semin Oncol* 1987;**14**:282–91.

151 Bloom SR, Long RG, Bryant MG, Mitchell SJ, Polak JM. Clinical, biochemical and pathological studies on 62 VIPomas. *Gastroenterology* 1980;**78**:1143.

152 Verner JV, Morrison AB. Endocrine pancreatic islet disease with diarrhea—report of a case due to diffuse hyperplasia of non-beta islet tissue with a review of 54 additional cases. *Arch Int Med* 1974;**113**:492–500.

153 Krejs G. Vipoma syndrome. *Am J Med* 1987;**82**(Suppl. 5B): 37–48.

154 Bronner F. Gastrointestinal absorption of calcium. In: Nordin BEC, ed. *Calcium in Human Biology*. London: Springer Verlag, 1988;93–123.

155 Maklouf GM, Said SI, Yau WM. Interplay of vasoactive intestinal polypeptide (VIP) and synthetic VIP fragments with secretin and octapeptide of cholecystokinin (octa CCK) on pancreatic and biliary secretion. *Gastroenterology* 1974; **66**:737–42.

156 Hohmann EL, Levine L, Tashjian AH. Vasoactive intestinal peptide stimulates bone resorption via a cyclic adenosine 3′,5′-monophosphate-dependent mechanism. *Endocrinology* 1983;**112**:1233–9.

157 Lemann J Jr, Litzow JR, Lennon FJ. The effects of chronic acid loads in normal man: further evidence for the participation of bone mineral in the defense against chronic metabolic acidosis. *J Clin Invest* 1966;**45**:1608–14.

158 Kumar R. The metabolism and mechanism of action of 1,25-dihydroxyvitamin D_3 [Editorial review]. *Kidney Int* 1986;**30**: 793–803.

159 Reichel H, Koeffler HP, Norman AW. The role of the vitamin D endocrine system in health and disease. *N Engl J Med* 1989;**320**:980–91.

160 Burnatowska MA, Harris CA, Sutton RAL, Seely JF. Effect of vitamin D on renal handling of calcium, magnesium and phosphate in the hamster. *Kidney Int* 1985;**27**:864–70.

161 Friedman PA, Gesek FA. Vitamin D_3 accelerates PTH-dependent calcium transport in distal convoluted tubule cells. *Am J Physiol* 1993;**265**:F300–8.

162 Tanaka Y, Castillo L, DeLuca HF. The 24-hydroxylation of 1,25-dihydroxyvitamin D_3. *J Biol Chem* 1977;**252**:1421–4.

163 Kream BE, Eisman JA, DeLuca HF. Intestinal cytosol binders for 1,25-dihydroxyvitamin D_3: use in competitive binding protein assay. In: Norman AW, Schaefer K, Coburn JW *et al*., eds. *Vitamin D: Biochemical, Chemical and Clinical Aspects Related to Calcium Metabolism*. New York: Walter de Gruyter, 1977:501–10.

164 Harrell GT, Fisher S. Blood chemical changes in Boeck's sarcoid with particular reference to protein, calcium and phosphatase values. *J Clin Invest* 1939;**18**:687–93.

165 Adams JS, Sharma OP, Gacad MA, Singer FR. Metabolism of 25-hydroxyvitamin D_3 by cultured pulmonary alveolar macrophages in sarcoidosis. *J Clin Invest* 1983;**72**:1856–60.

166 Basile JN, Liel Y, Shary J, Bell NH. Increased calcium intake does not suppress circulating 1,25-dihydroxyvitamin D in normocalcemic patients with sarcoidosis. *J Clin Invest* 1993;**91**:1396–8.

167 McCurley T, Salter J, Glick A. Renal insufficiency in sarcoidosis. *Arch Pathol Lab Med* 1990;**114**:488–92.

168 Casella FJ, Allon M. The kidney in sarcoidosis. *J Am Soc Nephrol* 1993;**3**:1555–62.

169 Muther RS, McCarron DA, Bennet WM. Renal manifestation of sarcoidosis. *Arch Intern Med* 1981;**141**:643–5.

170 Edelson GW, Talpos GB, Bone HG III. Hypercalcaemia associated with Wegener's granulomatosis and hyperparathyroidism: etiology and management. *Am J Nephrol* 1993;**13**:275–7.

171 Breslau NA, McGuire SL, Zerwekh JE, Frenkel EP, Pak CYC.

Hypercalcaemia associated with increased serum calcitriol levels in three patients with lymphoma. *Ann Intern Med* 1984;**100**:1–7.

172 Davies M, Hayes ME, Mawer EB, Lumb GA. Abnormal vitamin D metabolism in Hodgkin's lymphoma. *Lancet* 1985;**1**:1186–8.

173 Kozeny GA, Barbato AL, Bansal VK, Vertuno LL, Hano JE. Hypercalcaemia associated with silicone-induced granulomas. *N Engl J Med* 1984;**311**:1103–5.

174 Gray TK, Lowe W, Lester GE. Vitamin D and pregnancy: the maternal–fetal metabolism of vitamin D. *Endocr Rev* 1981;**2**:264–74.

175 Coe FL, Parks JH, Lindheimer MD. Nephrolithiasis during pregnancy. *N Engl J Med* 1978;**298**:324–6.

176 Sutton RAL. 25-hydroxyvitamin D_3 (25(OH)D_3) enhancement of distal tubular calcium reabsorption in the dog [Abstract]. *Kidney Int* 1975;**8**:404.

177 Bataille P, Achard JM, Fournier A *et al.* Diet, vitamin D and vertebral mineral density in hypercalciuric calcium stone formers. *Kidney Int* 1991;**39**:1193–205.

178 Hennemann PH, Dempsey EF, Carroll EL, Albright F. The cause of hypercalciuria in sarcoid and its treatment with cortisone and sodium phytate. *J Clin Invest* 1956;**35**:1229–42.

179 Salmeron G, Lipsky PE. Immunosuppressive potential of antimalarials. *Am J Med* 1983;**75**:19–24.

180 O'Leary TJ, Jones G, Yip A *et al.* The effects of chloroquine on serum 1,25-dihydroxyvitamin D and calcium metabolism in sarcoidosis. *N Engl J Med* 1986;**215**:727–30.

181 Taylor A, Bikle DD, Norman ME. Serum dihydrotachysterol levels and biological action in normal man. *J Clin Endocrinol Metab* 1988;**67**:198–202.

182 Smith LH. Medical evaluation of urolithiasis: etiologic aspects and diagnostic evaluation. *Urol Clin North Am* 1974;**1**:241–60.

183 Dahlberg PJ, Van den Berg CJ, Kurtz SB, Wilson DM, Smith LH. Clinical features and management of cystinuria. *Mayo Clin Proc* 1977;**52**:533–42.

184 Wasserstein AG, Stolley PD, Soper KA *et al.* Case-control study of risk factors for idiopathic calcium nephrolithiasis. *Miner Electrolyte Metab* 1987;**13**:85–95.

185 Rao PN, Buxton A, Prendiville V, Blacklock NJ. Do stone formers accept dietary advice? In: Schwille PO, Smith LH, Robertson WG, Vahlensieck W, eds. *Urolithiasis and Related Clinical Research.* New York: Plenum Press, 1985:457–60.

186 Schwille PO, Rümenapf G, Köhler R. Blood levels of glucometabolic hormones and urinary saturation with stone forming phases after an oral test meal in male patients with recurrent idiopathic calcium urolithiasis and in healthy controls. *J Am Coll Nutr* 1989;**8**:557–66.

187 Duranti E, Sasdelli M. Effects of dietary sodium on lithogenic risk factors. In: Walker VR, Sutton RAL, Cameron ECB, Pak CYC, Robertson WG, eds. *Urolithiasis.* Plenum Press: 1989: 747–8.

188 Ackermann D, Baumann JM, Futterlieb A, Zingg EJ. Influence of calcium content in mineral water on chemistry and crystallization conditions in urine of calcium stone formers. *Eur Urol* 1988;**14**:305–8.

189 Krebs T, Ackermann D, Danuser HJ, Hess B. Beziehung zwischen 24 h-Urinmenge, spezifischem Gewicht und relativer Übersättigung bei harnsteinbildenden Patienten [Abstract]. *Urologe [A]* 1992;**45**(Suppl.).

190 Oreopoulos DG, Husdan H, Leung M, Reid DBW. Urine oxalic acid relation to urine flow [Letter]. *Ann Int Med* 1976;**85**:617.

191 Tiselius HG, Ahngard LE. The diurnal urinary excretion of oxalate and the effect of pyridoxine and ascorbate on oxalate excretion. *Eur Urol* 1977;**3**:41–6.

192 DeWardener HE. The control of sodium excretion. In: Orloff J, Berliner RW, Geiger SR, eds. *Handbook of Physiology. Section 8, Renal Physiology.* Washington DC: American Physiological Society, 1973:677–720.

193 Hess B, Casez JP, Takkinen R, Ackermann D, Jaeger P. Relative hypoparathyroidism and calcitriol up-regulation in hypercalciuric renal stone formers—impact of nutrition. *Am J Nephrol* 1993;**13**:18–26.

194 Sakhae K, Harvey JA, Padalino JK, Whitson P, Pak CYC. The potential role of salt abuse on the risk for kidney stone formation. *J Urol* 1993;**150**:310–12.

195 Jaeger P, Lippuner K, Casez JP *et al.* Low bone mass in idiopathic renal stone formers: magnitude and significance. *J Bone Miner Res* 1994;**9**:1525–32.

196 Yendt ER, Cohanim M. Increased urinary glycollate in idiopathic calcium-oxalate nephrolithiasis. In: Walker VR, Sutton RAL, Cameron ECB, Pak CYC, Robertson WG, eds. *Urolithiasis.* New York: Plenum Press, 1989:439–41.

197 Lindsjö M. Oxalate metabolism in renal stone disease, with special reference to calcium metabolism and intestinal absorption. *Scand J Urol Nephrol Suppl* 1989;**119**:V:2–22.

198 Scholz D, Schwille PO, Sigel A. Double-blind study with thiazide in recurrent calcium lithiasis. *J Urol* 1982;**128**:903–7.

199 LaCroix AZ, Wienpahl J, White LR. Thiazide diuretic agents and the incidence of hip fracture. *N Engl J Med* 1990; **322**:286–90.

200 Ahlstrand C. Biochemical studies in calcium oxalate stone formers, with special reference to the effects of thiazide treatment. *Linköping Univ Med Dissert* 1984;**172**:6–73.

201 Woelfel A, Kaplan RA, Pak CYC. Effect of hydrochlorothiazide therapy on the crystallization of calcium oxalate in urine. *Metabolism* 1977;**26**:201–5.

202 Ahlstrand C, Tiselius NG, Larsson L, Hellgren E, Clinical experience with long-term bendroflumethiazide treatment in calcium oxalate stone-formers. *Br J Urol* 1984;**56**:255–62.

203 Brocks P, Dahl C, Wolf H, Transböl I. Do thiazides prevent recurrent idiopathic renal calcium stones. *Lancet* 1981; **2**:124–5.

204 Ettinger B, Citron JT, Livermore B, Dolman LI. Chlorthalidone reduces calcium oxalate calculous recurrence but magnesium hydroxyde does not. *J Urol* 1988;**139**:679–84.

205 Marshall RW, Barry H. Urinary saturation and the formation of calcium-containing renal calculi: the effects of various forms of therapy. In: Cifuentes DeLatte L, Rapado A, Hodgkinson A, eds. *Urinary Calculi: Recent Advances in Aetiology, Stone Structure and Treatment.* Basel: S Karger, 1973:164–9.

206 Pak CYC. Quantitative assessment of various forms of therapy for nephrolithiasis. In: Cifuentes DeLatte L, Rapado A, Hodgkinson A, eds. *Urinary Calculi: Recent Advances in Aetiology, Stone Structure and Treatment.* Basel: S Karger, 1973:177–87.

207 Pak CYC, Nicar M, Northcutt C. The definition of the mechanism of hypercalciuria is necessary for the treatment of recurrent stone formers. *Contrib Nephrol* 1982;**33**:136–51.

208 Hayashi Y, Kaplan RA, Pak CYC. Effect of sodium cellulose

phosphate therapy on crystallization of calcium oxalate in urine. *Metabolism* 1975;**24**:1273–8.

209 Rapado A, Cifuentes DeLatte L, Villarino JA, Sanchez Martini JA. Tratemiento de le hipercalciuria idiopática con cellulosa fosfato sodica. *Rev Clin Esp* 1970;**119**:61–6.

210 Scholz D, Schwille PO, Herzog T, Sigel A. Effects of a cation exchange resin on intestinal calcium absorption and urinary calcium in calcium stone formers. *Urol Res* 1981;**9**: 263–9.

211 Butz M. Oxalatsteinprophylaxe durch Alkali-Therapie. *Urologe [A]* 1982;**21**:142–6.

212 Pak CYC, Sakhae K, Fuller CJ. Physiological and physico-chemical prevention of calcium-stone formation by potassium citrate therapy. *Trans Assoc Am Physicians* 1983;**96**: 294–305.

213 Pak CYC. Citrate and renal calculi. *Miner Electrolyte Metab* 1987;**13**:257–66.

214 Barcelo P, Wuhl O, Servitge E, Rousaud A, Pak CYC. Randomized double blind study of potassium citrate in idiopathic hypocitraturic calcium nephrolithiasis. *J Urol* 1993;**150**:1761–4.

215 Schwille PO, Weippert JH, Bausch W, Rümenapf G. Acute oral alkali citrate load in healthy humans—response of blood and urinary citrates, mineral metabolism, and factors related to stone formation. *Urol Res* 1985;**13**:161–8.

216 Lindberg J, Harvey J, Pak CYC. Effect of magnesium citrate and magnesium oxide on the crystallization of calcium salts in urine: changes produced by food–magnesium interaction. *J Urol* 1990;**143**:248–51.

217 Smith LH. Hyperoxaluric states. In: Coe FL, Favus MJ, eds. *Disorders of Bone and Mineral Metabolism*. New York: Raven Press, 1992:707–27.

218 Levine BS, Rodman JS, Wienerman W *et al.* Effect of calcium supplementation on urinary calcium oxalate saturation in female stone formers: implications for prevention of osteoporosis. *Am J Clin Nutr* 1994;**60**:592–6.

219 Harrison AR, Kasidas GP, Rose GA. Hyperoxaluria and recurrent stone formation apparently cured by short courses of pyridoxine. *Br Med J* 1981;**282**:2087–98.

220 Murthy MSR, Farooqui S, Talwar HS *et al.* Effect of pyridoxine supplementation on recurrent stone formers. *Int J Clin Pharmacol Ther Toxicol* 1982;**20**:434–7.

221 Rattan V, Sidhu H, Vaidyanathan S, Thind SK, Nath R. Effect of combined supplementation of magnesium oxide and pyridoxine in calcium-oxalate stone formers. *Urol Res* 1994;**22**:161–5.

222 Rattan V, Thind SK, Sethi RK, Sidhu H, Nath R. Oxalate metabolism in magnesium-deficient rats. *Magnes Res* 1993;**6**:125–31.

223 Hallson PC, Kasidas GP. Hyperoxaluria in calcium oxalate urolithiasis. In: Wickham JEA, Buck AC, eds. *Renal Tract Stone. Metabolic Basis and Clinical Practice*. Edinburgh: Churchill Livingstone, 1990:271–84.

224 Watts RWE. Hyperoxaluric states. In: Wickham JEA, Buck AC, eds. *Renal Tract Stone. Metabolic Basis and Clinical Practice*. Edinburgh: Churchill Livingstone, 1990:387–400.

225 Caudarella R, Tolomelli B, Berveglieri F *et al.* Vitamin B_6 status and oxalate excretion in patients with calcium lithiasis. In: Walker VR, Sutton RAL, Cameron ECB, Pak CYC, Robertson WG, eds. *Urolithiasis*. New York: Plenum Press, 1989:849–50.

226 Dominquez JH, Gray RW, Lemann J Jr. Dietary phosphate deprivation in women and men: effects on mineral and acid balances, parathyroid hormone, and the metabolism of 25-OH-vitamin D. *J Clin Endocrinol Metab* 1976;**43**: 1056–68.

227 Nordin BEC, Hodgkinson A, Peacock M. The measurement and the meaning of urinary calcium. *Clin Orthop Rel Res* 1967;**52**:293–322.

228 Van den Berg C, Kumar R, Wilson DM, Heath III H, Smith LH. Orthophosphate therapy decreases urinary calcium excretion and serum 1,25-dihydroxyvitamin D concentrations in idiopathic hypercalciuria. *J Clin Endocrinol Metab* 1980;**51**: 998–1001.

229 Portale AA, Halloran BP, Murphy MM, Morris RC Jr. Oral intake of phosphorus can determine the serum concentration of 1,25-dihydroxyvitamin D by determining its production rate in humans. *J Clin Invest* 1986;**77**:7–12.

230 Pak CYC. Effects of cellulose phosphate and of sodium phosphate on the formation product and activity product of brushite in urine. *Metabolism* 1972;**21**:447–55.

231 Pak CYC, Eanes ED, Ruskin B. Spontaneous precipitation of brushite in urine: evidence that brushite is the nidus of renal stones originating as calcium phosphate. *Proc Natl Acad Sci USA* 1971;**68**:1456–60.

232 Schwille PO, Rümenapf G, Wölfel G, Köhler R. Urinary pyrophosphate in patients with recurrent calcium urolithiasis and in healthy controls: a re-evaluation. *J Urol* 1988;**140**: 239–45.

233 Butz M, Dulce HJ. Enhancement of urinary citrate in oxalate stone formers by the intake of alkali salts. In: Smith LH, Robertson WG, Finlayson B, eds. *Urolithiasis. Clinical and Basic Research*. New York: Plenum Press, 1981:881–4.

234 Pak CYC, Skurla C, Brinkley L, Sakhae K. Augmentation of renal citrate excretion by oral potassium citrate administration: time course, dose frequency schedule, and dose-response relationship. *J Clin Pharm* 1984;**24**:19–26.

235 Schwille PO, Schmiedl A. Citrate in the treatment of idiopathic recurrent calcium urolithiasis (RCU)—an overview. In: Rao PN, Kavanagh J, Tiselius HG, eds. *Urolithiasis. Consensus and Controversies*. Proceedings of the Fifth European Urolithiasis Symposium, Manchester, 21–23 April 1994. South Manchester University Hospitals, Manchester, 1995:151–61.

236 Rümenapf G, Schwille PO. The influence of oral alkali citrate on intestinal calcium absorption in healthy men. *Clin Sci* 1987;**73**:117–21.

237 Schwille PO, Herrmann U, Wolf C, Berger I, Meister R. Citrate and recurrent idiopathic urolithiasis. A longitudinal pilot study on the metabolic effects of oral potassium citrate administered over the short-, medium- and long-term to male stone patients. *Urol Res* 1992;**20**:145–55.

238 Herrmann U, Schwille PO, Schwarzlaender H, Berger I, Hoffmann G. Citrate and recurrent idiopathic calcium urolithiasis. A longitudinal pilot study on the metabolic effects of oral potassium-sodium citrate administered over the short-, medium- and long-term to male stone patients. *Urol Res* 1992;**20**:347–53.

239 Goldberg H, Grass L, Vogl R, Rapoport A, Oreopoulos DG. Urinary citrate and renal stone disease. *Can Med Assoc J* 1989;**141**:217–21.

240 Curhan GC, Willett WC, Rimm EB, Stampfer MJ. A

prospective study of dietary calcium and other nutrients and the risk of symptomatic kidney stones. *N Engl J Med* 1993;**328**:833–8.

241 Schwille PO, Siegert R, Schick CH *et al.* Orchiectomy-induced osteopathy in the rat—preliminary report on the state of mineral and bone metabolism, and its response to oral calcium-sodium citrate. *Med Sci Res* 1994;**22**:529–31.

242 Martinez ME, Villa E, Martul MV *et al.* Influence of calcium intake on calcitriol levels in idiopathic hypercalciuria in children. *Nephron* 1993;**65**:36–9.

243 Ackermann D, Baumann JM, Siegrist P. Sulfatgehalt von Mineralwasser und Sulfaturie. *Fortschr Urol Nephrol* 1988;**26**: 254–6.

244 Krizek V, Sadilek L. Trinkkuren mit Mineralwässern bei Harnsteinleiden. *Fortschr Urol Nephrol* 1985;**23**:147–59.

245 Pizzarelli F, Peacock M. Effect of chronic administration of ammonium sulfate on phosphatic stone recurrence. *Nephron* 1987;**46**:247–52.

246 Gault MH, Parfrey PS, Robertson WG. Idiopathic calcium phosphate nephrolithiasis. *Nephron* 1988;**48**:265–73.

247 Schwille PO, Rümenapf G, Köhler R, Weippert JH. Fasting gastrinemia and elevated supersaturation with hydroxyapatite of fasting urine—observations in renal calcium stone patients and controls. *Urol Res* 1987;**15**:99–104.

248 Herrmann U, Schwille PO, Manoharan M, Gruber H, Wenig A. Oral cimetidine in humans—evidence for urine acidification and inhibition of calcium oxalate crystallization. In: Ryall R, Bais R, Marshall VR, Rofe AM, Smith LH, Walker VR, eds. *Urolithiasis and Related Clinical Reseach.* New York: Plenum Press, 1994:223–4.

249 Gruber H. *Orales Cimetidin beim Gesunden—eine Dosis-Wirkungsstudie zu Plasmaspiegeln, Gastrinämie, Netto-Ausscheidung von Säure im Urin, und die Kristallisation von Calciumoxalat.* PhD Thesis, University of Erlangen, 1995.

250 Churchill DN. Medical treatment to prevent recurrent calcium urolithiasis. A guide to critical appraisal. *Miner Electrolyte Metab* 1987;**13**:294–304.

251 Peacock M. The mechanisms of hypercalciuria are unnecessary for treatment of recurrent renal calcium stone formers. *Contrib Nephrol* 1982;**33**:152–62.

61 Surgical Management of Renal Stones
H.N.Whitfield

Introduction

Urinary tract stone disease has a history that goes back as far as any other recorded disease. In spite of modern methods of diagnosis and treatment, stones are still a cause of major morbidity and mortality throughout the world. The advent of revolutionary techniques in the surgical approach to the management of renal stones has not been matched by any similar advances in either the understanding of the aetiology of many types of stone or in the prophylaxis and medical treatment. Although attempts have been made to classify renal stones [1–3], the variations and combinations in intrarenal anatomy, age, sex, stone composition, stone burden, renal function, biochemistry and urinary infection combine to make a clinically relevant classification impossible to devise.

These different aspects of renal tract stone disease highlight the importance of a multidisciplinary approach. A comprehensive team would consist of a nephrologist, a biochemist and a radiologist as well as a urological surgeon. Only by taking this broad view can patients be offered the greatest potential benefits in the management of their stones. In addition to the factors already mentioned, the age, occupation and fitness of the patient, their symptoms and the availability of equipment and expertise in the varying aspects of stone management will all have a bearing on the approach to any individual.

The advances in minimally invasive approaches to the management of stone disease have changed patients' expectations, sometimes in unrealistic ways. At a time when there were few, if any, alternatives to open surgery for the management of stone disease decisions were easier to make than now, when so many new treatment modalities are available either alone or in combination. The high capital cost of equipment that is needed to provide a comprehensive stone service has led to the development of stone centres, which must be in the interests of patients, though depriving many urologists of the opportunity to treat what remains a very common urological disorder. In this chapter treatment options will be discussed with the assumption that there is no restriction on the availability of technical resources and surgical expertise.

Clinical features

Pain

The occurrence of pain is very variable and not infrequently the severity of the pain is in inverse relationship to the size of the stone. Small calculi which are mobile within the renal pelvis can cause intermittent obstruction which results in classic renal colic. A small stone trapped in a calyx with a narrow calyceal neck may also give rise to pain of similar severity, so-called calyceal colic.

A stone which is not causing acute obstruction may be the cause of a more persistent dull aching pain in the loin, but sometimes even staghorn calculi may be entirely asymptomatic. It is not uncommon to encounter a patient with a non-functioning kidney secondary to a staghorn stone of infective origin who denies any symptoms. Nevertheless, on removal of the affected kidney the patient may be surprised to find a significant improvement in his or her general well-being.

Haematuria

Bleeding from the urothelium may arise, particularly when a mobile stone is present within the collecting system. On occasions, such haematuria may be quite heavy but at other times only microscopic haematuria is present. A mobile stone may cause exercise-induced haematuria.

Urinary infection

When renal stones are associated with chronic upper urinary tract infection the patient may complain of a persistent dull ache together with a general feeling of malaise. When there is an element of obstruction from the stone a midstream specimen of urine (MSU) may not always reveal the presence of infection.

The combination of acute obstruction and upper urinary tract infection is an emergency. The presence of severe loin pain and tenderness, pyrexia, tachycardia and leucocytosis should immediately raise clinical suspicion of the diagnosis. On ultrasound, however, there may sometimes be only a minor degree of pelvicalyceal dilatation. Organisms may not appear in or be grown from the urine because of the presence of obstruction.

Conservative management

The acute case

Patients who present with renal colic from a stone causing obstruction either at the pelviureteric junction or, very occasionally, to the neck of a calyx, may be safely managed conservatively unless there is evidence of infection coincidentally.

Pain relief

Renal colic produces very severe pain and strong analgesia is required to relieve it. The most popular treatment is parenteral pethidine because it is widely believed that morphine causes spasm of the renal pelvis and ureter and may provoke further colic. However, there is very little pharmacological evidence to corroborate this view and it may be that the nausea and vomiting that is so frequently an accompaniment of acute renal colic may, in part, be provoked by pethidine. Both morphine and diamorphine are stronger analgesics and may provide better relief.

Antispasmodics do not affect ureteric or pelvic wall motility, although drugs such as propantheline hydrochloride are very commonly prescribed in the hope that they will reduce colic and thereby relieve pain. Organ bath experiments do not, however, provide any evidence that this is so. All such drugs have unpleasant side effects, e.g. dry mouth and blurred vision. Additionally, it has not yet been established whether spontaneous passage of stones is promoted by peristalsis or whether renal pelvic and ureteric relaxation encourages onward progression of a stone. For these reasons it is hard to recommend anticholinergic drugs in this situation [4,5].

In an attempt to encourage spontaneous passage of an obstructing stone, a diuresis is often encouraged. There is no evidence that this will increase the chances that a stone will pass spontaneously and there is experimental evidence that the increased intratubular pressure which will be induced causes greater nephron damage [6].

The decision whether to persevere with conservative management will depend on the severity of the patient's symptoms and the assessment of renal function. It is usual that the acute pain subsides over 48 h but a dull loin ache may remain. Although the intravenous urogram (IVU) is the method of choice in making the initial diagnosis, renography provides a more accurate method of monitoring renal function subsequently [7].

The decision as to whether surgery will ultimately be required will depend on the frequency with which episodes of colic occur, the size of the stone and therefore the likelihood of it passing spontaneously, the age and fitness of the patient and whether or not there is a urinary tract infection. The timing of surgery is not critical in the absence of infection. Complete functional recovery can be anticipated even after complete obstruction which has lasted for as long as 10 days. However, when an infection exists above an obstruction, renal function is permanently impaired quickly and, therefore, there must be no delay in removing the obstructing stone.

Stone dissolution

Pure cystine stones may be dissolved by medical treatment and the details of this are referred to in Chapter 59. Uric acid stones also dissolve if the urine is alkalinized using sodium bicarbonate 650 mg every 6–8 h. If this is combined with the administration of acetazolamide 250 mg daily, cardiovascular problems secondary to sodium overload are minimized [8,9]. Alkalinization therapy should be combined with allopurinol in a dose of 300–600 mg/day. In the case of both cystine and uric acid stones, medical treatment will fail if there has been any deposition of calcium in the stone.

Stones which are composed of struvite and which are infective in origin may sometimes be dissolved using hemiacidrin, which was first described in 1959 [10]. Since that time irrigation with a solution of hemiacidrin has been performed postoperatively for residual calculi [11], and as a primary manoeuvre either through a percutaneous nephrostomy [12] or via a ureteric catheter [13]. Such treatment is not without risks and careful monitoring is necessary. Episodes of septicaemia may occur and careful bacteriological supervision is necessary. While the stone is being dissolved the urine becomes loaded with debris and it is important that there should be no obstruction to urine outflow. The hydrostatic pressure used for the infusion must be carefully monitored. For all these reasons this form of treatment is used infrequently.

Surgical management

The surgical management of renal stones has undergone a revolution since 1976 when percutaneous renal surgery was first introduced. Since that time the advent of extracorporeal shockwave lithotripsy (ESWL) [14] has added a further dimension and the combination of these two methods of treatment has made it now unnecessary to contemplate open surgery for renal stones in the vast majority of patients. Open surgery for staghorn calculi remains the treatment of choice when the bulk of the stone lies within calyces rather than within the renal pelvis. Some patients in whom there is a disorder of the outflow tract which would need correction at the same time as the removal of the stone may also be best treated by open surgery, though endoscopic methods of treatment of pelviureteric junction obstruction have been developed [15,16]. Complications of both percutaneous renal surgery and of ESWL on rare occasions may also require an open procedure. However, whatever kind of surgical intervention is performed certain investigations must be undertaken preoperatively.

Preoperative investigations

Urine analysis

All patients will require careful bacteriological monitoring and an MSU should be cultured. If, on clinical grounds, it is thought that the stone is infective in origin, antibiotics should be given prophylactically with the premedication even if there is no growth on urine culture.

Radiology

Intravenous urography

A preoperative IVU is a prerequisite for all types of surgery for renal stones. The relationship of the stone to the collecting system will influence the particular operation which is performed. It is essential, in addition to a preoperative urogram, to take a plain abdominal X-ray of the patient on the day that surgery is planned. All urologists can recount stories of patients in whom unexpected things have happened to stones and there is no more disastrous an occurrence than to explore a kidney only to discover that the stone has previously passed spontaneously.

Computed tomography scan

It is not always possible to determine from an IVU the precise localization of a stone within the collecting system. If a solitary calyceal stone is present it is very important for the surgeon to know whether such a calyx is placed anteriorly, posteriorly or in the mid-axis of the kidney. Oblique films may help to define this but a more accurate method of localization has been described in which a computed tomography (CT) scan is used for stone localization [17]. More recently the use of spiral CT has been described, enabling a three-dimensional image to be built up, though it is too early to decide whether this method of imaging will improve the results of subsequent surgery [18,19]. A CT scan plays an important part in

defining the presence of non-opaque stones and their relationship to intrarenal anatomy.

Renal arteriography

Selective renal angiography has been described as providing additional useful information, particularly if congenital anomalies of arterial supply or malrotation are suspected. If a lower pole partial nephrectomy is planned there may be an advantage in defining renal arterial anatomy preoperatively [20]. However, such information is now obtainable less invasively with the use of spiral CT.

Ultrasound

Although renal stones are frequently imaged by ultrasound during ESWL, ultrasound is not a good way of primarily identifying renal stones nor of relating the stone to intrarenal pelvicalyceal anatomy. It is not possible to differentiate a stone within a calyx from a stone within a calyceal diverticulum or cyst, for example. In renal stone disease ultrasound is best reserved for the demonstration of acute obstruction when there is no contrast excretion during IVU or as an adjunct to plain radiography, particularly for stones which are poorly radio-opaque.

Measurement of renal function

Preoperatively it is essential to know the overall renal function in terms of blood urea, serum creatinine and preferably creatinine clearance. It is also extremely important to have a measure of differential renal function and this can only be satisfactorily provided by a radioisotopic measurement. Not only will it be possible to ascertain the contribution of each kidney to total function but the presence of outflow obstruction will also be revealed [21]. When the overall and differential renal function are known the decision can be made as to which kidney should be operated upon first in cases of bilateral stone disease, and at other times the decision can be made whether conservative or ablative surgery is indicated. When a kidney is contributing less than 10% to overall renal function nephrectomy is usually the best choice. Where a kidney is contributing more than 20% to overall function then a conservative approach should be adopted. Various circumstances will influence the decision when the differential renal function lies between 10 and 20%.

Biochemical investigations

It is usually preferable to await the results of stone analysis before embarking on investigations to determine the metabolic disorder which might be underlying stone formation. However, prior to ESWL it can be useful to define stone composition which can help in the planning of lithotripsy. A technique originally described for looking at urine crystals after ESWL combining scanning electron microscopy (SEM) with X-ray energy dispersive spectroscopy [22] can also be used for identifying stone composition prior to ESWL.

Pyelolithotomy

For mobile calyceal stones and for pelvic stones, a simple pyelolithotomy is indicated. Full mobilization of the kidney is not necessary; following a pyelotomy the stone should be readily removed. Such surgery is only indicated if facilities for ESWL or percutaneous renal surgery are not available.

Coagulation pyelolithotomy

The difficulty of removing multiple small stone fragments led to the development of coagulation pyelolithotomy in which a fibrin coagulum made by a mixture of thrombin and fibrinogen is introduced into the renal pelvis. The mixture of thrombin and fibrinogen forms a firm clot in which small stone fragments become embedded and these can be extracted along with the coagulum. Any coagulum which remains is dissolved by the urine over the subsequent 24 h. The technique is an attractive one but requires careful control to reproduce a stable, firm coagulum. Encouraging results have been reported [23].

Extended pyelolithotomy

When a large stone fills the renal pelvis and calyces surgical access can be greatly increased by dissecting the renal sinus between the renal pelvis and the renal parenchyma—the Gil-Vernet approach [24]. It is often possible to dissect up to the calyceal necks and an incision into the renal pelvis will then give access not only to the renal pelvic portion of a staghorn calculus but also sometimes to the clubbed calyceal extensions. This provides a very satisfactory, atraumatic approach, bearing in mind only that the posterior branch of the renal artery runs across the back of the renal pelvis and will have to be retracted. It may be necessary to remove calyceal extensions of a staghorn calculus via separate nephrostomy incisions if adequate exposure cannot be obtained. The technique is employed by most surgeons who are operating on staghorn calculi, but whether it is the sole method of access or the main one to which nephrotomies are added will depend on the shape and size of the stone within the kidney and the experience and preference of the surgeon.

Nephrotomy

Anatrophic nephrolithotomy

It is well recognized that an incision along the Brodel's convex border of the kidney (bloodless 'plane'), which bivalves a kidney, results in very considerable renal damage because the vascular supply of the kidney is such that the posterior branch of the renal artery supplies the posterior two-thirds of the renal parenchyma and the anterior renal artery branches supply the remainder of the kidney. If an incision is to be made which avoids dividing interlobar end arteries then the incision has to be placed on the posterior surface of the kidney at the junction of the areas supplied by the anterior and posterior branches of the renal artery. The line of division can be identified by clamping the posterior segmental artery and administering an intravenous dose of 20 ml of methylene blue. The incision is carried through the parenchyma and down towards the hilum, intersecting the structures at the base of the posterior infundibulum [25].

Radial nephrotomy

Access to the calyceal portions of a staghorn calculus may be obtained by nephrotomies arranged radially on the posterior aspect of the kidney as far away from the hilum as is possible, to avoid damage to pericalyceal veins which are placed anteriorly. The main portion of a staghorn calculus can be removed through a pyelotomy and residual stone fragments through as many radially placed nephrotomies as necessary. This approach has been popularized by Wickham [26].

Preservation of function during renal ischaemia

When radial nephrotomies or the anatrophic nephrotomy are performed it will be necessary to clamp the renal artery to allow satisfactory vision and to prevent blood loss. If the renal artery is clamped for more than 30 min irreversible ischaemic damage is likely. Methods of renal preservation have been developed; several different techniques of cooling the kidney are available and there is no doubt that renal function is very safely preserved for up to 2 h if the kidney is cooled to about 20°C. Graves [27] described a simple method in which a plastic bag was filled with ice-cold saline and invaginated around the kidney. Wickham and colleagues developed a pair of coiled saucer-shaped discs which are placed either side of the kidney and ice-cooled water is pumped around the coils [28]. Boyce has employed crushed sterile ice to pack around the kidney [29] while Marberger and Georgi have described a method of intra-arterial perfusion of the kidney with a cooled perfusate through a Swan–Ganz catheter introduced into the renal artery by the Seldinger technique of femoral arterial puncture [30]. Whatever method is used, the parenchymal temperature must be monitored by a telethermometer probe.

An alternative method of preserving renal function was described by Fernando *et al.* in 1976 [31]; they demonstrated that inosine, a purine nucleotide, if given intravenously, enabled the renal artery to be clamped with safety for up to 1 h [32].

Peroperative X-rays

Radiology is vitally important to any surgeon undertaking renal stone surgery and contact films provide evidence of whether or not complete stone clearance has been achieved. The aim of stone surgery must be to clear the kidney of all stones and stone fragments as without complete clearance stone recurrence is almost inevitable. A method of building up a three-dimensional image of the kidney by contact X-rays taken in two planes has been described by Gil-Vernet [24].

Partial nephrectomy

It has been claimed that the risk of recurrent stone formation is decreased if, at the time of stone removal, that part of the kidney is also removed which is considered to be important in the aetiology of formation of that stone [33]. Such pathological conditions would include localized pyelonephritis, calyceal diverticula and the presence of Randall's plaques in the renal parenchyma surrounding the calyx in which a stone is lodged. A long-term follow-up study [34] showed that stone recurrence rates were equal on the operated and contralateral kidney suggesting that partial nephrectomy had successfully prevented anatomical factors from giving rise to a higher recurrence rate on the previously operated side. The technique certainly has its place, particularly where a calyceal stone is associated with some localized disease process of the kidney.

Bench surgery

In some cases of recurrent staghorn calculus formation extracorporeal renal surgery improves the chances of achieving a complete stone clearance because of improved illumination, extended ischaemia time and improved intraoperative radiology [35]. By definition, any such patient in whom this technique is considered will be a formidable operative challenge because recurrent surgery for staghorn calculus disease is never easy; there may also be occasional indications for performing bench surgery as a primary manoeuvre in a patient with very extensive stone disease. Great care must be taken not to devascularize the renal pelvis, the ureter or the major venous and arterial branches. Athough *in situ* surgery can be performed very satisfactorily in the majority of patients with renal stone disease there are occasions when bench surgery followed by autotransplantation into the renal fossa may be the better technique. Such procedures, however, should not be performed outside major centres in which dialysis facilities are available.

Nephrectomy

All urologists have encountered the dilemma which arises when a patient presents with a large stone in a solitary kidney. Not infrequently the opposite kidney has been removed some time previously for stone disease. The recurrent stone formation rate is known to be high and therefore a kidney should not be ablated unless there is evidence of the absence of worthwhile function and unless it is considered that no useful function will return on stone removal. As a general rule any kidney which produces less than 10% of overall renal function is unlikely to provide worthwhile function on de-stoning.

Laparoscopic nephrectomy has been described as an alternative to open surgery but most authors have recommended that patients with non-functioning kidneys secondary to stone disease are not suitable because surrounding adhesions make dissection too difficult [36].

Postoperative complications

Residual stones

Residual renal stones are likely to present difficult problems postoperatively. The decision has to be made whether the stone is of the kind which could possibly respond to some form of dissolution *in situ*. Cystine, uric acid and struvite stones are the only ones which are likely to respond to this kind of treatment. Inevitably, residual stones increase the risk of persisting infection and stone recurrence and an alternative approach is to remove them percutaneously. If a nephrostomy tube has been left *in situ* and the track is not too crooked it may be possible to dilate the nephrostomy track sufficiently to enable the inside of the kidney to be inspected and any residual stones removed.

Infection

After complete stone clearance, residual infection is likely to continue to be present for some considerable time if the stone was of an infective origin. For this reason long-term prophylactic antibiotics should be give postoperatively for a minimum of 3 months and then continuing careful monitoring of urine cultures should be made at monthly intervals. Unless great attention is paid to maintain the urine sterile it is likely that recurrent stones will form.

Obstruction

Following a pyelolithotomy for stone disease, postoperative stenosis of the pelviureteric junction may occur. This is particularly likely if there has been urinary extravasation and infection postoperatively, and the chances are increased still further if an extensive pyelotomy has been made which will tend to devascularize the renal pelvic wall. Not uncommonly the presence of such a stenosis is first revealed at the time of a follow-up IVU 3 months postoperatively. Each case must be treated on its merits but it is likely that if objective evidence of significant obstruction is demonstrated some form of reconstructive surgery will be required. A percutaneous approach to incise the pelviureteric junction may be an alternative.

Percutaneous nephrolithotomy

There are a number of reports describing patients in whom stones were removed through a pre-existing nephrostomy track. However, these earliest reports all describe the procedure in patients in whom the nephrostomy track had been established at open operation but who had remaining residual stones [37–39]. Credit for the first planned percutaneous nephrolithotomy (PCNL) must go to Fernström who demonstrated the possibility of removing renal calculi percutaneously through a nephrostomy track formed for the purpose [40]. Subsequently, the technique was further developed in Germany and the United Kingdom [41–44]. The possibility of establishing a percutaneous track between the collecting system and the skin had first been demonstrated by Goodwin and Casey [45]. During PCNL such a track is subsequently dilated to a size which will accommodate whatever endoscopic instrument is needed to remove the stone. In practice this means that a track must be between 24 and 30 F. Subsequently, the stone(s) is removed.

Stones which are too large to be removed intact can be disintegrated either by ultrasound, electrohydraulically or with the more recently introduced pneumatic stone disintegrator. Both the ultrasound and the pneumatic disintegrators incorporate a suction channel. The stone is disintegrated and stone particles are either removed by suction or with suitable grasping forceps. The relative merits of these different forms of disintegration are debatable. The ultrasound probe is safe, because only the stone is affected by the ultrasound and the urothelium is not damaged unless the tip of the instrument becomes overheated. Electrohydraulic lithotripters will sometimes fragment stones which are too hard to be disintegrated by ultrasound. However, the number of fragments created may be quite large and the time taken to remove them can be quite prolonged. Stone fragments can be dispersed into part of the collecting system to which access is difficult. The tip of the electrohydraulic probe must not been left in contact with the urothelium but should be pressed firmly against the stone if urothelial damage is to be avoided. The pneumatic probe can only damage the collecting system if inappropriate mechanical pressure is applied to the urothelium either directly or via the stone.

Complications

All surgical procedures carry some risk and percutaneous renal surgery is no exception. Nevertheless, it is recognized that the morbidity associated with percutaneous surgery is significantly lower than with conventional open operations [46].

Haemorrhage

Bleeding may occur during dilatation of the track. This is usually because a vein in the region of a calyceal neck has been breached. Tamponade with an Amplatz sheath during the second stage of the procedure is usually enough to reduce the bleeding so that the second stage can be performed. Methods of stone destruction can provoke bleeding, particularly electrohydraulic disintegration. Even a small amount of bleeding can obscure vision and under such circumstances it is best to abandon the procedure, leaving a large-sized nephrostomy tube *in situ*. Stone removal can be completed at a subsequent operation.

Very severe bleeding may occasionally necessitate highly selective renal arterial embolization. If this fails to control the bleeding fully then in the last resort a nephrectomy may be required.

Infection

All renal stones, even those which are primarily metabolic in origin, have a potential for being associated with infection. Patients undergoing PCNL should, therefore, be treated prophylactically with an appropriate antibiotic immediately prior to surgery. Patients whose stones are infective in origin are at particular risk and will require long-term antibiotics after stone removal to ensure that any infection is eliminated and not merely suppressed.

Irrigant extravasation

If the collecting system is injured, fluid that is used for irrigation may either leak into the perinephric tissues or, much more seriously, be infused intravenously. Breaches of the pleura or peritoneum are very uncommon but in such circumstances large volumes of fluid can be lost in a short space of time. It is therefore mandatory to monitor continuously during the procedure the volume of fluid irrigated and the volume retrieved. If a discrepancy of more than 2 l is found the procedure should be stopped. If large quantities of fluid are extravasated a 'transurethral resection-like' reaction can occur [47].

Residual stones

There are different reasons why, following PCNL, stone clearance may be incomplete. Sometimes fragments of stone break off and enter inaccessible parts of the pelvicalyceal system. At other times it is not easy to identify preoperatively whether a stone will be accessible through the planned track, which enters through a posterior calyx. A 'parallel lie' situation can arise with a lower pole stone in an anterior lower calyx which remains inaccessible through a posteriorly placed track. Middle calyces may also prove to be inaccessible and if the only stone is lying within a middle calyx a direct puncture may be necessary. On other occasions, the majority of calculi can be left with the knowledge that any residual fragments or stones can be treated subsequently by ESWL. Stone fragments which fall down the ureter provoke the greatest risk of complications. On occasions it is worthwhile inserting an indwelling JJ stent to prevent such an occurrence.

Perforation of adjacent organs

There are reports of perforation of the large bowel, duodenum, inferior vena cava, peritoneal cavity, pleural cavity and the pleura. Such events are usually due to poor technique and are rare [48].

Extracorporeal shockwave lithotripsy

The development of ESWL for the management of urinary tract stones has been responsible for a revolution in urology over the last 10 years, the effects of which are still in evidence. The technique was developed in Germany and the first clinical applications were reported in the early 1980s [14]. The principle of the method was that shockwaves were generated by an underwater spark discharge from an electrode that was localized in the first geometric focus of an elipsoidal reflector. These shockwaves were then collected in the second focus which was the area of highest energy density. In order to destroy a calculus the patient had to be positioned in such a way that the calculus was situated in the second focus. Precise localization of the calculus was achieved by a two-dimensional X-ray imaging system. Under epidural or general anaesthesia the patient was placed in a water-filled tub to ensure that the shockwave energy was transmitted directly to the calculus and not to the skin surface. Initially, ESWL was confined to the treatment of stones which were less than 2 cm in diameter and which were lying within the renal pelvis. The potential

for widening the scope of stones treated was first exploited by Eisenberger et al. [49]. They described the integration of percutaneous renal surgery and lithotripsy and the principles which they defined have become widely accepted. Since that time a large number of lithotripters from a wide variety of manufacturers has become available.

The objective is to enable treatment to be performed on an outpatient basis with a minimum of analgesia or sedation. Although first described for the management of renal stones, ESWL is now widely accepted as being the method of choice for many ureteric stones and some bladder stones. Lithotripter manufacturers had anticipated that stones in the gallbladder would also be suitable for treatment but the advent of laparoscopic cholecystectomy has drastically reduced the indications for gallstone lithotripsy. There are still occasions on which, however, ESWL is valuable for stones within the common bile duct.

Principles of lithotripsy

All lithotripters require three components: (i) there must be a method of generating shockwaves which can be brought to a focus; (ii) the stone must be imaged either by ultrasound or radiologically; and (iii) there must be a mechanism to bring the stone to the shockwave focus, either by moving the patient or by moving the shockwave generator and thereby the stone focus. The shockwave must be coupled to the patient in a way that prevents pain at the site of entry and avoids dissipating the shockwave energy. This coupling is produced either through a water bath or a shockwave cushion, depending on the individual lithotripter.

Shockwaves

The original Dornier HM3 and many subsequent lithotripters have relied on generating underwater a high tension spark which is discharged across two electrodes. This shockwave is produced at the first focus of a hemi-elipsoid and the reflection from the sides of this then brings the shockwaves to a second focus where the stone will be located. All lithotripters in common use today which rely on this method of shockwave generation can be used without general or epidural anaesthesia, because the diameter of the hemi-elipsoid has been increased sufficiently to ensure that the angle of entry of the shockwaves at the skin surface is as oblique as possible and that the area of skin surface over which the shockwave enters is as wide as possible.

An alternative way of producing a shockwave is with the piezoelectric principle. A mosaic of piezoelectric crystals covers a water-filled dish in which the patient's loin is submerged. The shockwaves generated are brought to a small focus. More repeat treatments are required with piezoelectric lithotripsy than with other forms of shock-wave generation.

An electromagnetic method of shockwave generation can also be used. A magnetic field is produced which moves a flexible membrane to produce a pressure wave which is then focused.

No one method of shockwave production is inherently better than another. Unanswered questions remain about the relative safety of the different methods. What is beyond doubt is that the range of peak focal pressures available with different lithotripters varies enormously (Fig. 61.1).

Imaging

The Dornier HM3 used two-dimensional radiological imaging which was very satisfactory for most cases. However, there was some risk from radiation exposure both to the patient and the operators. Poorly opaque and radiolucent stones were difficult to treat but progress of stone disintegration could be monitored during treatment with some accuracy. Most lithotripters now incorporate ultrasound imaging, either alone or in combination with radiological imaging. Ultrasound has the advantage that during treatment the stone can be imaged constantly, increasing the accuracy of stone treatment. In lithotripters with dual facilities for imaging, X-ray localization is usually confined to the treatment of stones within the ureter. Depending on the particular lithotripter and the expertise of the operator most stones within the ureter can now be visualized and treated.

Complications

The two complications which occur most frequently are infection and obstruction. As has been stated previously, many stones which are metabolic in origin may also have an infective component. Although controversy surrounds the need for prophylactic antibiotics, in the author's opinion these are mandatory, particularly as most patients are treated on an outpatient basis and may travel quite large distances to a stone centre.

To reduce the chances of ureteric obstruction, stones which are larger than 2–2.5 cm in diameter should not be treated without some adjuvant intervention. The larger the stone the greater the number of stone particles which will be produced and, therefore, the higher the incidence of ureteric obstruction by stone fragments, the so-called 'stein strasse' [50] (Fig. 61.2).

Integrated stone management

Although the need for open stone surgery has diminished since the advent of ESWL there remains the need for considerable expertise, not only in defining the most appropriate form of treatment, but also in practising the endoscopic manoeuvres which are now commonly required. The margin for error in any minimally invasive procedure of this kind is much smaller than with open surgery and a meticulous technique is essential. As with other endoscopic procedures, the learning curve is slower than with open surgery and difficult to teach as well as to learn.

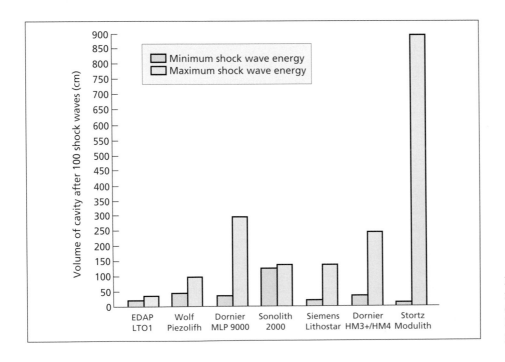

Fig. 61.1 A comparison of the minimum and maximum shock wave energies available from different lithotripters. (Reproduced by kind permission of J Rassweiler.)

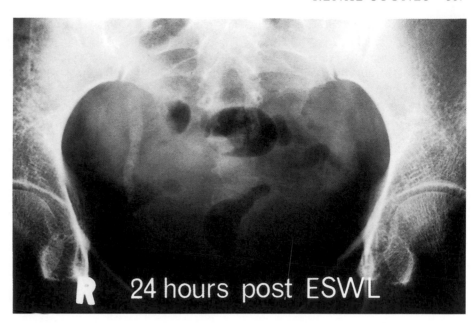

Fig. 61.2 An accumulation of stone fragments 'stein strasse' at the lower end of the right ureter 24 hours post-lithotripsy.

It is impossible to lay down rigid rules about the management of stones in individual patients because there are so many variables. Broad guidelines, however, can be stated.

Simple renal pelvic stones

Any stone which is less than 2.5 cm in diameter can be treated effectively by ESWL provided that there is no outflow obstruction. However, the combination of a renal pelvic stone and a pelviureteric junction obstruction requires an endoscopic approach in which not only is the stone removed but the pelviureteric junction is treated as well.

Lucent stones

Although radiolucent stones can be imaged with ultrasound, such stones are necessarily composed of uric acid which is relatively hard and resistant to disintegration. Furthermore, it is very difficult to monitor the results of disintegration, not only within the kidney but more particularly if fragments enter the ureter. For this reason a percutaneous approach may be preferable for uric acid stones.

Renal stones in the obese patient

All forms of stone management become more difficult and are associated with a higher morbidity when the patient is obese. With ESWL the distance between the skin surface and the kidney may be increased to such a depth that bringing the stone to the shockwave focus is impossible.

However, this is only likely to occur when the patient weighs more than 135 kg.

The distance between the pelvicalyceal system and the skin may also prove a problem during percutaneous surgery. The standard length of an Amplatz sheath is 6 cm and this may, on occasion, be too short. Even the standard nephroscope shaft may occasionally prove to be too short to provide intrarenal access; although it would theoretically be possible to define this prior to surgery using ultrasound this is not always the case.

Open renal surgery in any obese patient carries with it increased risks of general complications such as deep vein thrombosis, pulmonary embolism and chest infection. Renal access may be impaired, particularly in women where the distance between the costal margin and the iliac crest is small.

Calculi in horseshoe kidneys

This is one of the commonest anomalies encountered and patients who have a horseshoe kidney are at greater risk than average of stone formation because there is often a degree of impaired drainage of the renal pelvis. Furthermore, because the ureter tends to take off from higher up the renal pelvis and not from the most dependent part, ESWL may not be the method of choice for treating pelvic stones as clearance of the stone fragments after lithotripsy is less satisfactory than in a normal kidney [51].

Although horseshoe kidneys are associated with anomalies of arterial and venous anatomy, a percutaneous approach may nevertheless be achieved successfully and offer the best solution.

Calyceal stones

The management of calyceal stones has been revolutionized by the advent of ESWL. Patients would not have been offered even percutaneous renal surgery for stones of 5 mm or less which could be expected to pass spontaneously [52]. However, during their passage down the ureter such stones can cause disabling renal colic and there is now a very good case for offering such patients prophylactic ESWL. The success of lithotripsy in this situation depends on the anatomy of the calyceal neck. If the calyx is drained by a wide infundibulum uncomplicated lithotripsy is the rule, with the passage of stone fragments occurring quickly and painlessly even from lower calyces in the majority of patients. However, when there is a narrow calyceal neck or more particularly when there is a calyceal cyst from which no obvious drainage occurs, lithotripsy becomes a much more speculative procedure. The concept of calyceal colic is a real clinical entity and even if there is impaired drainage from the stone-bearing calyx, nevertheless, patients may experience pain relief even in the absence of stone clearance [53].

In many series cystinuria accounts for up to 5% of renal stones that are encountered. This common inherited disorder is more fully described in Chapter 59 and cystine stones are almost certainly one of the few metabolic stones which can be successfully treated medically. However, if there is any calcium deposit on the surface of the stone, medical treatment is not likely to be successful. Stones composed of cystine have a reputation for being harder than many others and resistant to ESWL disintegration. For this reason, and because stones composed of cystine are often only encountered when they have grown to a significant size, percutaneous surgery may be the most appropriate. Even then, disintegrating these stone can prove difficult [54].

Staghorn calculi

Controversy continues about the best method of management of staghorn stones. There are occasions, particularly when the bulk of the stone lies within calyces, when open renal surgery provides the best opportunity for complete stone clearance within the shortest time span. The increased morbidity from an open operation must be balanced against the morbidity which would occur after several endoscopic procedures and several intrarenal tracks. The management of staghorn stones with monotherapy ESWL has been reported by some centres, though has not gained universal acceptance [55]. One real drawback of open renal surgery is that the opportunity to acquire the appropriate surgical expertise is available only in a limited number of centres which offer particular expertise in stone management.

The combination of percutaneous renal surgery and lithotripsy is an effective approach. Following initial debulking, residual stone fragments can be disintegrated by lithotripsy (Fig. 61.3). Alternatively, a second track could be placed to the upper calyceal group but it is not easy to avoid a pleural puncture, nor is it easy to ensure complete stone clearance of a complex calyceal group.

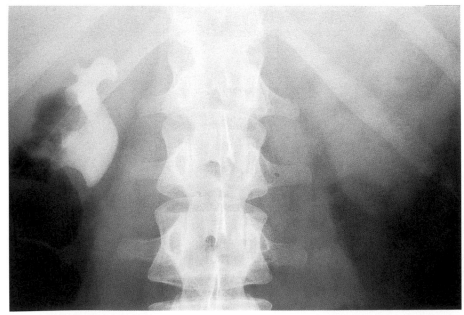

(a)

Fig. 61.3 An illustration of combined PCNL and ESWL for a staghorn calculus. (a) A control film; (b) after contrast; (c) one day post-PCNL; (d) one day post-ESWL, four days post-PCNL; (e) six days post-PCNL, three days post-PCNL.

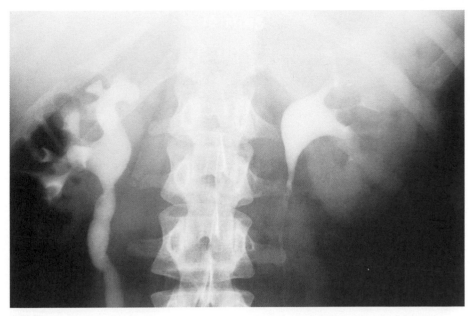

(b)

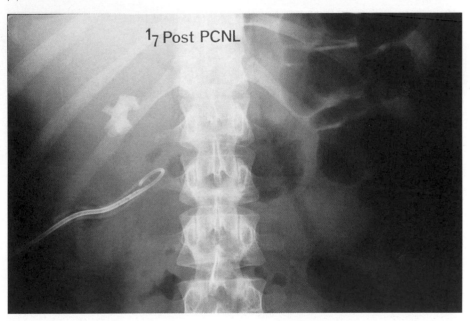

1₇ Post PCNL

(c)

Fig. 61.3 *Continued.*

Biochemical investigations

Every patient who has been operated on for renal stone disease should be fully investigated to determine any underlying predisposing cause for stone formation. The stone which has been removed should be sent for analysis and for culture. Following chemical analysis of the stone the most appropriate biochemical tests will become apparent, but the possibility of coincidental infection together with a metabolic disorder must not be overlooked. A scheme for the investigation of a patient who has had a renal stone is shown in Table 61.1. The treatment of the patient must continue following removal of the stone and the aim must be to prevent further stone formation. Particular advice about the measures to be followed is detailed in previous chapters, but there is no doubt at all that whenever a patient has formed one stone he or she is at significant risk of forming another. In the majority of patients the main prophylactic measure will be to maintain adequate fluid intake. The surgeon must also be prepared to undertake the medical treatment of any predisposing metabolic disorder which may be revealed as a result of stone analysis and biochemical investigations.

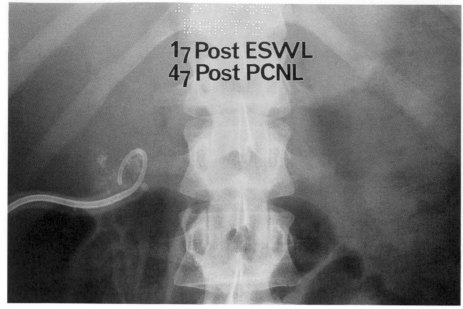

(d)

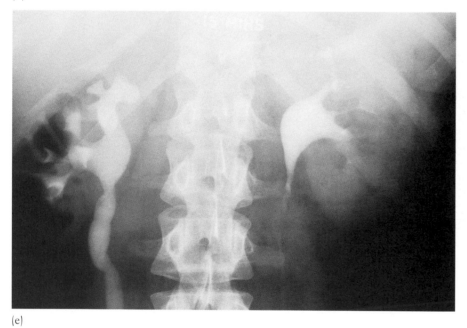

(e)

Fig. 61.3 *Continued.*

Table 61.1 A scheme for the metabolic evaluation of a patient with renal stone disease.

Blood	Urea, creatinine, electrolytes
	Calcium, phosphate, alkaline phosphatase
	Urate
	Glucose
Urine 24 hour acidified collection	Creatinine
	Calcium
	Oxalate
	Sodium
	Citrate
Random fresh sample	Cystine screen
	pH
	Protein/creatinine ratio
	Urine culture
Stone	Any available material must be analysed

References

1 Wickham JEA. The surgical treatment of renal lithiasis. In: Wickham JEA, ed. *Urinary Calculous Disease*. Edinburgh: Churchill Livingstone, 1979:106–9.

2 Rocco F, Mandressi A, Larcher P. Surgical classification of renal calculi. *Eur Urol* 1984;**10**:121–3.

3 Griffith DP, Valiquette L. PICA/Burden: a staging system for upper tract urinary stones. *J Urol* 1987;**138**:253–7.

4 Andersson KE, Ulmsten U. Effects of spinal anaesthesia, lidocaine and morphine on the motility of the human ureter *in vivo*. *Scand J Urol Nephrol* 1975;**9**:236.

5 Ross JA, Edmond P, Kirkland IS. *Behaviour of the Human Ureter in Health and Disease*. Edinburgh: Churchill Livingstone, 1972.

6 Osbourne DE, Lee J, Williams G. Experimental ureteric obstruction. *Br J Urol* 1974;**46**:15.

7 Holm-Nielsen A, Jorgensen T, Morgensen P, Fogh J. The prognostic value of probe renography in ureteric stone obstruction. *Br J Urol* 1981;**53**:504–7.

8 Drach GW. Urolithiasis. In: Conn HF, ed. *Current Therapy*. Philadelphia: WB Sanders, 1976:552.

9 Drach GW, Smith MJD, Boyce WH. Medical therapy of renal calculi. *J Urol* 1970;**104**:635–9.

10 Mulvaney WP, A new solvent for certain urinary calculi; a preliminary report. *J Urol* 1959;**82**:546–8.

11 Jacobs SC, Gilles RF. Dissolution of residual renal calculi with Hemiacidrin. *J Urol* 1976;**115**:2.

12 Dretler GW, Pfister RC, Newhouse JH. Renal stone dissolution via percutaneous nephrostomy. *N Engl J Med* 1979;**300**:341–3.

13 Nemoy NJ, Stamey TA. Use of hemiacidrin in management of infected stones. *J Urol* 1976;**116**:693–5.

14 Chaussy CH, Schmiedt E, Jocham D *et al*. First clinical experience with extracorporeally induced destruction of kidney stones by shock waves. *J Urol* 1982;**127**:417–19.

15 Whitfield HN, Mills V, Miller RA, Wickham JEA. Percutaneous pyelolysis: an alternative to pyeloplasty. *Br J Urol* 1983;**55** (Suppl.):93–6.

16 Ramsay JWA, Miller RA, Kellett MJ *et al*. Percutaneous pyelolysis: indications, complications and results. *Br J Urol* 1984;**56**:586–8.

17 Wickham JEA, Fry IK, Wallace DMA. Computerised tomography localisation of intrarenal calculi prior to nephrolithotomy. *Br J Urol* 1980;**52**:422–5.

18 Smith RC, Rosenfield AT, Choe KA *et al*. Acute flank pain: comparison of non-contrast-enhanced CT and intravenous urography. *Radiology* 1995;**194**:789–94.

19 Katz DS, Lane MJ, Sommer FG. Unenhanced helical CT of ureteral stones: incidence of associated urinary tract findings. *AJR* 1996:1319–22.

20 Drach GW. Urinary lithiasis—renal angiography. In: Harrison JH, Gittes RF, Perlmutter AD, Stamey TA, Walsh PC, eds. *Campbell's Urology*. London: WB Saunders, 1978:779–878.

21 Britton KE, Whitfield HN. Radionuclide measurement of disordered renal function. In: Chisholm GD, Williams DI, eds. *Scientific Foundations of Urology*. 2nd edn. London: Heinemann, 1982:65–74.

22 Bowsher WG, Crocker RP, Ramsay JWA, Whitfield HN. Single urine sample diagnosis. A new concept in stone analysis. *Br J Urol* 1990;**65**:236–9.

23 Patel VJ. Coagulum pyelolithotomy. *Br J Surg* 1973;**60**:230–6.

24 Gil-Vernet JN. New surgical concepts in removing renal calculi. *Urol Int* 1965;**20**:255–88.

25 Boyce WH, Elkins IB. Reconstructive renal surgery following an atrophic nephrolithotomy—follow-up of 100 consecutive cases. *J Urol* 1974;**11**:307–12.

26 Wickham JEA, Coe N, Ward JP. 100 cases of nephrolithotomy under hypothermia. *J Urol* 1974;**112**:702–5.

27 Graves FT. Renal hypothermia: an aid to partial nephrectomy. *Br J Surg* 1963;**50**:362–7.

28 Wickham JEA, Hanley HG, Joekes AM. Regional renal hypothermia. *Br J Urol* 1967;**38**:727–43.

29 Boyce WH. Surgery of urinary calculi in perspective. *Urol Clin North Am* 1983;**10**:584–94.

30 Marberger M, Georgi M. Balloon occlusion of the renal artery in tumour nephrectomy. *J Urol* 1975;**14**:360–3.

31 Fernando AF, Armstrong DMG, Griffiths JF *et al*. Enhanced preservation of the ischaemic kidney with inosine. *Lancet* 1976;**1**:555–7.

32 Fitzpatrick JM, Wallace DMA, Whitfield HN *et al*. Inosine in ischaemic renal surgery: long-term follow-up. *Br J Urol* 1981;**53**:524–7.

33 Stewart HH. The surgery of the kidney in the treatment of renal stone. *Br J Urol* 1960;**32**:392–413.

34 Rose MB, Follows OJ. Partial nephrectomy for stone disease. *Br J Urol* 1977;**49**:605–10.

35 Novick AC, Stewart HH, Straffon RA. Extracorporeal renal surgery and auto-transplantation: indications, techniques and results. *J Urol* 1980;**123**:86.

36 Eraky I, El-Kappany HA, Ghoneim MA. Laparoscopic nephrectomy: Mansoura experience with 106 cases. *Br J Urol* 1995;**75**:271–5.

37 Rupel E, Brown R. Nephroscopy with removal of stone following nephrostomy for obstructive calculus. *J Urol* 1941;**46**:177–82.

38 Bartley O, Chidekel N, Radber GC. Percutaneous drainage of the renal pelvis for uraemia due to obstructed urinary flow. *Acta Chir Scand* 1965;**129**:443–6.

39 Bissada NK, Meacham KR, Redman JF. Nephroscopy with removal of renal pelvic calculi. *J Urol* 1974;**112**:414–16.

40 Fernström I, Johansson B. Percutaneous pyelolithotomy: a new extraction technique. *Scan J Urol Nephrol* 1976;**10**: 257–9.

41 Thüroff JW, Hutschenwreiter GC. Fallbericht: Perkutane Nephrostomie und Instrumentelle Steinentfernung. *Lokalanaesth Urol Int* 1980;**35**:375–80.

42 Wickham JEA, Kellett MJ. Percutaneous nephrolithotomy. *Br J Urol* 1981;**53**:297–9.

43 Whitfield HN. Percutaneous nephrolithotomy. *Br J Urol* 1983;**55**:609–12.

44 Alken P, Hutschenwreiter G, Gunter R. Percutaneous kidney stone removal. *Eur Urol* 1982;**8**:304–11.

45 Goodwin WE, Casey WC. Percutaneous trocar. Nephrostomy in hydronephrosis. *J Am Med Assoc* 1955;**157**:891–4.

46 Rittenberg MH, Koolpe H, Keeler L, McNamara T, Bagley DH. Pain control: comparison of percutaneous and operative nephrolithotomy. *Urology* 1985;**25**:468–71.

47 Miller RA, Whitfield HN. Absorption of 1.5% glycine after percutaneous ultrasonic lithotripsy for renal stone disease. *Br Med J* 1985;**291**:967.

48 Netto NR, Lemos GC, Fruza JL. Perforation following percutaneous nephrolithotomy. *Urology* 1981;**32**:223–4.

49 Eisenberger F, Fuchs G, Miller K, Bub P, Rassweiler J.

Extracorporeal shock wave lithotripsy (ESWL) and endo-urology: an ideal combination for the treatment of kidney stones. *World J Urol* 1985;**3**:41–7.

50 Coptcoat MJ, Webb DR, Kellett MJ, Whitfield HN, Wickham JEA. The Stein Strasse: a legacy of extracorporeal lithotripsy? *Eur Urol* 1988;**4**:83–5.

51 Smith JE, Van Arsdalen KN, Hanno PM, Pollack HM. Extracorporeal shock wave lithotripsy treatment of calculi in horseshoe kidneys. *J Urol* 1989;**142**:683–6.

52 Andersson L, Sylven M. Small renal caliceal calculi as a cause of pain. *J Urol* 1983;**130**:752–3.

53 Mee SL, Thüroff JW. Small caliceal stones: is extracorporeal shock wave lithotripsy justified? *J Urol* 1988;**139**:909–10.

54 Bhatta KM, Prien EL Jr, Dretler SP. Cystine calculi - rough and smooth: a new clinical distinction. *J Urol* 1989;**142**:937–40.

55 Segura JW, Preminger GM, Assimos DG *et al.* Nephrolithiasis clinical guidelines panel summary report on the management of staghorna calculi. *J Urol* 1994;**151**:1648–51.

62 Surgical Management of Ureteric Stones

H.N.Whitfield

Introduction

Many studies have been performed which highlight the importance of upper urinary tract stone disease. Epidemiological studies play an important part in defining the size of the problem in any given population as well as raising questions about the reasons behind widely differing reported rates of incidence. The economic implications are fundamentally important particularly in the era of an ever increasing technological revolution in the management of urinary tract stones. There is no obvious link between the varying rates of incidence in different countries and within different countries in climate, geographical latitude and water hardness [1–5]. All studies confirm the higher incidence of ureteric stones in men in the ratio of 2:1. Most patients who develop pain from the passage of a ureteric stone will present to a hospital and a significant workload will result.

Clinical features

The patient classically presents with a very severe intermittent colicky pain, the site of which can vary between the loin and the groin. The precise location of maximum pain is a poor guide to the site of the stone. Although there are exacerbations and remissions in the intensity of the colicky pain, a dull background ache remains at all times for 24–48 h unless the stone has been passed within that time. The severity of the pain has been likened to childbirth and the pain is often accompanied by a high degree of anxiety in patients who have not experienced renal colic previously. The pain may radiate to the scrotum or labia and occasionally down to the thigh. Unless there is associated infection above the impacted stone the patient will not be pyrexial, though there may be sweating and a tachycardia because of the pain. Vomiting has always been reported as a common feature, but this may often be due to the treatment that has been given, pethidine, rather than to the severity of the pain itself.

Abdominal examination will usually reveal tenderness in the loin, the hypochondrium or the groin or any combination of these. However, the degree of tenderness is not great unless there is associated infection.

Investigations

Urine

The urine should be tested by dipstick for the presence of blood; if absent the diagnosis should be questioned very strongly. Urine microscopy, if available, may confirm the presence of red blood cells and may show organisms. Urine should be sent off for culture and sensitivity testing.

Imaging

It is essential that the clinical diagnosis of ureteric colic occurring for the first time should be confirmed on an intravenous urogram (IVU). A plain abdominal X-ray together with ultrasound gives insufficient information on which to base management decisions. Although a plain abdominal X-ray may reveal calcification in the line of the urinary tract, ultrasound is not a reliable way of confirming whether such calcification lies within the collecting system.

Emergency intravenous urogram

An emergency IVU is mandatory in all patients presenting with renal colic. The investigation should be performed as soon as possible, while the patient is in pain. A plain control film (or two) is taken, followed by the injection of an adequate volume of contrast. This may need to be higher than in an elective IVU performed on a prepared patient. A film taken immediately after the injection of contrast will classically show a delay in the appearance of the nephrogram. The subsequent appearance of contrast within the pelvicalyceal system and ureter on the side of the colic will depend on the site and degree of obstruction. Later films should therefore be taken at appropriate intervals depending on individual circumstances. When the suspected calculus lies in the intramural part of the ureter, it is essential to ask the patient to empty his or her bladder before taking the films because a full bladder can obscure a contrast-filled ureter. On occasions very delayed films must be taken before the site of obstruction can be confirmed.

Immediate management

Hospitalization

It is common for most patients presenting to an accident and emergency department with renal colic to be admitted. However, this may not always be necessary if the diagnosis can be made and the patient offered adequate analgesia and medical support at home by his or her general practitioner.

Analgesia

Parenteral narcotic analgesics such as pethidine are often given to relieve the very severe pain of renal/ureteric colic. Intravenous, intramuscular or oral administration can be used. Diclofenac has also been shown to be effective in providing pain relief [6]. This is one of the non-steroidal anti-inflammatory drugs which exert their effects through inhibition of prostaglandin synthesis. The cyclo-oxygenase enzyme responsible for converting arachidonic acid into prostaglandins is inhibited, suggesting that prostaglandin release is responsible for the pain which occurs in ureteric colic.

Antispasmodics

Antispasmodics do not have a useful part to play in ureteric colic. There is no evidence that in the pharmacological doses used ureteric spasm is reduced. In any event, the best way of encouraging the passage of a ureteric stone is by promoting ureteric peristalsis.

Conservative management

With the advent of newer minimally invasive methods of treating ureteric stones the fact must not be forgotten that 80% of such stones will pass spontaneously [7]. Most stones less than 5 mm in diameter will pass spontaneously within a 6-week period. It has long been established [8,9] that stones less than 4 mm in diameter in the lower half of the ureter pass spontaneously more often than those in the upper half and that stones above 6 mm, whether in the lower or the upper ureter, rarely pass spontaneously. The importance of including conservative treatment as an option has been emphasized more recently by Morse and Resnick [10]. In a series of 378 patients, 60% passed their

stones spontaneously overall: 22% from the proximal, 46% from the middle and 71% from the distal ureter.

Interventional therapy

Indications

Pain

It is usual that the acute pain of ureteric colic subsides spontaneously within 48–72 h. However, some patients continue to experience intermittent episodes of severe colic quite frequently. Others complain of a continuous aching discomfort in the loin. In either event, intervention is indicated at an earlier stage than in the asymptomatic patient.

Size and site of stone

Any stone which is more than 5 mm in diameter has only a small chance of passing spontaneously. The higher up the ureter the stone remains, the lower the chances of spontaneous elimination. The three well-recognized areas of maximum ureteric narrowing occur at the pelviureteric junction, at the pelvic brim where the ureter crosses the bifurcation of the common iliac artery and in the intramural portion of the ureter.

Infection

Any evidence that the patient has developed a urinary tract infection above the site of obstruction is an indication for urgent intervention. The usual clinical features are that the patient experiences a more severe loin ache than is associated with a quiescent calculus and that he or she becomes pyrexial. Confirmation of infection may be difficult to provide. The urine may show relatively few abnormalities as the red cells, white cells and organisms which are situated above the obstruction do not enter the bladder. A raised white blood cell count is common, however.

If the diagnosis is suspected an ultrasound should be performed to define the degree of upper tract dilatation and a percutaneous nephrostomy should be inserted and left *in situ*. At the time of stent insertion no attempt should be made to delineate the anatomy by a nephrostogram, as this risks provoking a more profound septicaemia. Urine should be taken from the renal pelvis and sent urgently for culture and the patient should be started on a best-guess parenteral antibiotic. It cannot be overemphasized that the combination of infection and obstruction will result in irreversible renal damage within a matter of hours. It is the role of the urologist to be sensitive to this complication and to institute early effective intervention.

Non-progression of the stone

On the basis of symptoms and renal ultrasound it is not possible to establish whether renal impairment is occurring. The only safe way to pursue a conservative policy of management is to monitor renal function by an isotope renogram. Any evidence of deterioration is an indication for intervention.

Patient occupation

It is unwise for patients to travel abroad knowing that they have a ureteric calculus. On occasions, therefore, even though renal function remains stable and the patient has no symptoms intervention is advisable.

Treatment options

It is rare for open surgery to be the primary treatment option for any ureteric stone. Uncommonly, the resolution of complications from other forms of treatment may require an open procedure and the choice of treatment most often depends on the facilities available and the expertise of the urologist.

Stone basketry

In their study, Morse and Resnick [10] treated 62 of 79 (78%) of stones in the lower third of the ureter by basketing under fluoroscopic control, recording a success rate of 49 out of 62 (79%). However, only stones 5 mm or smaller could be removed by this technique, which was associated with a complication rate of 1.6%. There is no doubt that this well-tried method of treatment is safe and effective, but certain rules must be remembered. The stone should not be greater than 5 mm in diameter nor higher within the ureter than the lower third. Fluoroscopic control must always be available. The longer the time for which the stone has been present, the lower the success rate.

Extracorporeal shockwave lithotripsy

Extracorporeal shockwave lithotripsy (ESWL) has become the treatment of choice for stones in the upper third of the ureter. Controversy and debate continue over the question of whether in situ treatment yields results which are as good as those achieved after the stone has been pushed back into the renal pelvis and a JJ stent inserted. It is very difficult to compare reported success rates because the variables in terms of stone size, stone composition, degree and length of time of impaction are variable. Stone-free rates at 3 months both after in situ lithotripsy alone and following stone manipulation are comparable (81–96 and 88–91%, respectively) [11,12]. The evidence that an indwelling ureteric stent improves the passage of stone fragments either following renal or ureteric lithotripsy is conflicting [13,14].

Most second-generation lithotripters can be used to treat stones in the lower third of the ureter either using X-ray or ultrasound localization. Most centres have reported that an increased number of shockwaves at a higher voltage and a greater number of treatment sessions are required for the successful treatment of ureteric stones when compared to renal stones. Although there may be some learning curve to overcome in imaging stones throughout the ureter, overall success rates of well over 90% are reported so consistently that this would seem to be the method of choice for initial treatment of all ureteric stones for which intervention is required [15,16].

Ureteroscopy

Ureteroscopy has an important part to play in patients who have stones which have not responded to less invasive methods of treatment or those in whom the stone is associated with some degree of impaction or ureteric obstruction. The most modern ureteroscopes are of a smaller calibre than those originally described. Watson et al. [17] reported a series in which the first 100 patients were treated with ureteroscopes of 11.5 F. Access was only possible in 73% and the complications were quite significant, with 3% developing strictures, 12% requiring nephrostomy drainage and a 7% ureteric perforation rate. In a subsequent series of 200 patients in whom a miniaturized ureteroscope was employed, access was successful at the first attempt in 99% and none of the complications mentioned previously were encountered.

Ureteroscopy for ureteric stones is performed in conjunction with some form of stone disintegration. Electrohydraulic fragmentation technology has been available for over 40 years, having first been described for the disintegration of bladder stones. The size of the probes has been reduced progressively so that they can now be used with almost any ureteroscope. High-frequency ultrasound probes are also available but being rigid the range of ureteroscopes with which they can be used is correspondingly reduced. The amount of power that is available in the small probes is small and often inadequate to achieve stone disintegration. Laser lithotripsy, using either the pulsed dye laser, neodymium-yttrium aluminium garnet (Nd-YAG) and alexandrite lasers are all commercially available. As the fibres are all very small (200–600 nm diameter) they can be used with the smallest flexible ureteroscopes [17,18]. The main disadvantages of laser lithotripsy are its high capital cost and its relatively low power, making it impossible to disintegrate very hard stones.

A recently introduced pneumatic lithotripsy probe has

been introduced for use in both the kidney and the ureter and has been shown to be effective in fragmenting large hard stones within the ureter that have been resistant to laser disintegration [19,20].

The relative safety of the different methods of disintegration has been examined in a recent report by Wu *et al.* [21]. They conclude that direct contact of the laser beam or the electrohydraulic spark with the urothelium should be avoided. Pneumatic lithotripsy would seem to be safer because only direct puncture of the ureteric wall poses a potential hazard.

Retroperitonoscopy

The technique that has been described by Gaur [22] has provided another significant advance in the approach to minimally invasive surgery in the urinary tract. Stones in the middle third of the ureter have always provided the greatest challenge and using the retroperitoneal approach that he describes, it is possible to expose the ureter with a laparoscopic technique used retroperitoneally. Through a small trochar incision in the flank a subcutaneous space is created into which a balloon is placed. The balloon is then filled with 500 ml of saline and left inflated for a few minutes. Subsequently, a telescope can be introduced through which it is possible to visualize the ureter and its contained stone. Using conventional laparoscopic techniques the ureter can be opened and the stone removed. Reports of the success of this new method of treatment are increasing.

Conclusion

A large proportion, perhaps up to 80%, of ureteric stones less than 5 mm in diameter will pass spontaneously. Conventional endoscopic basketry provides a safe method of removing stones of 5 mm or less in the lower third of the ureter, providing that fluoroscopic monitoring is employed. Lithotripsy *in situ* for other stones in the ureter is associated with success rates of over 90%, comparable to the success rates reported following either retrograde stone manipulation and/or insertion of a ureteric stent. Ureteroscopy which normally requires a general anaesthetic, should be reserved for those stones which cannot be removed by simpler, less invasive methods of treatment. Of the different methods of stone disintegration, the recently introduced pneumatic disintegrator has the advantages of being safe, economical and effective.

References

1 Power C, Barker DJP, Blacklock MJ. Incidence of renal stones in 18 British towns. *Br J Urol* 1987;**59**:105–10.
2 Scott R. Epidemiology of stone disease. *Br J Urol* 1985;**57**: 491–7.
3 Johnson CM, Wilson DM, O'Fallon WA, Malek RS, Kurland LT. Renal stone epidemiology: a 25 year study in Rochester, Minnesota. *Kidney Int* 1979;**16**:624–31.
4 Hiatt RA, Dales LG, Friedman GD, Hunkeler EM. Frequency of urolithiasis in a pre-paid medical care program. *Am J Epidemiol* 1982;**115**:255–65.
5 Shuster J, Finlayson B, Scheaffer R *et al*. Water hardness and urinary stone disease. *J Urol* 1982;**128**:422–5.
6 Sandhu DPS, Iacovou JW, Fletcher MS *et al*. A comparison of intramuscular ketorolac and pethidine in the alleviation of renal colic. *Br J Urol* 1994;**74**:690–3.
7 O'Flynn JD. The treatment of ureteric stones. Report on 1120 patients. *Br J Urol* 1980;**52**:436–8.
8 Sandegard E. Prognosis of stone in the ureter. *Acta Chir Scand Suppl* 1956:219.
9 Ueno A, Kawamura T, Ogawa A, Takayasu H. Relation of spontaneous passage of ureteral calculi to size. *Urology* 1977; **10**:544.
10 Morse RM, Resnick MI. Ureteral calculi: natural history and treatment in an era of advanced technology. *J Urol* 1991;**145**: 263–5.
11 Danuser H, Ackermann DK, March DC, Studer AE, Zingg EJ. Extracorporeal shock wave lithotripsy *in situ* or after push-up for upper ureteral calculi: a prospective randomized trial. *J Urol* 1993;**150**:824–6.
12 Hendrikx AJM, Bierkens AF, Oosterhof GON, Debruyne FMJ. Treatment of proximal and midureteral calculi: a randomized trial of *in situ* and pushback extracorporeal lithotripsy. *J Endourol* 1990;**4**:353–61.
13 Fetner CD, Preminger GM, Seger J, Lea TA. Treatment of ureteral calculi by extracorporeal shock wave lithotripsy at a multi-use centre. *J Urol* 1988;**139**:1192.
14 Preminger GM, Kettelhut MC, Elkins SL, Seger J, Fetner CD. Ureteral stenting during extracorporeal shock wave lithotripsy: help or hindrance? *J Urol* 1989;**142**:32–6.
15 Talati J, Khan LA, Noordzij JW *et al*. The scope and place of ultrasound-monitored extracorporeal shock wave lithotripsy in a multimodality setting and the effects of experimental, audit-evoked changes on the management of ureteric calculi. *Br J Urol* 1994;**73**:480–6.
16 Frabboni R, Santi V, Ronchi M *et al*. *In situ* echoguided extracorporeal shock wave lithotripsy of ureteric stones with the Dornier MPL 9000: a multicentre study group. *Br J Urol* 1994;**73**:487–93.
17 Watson GM, Landers B, Nauth-Misir R, Wickham JEA. Developments in the ureteroscopes, techniques and accessories associated with laser lithotripsy. *World J Urol* 1993;**11**: 19–25.
18 Zerbib M, Flam R, Belas M, Debre B, Steg A. Clinical experience with a new pulsed dye laser for ureteral stone lithotripsy. *J Urol* 1990;**143**:483–4.
19 Naqvi SAA, Khaliq M, Zafar MN, Rizvi SAH. Treatment of ureteric stones. Comparison of laser and pneumatic lithotripsy. *Br J Urol* 1994;**74**:694–8.
20 Wadhwa SN, Hemal AK, Sharma RK. Intracorporeal lithotripsy with the Swiss lithoclast. *Br J Urol* 1994;**74**:699–702.
21 Wu TT, Hsu TH, Li AF, Chen MT, Chang LS. Morphological change in the urothelium after electrohydraulic versus pulsed dye laser lithotripsy. *Br J Urol* 1994;**74**:685–9.
22 Gaur RP. Retroperitoneal laparoscopy: some modifications. *Br J Urol* 1996;**77**:304–6.

63 Management of Bladder and Urethral Calculi

M.Bhandari and R.Ahlawat

Introduction

Descriptions of procedures for the removal of bladder calculi are as old as the history of urology itself. Ancient bladder stones formed over the foreign bodies used for sexual gratification could fill a museum. The performance of crude transurethral procedures as early as the third century BC by Ammonios and suprapubic removal of calculi described in India about 2000 BC [1] are a testimony to this fact. In the sixth century BC the famous Indian surgeon Sushruta stated that the art of extracting bladder stones 'should be taught by withdrawing seeds from the kernel of a vimbi, vilva or jackfruit' [2]. Open surgical techniques for stone removal attained a peak of popularity during the eighteenth century, while the transurethral approach to bladder calculi has almost replaced open surgery during the last century.

Masterly transurethral removal of bladder stones started with blind lithotripsy under tactile guidance [3], a technique which had its proponents until as late as the early 1970s. The introduction of fibre optic systems for endoscopic illumination and visualization was the key factor responsible for the revolution in the technique of transurethral removal of bladder stones under vision. Mechanical grinding of big calculi before their removal progressed to quick disintegration within the bladder by the application of a variety of energies. Today ultrasonic, electrohydraulic and, lately, lithoclast energies have made the removal of bladder stones per urethram straightforward.

Aetiology

Bladder calculous disease can be broadly divided into: (i) a primary endemic variety, occurring in children; and (ii) calculi secondary to bladder outlet obstruction, lower urinary tract infection or foreign bodies such as indwelling urethral catheters. Secondary calculi may also drop to the bladder as a result of migration from the upper tract, the bladder acting only as a catchment area where the stone may grow further.

Primary disease

Primary bladder stone disease affects children under 10 years of age, and has a strong predilection for males. It is a distinct entity and is not associated with upper urinary tract calculus disease. There is no evidence of lower urinary tract obstruction or dysfunction in these children and 80% of the bladders on operation are found to have near normal bladder mucosa devoid of any evidence of bladder hypertrophy, cystitis or other gross bladder changes [4]. Such stones are usually solitary with a variable composition and have a well-defined nucleus surrounded by concentric laminations.

The geographical distribution of the disease has changed with time. The disease has disappeared from affluent industrialized societies. In Europe, the incidence has now dropped to 10% of all urolithiasis cases from a high of 80% in the nineteenth century. An endemic bladder stone disease zone presently extends from southern Russia, Egypt, Turkey, Israel, Lebanon and Syria to China, Thailand and Indonesia including Iran, Pakistan and India. However, they are uncommon in south and central Africa as well as in South and Central America. Within the countries of high incidence there appears to be a great variance in the prevalence rate from one area to another, with a high incidence in non-industrialized and rural zones.

The geographical distribution of primary bladder stones in children has revealed that the incidence is highest in areas of mild to moderate protein energy malnutrition (PEM) but falls significantly in areas with a severe degree of PEM [5]. Evidence of keratinization of the bladder mucosa as expected in vitamin A deficiency, implicated as a cause of these stones in the past, has been found lacking on careful examination of urothelium at the time of surgery; up to 85% of patients have normal-looking urothelium.

Composition of these stones has been shown to be predominantly ammonium acid urate (AAU) and calcium oxalate in an X-ray diffraction study of primary bladder stones in Indian children [6]. In some areas, stones are predominantly formed of AAU and phosphates, whereas in certain parts of the world pure urate calculi predominate. A high concentration of uric acid and ammonia is necessary to form AAU at normal urinary pH in sterile urine [7]. While precipitates below pH 5.8 mainly consist of uric acid, AAU predominates as the pH rises above 6.3. The requirement of ammonia to form AAU crystals has been shown to decrease significantly after some urate crystals have initially formed [8]. While consumption of whole wheat as a staple food has been cited as a cause of increased saturation of uric acid in the urine of these children, dehydration and acidosis from fever and diarrhoea may raise the concentration of ammonium ions, apart from further supersaturating the urine with uric acid. A deficiency of dietary phosphate, chronic dehydration and excessive protein and oxalate consumption have been implicated as other possible aetiological factors [9].

Secondary disease

In sharp contrast, adult bladder stone disease is secondary to urinary stasis due to bladder outflow obstruction. Infection often plays a major part in the formation, growth and recurrence of this secondary bladder stone disease. Truly migratory stones from the upper tract, having passed through the ureterovesical junction, generally continue their journey to the exterior rather than settling and growing further in the bladder, unless there is some functional or anatomical infravesical obstruction. The composition of migrated stones is, obviously, similar to those in the kidney, while the type of further growth locally is dependent upon the local environment, pH and the presence or absence of infection.

The propensity of foreign bodies to induce stone formation by acting as a nidus for calculus encrustation in the bladder (Fig. 63.1) even in the absence of infection has long been recognized. The introduction of a foreign body into the bladder is a standard experimental method to study nucleation and growth characteristics of calculi [10]. In these cases, the initial factor in stone formation is phosphate deposition over the surface of the foreign body. The commonest example of stone formation over a foreign body is encrustation over longstanding catheters and self-retaining stents.

Diagnosis

Primary bladder stone disease is predominantly found in male children between the ages of 1 and 8 years, with a peak incidence at the age of 3 years. Urine may often be passed more comfortably in odd postures and children often present with vague abdominal pain, abrupt interruption of the urinary stream and crying during urination. Pulling and rubbing of the prepuce and the passage of cloudy urine that leaves a white sandy residue is often reported by the parents. While such symptoms are diagnostic of bladder calculi in children in endemic areas, such symptoms are usually missing in adults with secondary calculi, the commonest patients in most urological practices. The symptoms of associated urinary stasis with or without urinary tract infection in the latter patients dominate the

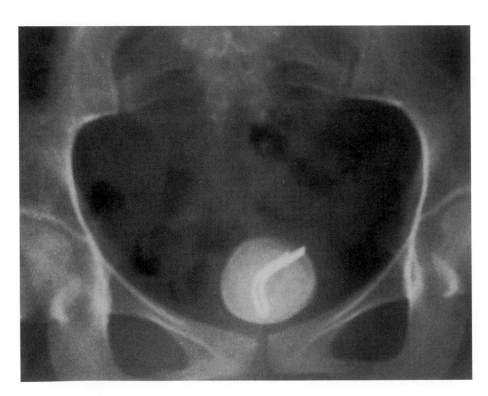

Fig. 63.1 A 17-year-old female with a bladder calculus: a plain X-ray of the pelvis showed a hairpin embedded in the stone, the pointer to its aetiology. The girl, in retrospect, admitted to have inserted it 'inadvertently'.

picture, although the clinical diagnosis is usually made with some secondary clues. Males with anatomical bladder outlet obstruction and those with functional neurogenic vesicourethral dysfunction comprise the high-risk groups. In a patient with outlet obstruction, symptoms such as terminal haematuria, episodic pain referred to the tip of the penis or pain and sudden interruption of the urinary stream in the sitting or erect posture may indicate an underlying bladder stone. Patients with neglected neurogenic vesico-urethral dysfunction presenting with massive phosphaturia and the passage of large amounts of debris per urethram also indicate the presence of bladder stones. A careful history of the possibility of a foreign body such as the use of an indwelling catheter or a ureteric stent will facilitate the diagnosis of stones formed over foreign bodies. However, stones formed over foreign bodies deliberately introduced through the urethra are only diagnosed on imaging or during a careful history bringing out a confession that the foreign body has been inserted.

Stones may also be formed over non-absorbable suture material used in the bladder, as happened in one of the author's experience in one female patient following the successful repair of a difficult vesicovaginal fistula via the vaginal route. During the follow-up period the patient continued to have infection and investigations revealed a bladder stone which on exploration was found to be stuck to the bladder mucosa over the suture line within the bladder. Evidence of the Prolene suture in the substance of the stone confirmed its formation over sutures used for the closure of the vaginal layer.

Occasionally very large calculi (Fig. 63.2) may be palpated abdominally or vaginally. Palpation of a stone on bimanual examination in a child, when the child relaxes the abdominal muscles during crying, is a reliable sign of a bladder stone. This finding in children is possible mainly on account of a thin abdominal wall muscle mass and the absence of a prostate. There are no reliable physical findings for the specific diagnosis of bladder stone associated with prostatic hypertrophy or neurogenic bladder in adults.

Biochemical studies are normal. Impairment of renal function is usually the result of underlying pathology such as intrinsic renal disease or obstructive uropathy. Urinalysis reveals microscopic haematuria and heavy pyuria. Infection may or may not be present. The cornerstone of diagnosis, however, is imaging. Ultrasonographic examination reveals an acoustic shadow cast by the stone irrespective of its radiodensity. Stones with a large amount of uric acid may not be seen on a plain radiograph and appear as filling defects in the bladder films of an intravenous pyelogram or cystography or as an acoustic shadow on ultrasound. At times, stones in a pelvic kidney or a ureterocele may appear to be within the bladder on plain radiography (Fig. 63.3), while carcinoma of the bladder, ureterocele or a clot may cast a filling defect in the cystogram. A fixed position of the shadow on different films on the same side of the midline should arouse such suspicion, which may be confirmed by an ultrasound examination. Computed tomography is very rarely required to establish the diagnosis. The passage of a metal dilator to

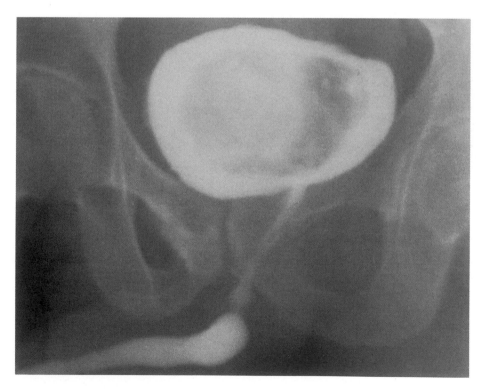

Fig. 63.2 A giant bladder calculus occupying almost the whole of the bladder is seen as a negative shadow in this cystourethrogram. The stone was palpable on rectal examination.

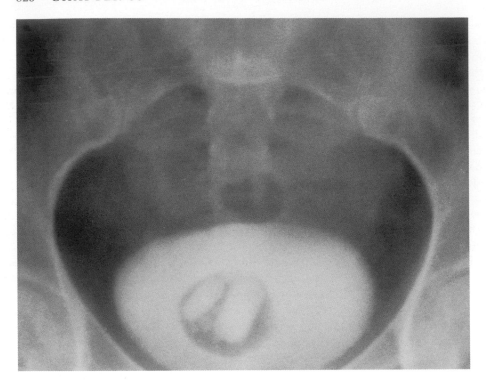

Fig. 63.3 Multiple calculi within the bladder area were found to be present within a ureterocele. Existence of the ureterocele had been suspected because of the persistence of all the calculi to appear together at a similar location in two successive plain X-rays.

sound the stone as a diagnostic tool is mentioned only to be condemned. Cystoscopic examination is the definitive investigation to diagnose bladder stones, although bladder calculi embedded within the bladder wall due to associated cystitis glandularis mimicking carcinoma of the bladder have been reported.

Management

The management of a bladder stone cannot be isolated from the treatment of the underlying disease. As far as possible, the method chosen should be able to treat the stone as well as the underlying condition predisposing to the stone. The bladder may be approached transurethrally or through the suprapubic route. With the advent of advances in endoscopic techniques and the availability of various energy sources for intracorporeal destruction of stones, the per urethral approach under vision is more popular with urologists. While approaching the stone transurethrally, the factors that have to be kept in mind are the calibre of the urethra, the size of the instrument that is chosen, as well as the likely duration of the contact between the instrument and the urethra. The importance of an instrument with a calibre smaller than the urethra and completion of the procedure within an acceptable period to keep the iatrogenic insult to the urethra to a minimum cannot be over emphasized. The calibre of the instrument largely depends upon the method of disintegration. The duration of the procedure, however, depends not only upon the efficacy of the energy source, but also to a large extent upon the size

and the composition of the stone. The suprapubic route, besides being popular for open surgical removal of large bladder stones, is also being increasingly utilized for percutaneous disintegration and retrieval of large stones, especially when the urethra may not be suitable for endoscopic procedures. Chemodissolution and extracorporeal shockwave lithotripsy of bladder stones are alternative methods of management where the invasion may be minimal but the treatment time may be long and tedious. The best treatment is minimally invasive as well as quick.

Transurethral approach

Classic blind litholapaxy

Blind lithotripsy using the Bigelow technique is a fading art. The safe accomplishment of stone destruction and removal by this method requires considerable surgical dexterity. Experts were able to produce extremely good results [11], and the technique was described in detail by Swift-Joly in 1929. The instrument needs to be removed intermittently for visualization and evacuation of fragments. However, the potential for causing severe bladder damage in the hands of an inexperienced urologist has rendered the technique obsolete. The high incidence of bladder injury is on account of gradual emptying of the bladder during the procedure escaping the attention of the surgeon and inexperienced tactile guidance in grasping the stone with the jaws of the lithotrite while trying to avoid entrapment of the bladder wall.

Endoscopic mechanical lithotripsy

The introduction of optical systems made possible the undertaking of the entire procedure under vision, thus improving the safety of mechanical lithotripsy; however, incorporation of the optics within the same calibre instrument resulted in a loss of strength of the crushing jaws. The technique works well with small stones up to 2–2.5 cm diameter. Deterioration of the endoscopic vision as and when haematuria develops during a prolonged procedure while disintegrating a large stone, necessitates periodic emptying of the bladder resulting in frequent interruptions. A variety of lithotrites is available which allow direct visual control (Lowsley, Hendrickson, Mauermyer). They work on a common principle, enabling a stone to be grasped and destroyed under vision, followed by the complete removal of fragments under visual monitoring either by using an Ellick evacuator, a Toomey syringe or by using various grasping instruments. The availability of intracorporeal lithotripsy has restricted the use of mechanical lithotripters to smaller stones only.

Endoscopic lithotripsy with intracorporeal stone disintegration devices

An ultrasonic lithotripter (Fig. 63.4) comprises a purpose-built lithotripter, ultrasound transducer, a hollow sonotrode and an external generator. A foot switch operates a roller pump which is incorporated for simultaneous evacuation of stone fragments as well as cooling of the sonotrode. Ultrasound energy of 20–27 kHz disintegrates urinary calculi through a drill-like action. Longitudinal and transverse vibrations result in a jackhammer impact of the hollow sonotrode probe. However, the rigid nature of the sonotrode requires a straight working channel and an angled eye-piece for vision. Such a lithotripter has proved to be effective for the disintegration of bladder stones and

the design has been modified to deal with a larger bulk by engaging the stones [12]. However, the ultrasonic generator is more commonly used for the disintegration of upper urinary tract stones. The ultrasonic lithotrite has been found to be valuable in patients with struvite calculi. Calcium monohydrate and calcium phosphate stones can be too hard to fragment; urate stones are also resistant to ultrasound fragmentation. This technique is best restricted to stones less than 3 cm in diameter. Though the energy is relatively weak, there are certain advantages of this technique over electrohydraulic fragmentation: ultrasound energy does not damage the bladder wall and the stone is drilled systematically and does not jump around the bladder, which may happen with electrohydraulic disintegration.

Goldberg applied the destructive property of electro-hydraulic shockwaves on stones within a liquid medium for the treatment of bladder stones [13]. The equipment (Fig. 63.5) consists of a pulse generator, electrodes and a foot pedal to activate the probe. The Calcutript (manufactured by Storz, Germany) works at a maximum pressure of 1020 bar. The size of the flexible electrodes used ranges from 3 to 9 F and may be used through the side channel of a cystoscope. The equipment has the potential for providing pulses at various power levels at frequencies ranging from a single shot to 70 shots/s and the duration of the pulses can be varied between 1 and 5 s. The stone is exposed to pulses of hydraulic shockwaves which are produced by high voltage, underwater discharges in one-sixth normal saline. The pressure curve of the electrohydraulic waves decays from the point of discharge, hence it is necessary to keep the calculus close to the probe. The pressure front of the impulse is partially reflected by the calculus, resulting in a rebound phase and, subsequently, additional high strain forces and cavitation phenomena within the stone. Strict adherence to electrical safety precautions is necessary and the probe must be

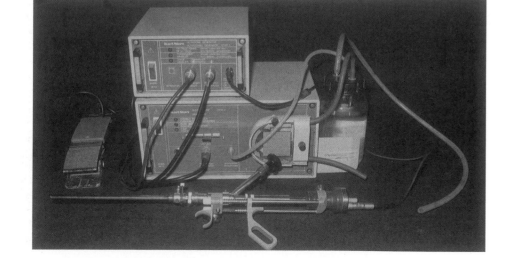

Fig. 63.4 Ultrasonic lithotripter for intracorporeal stone disintegration, complete with an ultrasonic generator and roller pump. The purpose-built cystoscope sheath can be seen in the foreground with the facility to mount the transducer and sonotrode in the bracket at the back.

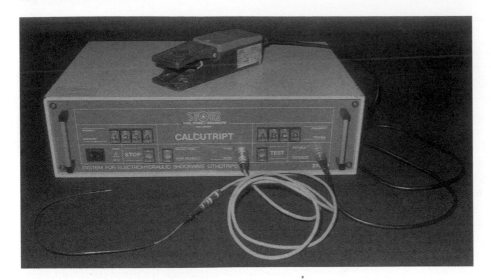

Fig. 63.5 An electrohydraulic shockwave generator. Note the flexible probe which can be passed through the catheter channel of a standard cystoscope.

kept at least 5 mm away from the bladder wall, as any tissue within 5 mm of the point of discharge is hit by the full impact of the shockwave, resulting in the disruption of tissue. Furthermore, the lens of the telescope may be damaged if the end of the probe is too close at the time of discharge. Electrohydraulic energy is powerful and effective in fragmenting bladder calculi in most cases [14,15].

The poor response of hard stones larger than 3 cm in diameter and safety concerns when using electrohydraulic energy were indications for investigating other safer energy sources. While some, like the Q-switched pulsed dye laser, were found to be too weak, others like the microexplosion technique were too complex and cumbersome. The latter technique was used for the treatment of bladder stones by Watanabe *et al.* [16]. Through a cystoscope made for the purpose, 2–10 mg of lead azide was used to disintegrate the stone by creating an explosion chamber in a special detonator catheter. For larger stones it was necessary to

drill holes and four to six detonations were required to ensure total fragmentation. A new energy source, the Swiss Lithoclast (Fig. 63.6), designed on a pneumatic principle and primarily for upper urinary tract stones, holds promise for bladder calculi [17]. This energy source combines safety to tissues, as in conventional ultrasound, with much more power, as needed for quick disintegration of large bladder stones. Energy may be delivered via 0.8–2 mm rigid and semirigid probes through standard nephroscopes and ureteroscopes.

Percutaneous cystolithotripsy

With the refinements of percutaneous surgery for renal stones, the percutaneous technique has also found an application in the treatment of large bladder stones [18]. The equipment required for this technique is the same as that used for the upper tract. The bladder is punctured suprapubically and a tract is established using dilators. The

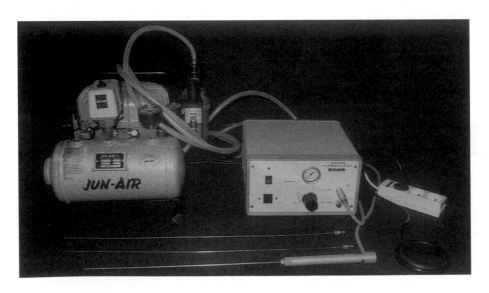

Fig. 63.6 The Swiss Lithoclast with shockwave generator and compressor. Though the thick probes are rigid, the thin probes meant for ureteric use are semirigid and can also be passed through the side channel. The angulation, however, reduces the energy at the tip of the probe.

track is held open using an Amplatz sheath. The stone is destroyed using any of the disintegration devices mentioned above. This approach is preferred over the transurethral route in a situation when the urethra is narrowed by a stricture or is of inadequate size and in patients with a suprapubic cystostomy which has already been established. The only problem encountered is the evacuation of fragments in elderly patients; it has been found that the evacuators cannot be used effectively through the suprapubic route. There is a tendency for the fragments to settle in the retroprostatic space. By using this technique with larger stones it is possible to avoid trauma to the urethra induced by prolonged contact of the instrument within the urethra and frequent removal and insertion of the instrument, which may lead to a high incidence of stricture of the urethra.

Open cystolithotomy

Despite the availability of various endoscopic techniques, open cystolithotomy may still be a wise, safe and efficient choice in some patients. A very large stone, a contracted bladder, the need to remove a large prostate simultaneously or even staging the management of the bladder neck or urethral condition transurethrally (prostate resection, visual urethrotomy) for a later date may all be indications for such a decision.

Extracorporeal shockwave lithotripsy

Despite being the least invasive technique available to date,

the application of this modality to manage bladder stones has not gained popularity. While one of the reasons is the ease with which the urinary bladder, a hollow organ with direct access to the exterior, can be approached per urethram, there is a technical concern too. A stone in the bladder, when subjected to lithotripsy, is likely to jump around freely in the bladder and would need to be refocused repeatedly. The value of the technique's non-invasive nature is further lost as even after fragmentation it may well be necessary to evacuate the stone fragments, either with the help of an endoscope introduced through the urethra or through an indwelling catheter in the bladder, as bladder outlet pathology is often co-existent.

Urethral calculi

The common urethral calculi encountered are the migratory non-urethral calculi from the upper tract or bladder which become lodged, usually in the prostatic urethra or at the fossa navicularis. Calculi formed within the urethra are uncommon but not rare and may form in a dilated prostatic urethra proximal to an obstruction, e.g. stricture disease (Fig. 63.7) or in a urethral diverticulum. Asymptomatic small stones are not uncommonly found over the hair following skin inlay urethroplasties when hair-bearing scrotal skin has been used.

Fixed stones over hair in urethroplasty patients and impacted stones in a dilated proximal urethra in patients with stricture disease, especially those on supravesical diversion, may be incidental discoveries. Migratory calculi in the urethra usually present as an emergency as painful

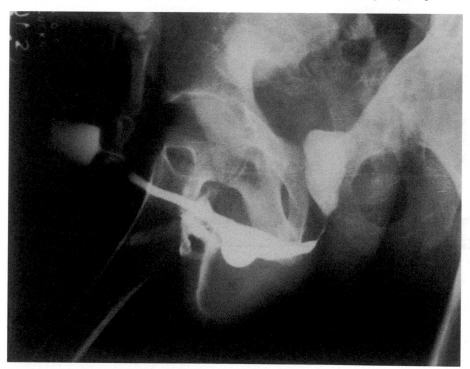

Fig. 63.7 A large urethral calculus impacted in a dilated posterior urethra proximal to a urethral stricture.

retention. Stones large enough to cause symptoms in the urethra may be palpable externally or on rectal examination, though some may be missed due to dense periurethral scarring. A plain X-ray may not include the urethra below the membranous region so radiologists must make sure to include this region. The presence of calculi in the upper urinary tract should always be looked for.

Spontaneous passage of the majority of urethral calculi has been reported following per urethral instillation of 2% lignocaine jelly [19] and is initially worth trying if the urologist is sure of the migratory nature of the calculus. The calculus may also be flushed back with saline or pushed back into the bladder while attempting to catheterize the patient with painful retention. If catheterization has been successful in disimpacting the stone into the bladder, the emergency is averted and the catheter may be left indwelling until the urethral calculus, now a bladder stone, is managed electively.

The type of intervention that becomes necessary when these initial manoeuvres fail would largely depend upon the size of the calculus, the calibre of the urethra and the site of impaction, apart from the status of the associated urethral disease if present. Successful milking of calculi impacted in the navicular fossa with or without the use of a meatotomy and the use of a Fogarty catheter for their extraction [20] have been reported. Endoscopic manipulation of proximal urethral calculi back into the bladder before disintegration and evacuation as bladder stones is likely to be the management favoured by most urologists. Associated urethral pathology may be treated at the same time. If disimpaction fails, ultrasonic disintegration of large urethral calculi may be accomplished within the urethra without any adverse effect to the urethral mucosa [21]. A new generation of imaginative, non-invasive urologists may find a place for extracorporeal shockwave lithotripsy in the treatment of urethral calculi [22]. Urethrotomy with subsequent removal of the calculus may be a safe option in infants or young children where the urethral calibre is a matter of concern for instrumentation.

References

1 Clark ES. A history of the stone. *Br J Hosp Med* 1968;**2**: 1054–7.

2 Sushruta. *Sushruta Samhita* (an English translation based on the original Sanskrit text, edited and published by Kaviraj Kunja Lal Bhishagratna in 3 volumes), Vol. 1. Calcutta: Wilkins Press, 1907:30.

3 Bigelow HJ. Lithotrity—a single operation. *Boston Med Surg J* 1879;**98**:259.

4 Aurora AL, Taneja OP, Gupta DN. Bladder stone disease of childhood—a clinicopathological study. *Acta Ped Scand* 1970; **59**:385–98.

5 Teotia M, Teotia SPS. Inhibitors of crystallisation in bladder stone in children. *Lancet* 1972;**1**:599.

6 Rao MVR, Agarwal JS, Taneja OP. Studies in urolithiasis II. X-ray diffraction analysis of calculi from Delhi region. *Indian J Med Res* 1976;**132**:1117–20.

7 Teotia M, Sutor DJ. Crystallisation of ammonium acid urate and other uric acid derivatives of urine. *Br J Urol* 1971;**43**: 381–6.

8 Brockis JG, Boyyer RC, McCullock RK *et al.* Pathophysiology of endemic bladder stones. In: Brockis GJ, Finlayson B (eds) *Urinary Calculus.* Littleton, MA: PSG Publishing, 1981:237.

9 Van Reen R. Idiopathic urinary bladder stones of childhood. *Aust NZ J Surg* 1980;**50**:18.

10 Khan SR, Finlayson B, Hackett RL. Microstructure of calcium oxalate foreign body stones produced in rat bladder. *Urol Res* 1984;**12**:54.

11 Hadley HL, Barnes RW, Rosenquist RC. Tactile litholapaxy—safe and efficient. *Urology* 1977;**9**:263–5.

12 El Fahiq S, Wallace DM. Ultrasonic lithotripsy for urethral and bladder stones. *Br J Urol* 1978;**50**:255–6.

13 Goldberg VV. On the history of electrohydraulic lithotripsy method. *Urol Nefrol (Moscow)* 1974;**50**:90.

14 Comisarow RH, Barkin M. Electrohydraulic cystolitholapaxy. *Can J Surg* 1979;**22**:525–6.

15 Raney AM. Electrohydraulic cystolithotripsy. *Urology* 1976;**7**: 379–81.

16 Watanabe H, Watanabe K, Shiino K *et al.* Microexplosion cystolithotripsy. *J Urol* 1983;**129**:23.

17 Wisard M, Jichlinski P, Languetin JM *et al.* Première evaluation clinique du lithoclaste CHUV à enegie blastique. *Helv Chir Acta* 1991;**58**:318–21.

18 Miller RA, McNicholas TA, Carter S *et al.* Percutaneous vesical endoscopy and local anaesthetic rigid endoscopy: two new techniques. *J Endourol* 1987;**1**:317–23.

19 El Sherif AE, El Hafi R. Proposed new method for nonoperative treatment of urethral stones. *J Urol* 1991;**146**:1546–7.

20 Jackson RS. Urethral stone managed with fogarty catheter. *N Engl J Med* 1971;**285**:1469.

21 Durazi MH, Samiei MR. Ultrasonic fragmentation in the treatment of male urethral calculi. *Br J Urol* 1981;**62**:443–4.

22 Kramolowsky EV, Leoning SA. Extracorporeal shock wave lithotripsy: noninvasive treatment for the treatment of bulbous urethral stones. *J Urol* 1988;**139**:362–3.

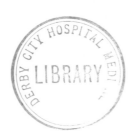

64 Horizons in Urolithiasis

F. Eisenberger and A. S. Schmidt

Introduction

The treatment of urolithiasis has undergone enormous developments within the last 15 years. The 'gold standard' of open surgery was replaced by less invasive methods like extracorporeal shockwave lithotripsy (ESWL), ureteroscopy and percutaneous nephrolithotomy. During the last few years these new treatment modalities have themselves been improved and new technical developments like laser lithotripsy have been introduced, which has opened up new options for the treatment of different stone entities. Furthermore, in recent years political pressure has developed on the health care systems of all industrial countries to improve the cost effectiveness of treatment. This is an appropriate time to summarize the current status of stone therapy and to discuss possible developments and trends for the future.

The future of extracorporeal shockwave lithotripsy

Since the introduction of ESWL into clinical use for the treatment of urolithiasis 10 years ago, lithotripter technology has undergone many technical developments. Initially, the Dornier HM3 lithotripter used an underwater spark discharge for the generation of shockwaves which were directed and coupled into the body via a complete water bath, while the stone was focused with biplanar fluoroscopy systems. Subsequently, different shockwave sources were established, either using an electromagnetic membrane configured plane (Siemens Lithostar, Dornier Compact) or cylindrically (Storz Modulith), or spherically aligned piezoelectric elements (Wolf Piezolith, EDAP, Diasonic). Shockwave coupling is achieved using a water-filled cushion and ultrasound is used for stone location. Many papers have been published to prove the feasibility of these new so-called 'second-generation' lithotripters in clinical routine, emphasizing the advantages in handling, reduced costs and reduction of pain sensation during treatment, making anaesthesia unnecessary in the majority of cases. On the other hand, treatment results in terms of stone disintegration and total stone clearance requiring minimal numbers of treatment sessions have not been as good as those published initially with the unmodified Dornier HM3 device—reporting 72% stone-free patients and 95% with fragments less than 5 mm in diameter with a retreatment rate of 1.44 [1].

Virgili et al. [2] reported the results of treatment in 930 patients using a Wolf Piezolith 2300, with complete disintegration in 90.1% of cases, achieving a stone-free status in 77.5%, but requiring 2.4 sessions per patient on average. Psihramis et al. [3] published the results of the first 1000 cases treated with a Siemens Lithostar: satisfactory disintegration occurred in 72%, the stone-free rate was 55.7% and the retreatment rate was 1.18. Nevertheless, the comparison of treatment data from different centres is difficult due to different stone populations, stone composition, individual treatment strategies and national health care systems. A Dutch study group tried to compare the efficacy and complications of five different second-generation lithotripters (Siemens Lithostar, Dornier HM4, Wolf Piezolith 2300, Direx Tripter X-1, Breakstone Lithotripter) [4]. While the success rate of 75% in terms of complete fragmentation was astonishingly constant for all the tested devices, significant differences were found for retreatment rates, between 1.1 for the Dornier HM4 and 1.34 for the Wolf Piezolith 2300. The number of shockwaves applied ranged from 3546 with the Siemens Lithostar to 1287 with the Breakstone Lithotripter. The need for anaesthesia also differred: 90% of patients treated with the Dornier HM4 and 97% with the Wolf Piezolith 2300 did not receive any anaesthesia at all, while 44% of patients treated with the Direx Tripter X-1 and 25% with the Breakstone Lithotripter received general anaesthesia. These clinical findings are reproducible in an experimental setting using artificial stones; with the same number of shocks, stone volume loss was greatest with the electrohydraulic machine (Dornier HM4), followed by the electromagnetic (Siemens Lithostar) and piezoelectric (Wolf Piezolith 2300) lithotripters for both low- and high-intensity settings [5].

Increasing experience with ultrasound-guided litho-tripters proved that particular advantages of ultrasound (e.g. cost reduction, permanent monitoring, lack of exposure to ionizing radiation) could not cancel out certain dis-advantages, such as difficulties in locating ureteric calculi, control of disintegration and stone location in obese patients or those with horseshoe kidneys. On the other hand, the drawbacks of pure fluoroscopic stone visualiza-tion are well known: focusing of radiolucent stones and—though in the days of laparoscopic cholecystectomy less important—the treatment of gall stones. Therefore, a combination of both stone-locating systems is a major demand of clinicians to the manufacturers of lithotripters. Different solutions to this problem have been found.

Siemens integrated a new overhead module in the Lithostar, with an in-line ultrasound unit in the centre of the electromagnetic membrane, with a larger aperture to increase the pressure within a smaller area, because gall stones require higher shockwave pressures for fragmenta-tion. The Mainz group reported 75 patients treated within 15 months with this device. They found a disintegration rate of 86% and a stone-free rate after 3 months of 78% [6]. Netto et al. emphasized the impact of the Lithostar Plus in the treatment of 23 radiolucent calculi with a stone-free rate of 76.4%, evaluated with excretory urography and ultrasound [7].

The Storz Modulith SL20 provides ultrasound and fluoroscopic imaging by the use of an in-line ultrasound scanner within the shockwave source and an external C-arm after moving the patient along the unit's longitudinal axis. Liston et al. reported the results of treating 500 patients with this unit achieving a stone-free rate after 3 months of 77.6% and complete disintegration in 92.3% of patients [8]. The treatment was performed in the majority of cases without any anaesthesia or analgesia, with less than 2% of patients receiving general anaesthesia, although the retreatment rate of 1.4 have to be considered relatively high [8]. Similar data have been obtained using the Therasonic lithotripter, a device with a piezoelectric shockwave source, in-line ultrasound scanner and an external X-ray unit [9].

The new Dornier Lithotripter features an endoscopic table with the fluoroscopy unit mounted on a C-arm while the therapy unit consists of an electromagnetic membrane and in-line ultrasound which is applied in an oblique position. Shockwave coupling is performed using a conical water bag thereby avoiding interference with the X-ray system. The shockwave source provides a maximum pressure of 80 MPa with a –6 dB focal size of 58 mm by 2.5 mm. After the first 775 treatments complete disintegra-tion was achieved in 94% of cases requiring a retreatment rate of 1.28. At the 3-month follow-up a stone-free status was found in 85.9% of patients. These figures prove the efficacy of a combination of ultrasound and fluoroscopy for

stone location and a high shockwave pressure for stone disintegration [10].

On the other hand, the application of high energy shockwaves raises the question of biological side effects. In clinical practice haematuria is a common finding after ESWL. In nuclear magnetic tomographic studies, intrarenal fluid collections have been detected in up to 74% [11]. Severe side effects, e.g. perirenal haematoma, are seen in 1–2% of cases. Very rarely, complications such as pancreatitis, arrhythmia or intestinal bleeding have been reported [12]. Animal experiments have been reported to evaluate the relationship of renal lesions to the number of shockwaves, shockwave energy and application frequency. A classification of shockwave-induced renal trauma has been proposed. In the very low energy range no vascular lesions are detectable. Histological investigations reveal sporadic necrosis of tubules (grade 0 lesion). In the low energy range petechial bleeding in the medullary region is detectable microscopically. Histologically, intratubular bleeding is found (grade I lesion). In the medium energy range, focal cortical haematoma are found. Histologically, rupture of the venules and arterioles was detected (grade II lesion). In the high energy range, perirenal haematoma caused by rupture of the arteriae interlobulares were found (grade III lesion) [13].

The relationship between renal trauma and the mechanism of shockwave generation remains unresolved if the different numbers of shockwaves that are necessary for comparable clinical results of each lithotripter are taken into account. Therefore, the question of the optimal shock-wave source that would combine high disintegration capabilities and minimal damage to surrounding tissues is still unanswered, as neither the mechanisms of stone disintegration nor the mechanism of tissue damage are yet fully understood [14]. Nevertheless, the clinical impact of these findings seems to be minor, because even after shockwave treatment in children no changes in renal size and function were found after a follow-up of 149 weeks [15]. On the other hand, it has to be conceded that efficient shockwave disintegration is associated with a potential risk of renal trauma.

More recently, the speed of innovation in ESWL has reduced, suggesting that the technical improvements may be exhausted; a breakthrough in improving stone dis-integration seems to be unlikely. Efforts to improve the technology will be focused on lithotripter handling, multifunctional use and lowering treatment costs, without opening up new treatment options.

Extracorporeal shockwave lithotripsy for ureteric calculi

ESWL, originally designed for the treatment of renal stones, has also been used to treat ureteric calculi. Complete disintegration has been achieved *in situ* in 80% of patients only [16]. Reasons for these reduced success rates are: (i) the attenuation of shockwave energy by 14% when compared to renal ESWL because of reflection of the shockwaves by bones or soft tissues [17]; (ii) the lack of an expansion chamber inhibits the dispersion of fragments leading to a shell formation, which reflects the shockwave energy, retarding further disintegration [18]; and (iii) the lack of a fluid interphase around the stone prevents the generation of cavitation effects [19]. Furthermore, the localization of ureteric stones may be restricted, in the case of the Dornier HM3, by the oblique arrangement of the X-ray tubes; additionally, the detection of stones by ultrasound is limited to either the upper ureter when there is significant dilatation or to the prevesical part of the ureter. In an experimental investigation, Parr *et al.* [20] compared the fragmentation rate of artificial calculi placed freely in a latex bag with the fragmentation rate after confining the stone in a latex tube with or without external tension. They found a fragmentation rate five times higher for free stones in comparison to confined stones; further constriction led to a less significant diminution. Interestingly, the placement of a stent along the impacted stone did not lead to improved fragmentation. In clinical practice using a Wolf Piezolith 2300 with ultrasonic stone location, complete stone disintegration without auxiliary endoscopic measures occurred only in 63%, and even then a large number of shockwaves (mean 6271) was administered [20]. Mashimo *et al.* [21] reported successful treatment of 15 of 79 patients with mid-ureteric stones with another ultrasound-guided device, the EDAP LT-01 lithotripter [21]. After *in situ* ESWL of ureteric calculi using the Siemens Lithostar and the Storz Modulith SL20, complete disintegration was found in 90 and 85%, respectively, of patients requiring 1.5 and 1.15 treatments on average [22,23]. Using the Dornier MPL 9000X, equipped with an integrated C-arm, successful *in situ* treatment of ureteric stones was achieved in 86.7% of patients [24]. These data support the role of *in situ* ESWL of ureteric stones as the minimal invasive therapy of first choice under particular preconditions: fluoroscopic stone detection, prone positioning for mid-ureteric stones and high shockwave energy.

Ureteroscopy for ureteric calculi

Based on the pioneering work of Lyon *et al.* [25] and Perez-Castro and Martinez-Pineiro [26] in 1979, the development of ESWL was paralleled by improvements in ureteroscopy. Initially, instruments with an outer diameter of 9.5 F were available using rod lenses. While access to the distal third of the ureter was possible in most cases, more difficulties were encountered in the upper parts of the ureter. With the development of fibreoptic ureteroscopes providing smaller outer diameters of less than 6 F at the tip and semi-rigidity

(i.e. a clear view even if the instrument became slightly bent) a ureteroscopic approach to the entire ureter became possible in almost every case. Unfortunately, these miniaturized instruments provide only a small working channel of 3 F or even less, compromising irrigation flow and the feasibility of using instruments for stone retrieval or intraureteric lithotripsy [27].

Different methods for stone disintegration have been used within the last decade. Initially, ultrasound via rigid probes was used. One disadvantage was that the rigid probe necessitated an oblique view into the ureteroscope, with difficult instrumentation in the upper tract in particular. Also the use of ultrasound provoked the risk of ureteric damage because of high temperatures at the tip of the probe, especially if irrigation was not sufficient. Electrohydraulic lithotripsy underwent significant improvements, enabling the use of thin flexible probes via semirigid or flexible instruments with more selective energy settings [28]; however, the unselective energy absorption of mucosa and stone can result in ureteric trauma.

A relatively new and effective method for intraluminal lithotripsy is the Swiss Lithoclast. Stone disintegration is performed with a pneumatically driven ballistic system. Advantages of the device are the extraordinary reliability and easy handling of the system; the disadvantages are the rigidity of the probe requiring an almost straight working channel, and an energy application parallel to the ureter causing stone migration into upper parts of the collecting system [29].

Since the 1980s, lasers have been developed for the intraluminal destruction of urinary calculi. Solid state systems (neodymium-yttrium aluminium garnet (Nd-YAG), alexandrite) have been utilized as well as pulsed dye lasers (coumarin, rhodamine) providing disintegration rates between 80 and 90% [30–35]. Basically, all these devices generate a plasma bubble between the fibre tip and the stone; the ultrathin fibres, with diameters between 200 and 300 μm, can be introduced even through flexible ureteroscopes. As the energy absorption of stone and tissue is different selective energy application is possible, destroying the stone and sparing the ureter. Disadvantages of all lasers are the high costs of the devices (approximately US$200 000) and the time-consuming procedure.

Further development of rigid or semirigid ureteroscopy seems unlikely, as a further diminution of the calibre of the instrument will compromise stability of the instrument, reduce visibility due to reduced irrigation, and render stone disintegration or retrieval less effective because a minimal mechanical strength of the devices is mandatory. The development of flexible, steerable ureteroscopes may open new possibilities, especially regarding anaesthesia-free use, but the limitations due to miniaturized irrigation and working ports are obvious.

Extracorporeal shockwave lithotripsy or percutaneous nephrolithotomy for staghorn calculi

Although initially established for the therapy of smaller renal stones, the success of ESWL treatment encouraged urologists to utilize this non-invasive method for the treatment of larger stones also. Wirth *et al.* [36] reported 186 patients with partial, and 55 patients with complete staghorn stones undergoing multistage ESWL monotherapy. After 1 year of follow-up 55% of all patients and 46% of patients with complete staghorn calculi were rendered stone-free. Although the rate of auxiliary measures at 50% was relatively high, severe complications were rare and the rate of urinary tract infection dropped from 50.6% initially to 22.5% post-treatment [36]. These results are comparable to those gained with a percutaneous or a combined approach for staghorn stones [37]. On the other hand, the variable classification of large renal calculi into two groups, partial and complete staghorn calculi, makes any comparison of treatment results difficult.

Lam *et al.* [38] introduced a stone classification by measuring the stone surface area. After stratification of their material, a stone-free rate of 94.4% was achieved after combination therapy of percutaneous nephrolithotomy and ESWL compared with 63.2% after ESWL monotherapy for stones with a surface smaller than 500 mm², and for stones with a surface area between 501 and 1000 mm² the figures were 86 and 45.7%, respectively. For even larger stones, stone-free rates of 82.4% after combination therapy and 22.2% after ESWL monotherapy were seen, which underlines the superiority of a primary percutaneous approach to large stones in terms of total stone clearance. Although the morbidity after this more invasive procedure was significantly higher, severe complications were avoided [38]. Therefore percutaneous nephrolithotomy remains an important tool in the management of staghorn stones, although the impact of ESWL increases.

Non-urological indications for shockwave application

Biliary lithotripsy

In 1985 shockwave lithotripsy was introduced for the treatment of gallstones. Ideal candidates for biliary lithotripsy were the so-called '4-S stones': symptomatic, solitary (smaller than 20 mm), sonolucent, sufficiently contractile gallbladder [39]. Under adjuvant oral chemolysis with ursodeoxycholic acid and chenodeoxycholic acid, stone-free rates after 1 year of 61–90% were achieved [40]. Reasons for the wide range of success rates were accuracy and experience in detecting residual fragments with ultrasound and the initial stone selection, excluding non-

pure cholesterol stones. As these conditions are fulfilled by only 10% of all gallstones, alternative concepts were introduced into clinical practice: regardless of stone composition and size all gallstones were subjected to ESWL treatment with high energy, a large number of shockwaves and a high rate of retreatments. Under these circumstances, a stone-free rate after 1 year of 75% has been reported [41], requiring a median of three treatments (ranging from one to 21) and 4000 shockwaves (ranging from 1000 to 16 000) per treatment. Complications of this regimen were relatively rare: biliary colic in 13.8% and pancreatitis in less than 1% [41]. On the other hand, laparoscopic cholecystectomy offers a minimally invasive treatment for gallstones without the risk of stone recurrence or the need for prolonged postoperative medical treatment. The role of biliary lithotripsy is therefore decreasing. Further technical improvements, like non-invasive stone analysis using computed tomography scan or ultrasound to eliminate unsuitable candidates for the treatment, could improve the impact of biliary lithotripsy for the treatment of gallstones.

Lithotripsy of pancreatic duct stones

Stones in the pancreatic duct are caused by alcohol provoked pancreatitis with concomitant strictures of the pancreatic duct [42]. Surgical therapy, including resection or drainage, can improve pain but compromises the function of the gland [43]. Since 1987 ESWL has been used as a supportive measure in combination with endoscopic procedures [44]. Stone location is performed with ultrasound or fluoroscopically after placement of a nasopancreatic tube [45,46]. Fragmentation was achieved in 75–100% of cases and pain relief in 45–75% of cases [47–49]. ESWL of pancreatic duct stones has thus gained some acceptance as an adjunct to modern endoscopic strategies to avoid or postpone major pancreatic surgery.

Shockwaves in the treatment of pseudarthrosis

During experimental investigations regarding the feasibility of shockwave application through bony tissue and possible bioeffects during shockwave treatment of ureteric calculi, increased osteoblastic activity was found [50]. This effect was introduced into clinical practice after basic research investigating fracture or wound healing in animal experiments [51,52]. In a preliminary series of 54 patients the generation of callus was induced in all cases, but fracture healing occurred in only two-thirds of patients. Because side effects were few and minor (petechial skin bleeding) this method represents a non-invasive tool in cases refractory to other forms of therapy. Changes in the treatment regimen may improve the results and further investigations in improving patient selection are necessary [53,54].

Shockwaves in the treatment of insertion tendinopathy

Based on the encouraging results of shockwave treatment of pseudarthosis this method has also been used for the therapy of chronic pain of soft tissue adjacent to bones due to tendinopathy with or without the formation of exostoses. This type of treatment has been used after the failure of physical treatment, antiphlogistic medication or even surgical resection of the exostosis. Without any analgesia, shockwaves are directed into the centre of pain sensation; 1200–3000 shockwaves are applied during one session, which were repeated from five to 30 times each day. The interval of pain relief ranged from 15 min to 2.5 months [55]. Shockwave therapy of tendinopathies is considered a valuable support of physical therapy, eliminating or at least reducing the need for antiphlogistic and analgesic medication.

Shockwaves in the treatment of malignant tumours

To study the effect of shockwaves on biological tissues, tumour cell lines were treated. *In vitro* studies on prostatic cancer (PC-3), SK-mel-28 melanoma and Dunning tumours revealed dose-related reduction of cell division and survival which differed for specific tumour entities [56,57]. Flowcytometric DNA analyses showed a characteristic lesion of tumour cells in the G2 and M phase of mitosis [56]. This effect could be used therapeutically if the tumour cells could be synchronised. Damage occurred mostly to the mitochondria. Possible mechanisms for the mitochondrial damage are direct mechanical lesions or the formation of free radicals which have an adverse effect on phosphorylation processes.

Growth delay and histological changes have also been found in *in vivo* studies of Dunning tumours. Besides a direct cytotoxic effect, vascular lesions leading to necrosis and haemorrhage may occur [58]. Additionally, an increased sensitivity to adjuvant medical treatment has been reported, which can again be explained by membrane defects which lead to increased diffusion of cytotoxic agents into the cell. *In vitro* studies have revealed an effect of cisplatinum on shockwave-treated tumour cells [59]. Interesting results have been found regarding the interaction of shockwaves and biological response modifiers like tumour necrosis factor or interferon α, leading to complete growth delay of implanted tumour cells [60].

Although these results are only preliminary and experimental, they show interesting trends which may open up new treatment modalities for malignant tumours.

References

1 Lingeman JE, Newman D, Mertz JHO *et al.* Extracorporeal shockwave lithotripsy: the Methodist Hospital of Indiana experience. *J Urol* 1986;**135**:1134–8.

2 Virgili G, Vespasiani G, Mearini E, Di Stasi SM, Micali F. Extracorporeal piezoelectric lithotripsy: experience in 930 patients. *J Endourol* 1992;**6**:309–14.

3 Psihramis KE, Jewett MA, Bombardier C, Caron D, Ryan M. Lithostar extracorporeal shockwave lithotripsy: the first 1000 patients. *J Urol* 1992;**147**:1006–9.

4 Bierkens A, Hendrikx A, De Kort V *et al.* Efficacy of second generation lithotriptors: a multicenter comparative study of extracorporeal shockwave lithotripsy treatments with the Siemens Lithostar, Dornier HM4, Wolf Piezolith 2300, Direx Tripter X-1 and Breakstone Lithotriptors. *J Urol* 1992;**148**: 1052–7.

5 Choung CJ, Zhong P, Preminger GM. A comparison of stone damage caused by different modes of shockwave generation. *J Urol* 1992;**148**:200–5.

6 Fichtner J, Bürger RA, Witsch U, Hohenfellner R. Extracorporeal shockwave lithotripsy with ultrasound-guided Lithostar Plus. *Eur Urol* 1992;**21**:192–4.

7 Netto NR, Claro JFA, Cortado PL. Extracorporeal shockwave lithotripsy of radiolucent urinary calculi using the Siemens Lithostar Plus. *J Urol* 1992;**148**:1112–13.

8 Liston TG, Montgomery BSI, Bultitude MI, Tiptaft RC. Extracorporeal shockwave lithotripsy with the Storz Modulith SL20: the first 500 patients. *Br J Urol* 1992;**69**:465–9.

9 Mykulak DJ, Grunberger I, Macchia RJ *et al.* Initial experience with Therasonic Lithotriptor. *Urology* 1992;**39**:346–51.

10 Schmidt A, Volz C, Eisenberger F. The Dornier-Lithotripter U30—first clinical experience. *J Endourol* 1995;**9**:363–6.

11 Kaude JV, Williams C, Millner M, Scott K, Finlayson B. Renal morphology and function immediately after extracorporeal shockwave lithotripsy. *Am J Radiol* 1985;**145**:305–13.

12 Chaussy C. ESWL: past, present and future. *J Endourol* 1988;**2**: 97–105.

13 Rassweiler J, Köhrmann, Marlinghaus E, Heine G, Alken P. Threshold of shockwave energy for different degrees of renal trauma in the canine kidney model. *J Urol* 1991;**145**:255A (abstr. 171).

14 Eisenberger F, Schmidt A. ESWL and the future of stone management. *World J Urol* 1993;**11**:2–6.

15 Thomas R, Frentz JF, Harmon E, Frentz GD. Effect of extracorporeal shockwave lithotripsy on renal function and body height in pediatric patients. *J Urol* 1992;**148**:1064–6.

16 Schmidt AS, Rassweiler JJ, Gumpinger R, Mayer R, Eisenberger F. Minimally invasive treatment of ureteric calculi using modern techniques. *Br J Urol* 1990;**65**:242–9.

17 Schmidt AS, Müller M, Wilke J, Eisenberger F. Intrakorporale Druckmessungen in Nierenbecken und Harnleiter während der extrakorporalen Stoßwellenlithotripsie. *Urologie Poster* 1990; **4**:264–5.

18 Mueller SC, Wilbert D, Thueroff JW, Alken P. Extracorporeal shockwave lithotripsy of ureteral stones: clinical experience and experimental findings. *J Urol* 1986;**135**:831–5.

19 Crum LA. Cavitation microjets as a contributory mechanism for renal calculi disintegration in ESWL. *J Urol* 1988;**140**: 1587–91.

20 Parr NJ, Pye SD, Ritchie AWS, Tolley DA. Mechanisms responsible for diminished fragmentation of ureteral calculi: an experimental and clinical study. *J Urol* 1992;**148**:1079–83.

21 Mashimo S, Suyama K, Goh M *et al.* Middle ureter stones:

results of *in situ* extracorporeal shockwave lithotripsy with EDAP LT01 Lithotripters. *J Endourol* 1992;**6**:319–22.

22 El-Gammal M, Fouda A, Meshref A *et al.* Management of ureteral stones by extracorporeal shockwave lithotripsy using Lithostar Lithotriper. *J Urol* 1992;**148**:1086–7.

23 Rassweiler J, Henkel T, Joyce A *et al.* Extracorporeal shockwave lithotripsy of ureteric stones with the Modulith SL 20. *Br J Urol* 1992;**70**:594–9.

24 Rauchenwald M, Colombo T, Petritsch P, Vilits P, Hubmer G. *In situ* extracorporeal shockwave lithotripsy of ureteral calculi with the MPL-9000X Lithotriptor. *J Urol* 1992;**148**:1097–101.

25 Lyon ES, Banno JJ, Schoenberg HW. Transurethral ureteroscopy in men using juvenile cystoscopy equipment. *J Urol* 1979;**122**: 152–3.

26 Perez-Castro EE, Martinez-Pineiro JA. Transurethral ureteroscopy: a current urological procedure. *Arch Esp Urol* 1980;**33**: 445–52.

27 Schmidt A, Eisenberger F. Laser lithotripsy of ureteral calculi using a pulsed dye laser with automatic shut off after tissue contact. *J Endourol* 1993;**7**:201–4.

28 Vorreuther R, Engelking R. Features and acoustic output of five electrohydraulic lithotripters for endoureteral stone treatment. *J Endourol* 1992;**6**:41–5.

29 Denstedt JD, Eberwein PM, Singh RR. The Swiss Lithoclast—a new device for intracorporeal lithotripsy. *J Urol* 1992;**148**: 1088–90.

30 Fugelso P, Neal P. Endoscopic laser lithotripsy: safe, effective therapy for ureteral calculi. *J Urol* 1991;**145**:949–51.

31 Govier F, Gibbons R, Correa R *et al.* Pulsed dye laser fragmentation of ureteral calculi: a review of the first 50 cases at Virginia Mason Medical Center. *J Urol* 1990;**143**:685–6.

32 Psihramis K. Laser lithotripsy of difficult ureteral calculus: results in 122 patients. *J Urol* 1992;**147**:1010–12.

33 Watson G, Murray S, Dretler S, Parrish J. Pulsed dye laser fragmentation of ureteral calculi: initial urological experience. *J Urol* 1987;**138**:195–8.

34 Weber H, Miller K, Rüschoff J, Gschwend R, Hautmann R. Experimentelle Ergebnisse und erste klinische Erfahrungen mit dem Alexandrit-Laserlithotripter. *Urologe [A]* 1990;**29**:304–8.

35 Zerbib M, Flam T, Belas M, Debre B, Steg A. Clinical experience with a new pulsed dye laser for ureteral stone lithotripsy. *J Urol* 1990;**143**:483–4.

36 Wirth MP, Theiss M, Frohmueller HGW. Primary extracorporeal shockwave lithotripsy of staghorn renal calculi. *Urol Int* 1992;**48**:71–5,

37 Eisenberger F, Rassweiler JJ, Bub P, Kallert B, Miller K. Differentiated approach to staghorn calculi using extracorporeal shockwave lithotripsy and percutaneous nephrolithotomy: an analysis of 151 consecutive cases. *World J Urol* 1987;**5**:248–52.

38 Lam SH, Lingeman JE, Barron M *et al.* Staghorn calculi: analysis of treatment results between initial percutaneous nephrostolithotomy and extracorporeal shockwave lithotripsy monotherapy with reference to surface area. *J Urol* 1992;**147**: 1219–25.

39 Sauerbruch T, Delius M, Paumgartner G. Fragmentation of gallstones by extracorporeal shockwaves. *N Engl J Med* 1986; **314**:818–23.

40 Sackman M. Gallbladder stones: shockwave therapy. *Baillières Clin Gastroenterol* 1992;**6**:697–702.

41 Nam VC, Soehendra N. Extrakorporale Stoßwellenlithotripsy als Monotherapie zur Behandlung der Gallenblasensteine. In: Chaussy C, Eisenberger F, Jocham D, Wilbert D, eds. *Stoßwellenlithotripsie—Aspekte und Prognosen.* Tübingen: Attempto-Verlag, 1993:63–70.

42 Sarles H, Bernard JP, Gullo L. Pathogenesis of chronic pancreatitis. *Gut* 1990;**31**:629–32.

43 Malfertheiner P, Büchler M. Indications for endoscopic or surgical therapy in chronic pancreatitis. *Endoscopy* 1991;**23**: 185–8.

44 Sauerbruch T, Holl J, Sackmann M *et al.* Disintegration of a pancreatic duct stone with extracorporeal shockwaves in a patient with chronic pancreatitis. *Endoscopy* 1987;**23**:207–10.

45 Kerzel W, Ell C, Schneider H *et al.* Piezoelectric shockwave lithotripsy of multiple pancreatic duct stones under ultrasonographic control. *Endoscopy* 1989;**21**:229–31.

46 Sauerbruch T, Holl J, Sackmann M, Paumgartner G. Extracorporeal shockwave lithotripsy of pancreatic duct stones. *Gut* 1989;**30**:1406–10.

47 Soehendra N, Grimm H, Meyer HW, Schreiber HW. Extrakorporale Stoßwellenlithotripsie bei chronischer Pankreatitis. *Dtsch Med Wochenschr* 1989;**114**:1402–6.

48 Neuhaus H. Fragmentation of pancreatic duct stones by extracorporeal shockwave lithotripsy. *Endoscopy* 1991;**23**: 161–5.

49 Den Toom R, Nus HGT, Van Blankenstein M *et al.* Extracorporeal shockwave lithotripsy of pancreatic duct stones. *Am J Gastroenterol* 1991;**86**:1033–6.

50 Graff J, Richter KD, Pastor J. Effect of high energy shockwaves on bony tissue. *Urol Res* 1988;**16**:252–7.

51 Haupt G, Chapvil M. Effect of shockwaves on the healing of partial-thickness wounds in piglets. *J Surg Res* 1990;**49**:45–8.

52 Haupt G, Haupt A, Gerety B, Chapvil M. Enhancement of fracture healing with extracorporeal shockwaves. *J Urol* 1990;**143**:230A.

53 Haupt G, Haupt A, Senge T. Die Behandlung von Knochen mit extrakorporalen Stoßwellen-Entwicklung einer neuen Therapie. In: Chaussy C, Eisenberger F, Jocham D, Wilbert D, eds. *Stoßwellenlithotripsie—Aspekte und Prognosen.* Tübingen: Attempto-Verlag, 1993:120–6.

54 Witsch U, Bürger RA, Karnoski V, Haist J. Hochenergie-Stoßwellenbehandlung—eine Methode zur Therapie von Pseudarthrosen. *Urologe [A]* 1992;**31**:A43.

55 Dahmen GP, Meiss L, Nam VC, Skruodies B. Extrakorporale Stoßwellentherapie (ESWL) im knochennahen Weichteilbereich an der Schulter. *Extracta Orthop* 1992;**111**:25–8.

56 Russo P, Stevenson RA, Mies C *et al.* High energy shock waves suppress tumor growth *in vitro* and *in vivo*. *J Urol* 1986; **135**:626–32.

57 Jones BJ, McHale AP, Butler MR. Effect on high-energy shock wave frequency on viability of malignant cell line *in vitro*. *Eur Urol* 1992;**22**:70–4.

58 Debus J, Peschke P, Hahn EW, Lorenz WJ. Treatment of the Dunning prostate rat tumor R 3327-AT 1 with the pulsed high energy ultrasound shockwaves (PHEUS): growth delay and histomorphological changes. *J Urol* 1992;**146**:1143–8.

59 Gambihler S, Delius M. *In vitro* interaction of lithotripter shockwaves and cytotoxic drugs. *Br J Cancer* 1992;**66**:69–73.

60 Oosterhof GON, Smiss GAH, De Ruyter AE, Schalken JA, Debryune FMJ. Effects of high-energy shockwaves combined with biological response modifiers in different human kidney cancer. *Ultrasound Med Biol* 1991;**17**:391–400.

Index